IMMUNOBIOLOGY
OF
TRANSFUSION
MEDICINE

IMMUNOBIOLOGY
OF
TRANSFUSION
MEDICINE

EDITED BY
GEORGE GARRATTY

American Red Cross Blood Services
and University of California, Los Angeles
Los Angeles, California

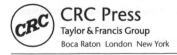

CRC Press
Taylor & Francis Group
Boca Raton London New York

CRC Press is an imprint of the
Taylor & Francis Group, an **informa** business

CRC Press
Taylor & Francis Group
6000 Broken Sound Parkway NW, Suite 300
Boca Raton, FL 33487-2742

First issued in paperback 2019

ISBN-13: 978-0-8247-9122-3 (hbk)
ISBN-13: 978-0-367-40228-0 (pbk)

Library of Congress Cataloging-in-Publication Data

Immunobiology of transfusion medicine / edited by George Garratty.
     p. cm.
   Includes bibliographical references and index.
   ISBN 0-8247-9122-3 (alk. paper)
   1. Blood--Transfusion--Immunological aspects. 2. Immunohematology. I. Garratty,
George.
   [DNLM: 1. Blood Transfusion--adverse effects. 2. Blood Groups--immunology.
3. Blood Cells--immunology. WH 140 I33 1993]
RM171.I457   1993
615'.39--dc20
DNLM/DLC
for Library of Congress   93-27707
                                            CIP

Visit the Taylor & Francis Web site at
http://www.taylorandfrancis.com

and the CRC Press Web site at
http://www.crcpress.com

Preface

Although transfusion medicine can be said to go back to the seventeenth century, the immunological aspects date from Landsteiner's discovery of the first blood group system in 1900. One could say that this was the birth of immunogenetics and immunohematology. Since Landsteiner's discovery of the A and B antigens on red blood cells (RBCs), over 600 other RBC blood group antigens have been described. Over 100 have been described as being associated with white cells and platelets. A corresponding plethora of antibodies to these antigens has also been described. Apart from the very practical problems of providing "compatible" cellular products to patients who develop such antibodies, the basis of the immune reactions involved provides an intriguing model for immunologists. Knowledge of the chemistry of blood group antigens is still in its infancy. Although a great deal of knowledge concerning the glycoproteins and glycolipids associated with ABH, Lewis, Ii, and P antigens was accumulated in the 1960s and 1970s, it is only during the last decade that we have begun to understand the structure of some other blood group antigens. These findings may have wide-ranging implications as it is still not known if blood group antigens, as detected on red cells, white cells, or platelets, have a biological role. It would be surprising if such polymorphic systems do not have an important immunobiological role. For many years statistical associations between certain blood groups and certain diseases have been noted, but only recently has a more scientific basis for these associations begun to emerge. Some antigens, such as ABH, I, i, Lewis, T, and Tn were first detected on red cells, but are widely distributed in many tissues. It is becoming obvious that many of the antigens studied by tumor immunologists are very similar, if not identical, to red cell antigens already described.

Avoiding the immune destruction of circulating cells such as erythrocytes, leukocytes, and platelets is one of the major goals of transfusion medicine. The in vivo and in vitro reactions involved in these immune reactions provide easily studied human models for complement- and macrophage-mediated cell destruction, autoimmunity, and drug-induced immune destruction of cells. Although complement-mediated cell destruction is understood quite well, many aspects of the more common extravascular destruction of blood cells are still not understood. Over the last four decades we have learned that important factors such as immunoglobulin class and subclass, complement-activating ability of the antibody, quantity of cell-bound antibody and complement components, affinity of the antibody, and activity of the mononuclear phagocyte system all play a role, but there are still many anomalies between the observed in vivo destruction and our in vitro results. We need to reconcile these differences before in vitro assays can be improved and to forecast accurately the survival of transfused cellular components.

Finally, transfusion has recently been found to have significant direct and indirect effects on the immune response. This has had very practical effects on the management of patients undergoing renal transplantation, where rejection of transplanted kidneys has been shown to relate directly to the pretransplantation transfusion schedule. There is a growing controversy on whether transfusion creates a predisposition to recurrence of solid tumors and susceptibility to bacterial and viral infection. It has been known for some years that lymphocytes can survive in stored donor blood and that acute graft-versus-host disease (GVHD) can occur in immunocompromised hosts (e.g., fetuses), but recent studies suggest that chronic GVHD may be occurring on a much larger scale in transfused patients. Without doubt, the biggest impact on transfusion medicine in the last decade has been the transmission of infectious disease. Retroviral infections associated with human immunodeficiency virus (HIV) and human T-cell leukemia virus (HTLV) are associated with profound immunological changes. Studies on transfusion-transmitted retroviral infections have led to an explosion of knowledge on the effect of these retroviruses on the immune system.

It is hoped that this book will not only update blood transfusion scientists on the immunobiology of transfusion medicine, but will stimulate immunologists to realize that the immunobiological models provided by the immune reactions of red cells, white cells, and platelets are understudied by immunologists and provide a rich field for cooperative basic and applied research.

George Garratty

Contents

Preface iii
Contributors ix

Part I Immunochemistry of Antigens on Erythrocytes, Leukocytes, and Platelets

1. Carbohydrate-Associated Blood Group Antigens: The *ABO*, *H/Se*, and *Lewis* Loci   3
    John B. Lowe

2. Glycophorins: Structures and Antigens   37
    Dominique Blanchard and Wolfgang Dahr

3. Sialic Acid-Dependent Red Blood Cell Antigens   69
    Dieter Roelcke

4. Erythrocyte Blood Group Antigens Associated with Phosphatidylinositol Glycan-Linked Proteins   97
    Marilyn J. Telen

5. The Rh Blood Groups   111
    Peter D. Issitt

6. Platelet and Neutrophil Alloantigens: Their Nature and Role in Immune-Mediated Cytopenias   149
    A. E. G. Kr. von dem Borne, S. Simsek, C. E. van der Schoot, and R. Goldschmeding

v

7. Cellular and Molecular Biology of Senescent Cell Antigen   173
   Marguerite M. B. Kay

Part II   Associations of Blood Groups with Disease

8. Do Blood Groups Have a Biological Role?   201
   George Garratty

9. Associations of Red Blood Cell Membrane Abnormalities with Blood Group
   Phenotype   257
   Marion E. Reid

10. Association of Blood Group Antigens with Immunologically Important Proteins   273
    Joann M. Moulds

11. Use of Hematopoietic Cells and Markers for the Detection and Quantitation of
    Human In Vivo Somatic Mutation   299
    Stephen G. Grant and Ronald H. Jensen

Part III   Red Cell Antibodies

12. Immunological and Physicochemical Nature of Antigen–Antibody Interactions   327
    Carel J. van Oss

13. Monoclonal Antibodies to Human Red Blood Cell Blood Group Antigens   365
    Marion L. Scott and Douglas Voak

14. Structural Analyses of Red Blood Cell Autoantibodies   387
    Don L. Siegel and Leslie E. Silberstein

Part IV   Immune Destruction of Cells

15. Complement in Transfusion Medicine   403
    John Freedman and John W. Semple

16. Macrophage-Mediated Cell Destruction   435
    Peter Horsewood and John G. Kelton

17. Cellular Immunoassays and Their Use for Predicting the Clinical Significance
    of Antibodies   465
    Barbara Żupańska

18. Autoimmune Hemolytic Anemia   493
    George Garratty

19. Drug-Induced Immune Hemolytic Anemia   523
    George Garratty

Contents

20. Hemolytic Disease of the Newborn   553
    John M. Bowman

21. Alloimmune Refractoriness to Transfused Platelets   597
    Sherrill J. Slichter

Part V   The Effect of Transfusion on the Immune Response

22. Transfusion-Induced Graft-Versus-Host Disease   631
    Kathleen Sazama and Paul V. Holland

23. Retroviral Infections and the Immune Response   657
    Harry E. Prince

Index   699

Contributors

Dominique Blanchard, Ph.D. Biotechnology Laboratory Manager, Centre Regional de Transfusion Sanguine, Nantes, France

John M. Bowman, O.C., M.D., C.R.C.P., F.R.S.C. Professor of Pediatrics and Child Health and of Obstetrics, Gynecology, and Reproductive Sciences, and Medical Director, Rh Laboratory, Faculty of Medicine, University of Manitoba Health Sciences Centre, Winnipeg, Manitoba, Canada

Wolfgang Dahr, Prof. Dr. med. Scientific Consultation and Translations, Bergish Gladbach, Germany

John Freedman, M.D., F.R.C.P.(C.) Associate Professor, Department of Medicine, University of Toronto, Toronto, Ontario, Canada

George Garratty, Ph.D., F.I.M.L.S., F.R.C.Path. Scientific Director, American Red Cross Blood Services, and Clinical Professor of Pathology, University of California, Los Angeles, Los Angeles, California

R. Goldschmeding, M.D., Ph.D. Head, Leukocyte Platelet Laboratory, Immunohematology Department, Central Laboratory of the Netherlands Red Cross Blood Transfusion Service, Amsterdam, The Netherlands

Stephen G. Grant, Ph.D. Assistant Research Scientist, Departments of Radiology, Pediatrics, and Obstetrics, Gynecology, and Reproductive Sciences, University of California, San Francisco, San Francisco, California

Paul V. Holland, M.D. Medical Director and Chief Executive Officer, Sacramento Medical Foundation, Sacramento, California

Peter Horsewood, Ph.D.   Assistant Professor, Department of Pathology, McMaster University Medical Centre, Hamilton, Ontario, Canada

Peter D. Issitt, Ph.D., F.I.M.L.S., F.I.Biol., F.R.C.Path.   Associate Professor of Pathology, Transfusion Service, Duke University Medical Center, Durham, North Carolina

Ronald H. Jensen, Ph.D.   Professor, Division of Molecular Cytometry, Department of Laboratory Medicine, University of California, San Francisco, San Francisco, California

Marguerite M. B. Kay, M.D.   Departments of Microbiology and Immunology, and Medicine, University of Arizona College of Medicine, Tucson, Arizona

John G. Kelton, M.D.   Professor, Departments of Medicine and Pathology, McMaster University Medical Centre, Hamilton, Ontario, Canada

John B. Lowe, M.D.   Associate Professor and Associate Investigator of the Howard Hughes Medical Institute, Department of Pathology, University of Michigan Medical School, Ann Arbor, Michigan

Joann M. Moulds, Ph.D.   Assistant Professor, Rheumatology and Clinical Immunogenetics, University of Texas Medical School, Houston, Texas

Harry E. Prince, Ph.D.   Head, Division of Cellular Immunology, Research Department, American Red Cross Blood and Tissue Services, Los Angeles, California

Marion E. Reid, Ph.D.   Director of Immunohematology, Immunohematology Laboratory, The New York Blood Center, New York, New York

Dieter Roelcke, Prof. Dr.   Institute for Immunology and Serology, University of Heidelberg, Heidelberg, Germany

Kathleen Sazama, M.D., J. D.   Associate Professor and Director of Clinical Pathology, Pathology Department, University of California, Davis, Sacramento, California

Marion L. Scott, B.Sc., Ph.D.   Research and Development Manager, International Blood Group Reference Laboratory, Bristol, England

John W. Semple, Ph.D.   Assistant Professor, Departments of Pharmacology and Medicine, University of Toronto, Toronto, Ontario, Canada

Don L. Siegel, Ph.D., M.D.   Assistant Professor, Departments of Pathology and Laboratory Medicine, University of Pennsylvania School of Medicine, Philadelphia, Pennsylvania

Leslie E. Silberstein, M.D.   Associate Professor and Director of Blood Bank/Transfusion Medicine Section, Departments of Pathology and Laboratory Medicine, University of Pennsylvania School of Medicine, Philadelphia, Pennsylvania

S. Simsek, M.D.   Junior Investigator, Immunohematology Department, Central Laboratory of the Netherlands Red Cross Blood Transfusion Service, Amsterdam, The Netherlands

Sherrill J. Slichter, M.D.   Director, Medical and Research Division, Puget Sound Blood Center, and Professor of Medicine, Hematology Division, University of Washington School of Medicine, Seattle, Washington

Marilyn J. Telen, M.D.   Associate Professor, Department of Medicine, Duke University Medical Center, Durham, North Carolina

C. E. van der Schoot, M.D. Ph.D.   Head, Immunocytology Laboratory, Immunohematology Department, Central Laboratory of the Netherlands Red Cross Blood Transfusion Service, Amsterdam, The Netherlands

Carel J. van Oss, Ph.D.   Professor of Microbiology and Adjunct Professor of Chemical Engineering, Department of Microbiology, School of Medicine and Biomedical Sciences, State University of New York at Buffalo, Buffalo, New York

Douglas Voak, B.Sc., Ph.D., F.R.C.Path.   Top Grade Scientific Officer, East Anglican Blood Transfusion Centre, and Division of Transfusion Medicine, University of Cambridge, Cambridge, England

A. E. G. Kr. von dem Borne, M.D., Ph.D.   Head, Department of Hematology, Academic Medical Centre, University of Amsterdam, and Department of Immunohematology, Central Laboratory of the Netherlands Red Cross Blood Transfusion Service, Amsterdam, The Netherlands

Barbara Żupańska, M.D., Ph.D.   Professor of Hematology, Department of Serology, Institute of Hematology and Blood Transfusion, Warsaw, Poland

I

Immunochemistry of Antigens on Erythrocytes, Leukocytes, and Platelets

1

Carbohydrate-Associated Blood Group Antigens:
The *ABO*, *H/Se*, and *Lewis* Loci

JOHN B. LOWE
Howard Hughes Medical Institute
University of Michigan Medical School
Ann Arbor, Michigan

I. INTRODUCTION

The human ABO, H, and Lewis blood group determinants were initially defined with serological techniques, in the context of investigating genetic polymorphisms in the expression of these antigens, and their roles in mediating red blood cell destruction. Since the discovery of these determinants earlier in this century, the structural nature of these molecules, and the genetic basis for polymorphism in their expression, have been the subject of intense study. These investigations have yielded a rather high resolution picture of the chemical nature of these molecules and their biosynthetic paths, and they have yielded consistent hypotheses concerning the nature of the genes that determine the expression of these structures. As will be discussed in detail below, the A, B, H, and Lewis blood group active antigens are now known to be oligosaccharide molecules whose synthesis is catalyzed by the sequential action of enzymes known as glycosyltransferases. Recent investigative activities in this field have centered on the isolation and characterization of the genes that encode these enzymes. These efforts have been successful in several instances; such genetic sequences represent tools that are now in use in studies designed to define the molecular basis for the expression patterns of these oligosaccharide-based blood groups and to define the genetic basis for polymorphism in their expression.

This chapter includes an overview of information concerning the chemical nature of the ABO, H, and Lewis blood group determinants, their biosynthetic pathways, and their clinical significance. Where more detailed information on these subjects is desired, the reader should consult recent reviews pertinent to these issues that will be cited at appropriate places in the text. The major focus of this chapter, however, is to summarize recent work involving the molecular cloning of the ABO, H, and Lewis blood group loci and to discuss the implications of this work in providing molecular confirmation of previous hypotheses concerning the genetic basis for polymorphisms at these loci.

II. STRUCTURE AND SYNTHESIS OF THE ABH BLOOD GROUP DETERMINANTS

The system of genetically polymorphic red blood cell surface antigens known as the ABO blood group system was first discovered at the turn of the century by Landsteiner and colleagues and

3

others (1–3). This work demonstrated that humans could be segregated into distinct groups based on the presence of agglutinating substance in sera that recognized red cells from humans of other groups. These initial observations were quickly put to practical use in the formation of rational approaches to blood typing and blood transfusion practices. Nonetheless, the chemical and genetic basis for antigenic differences determined by the *ABO* locus have taken the remainder of this century to determine. These studies have also demonstrated that the A, B, and H molecules, which represent the component antigens of the ABO system, are not restricted in their expression to the erythrocyte but are in fact displayed by a variety of tissues, including endothelial cells and the epithelial cells that line glands and internal organs, for example (reviewed in refs. 4 and 5). Moreover, water-soluble forms of these antigens exist. As is discussed in detail below, the expression of soluble ABH-active blood group substances is determined by a discrete genetic locus (the *Se* locus) that most probably corresponds to a specific α(1,2)fucosyltransferase gene.

Early efforts to define the nature of red cell A, B, and H substances were restricted to those designed to extract this material from red cell membranes using both polar and apolar solvents (reviewed in ref. 6). Early work involving the isolation of ABH reactive material from tissue fluids and by protease treatment of fluids and tissues has been reviewed (7).

These early studies indicated that the A, B, and H determinants consist of carbohydrate molecules, based largely on evidence that complex carbohydrate-rich components of tissues or fluids could inhibit agglutination of red cells by antibodies or lectins (8,9). The chemical structures of the determinants that specify the A, B, and H blood group molecules and the related Lewis blood group determinants was reported in the 1950s and 1960s from the laboratories of Morgan and Watkins (10,11) and Kabat (12). This work was done largely on soluble blood group substances isolated from human ovarian cyst fluid (7) and demonstrated that the antigenic determinants of the ABO blood group system are oligosaccharides (Fig. 1). The antigenic trisaccharide components of the B and H determinants have since been created by organic synthetic methods (13,14; reviewed in ref. 15). The chemical and biological properties of these synthetic molecules are virtually identical to those of the natural ones, thus providing an independent confirmation of the structural analyses performed on natural blood group–active glycoconjugates.

The antigenic determinants of the ABO blood group system represent terminal components of structurally complex oligosaccharide moieties displayed by soluble glycosphingolipids, free oligosaccharides, and membrane-associated molecules. These latter entities include integral membrane proteins, as well as membrane-associated glycolipids, that are expressed at the surfaces of red cells and other tissues (reviewed in refs. 5 and 16). As shown in Figure 2, the synthesis of the A, B, and H substances is determined by the sequential action of glyco-syltransferases encoded by distinct genetic loci. The penultimate step in this biosynthetic pathway is catalyzed by α(1,2)fucosyltransferases acting upon specific disaccharide precursors. Four well-characterized types of disaccharide precursors are known to be expressed in human tissues (see Fig. 1). Types 1 and 2 chains are located at the periphery of oligosaccharides in both O- and N-linkage to proteins and also in lipid-linked oligosaccharides. Type 3 chains represent components of O-linked oligosaccharides, and type 4 chains are found only on lipids. Synthesis of type 1 molecules is generally restricted to endodermally derived tissues, including epithelia that line the respiratory, digestive, urinary, and reproductive tracts and some exocrine glands (4). Type 1 molecules represent the major carriers of ABH determinants found on proteins and lipids in body fluids and secretions. Type 2 ABH determinants are expressed by mesodermally derived tissues like erythrocytes or in ectodermally derived tissues like the epidermis (reviewed in refs. 4 and 5). The majority of ABH determinants on erythrocytes represent type 2 oligosaccharide moieties (4–6). Type 3 chains represent molecules in which the ABH antigens are displayed by relatively short oligosaccharide chains lined to proteins via

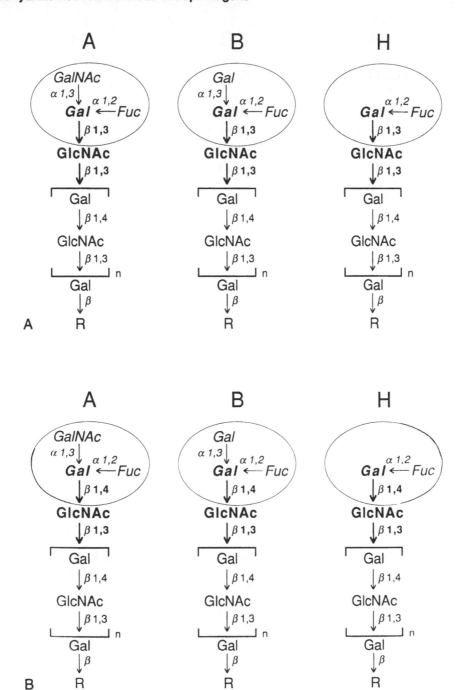

Figure 1 Structures of A, B, and H determinants. The immunodominant portion of each molecule is circled and is composed of the italicized monosaccharide components. The portions of each molecule that determines whether it is classified as type 1, 2, 3, or 4 are denoted by component monosaccharides displayed in bold type. Panels A and B show, respectively, type 1 and type 2, A, B, and H determinants. R denotes the underlying glycoconjugate backbone of an N-linked, O-linked, or lipid-linked substructure (see Fig. 3). The moiety in brackets represents a single lactosamine unit. This unit may not be found at all ($n = 0$) or may be represented many times as a component of a linear polymer, where n may be 1 to more than 5. Not shown are the β1,6 branch points that give rise to I antigenic determinants and also to multiple A,

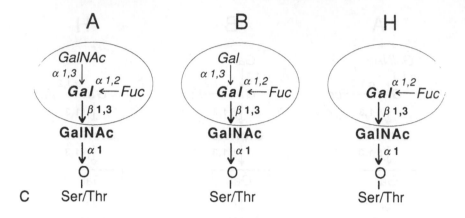

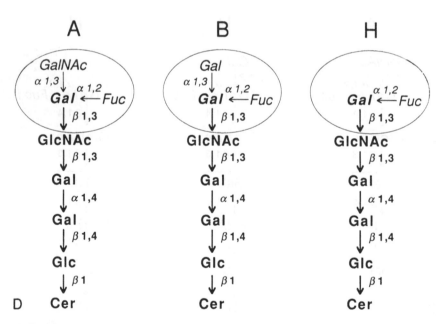

Figure 1 Continued   B, and H determinants on an arborized oligosaccharide (see Fig. 3 for the positions of such branch points). Panel C, type 3 A, B, and H determinants. These oligosaccharides are attached to some proteins via an N-acetylgalactosamine moiety in alpha anomeric linkage to some serines (Ser) or threonines (Thr). Panel D, type 4 A, B, and H determinants. The globo-series ABH glycolipid antigens are shown here. Component monosaccharides that make up the globo-series backbone are indicated by boldface type. These molecules are anchored within the erythrocyte membrane via a ceramide (Cer) moiety. Analogous structures based upon ganglio-series glycolipid precursors (Galβ1,3GalNAcβ1,3Galβ 1,4Blcβ1-Cer) may also exist in human tissues (reviewed in ref. 44).

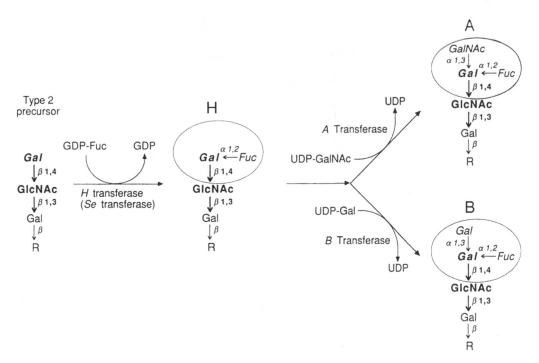

Figure 2 Biosynthesis of H, A, and B determinants. A precursor oligosaccharide (type 2 shown here) is first fucosylated by an α(1,2)fucosyltransferase that utilizes GDP-fucose as its substrate. This enzyme may be either the *H* transferase encoded by the *H* blood group locus or by the transferase encoded by the *Secretor* locus, indicated in parentheses. The product of this reaction, the H determinant, may then be utilized by the glycosyltransferase encoded by the *A* blood group locus (*A* transferase; α(1,3)N-acetylgalactosaminyltransferase), or by the *B* blood group locus (*B* transferase; α(1,3)galactosyltransferase), to form, respectively, the A or B blood group determinant. The *A* transferase utilizes UDP-N-acetylgalactosamine (UDP-GalNAc) as the sugar nucleotide donor, whereas the *B* transferase utilizes UDP-galactose (UDP-Gal). Biosynthesis of types 1, 3, and 4 A, B, and H determinants is formally analogous to the reactions shown here. R denotes the glycoconjugate substructures of N-linked, O-linked, or lipid-linked oligosasaccharide precursors.

serine or threonine residues. Type 3 ABH-active chains have been best characterized as components of mucins isolated from ovarian cyst fluid or gastric mucosa (reviewed in ref. 17). These types of ABH determinants are most likely not expressed by human erythrocytes (18,19). By contrast, however, so-called "A-associated" type 3 chains (Fig. 3) have been found to be significant components of the glycolipids extracted from the red cells of blood group A individuals (18,19). ABH determinants constructed from type 4 chains have been described as components of human red cell glycolipids (20,21).

These oligosaccharide precursors serve as substrates, along with a second, nucleotide sugar substrate (GDP-fucose), in a transglycosylation reaction catalyzed by α(1,2)fucosyltransferases. In this reaction, GDP-fucose serves to donate a fucose moiety that is covalently attached in alpha anomeric linkage to carbon 2 of the galactose molecule at the oligosaccharide's nonreducing end. This reaction yields the blood group H determinant, formally defined as a Fucα(1,2)Galβ- linkage (5). As will be discussed in more detail below, genetic and biochemical evidence indicates that the human genome encodes two distinct α(1,2)fucosyltransferases representing, respectively, the product of the *H* and the *Secretor* (*Se*) blood group loci. The *H* and *Se* α(1,2)fucosyltransferases exhibit distinct tissue-specific expression patterns and different

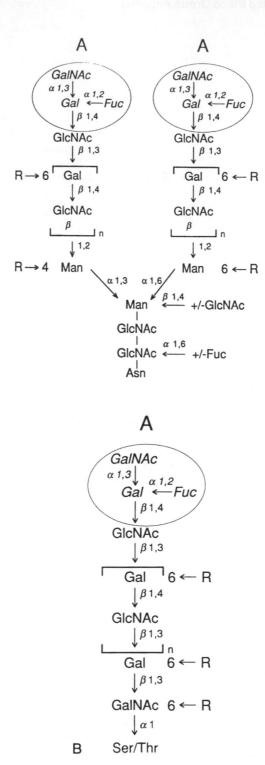

Figure 3 N-linked oligosaccharides, O-linked, and lipid-linked oligosaccharide molecules that display ABH blood group determinants. Panel A illustrates a typical asparagine-linked (N-linked) A-active molecule. Panel B shows a typical serine/threonine–linked (O-linked) A-active molecule. A typical lipid-linked A-active molecule is shown in panel C. Panel D displays an example of the type 3 precursor to an "A-associated" type 3 glycolipid chain. Note that the terminal disaccharide unit is identical to the

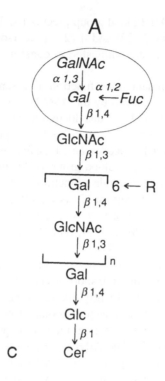

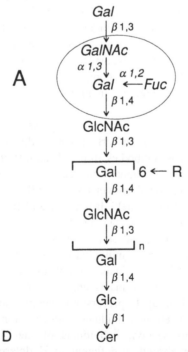

disaccharide unit of a type 1 precursor chain (see Fig. 1A). This may be fucosylated by the *H* fucosyltransferase or the *Se* fucosyltransferase to generate a type 1 H determinant (see Fig 2 and 4) and then further modified by the A_1 transferase (see Figs. 2 and 4) to yield repeating A-active trisaccharide units (repetitive A units; Fig. 4). R denotes branching oligosaccharide chains linked via β-linked GlcNAc residues. Lactosamine units that may be polymerized (n = 0 to 5 or more) are enclosed in brackets.

affinities for different types of ABH blood group precursors. Thus, it is generally believed that the *H* enzyme operates on types 2 (22) and 4 (23) precursors to form type 2 and type 4 H molecules, whereas the *Se* α(1,2)fucosyltransferase constructs type 1 (22) and type 3 (19) H determinants (see Fig. 2).

Types 2 through 4 H determinants then function as essential precursors for the action of codominant glycosyltransferases encoded by the *ABO* blood group locus (reviewed in ref. 5). Individuals who maintain an *A* allele at this locus encode an α1,3N-acetylgalactosaminyl-transferase that acts upon H determinants to form blood group A molecules (see Fig. 2). Similarly, the blood group *B* allele encodes an a1,3galactosyltransferase that utilizes the H oligosaccharide precursor to construct a blood group B determinant (see Fig. 2). By contrast, the *O* allele at the *ABO* locus does not encode a functional glycosyltransferase capable of further modifying the H oligosaccharide determinant. Consequently, depending upon the alleles present at the *ABO* locus, it is possible to construct A determinants only (genotype *AA* or *AO*), B determinants exclusively (genotype *BB* or *BO*), both A and B determinants (genotype *AB*), or neither A nor B determinants (genotype *OO*).

It has been estimated that approximately 80% of the ABH determinants expressed on erythrocytes are displayed by the anion transport protein (band 3) (approximately 1–2 million ABH determinants per red cell; ref. 6). Slightly smaller numbers of the oligosaccharide moieties are expressed by the red cell glucose transport protein (band 4.5) (approximately 5×10^5 determinants (25,26). Each of these two integral membrane proteins displays a single N-linked oligosaccharide determinant (26,27). The ABH determinants on these proteins are present at the termini of a highly branched poly N-acetylgalactosaminoglycan attached to this single N-linked site (see Fig. 3) (28). Lesser numbers of ABH determinants are expressed by other red cell membrane glycoproteins, including the Rh-related proteins, for example (29). Although the termini of these oligosaccharides display ABH determinants, the remaining portions of these glycan moieties are not well defined. The remaining red cell ABH determinants (approximately 5×10^5) are displayed by poly N-acetylactosaminoglycans attached to glycolipids (30). These latter molecules have been termed polyglycosylceramides or macroglycolipids (31,32) (see Fig. 3). ABH determinants are also found as components of so-called O-linked oligosaccharides (17) attached to secretory glycoproteins, including mucins, via some serine and threonine residues (see Fig. 3).

The genetically determined structural polymorphisms in these oligosaccharides have important clinical implications (33). In early infancy, the immune system generates potent immunoglobulin M (IgM)–type antibodies directed against the ABO oligosaccharide deter-minant(s) *not* expressed by the individual's red cells or tissues. This presumably occurs via exposure to environmental microbial antigens structurally similar or identical to the A and B determinants. Thus, type O individuals, lacking A and B determinants, normally maintain significant levels of naturally occurring IgM antibodies (isoagglutinins) specific for A and B blood group structures. Similarly, the sera of blood group A individuals contain potent IgM-type B isoagglutinins, and type B individuals maintain potent anti-A isoagglutinin titers. By contrast, blood group AB individuals do not make anti-A or anti-B isoagglutinins. (Antibodies directed against H determinants are not formed in most individuals because a significant fraction of blood group H precursor molecules are not enzymatically converted to A and/or B determinants even in individuals with functional A or B alleles. Nonetheless, as is discussed later in this section, individuals of the rare Bombay and para-Bombay phenotypes are relatively or absolutely deficient in H determinants and thus typically also generate anti-H antibodies.)

The high titer of these naturally occurring IgM isoagglutinins, and their ability to fix complement, allow them to rapidly lyse transfused red cells displaying their cognate antigen. Naturally, this yields a brisk intravascular hemolysis along with the other clinical manifestations of an immediate or acute transfusion reaction (33–35). Routine ABO blood group typing and cross-matching procedures implemented earlier in this century are designed to ensure ABO blood group compatibility during transfusion of either red cells or plasma so as to prevent this circumstance.

III. SUBGROUPS OF A AND B—ENZYMES AND OLIGOSACCHARIDES

Serological procedures related to those used to ensure ABH blood group compatibility may be used also to demonstrate variants of blood group A determinants, known as subgroups of A (34). For instance, the lectin *Dolichos biflorus*, at an appropriate dilution, will agglutinate some but not all group A red cells (36); the former are termed A_1 cells and the latter A_2. To further emphasize that these subgroups represent related, but nonetheless distinct, antigens, it should be noted that antibody specific for A_1 cells may be prepared from B or O sera by absorption with A_2 cells, whereas anti-A_2 antibody cannot be similarly prepared by absorption with A_1 cells (34). Likewise, red cells from AB individuals may be classified as A_1B or A_2B. The frequency of the A_1 or A_2 trait varies among different ethnic populations (37). For example, in Germany, 32.5% of group A individuals have red cells with the A_1 trait, whereas 9.4% are A_2. By contrast, the A_2 trait was not detected in a series of some 220 Vietnamese individuals. Genetic considerations suggested that A_1 and A_2 traits correspond to distinct, codominant alleles at the *ABO* locus (5). This notion is supported by studies demonstrating that the *A* allele-determined α1,3N-acetylgalactosaminyltransferase in the plasma of A_1 individuals and the analogous enzyme in A_2 plasma differ in their pH optima, isoelectric points, metal ion requirements, and substrate affinities (reviewed in ref. 5). Other subgroups of A have also been described (reviewed in ref. 38), each with distinct antigenic characteristics and transferase activities. Weakly reactive B antigens have also been described (34,38) and are most probably analogous to the subgroups of A.

The structural consequences of the enzymatic differences among the different transferase subgroups remain incompletely defined. Thus, although the immunodominant antigenic determinant on A1 and A2 cells is essentially identical, the molecular basis for differences in antigenic reactivity, as assessed with antibodies or lectins, is poorly understood. Evidence exists to support the notion that A1 and A2 subgroups differ both in the absolute number of immunodominant antigen molecules (39,40) and also in their molecular structure (39,41–43). It has been proposed that a major reason for the antigenic differences between A1 and A2 red cells may be ascribed to the abundance of repetitive type 3 A determinants on A1 cells relative to A2 cells (reviewed in ref. 44). In this model, in A1 red cell precursors, lipid-linked type 3 A-associated molecules are extended first to H-active type 3 chains, which are in turn efficiently utilized by the A1 transferase to yield type 3 A (and repetitive A) determinants. By contrast, in A2 red cell precursors, lipid-linked H-active type 3 chains are not extended to A-active type 3 molecules (Fig. 4). Similar outcomes would presumably occur with type 4 chain precursors. This hypothesis is supported by in vitro experiments demonstrating that the *A*1 transferase is substantially more efficient than the *A*2 transferase at converting H-active types 3 and 4 chains into types 3 and 4 A determinants (23,45) and by the observation that H types 3 and 4 chain glycolipids are more abundant in A2 cells relative to A1 cells (23). It remains to be determined if this mechanism is responsible for all of the phenotypic differences between A1 and A2 cells and if analogous mechanisms are operative in other A (and B) subgroups. The recent molecular cloning of the *ABO* locus (discussed below) will provide the tools to correlate the differences in kinetic characteristics of the various *A* subgroup transferases with differences in their respective peptide sequences.

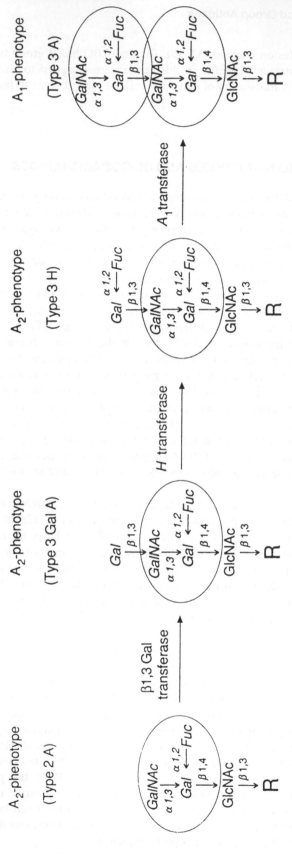

Figure 4 Proposed basis for structural differences between antigens constructed by the A₁ and A₂ subgroup transferases. Both A₁ and A₂ subgroup transferases can construct type 2 A determinants (far left) to yield molecules representative of the A₂ phenotype. This structure is then modified by a β1,3galactosyltransferase (β1,3Gal transferase) that forms a type 3 precursor (type 3 Gal A), which is also representative of the A₂ phenotype. The α(1,2)fucosyltransferase encoded by the H locus (H transferase) fucosylates this precursor to form type 3 H determinant. This molecule is efficiently utilized by the A₁ transferase (but not by the A₂ transferase) to form a type 3 A determinant, with repetitive A-reactive units. This structure is proposed to be responsible for the A₁ phenotype. R denotes the underlying glycosphingolipid substructure analogous to the molecule illustrated in Figure 3C. A-reactive portions of the molecule are circled, and the component monosaccharides of these moieties are italicized.

IV. THE CIS-AB PHENOTYPE

Rare pedigrees have been described wherein the ability to display both A and B determinants is inherited from a single parent (i.e., via a single chromosome) (46–48). In most individuals with the cis-AB phenotype, the A antigen reacts in a manner analogous to A_2 cells and the B antigen is only weakly reactive. Two general mechanisms may be considered to explain this phenotype. First, it seems possible that a single intrachromosomal gene duplication event could have yielded a pair of tandemly reiterated transferase loci; subsequent mutation within one or both of the duplicated alleles could then give rise to the inheritance of two closely linked loci that encode separate transferases, one with *A*-like activity and one with *B*-like activity. Support for this mechanism comes from studies of a cis-AB family wherein biochemical studies demonstrated that the *A*-like and *B*-like cis-inherited transferase activities could be physically separated (49).

In an alternative mechanism, mutagenesis of a wild-type *A* or *B* transferase (via point mutation, gene conversion, or intragenic crossover) could in theory yield a hybrid enzyme capable of utilizing the nucleotide sugar substrates for both the *A* and *B* transferases and thus also capable of constructing both A and B determinants. In this context, it should be noted that biochemical studies have demonstrated that group *B* $\alpha(1,3)$galactosyltransferase may under some circumstances utilize UDP-GalNAC to form A determinants (50). This observation is perhaps not surprising when one considers that the substrates UDP-galactose and UDP-N-acetylgalactosamine are structurally similar compounds, and suggests the possibility that a hybrid enzyme capable of cis-AB–like activity might arise from the *A* or *B* transferase allele after a rather small number of amino acid alterations. Support for a hybrid enzyme mechanism comes from studies of cis-AB pedigrees where it has not been possible to physically dissociate the cis-inherited AB transferase activity into component A and B transferase activities (51,52). These latter studies thus imply that in some cis-AB pedigrees, a single allele gives rise to a bifunctional enzyme that can utilize UDP-GalNAc and UDP-Gal with comparable, though not equal, efficiencies to yield both A and B structures (51).

V. MOLECULAR CLONING OF THE *ABO* LOCUS

Isolation and characterization of the deoxyribonucleic acid (DNA) sequences corresponding to the *ABO* locus represent a major and largely final step toward a molecular confirmation of the hypothesis that this locus encodes a series of allelic glycosyltransferases and thus determines red cell ABO phenotype. Early efforts toward this end included attempts to isolate the *A* or *B* transferases from human serum (53,54) and human urine (reviewed in ref. 17). These enzymes, like other mammalian glycosyltransferases, are typically found in vanishingly small amounts in these fluids, and purification efforts from these sources yielded transferase protein in an impure state or in amounts too small to be useful. Recently, however, the human A enzyme has been isolated in sufficient quantity and purity for molecular cloning purposes (55). Human lung served as the source of enzyme for this purification in a multistep chromatography protocol that achieved a 600,000-fold purification. The soluble enzyme obtained with this approach was virtually homogeneous and was subjected to protein sequencing procedures. The partial amino acid sequence so obtained was used to construct a series of corresponding synthetic deoxy-oligonucleotides; these were in turn used with the polymerase chain reaction to isolate a cloned complementary DNA (cDNA) corresponding to the *A* blood group $\alpha(1,3)N$-acetylgalac-tosaminyltransferase (56). The DNA sequence of this cDNA predicts a corresponding 353–amino acid long protein. This protein is predicted to be a membrane-spanning protein by virtue of an extremely hydrophobic 24–amino acid segment near its amino terminus. This hydrophobic segment is preceded by a 15-residue amino terminal segment and is followed by some 314 amino acids at the carboxy terminus. This type of sequence organization is topologically analogous to that previously described for several other mammalian glyco-syltransferases (reviewed in ref. 57) and yields a so-called type II transmembrane orientation (Fig. 5). This topology (58) places the short amino terminus of the protein in the cytosol and the longer COOH terminal segment within the lumen of the Golgi apparatus. It is in the Golgi lumen and also in distal membrane-delimited compartments between the Golgi and the exterior of the cell, collectively called the trans-Golgi network (59), that virtually all terminal glycosylation reactions occur (60). It therefore follows that this large COOH terminal segment corresponds to the catalytically active portion of the enzyme, as has been demonstrated experimentally for other mammalian glycosyltransferases (61,62). The protein contains a single potential consensus sequence for asparagine-linked glycosylation (60), suggesting that this enzyme, like other mammalian glycosyltransferases (57), is synthesized as a glycoprotein. Evidence supporting the assignment of the cloned cDNA to the transferase enzyme itself includes that fact that peptide sequence information derived from the purified enzyme corresponds with near perfection to several positions in the predicted sequence (56).

As noted above, the cDNA predicts a membrane-bound enzyme, whereas the A transferase was isolated as a soluble entity (55). This apparent discrepancy may be resolved when considering the fact that the amino terminus of the soluble purified enzyme corresponds to an alanine residue at residue 54, as predicted by the cDNA sequence. This observation demonstrates that the biogenesis of the A transferase is similar to that described for other mammalian

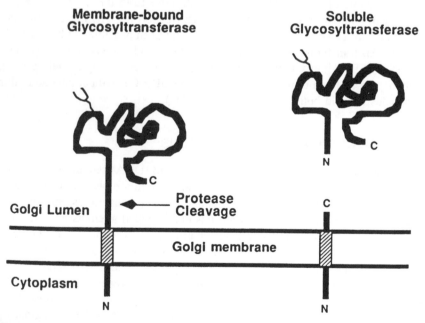

Figure 5 Topological schematic of the type II transmembrane orientation of mammalian glycosyl-transferases, including the A and B blood group glycosyltransferases. The amino terminus (N) of the intact enzyme is located within the cytosplasm, whereas the larger carboxy terminal portion (C), corresponding to the catalytic domain, is found in the lumen of the Golgi apparatus. The enzyme is anchored within the Golgi membrane by a short, hydrophobic transmembrane segment (hatched box). The A and B transferases are predicted to contains a single potential N-linked glycosylation site, which, if utilized, would imply that the enzyme is a glycoprotein (this oligosaccharide is denoted by the branched motif attached to the protein backbone). Soluble, catalytically active forms of mammalian glycosyltransferases are believed to be derived from their membrane-bound precursors by a proteolytic event that releases the catalytic domain from the membrane tether.

glycosyltransferases in that its soluble, catalytically active form is derived from a transmembrane precursor by a specific proteolytic cleavage (see Fig. 5). This process presumably accounts for the soluble, catalytically active A and B transferase activities that may be detected in human serum (53,54), for example.

The A transferase cDNA represents a tool with which to investigate the molecular basis for polymorphism at the ABO locus via molecular analysis of A, B, and O alleles (63). In outline, the first of these studies entailed DNA sequence analysis of cDNAs derived from cultured human cell lines that exhibited various ABO phenotypes. In cloned cDNAs derived from O phenotype cell lines, DNA sequencing analysis determined that they each contained a single base pair deletion relative to the A transferase cDNA. This deletion corresponds to one of the base pairs within the codon for amino acid residue 87 of the A transferase. This single base pair deletion shifts the translational reading frame and consequently yields a polypeptide whose amino acid sequence is completely different from the A transferase amino acid sequence in a region distal to amino acid residue 86. Furthermore, the frameshifted translational reading frame then yields a termination codon corresponding to position 117 of the A transferase (Fig. 6). Thus, the consequence of this single base pair deletion in the O allele, and its associated alterations in the predicted polypeptide sequence, is that the O allele is predicted to give rise to an messenger ribonucleic acid (mRNA) transcript that, if translated, would yield an altered and shortened polypeptide without a functional catalytic domain. This protein would presumably be incapable of exhibiting any transferase activity, a prediction that is in keeping with the observation that homozygous O individuals display no detectable A or B determinants on their red cells, nor is it possible to demonstrate A or B transferase activities in their sera.

To determine the molecular basis for the differences between the A and B transferase alleles, transferase cDNAs were isolated from cell lines with A and/or B phenotypes (63). Comparisons of the DNA sequences of these molecules identified seven nucleotide sequence differences between their respective protein-coding portions. These differences yield four consistent and distinct amino acid differences between the A and B enzymes, in addition to several presumably functionally neutral amino acid sequence polymorphisms (Fig. 6) (63). The consistent differences represent either arginine (A) or glycine (B) at amino acid position 176, glycine (A) or serine (B) at position 235, leucine (A) or methionine (B) at position 266, and glycine (A) or alanine (B) at position 268. The polymerase chain reaction was used to confirm that the DNA sequence differences found in the cDNAs also exist at the genomic DNA level in individuals of known ABO phenotype. These observations indicate that the nature of specific amino acid residues at as few as four positions, in a transferase consisting of 353 amino acids, can determine the efficiency with which the enzyme can utilize a nucleotide sugar substrate, and thus also determine which of two different oligosaccharide structures will be displayed on the surface of a red cell. Thus, for the A and B transferases, these four amino acid sequence differences, in isolation or in combination, can determine if the transferase will utilize UDP-GalNAc (A transferase) or UDP-Gal (B transferase) (63).

A subsequent study has explored the relationship between these four polymorphic amino acid pairs and the ability of the corresponding enzyme to utilize UDP-GalNAc and UDP-Gal (64). In this study, chimeric cDNAs were constructed so as to yield transferase polypeptides in which all possible combinations of the four polymorphic pairs were represented (64). Each chimeric cDNA was then tested for its ability to yield surface-localized A and/or B antigen expression, when expressed after transfection in HeLa cells, an O phenotype–cultured human cell line. These experiments demonstrated that the arginine (A) or glycine (B) polymorphism at amino acid position 176 has little, if any, influence on the enzymes' abilities to discriminate between UDP-GalNAc and UDP-Gal. By contrast, substrate discrimination is strongly influenced by the polymorphisms at positions 266 and 268. Specifically, the A transferase genotype at these two positions (leucine at position 266; glycine at position 268) yields an A phenotype regardless of the polypeptide sequence (*A* or *B*) at the other two polymorphic residues. Likewise, *B* transferase genotype (methionine at position 266; alanine at position 268) at these two positions yields a B phenotype regardless of the sequence at the other two polymorphic positions.

In a more complex combination (64), a chimera containing the *A*-type residue at 266 (leucine) and the *B*-type residue at 268 (alanine) functions only as an *A* transferase when position 235 is occupied by an *A*-type residue (glycine) at position 235. By contrast, a similar chimera, containing the *A*-type residue at 266 and the *B*-type residue at 268, but instead containing a *B*-type residue (serine) at position 235, will express a low level of *B* enzyme activity in addition to essentially normal *A* enzyme activity. This latter chimeric enzyme thus represents a single polypeptide with "AB" activity. Four other chimeric enzymes constructed in this study also exhibited AB activity. These chimeras have in common the *B*-specific amino acid at position 266 (methionine) and the *A*-specific residue at positions 268 (glycine). These observations provide support for the hypothesis that the AB activity in some cis-AB pedigrees is manifest by naturally occurring chimeric transferase capable of utilizing both UDP-GalNAc and UDP-Gal (51). It can be expected that a confirmation of this hypothesis, and of alternative ones, will be obtained using approaches similar to those described above. Likewise, these methods should prove useful in exploring the molecular basis for differences in substrate affinities exhibited by the transferases encoded by *A* and *B* subgroup alleles and may in turn yield a better understanding of the molecular differences between the oligosaccharide products constructed by the variant *A* and *B* transferases.

VI. THE HUMAN *H* AND *Se* BLOOD GROUP LOCI

As outlined above, the transferases encoded by the *ABO* locus operate upon H blood group–active oligosaccharide precursors (see Fig. 2). H-active precursors are essential substrates for the A and B transferases, which will not utilize oligosaccharide substrates without terminal Fucα1,2Galβ linkages (5). Likewise, Fucα1,2Galβ linkages represent integral components of A and B antigenic determinants, since, for example, the B-like antigen Galα(1,3)Galβ 1,4GlcNAc-R does not react with antisera directed against bona fide blood group A determinants (65).

As shown in Figure 2, H-active Fucα1,2Galβ linkages are constructed by the action of α(1,2)fucosyltransferases (GDP-Fuc:Galβ 2-α-L-fucosyltransferase, E.C. 2.4.1.69). These enzymes may act upon type 1, 2, 3, or 4 glycoprotein or glycolipid precursors (reviewed in ref. 5) or even on free β-D-galactosides (66). In humans, a rather common genetic polymorphism exists at a locus termed the *Secretor* (*Se*) locus, which in turn determines the expression of α(1,2)fucosyltransferase activity, and thus H antigen, in tissues that elaborate secreted, soluble blood group–active glycoproteins, glycophingolipids, and free oligosaccharides. This trait is classically determined by testing saliva for the presence of blood group–active substances with hemagglutination-inhibition procedures (34). The bulk of blood group–active material (largely based upon type 1 precursors; reviewed in ref. 4) is apparently produced by submaxillary glands and sublingual glands, with substantially lesser amounts being made by the parotid gland (67,68). Consequently, because of the essential role for H determinants in the synthesis of A and B determinants, this locus also determines whether or not an individual with a functional *A* and/or *B* allele will synthesize and release soluble A- and/or B-active blood group substance in these tissues. Thus, in Secretor individuals, which represent roughly 80% of most populations (69), H-active blood group substance is detected in saliva, as is also A- and/or B-active substance, depending upon the alleles present at the *ABO* locus. By contrast, the salivary glands of non-Secretors do not synthesize H-active determinants, nor A or B determinants, despite the fact that the *A* or *B* transferases may be present in those tissues.

Genetic polymorphisms also exist at a second, apparently distinct locus, termed the *H* locus, that also determines expression of α(1,2)fucosyltransferase activity (reviewed in ref. 4 and 5). It is the *H* locus that is believed to encode the α(1,2)fucosyltransferase that acts in erythrocyte precursors to generate type 2 H determinants on red cells. Rare individuals, of the Bombay (O$_h$), phenotype (first described in ref. 70), represent examples of homozygosity for two null alleles at the *H* locus. The red cells of persons with this phenotype are deficient in H (and thus also A and B) determinants. The secretory tissues of individuals with the Bombay phenotype are also deficient in H determinants. These individuals consequently develop potent isoagglu-tinins directed against H, A, and B determinants, presumably by virtue of exposure to structurally analogous environmental antigens, and they are thus cross-match incompatible with all donors except those also deficient in the synthesis of H determinants (34,35).

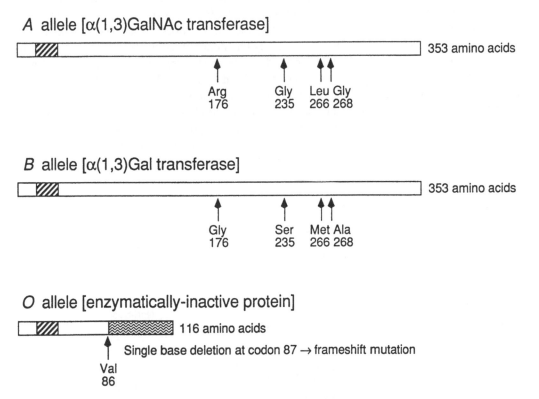

A allele [α(1,3)GalNAc transferase]

353 amino acids

Arg 176   Gly 235   Leu 266   Gly 268

B allele [α(1,3)Gal transferase]

353 amino acids

Gly 176   Ser 235   Met 266   Ala 268

O allele [enzymatically-inactive protein]

116 amino acids

Single base deletion at codon 87 → frameshift mutation

Val 86

Figure 6 Functionally significant structural differences between the polypeptides encoded by the *A*, *B*, and *O* alleles of the *ABO* blood group locus. Linear representations of the ABO polypeptides are displayed as boxes. The left border of each box corresponds to the amino terminus of that protein, and the right borders of each correspond to their respective carboxy termini. The hatched portion of each box denotes the transmembrane segment of the proteins. The *A* locus encodes a 354–amino acid long protein (top) that exhibits α(1,3)N-acetylgalactosaminyltransferase activity. The *B* locus encodes a protein of identical length (middle), which functions as an α(1,3)galactosyltransferase. The A and B enzymes differ at the four amino acid positions indicated by the numbered arrows. The amino acids at these positions are indicated above the numbers. The *O* allele encodes a truncated, enzymatically inactive protein with a length of 116 amino acids. The sequence of the *O* allele–encoded protein is identical to the sequences of A and B transferases through a valine residue at amino acid position 86 but differs at the 30 subsequent positions (indicated by the wavy lines within the box representing the *O*-encoded protein). These latter amino acids, and the termination codon that truncates the protein at 116 residues, are the consequence of a single base deletion in the DNA sequence corresponding to codon 87 of the *A* and *B* alleles (see text for additional detail).

In an attempt to construct a genetic model that unified the observations regarding the Secretor/non-Secretor phenotypes and the Bombay phenotypes, it was proposed that the *H* locus corresponds to a structural gene that encodes the α(1,2)fucosyltransferase found both in red cell precursors and in secretory epithelia, and that the *Se* locus represents a regulatory gene that controls expression of the *H* gene in secretory tissues (reviewed in ref. 5). Although this model was consistent with the phenotypes that had been studied at the time, it was not necessarily concordant with subsequent descriptions of the so-called para-Bombay phenotype (71). These individuals have H-deficient red cells, but they maintain an essentially normal amount of salivary H blood group substance (12). A complicated genetic model invoking a third locus (Z) that controls expression of the *H* gene in some tissues, has been put forth to explain the para-Bombay phenotype (reviewed in ref. 5).

To account for all of these observations, Oriol and his colleagues have instead postulated that the *H* and *Se* loci actually represent distinct structural genes that encode different α(1,2)fucosyltransferases (72). In this model (Fig. 7), the *H* locus is restricted in its expression to cells of the erythroid lineage (4), the epidermis (4,44), and primary sensory neurons of the peripheral nervous system (73). The α(1,2)fucosyltransferase encoded by the *Se* locus, is, in contrast, expressed by the epithelia that line the digestive, respiratory, biliary, and urinary tracts (74,75). One or two functional alleles at both the *H* and *Se* loci yield the Secretor phenotype. Homozygosity for null alleles at the *Se* locus, however, with one or two functional *H* alleles, yields the less common non-Secretor phenotype. Two null alleles at the *H* locus with at least one functional *Se* allele generates the para-Bombay phenotype, whereas Bombay phenotypic individuals maintain two null alleles at both loci. This is a more economical model than the regulatory locus models, and it is supported by an extensive analysis of a large series of

Genotype	Phenotype	Phenotype (trivial name)
HH or *Hh*	H (A&B) on red cells	
Sese or *SeSe*	H (A&B) in secretions	Secretor
HH or *Hh*	H (A&B) on red cells	
sese	H (A&B) absent from secretions	Non-Secretor
hh	weak or absent H (A&B) on red cells (antigens adsorbed from plasma)	
Sese or *SeSe*	H (A&B) in secretions	para-Bombay
hh	H (A&B) absent from red cells	
sese	H (A&B) absent from secretions	Bombay, or O$_h$

Figure 7   The two-locus hypothesis for H and Se phenotypes. The two-locus hypothesis of Oriol et al. (72) proposes that the *H* and *Se* loci represent distinct, autosomal (chromosome 19) α(1,2)fucosyltransferase genes with different tissue-specific expression patterns. This figure displays the antigenic phenotypes, for red cells and in secretions, predicted by this model for various genotypes at the two loci. A and B antigens are included in parentheses to indicate that they will be displayed also only if the individual also expresses a functional *A* or *B* transferase. H (and A or B) antigens are expressed weakly, or not at all, on the red cells of para-Bombay phenotypic individuals because they are acquired from glycosphingolipid-based antigens circulating in the plasma.

H-deficient pedigrees (72,76). It is furthermore supported by studies that have demonstrated substantial catalytic differences between the α(1,2)fucosyltransferase activity determined by the *H* locus and the α(1,2)fucosyltransferase activity determined by the *Se* locus (77–82). These studies have shown, for example, that the *Se*-determined enzyme maintains a substantially higher affinity for type 1 precursors than does the *H*-determined enzyme. This latter observation is consistent with other studies showing that the blood group substances found in secretory epithelium (where the *Se* locus is operative) are composed largely of type 1 molecules, whereas the bulk of red cell H determinants (constructed by the *H* locus) are formed from type 2 precursors (4). This model and its consequences are also consistent with the notion that the stereochemical differences between type 1 and type 2 precursors are so sufficiently large as to have required the evolution of a distinct α(1,2)fucosyltransferase for each (15). Genetic linkage analyses indicate that the *H* and *Se* loci are tightly linked on chromosome 19 (83), suggesting the possibility that the two genes evolved from a common ancestor by gene duplication mechanisms.

VII. MOLECULAR CLONING OF THE *H* BLOOD GROUP LOCUS

Recent molecular cloning work has elucidated the structure of a human α(1,2)fucosyltransferase gene and its cognate enzyme (82,84,85). This gene was isolated with a mammalian gene transfer system, in which a cultured murine cell line was used as a host for receipt of transfected human genomic DNA (84). This murine host did not express detectable α(1,2)fucosyltransferase activity nor surface-localized H blood group determinants. Nonetheless, these cells were shown to express surface-localized β-galactoside–terminating oligosaccharides that could function as acceptor molecules for α(1,2)fucosyltransferase, and were also shown to be able to synthesize fucosylated oligosaccharides. It was thus predicted that transfer of a functional human α(1,2)fucosyltransferase gene into these H antigen–negative murine cells would cause them to become H-antigen positive.

The source of transfected genetic material in this system was large (~100 kb), heterogeneous segments of human genomic DNA, which were introduced into the murine host by calcium phosphate–mediated transfection (84). It could be expected that transfer of the α(1,2)fucosyltransferase gene with this approach would occur at low frequency, since this gene would represent only a small fraction of the total number of human genes that would be transferred. Nonetheless, it was expected that these events, which would yield H-positive transfected cells, could be rescued by their adherence to plastic culture plates coated with an anti-H antibody. Several different H-positive transfectants were ultimately isolated with this approach (84). Southern blot analyses of these cell lines, using a probe specific for human *Alu*I repetitive DNA segments, disclosed that the genome of each contained two human DNA restriction fragments. Molecular cloning approaches were then used to isolate these two human DNA fragments from one of the H-positive transfectant cell lines. The larger of these two fragments was subsequently shown to determine expression of an α(1,2)fucosyltransferase when expressed in a cultured cell line (82).

Subsequent efforts have allowed the isolation and characterization of a cloned cDNA corresponding to this gene (85). This cDNA corresponds to a 3.6-kb transcript in human cells and contains an open reading frame that predicts the synthesis of a 365–amino acid long protein. This polypeptide, like the *A* and *B* transferases, is predicted to maintain the characteristic type II transmembrane topology typical of mammalian glycosyltransferases. This topology places the enzyme's amino terminal 8 residues within the cytosol, the next 17, relatively hydrophic residues within the Golgi membrane, and the remaining carboxy terminal 340 amino acids within the lumen of the Golgi apparatus (Fig. 8). Two potential N-glycosylation sites are found within this latter domain, suggesting that this enzyme is itself glycosylated. Despite its

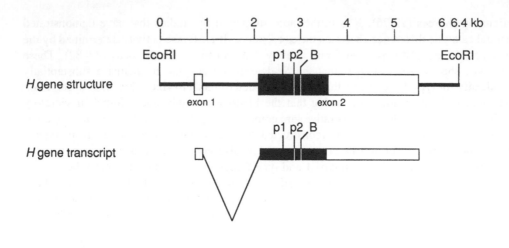

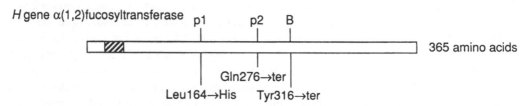

Figure 8 Structure of the *H* blood group gene, transcript, and fucosyltransferase and functionally significant mutations in Bombay and para-Bombay alleles. The human *H* gene (top) is contained within a 6.4-kb pair *Eco*RI DNA restriction fragment. It consists of two exons; exon 2 contains the entire coding region (solid region). The gene yields a 3.6-kb mRNA transcript (middle). The positions of inactivating mutations in the Bombay (B) and para-Bombay (p1 and p2) pedigrees discussed in the text are indicated on the gene structure and its transcript. The gene and its transcript are drawn to the scale indicated at the top of the figure. The transcript is translated to yield a 365–amino acid type 2 transmembrane protein (bottom, not to scale; transmembrane segment indicated by the hatched segment). The positions and identities of the amino acids corresponding to inactivating mutations in the Bombay and para-Bombay alleles are indicated above and below the schematic of the α(1,2)fucosyltransferase.

topological similarity to the *A* and *B* transferases, and other mammalian glycosyltransferases, this enzyme does not share any significant primary sequence similarity to any known polypeptides. Gene fusion experiments have been used to confirm that this cDNA does in fact encode an α(1,2)fucosyltransferase, and they indicate that the enzyme's COOH terminal 333 amino acids are sufficient to generate catalytic activity (85).

Analyses of the kinetic properties of the enzyme encoded by this cDNA are consistent with the notion that it corresponds to the human *H* blood group locus. Thus, as expressed in transfected cell lines (82,85), this α(1,2)fucosyltransferase displays affinities for donor and acceptor substrates (GDP-fucose, apparent K_m's between 12.4 and 17.5 mM; phenyl-β-D-galactoside, apparent K_m's between 2.0 and 4.4 mM) that are virtually indistinguishable from those exhibited by the human *H* α(1,2)fucosyltransferase (77–81). By contrast, these properties are significantly different from the properties ascribed to the α(1,2)fucosyltransferase activity believed to be encoded by the *Se* locus. Moreover, Southern blot techniques have localized this gene to human chromosome 19 (85), where the human *H* locus is known to reside (83).

VIII. MOLECULAR BASIS FOR BOMBAY AND PARA-BOMBAY PHENOTYPES

In recent studies designed to provide genetic confirmation that this gene corresponds to the *H* locus, the structure and function of this locus has been examined in Bombay and para-Bombay pedigrees (86). These studies were simplified by the observation that the coding portion of this rather small (less than 9 kb) gene is encompassed within a single 1.1-kb exon (see Fig. 8) (86). Sequence analysis of one allele of this gene in an individual with the Bombay phenotype identified six nucleotide sequence differences relative to a wild-type allele. One of these differences was located within the coding portion of the gene and creates a termination codon corresponding to a tyrosine residue at amino acid position 316 of the wild-type $\alpha(1,2)$fucosyltransferase (Tyr316→ter) (see Fig. 8). The coding region of this Bombay allele is thus predicted to yield a polypeptide whose COOH terminus is truncated by 50 amino acids relative to the wild-type enzyme. By contrast, the other sequence differences were located at positions that did not correspond to any obviously essential sites. To confirm that the coding sequence difference is responsible for inactivating this Bombay allele, mutagenesis procedures were used to move this DNA sequence difference and each of the others into the wild-type sequence background. The mutant sequences were then each tested for function by transfection into an $\alpha(1,2)$fucosyltransferase–deficient mammalian host (COS-1 cells). The construct containing the Tyr316→ter mutation generated no detectable $\alpha(1,2)$fucosyltransferase activity when tested in this manner, whereas each of the other mutant constructs yielded essentially normal activities. Finally, when the Tyr316→ter mutation in the Bombay allele was changed back to the wild-type tyrosine codon, full enzyme activity was restored. These results demonstrate that the Tyr316→ter mutation is responsible for inactivity of this allele, and they further indicate that the other DNA sequence differences represent functionally neutral DNA sequence polymorphisms.

Because the recessive Bombay phenotype is extremely rare (5,87), and because consanguinity is not infrequently observed in Bombay pedigrees (5,88), efforts were made to determine if the Bombay phenotypic individual was homozygous for the Tyr316→ter mutation. This sequence difference yields restriction site cleavage polymorphisms for a *Bst*N1 site (cleaves the wild-type allele) and an *Alu*I site (cleaves Bombay allele). The authors used the polymerase chain reaction to generate the segment of the coding region that encompasses this DNA sequence difference, using genomic DNA isolated from individuals in the pedigree. Restriction endonuclease cleavage analysis of this fragment was then used to assign alleles at this position. These analyses demonstrated that the Bombay phenotypic individual inherited the Tyr316→ter mutant allele from each (heterozygous) parent and is thus homozygous for the Tyr316→ter mutation. The other living siblings are not erythroid H deficient and were shown to be either heterozygous for the Tyr316→ter allele or homozygous for the wild-type sequence at this position. The Tyr316→ter allele was not detected with this approach in more that 100 alleles from unrelated H-positive individuals, thus demonstrating that it represents a rare sequence alteration. These data indicate that the Tyr316→ter mutation is responsible for the H-deficient phenotype of the propositus, and they also support the hypothesis that this gene corresponds to the human *H* blood group locus.

To directly test the hypothesis that the *H* and *Se* loci represent distinct $\alpha(1,2)$fuco-syltransferase genes, the authors studied both alleles of the cloned $\alpha(1,2)$fucosyltransferase gene in a Secretor-positive, erythroid H–deficient individual (para-Bombay phenotype; ref. 71). The coding region of each para-Bombay allele was found to contain a single base sequence alteration relative to corresponding positions in the wild-type $\alpha(1,2)$fucosyltransferase gene. One of the sequence differences yields a termination codon at a position corresponding to amino acid residue 276 (Gln276→ter) (see Fig. 8). This alteration is predicted to generate a protein that is truncated at a position 90 amino acids from the carboxy terminus of the wild-type $\alpha(1,2)$fucosyltransferase. The truncated protein derived from the Gln276→ter mutation was inactive as an $\alpha(1,2)$fucosyltransferase when tested by transfection. The DNA sequence found on the other allele represents a missense mutation at codon 164. This sequence difference substitutes a histidine for the leucine found at this position in the wild-type protein (Leu164→His) (see Fig. 8). This protein also yields undetectable $\alpha(1,2)$fucosyltransferase activity when tested by transfection.

Thus, since the para-Bombay phenotypic individual possessing these two inactive alleles expresses a functional *Se*-determined $\alpha(1,2)$fucosyltransferase (but not an *H*-determined $\alpha(1,2)$fucosyltransferase), the authors concluded that the human genome must contain a second $\alpha(1,2)$fucosyltransferase gene distinct from the *H* $\alpha(1,2)$fucosyltransferase locus, and that this second gene most likely corresponds to the *Se* locus. These results are consistent with the two-locus model of Oriol et al. (72), indicate that inactivating point mutations in the coding sequence of this cloned $\alpha(1,2)$fucosyltransferase gene are responsible for H blood group antigen deficiency in some Bombay and para-Bombay phenotypic individuals, and provide confirmatory evidence for biochemical (82,85) and chromosomal localization (85) studies that assign this gene to the human *H* blood group locus.

Future efforts in this area will most likely center on attempts to isolate the human *Se* blood group locus; on defining, at the molecular level, the tissue-specific expression patterns of the *H* and *Se* genes; and, ultimately, on identifying the functions, if any, for these genes and their cognate oligosaccharide products.

IX. THE HUMAN LEWIS BLOOD GROUP SYSTEM

The human Lewis blood group was first described in the context of an investigation into two cases of hemolytic disease of the newborn (Lewis was the surname of one of the women with the antibodies) (89). Although these studies indicated that the anti-Lewis antibodies apparently played no role in the disease process itself, they nonetheless demonstrated that the antigens represented a previously undescribed blood group antigen system that appeared to be inherited in a dominant manner. Subsequent studies demonstrated that the antigenic portion of the Lewis-active molecules is composed of carbohydrate and elucidated their molecular structures (Fig. 9) and their biosynthesis (Fig. 10) (90,91; reviewed in ref. 5).

As discussed below, human red cells display Le^a or Le^b antigens or no Lewis antigens at all depending upon an individual's *Lewis* (*Le*) and *Se* genotype. Red cell Le^a and Le^b antigens are not synthesized by the red cell precursors but are instead acquired by the erythrocyte membrane via an apparently passive adsorptive process that transfers Lewis-active molecules from the plasma where they normally circulate (92). The structures of the circulating Le^a- and Le^b-active molecules have been determined in fine detail (93,94) (see Fig. 9). These represent glycosphingolipids that are apparently transported in the plasma complexed with both low-density and high-density lipoproteins or as aqueous dispersions (92).

In most instances, anti-Lewis antibodies are apparently naturally occurring (34). They represent a rather common specificity in blood group serology; whereas potent anti-Le^a antibodies have been implicated in clinically significant hemolytic transfusion reactions, anti-Le^b antibodies have not generally been associated with this problem. Transfused plasma containing soluble Le^a or Le^b substances effectively neutralizes circulating Lewis antibodies (95). Moreover, Lewis antigen–positive red cells lose these antigens after they are introduced into a transfusion recipient (96) by a reversal of the adsorptive process through which they acquired these molecules in the donor.

The red cells of newborns are almost invariably deficient in Lewis antigens, but they acquire these determinants (Le^a initially in Lewis-positive infants) beginning about 10 days after birth

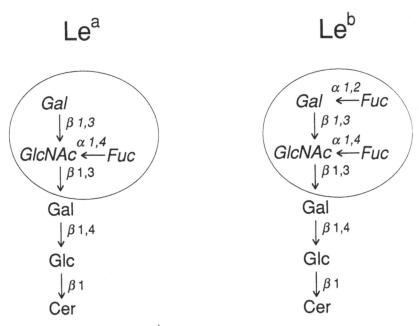

Figure 9   Structures of the Le^a and Le^b blood group glycosphingolipids. The immunodominant portion of each molecule is circled, and the component monosaccharides are italicized. The molecule associates with the red cell membrane via the ceramide (Cer) moiety.

(97). Full phenotypic expression of red cell Lewis antigens is achieved by about 24 months (98).

Genetic and biochemical studies have demonstrated that synthesis of the Le^a and Le^b antigens is under the control of both the *Se* and *Le* blood group loci (reviewed in refs. 4 and 5) (see Figs. 9 and 10). The *Le* blood group locus is believed to correspond to a structural gene that encodes an α(1,3/1,4)fucosyltransferase capable of utilizing a variety of oligosaccharide precursors (99–102) (see Fig. 9). This enzyme can operate upon unsubstituted type 1 oligosaccharide precursors to yield the Le^a determinant, and it can operate upon type 1 H determinants to generate the Le^b determinant (99–101). Histochemical studies and biochemical analysis of body fluids indicate that the *Lewis* fucosyltransferase is expressed with a tissue specificity that mirrors that of the *Se* locus. Thus, it is possible to identify *Lewis* locus–dependent expression of Le^a and Le^b antigens on the epithelia that line the digestive, respiratory, and urinary tracts, on bile ducts, and in salivary glands (reviewed in refs. 4 and 5). These tissues are largely of endodermal origin and generally correspond to the tissue types that express type 1 H determinants under the control of the *Se* locus.

Because the *Se* and *Le* loci are expressed in many of the same tissues, and because the *Lewis* enzyme can act upon the oligosaccharide product of the *Se* locus, an individual's genotype at both of the two loci determines if that individual will express Le^a molecules, Le^b molecules, or neither Le^a nor Le^b molecules. Thus, in secretory epithelia of Secretor-positive persons (where the *Se* α(1,2)fucosyltransferase is active), type 1 precursors are first converted to type 1 H determinants. These molecules are in turn converted to Le^b-active molecules by the action of the *Lewis* fucosyltransferase (Fig. 10A). In non-Secretors, however, type 1 H determinants are not synthesized, so that the unsubstituted type 1 precursors are converted by the *Lewis* enzyme into Le^a-active molecules (Fig. 10C). Naturally, in individuals homozygous for null alleles at the *Le* locus (Lewis-negative phenotype), but with at least one functional *Se* allele

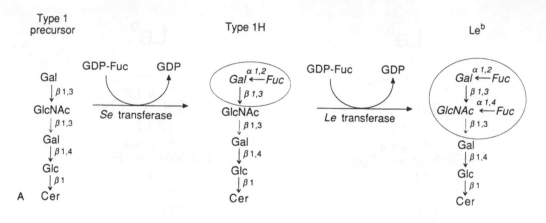

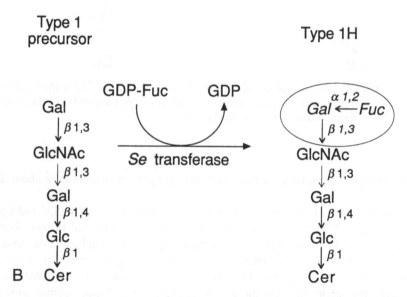

Figure 10 Biosynthesis of the Le[a] and Le[b] determinants. The α(1,2)fucosyltransferase determined by the *Secretor* locus (*Se* transferase) and the α(1,3/1,4)fucosyltransferase encoded by the *Lewis* locus (*Le* fucosyltransferase) operate singly, or sequentially, on type 1 glycosphingolipid precursors. The final product thus will depend upon the genotype at both loci (see text for details). The oligosaccharide products of each of the four possible phenotypes are indicated in panels A through D. The immunodominant portion of each molecule is circled, and component monosaccharides are italicized.

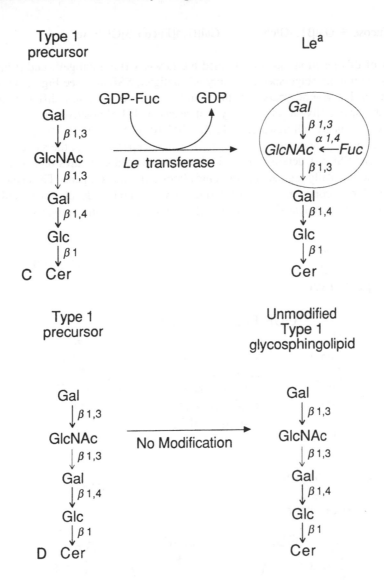

(Secretor-positive phenotype), type 1 H determinants will be synthesized but will remain unconverted to Le^b molecules (Fig. 10B). Similarly, in Secretor-negative, Lewis-negative individuals, only unsubstituted type 1 molecules will be made, and these will not be converted to Le^a-active molecules (Fig. 10D).

X. MOLECULAR CLONING OF *LEWIS* BLOOD GROUP LOCUS

Studies of the *Lewis* fucosyltransferase purified from human milk demonstrated that it is capable of constructing both Le^a and Le^b determinants and also a set of isomeric oligosaccharide molecules based on type 2 precursors (99,100) (Fig. 11). The Lewis enzyme thus represents an exception to a hypothesis that each mammalian glycosyltransferase is capable of constructing a single type of glycosidic linkage (103). Other biochemical studies (104) indicate that the Lewis enzyme is an example of a group of distinct of α(1,3)fucosyltransferases (GDP-Fuc:N-acetylglucosaminide 3-α-L-fucosyltransferases, E.C. 2.4.1.65) that can each catalyze the following general reaction using type 2 precursors:

$$\text{GDP-L-fucose} + \text{Gal}\beta1,4\text{GlcNAc-} \rightarrow \text{Gal}\beta1,4[\text{Fuc}\alpha1,3]\text{GlcNAc}$$

The product of this reaction has been termed the Lewis x (Le^x) antigen, and it has also been described as the murine stage-specific embryonic antigen, SSEA-1 (see Fig. 11) (105,106). (It should be noted that several years ago, the term Lewis x was used in a different context; i.e., to describe the specificity of an antibody that reacts with Le^a-positive, and Le^b-positive red cells and also with nearly all newborn red cells [107,108]. Although the antigen recognized by this type of antibody remains poorly characterized, it is apparently not the same as the SSEA-1 antigen [4]). The SSEA-1 determinant and related fucosylated structures represent members of a class of developmentally regulated embryonic oligosaccharide antigens. These molecules have been implicated in morphogenetic events during early mammalian development and thus impart a more generalized biological significance to the Lewis blood group antigens (reviewed in ref. 109).

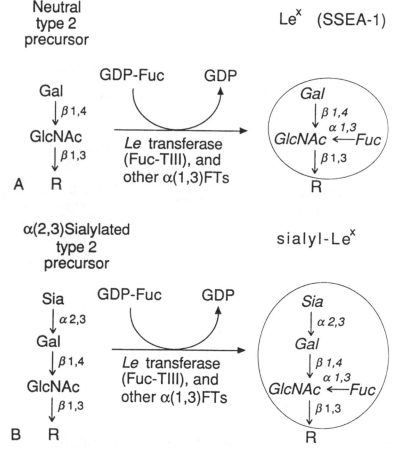

Figure 11 Le^x, sialyl-Le^x, sialyl-Le^a, and Le^y structures and biosynthesis. The Le^x determinant may be formed by $\alpha(1,3)$fucosylation of neutral 2 precursors (panel A). The *Lewis* fucosyltransferase and other human $\alpha(1,3)$fucosyltransferases ($\alpha(1,3)$FTs) are each competent to complete this reaction. The sialyl-Le^x molecule is formed by $\alpha(1,3)$fucosylation of type 2 precursors previously substituted with sialic acid (Sia) in $\alpha(2,3)$linkage (panel B). The *Lewis* fucosyltransferase and other human $\alpha(1,3)$fucosyltransferases ($\alpha[1,3]$FTs) can also complete this reaction. The sialyl-Le^a molecule is formed (panel C) in a manner analogous to the formation of sialyl-Le^x from type 1 precursors previously substituted with sialic acid in $\alpha(2,3)$linkage. The *Lewis* enzyme is most likely the only human fucosyltransferase capable of efficiently catalyzing this fucosylation reaction. The Le^y molecule is formed from type 2 H determinants (panel D)

A gene transfer approach has been used to isolate a cloned cDNA tentatively assigned to the *Lewis* blood group locus (101). The host for this approach was a cultured primate kidney cell line (COS-1) naturally deficient in endogenous $\alpha(1,3)$fucosyltransferases activity. These cells are thus also deficient in cell surface Lewis antigens, but they do construct surface-localized type 2 oligosaccharide molecules that can serve as precursors for the action of $\alpha(1,3)$fucosyltransferase activity encoded by exogenous genetic material in the form of a mammalian cDNA expression library. It was thus anticipated that transfection of the cDNA expression library into this cell line would yield rare transfectants that expressed surface-localized Le^x epitopes by virtue of their receipt and expression of a functional $\alpha(1,3)$fucosyltransferase cDNA. It was further expected that these particular Le^x-positive transfectants could be rescued from the other

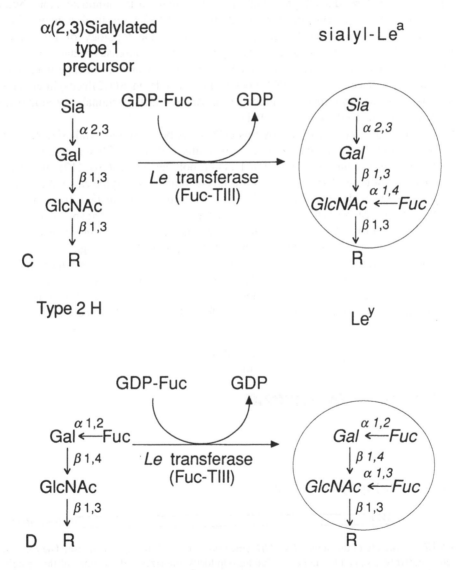

in a manner analogous to the synthesis of Le^b determinants from type 1 H determinants (see Fig. 10A). R denotes underlying the glycoconjugate substructure, which may consist of a protein- or lipid-linked oligosaccharide or free oligosaccharide. Immunodominant portions of these four molecules are circled, and the monosaccharide components of each epitope are italicized.

Le^x-negative cells in the population because they would adhere to plates coated with an anti-Le^x antibody. Episomal vector molecules, containing cloned α(1,3)fucosyltransferase cDNAs, could then be rescued from these Le^x-positive adherent cells.

This cell line was therefore transfected with a mammalian cDNA expression library prepared from a human cell line (A431 cells) that displays cell surface Lewis antigens (110), and that also expresses relatively high levels α(1,3)fucosyltransferase activity. The library was prepared in a mammalian expression vector (111) capable of efficiently transcribing the cloned cDNAs and also capable of replicating in both prokaryotic *(Escherichia coli)* and mammalian (COS-1 cells) hosts. The transfected COS-1 cells were first screened for transfected, Le^x-positive cells and later with an α(1,3)fucosyltransferase assay and a procedure known as "sib selection." This approach yielded a cloned cDNA whose sequence predicted a 361–amino acid long type II polypeptide with a 15-residue NH$_2$ terminal cytosolic domain, a 19–amino acid long hydrophobic membrane spanning segment, and a 327-residue COOH terminal domain (Fig. 12). Biochemical studies confirmed the predicted transmembrane topology of the protein and demonstrated that the two asparagine-linked glycosylation consensus sequences within the protein are utilized to yield a glycosylated fucosyltransferase. Gene fusion experiments reported in this paper confirmed that the cDNA does in fact encode an α(1,3)fucosyltransferase and indicate that sequence information within the enzyme's COOH-terminal 319 amino acids is sufficient to generate catalytic activity (101).

The recombinant enzyme encoded by this cDNA has been used to synthesize several types of α(1,3)- and α(1,4)fucosylated molecules, including Le^a, Le^b, SSEA-1 or Le^x, sialyl-Le^a, and sialyl-Le^x determinants (see Figs. 9 and 11) on both analytical (101,112) and preparative (113) scales. The oligosaccharide products that this recombinant enzyme can make mirror those made by the Lewis blood group α(1,3/1,4)fucosyltransferase purified from human milk (100,114) and provide very strong evidence that the cloned cDNA corresponds to the human *Lewis* blood group locus. This cDNA localizes to a gene on human chromosome 19, where the *Lewis* locus is known to reside (83,115), in further support of this assignment. It should be emphasized, however, that this remains a provisional assignment; confirmation will require formal linkage of this gene to the Lewis blood group phenotype in pedigrees informative for this locus. This cloned cDNA and its corresponding genomic sequences should also facilitate studies designed to determine the molecular basis for null alleles at this locus. Like the *H* locus,

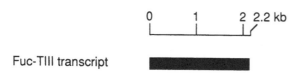

Fuc-TIII [α(1,3/1,4)fucosyltransferase]

361 amino acids

Figure 12   Structure of the human *Fuc-TIII* gene transcript, and fucosyltransferase. The *Fuc-TIII* gene has been tentatively assigned to the *Lewis* blood group locus; the sizes and positions of this gene's intron and exons have not yet been defined. Its transcript is drawn to the scale indicated at the top of the figure. The coding portion of this transcript (solid region) encodes a 361–amino acid type 2 transmembrane protein that functions as an α(1,3/1,4)fucosyltransferase (bottom, not to scale; transmembrane segment indicated by the hatched segment).F12

this gene contains a single coding exon (J.B. Lowe, unpublished data), which should simplify these types of analyses. The enzyme encoded data by this gene has recently been termed Fuc-TIII (116) in an attempt to simplify the nomenclature of the human $\alpha(1,3)$fucosyltransferase genes and to avoid referring to it as the *Lewis* enzyme until this assignment has been confirmed.

XI.   THE *Fuc-TIII* GENE IS A MEMBER OF AN $\alpha(1,3)$FUCOSYLTRANSFERASE GENE FAMILY

Biochemical and genetic studies indicated that the human genome encodes at least four, and perhaps more, distinct $\alpha(1,3)$fucosyltransferase activities (104,117–122). One of these corresponds to the enzyme believed to be encoded by the *Lewis* locus. Recent molecular cloning studies have begun to illuminate the structural and functional properties of the other $\alpha(1,3)$-fucosyltransferase genes, and their relationship to the *Fuc-TIII* gene described in the section above, which has been tentatively assigned to the *Lewis* locus. These studies have identified and characterized three additional human $\alpha(1,3)$fucosyltransferase genes (112,116,123–125). One of these, termed *Fuc-TIV* (112,116,124), or *ELFT* (123), is apparently expressed in myeloid cells, and localizes to human chromosome 11 (116). Its corresponding enzyme is encoded by a single exon and shares approximately 60% amino acid sequence identity with Fuc-TIII. The two other distinct human $\alpha(1,3)$fucosyltransferase genes that have been isolated encode enzymes termed Fuc-TV and Fuc-TVI. Like *Fuc-TIII*, these genes are found on human chromosome 19, and maintain single coding exons (116,125). Their corresponding enzyme products share more than 90% amino acid sequence identity with each other and with Fuc-TIII. Southern blot analyses indicate that the *Fuc-TIV*, *-V*, and *-VI* genes fully represent all existing human genes with substantial DNA sequence similarity to the *Fuc-TIII* gene. By contrast, these analyses have identified as yet uncloned human DNA sequences that cross-hybridize with the *Fuc-TIV* gene, which may represent additional fucosyltransferase genes whose protein sequences may be more similar to *Fuc-TIV* than to the chromosome 19-localized genes *Fuc-TIII*, *-V*, and *-VI*.

These observations suggest the possibility that a relatively distant gene duplication event generated two distinct ancestral $\alpha(1,3)$fucosyltransferase genes on two different chromosomes and that they have subsequently undergone substantial sequence divergence. In turn, more recent duplicative events may have generated the family of structurally similar chromosome 19-localized $\alpha(1,3)$fucosyltransferase genes, that have not yet experienced substantial sequence divergence, and that remain physically linked on chromosome 19. This hypothesis is consistent with analyses of pedigrees containing individuals deficient in $\alpha(1,3)$fucosyltransferase activities, wherein an inherited deficiency in the ability to express a plasma-type $\alpha(1,3)$fucosyltransferase activity is genetically linked to the Lewis blood group–negative phenotype (120). Preliminary Southern blot analyses, which suggest that the chromosome 19-localized $\alpha(1,3)$fucosyl-transferase genes maintain close physical linkage (B.W. Weston, unpublished data), also support this proposal. Confirmation of this hypothesis will require the completion of ongoing efforts to define precisely the physical relationship of these genes.

XII.   LEWIS-TYPE OLIGOSACCHARIDES FUNCTION AS LIGANDS FOR CELL ADHESION RECEPTORS IN INFLAMMATION

Recent work has demonstrated that members of the Lewis family of oligosaccharide determinants play important, essential roles in the process whereby immune cells leave the vascular tree to arrive at inflammatory foci. It has been known for some time that an initial step in this process involves adherence of myeloid-lineage cells (neutrophils and monocytes) to the vascular endothelium within an inflammatory focus (reviewed in ref. 126). Vascular endothelial cells express an adhesion receptor, known as endothelial leukocyte adhesion molecules 1 (ELAM-1) (127), or E-selectin (128), through which myeloid cells bind to the vascular wall. The structure of E-selectin indicates that it is a member of a family of carbohydrate-binding proteins (127), or lectins (129), and has suggested that it binds to myeloid cells via specific, surface-localized oligosaccharide counter-receptor molecules. Several groups have now confirmed this hypothesis, and have demonstrated that E-selectin binds with high affinity to sialyl-Le^x determinants (see Fig. 11) expressed on myeloid cells (102,130–132). Likewise, it has been shown that E-selectin can also bind with high affinity to sialyl-Le^a determinants (132–134) (see Fig. 11), which are "aberrantly" expressed by some types of cancer cells (135). Sialyl-Le^x determinants also may be "aberrantly" expressed in some malignancies; these observations have prompted suggestions that sialyl-Le^a and sialyl-Le^x oligosaccharides expressed by malignant cells may function to promote E-selectin–dependent metastasis (102,133,134). These oligosaccharide molecules may also function as counter-receptors for two other members of the selectin family of lectinlike cell adhesion receptors, P-selectin (136,137) and L-selectin (138), and thus may play roles in lymphocyte trafficking (via L-selectin) and in acute inflammation (via P-selectin) (reviewed in ref. 139). In these contexts, it should be noted that the *Fuc-TIII* gene, tentatively assigned to the *Lewis* blood group locus, encodes an enzyme that can participate in the synthesis of both sialyl-Le^x and sialyl-Le^a molecules (101,102) (see Fig. 11). Thus, it may predicted that an individual's *Lewis* genotype may influence the likelihood of selectin-dependent spread of malignancies.

XIII. CONCLUSIONS

Experimental exploration of the ABO, H/Se, and Lewis blood groups has evolved from serological descriptions of the antigens, to determination of their chemical structures, and, more recently, to the isolation and characterization of the genes that are responsible for their biosynthesis and expression. These latter efforts are now beginning to define the molecular genetic basis for polymorphisms at these loci. Nonetheless, the biological functions, if any, of these blood group oligosaccharide determinants remain undefined. Homozygosity for null alleles at each of these loci is apparently unaccompanied by any obvious and serious detrimental phenotype (excepting in the context of a mismatched blood transfusion). This would suggest that these molecules do not now participate in essential functions in humans even though they may have done so in the evolutionarily distant past. Nonetheless, the functions recently assigned to the sialylated Lewis molecules indicate that these types of oligosaccharides do play important roles in essential biological processes. In this context, it seems possible that the now (apparently) vestigial functions for the Le^a and Le^b, and the ABH determinants, might be discerned through studies of these molecules in lower species, where they may retain essential functions. These efforts will be facilitated by the use of cloned glycosyltransferase gene segments, whose isolation was made possible by the pioneering work of those scientists involved in the determination of the chemical nature and biosynthesis of these antigens.

ACKNOWLEDGMENTS

I thank Becky Stone and Thien Nguyen for their assistance in preparing this manuscript. The author is an Associate Investigator of the Howard Hughes Medical Institute.

REFERENCES

1. Landsteiner K. Zur Kenntnis der antifermentativen, lytischen und agglutinierenden Wirkungen des Blutserums und der Lymph. Zbl Batk 1900; 27:367.

2. Landsteiner K. Uber agglutinationserscheinungen normalen menschlichen Blutes. Wien Klin Wochenschr 1901; 14:1132.
3. von Decastello A, Sturli A. Uber die isoagglutinine im serum gesunder und kranker menschen. Munch Med Wochschr 1902; 49:1090.
4. Oriol R, Le Pendu J, Mollicone R. Genetics of ABO, H, Lewis, X and related antigens. Vox Sang 1986; 51:161.
5. Watkins WM. Biochemistry and Genetics of the ABO, Lewis, and P blood group systems. Adv Hum Genet 1980; 10:1.
6. Laine RA, Rush JS. Chemistry of human erythrocyte polylactosamine glycopeptides (erythroglycans) as related to ABH blood group antigenic determinants. Adv Exp Med Biol 1988; 228:331.
7. Kabat EA. Specific polysaccharides of blood. In: Blood Group Substances. New York: Academic Press, 1956:15.
8. Watkins WM, Morgan WTJ. Neutralization of the anti-H agglutinin in eel serum by simple sugars. Nature 1952; 169:852.
9. Morgan WTJ, Watkins WM. Inactivation of the H-receptor on human erythocytes by an enzyme obtained from Trichomonas foetus. Br J Exp Pathol 1953; 34:94.
10. Morgan WTJ, Watkins WM. Genetic and biochemical aspects of human blood group A-, B-, H-, Le^a- and Le^b-specificity. Br Med Bull 1969; 25:30.
11. Morgan WTJ, Watkins WM. The product of the human blood group A and B genes in individuals belonging to group AB. Nature 1956; 177:21.
12. Kabat EA. Immunochemical studies on the carbohydrate moiety of water-soluble blood group A, B, H, Le^a, and Le^b substances and their precursor I antigens. Carbohydrates in Solution. Adv. Chem. Ser. 117, Washington, D.C.: American Chemical Society, 1973:334.
13. Lemieux RU, Driguez H. The chemical synthesis of 2-O-(α-L-fucopyranosyl)-3-O(α-D-galactopyranosyl)D-galactose. The terminal structure of the blood-group B antigenic determinant. J Am Chem Soc 1975; 97:4069.
14. Jacquinet JC, Sinäy P. Synthèse des substances de groups sanguin IV. Synthèse du 2-acetamido-2-deoxy-4-O-[2-O-(α-L-fucopyranosyl)-β-D-galacto-pyranosyl]-D-glucopyranose, porteur de la spècificitè H. Tetrahedron 1976; 32:1693.
15. Lemieux RU. Human blood groups and carbohydrate chemistry. Chem Soc Rev 1978; 7:23.
16. Hakomori S. Blood group ABH and Ii antigens of human erythrocytes: chemistry, polymorphism, and their developmental change. Semin Hematol 1981; 18:39.
17. Sadler JE. Biosynthesis of glycoproteins: formation of O-linked oligosaccharides. In: Ginsburg, Robbins, eds. Biology of Carbohydrates. Vol. 2. New York: Wiley, 1984:199.
18. Clausen H, Levery SB, Nudelman E, Tsuchiya S, Hakomori S. Repetitive A epitope (type 3 chain A) defined by blood group A$_1$-specific monoclonal antibody TH-1: chemical basis of qualitiative A$_1$ and A$_2$ distinction. Proc Natl Acad Sci USA 1985; 82:1199.
19. Le Pendu J, Lambert F, Samuelsson BE, Breimer ME, Seitz RC, Urdaniz MP, Suesa N, Ratcliffe M, Francoise A, Poschmann A, Vinas J, Oriol R. Monoclonal antibodies specific for type 3 and type 4 chain-based blood group determinants: relationship to the A1 and A2 subgroups. Glycoconjugate J 1986; 3:255.
20. Clausen H, Levery SB, Nudelman E, Baldwin M, Hakomori S. Further characterization of type 2 and type 3 chain blood group A glycosphingolipids from human erythrocyte membranes. Biochemistry 1986; 25:7075.
21. Kannagi R, Levery SB, Hakomori S. Blood group H antigen with globo-series structure: isolation and characterization from human blood group O erythrocytes. FEBS Lett. 1984; 175:397.
22. Betteridge A, Watkins WM. Acceptor substrate specificities of human α-2-L-fucosyltransferases from different tissues. Biochem Soc Trans 1986; 13:1126.
23. Clausen H, Holmes E, Hakomori S. Novel blood group H glycolipid antigens exclusively expressed in blood group A and AB erythrocytes (type 3 chain H). II. Differential conversion of different H substrates by A$_1$ and A$_2$ enzymes, and type 3 chain H expression in relation to secretor status. J Biol Chem 261:1388.
24. Steck TL. The organization of proteins in the human red blood cell membrane. J Cell Biol 1974; 62:1.
25. Allard WJ, Lienhard GE. Monoclonal antibodies to the glucose transporter from human erythrocytes. J Biol Chem 1985; 160:8668.

26. Tanner MJA, Martin PG, High S. The complete amino acid sequence of the human erythrocyte membrane anion-transport protein deduced from the cDNA sequence. Biochem J 1988; 256:703.

27. Mueckler M, Caruso C, Baldwin SA. Sequence and structure of a human glucose transporter. Science 1985; 229:941.

28. Fukuda M, Fukuda MN. Changes in cell surface glycoproteins and carbohydrate structures during the development and differentiation of human erythroid cells. J Supramol Struct 1974; 17:313.

29. Moore SJ, Green C. The identification of Rhesus polypeptide-blood group ABH-active glycoprotein complex in the human red cell membrane. Biochem J 1987; 244:735.

30. Koscielak J, Miller-Podruza H, Kranze R. Isolation and characterization of (poly-glycosyl) ceramides (megaloglycolipids) with A, H, I blood group activities. Eur J Bichem 1976; 71:9.

31. Dejter-Juszynski M, Harpaz N, Flowers HM, Sharon N. Blood-group ABH-specific macro-glycolipids of human erythrocytes: isolation in high yield from a crude membrane glycoprotein fraction. Eur J Biochem 1978; 83:363.

32. Koscielak J, Miller-Podraza H, Krauze R, Piasek A. Isolation and characterization of poly(glycosyl)-ceramides (megaloglycolipids) with A, H, and I blood-group activities. Eur J Biochem 1976; 71:9.

33. In Petz LE, ed. Clinical Practice of Blood Transfusion. (Petz, L.E., ed.), New York: Churchill Livingstone, 1981.

34. Mollison PL. Blood Transfusion in Clinical Medicine. 8th ed. Oxford, England: Blackwell Scientific, 1987.

35. In: Rossie EC, Simon TL, Moss GS, eds. Principles of Transfusion Medicine. Baltimore: Williams & Wilkins, 1991.

36. Bird GWG. Haemagglutinins in seeds. Br Med Bull 1959; 15:165.

37. Mourant AE, Kopèc AC, Domaniewska-Sobczak K. The Distribution of the Human Blood Groups and Other Biochemical Polymorphisms. 2nd ed. Oxford, England: Oxford University Press, 1976.

38. Salmon CH, Cartron JP. ABO phenotypes. In: Greenwalt TJ, Steane EA, eds. CRC Handbook Series in Clinical Laboratory Science, Section D; Blood Banking. Vol. 1. Cleveland, OH: CRC Press, 1977:71.

39. Economidou J, Hughes-Jones NC, Gardner B. Quantitative measurements concerning A and B antigen sites. Vox Sang 1967; 12:321.

40. Mäkela O, Ruoslahti E, Ehnholm C. Subtypes of human ABO blood groups and subtype-specific antibodies. J Immunnol 1969; 10:763.

41. Kisailus EC, Kabat EA. Immunochemical studies on blood groups. LXVI. Competitive binding assays of A_1 and A_2 blood group substances with insolubilized anti-A serum and insolubilized A agglutinine from *Dolichos biflorus*. J Exp Med 1978; 147:830.

42. Mohn JF, Cunningham RK, Bates JF. Qualitative distinctions between subgroups A_1 and A_2. In: Mohn JF, Plunkett R, Cunningham RK, Lambert R, eds. Human Blood Groups. New York: Karger, 1977:316.

43. Moreno C, Lundblad A, Kabat EA. Immunochemical studies on blood groups. LI. A comparative study of the reaction of A_1 and A_2 blood groups glycoproteins with human anti-A. J Exp Med 1971; 134:439.

44. Clausen H, Hakomori S. ABH and related histo-blood group antigens: immunochemical differences in carrier isotypes and their distribution. Vox Sang 1989; 46:1.

45. Breimer ME, Samuelsson BE. A specific distribution of glycolipid based blood group A antigens in human kidney related to A_1/A_2, Lewis and secretor status of single individuals. Transplantation 1986; 42:88.

46. Yamaguchi H, Okubo Y, Hazama F. Another Japanese A_2B_3 blood-group family with the propositus having O-group father. Proc Jpn Acad 1966; 42:417.

47. Seyfried H, Walewska I, Verblinska B. Unusual inheritance of ABO group in a family with weak B antigens. Vox Sang 1964; 9:268.

48. Lopez M, Liberge G, Gerbal A, Brocteur J, Salmon C. Cis AB blood groups. Immunologic, thermodynamic and quantitative studies of ABH antigens. Biomedicine 1976; 24:265.

49. Yoshida A, Yamaguchi H, Okubo Y. Genetic mechanism of cis-AB inheritance. I. A case associated with unequal chromosomal crossing over. Am J Hum Genet 1980; 32:332.

50. Greenwell P, Yates AD, Watkins WM. UDP-N-acetyl-D-galactosamine as a donor substrate for

the glycosyltransferase encoded by the B gene at the human blood group ABO locus. Carbohydr Res 1986; 149:149.

51. Yoshida A, Yamaguchi H, Okubo Y. Genetic mechanism of Cis-AB inheritance. II. Cases associated with structural mutation of blood group glycosyltransferases. Am J Hum Genet 1980; 32:645.

52. Watkins WM, Greenwell P, Yates AD. The genetic and enzymatic regulation of the synthesis of the A and B determinants in the ABO blood group system. Immunol Commun 1981; 10:83.

53. Nagai M, Dave V, Kaplan BE, Yoshida A. Human blood group glycosyltransferases. I. Purification of N-acetylgalactosaminyltransferase. J Biol Chem 1978; 253:377.

54. Carne LR, Watkins WM. Human blood group B gene-specified alpha-3-galactosyltransferase: purification of the enzyme in serum by biospecific adsorption onto blood group O erythrocyte membranes. Biochem Biophys Res Commun 1977; 77:700.

55. Clausen H, White T, Takio K, Titani K, Stroud M, Holmes E, Karkov J, Thim L, Hakomori S. Isolation to homogeneity and partial characterization of a histo-blood group A defined Fuc α1->2Gal α1->3-N-acetylgalactosaminyltransferase from human lung tissue. J Biol Chem 1990; 265:1139.

56. Yamamoto F-I, Marken J, Tsuji T, White T, Clausen H, Hakomori S-I. Cloning and characterization of DNA complementary to human UDP-GalNAc:Fucα1->2Gal α1->3GalNAc transferase (histo-blood group A transferase) mRNA. J Biol Chem 1990; 264:1146.

57. Lowe JB. Molecular cloning, expression, and uses of mammalian glycosyltransferases. Semin Cell Biol 1991; 2:289.

58. Wickner WT, Lodish HF. Multiple mechanisms of protein insertion into and across membranes. Science 1985; 230:400.

59. Griffiths G, Simons K. The trans Golgi network: sorting at the exit site of the Golgi complex. Science 1986; 234:438.

60. Kornfeld R, Kornfeld S. Assembly of asparagine-linked oligosaccharides. Annu Rev. Biochem 1985; 54:631.

61. D'Agostaro G, Bendiak B, Tropak M. Cloning of cDNA encoding the membrane-bound form of bovine β1, 4-galactosyltransferase. Eur J Biochem 1989; 183:211.

62. Weinstein J, Lee EU, McEntee K, Lai P-H, Paulson JC. Primary structure of β-galactoside α2,6-sialyl-transferase. Conversion of membrane-bound enzyme to soluble forms by cleavage of the NH_2-terminal signal anchor. J Biol Chem 1987; 262:17735.

63. Yamamoto F-I, Clausen H, White T, Marken J, Hakomori S-I. Molecular genetic basis of the histo-blood group ABO system. Nature 1990; 345:229.

64. Yamamoto F-I, Hakomori S-I. Sugar-nucleotide donor specificity of histo-blood group A and B transferases is based on amino acid substitutions. J Biol Chem 1990; 265:19257.

65. Galili U. The natural anti-Gal antibody: evolution and autoimmunity in man. Immunol. Ser 1991; 55:355.

66. Chester MA, Yates AD, Watkins WM. Phenyl-β-D-galactopyranoside as an acceptor substrate for the blood-group H gene associated guanosine diphosphate L-fucose:β-D-galactosyl α-2-L-fucosyl-transferase. Eur J Biochem 1976; 69:583.

67. Wolf RO, Taylor LL. The concentration of blood-group substances in the parotid, sublingual and submaxillary salivas. J Dent Res 1964; 43:272.

68. Milne RW, Dawes C. The relative contributions of different salivary glands to the blood group activity of whole saliva in humans. Vox Sang 1973; 25:298.

69. Gaensslen RE, Bell SC, Lee HC. Distribution of genetic markers in United States populations: I. Blood group and secretor systems. J Forensic Sci 1987; 32:1016.

70. Levine P, Robinson E, Celano M, Briggs O, Falkinburg L. Gene interaction resulting in suppression of blood group substance B. Blood 1955; 10:1100.

71. Solomon J, Waggoner R, Leyshon WC. A quantitative immunogenetic study of gene suppression invoking A_1 and H antigens of erythrocyte without affecting secreted blood group substance. The A^hm and O^hm. Blood 1965; 25:470.

72. Oriol R, Danilovs J, Hawkins BR. A new genetic model proposing that the Se gene is a structural gene closely linked to the H gene. Am J Hum Genet 1981; 33:421.

73. Mollicone R, Davies DR, Evans B, Dalix AM, Oriol R. Cellular expression and genetic control

of ABH antigens in primary sensory neurons of marmoset, baboon and man. J Neuroimmunol 1986; 10:255.

74. Szulman AE. The ABH and Lewis antigens of human tissues during prenatal and postnatal life. In: Mohn JF, Plunkett R, Cunningham RK, Lambert R, eds. Human Blood Groups. Basel: Karger, 1977:426.

75. Rouger P, Poupon R, Gane P, Mallissen B, Darnis F, Salmon C. Expression of blood group antigens including HLA markers in human adult liver. Tissue Antigens 1986; 27:78.

76. Gerard G, Vitrac D, Le Pendu J, Muller A, Oriol R. H-deficient blood groups (Bombay) of Reunion Island. Am J Hum Genet 1982; 34:937.

77. Le Pendu J, Cartron JP, Lemieux RU, Oriol R. The presence of at least two different H-blood-group-related βDGal α-2-L-fucosyltransferases in human serum and the genetics of blood group H substances. Am J Hum Genet 1985; 37:749.

78. Kumazaki T, Yoshida A. Biochemical evidence that secretor gene, *Se*, is a structural gene encoding a specific fucosyltransferase. Proc Natl Acad Sci USA 1984; 81:4193.

79. Betteridge A, Watkins WM. Acceptor substrate specificities of human α-2-L-fucosyltransferases from different tissues. Biochem Soc Trans 1986; 13:1126.

80. Sarnesto A, Kohlin T, Thurin J, Blaszczyk-Thurin M. Purification of *H* gene-encoded β-galactoside α1-2fucosyltransferase from human serum. J Biol Chem 1990; 265:15067.

81. Sarnesto A, Kohlin T, Hindsgaul O, Thurin J, Blaszczyk-Thurin M. Purification of the secretor-type beta-galactoside alpha 1->2-fucosyltransferase from human serum. J Biol Chem 1992; 267:2737.

82. Rajan VP, Larsen RD, Ajmera S, Ernst LK, Lowe JB. A cloned human DNA restriction fragment determines expression of a GDP-L-fucose:β-D-galactoside 2-α-L-fucosyltransferase in transfected cells. J Biol Chem 1991; 24:1158.

83. Ball SP, Tongue N, Gibaud A, Le Pendu J, Mollicone R, Gerard G, Oriol R. The human chromosome 19 linkage group FUT1 (H), Fut2 (SE), LE, LU, PEPD, C3, APOC2, D19S7, and D19S9. Ann Hum Genet 1991; 55(pt 3):225.

84. Ernst LK, Rajan VP, Larsen RD, Ruff MM, Lowe JB. Stable expression of blood group H determinants and GDP-L-fucose:β-D-galactoside 2-α-L-fucosyltransfease in mouse cells after transfection with human DNA. J Biol Chem 1989; 264:3436.

85. Larsen RD, Ernst LK, Nair RP, Lowe JP. Molecular cloning, sequence, and expression of human GDP-L-fucose:β-D-galactoside 2-α-L-fucosyltransfease cDNA that can form the H blood group antigen. Proc Natl Acad Sci USA 1990; 87:6674.

86. Kelly RJ, Ernst LK, Larsen RD, Bryant JG, Robinson JS, Lowe JB. Molecular basis for H blood group deficiency in Bombay (O$_h$) and para-Bombay individuals. In preparation.

87. Race RR, Sanger R. Blood Groups in Man. 6th ed. Oxford, England: Blackwell Scientific, 1975.

88. Bhatia HM, Sathe MS. Incidence of "Bombay" (Oh) phenotype and weaker variants of A and B antigen in Bombay (India). Vox Sang 1974; 27:524.

89. Mourant AE. A 'new' human blood group antigen of frequent occurrence. Nature 1946; 158:237.

90. Rege VP, Painter TJ, Watkins WM, Morgan WTJ. Isolation of a serologically active fucose containing trisaccharide from human blood group Le[a] substrate. Nature 1964; 240:740.

91. Marr AMS, Donald ASR, Watkins WM, Morgan WTJ. Molecular and genetic aspects of human blood-group Le[b] specificity. Nature 1967; 215:1345.

92. Marcus DM, Cass LE. Glycosphingolipids with Lewis blood group activity: uptake by human erythrocytes. Science 1969; 164:553.

93. Hanfland P, Graham H. Immunochemistry of the Lewis blood group system: partial characterization of Le[a], Le[b] and H type 1 (Le[dh]) blood group active glycosphingolipids from human plasma. Arch Biochem Biophys 1981; 220:383.

94. Hanfland P, Kardowicz M, Peter-Katalinic J, Pfannschmidt G, Crawford RJ, Graham HA, Egge H. Immunochemistry of the Lewis blood group system: isolation and structures of the Lewis c active and related glycosphingloipids from the plasma of blood-group OLe(a-b-) nonsecretors. Arch Biochem Biophys 1986;246:655.

95. Mollison PL, Polley MJ. Temporary suppression of the Lewis blood-group antibodies to permit incompatible transfusion. Lancet 1963; 1:909.

96. Mollison PL. Blood Transfusion in Clinical Medicine. 6th ed. Oxford, England: Blackwell, 1979.

97. Andresen PH. Blood groups with characteristic phenotypical aspects. Acta Pathol Microbiol Scand 1948; 24:616.
98. Grubb R, Morgan WTJ. The 'Lewis' blood group characters of crythrocytes and body fluids. Br J Exp Pathol 1949; 30:198.
99. Johnson PH, Yates AD, and Watkins WM. Human salivary fucosyltransferases: evidence for two distinct α-3-L-fucosyltransferase activities, one of which is associated with the Lewis blood group *Le* gene. Biochem Biophys Res Commun 1981; 100:1611.
100. Prieels JP, Monnom D, Dolmans M, Beyer TA, Hill RL. Copurification of the Lewis blood group N-acetylglucosaminide α 1->4 fucosyltransferase and an N-acetylglucosaminide α 1->3 fucosyl-transferase from human milk. J Biol Chem 1981; 256:10456.
101. Kukowska-Latallo JF, Larsen RD, Nair RP, Lowe JB. A cloned human cDNA determines expression of a mouse stage-specific embryonic antigen and the Lewis blood group α(1,3/1,4)fuco-syltransferase. Genes Dev 1990; 4:1288.
102. Lowe JB, Stooolman LM, Nair RP, Larsen RD, Berhend TL, Marks RM. ELAM-1–dependent cell adhesion to vascular endothelium determined by a transfected human fucosyltransferase cDNA. Cell 63:475.
103. Hagopian A, Eylar EH. Glycoprotein biosynthesis: studies on the receptor specificity of the polypeptidyl: N-acetylgalactosaminyl transferase from bovine submaxillary glands. Arch Biochem Biophys 1968; 128:422.
104. Mollicone R, Gibaud A, Francois A, Ratcliffe M, Oriol R. Acceptor specificity and tissue distribution of three human α-3-fucosyltransferases. Eur J Biochem 1990; 191:169.
105. Gooi HC, Feizi T, Kapadia A, Knowles BB, Solter D, Evans MJ. Stage-specific embryonic antigen involves a 1->3 fucosylated type 2 blood group chains. Nature 1981; 292:156.
106. Solter D, Knowles BB. Monoclonal antibody defining a stage-specific mouse embryonic antigen (SSEA-1). Proc Natl Acad Sci USA 1978; 75:5565.
107. Arcilla MB, Sturgeon P. Le^X, the spurned antigen of the Lewis blood-group system. Vox Sang 1974; 26:425.
108. Andresen PH, Jordal K. An incomplete agglutinin related to the L (Lewis) system. Acta Pathol Microbiol Scand 1949; 26:636.
109. Feizi T. Demonstration by monoclonal antibodies that carbohydrate structures of glycoproteins and glycolipids are onco-developmental antigens. Nature 1985; 314:53.
110. Childs RA, Gregoriou M, Scudder P, Thorpe SJ, Rees AR, Feizi T. Blood group-active carbohydrate chains on the receptor for epidermal growth factor of A431 cells. EMBO J 1984; 3:2227.
111. Seed B, Aruffo A. Molecular cloning of the CD2 antigen, the T-cell erythrocyte receptor, by a rapid immunoselection procedure. Proc Natl Acad Sci USA 1987; 84:3365.
112. Lowe JB, Kukowska-Latallo JF, Nair RP, Larsen RD, Marks RM, Macher BA, Kelly RJ, Ernst LK. Molecular cloning of a human fucosyltransferase gene that determines expression of the Lewis x and VIM-2 eiptiopes but not ELAM-1–dependent cell adhesion. J Biol Chem 1991; 266:17467.
113. Dumas DP, Ichikawa Y, Wong CH, Lowe JB, Nair RP. Enzymatic synthesis of sialyl Le^x and derivatives based on a recombinant fucosyltransferase. Bioorg Med Chem Lett 1991; 1:425.
114. Palcic MM, Venot AP, Murray Ratcliffe R, Hindsgaul O. Enzymic synthesis of oligosaccharides terminating in the tumor-associated sialyl-Lewis-a determinant. Carbohydrate Res 1989; 190:1.
115. Le Beau MM, Ryan D, Jr, Pericak-Vance MA. Report of the committee on the genetic constitution of chromosomes 18 and 19, Human Gene Mapping 10: Tenth International Workshop on Human Gene Mapping. Cytogenet Cell Genet 1989; 51:338.
116. Weston BW, Nair RP, Larsen RD, Lowe JB. Isolation of a novel human (α(1,3)fucosyltransferase gene and molecular comparison to the human Lewis blood group α(1,3/1,4)fucosyltransferase gene. J Biol Chem 1992; 267:4152.
117. Tetteroo PAT, de Heij HT, Van den Eijnden DH, Visser FJ, Schoenmaker E, Geurts van Kessel AHM. A GDP-fucose:[Gal beta 1->4]Glc NAc alpha 1->3-fucosyltransferase activity is correlated with the presence of human chromosome 11 and the expression of the Lex, Ley, and sialyl-Lex antigens in human-mouse cell hybrids. J Biol Chem 1987; 262:15984.
118. Potvin B, Kumar R, Howard DR, Stanley P. Transfection of a human alpha-(1,3)fucosyltransferase gene into Chinese hamster ovary cells. Complications arise from activation of endogenous alpha-(1,3)fucosyltransferases. J Biol Chem 1990; 265:1615.

119. Foster CS, Gillies DRB, Glick MC. Purification and characterization of GDP-L-Fuc-N-acetyl-beta-D-glucosaminide alpha 1->3 fucosyltransferase from human neuroblastoma cells. Unusual substrate specificities of the tumor enzyme. J Biol Chem 1991; 266:3726.

120. Caillard T, LePendu J, Ventura M, Mada M, Rault G, Mannoni P, Oriol R. Failure of expression of alpha-3-L-fucosyltransferase in human serum is coincident with the absence of the X (or Le(x)) antigen in the kidney but not on leucocytes. Exp Clin Immunogenet 1988; 5:15.

121. Mollicone R, Candelier JJ, Mennesson B, Couillin P, Venot AP, Oriol R. Carbohydrate Res 228:265.

122. Couillin P, Mollicone R, Grisard MC, Gibaud A, Ravise N, Feingold J, Oriol R. Chromosome 11q localization of one of the three expected genes for the human alpha-3-fucosyltransferases, by somatic hybridization. Cytogenet Cell Genet 1991; 56:108.

123. Goelz SE, Hession C, Goff D, Griffiths B, Tizard R, Newman B, Chi-Rosso G, Lobb R. ELFT: a gene that directs the expression of an ELAM-1 ligand. Cell 1990; 63:1349.

124. Kumar R, Potvin B, Muller WA, Stanley P. Cloning of a human $\alpha(1,3)$fucosyltransferase gene that encodes ELFT but does not confer ELAM-1 recognition on CHO transfections. J Biol Chem 1991; 266:21777.

125. Weston BW, Smith PL, Kelly RJ, Lowe JB. Molecular cloning of a fourth member of a human $\alpha(1,3)$fucosyltransferase gene family: multiple homologous sequences that determine expression of the Lewis x, sialyl Lewis x, and difucosyl sialyl Lewis x epitopes. J Biol Chem 1992; 267:4152.

126. Springer TA. Adhesion receptors of the immune system. Nature 1990; 346:425.

127. Bevilacqua MP, Stengelin S, Gimbrone MA, Seed B. Endothelial leukocyte adhesion molecule 1: an inducible receptor for neutrophils related to complement regulatory proteins and lectins. Science 1989; 243:1160.

128. Bevilacqua M, Butcher E, Furie B, Furie B, Gallatin M, Gimbrone M, Harlan J, Kishimoto K, Lasky L, McEver R, et al. Selectins: a family of adhesion receptors. Cell 1991; 67:233.

129. Drickamer K. Two distinct classes of carbohydrate-recognition domains in animal lectins. J Biol Chem 1988; 263:9557.

130. Phillips ML, Nudelman E, Gaeta FC, Perez M, Singhal AK, Hakomori S, Paulson JC. ELAM-1 mediates cell adhesion by recognition of a carbohydrate ligand, sialyl-Lex. Science 1990; 250:1130.

131. Walz G, Aruffo A, Kolanus W, Bevilacqua M, Seed B. Recognition by ELAM-1 of the sialyl-Lex determinant on myeloid and tumor cells. Science 1990; 250:1132.

132. Tyrrel D, Pames P, Rao N, Foxall C, Abbas S, Dasgupta F, Nashed M, Hasegawa A, Kiso M, Asa D, Kidd J, Brandley BK. Structural requirements for the carbohydrate ligand of E-selectin. Proc Natl Acad Sci USA 1991; 88:10372.

133. Berg EL, Robinson MK, Mansson O, Butcher EC, Magnani JL. A carbohydrate domain common to both sialyl Lea and sialyl Lex is recognized by the endothelial cell leukocyte adhesion molecule ELAM-1. J Biol Chem 1991; 266:14869.

134. Takada A, Ohmori K, Takahashi N, Tsuyuoka K, Yago A, Zenita K, Hasegawa A, Kannagi R. Adhesion of human cancer cells to vascular endothelium mediated by a carbohydrate antigen, sialyl Lewis A. Biochem Biophys Res Commun 1991; 179:713.

135. Kim YS, Itzkowitz S. Carbohydrate antigen expression in the adenoma-carcinoma sequence. Prog Clin Biol Res 1988; 279:241.

136. Zhou, Q, Moore KL, Smith DF, Varki A, McEver RP, Cummings RD. The selectin GMP-140 binds to sialylated, fucosylated lactosaminoglycans on both myeloid and nonmyeloid cells. J Cell Biol 1991; 115:557.

137. Polley MJ, Phillips ML, Wayner E, Nudelman E, Singhal AK, Hakomori S-I, Paulson JC. CD62 and endothelial cell-leukocyte adhesion molecule 1 (ELAM-1) recognize the same carbohydrate ligand, sialyl-Lewis x. Proc Natl Acad Sci USA 1991; 88:6224.

138. Brandley BK, Watson SR, Dowbenko D, Fennie C, Lasky LA, Hasegawa A, Kiso M, Foxall C. The sialyl Lewis x oligosaccharide is a ligand for L-selectin. FASEB J 1992; A1890.

139. Lowe JB. Specificity and expression of carbohydrate ligands. In: Wegner CD, ed. The Handbook of Immunopharmacology. Orlando, FL, Academic Press, 1992. In press.

2

Glycophorins: Structures and Antigens

DOMINIQUE BLANCHARD
Centre Regional de Transfusion Sanguine
Nantes, France

WOLFGANG DAHR
Scientific Consultation and Translations
Bergisch Gladbach, Germany

I. INTRODUCTION

The predominant antithethic and polymorphic antigens (M and N) that are located on the glycophorins (GPs) or sialoglycoproteins (SGPs) in human red blood cell (RBC) membranes were discovered about 65 years ago using rabbit antibodies. M and N were shown to be encoded by codominant alleles—however, it was noticed that M+N− RBCs (genotype *MM*) exhibit a weak N antigen (now denoted as "N"). About 25 years after the discovery of M and N, two other antithetic and polymorphic antigens (S and s) were found and shown to be encoded by genes that are genetically linked to *M* and *N*, thus generating four possible haplotypes: *MS, Ms, NS, Ns*.

The serological and genetic complexity of the MNSs system has further increased by the definition of (1) quantitative and qualitative variants of the major antigens; (2) high- or low-frequency antigens that are either genetically (encoded by the same or an adjacent gene) or biochemically (common synthethic pathway) associated with the MNSs system; and (3) GP variants characterized solely on the basis of biochemical studies. About 30 antigens of the MNSs system have been accepted as being unique and numbered by the blood group nomenclature recommended by the International Society of Blood Transfusion (1,2)—several additional ones exist. The serology and the conventional genetics of the MNSs system have been reviewed by Race and Sanger (3), Issitt (4), and Salmon et al. (5). The *MNSs* locus is now known to encode the amino acid (AA) sequences of three members of the GP family (GP A, GP B, GP E), the genes of which are denoted as *GYPA*, *GYPB*, and so forth.

During the last decade, it became apparent that the antigens of the Gerbich (Ge) blood group system are located on two minor GPs (GP C, GP D), the AA sequences of which are encoded by the *Ge* locus (*GYPC* gene). Thus, the MNSs and Ge systems exhibit a biochemical but no known genetic relationship. Since the extracellular portions of the GPs are heavily glycosylated, it is understandable that the epitopes of many MNSs- or Ge-related antibodies comprise protein as well as carbohydrate. In addition, all GPs carry several antigens that consist solely of carbohydrate. These antigens are encoded by the genes for glycosyl-transferases and not by the *GYP* loci.

The majority of the antigens on the GPs are defined by antibodies, stimulated by blood transfusion or pregnancy. Some antigens may be detected by alloantibodies that occur naturally in human sera without any apparent immunization or by autoantibodies found in patients with autoimmune hemolytic anemia or cold agglutinin disease.

Reagents for the determination of the M and N blood type are available from several sources: human allo- and autoantibodies and antibodies prepared by immunization of rabbits, rats, or cows as well as agglutinins (lectins) occurring in certain plant seeds. During the last decade, several examples of mouse monoclonal anti-M and anti-N have been described. Gradually, mouse monoclonal antibodies against additional antigens on the GPs (S, Wr[b], En[a]KT, En[a]TS, Ge3, Ge4, T, Tn) are also emerging.

Biochemical characterization of the GPs and their antigens has always been critically influenced by the availability of suitable methods. Initially, the M and N antigens were shown to be located on sialic acid (Neu$N$Ac-)–rich (approximatively 20% by weight) glycoproteins (MN mucoids), extracted from RBC membranes by hot liquid phenol by the groups of Hohorst, Lisowska, Uhlenbruck, Springer, and Winzler. Three phenomena supported the wrong concept that the structural difference between the M and N antigens resides in the carbohydrate moiety of the GPs and that N represents a biosynthetic precursor of M: (1) the destruction of the M and N antigens by removal of Neu$N$Ac; (2) the occurrence of a weak N antigen (now denoted as "N") in M+N– RBCs; and (3) the discovery that some lectins, generally directed against carbohydrate residues, exhibit anti-M or -N specificity.

The advent of methods for the fractionation of membrane proteins on an analytical (dodecylsulfate polyacrylamide gel electrophoresis, SDS-PAGE) and preparative (chromatography in detergent solutions), as well as the development of methods for the AA sequence analysis of multiply glycosylated proteins by Marchesi's group, who created the term *glycophorin* (for carbohydrate carrier), paved the way for a different concept of the MNSs system. Cleve and coworkers made the fundamental observation that GP A exhibits M and/or N activity, whereas a minor component (now denoted as GP B) carries S, s, and "N" but no M antigen. Based on these and other data, the groups of Lisowska and Dahr proposed a different concept of the MNSs system about 15 years ago: (1) the *MNSs* locus encodes the AA sequences of GP A and GP B; (2) the genes for these two GPs are adjacent and homologous; (3) carbohydrate represents only a nonspecific part of some of the antigens of the MNSs system. The structural characterization of numerous antigens on the GPs has followed these hypotheses.

About 6 years ago, analyses of cDNA clones for GP A and GP C by the groups of Cartron and Fukuda opened a new chapter of the glycophorin story; i.e., molecular biology. The full repertoire for the analysis of the GPs and their antigens at the phenotypic (membrane), biosynthetic (messenger ribonucleic acid [MRA], glycosylation, and so forth) and genomic (chromosomes) levels is now available, thus guaranteeing a rather rapid progress of research.

The biochemistry and immunochemistry of the GPs has been reviewed by Anstee (6), Dahr (7), Reid (8), Lisowska (9), Moulds and Dahr (10), Blanchard (11), Huang et al. (12), Unger (13), and Rolih (14). Cartron et al. (15) have focused on the molecular biology. This chapter represents another attempt to review the ever-increasing knowledge of the GPs and their antigens.

II. NOMENCLATURES AND GENERAL FEATURES OF GLYCOPHORINS

Various nomenclatures and several features of the GPs are summarized in Table 1. All GPs exhibit a N terminal, glycosylated domain that carries several oligosaccharides (predominantly tetrasaccharides consisting of two Neu$N$Ac, one galactose (Gal), and one N-acetylgalactosamine (Gal$N$ac residue) attached O-glycosidically to Ser (= S) and Thr (= T) residues. GP A and GP C also exhibit one complex carbohydrate unit linked N glycosidically to an Asn (= N) residue.

The glycosylated domains of the GPs are exposed at the external RBC surface, carry the various antigens, and can be cleaved by treatment of intact RBCs with certain proteinases. By virtue of their high NeuNAc contents, the GPs can be specifically detected by periodic acid–Schiff (PAS) staining after separation of RBC membranes by SDS-PAGE. The distribution of stain among the bands reflects their NeuNAc contents.

All GPs exhibit a hydrophobic peptide stretch of about 20 AA residues that traverses the lipid bilayer of the membrane and interacts with lipids. This lipophilic portion of the GPs is responsible for self-aggregation of these molecules after extraction of membranes with organic solvents, such as phenol: after extraction, the GPs form aggregates containing about 10–30 monomers in detergent-free, aqueous solutions. Since dimers as well as monomers of the GPs are detectable when membranes are subjected to SDS-PAGE, it is conceivable that at least GP A exists as a dimer in intact membranes. However, direct evidence for the aggregational status of the GPs in situ is lacking. The intramembraneous or the adjacent portions of the GPs might also bind to other integral membrane proteins: there is evidence that GP A forms a complex with the major RBC membrane protein (= anion channel protein = "band 3") (16–19). Conversely, it is likely that GP B interacts with proteins related to the Rh blood group system (20–22).

All GPs exhibit a hydrophilic, but carbohydrate-free, C terminal portion of variable length that is exposed at the internal surface of the RBC membrane. The C terminal domains of GP C and GP D bind firmly to the linking protein "band 4.1." Glycophorin A also appears to interact with this component (23–26). The interaction of GP C and GP D with band 4.1 is not disrupted by nonionic detergents such as Triton X-100. Therefore, GPs A, B, and C may be purified by Triton X-100 solubilization of membranes followed by hot phenol/saline extractions and gel filtration of the pellet and supernatant fractions (27; W. Dahr, unpublished data). However, in our hands (28), the following method represents the best procedure to purify the GPs: (1) extraction of membranes by the hot phenol/saline procedure (29) followed by gel filtration (30,31) to separate GP A from the minor GPs; (2) purification of GP B by high performance liquid chromatography (HPLC)–ion exchange chromatography of the minor GP fraction in the presence of Triton X-100 (28); and (3) purification of GP C by subsequent HPLC-gel permeation chromatography in the presence of Triton X-100 (28). The above procedure permits the purification of sufficient material (GP A, about 1 µmol; GP B, about

Table 1 Nomenclature and Some Properties of Red Cell Membrane Glycophorins

Designation of molecules	GP A	GP B	GP E	GP C	GP D
Synonyms	α	δ	ι	β	γ
	MN SGP	Ss SGP		D SGP	E SGP
Properties					
Major antigens	M, N	S, s	M(?)	Ge 3	Ge 2,3
Blood group locus	MN	Ss	?	Ge	Ge
Encoding gene	GYPA	GYPB	GYPE	GYPC	GYPC
PAS-positive material (%)	85	10	?	4	1
Apparent molecular mass (kDa)	36	20	17(?)	32	23
Copies/Cell ($\times 10^3$)	900	200	<5	50–100	20
Polypeptide chain (aa res.)	131	72	59	128	106(?)
O-linked sugar chains	15	11	11(?)	12	8(?)
N-linked sugar chains	1	0	0	1	0

200 nmol; GP C, about 100 nmol) from a single blood unit for structural studies. Glycophorin D aggregates during hot phenol/saline extraction (31). This molecule could be purified in small quantities by Triton X-100 extraction of membranes followed by butanol extraction of the pellet and subsequent preparative SDS-PAGE (32).

III. GLYCOPHORINS A, B, AND E AND THE MNSs BLOOD GROUP SYSTEM

A. Structure and Antigens of Glycophorin A

1. Structure of GP A

Large quantities (up to 1 μmol) of pure GP A can be obtained from one blood unit. This allowed the elucidation of its complete AA sequence comprising 131 residues and its glycosylation sites. The attachement of the O-glycans to certain positions was found to be incomplete, in particular, in proximity to the lipid bilayer (33–36). More recently, the AA sequence of GP A was confirmed by sequencing of complementary deoxyribonucleic acid (cDNA) clones obtained from K562 cells or human fetal liver libraries (37–39).

The structure of GP A is characteristic of a transmembrane glycoprotein organized in three domains: (1) a glycosylated extracellular region (residues 1–72) containing cleavage sites for trypsin and papain that is only partially cleaved by chymotrypsin in intact cells; (2) an intramembraneous portion (residues 73–92) that may interact with neighboring lipids and with other integral membrane proteins such as band 3; (3) a nonglycosylated cytoplasmic region (residues 93–131) connected to the membrane skeleton (Fig. 1).

The extracellular domain is heavily glycosylated and carries an average of about 15 O-glycans, mainly corresponding to disialo-tetrasaccharides exhibiting the following structure (40):

NeuNAcα2-3Galβ1-3(NeuNAcα2-6)GalNAc-Ser (-Thr)

The structure of the biantennary type N-glycan with a bisecting GlcNAc residue and a side chain Fuc residue attached to Asn^{26} comprises about 13 monosaccharides (41,42).

2. M and N Antigens

The extracellular domain of GP A carries its various antigens. The M and N antigens were found to be located on N terminal octapeptides that could be obtained by cyanogen bromide treatment. A polymorphism at positions 1 and 5 was observed depending whether on the molecule was purified from M+N–, M+N+, or M–N+ RBCs (43–49). Glycophorin A from M+N– or M–N+ cells is denoted as GP A^M or GP A^N, respectively, and possesses the AA residue Ser^1/Gly^5 or Leu^1/Glu^5, respectively (see Fig. 1).

O-glycans are also involved in the M or N antigenic structures recognized by the majority of anti-M or anti-N antibodies (50). Most of the polyclonal and murine monoclonal antibodies require NeuNAc residues located on the tetrasaccharides or trisaccharides at the second, third, and/or fourth positions for binding. A detailed characterization of epitopes has been prevented by the lack of availability of a series of model peptides exhibiting a defined oligosaccharide(s) at (a) particular position(s). Either NeuNAcα2-3Gal, NeuNAcα2-6GalNAc, or both structures of the O-glycosidically linked oligosaccharides may be involved in the epitopes of the NeuNAc-dependent antibodies, as revealed by experiments involving resialylation of desialylated RBCs with purified sialyl-transferases (51). Apart from NeuNAc residues, the Galβ1-3GalNAc units may be involved in the M and N epitopes as shown for monoclonal anti-N antibodies (52,53) and polyclonal rabbit anti-M and anti-N that react specifically with desialylated RBCs (54; W. Dahr, unpublished data).

The involvement of the AA residues 1 and 5 in the M and N antigenic determinants could

GLYCOPHORIN A

```
                   M
                   -----
                            ----EnaTS-------  ----EnaFS---          -EnaFR, Wr-b-
                   N
                   ***  ******* * * ** *0 *   *   *    *    *    *
SSTTGVAMHTSTSSSVTKSYISSQTNDTHKRDTYAATPRAHEVSEISRVTVYPPEEETGERVQLAHHESEPEITLIFGVMAGVIGTILLISYGIRRLI
L E    10      20       30       40       50       60       70       80       90
------ exon A2--------/------------------exon A3--------/-------------/------exon A4--/------------/------exon A5-------

KKSPSDVKPLPSPDTDVPLSSVEIENPETSDQ
100   110   120   131
-/------exon A6------------/-exon A7
```

GLYCOPHORIN B

```
                   S
--N----      ----s------
***  ******* * * ** *
LSTTEVAMHTSTSSSVTKSYISSQTNGEMGQLVRPETVPAPVVIILILCVMAGIIGTILLISYSIRRLIKA
1      10       20      T30       40       50       60       72
------exon B2-------------/-------------------exon B4--------------/-exon B5
```

GLYCOPHORIN E

```
--M----
SSTTGVAMHTSTSSSVTKSYISSQTNGITLINWWAMARVIFEVMLVVVGMILLISYCIR
1      10       20       30       40       50       59
-----exon E2--------------/--------exon-E3----------------
```

Figure 1 Amino acid sequences (1-letter code), oligosaccharide attachment sites (* or O), major antigens, and alignment of exons of GP A, GP B, and GP E. Boldface letters represent the intramenbraneous domains. Residues that are identical are underlined.

be determined using rare RBCs that have a GP A or a GP B with an altered N terminal sequence. Agglutination tests with RBCs carrying the M^c or He antigens (structures in Table 2; see below) suggest that two major epitopes centered around the region of the first or fifth AA residue can be distinguished (reviewed in ref. 9). In addition, chemical modifications or removal of the N terminal AA residues showed that some antibodies require Ser^1 or Leu^1, whereas others are more dependent on the fifth residue (Gly^5 or Glu^5). The complexity of the M and N receptors is now well documented since the epitopes for several murine monoclonal antibodies have been investigated in detail (reviewed in refs. 7, 9, 55, and 56).

The diversity of the antibodies directed against the M and N determinants is further increased by (1) the anti-N formed by patients subjected to renal dialysis whose RBCs were modified by the formaldehyde used to sterilize the dialysis membranes; and (2) glucose-dependent anti-M or anti-N discovered in normal and diabetic sera. Formaldehyde as well as glucose were found to create modified N or M antigens by reacting with the amino group of the N terminal Leu or Ser residue (57–60).

The complexity of the M and N antigens is illuminated further by data on the M- or N-specific lectins. Studies with model compounds indicate that the agglutinins from *Bauhinea purpurea* (anti-N), *Moluccella laevis* (anti-N plus anti-A), *Iberis amara* (anti-M) (all GalNac specific), and *Vicia graminea* (anti-N, specific for Galβ1-3GalNAc) exhibit only a rather weak affinity for the tetrasaccharide (61,62). Such a peculiar behavior is necessary in order to prevent the lectins from reacting with several O-glycans on the GPs and, thus, to ensure blood group M or N specificity. In line with this, removal of the *N* terminal Leu residue strongly decreased the binding of anti-N from *Vicia graminea* (46,63).

Finally, it should be emphasized that the serological variability of the M and N antigens of RBCs is in part caused by the N antigen on GP B and M or N antigens on hybrid molecules.

Table 2 Partial Structures of Some Glycophorin Variants

Red cell variant	Abnormalities	Associated antigens
M^g	Altered GP A: L-S-T-N-E 　　　　　　　1　　　5	M^g
M^c	Altered GP A: S S̃-T-T̃-E 　　　　　　　1　　　5	
Mi.I	Altered GP A: -T̃-N-D-M-H 　　　　　　　　26　　29	Mi^a, Vw
Mi.II	Altered GP A: -T̃-N-D-L-H 　　　　　　　　26　　29	Mi^a, Hut
Mi.VII	Altered GP A: -T̃-T̃-V-S-P 　　　　　　　　50　52	Anek, Raddon Lane
Mi.VIII	Altered GP A: -T̃-T̃-V-Y-P 　　　　　　　　50　52	Anek, Raddon Lane
He	Altered GP B: W-S̃-T̃-S̃-G 　　　　　　　1　　　5	He
M^v	Altered GP B: abnormal N-terminal octapeptide	M^v

Variants of the M and N antigens resulting from alterations of the O-glycans are also described below.

3. En^a and Wr^b Antigens

The high-frequency En^a and Wr^b antigens are associated with residues 27–72 of GP A and detected by human alloantibodies and autoantibodies as well as mouse monoclonal reagents. The En^a antigens were classified according to their susceptibility to proteolytic treatments of RBCs (64): En^{a}TS or En^{a}FS are inactivated by trypsin or ficin, respectively, whereas En^{a}FR is resistant to ficin and (papain) treatment of intact RBCs. The En^{a}TS determinants are structurally heterogenous and correspond to about 5–10 AA residues within the positions 28–42 of GP A, whereas the En^{a}FS epitopes are more homogenous and are located within residues 46–56 of the molecule (36,65). Most of the antibodies require O-glycans for binding, and the oligosaccharide attached to Thr^{50} was shown to be essential for anti-En^{a}FS. However, two examples of human anti-En^{a}TS were found to react only with the proportion of GP A that is not glycosylated at Thr^{33} (36).

Several data suggest that the En^{a}FR and Wr^b antigens are located on, or associated with, GP A, in close proximity to the membrane (residues 62–72) and require lipids for complete expression of antigenic activity (17,19,65–68). They represent labile structures denatured by organic solvent extraction of RBC membranes. In contrast to anti-En^{a}FR, anti-Wr^b fails to react with rare Wr(a$^+$b$^-$) RBCs (69) that do not exhibit any AA sequence alteration of GP A (17). The suggestion that the Wr^b antigen corresponds to a complex structure involving GP A, band 3 and lipids (17) was confirmed recently by the finding that some monoclonal anti-Wr^b coimmunoprecipitate GP A *and* band 3 (19). One antibody was shown to react (albeit with a lower affinity; W. Dahr and M. Moulds, unpublished data) with RBCs lacking GP A and to immunoprecipitate band 3 from such cells (19). Data on the Wr^a antigen from Triton extractions of membranes (17) are also consistent with the assumption that the Wr^a/Wr^b polymorphism (70) is determined by a variability of the AA sequence of band 3.

4. Structure of GP A from M^g and Mc Erythrocytes

Glycophorin A from M^g and M^c RBCs shows alterations within the N terminal region of the molecule (Table 2).

The structure of the M^g-specific GP A is similar to that of GP A^N with an exchange at position 4 (Asn instead of Thr) that prevents glycosylation of residues 2, 3, and 4 (71–73). Therefore, GP A^{Mg} exhibits a slightly increased molecular mass in SDS-PAGE (74,75). The abnormal molecule is recognized by a specific antibody (anti-M^g) that does not agglutinate M$^+$N$^-$ or M$^-$N$^+$ RBCs. The specificity of anti-M^g was studied by chemical modifications of GPs and the use of several synthetic peptides (74,76).

In contrast, the M^c antigen is not defined by a specific antibody. The M^c-specific GP A represents a structure intermediate between those of GP A^M and GP A^N and exhibits a Ser or a Glu residue at positions 1 or 5, respectively (73,77). The N terminal region of the molecule is normally glycosylated and, according to the its structure, M^c RBCs are agglutinated by most anti-M and some anti-N. The M^c-specific GP A is considered to represent the evolutionary link between GPA^M and GPA^N.

5. Mi.I, Mi.II, Mi.VII, and Mi.VIII RBCs

The low-incidence Mi.I, Mi.II, Mi.VII, and Mi.VIII RBCs belong to the Miltenberger subsystem (see below). Mi.I and Mi.II RBCs carry the Mi^a and Vw or Mi^a and Hut antigens, respectively, which are defined by specific human alloantibodies and are located on abnormal GP A molecules (78–80). Mi.I- and Mi.II-specific GP A exhibit AA exchanges at position 28: Thr of normal GP A is replaced by a Met or a Lys residue, respectively (79). Owing to the absence of the consensus sequence required for N-glycosylation, Mi.I- and Mi.II-specific GP

A molecules are not glycosylated at Asn^{26} and exhibit a decreased molecular mass (about 2 kd) as compared with that of the normal counterpart.

The reactivity of RBCs with sera of the Anek, Raddon, or Lane type is the basis for the classification of Mi.VII and Mi.VIII cells. The Anek antigen was found to be associated with altered GP A molecules whose structure showed punctual AA exchanges at positions 49 and 52 (81,82) (Table 2). As compared with normal GP A, the Mi.VIII-specific GP A exhibits one AA exchange (Thr^{49} instead of Arg^{49}), whereas the Mi.VII-specific GP A shows two exchanges (Thr^{49} or Ser^{52} instead of Arg^{49} or Tyr^{52}, respectively), suggesting that the Mi.VIII-specific molecule might represent the evolutionary link between normal and Mi.VII-specific GP A (82). In both structures, Arg^{49} is replaced by a glycosylated Thr residue that appears to be essential for the Anek epitope. Although sera of the Raddon and Lane types have not been studied, it is reasonable to assume that they recognize similar epitopes. It is noteworthy that a *Mi.VII* homozygote made an alloanti-$En^{3}FS$, denoted as anti-$En^{a}KT$, reacting with normal GP A (83). All known examples of anti-$En^{a}FS$, already described above, fail to react with RBCs from the *Mi.VII* homozygote and react more weakly with those from *Mi.VII* or *Mi.VIII* heterozygotes. Therefore, they also exhibit anti-$En^{a}KT$ specificity.

No data on the structures of the DNA for Mi.II-, Mi.VII-, and Mi.VIII-specific GP A molecules are available. However, it has been postulated that these glycophorins might be hybrid molecules encoded by *GYPA-B-A* genes rather than by *GYPA* genes with point mutations (12,84).

B. Structure and Antigens of Glycophorin B

1. Structure of GP B

Glycophorin B represents about 10% of the glycophorins, as judged from PAS staining and could not be purified easily on a large scale by conventional chromatographic procedures. Tryptic peptides were at first prepared from the mixture of minor glycophorins obtained by gel permeation, thus allowing the determination of the AA residues 1–35 and the glycosylation sites (35,48,85). More recently, large-scale purification of GP B from $S^{+}s^{-}$ and $S^{-}s^{+}$ RBCs could be achieved by anion exchange chromatography using a HPLC system (28). Amino acid sequencing showed that the molecule is composed of at least 71 residues. No difference apart from the already known polymorphism at position 29 (Met or Thr for GP B^{S} or GP B^{s}, respectively), which determines S or s specificity, respectively, was found.

Ultimately, the complete AA sequence was deduced from the cDNA analysis of clones obtained from K562 cells (86) and from a human fetal liver library (39). Glycophorin B comprises 72 AA residues (see Fig. 1), of which Cys^{50} and the C terminal Ala^{72} were not identified by protein sequencing. The extracellular portion carries an average of 11 O-glycosidically linked oligosaccharides, but Asn^{26} is not glycosylated because the consensus sequence Asn-Xaa-Thr/Ser is lacking. The residues about 40–66 correspond to the hydrophobic domain of GP B that spans the membrane bilayer. The C terminal cytoplasmic domain of GP B is very short and is presumably not linked to the membrane cytoskeleton.

Comparison of the AA sequences of GP A and GP B indicates strong homologies, as outlined in Figure 1. Residues 1–26 are identical to residues 1–26 of GP A^{N} with a Leu or a Glu residue at position 1 or 5, respectively, which defines blood group N specificity. Apart from this identity of the N terminal portions of the molecules, residues 27–35 of GP B are rather homologous with residues 59–67 of GP A, and residues 46–71 of GP B are strickingly similar to residues 72–100 of GP A. This homology suggested that the gene coding for GP B was derived from the *GYPA* gene during evolution. Studies at the genomic level have lent further support to this hypothesis, as discussed below.

2. The "N" Antigen

As mentioned above, GP B carries the N, S, and s antigens. The trypsin-resistant and chymotrypsin-sensitive high-frequency N antigen on GP B is denoted as "N" in order to distinguish it from the polymorphic N antigen on GP A (87). Anti-N reagents react similarly with N terminal peptides from GP A^N and GP B (88). However, in agglutination assays, the "N" antigen in M+N− RBCs is usually only weakly reactive, thus permitting the determination of the MN phenotype. The major reason for this appears to be that the extracellular domain of GP B is much shorter than that of GP A. This conclusion is supported by data on rare RBCs (Finnish En(a-), Dantu^{NE}) described below.

3. S and s Antigens

Met or Thr residues at position 29 determines S or s specificity, respectively (28,35). Chemical modifications of the molecule and studies with synthetic peptides suggest that surrounding residues (the glycosylated Thr^{25}, Glu^{28}, His^{34}, and Arg^{35}) are also involved in the epitopes recognized by polyclonal antibodies (89,90).

The quantity of GP B in S+s+RBCs is about 1.5-fold higher than that in S−s+cells and intermediate in those with the phenotype S+s+ (47,88,91,92). To account for these data, it might be assumed that AA residues around position 29 are involved in the complex of GP B and Rh proteins or Rh-related glycoproteins (see below). Such an aggregate that appears to facilitate the incorporation of GP B into the membrane might be more stable with a Met instead of a Thr residue at position 29. However, other possibilities cannot be ruled out at present.

4. U and Duclos Antigens

Although it was assumed that the high-frequency U antigen is not located on GP B (93), there is strong evidence that it is located on a labile structure within residues approximately 33–40 of this molecule (94). In analogy to the En^aFR and Wr^b antigens, the U antigen requires lipids for optimal expression of activity and is destroyed by extraction of membranes by organic solvents.

Using papain treatment of RBCs, Issitt et al. (95) could distinguish two forms of the U antigen, UPS and UPR, that are sensitive or resistant toward this proteinase. The UPR antigen was found to be destroyed by certain hydrophobic sulfhydryl reagents. It remains to be elucidated whether this effect is due to modification of the Cys residue in the intramembraneous domain of GP B or to modification of proteins that complex with GP B.

Studies on Rh_{null} RBCs that lack the Rh proteins owing to apparently silent alleles at the *Rh* locus (amorphic type) or to regulatory gene(s) (regulator type) revealed that the quantity of GP B is decreased by about two thirds, regardless of whether the U antigen is roughly normal or strongly decreased (20). The latter RBC type has been denoted as "$Rh_{null}U−$" by some authors. In order to account for this finding, it has been proposed that the formation of a complex involving GP B and a different(s) protein(s) is necessary for optimal incorporation of GP B into the membrane and for optimal expression of the U antigen (20).

U^x and U^z are two different high-frequency antigens defined by human polyclonal antibodies. U^x is presumably located on the homologous, glycosylated N terminal domains of GP A and GP B (7,88). However, it is not clear why anti-U^x reacts preferentially with GP B. The U^z antigen is located within the AA residues approximately 29–36 of GP B, as judged from the effects of V8 proteinase and chymotrypsin (7,94). Since the quantity of GP B in RBCs depends on their Ss phenotype, the expression of the U^x and U^z antigens (as well as "N") is variable: S^+s^- cells exhibit stronger antigens than S^-s^+ RBCs (96).

A peculiar antibody (anti-Duclos) was discovered in the serum of a woman with the surname of Duclos (97), whose RBCs exhibit normal Ss and Rh antigens but a rather weak U antigen. Investigations on cells lacking GP B or the Rh proteins (Rh_{null} cells) suggested that the antibody recognizes an epitope involving a complex of GP B and a protein(s) absent from "$Rh_{null}U^-$" RBCs (20). Further analyses indicated that the proteinase-resistant portion of GP B is required for the binding of anti-Duclos (94).

A mouse monoclonal antibody, denoted as MB-2D10, exhibits anti-Duclos–like specificity in that it fails to agglutinate "$Rh_{null}U^-$" cells (21). However, the Duclos and MB-2D10 antigens are not identical, since MB-2D10 reacts with Duclos's cells and the MB-2D10 epitope is destroyed by chymotrypsin. Immunoblotting and immunoprecipitation experiments identified the antigen for MB-2D10 as the Rh-related glycoproteins (21,22). These components coimmunoprecipitate with the Rh proteins when anti-Rh sera (anti-D, anti-c or anti-E) are used (98,99). The immunoprecipitates obtained with MB-2D10 also contain the 30- to 32-kd Rh proteins and most probably GP B, thus providing direct evidence that at least three different proteins form an aggregate within the RBC membrane. The data on MB-2D10 suggest that the Duclos antigen might also be located on the Rh-related glycoproteins. In addition, these components, rather than the Rh proteins, appear to be necessary for optimal expression of the U antigen on GP B.

5. He and M^v Antigens

The low-frequency He antigen was found to be located in the N terminal region of an altered GP B (100) whose AA sequence is modified at positions 1, 4, and 5: Trp^1, Ser^4, or Gly^5 replace Leu, Thr, or Glu, respectively (Table 2). It is assumed that the He-specific GP B was generated by an inversion of the gene segment encoding the N terminal five residues. GP B^{He} lacks "N" activity (101) and is normally glycosylated at positions 2, 3, and 4. The He epitope recognized by human anti-He involves the NH_2 terminal Trp and NeuNAc residues (100).

Interestingly, some antibodies (denoted as anti-M^e) react with both the M antigen of GP A and the He antigen on GP B, suggesting that Gly^5 is the predominant AA residue in the structures of their epitopes (100).

The low-frequency M^v antigen is located within the N terminal eight residues of an altered GP B, but its structure has not been yet elucidated (102). One anti-M^v serum (Arm) was found to react with the M^v as well as the N and "N" antigens. Immunochemical investigations indicated that human polyclonal anti-M^v require the N terminal residues and sialic acid(s) for binding. Interestingly, it was observed that the abnormal GP B in M^v RBCs is produced in small quantity (about 20% of normal GP B) (103).

C. Genes Encoding Glycophorins A, B, and E

The first investigations on the molecular biology of glycophorins showed that GP A and GP B are encoded by separate single-copy genes coordinately regulated by a tumor-promoting phorbol ester (104).

The genomic structures encoding GP A and GP B were investigated using DNA libraries constructed from the human erythroleukemia cell line K562 (105) and from human leukocytes (106, 107). Restriction maps obtained with endonucleases and oligonucleotides as probes showed that *GYPA* or *GYPB* is composed of seven or five exons, respectively (reviewed in refs. 12 and 15). The exons encoding mature GP A are depicted in Figure 1.

Exon A1 codes for the major part of the leader peptide that is absent from the mature form of GP A. Exon 2 encodes the remainder of this peptide (residues −7 to −1) and the N terminal sequence of GP A (up to Asn^{26}) carrying the polymorphisms at positions 1 and 5 (M and N blood group antigens). Exons 3 and 4 correspond to the remaining extracellular portion of GP A: residues 27–58 or 59–71, respectively. The intramembraneous portion is encoded by exon 5 (codons 72–100), whereas the cytoplasmic segment is mainly encoded by exon 6 (codons 101–126). Amino acid residues 127–131, corresponding to the C terminal end of GP A, are encoded by exon 7, which also contains the 3′-untranslated region.

Exons B1 and B2, encoding the leader peptide and the N terminal portion of GP B, are identical with their counterparts A1 and A2 of the *GYPA* gene coding for N-specific GP A (Leu[1]/Glu[5]). The nucleotide sequence of *GYPB* is very similar to that of the *GYPA* gene and contains the sequence corresponding to exon A3 (coding for residues 27–58) that is not translated into GP B owing to a substitution at the first nucleotide of the 5′ consensus splicing signal sequence in intron B3 (105). Consequently, the AA residues 27–58 of GP A are lacking in GP B. This unexpressed exon B3 is designated as pseudoexon because it is homologous to exon A3 and is expressed in a number of glycophorin variants (12).

Exon B3 codes for residues 27–39 of GP B containing the polymorphism at position 29 (S and s blood group antigens), whereas exons B4 and B5 encode the majority of the intramembraneous portion of GP B (residues 40–71).

A third, related gene, at first described as invariant gene (108), and now designated *GYPE*, was identified during the investigations on *GYPA* and *GYPB* genes (109,110). *GYPE* contains four exons (E1–E4) and a large intronic sequence, partially used as exons in the *GYPA* and *GYPB* genes. Exon E1 encodes the major part of a leader sequence comprising 19 residues that is very similar with that of GP A and GP B, whereas exon 4 codes for the 3′-untranslated sequence. Exons 2 and 3 of the *GYPE* gene encode a novel glycophorin exhibiting 59 AA residues (expected molecular mass about 17 kd; see Fig. 1) that has not yet been identified with certainty at the membrane level. It is noteworthy that GP E would express the blood group M antigen (Ser[1]/Gly[5]) and that several attempts to visualize the protein on blots using anti-M were unsuccessful (12; Blanchard D. and Cartron J.P., unpublished data). However, Anstee reported an anti-M–reactive band exhibiting a molecular mass of about 20 kd that might correspond to GP E (111). Glycophorin E might correspond to the minor (about 0.2% of total stain) component J, detectable by SDS-PAGE and PAS staining of extracted GPS, that has been assumed to represent a further unique GP (18,20).

The three genes coding for GP A, GP B, and GP E are members of a single gene family and show over 90% homology, suggesting that *GYPB* and *GYPE* were derived from an ancestral *GYPA* gene by gene duplication, recombination through Alu repeats, and point mutations of the duplicated genes (105,109,110). In agreement with previous data obtained by linkage analysis (112), the structural gene for GP A was assigned to chromosome 4 in the region 4q28-q21 using DNA probes (38). *GYPE* was also located on chromosome 4 to an adjacent site (110).

D. Absence of Glycophorins A and/or B and Lepore-Type Hybrids

1. En(a–), M[k] and S–s–U– Variants

Red blood cells exhibiting the En(a–) phenotype from individuals homozygous for the rare gene *En* were found to lack GP A and all antigens associated with this molecule (M or N, En[a]TS, En[a]FS, En[a] FR, Wr[b]) (47,113–122).

Conventional genetic analysis suggested that the En(a–) phenotype, of which two varieties (Finnish and English) are known, is caused by a silent allele at the *MN/En* (*GYPA*) locus. Consistent with this conclusion, En(a⁻) RBCs of the Finnish type were found to exhibit a normal quantity of GP B associated with "N," s, and U antigens. However, the English variety of the En(a–) RBC phenotype was shown to possess an unusual (trypsin-resistant) M antigen as well as S and U antigens associated with a decreased quantity of GP B. These findings suggested that this molecule might represent a GP A-B hybrid of the Lepore type (see below). Apart from this, English En(a–) phenotypic individuals were shown to exhibit a further abnormality; i.e., the genotype *En/M[k]* rather than *En/En*.

Analysis of genomic DNA indicates that the exons A2–A7 and B1 are absent from the genome of Finnish En(a–) phenotypic individuals (38,110,123). Thus, a *GYPA-B* hybrid (exon 1 derived from the *GYPA* gene) appears to occur in these individuals. The genome of English

En(a⁻) phenotypic individuals was shown to lack a major portion of the *GYPA* gene (110). The available data suggest, but do not prove unambiguously, that the English *En* gene complex encodes a *GYPA-B* hybrid gene comprising exons 1 and 2 from a *GYPA* gene and exons 3–5 from a *GYPB* gene.

Red blood cells exhibiting the S⁻s⁻U⁻ phenotype from individuals homozygous for the *u* gene were found to lack GP B and all antigens ("N," S or s, U) associated with this molecule (120,124–128). Analyses of genomic DNA have shown that the *GYPB* region encoding mature GP B is deleted in most S⁻s⁻U⁻ phenotypic individuals (110,123,128). However, only a partial deletion or alteration of the *GYPB* gene was detected for some *uu* individuals (129), thus indicating a heterogeneous genetic background of the S⁻s⁻U⁻ phenotype. A deletion involving exons B2–B5 and E1 has been found for one S⁻s⁻U⁻ phenotypic individual, suggesting the possibility of the occurrence of a hybrid gene comprising exons B1 and E2–E4 (110).

SDS-PAGE analysis of membranes from RBCs exhibiting the S⁻s⁻U⁺ (weak or variant) phenotype failed to reveal any GP B. However, SDS-PAGE of large quantities of extracted GPs disclosed small quantities of GP B or a GP B–like molecule (120,124,125). Further characterization of the heterogenous S⁻s⁻ phenotype will require more detailed analyses of genomic DNA.

M^k denotes a gene complex silent at the *MN* and *Ss* loci (3–5). Initially, SDS-PAGE analyses of RBC membranes from M^k heterozygotes revealed that the contents of GP A and GP B are decreased by about 50% (75,130). SDS-PAGE analyses of RBC membranes from individuals heterozygous for two rare genes (En/M^k, $Mi.III/M^k$, $Mi.V/M^k$) served to show that M^k produces neither mature GP A nor GP B (103,119,131,132). Later on, M^k homozygotes were detected and their RBCs were shown to lack GP A and GP B as well as all antigens associated with these molecules (133,134). Analysis of genomic DNA from one M^k homozygote revealed a large deletion involving exons A2–A7, B1–B5, and E1. Thus, a hybrid gene comprising exons A1 and E1–E4 might occur in this individual (110,123).

2. Lepore-Type Hybrids

As described above, GP A, GP B, and GP E are homologous proteins and their genes are presumably directly adjacent on chromosome 4. Investigations of the family of hemoglobin proteins have shown that similarities of DNA sequences of adjacent genes may trigger a misalignment of homologous chromotids at synapsis (during meiosis) (reviewed in ref. 135). A subsequent deletion may create a new hybrid gene of the Lepore type encoding a portion of *both* parental proteins. In addition, crossing over of chromatids within nonallelic genes, followed by recombination, may create a gene of the Lepore type as well as an anti–Lepore-type gene complex encoding both parental genes as well as an anti–Lepore-type hybrid gene (or protein) (for a schematic representation of these genetic events see Fig. 2 in ref. 10). Some of the *MNSs* gene complexes that might represent variants of the Lepore type have already been described above. Further possible Lepore-type hybrids and gene complexes of the anti–Lepore type are described below.

SDS-PAGE analysis of RBC membranes from *Mi.V* heterozygotes revealed an approximate 50% decrease of GP A and GP B as well as a new component with a molecular mass intermediate between those of GP A and GP B. The quantity of the new component was found to be roughly comparable to that of GP B (75,103,127,131). Subsequent SDS-PAGE studies on *Mi.V* homozygotes showed only the new component and complete absence of GP A and GP B (136,137). The phenotype of the new molecule and that of Mi.V RBCs (M or N, En^aTS, En^aFS, s, Hil, U) suggested that it represents a hybrid of the Lepore type comprising a N terminal portion from GP A and a C terminal portion from GP B (131,136,137).

Analyses of genomic DNA have elucidated the exact structure of the Mi.V hybrid (106,138): It comprises the residues 1–58 from GP A and the residues 27–72 from GP B. The sequence of the protein in the region of the gene fusion is shown in Table 3. As one might expect, a synthetic peptide covering this region was recently found to inhibit anti-Hil (139). The exact DNA sequence of the gene fusion occurring in intron 3 has been determined for one Mi.V individual (138). Detailed studies on another Mi.V individual suggest that the *Mi.V*-specific genome comprises exons B1, A2–A3, and B3–B5 as well as the gene encoding GP A (106). Thus, the Mi.V-specific molecule (in that particular donor) represents a GP B-A-B hybrid, although this is not apparent from the structure of the mature protein (lacking the leader sequence encoded in part by exon B1). The data described above indicate that, in the particular case described above, the *Mi.V* gene does not represent a hybrid of the Lepore type but a fusion product resulting from gene conversion in which *GYPA* and *GYPB* served as donor and recipient, respectively. Further possible examples of variants resulting from gene conversion will be described below.

The variants J.R. and J.L. (also denoted as Mi.V (J.L.) or Mi.V*) appear to be rather similar to the Mi.V variant described above, except for a S instead of a s antigen and the absence of the Hil activity (138,140–142), and might represent further Lepore-type hybrids. Structural studies of the J.L. variant have disclosed that its AA sequence is identical with that of the Mi.V hybrid except for a Met residue (determining S specificity) at position 61 (138,142). The sequence in the region of the fusion is shown in Table 3. Recently, an antibody (anti-TSEN) reacting with J. L. and J. R. as well as Mi.IV RBCs was found to be inhibited by a synthetic peptide covering the residues 54–67 of the J.L. hybrid (143). Therefore, the umbrella designation Mi.XI appears to be justified for the J.R. and J.L. variants. A further antibody (anti-MINY) was shown to be inhibited by the Mi.V- and J.L.-specific peptides (residues 54–67) (144). Apparently, anti-MINY, which agglutinates Mi.III, Mi.IV, Mi.V, Mi.VI, and Mi.XI RBCs, does not distinguish between a Met or a Thr residue at position 61.

Recently, Daniels et al. (145) have described a further possible variant (TK) of the Lepore type associated with the novel low-frequency antigen SAT. Red blood cells from a *TK* homozygote were found to exhibit the phenotype M^-, N^+weak, En^aTS^+, En^aFS^+, EN^aFR^-, Wr^{b-}, S^-, s^-, U^-. They lack normal GP A and GP B and contain a new molecule with intermediate mobility in SDS-PAGE. It remains to be elucidated whether the C terminal domain of the molecule is derived from GP B, GP E, or GP A. Interestingly, the SAT antigen in a different family (Sat) was found to be associated with a weak M antigen that is located on a component migrating at the position of GP A in SDS-PAGE.

Table 3 Partial Structures of Lepore and Anti-Lepore Type Hybrid Glycophorins

GP variant	Partial ab sequence× [a]	Associated antigens
Mi. V	-PEEET0GETGQLVHR- 54 67	Hil, MINY
I.L (Mi.XI)	-PEEETGEMGQLVHR- 54 67	TSEN, MINY
St[a]	** * -YISSQTNGERVOLA- 20 33	St[a]
Dantu	-VHRITVPEITLIIL- 33 46	Dantu

(a) Residues corresponding to the sequence of GPA are underlined.

E. Anti–Lepore-Type Hybrids and Other Hybrid Molecules

1. Anti–Lepore-Type Hybrids

Red blood cells carrying the St^a antigen were presumed to carry a hybrid of the anti–Lepore type (146–149). SDS-PAGE of RBCs membranes from heterozyotes and a homozygote revealed a new molecule with a mobility intermediate between GP A and GP B, in addition to normal GPA and GP B. The quantity of GP A in membranes from St^a heterozygotes and one homozygote was found to be decreased by about 20, or about 50%, respectively (150). The new molecule was shown to carry N and St^a antigens (146,149). Amino acid sequence analysis revealed that it comprises 99 residues (149). The residues 27–99 correspond to the residues 59–131 of GP A, whereas the residues 1–26 correspond to the residues 1–26 of GP B *and* of the blood group N–specific GP A. Therefore, AA sequence analysis could not prove the presumed GP B-A hybrid nature of the molecule; i.e., a GP A variant resulting from a deletion of exon 3 (encoding residues 27–58) could not be ruled out (149). The sequence of the St^a-specific molecule in the region of the gene fusion or deletion carrying the St^a antigen is shown in Table 3.

Analyses of genomic DNA have ultimately established the GP B-A hybrid nature of the St^a-specific molecule (138,151–153). The fusion between the two genes was found to occur within intron 3, and three different mutations have been characterized at the genomic level (153), thus indicating a heterogeneous genetic background of the St^a phenotype.

A further rare variety of the St^a phenotype, i.e., M^Z, described by Metaxas et al. (154), was investigated by Dahr et al. (150). Studies on two related M^Z heterozygotes suggest that the M^Z gene complex encodes blood group N–specific GP A and blood group s–specific GP B, in addition to a novel, St^a-specific molecule. However, SDS-PAGE revealed a pattern comparable to that of a St^a homozygote: the quantity of the novel molecule was found to be higher than in a common St^a heterozygote. Furthermore, the quantity of GP A was found to be decreased by about 50%. Structural analysis suggest that the M^Z-specific molecule is almost identical with the hybrid occurring in common St^a phenotypic individuals. However, it exhibits the blood group M–specific sequence (Ser or Gly at positions 1 or 5, respectively) (150). A complete understanding of the new molecule in M^Z RBCs must await studies at the genomic DNA level: It might be encoded by a *GYPA* gene exhibiting a deletion of exon 3. Alternatively, it is also possible that the molecule is encoded by a hybrid gene comprising exons E2 and A4–A7. In view of the large quantity of the new molecule and the strong decrease of the GP A content in M^Z RBC membranes as well as the findings on Dantu RBCs, described below, it is conceivable that the genome of M^Z heterozygotes contains two genes encoding the new molecule.

Individuals whose RBCs carry the low-frequency antigen Dantu (155) were also found to exhibit gene complexes of the anti-Lepore type. Three varieties of the *Dantu* gene complex have been discovered: Dantu^{Ph} (137,156), Dantu^{NE} (18,157–159), and Dantu^{MD} (160). The *Dantu*^{MD} gene complex, detected in one white heterozygote, was found to encode GP A (slightly decreased) and a GP B-A hybrid molecule comprising the residues 1–39 from GP B (s-specific) and the residues 72–131 from GP A, as judged from studies at the phenotypic level (160). The Dantu-specific sequence stretch, assumed to carry the Dantu antigen (18,159), is shown in Table 3. The structure of the mature Dantu-specific molecule suggests that it is encoded by a hybrid gene comprising exons B2, B3, and A5–A7.

The *Dantu*^{Ph} gene complex, detected in one Zimbabwean family (137,156), gives rise to a SDS-PAGE pattern similar to that of *Dantu*^{MD} described above. However, *Dantu*^{Ph} does not produce any GP B, as judged from the absence of this molecule from the RBC membranes of *Dantu*^{Ph}/u heterozygotes (156).

The *Dantu* gene complex of the NE variety, not uncommon among blacks, was found to encode blood group M–specific GP A as well as the Dantu-specific GP B-A hybrid, but no GP B, as judged from the absence of the latter molecule from the RBC membranes of *Dantu*$^{NE/u}$

heterozygotes (18,157). SDS-PAGE of RBC membranes from $Dantu^{NE}$ heterozygotes disclosed a pattern similar to those of the M^Z heterozygotes and the homozygote of the common St^a variety described above: the level of GP A was decreased by about 55% and large quantities (molar ratio to GP A about 2:1) of the hybrid were detected (157). Studies of genomic DNA have confirmed the observations made at the phenotypic level and added the important piece of evidence that the genome of a $Dantu^{NE}$ heterozygote contains two copies encoding the GP B-A hybrid molecule (161, 162). In view of this finding, it is rather tempting to speculate that the genome of M^Z heterozygotes also contains two copies encoding the St^a-specific molecule, as already mentioned above.

As described above, the quantity of GP A was found to be slightly (about 20%) decreased in all RBC membranes exhibiting a low (molar ration to GP A about 0.8:1.0) quantity of a St^a- or Dantu-specific molecule. In all RBC membranes exhibiting larger quantities of these St^a- or Dantu-specific molecules, the membrane level of GP A was shown to be decreased to a significant extent (about 50–55%). In order to account for these data, it has been suggested (18,150,157) that GP A forms a complex with "band 3" during membrane biosynthesis and that the formation of this GP A–band 3 complex represents the prerequisite for optimum incorporation of GP A into the membrane.

2. Other Hybrid Molecules

SDS-PAGE of RBC membranes from *Mi.III*, *Mi.IV*, and *Mi.VI* heterozygotes revealed a decrease of normal GP B (about 50%) and an abnormal GP B exhibiting an increased molecular mass (about 5,000 d) (103,127,131,163). SDS-PAGE analyses of membranes from *MiIII/M^k*, *Mi.III/Mi.III*, and *Mi.III/Dantu^{NE}* heterozygotes disclosed the complete absence of normal GP B (103, 127,131,161). Inhibition tests with GP fractions and immunoblotting established that the abnormal GP B carries N (Mi.III, Mi.IV, Mi.VI), Mi^a (Mi.III, Mi.IV, Mi.VI), Anek (Mi.VI) and En^aKT (Mi.III) antigens (80,83,127,164,165). As judged from serological studies, the abnormal GP B in Mi.III and Mi.VI or Mi.IV RBCs exhibits a qualitatively altered s or S antigen, respectively (3,4).

The data described above suggested that Mi.III, Mi.IV, and Mi.VI RBCs carry a GP B-A-B hybrid molecule (83). Indeed, recent studies of genomic DNA (166) have shown that the Mi.III- and Mi.VI-specific molecules represent hybrids resulting from gene conversions involving *GYPA* and *GYPB* as donor and recipient, respectively. Since a portion of intron 3 from *GYPA* is also transfered, a part of the sequence of the "pseudoexon" of *GYPB* is expressed in the mature hybrid molecules (see Fig. 2).

Elucidation of the Mi.III and MI.IV variants provides a basis for the understanding of the various antigens of the Mi subsystem (84) that was originally defined as a collection of four (I–IV) cell classes reacting with the serum from a woman with the surname of Miltenberger (anti-Mi^a) (3,4,167). Anti-Mi^a appears to be directed against the sequence QTNDM(or K)HKRDTY occurring in the Mi.I-, Mi.II-, Mi.III-, and Mi.VI-specific GPs (84). The specificities of other antibodies related to the Mi subsystem may also be predicted from the structures of the Mi. variant GPs (84): Anti-Vw and anti-Hut appear to be directed against the sequences QTNDMHKR and QTNDKHKRDTYAATP, respectively. Anti-Vw+Hut seems to react with the latter sequence, regardless of whether there is a Met or a Lys residue at position 28. Anti-Hut+Mur might recognize the sequence QTNDKHKRDTY occurring in Mi.II-, Mi.III-, and Mi.VI-specific GPs. Anti-Mur is assumed to bind to the sequence YPAHTANE, encoded by the GP B-pseudoexon, that occurs in Mi.III- and Mi.VI-specific GPs. The sequence of the Mi.III-specific GP within the residues 45–55 is identical to that of normal GP A, explaining the En^aKT specificity of the molecule. Conversely, the residues 45–55 of the Mi.VI-specific GP are identical to the residues 46–56 of Mi.VIII-specific GP A, thus providing an explanation for the Anek antigen on both molecules. However, it is not clear why Mi.VI RBCs are nonreactive with Lane serum. The residues 54–64 of the Mi.III- and Mi.VI-specific molecules are identical to the residues 55–65 of the Mi.V-specific GP. This finding explains the occurrence of the Hil, MINY, and s (qualitatively altered) antigens on all these molecules.

Mi.IV RBCs are rather similar to Mi.VI RBCs except for TSEN and a S (qualitatively) altered antigen instead of Hil and s antigens. Therefore, it has been suggested that the structure of the Mi.IV-specific GP is almost identical to that of the Mi.VI-specific GP except for a Met instead of a Thr residue at position 60 (84).

A further related GP B-A-B variant, denoted as Mi.X, which has been described recently (168), is also shown in Figure 2. Mi.X RBCs exhibit the phenotype Vw⁻, Hut⁻, Mur⁻, Hut plus Mur⁺, Hil⁺, Anek⁻, Lane⁻. It is not clear why these cells are nonreactive with anti-Hut.

Recently, Skov et al. (169) have described the Mi.IX variant that is characterized by the Mur and DANE antigens as well as a trypsin-resistant GP A that lacks certain EnᵃTS antigens and exhibits a slightly decreased molecular mass. Since the Mur antigen appears to correspond to the sequence YPAHTANE, the Mi.IX-specific GP A appears to represent a GP A-B-A hybrid that contains a part of the GP B–pseudoexon (84). As judged from the hypothetical AA sequence determined by the GP B–pseudoexon (see Fig. 2), the Mi.II-, Mi.VII-, and Mi.VIII-specific GP A molecules might also represent GP A-B-A hybrids that were generated by gene conversion (12,84).

IV. GLYCOPHORINS C AND D AND THE ANTIGEN OF THE GERBICH BLOOD GROUP SYSTEM

A. Structure and Antigens of GPs C and D

1. Structure of GP C

The partial AA sequence of GP C and its glycosylation sites could be determined by analysis of its N terminal tryptic peptide (residues 1–48) (27,170) and the purified molecule obtained

Hypothetic residues
encoded by the 'GP B-
pseudoexon' :   DKHKRDTYPA-HTANEVSEISVTTVSPPEKKN

Partial structure   ** *
of normal GP B :   -ISSQTN--GETGQLVHR-
                        21   25   27 30   35

Partial structure   ** *0 *   *   *   * * *   *
of normal GP A :   -ISSQTNDTHKRDTYAATPRAHEVSEISVRTVYPPEEETGERVQLAHH-
                        21   25   30   35   40   45   50   55   60   65

                        *? *   *   *   ? * *
Mi.III (B-A-B) :   -ISSQTNDKHKRDTYPA-HTANEVSEISVRTVYPPEEETGETGQLVHR-
                        21   25   30   35   40   45   50   55   60   65

                        ?? ?   ?   ?   ? ? ??
Mi.VI (B-A-B) :   -ISSQTNDKHKRDTYPA-HTANEVSEISVTTVYPPEEETGETGQLVHR-
                        21   25   30   35   40   45   50   55   60   65

                        ?? ?   ?   ?   ? ? ?
Mi.X (B-A-B) :   -ISSQTNDKHKRDTYAATPRAHEVSEISVRTVYPPEEETGETGQLVHR-
                        21   25   30   35   40   45   50   55   60   65

Figure 2 Partial structures of GP A, GP B, and Mi.III-, Mi.VI-, and Mi.X-specific GPs. Amino acid residues that are identical with those of GP A are underlined. Hypothetical residues encoded by the "GP B–pseudoexon" are shown above the sequence of GP B.

on a large scale by preparative chromatography (up to residue 88) (28). Its complete sequence of 128 AA residues (Fig. 3) was deduced from the nucleotide sequence of cDNA isolated from human reticulocyte (171) or liver (172–174) cDNA libraries. The molecule is a type III transmembrane glycoprotein composed of three domains, since it is synthetized without a leader peptide and translation of the corresponding mRNA starts at Met[1] (172,174).

The N terminal extracellular region, comprising AA residues 1–56, carries an average of 12 O-glycans whose structures are similar to those of GP A and GP B and one N glycan attached to Asn[8]. The hydrophilic domain also carries various antigens (see below). Interestingly, a set of six AA residues at the positions 17–22 and 36–41 are identical, suggesting that an internal duplication occurred within the *GYPC* gene during evolution (27,171).

The intramembraneous hydrophobic domain of GP C corresponds to the residues 57–81, whereas the C terminal hydrophilic portion contains 47 residues that strongly interact with the membrane skeleton via band 4.1 (23–26). The cytoplasmic domain is longer than that of GP A and provides GP C with the functional property of regulating the mechanical stability of the RBC membrane (175). The four tyrosine residues of the molecule are located in this cytoplasmic domain. As a result of this, GP C cannot be labeled with [125]iodine in intact RBCs.

2. Structure of GP D

Glycophorin D is a minor component of the red cell membrane and represents only about 1% of the total GPs (Table 1). The molecule could be purified by preparative electrophoresis and sequenced partially. Its N terminus was found to be blocked, but the AA sequence of a large portion of the molecule could be obtained (32). The identified AA residues are identical with the residues 30–128 of GP C. The identity of the C terminal portions of GP C and GP D was also shown by peptide mapping experiments (32) and the demonstration that rabbit antisera raised against one of the molecules bind to both of them (32,176). More recently, a murine monoclonal antibody directed against a synthetic peptide (residues 106–121 of GP C) was obtained. As expected, the antibody (NaM57-1F6) bound to GP C and GP D in blotting

```
GLYCOPHORIN   C

                              Ge 3 antigen
                              --------------

   ** * O**      *        *   ***   ***            *
MWSTRSPNSTAWPLSLEPDPGMASASTTMHTTTTIAEPDPGMSGWPDGRMETSTPTIMDIVVIAG
1         10        20        30        40        50        60
----exon C1----/--- exon 2 C2-----/------- exon C3  -----------/-

VIAAVAIVLVSLLFVMLRYMYRHKGTYHTNEAKGTEFAESADAALQGDPALQDAGDSSRKEYFI
      70        80        90       100       110       120     128
--------------------------exon C4---------------------------------

GLYCOPHORINS   D  (proposed   sequence)

                   Ge 2 antigen      Ge 3 antigen
                   ------            ----------------
                   * ***   ***              *
            ASASTTMHTTTTIAEPDPGMSGWPDGRMETSTPTIMDIVVIAG

VIAAVAIVLVSLLFVMLRYMYRHKGTYHTNEAKGTEFAESADAALQGDPALQDAGDSSRKEYFI
```

Figure 3 Amino acid sequences (1-letter code), oligosaccharide sites (* or O), major antigens, and alignment of exons of GP C and GP D. Boldface letters represent the intramembraneous domains.

experiments (M. J. Loirat, J. P. Cartron, and D. Blanchard, unpublished data). Glycophorin D also binds firmly to the membrane skeleton (26,31,177), just like GP C. In addition, both GPs carry the Ge3 antigen, located within the residues about 41–55 of GP C (176,178). Glycophorin D lacks an N-glycan and does not react with monoclonal antibodies directed against the residues 1 to about 20 of GP C (173,177,179).

Analysis of genomic DNA from rare Gerbich and Yus individuals (see below) indicates that one unique gene encodes both C *and* GP D (173,180). To account for these findings and the lower molecular mass (24 kd) of GP D as compared with GP C (32 kd), it was proposed that GP D represents an abridged version of GP C (32,173,180). Glycophorin D might be generated by initiation of protein synthesis at the codon determining Met[22] of GP C. However, the N terminal Met residue of GP D appears to be cleaved and the new N terminal residue (Ala) seems to be blocked subsequently (possibly by an acetyl group).

3. High-Frequency Antigens of GP C and GPD

The Gerbich (Ge) blood group system comprises four high-frequency antigens (Ge1, Ge2, Ge3, and Ge4), defined by human alloantibodies (reviewed in ref. 13). The number 020 has been assigned to the system by the Working Party on Terminology for Red Blood Cell Surface Antigens of the International Society of Blood Transfusion (ISBT) (1,2). The numbers 020002, 020003, or 020004 denote Ge2, Ge3, or Ge4, respectively; Ge1 (number 020001) is obsolete, since anti-Ge1 is not now available. Red blood cells from common individuals exhibit the phenotype Ge:2,3,4. Rare RBCs lacking Ge antigens have been classified as Ge negative of Gerbich type (Ge:–2,–3,4), the Yus type (Ge:–2,3,4), or the Leach type (Ge:–2,–3,–4). Apart from the above-mentioned Ge antigens, the low-incidence antigens Wb (020005), Ls[a] (020006), An[a] (020007), and Dh[a] (020008) have been moved to the Ge system (1,2).

The antigens of the Ge blood group system were found to be located on GP C and D. Anti-Ge3 binds to both GPC and GP D, whereas anti-Ge2 reacts only with GP D (176,178). From its destruction by trypsin and chemical modifications, the Ge3 epitope was localized within the residues approximately 41–55 of GP C (178), corresponding to residues about 20–34 of GP D. NeuNAc residues of the O-glycan attached to Ser[42] of GP C are involved in many Ge3 epitopes. A mouse monoclonal antibody with a specificity comparable to that of the human anti-Ge3 alloantibodies was obtained recently (181).

Since the Ge2 antigen is carried by GP D that appears to be identical with the residues 23–128 of GP C (32,176,178), we have proposed that the Ge2 epitope is located at the N terminal end of GP D (178). In line with the assumption that the N terminal Met residues is cleaved from mature GP D and that the N terminus is blocked (32), chemical modification of Met residues or amino groups did not have any effect on the Ge2 activity of GPs (178). O-glycans attached to Ser or Thr residues are involved in all determinants recognized by the seven alloanti-Ge2 investigated (178).

The Ge4 antigen, defined by a human alloantibody discovered more recently (182), is located on the N terminal portion of GP C (residues 1–22) that is not present on GP D. Several murine monoclonal antibodies with anti-Ge4–like specificity (binding to GP C but not GP D) were obtained (55,56,177,179). Binding to GP C of the majority of these antibodies was prevented by chemical modification of the N-terminal Met residues or by desialylation (56,179), showing that Met[1] and NeuNAc residues, most probably those carried by the O-glycans attached to Ser[3] and Thr[4], are essential for the corresponding epitopes. However, one monoclonal antibody (APO 3) has a different specificity, since it does not require NeuNAc residues. Its epitope was localized within the residues about 15–20 of GP C. It involves Glu[17] and/or Asp[19] and the oligosaccharide attached to Ser[15] (179). Recently, we obtained two further murine monoclonal antibodies with specificity similar to that of APO 3 (M. J. Loirat and D. Blanchard, unpublished data). These antibodies are of interest to investigate the expression of GP C in nonerythroid cells, since GP C was found to be widely expressed in different cells and tissues but in a differently glycosylated form (15,183,184).

4. Genes for GP C and GP D

Clones of the *GYPC* gene have been isolated and analyzed in detail (174,180). The gene is organized in four exons separated by three introns: exons 1–3 encode the extracellular domain of GP C (residues 1–16, 17–35, or 36–63, respectively), whereas exon 4 codes for the intramembraneous and the cytoplasmic domains of the molecule (see Fig. 3). There is general agreement that the *GYPC* gene also encodes GP D. Exons 2, 3, and 4 are used for the synthesis of GP D. Using a DNA probe, the *GYPC* gene has been assigned to chromosome 2 in the region 2q14-Q21 (185). Its location is, therefore, on a different chromosome than the GYPA and *GYPB* genes.

B. Variants of GP C and GP D

1. Ge-Negative Variants of the Leach Type

Gerbich-negative RBCs of the Leach type do not express the Ge2, Ge3, and Ge4 antigens and are characterized by the total absence of both GP C and GP D (177). A proportion of the Leach cells are elliptocytic (177, 186) and exhibit altered membrane properties (mechanical stability and membrane deformability) (175).

Analysis at the genomic level showed that the *GYPC* gene from one individual (PL) with the Leach phenotype contains the 5' portion with exons 1 and 2 but totally lacks exons 3 and 4 and the 3' portion (180). Similar conclusions were obtained from the study of two additional individuals (Cud and WB) with the Leach phenotype. However, analysis of a fourth case (LN) showed a single nucleotide deletion in codon 45 of a largely intact *GYPC* gene (187). This mutation generates a stop codon before the domain encoding the transmembrane portion of GP C. The corresponding mRNA that has been detected in mononuclear blood cells would be translated into a truncated form of GP C/D. In the aforementioned four cases, the corresponding encoded proteins have not been detected in RBC membranes, suggesting that they cannot be inserted into the membrane.

2. Variants of the Ge and the Yus Types

In contrast to the Ge-negative RBCs of the Leach type, the cells of the Gerbich and Yus types are not elliptocytic (31,188). Both types of RBCs lack normal GP C and GP D and carry an unusual GP with features common to GP C and GP D (e.g., interaction with the membrane skeleton) that prevent the cells from becoming elliptocytic. The new GP of the Gerbich type, designated as GP C^{Ge}, carries the Ge4 antigen, is resistant to trypsin treatment of cells, and has an apparent molecular mass of 24–26 kd in SDS-PAGE. The GPC^{Yus} molecule has a slightly higher apparent molecular mass (25–28 kd), is cleaved by trypsin treatment of cells, and carries the Ge3 and Ge4 antigens. Glycophorin C^{Ge} and GP C^{Yus} exhibit the N terminal portion of GP C: they carry receptors for murine monoclonal antibodies with anti-Ge4–like specificity and for *Lens culinaris* lectin (173,176,178,188) that binds to the *N*-glycan attached to Asn^8 of GP C. they also share a common C terminal cytoplasmic portion with GP C and GP D, which reacts with rabbit antisera (176,178).

Analysis of genomic DNA showed that the *GYPC* gene in Gerbich individuals lacks exon 3 and, therefore, codes for a molecule comprising the residues 1–35 and 64–128 of GP C (173,174,180,189). The lack of the residues 36–63 containing the tryptic cleavage site (Arg^{48}) and the Ge3 epitope (residues 41–55) explains the characteristic features of GP C^{Ge}. The deletion of exon 3 in the Ge type was confirmed by sequencing of the GP C^{Ge} cDNA (190). It is noteworthy that a GP D^{Ge} molecule with about 73 AA residues has not been detected in RBC membranes of the Ge type. Since *GYPC* in individuals of the Ge type exhibits exon 2, one might expect the occurrence of such a molecule.

Similarly, a 57-bp deletion in cDNA fragments generated from the GP C^{Yus} mRNA was identified. This deletion corresponds to exon 3 of the *GYPC* gene (173,174,180,189,190). The GPC^{Yus} molecule lacks the residues 16–35 of GP C corresponding to the N terminal region of GP D.

From these observations, it was suggested that the genes encoding the GP C^{Ge} and GP C^{Yus} molecules represent two allelic forms of a unique ancestral *GYPC* gene. Unequal crossing overs between the homologous 3.4-kb repeat sequences of the *GYPC* gene might account for the two types of deletions: exon 2 for the Yus type and exon 3 for the Ge type (174,180,190).

3. Low-Frequency Antigens of the Ge System

The Wb antigen was found to be located on the N terminal, trypsin-sensitive portion of an abnormal GP C molecule, designated as GP C^{Wb} (191,192). The altered molecule has an apparent molecular mass approximately 2.7 kd lower than that of normal GP C resulting from the absence of the N-glycan normally attached to Asn^8. Sequencing of the GP C^{Wb} cDNA demonstrated an A-G substitution at nucleotide 23, resulting in the substitution of Asn^8 by a Ser residue (190). Endo-β-N-acetylglucosamineidase F–treated GP C exhibits a lower electrophoretic mobility than GP C^{Wb}, suggesting that Ser^8 of the abnormal component carries an O-glycan that might be involved in the epitope for anti-Wb.

Ls(a+) RBCs carry the low-frequency Ls^a antigen and contain GP C and GP D with increased apparent molecular masses (about 6 kd) (193). These molecules are presumably encoded by a *GYPC* gene containing an additional copy of exon 3 (189).

Immunoblotting experiments recently demonstrated that the low-incidence Dh^a antigen is located on an altered GP C (194). The epitope is carried by the N terminal, trypsin-sensitive portion of the molecule and comprises sialic acid residues, but it is not dependent on the N-glycan. Since GP C^{Dha} displays a normal mobility in SDS-PAGE, it has been suggested that the Dh^a variant arose from a single AA substitution (194), but this hypothesis awaits the proof by AA or DNA sequencing.

The low-frequency An^a antigen was found to be located on the trypsin-sensitive portion of GP D and shown to be destroyed by sialidase (195). Dosage studies suggest that An^a and Ge2 are antithetic antigens. However, the molecular basis for the An^a antigen has not yet been identified.

V. STRUCTURES AND ANTIGENS OF O-GLYCANS

A. Major Tetrasaccharide and Its Precursor

Apart from the major tetrasaccharide (structure [a] in Fig. 4), already mentioned above (40), normal RBCs were found to contain four additional O-glycans (structures [b]–[e]) that represent biosynthetic precursors of the tetrasaccharide (196). The linear trisaccharide (structure [b]) accounts for about one fifth of the O-glycans, whereas structures (c)–(e) were detected only in rather small quantities (196). As described above, structures (a)–(c) are involved in the epitopes for several antibodies related to the MNSs and Ge systems. Apart from this, structures (a)–(c) represent the antigens recognized by certain monoclonal autoantibodies (anti-Pr) occurring in cold agglutinin disease (197,198). The Pr antigens do not comprise the polypeptide chains of the GPs, and, therefore, these receptors are located on each of the GPs (199). Structure (e) occurs only in rather small quantity and accounts for the reaction of desialylated RBCs of GPs with the lectins from *Helix pomatia* and related snails (61,196). Removal of NeuNAc residues from structures (a)–(c) uncovers structure (d) that represents the T antigen (61,200). The

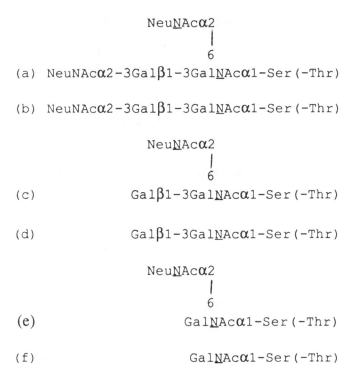

NeuNAcα2
|
6
(a) NeuNAcα2-3Galβ1-3GalNAcα1-Ser(-Thr)

(b) NeuNAcα2-3Galβ1-3GalNAcα1-Ser(-Thr)

NeuNAcα2
|
6
(c)   Galβ1-3GalNAcα1-Ser(-Thr)

(d)   Galβ1-3GalNAcα1-Ser(-Thr)

NeuNAcα2
|
6
(e)   GalNAcα1-Ser(-Thr)

(f)   GalNAcα1-Ser(-Thr)

Figure 4 Structures of major O-glycan and its biosynthetic precursors.

corresponding antibody (anti-T) occurs naturally in most human sera. Therefore, desialylated RBCs are polyagglutinable. Several examples of mouse monoclonal anti-T have been obtained recently (9,56; M. J. Loirat and D. Blanchard, unpublished data).

In Tn syndrome, an acquired condition of persistent mixed-field polyagglutinability, a proportion of RBCs exhibits a defect of UDP-Gal: GalNAc-β-3-D-galactosyl-transferase (201–203). Consequently, GalNAcα-Ser(-Thr) (structure [f]) representing the Tn antigen is exposed on these cells (204,205). The Tn antigen is detectable by antibodies occurring naturally in most human sera, by several GalNAc-specific lectins, and also by mouse monoclonal reagents (56,204,206). The galactosyl-transferase is presumably not completely absent from Tn RBCs, since sialylated derivatives of structure (d) were found to occur on these cells (203). The Tn disorder affects RBCs as well as platelets and granulocytes and, therefore, is thought to result from a defect in a common stem cell in bone marrow (207). Recently, structure (e) (sialyl-Tn antigen) has been identified as an additional, minor antigen of Tn RBCs (206).

B. Minor Variants of O-glycans

Apart from the major tetrasaccharide (structure [a]) and its precursors, several minor variants of the O-glycans have been identified in the GPs (Fig. 5). Two trisialopentasaccharides (structures [g] and [h]) result from the attachment of an additional NeuNAc residue to structure (a) (208). It is not known whether these pentasaccharides exhibit any significances for the antigens of the GPS.

In blood group O RBCs, a small percentage of structure (c) and (d) appears to be converted to structure (i) by the attachment of a Fuc residue. This blood group H-active O-glycan may

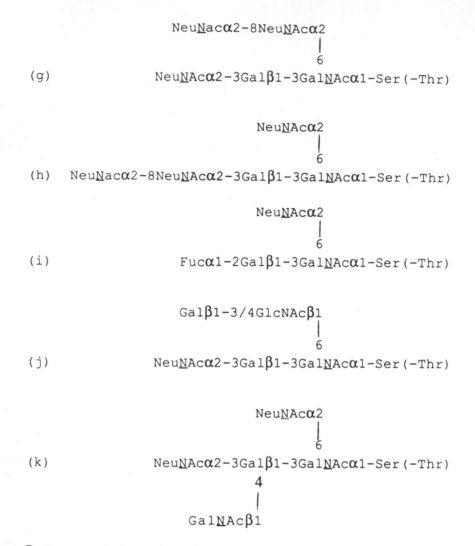

Figure 5 Structures of minor variants of the O-glycans.

be further modified by the attachment of a GalNAC or a Gal residue in blood group A or B individuals, respectively (209,210).

A series of additional minor O-glycans results from the attachment of GlcNAc and further sugar residue to structure (b). The major compound (structure [j], which may be further modified by the addition of Gal, GlcNAc, Fuc, or NeuNAc (71,211), is shown in Fig. 5. Remarkably, structure (j) and related O-glycans occur predominantly or exclusively in the N terminal region (residues 1–30) of GP A (212). Glycophorin A from most whites contains only small quantities (about 0.03–0.2 mol/mol of GP A). Larger quantities (up to about 5 mol) were detected in GP A from blacks possessing strong Tm, Sj, Sext, Hu, Can, and/or M_1 antigens (212). It is assumed that the corresponding antibodies are directed against the M- or N-specific AA residues at the first or fifth positions of GP A *and* the GlcNAc-containing O-glycans (212). The serological complexity of the aforementioned antigens is presumably caused by the following phenomena: (1) some antibodies are not completely specific for the M- or N-specific AA residues; (2) they appear to require different levels of GlcNAc-containing O-glycans for agglutination; (3) certain antibodies might react preferentially or exclusively with a particular oligosaccharide (s) within the family of structure (j) and related coumpounds; (4) some antibodies (anti-Can, anti-Tm, anti-M plus-M) might crossreact with structures ([a] and in particular [b] and [d]) devoid of GlcNAc.

In RBCs exhibiting the rare Cad phenotype, structures (a) and (b) are modified to variable extents (about 10–90%) by the attachment of a GalNAc residues (structure [k]) (213–215). A corresponding antibody (anti-Cad) is present in most human sera. Therefore, Cad RBCs are polyagglutinable. The Cad antigen may be regarded as a "super variant" in the Sd^a system. Structure (k) could not be detected in GPs from $Sd(a^+)$ RBCs (215). The Cad antigen was also found to be located on gangliosides (216), and since a transferase transferring GalNAc to gangliosides, but not to GPs, was detected in the kidney from $Sd(a^+)$ individuals (217), it was assumed that Sd^a antigen is located exclusively on gangliosides. Therefore, it is likely that the Cad phenotype results from a change in the acceptor specificty of this GalNAc-transferase.

REFERENCES

1. Lewis M, et al. Blood Group Terminology 1990. From the ISBT Working Party on Terminology for Red Cell Surface antigens. Vox Sang 1990; 58:152.
2. Lewis M., et al. ISBT Working Party on Terminology for Red Cell Surface Antigens: Los Angeles Report. Vox Sang 1991; 61:158
3. Race RR, Sanger R. Blood Groups in Man. 6th ed. Oxford, England: Backwell Scientific, 1975.
4. Issitt PD. Applied Blood Group Serology, 3rd ed. Miami: Montgomery Scientific, 1985.
5. Salmon C, Cartron JP, Rouger P. The Human Blood Groups. New York: Masson Publishing USA, 1884.
6. Anstee DJ. The blood-group MNSs-active sialoglycoproteins, Semin Hematol 1981; 18:13.
7. Dahr W. Immunochemistry of sialoglycoproteins in human red blood cell membrane. In: Vengelen-Tyler V, Judd WJ, eds. Recent Advances in Blood Group Biochemistry. Arlington, VA: American Association of Blood Banks, 1986:27.
8. Reid ME. Biochemistry and molecular cloning analysis of human red cell sialoglycoproteins that carry Gerbich blood group antigens. In: Unger PJ, Laird-Fryer B, eds. Blood Group Systems: MN and Gerbich. Arlington VA: American Association of Blood Banks, 1989:73.
9. Lisowska E. Antigenic properties of human eythrocyte glycophorins. In: Wu AM, ed. Molecular Immunology of Complex Carbohydrates. New York: Plenum Press, 1988:265.
10. Moulds JJ, Dahr W. MNSs and Gerbich blood group systems. In: Litwin SD, Scott DW, Flaherty L, Reisfeld RA, Marcus D, ed. Human Immunogenetics: Basic Principles and Clinical Application. New York: Marcel Dekker, Basel, 1989:713.
11. Blanchard D. Human red cell glycophorins: biochemical and antigenic properties. Trans Med Rev 1990; 4:170.
12. Huang CH, Johe KK, Seifter S, Blumenfeld OO. Biochemistry and molecular cloning of MNSs blood group antigens. Baillieres Clin Haematol 1991. In press.
13. Unger PJ. The Gerbich blood groups: distribution, serology and genetics. Unger PJ, Laird-Fryer B, eds. Blood Group Systems: MN and Gerbich. Arlington VA: American Association of Blood Banks, 1989:73.
14. Rolih S. Biochemistry of MN antigens. In: Unger PJ, Laird-Fryer B, eds. Blood Group Systems: MN and Gerbich. Arlington VA: American Association of Blood Banks, 1989:31.
15. Cartron JP, Colin Y, Kudo S, Fukuda M. Molecular genetics of human erythrocyte sialo-glycoproteins: glycophorins A, B, C, and D. In: Harris JR, ed. Blood Cell Biochemistry. New York: Plenum Press, 1990:299.
16. Nigg EA, Bron C, Girardet M, Cherry RJ. Band 3-glycophorin A association in erythrocyte membrane demonstrated by combining protein diffusion measurements with antibody-induced cross-linking. Biochemistry 1980; 19:1887.
17. Dahr W, Wilkinson S, Issitt P, Beyreuther K, Hummel M, Morel P. High frequency antigens of

human erythrocyte membrane sialoglycoproteins. III. Studies on the En^aFr, Wr^b and Wr^a antigens. Biol Chem Hoppe-Seyler 1986; 367:1033.

18. Unger P, Procter JL, Moulds JJ, Moulds MK, Blanchard D, Guizzo ML, McCall LA, Cartron JP, Dahr W. The Dantu erythrocyte phenotype of the NE variety. II. Serology, immunochemistry genetics, and frequency. Blut 1987; 54:33.

19. Telen MJ, Chasis JA. Relationship of the human erythrocyte Wr^a antigen to an interaction between glycophorin A and Band 3. Blood 1980; 76:842.

20. Dahr W, Kordowicz M, Moulds J, Gielen W, Lebeck L, Krüger, J. Characterisation of the Ss sialoglycoprotein and its antigen in RH_{null} erythrocytes. Blut 1987; 54:13.

21. von dem Borne AEG, Bos MJE, Lomas C, Tipett P, Bloy C, Hermand P, Cartron JP, Admiraal LG, van de Graaf J, Overbeeke MAM. Murine monoclonal antibodies against a unique determinant of erythrocytes, related to Rh and U antigens: expression on normal and malignant erythrocyte precursors and Rh_{null} red cells. Br J Haematol 1990; 75:254.

22. Mallison G, Anstee DJ, Avent ND, Ridgwell K, Tanner MJA, Daniels GL, Tipett P, von dem Borne AEG. Murine monoclonal antibody MB-2D10 recognizes Rh-related glycoproteins in the human red cell membrane. Transfusion 1990; 30:22.

23. Owens JW, Mueller TJ, Morrison M. A minor sialoglycoprotein of the human erythrocyte membrane. Arch Biochem Biophys 1980; 204:247.

24. Mueller TJ, Morrison M. Glycoconnectin (PAS 2), a membrane attachment site for the human erythrocyte cytoskeleton. In: Kruckeberg JE, Eaton JE, Brewer GJ, eds. Erythrocyte Membrane 2: Recent Chemical and Experimental Advances. New York: Liss, 1981:95.

25. Anderson RA, Lovrien RE. Glycophorin is linked by band 4.1 protein to the human erythrocyte membrane skeleton. Nature 1984; 307:655.

26. Sondag D, Alloisio N, Blanchard D, Ducluzeau MT, Colonna P, Bachir D, Bloy C, Cartron JP, Delaunay J. Gerbich reactivity in 4.1(−) hereditary elliptocytosis and protein 4.1 level in blood group Gerbich deficiency. Br J Haematol 1987; 65:43.

27. Dahr W, Beyreuther K, Kordowicz M, Kruger J. N-terminal amino acid sequence of sialoglycoprotein D (glycophorin C) from human erythrocyte membranes. Eur J Biochem 1982; 125:57.

28. Blanchard D, Dahr W, Hummel M, Latron F, Beyreuther K, Cartron JP. Glycophorins B and C from human erythrocyte membranes. Purification and sequence analysis. J Biol Chem 1987; 262:5808.

29. Glöckner WM, Newman RA, Dahr W, Uhlenbruck G. Alkali-labile oligosaccharides from glycoproteins of different erythrocyte and milk fat globule membranes. Biochim Biophys Acta 1976; 443:402.

30. Furthmayr H, Tomita M, Marchesi VT. Fractionation of the major sialoglycoproteins of the human red blood cell membrane. Biochem Biophys Res Commun 1975; 65:113.

31. Dahr W, Moulds JJ, Baumeister G, Moulds M, Kiedrowski S, Hummel M. Altered membrane sialoglycoproteins in human erythrocytes lacking the Gerbich blood group antigens. Biol Chem Hoppe-Seyler 1985; 366:201.

32. El Maliki B, Blanchard D, Dahr W, Beyreuther K, Cartron JP. Structural homology between glycophorins C and D of human erythrocytes. Eur J Biochem 1989; 183:639.

33. Tomita M, Marchesi VT. Amino acid sequence and oligosaccharide attachment sites of human erythrocyte glycophorin. Proc Natl Acad Sci USA 1975; 72:2964.

34. Tomita M, Furthmayr H, Marchesi VT. Primary structure of human erythrocyte glycophorin A. Isolation and characterisation of peptides and complete amino acid sequence. Biochemistry 1978; 17:4756.

35. Dahr W, Beyreuther K, Steinbach H, Gielen W, Kruger J. Structure of the Ss blood group antigens. II. A methionine/threonine polymorphism within the N-terminal sequence of the Ss glycoprotein. Hoppe-Seylers Z Physiol Chem 1980; 361:895.

36. Dahr W, Müller T, Moulds J, Baumeister G, Issitt PD, Wilkinson S, Garratty G. High frequency antigens of human erythrocyte membrane sialoglycoproteins. I. En^a receptors in the glycosylated domain of the MN sialoglycoprotein. Biol Chem Hoppe-Seyler 1985; 366:41.

37. Siebert PD, Fukuda M. Isolation and characterization of human glycophorin A cDNA clones using a synthetic oligonucleotide approach: Nucleotide sequence and mRNA structure. Proc Natl Acad Sci USA 1986; 83:1665.

38. Rahuel C, London J, d'Auriol L, Mattei MG, Tournamille C, Skrzynia C, Lebouc Y, Galibert F, Cartron JP. Characterization of cDNA clones for human glycophorin A. Use for gene localization and for analysis of normal glycophorin-A-deficient (Finnish type) genomic DNA. Eur J Biochem 1988; 172:147.

39. Tate CG, Tanner MJA. Isolation of cDNA for human erythrocyte membrane sialoglycoproteins α and δ. Biochem J 1988; 254:743.

40. Thomas DB, Winzler RJ. Structural studies on human erythrocyte glycoproteins. Alkali-labile oligosaccharides. J Biol Chem 1969; 244:5943.

41. Yoshima H, Furthmayr H, Kobata A. Structures of the asparagine-linked sugar chains of glycophorin A. J Biol Chem 1980; 255:9713.

42. Irimura T, Tsuji T, Tagami S, Yamamoto K, Osawa T. Structure of a complex-type sugar chain of human glycophorin A. Biochemistry 1981; 20:560.

43. Dahr W, Uhlenbruck G, Janssen E, Schmalisch R. Different N-terminal amino acids in the MN-glycoprotein from MM and NN erythrocytes. Hum Genet 1977; 35:335.

44. Wasnioswka K, Drzeniek Z, Lisowska E. The amino acids of M and N blood group glycopeptides are different. Biochem Biophys Res Commun 1977; 76:385.

45. Lisowska E, Wasnioswka K. Immunochemical characterization of cyanogen bromide degradation products of M and N blood-group glycopeptides. Eur J Biochem 1978; 88:247.

46. Dahr W, Uhlenbruck G. Structural properties of the human MN blood group antigen receptor sites. Hoppe-Seylers Z Physiol Chem 1978; 359:835.

47. Dahr W, Uhlenbruck G, Leikola J, Wagstaff W. Studies on the membrane glycoprotein defect of En(a–) erythrocytes. III. N-terminal amino-acids of sialoglycoproteins from normal and En(a–) red cells. J Immunogenet 1978; 5:117.

48. Furthmayr H. Structural comparison of glycophorins and immunochemical analysis of genetic variants. Nature 1978; 271:519.

49. Blumenfeld OO, Adamany AM. Structural polymorphism within the amino-terminal region of MM, NN and MN glycoproteins (glycophorins) of the human erythrocyte membrane, Proc Natl Acad Sci 1978; 75:2727.

50. Judd WJ, Issitt PD, Pavone BG, Anderson J, Aminoff D. Antibodies that define NANA-independent MN-system antigens. Transfusion 1979; 10:12.

51. Sadler JE, Paulson JC, Hill RL. The role of sialic acid in the expression of human blood group antigen. J Biol Chem 1979; 254:2112.

52. Wasnioswska K, Duk M, Steuden I, Czerwinski M, Wiedlocha A, Lisowska E. Two monoclonal antibodies recognizing different epitopes of blood group N antigen. Arch Immunol Ther Exp 1988; 36:623.

53. Jaskiewicz E, Lisowska E, Lunblad A. The role of carbohydrate in the blood group N-related epitopes recognised by three monoclonal antibodies. Glycoconjugate J 1990; 7:255.

54. Lisowska E, Kordowicz M. Immunochemical properties of M and N blood group antigens and their degradation products. In: Mohn F, ed. Human Blood Groups. Basel: Karger, 1977:188.

55. Rouger P, Anstee DJ, Salmon C. First International Workshop on Monoclonal Antibodies against Human Red Blood Cell and Related Antigens. Vol. II. Paris: Librairie Arnette, 1988:259.

56. Chester MA, Johnson U, Lundblad A, Löw B, Messeter L, Samuelson B. Proceedings of the Second International Workshop and Symposium on Monoclonal Antibodies Against Human Red Blood Cell and Related Antigens, Lund, 1990:93.

57. Dahr W, Moulds JJ. An immunochemical study on anti-N antibodies from dialysis patients. Immunol Commun 1981; 10:173.

58. Drzeniek Z. Purification of antibody recting with nonenzymatically glycosylated blood group M determinants. Immunol Lett 1983; 6:179.

59. Morel PA, Bergren MO, Hill V, Garatty G, Perkins HA. M and N specific agglutinins of human erythrocytes stored in glucose solutions. Transfusion 1981; 21:652.

60. Reid ME, Ellisor SS, Barker JM, Lewis T, Avoy DR. Characteristics of an antibody causing agglutination of M-positive non-enzymatically glycosylated human red cells. Vox Sang 1981; 41:85.

61. Dahr W, Uhlenbruck G, Bird GWB. Further characterization of some heterophile agglutinins reacting with alkali-labile carbohydrate chains of human erythrocyte glycoproteins. Vox Sang 1975; 28:133.

62. Prigent MJ, Verez Bencomo V, Sinay P, Cartron JP. Interaction of synthetic glycopeptides carrying clusters of O-glycosidic disaccharide chains (β-D-Gal(1-3)α-D-GalNAc) with β-D-Galactose-binding lectins. Glycoconjugate J 1984; 1:73.

63. Duk M, Lisowska E, Kordowicz M, Wasniowska K. Studies on the specificity of the binding site of *Vicia graminea* anti-N lectin. Eur J Biochem 1982; 123:105.

64. Issitt PD, Daniels G, Tippett P. Proposed new terminology for En[a] (letter), Transfusion 1981; 21:473.

65. Gardner B, Parsons SF, Merry AH, Anstee DJ. Epitopes on sialoglycoprotein α: evidence for heterogeneity in the molecule. Immunology 1989; 68:283.

66. Ridgwell K, Tanner MJA, Anstee DJ. The Wr[b] antigen, a receptor for *Plasmodium falciparum* malaria, is located on a helical region of the major membrane sialoglycoprotein of human red blood cells. Biochem J 1983; 209:273.

67. Rigwell K, Tanner MJA, Anstee DJ. The Wr[b] antigen in St[a] positive and Dantu positive human erythrocytes. J. Immunogenet 1984; 11:365.

68. Rearden A. Phospholipid dependence of Wr[b] antigen expression in human erythrocyte membrane. Vox Sang 1985; 49:346.

69. Adams J, Broviac M, Brooks W, Johnson NR, Issitt PD. An antibody, in the serum of a Wr(a+) individual, reacting with an antigen of very high frequency. Transfusion 1971; 11:290.

70. Wren MR, Issitt PD. Evidence that Wr[a] and Wr[b] are antithetical. Transfusion 1988; 28:113.

71. Blumenfeld OO, Adamany AM, Puglia KV. Amino acid and carbohydrate structural variants of glycoprotein products (M-N glycoproteins) of the M-N allelic locus. Proc Natl Acad Sci USA 1981; 78:747.

72. Dahr W, Beyreuther K, Gallasch E, Krüger J, Morel P. Amino acid sequence of the blood group Mg-specific major human erythrocyte membrane sialoglycoprotein. Hoppe-Seylers Z Physiol Chem 1981; 363:81.

73. Furthmayr H, Metaxas MN, Metaxas-Bühler M. Mutations within the amino-terminal region of glycophorin A. Proc Natl Acad Sci USA 1981; 78:631.

74. Dahr W, Metaxas-Bühler M, Metaxas MN, Gallasch E. Immunochemical properties of M[g] erythrocytes. J Immunogenet 1981; 8:79.

75. Anstee DJ, Tanner MJA. Genetic variants involving the major membrane sialoglycoprotein of human erythrocytes. Studies on erythrocytes of type M[K], Miltenberger class V and M[g]. Biochem J 1978; 175:149.

76. Cartron JP, Ferrari B, Huet M, Pavia AA. Specificity of anti-M[g] antibody—a study with synthetic peptides and glycopeptides. Exp Clin Immunogenet 1984; 1:112.

77. Dahr W, Kordowicz M, Beyreuther K, Krüger J. The amino acid sequence of the M[c]-specific major red cell membrane sialoglycoprotein—an intermediate of the M- and N-active molecule. Hoppe-Seylers Z Physiol Chem 1981; 362:363.

78. Blanchard D, Asseraf A, Prigent MJ, Cartron JP. Miltenberger class I and II erythrocytes carry a variant of glycophorin A. Biochem J 1983; 213:399.

79. Dahr W, Newman RA, Contreras M, Kordowicz M, Teesdale P, Beyreuther K, Krüger J. Structures of the Miltenberger class I and II specific major human erythrocyte membrane sialoglycoproteins. Eur J Biochem 1984; 138:259.

80. Herron B, Smith GA. Identification by immunoblotting of the erythrocyte membrane sialo-glycoproteins that carry the Vw and Mur antigens. Vox Sang 1991; 60:118.

81. Dahr W, Beyreuther K, Moulds JJ. Structural analysis of the major human erythrocyte membrane sialoglycoprotein from Miltenberger class VII cells. Eur J Biochem 1987; 166:27.

82. Dahr W, Vengelen-Tyler V, Dybjaer E, Beyreuther K. Structural analysis of glycophorin A from Miltenberger class VIII erythrocytes. Biol Chem Hoppe-Seyler 1989; 370:855.

83. Laird-Fryer B, Moulds JJ, Dahr W, Min YO, Chandanayingyong D. Anti-En[a]FS detected in the serum of a MiVII homozygote. Transfusion 1986; 26:51.

84. Dahr W. The Miltenberger sub-system of the MNSs blood group system: review and outlook. Vox Sang 1992; 62:129.

85. Furthmayr H. Glycophorins A, B and C: a family of sialoglycoproteins. Isolation and preliminary characterization of trypsin derived peptides. J Supramol Struct 1978; 9:79.

86. Siebert PD, Fukuda M. Molecular cloning of a human glycophorin B cDNA: nucleotide sequence and genomic relationship to glycophorin A. Proc Natl Acad Sci USA 1987; 84:6735.

87. Dahr W, Uhlenbruck G, Knott H. Immunochemical aspects of the MNSs blood group system. J Immunogenet 1975; 2:87.

88. Dahr W. Serology, genetics and chemistry of the MNSs blood group system. Rev Fr Transfu Immunohematol 1981; 24:53.

89. Dahr W, Gielen W, Beyreuther K, Kruger J. Structure of the Ss blood group antigens. I. Isolation of the Ss-active glycopeptides and differentiation of the antigens by modification of methionine. Hoppe-Seylers Z Physiol Chem 1980; 361:145.

90. Dahr W, Beyreuther K, Bause E, Kordowicz M. Structures and antigenic properties of human erythrocyte membrane sialoglycoproteins. Prot Biol Fluids 1982; 29:57.

91. Dahr W, Uhlenbruck G, Schmalisch R, Janssen E. Ss blood group associated PAS-staining polymorphism of glycoprotein 3 from human erythrocyte membranes. Hum Genet 1976; 32:163.

92. Dahr W, Weber W, Kordowicz M. The allele S^u in Caucasians—medico-legal, immunochemical and genetic aspects. In: Hummel, Gerchow J, eds. Biomathematical Evidence of Paternity. Berlin: Springer-Verlag, 1981; 131.

93. Ballas SK, Reilly PA, Murphy DL. The blood group U antigen is not located on glycophorin B. Biochim Biophys Acta 1986; 884:337.

94. Dahr W, Moulds JJ. High frequency antigens of human erythrocyte membrane sialoglycoproteins. IV. Molecular properties of the U antigen. Biol Chem Hoppe-Seyler 1987; 368:659.

95. Issitt PD, Marsh WL, Wren MR, Theuriere M, Mueller K. Heterogeneity of anti-U demeonstrable by the use of papain-treated red cells, Transfusion 1989; 29:508.

96. Booth PB. Two melanesian antisera reacting with SsU components. Vox Sang 1978; 34:212.

97. Habibi B, Fouillade MT, Duedar N, Issitt PD, Tippett P, Salmon C. The antigen Duclos, Vox Sang 1978; 34:302.

98. Moore S, Green C. The identification of specific Rhesus-polypeptide-blood-group-ABH-active-gly-coprotein complexes in the human red-cell membrane. Biochem J 1987; 244:735.

99. Avent N, Judson PA, Parsons SF, Mallinson G, Anstee DJ, Tanner MJA, Evans PR, Hodges E, Maciver A, Holmes C. Monoclonal antibodies that recognize different membrane proteins that are deficient in RH_{null} human erythocytes. Biochem J 1988; 251:499.

100. Dahr W, Kordowicz M, Judd WJ, Moulds J, Beyreuther K, Krüger J. Structural analysis of the Ss sialoglycoprotein specific for Henshaw blood group from human erythrocyte membrane. Eur J Biochem 1984; 141:51.

101. Judd WJ, Rolih SD, Dahr W, Oilshlager R, Miller FM, Lau P. Studies on the blood of an $MsHe/MS^u$ proposita and her family. Serological evidence that Henshaw-producing genes do not code for the 'N' antigen. Transfusion 1983; 23:382.

102. Dahr W, Longster G. Studies on M^v red cells. II. Immunochemical investigations. Blut 1984; 49:299.

103. Dahr W, Longster G, Uhlenbruck G, Schumacher K. Studies on Meltenberger class III, V, M^v and M^k red cells. I. Sodium-dodecyl sulphate polyacrylamide gel electrophoretic investigations. Blut 1978; 11:219.

104. Siebert PD, Fukuda M. Human glycophorin A and B are encoded by separate single copy genes coordinately regulated by a tumor-promoting phorbol ester. J Biol Chem 1986; 261:12433.

105. Kudo S, Fukuda M. Structural organization of glycophorin A and B genes: glycophorin B gene evolved by homologous recombination at *Alu* repeat sequences. Proc Natl Acad Sci USA 1989; 86:4619.

106. Vignal A, Rahuel C, El Maliki B, LeVanKim C, London J, Blanchard D, d'Auriol L, Galibert F, Blajchman MA, Cartron JP. Molecular analysis of glycophorin A and B gene structure and expression in homozygous Miltenberger class V (Mi.V) human erythrocytes. Eur J Biochem 1989; 184:337.

107. Rahuel C, Vignal A, London J, Hamel S, Romeo PH, Colin Y, Cartron JP. Structure of the 5'-flanking region of the glycophorin A gene and analysis of its multiple transcripts. Gene 1989; 85:471.

108. Rahuel C, London J, Vignal A, Cherif-Zahar B, Colin Y, Siebert P, Fukuda M, Cartron JP. Alterations of the genes for glycophorin A and B in glycophorin A deficient individuals. Eur J Biochem 1988; 177:605.

109. Kudo S, Fukuda M. Identification of a novel human glycophorin, glycophorin E, by isolation of

genomic clones and complementary DNA clones utilizing polymerase chain reaction. J Biol Chem 1990; 265:1102.

110. Vignal A, Rahuel C, London J, Cherif Zahar B, Schaff S, Hattab C, Okubo Y, Cartron JP. A novel gene member of the human glycophorin A and B gene family. Molecular cloning and expression. Eur J Biochem 1990; 191:619.

111. Anstee DJ. The nature and abundance of human red cell surface glycoproteins. J Immunogenet 1990; 17:219.

112. Cook PJL, Lindenbaum RH, Salonen R, De La Chapelle A, Daker MG, Buckton KE, Noades JE, Tippett P. The MNSs blood groups of families with chromosome 4 rearrangements. Ann Hum Genet 1981; 45:39.

113. Darnborough J, Dunsford I, Wallace JA. The En^a antigen and antibody. A genetical modification of human red cells affecting their blood grouping reactions. Vox Sang 1969; 17:241.

114. Furuhjelm U, Myllyla G, Nevanlinna HR, Nordling S, Pirkola A, Gavin J, Gooch A, Sanger R, Tippett P. The red cell phenotype En(a–) and anti-En^a: serological and physicochemical aspects. Vox Sang 1969; 17:256.

115. Gahmberg CG, Myllyla G, Leikola J, Pirkola A, Nordling S. Absence of the major sialoglycoprotein in the membrane of human En(a–) erythrocytes and increased glycosylation of band 3. J Biol Chem 1976; 251:6108.

116. Tanner MJA, Anstee DJ. The membrane change in En(a–) human erythrocytes. Biochem J 1976; 153:271.

117. Anstee DJ, Barker DM, Judson PA, Tanner MJA. Inherited sialoglycoprotein deficiencies in human erythrocytes of type En(a–). Br J Haematol 1977; 35:309.

118. Dahr W, Uhlenbruck G, Leikola J, Wagstaff W, Landfried K. Studies on the membrane glycoprotein defect of En(a–) erythrocytes. I. Biochemical aspects. J Immunogenet 1976; 3:329.

119. Dahr W, Uhlenbruck J, Wagstaff W, Leikola J. Studies on the membrane glycoprotein defect of En(a–) erythrocytes. II. MN antigenic properties of En(a–) erythrocytes. J Immunogenet 1976; 3:383.

120. Dahr W, Issitt P, Moulds J, Pavone B. Further studies on the membrane glycoprotein defects of S-s- and En(a–) erythrocytes. Hoppe-Seylers Z Physiol Chem 1978; 359:1217.

121. Metaxas MN, Metaxas-Bühler M. Rare genes of the MNSs system affecting the red cell membrane. In: Mohn, JF, ed. Human Blood Groups. Basel: Karger, 1977; 344.

122. Taliano V, Guevin RM, Hebert D, Daniels GL, Tippett P, Anstee DJ, Mawby WJ, Tanner MJA. The rare phenotype En(a–) in a French-Canadian family. Vox Sang 1980; 38:87.

123. Tate CG, Tanner MJA, Judson PA, Anstee DJ. Studies on human red-cell membrane glycophorin A and glycophorin B genes in glycophorin-deficient individuals. Biochem J 1989; 263:993.

124. Dahr W, Uhlenbruck G, Issitt PD, Allen FH Jr. SDS-polyacrylamide gel electrophoretic analysis of the membrane glycoproteins from S-s- erythrocytes. J Immunogenet 1975; 2:249.

125. Dahr W, Issitt PD, Uhlenbruck G. New concepts of the MNSs blood group system. In: Mohn F, ed. Human Blood Group. Basel: Karger 1977:197.

126. Sondag-Thull D, Girard M, Blanchard D, Bloy C, Cartron JP. S-s-U- phenotype in a caucasian family. Exp Clin Immunogenet 1986; 3:181.

127. Blanchard D, Asseraf A, Prigent MJ, Moulds J, Chandanayingyong D, Cartron JP. Interaction of Vicia graminea anti-N lectin with cell surface glycoproteins from erythrocytes with rare blood group antigens. Hoppe-Seylers Z Physiol Chem 1984; 365:469.

128. Huang CH, Johe K, Moulds JJ, Siebert PD, Fukuda M, Blumenfeld OO. δ Glycophorin (glycophorin B) gene deletion in two individuals homozygous for the S-s-U- blood group phenotype. Blood 1987; 70:1830.

129. Huang CH, Lu WM, Boots Macy E, Guizzo ML, Blumenfeld OO. Two types of δ glycophorin gene alterations in S-s-U- individuals. Transfusion 1989; 29:355.

130. Dahr W, Uhlenbruck G, Knott H. The defect of M^K erythrocytes as revealed by sodium dodecylsulfate-polyacrylamide gel electrophoresis. J Immunogenet 1977; 4:191.

131. Anstee DJ, Mawby WJ, Tanner MJA. Abnormal blood-group-Ss-active sialoglycoproteins in the membrane of Miltenberger class III, IV and V human erythrocytes. Biochem J 1979; 183:193.

132. Judd WJ, Geisland JR, Issitt PD, Wilkinson SL, Anstee DJ, Shin C, Glidden H. Studies on the blood of an Mi^v/M^k proposita and her family. Transfusion 1983; 23:33.

133. Tokunaga E, Sasakama S, Tamaka K, Kawamata H, Giles CM, Ikin EW, Poole J, Anstee DJ, Mawby W, Tanner MJA. Two apparently healthy japanese individuals of type MkMk have erythrocytes which lack both the blood group MN- and Ss-active sialoglycoproteins. J Immunogenet 1979; 6:383.

134. Okubo Y, Daniels GL, Parsons SF, Anstee DJ, Yamaguchi H, Tomita T, Seno T. A Japanese family with two sisters apparently homozygous for M^k. Vox Sang 1988; 54:107.

135. Bunn HF, Forget BG, Ranney HM. Thalassemia-like disorders associated with structurally abnormal globin chains. In: Human Haemoglobins. London: Saunders 1977:151.

136. Vengelen-Tyler V, Anstee DJ, Issitt PD, Pavone BG, Ferguson SJ, Mawby WJ, Tanner MJA, Blajchman MA, Lorque P. Studies on the blood of an MiV homozygote. Transfusion 1981; 21:1.

137. Mawby WJ, Anstee DJ, Tanner MJA. Immunochemical evidence for hybrid sialoglycoproteins of human erythrocytes. Nature 1981; 291:161.

138. Huang CH, Blumenfeld OO. Identification of recombination events resulting in three hybrid genes encoding human MiV, MiV(J.L.) and St^a glycophorins. Blood 1991; 8:1813.

139. Johe KK, Vengeler-Tyler V, Leger R, Blumenfeld OO. Synthetic peptides homologous to human glycophorins of the Miltenberger complex of variants of MNSs blood group system specify the epitopes for Hil, S^{JL}, Hop, and Mur antisera. Blood 1991; 78:2456.

140. Langley JW, Issitt PD, Anstee DJ, McMahan M, Smith N, Pavone BG, Tessel JA, Carlin MA. Another individual (JR) whose red blood cells appear to carry a hybrid MNSs sialoglycoprotein. Transfusion 1981; 21:15.

141. Morel PA, Vengelen-Tyler V, Williams EA, Anstee DJ, Parsons SF, Daniels GL. Another MNSs variant producing a hybrid MNSs sialoglycoprotein. Blood Transfu Immunohematol 1982; 34:597.

142. Johe KK, Smith AJ, Vengelen-Tyler V, Blumenfeld OO. Amino acid sequence of an α-δ-glycophorin hybrid. J Biol Chem, 1989; 164:17486.

143. Reid ME, Moore BPL, Poole J, Parker NJ, Asenbryl E, Vengelen-Tyler V, Lubenko A, Galligan B. TSEN: a novel MNSs-related blood group antigen. Vox Sang 1992; 63:122.

144. Reid ME, Poole J, Green C, Neill G, Banks J. MINY: a novel MNSs-related blood group antigen, Vox Sang 1992; 63:129.

145. Daniels GL, Green CA, Okubo Y, Seno T, Yamaguchi H, Ota S, Taguchi T. SAT, a 'new' low frequency blood group antigen, which may be associated with two different MNS variants. Transfu Med 1991; 1:39.

146. Blanchard D, Cartron JP, Rouger P, Salmon P. Pj variant, a new hybrid MNSs glycoprotein of the human red cell membrane. Biochem J 1982; 203:419.

147. Anstee DJ, Mawby WJ, Parsons SF, Tanner MJA, Giles CM. A novel hybrid sialoglycoprotein in St^a-positive human erythrocytes. J Immunogenet 1982; 9:51.

148. Blumenfeld OO, Adamany AM, Kikuchi M, Sabo B, McCreary J. Membrane glycophorins in St^a blood group erythrocytes. J Biol Chem 1986; 261:5544.

149. Blanchard D, Dahr W, Beyreuther K, Moulds J, Cartron JP. Hybrid glycophorins from human erythrocyte membranes. Isolation and complete structural analysis of the novel sialoglycoprotein from St(a+) red cells. Eur J Biochem 1987; 167:361.

150. Dahr W, Blanchard D, Chevalier C, Cartron JP, Beyreuther K, Fournet B. The M^Z variety of the St(a+) phenotype—a variant of glycophorin A exhibiting a deletion. Biol Chem Hoppe-Seyler 1990; 371:403.

151. Huang CH, Guizzo ML, Kikuchi M, Blumenfeld OO. Molecular genetic analysis of hybrid gene encoding St^a glycophorin of the human erythrocyte membrane. Blood 1989; 74:836

152. Rearden A, Phan H, Dubnicoff T, Kudo S, Fukuda M. Identification of the crossing-over point of a hybrid gene encoding human glycophorin variant St^a. Similarity to the crossing-over point in haptoglobin-related genes. J Biol Chem 1990; 265:9259.

153. Huang CH, Blumenfeld OO. Multiple origins of the human glycophorin St^a gene—identification of hotspots for independent unequal homologous recombinations. J Biol Chem 1991; 266-23306.

154. Metaxas MN, Metaxas-Bühler M, Ikin E. Complexities of the MN locus. Vox Sang 1968; 15:102.

155. Contreras M, Green C, Humphreys J, Tippett P, Daniels G, Teesdale P, Armitage S, Lubenko A. Serology and genetics of MNSs-associated antigen Dantu, Vox Sang 1984; 46:377.

156. Tanner MJA, Anstee DJ, Mawby WJ. A new human erythrocyte variant (Ph) containing an abnormal membrane sialoglycoprotein. Biochem J 1980; 187:493.

157. Dahr W, Moulds J, Unger P, Kordowicz M. The Dantu erythrocyte phenotype of the NE variety. I. Dodecylsulfate gel electrophoresis studies. Blut 1987; 55:19.

158. Merry AH, Thomson EE, Anstee DJ, Stratton F. The quantification of erythrocyte antigen sites with monoclonal antibodies. Immunology 1984; 51:793.

159. Dahr W, Beyreuther K, Moulds J, Unger P. Hybrid glycophorins from human erythrocyte membranes. I. Isolation and complete structural analysis of the hybrid sialoglycoprotein from Dantu-positive red cells of the N.E. variety. Eur J Biochem 1987; 166:31.

160. Dahr W, Pilkington PM, Reinke H, Blanchard D, Beyreuther K. A novel variety of the Dantu gene complex (Dantu^{MD}) detected in a Caucasian. Blut 1989; 58:247.

161. Huang CH, Puglia KV, Bigbee WL, Guizzo ML, Hoffman M, Blumenfeld OO. A family study of multiple mutations of alpha and delta glycophorins (glycoporins A and B). Hum Genet 1988; 81:26.

162. Huang CH, Blumenfeld OO. Characterization of a genomic hybrid specifying the human erythrocyte antigen Dantu: Dantu gene is duplicated and linked to a δ glycophorin gene deletion. Proc Natl Acad Sci USA 1988; 85:9640.

163. Anstee DJ. Blood group MNSs-active sialoglycoproteins of the human erythrocyte membrane. In: Sandler GS, Schanfield M, eds. Immunobiology of the Erythrocyte. New York: Liss, 1980:67.

164. King MJ, Poole J, Anstee DJ. An application of immunoblotting in the classification of the Miltenberger series of blood group antigens. Transfusion 1989; 29:106.

165. Dahr W, Newman RA, Contreras M, Chandanayingyong D, Kordowicz M. Immunochemical studies on the Miltenberger system. Congress Report of the 9th Congress of the Society of Forensic Haemogenetics Bern. Würzburg, Schmidt and Meyer, 1981:201.

166. Huang CH, Blumenfeld OO. Molecular genetics of human erythrocyte MiIII and MiVI glyco-phorins. J Biol Chem 1991; 266:7248.

167. Cleghorn TE. A memorandum on the Miltenberger blood groups. Vox Sang 1966; 11:219.

168. Huang CH, Kikuchi M, McCreary J, Blumenfeld OO. Gene conversion confined to a direct repeat of the acceptor splice site generates allelic diversity at human glycophorin (GYP) locus. J Biol Chem 1992; 267:3336.

169. Skov F, Green C, Daniels G, Khalid G, Tippett P. Miltenberger class IX of the MNS blood group system. Vox Sang 1991; 61:130.

170. Dahr W, Beyreuther K. A revision of the N-terminal structure of sialoglycoprotein D (glycophorin C) from human erythrocyte membranes. Biol Chem Hoppe-Seyler 1985; 366:1067.

171. Colin Y, Rahuel C, London J, Romeo PH, d'Auriol L, Galibert F, Cartron JP. Isolation of cDNA clones and complete amino acid sequence of human erythrocyte glycophorin C. J Biol Chem 1986; 261:229.

172. High S, Tanner MJA. Human erythrocyte membrane sialoglycoprotein β. The cDNA sequence suggests the absence of a cleaved N-terminal sequence. Biochem J 1987; 243:271.

173. Le Van Kim C, Coilin Y, Blanchard D, Dahr W, London J, Cartron JP. Gerbich blood group deficiency of the Ge:−1, −2, −3 and Ge:−1, −2, 3 types. Immunochemical study and genomic analysis with cDNA probes. Eur J Biochem 1987; 165:571.

174. Colin Y, Le Van Kim K, Tsapis A, Clerget M, d'Auriol L, London J, Galibert F, Cartron JP. Human erythrocyte glycophorin C. Gene structure and rearrangement in genetic variants. J Biol Chem 1989; 264:3773.

175. Reid ME, Chasis JA, Mohandas N. Identification of a functional role for human erythrocyte sialoglycoproteins β and γ Blood 1987; 69:1068.

176. Reid ME, Anstee DJ, Tanner MJA, Ridgwell K, Nurse GT. Structural relationships between human erythrocyte sialoglycoproteins β and and abnormal sialoglycoproteins found in certain rare human erythrocyte variants lacking the Gerbich blood-group antigen(s). Biochem J 1987; 244:123.

177. Anstee DJ, Parsons SF, Ridgwell K, Tanner MJA, Merry H, Thompson EE, Judson PA, Johnson P, Bates S, Fraser ID. Two individuals with elliptocytic red cells apparently lacking three minor erythrocyte membrane sialoglycoproteins. Biochem J 1984; 218:615.

178. Dahr W, Kiedrowski S, Blanchard D, Hermand P, Moulds J, Cartron JP. High frequency antigens of human erythrocyte membrane sialoglycoproteins. V. Characterisation of the Gerbich blood group antigens: Ge2 and Ge3. Biol Chem Hoppe-Seyler 1987; 368:1375.

179. Dahr W, Blanchard D, Kiedrowski S, Poschmann A, Cartron JP, Moulds J. High-frequency antigens

of human erythrocyte membrane sialoglycoproteins. VI. Monoclonal antibodies reacting with the N terminal domain of glycophorin C. Biol Chem Hoppe-Seyler 1989; 370:849.

180. Tanner MJA, High S, Martin PG, Anstee DJ, Judson PA, Jones TJ. Genetic variants of human red-cell membrane sialaoglycoprotein β. Study of the alterations occurring in the sialoglycoprotein-β gene. Biochem J 1988; 250:407.

181. Loirat MJ, Gourbil A, Frioux Y, Muller JY, Blanchard D. A murine monoclonal antibody directed against the Gerbich 3 blood group antigen. Vox Sang 1992; 62:45.

182. McShane K, Chung A. A novel human alloantibody in the Gerbich system. Vox Sang 1989; 57:205.

183. Villeval A, Rahuel C, El Maliki B, Le Van Kim C, London J, Blanchard D, d'Auriol L, Galibert F, Blajchman MA, Cartron JP. Molecular analysis of glycophorin A and B gene structure and expression in homozygous Miltenberger class V (Mi^V) human erythrocytes. Eur J Biochem 1989; 184:337.

184. Le Van Kim C, Colin Y, Mitjavila MT, Clerget M, Dubart A, Nakazawa M, Vainchenker W, Cartron JP. Structure of the promoter region and tissue specificity of the human glycophorin C. J Biol Chem 1989; 264:20407.

185. Mattei MG, Colin Y, Le Van Kim C, Mattei JF, Cartron JP. Localization of the gene for human erythrocyte glycophorin C to chromosome 2q14-q21. Hum Genet 1986; 74:420.

186. Daniels GL, Shaw MA, Judson PA, Reid ME, Anstee DJ, Colpitts P, Cornwall S, Moore BPL, Lee S. A family demonstrating inheritance of the Leach phenotype: a Gerbich-negative phenotype associated with elliptocytosis. Vox Sang 1986; 50:117.

187. Telen MJ, Le Van Kim C, Chung A, Cartron JP, Colin Y. Molecular basis for elliptocytosis associated with glycophorin C deficiency in the Leach phenotype. Blood 1991; 78:1603.

188. Anstee DJ, Ridgwell K, Tanner MJA, Daniels GL, Parsons SF. Individuals lacking the Gerbich blood group antigen have alterations in the human erythrocyte membrane sialoglycoproteins β and γ. Biochem J 1984; 221:97.

189. High S, Tanner MJA, McDonald EB, Anstee DJ. Rearrangements of the red-cell membrane glycophorin C (sialoglycoprotein β) gene. A further study of alterations in the glycophorin C gene. Biochem J 1989; 262:47.

190. Chang S, Reid ME, Conboy J, Kan YW, Mohandas N. Molecular characterization of erythrocyte glycophorin C variants. Blood 1991; 77:644.

191. Reid ME, Shaw AA, Rowe G, Anstee SDJ, Tanner MJA. Abnormal minor erythrocyte membrane sialoglycoprotein (β) in association with rare blood-group antigen Webb. Biochem J 1985; 232:289.

192. McDonald EB, Gerns LM. An unusual sialoglycoprotein associated with the Webb-positive phenotype. Vox Sang 1986; 50:112.

193. McDonald EB, Condon J, Ford D, Fisher B, Gerns LM. Abnormal beta and gamma sialoglycoprotein associated with the low-frequency antigen Ls^a. Vox Sang 1990; 58:300.

194. Spring FA. Immunochemical characterisation of the low-incidence antigen, Dh^a. Vox Sang 1991; 61:65.

195. Daniels G, Khalid G, Cedergren B. The low frequency red cell antigen An^a is located on glycophorin D. International Society of Blood Transfusion/American Association of Blood Banks 1990 Joint Congress, Los Angeles, Abstract S773, 194.

196. Lisowska E, Duk M, Dahr W. Comparison of alkali-labile oligosaccharide chains of M and N blood-group glycopeptides from human erythrocyte membrane. Carbohydrate Res 1980; 79:103.

197. Roelcke D. Pr and Gd antigens. Rev Fr Transfu Immunohematol 1981; 24:27.

198. Roelcke D, Kreft H. Characterization of various anti-Pr cold agglutinins. Transfusion 1984; 24:210.

199. Dahr W, Lichthardt D, Roelcke D. Studies on the receptor sites of the monoclonal anti-Pr and -Sa cold agglutinins. Prot Biol Fluids 1982; 29:365.

200. Vaith P, Uhlenbruck G. The Thomsen agglutination phenomenon: a discovery revisited 50 years later. Z Immun Forsch 1978; 154:1.

201. Cartron JP, Andreu G, Cartron J, Bird GWG, Salmon C, Gerbal A. Demonstration of T-transferase deficiency in Tn-polyagglutinable erythrocytes. Eur J Biochem 1978; 92:111.

202. Berger EG, Kozdowski I. Permanent mixed-field agglutinable erythrocytes lack galactosyltransferase activity. FEBS Lett 1978; 93:105.

203. Dahr W, Gielen W, Pierce S, Schaper R. UDP-GalNAc-β-3-D-Galactosyl-transferase deficiency in Tn syndrome. Glycoconjugates. In: Schauer R, Boer R, Buddecke E, Kramer MF, Vliegenthart

JFG, Wiegandt H, eds. Proceedings of the 5th International Symposium. Stuttgart: Thieme Verlag, 1979:272.

204. Dahr W, Uhlenbruck G, Bird GWG. Cryptic A-like receptor sites in human erythrocyte glycoproteins: proposed nature of Tn-antigen. Vox Sang 1974; 27:29.

205. Dahr W, Uhlenbruck G, Gunson HH, van der Hart M. Molecular basis of Tn-polyagglutinability. Vox Sang 1975; 29:36.

206. Kjeldsen T, Hakomori S, Springer GF, Desai P, Harris T, Clausen H. Coexpression of sialosyl-Tn (NeuAcα2-6GalNAcα1-O-Ser/Thr) and Tn (GalNAcα1-O-Ser/Thr) blood group antigens on Tn erythrocytes. Vox Sang 1989; 57:81.

207. Cartron JP, Blanchard D, Nurden A, Cartron J, Rahuel C, Lee D, Vainchenker W, Testa U, Rochant H. Tn syndrome: a disorder affecting red blood cell, platelet, and granulocyte cell surface components. In: Salmon C, ed. Blood Group and other Red Cell Surface Markers in Health and Disease. New York: Masson, 1982:39.

208. Fukuda M, Lauffenburger M, Sasaki H, Rogers ME, Dell A. Structures of novel sialylated O-linked oligosaccharides isolated from human erythrocyte glycophorins. J Biol Chem 1987; 262:11952.

209. Finne J, Krusius T, Rauvala H, Järnefelt J. Molecular nature of the blood-group ABH antigens of the human erythrocyte membrane. Rev Fr Transfu Immunohematol 1980; 23:545.

210. Takasaki S, Yamashita K, Kobata A. The sugar chain structures of the ABO blood group active glycoproteins obtained from human erythrocyte membrane. J Biol Chem 1978; 253:6086.

211. Adamany A, Blumenfeld OO, Sabo B, McCreary J. A carbohydrate structural variant of MM glycoprotein (glycophorin A). J Biol Chem 1983; 258:11537.

212. Dahr W, Knuppertz G, Beyreuther K, Moulds JJ, Moulds M, Wilkinson S, Capon C, Fournet B, Issitt PD. Studies on the structures of the Tm, Sj, M_1, Can, Sext and Hu blood group antigens. Biol Chem Hoppe-Seyler 1991; 372:573.

213. Cartron JP, Blanchard D. Association of human erythrocyte membrane glycoproteins with blood-group Cad specificity. Biochem J 1982; 207:497.

214. Blanchard D, Cartron JP, Fournet B, Montreuil J, van Halbeek H, Vliegenthart JFG. Primary structure of the oligosaccharide determinant of blood group Cad specificity. J Biol Chem 1983; 258:7691.

215. Blanchard D, Capon C, Leroy Y, Cartron JP, Fournet B. Comparative study of glycophorin A derived O-glycans from human Cad, Sd(a+) and Sd(a−) erythrocytes. Biochem J 1985; 232:813.

216. Blanchard D, Piller F, Gillard B, Marcus D, Cartron JP. Identification of a novel ganglioside on erythrocytes with blood group Cad specificity. J Biol Chem 1985; 260:7813.

217. Piller F, Blanchard D, Huet M, Cartron JP. Identification of a α-NeuAc-(2-3)-β-D-galactopyranosyl N-acetyl-β-D-galactosaminyltransferase in human kidney. Carbohydrate Res 1986; 149:171.

3

Sialic Acid–Dependent Red Blood Cell Antigens

DIETER ROELCKE
University of Heidelberg
Heidelberg, Germany

I. INTRODUCTION

A. Historical Data

In 1926–1930, the existence of sialic acid was reported by the serologists Hübener (1), Thomsen (2), and Friedenreich (3), who detected (1) and interpreted (2,3) the phenomenon of polyagglutination caused by the reaction of anti-T with the T antigen. Anti-T, present in almost all human sera, recognizes the T antigen that is masked by sialic acid on the intact red blood cell (RBC) surface but is liberated by the action of bacterial and viral sialidases. In this case, sialic acid serves to mask an antigen.

The first reports demonstrating that sialic acid could contribute to the construction of antigens, i.e. the MN blood groups, were presented by Mäkelä and Cantell (4) and Springer and Ansell (5) in 1958. We now know that the genetically defined differences between M and N antigens are differences in the peptide sequence and that sialic acid contributes to the antigens only facultatively.

In 1969, we detected (6) the first antigens; i.e. Pr_1, and so forth (formerly termed HD), where sialic acid contributes invariably and serves as the immunodominant component.

This chapter deals with sialic acid–dependent human RBC antigens. The role of sialic acid for the MN, En^a, and Ge antigens, which are recognized mainly by alloantibodies, is briefly discussed and the sialoantigens recognized by autoantibodies (cold autoagglutinins) are described. Introducing the sections on the antigens, some biochemical data on sialic acids and sialidases are presented.

B. Sialic (Neuraminic) Acid: Structure and Nomenclature

Neuraminic acid is the basic molecule of a group of about 30 naturally occurring acid aminosugars termed sialic acids. Its complete chemical designation is 5-amino-3,5-dideoxy-D-glycero-D-galacto-nonulosonic acid. As shown in Fig. 1, neuraminic acid consists of nine C atoms. It has a carboxyl group (C-1) and possesses a C-2 keto function and an amino group at C-5. In this form, the molecule is unstable owing to a reaction between the C-2 keto function

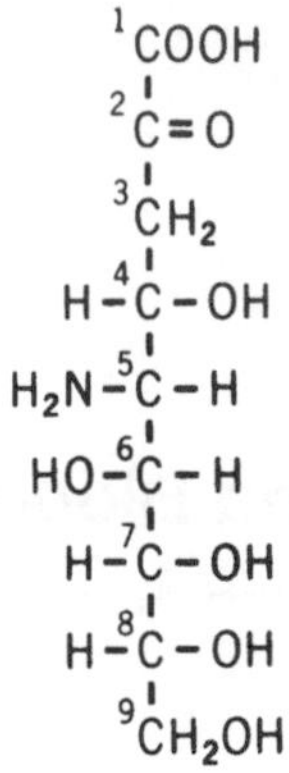

1 COOH
2 C=O
3 CH2
H-4C-OH
H2N-5C-H
HO-6C-H
H-7C-OH
H-8C-OH
9 CH2OH

Figure 1 Neuraminic acid.

and the C-5 amino group. Therefore, exclusively N-acylated derivatives, i.e., N-acylneuraminic acids, occur in nature. N-acetylneuraminic acid is the most common N-acylneuraminic acid. N-glycolylneuraminic acid is also found. N-acetylneuraminic acid is the sialic acid of the human RBC membrane.

In solution, N-acetylneuraminic acid, like other sialic acids, adapts a $^{2}C_5$H(1C) conformation (Fig. 2). Free N-acetylneuraminic acid has a high preference for the beta anomeric configuration as established by ^{1}H-NMR spectral analysis (7) (Fig. 2a). In contrast to the free molecule, glycosidically linked N-acetylneuraminic acid, as found, e.g., on glycoproteins and glycolipids (gangliosides) on the cell surface, has alpha configuration, as shown in figure 2b.

The general name *sialic acid* should be used if the exact structure of the sialic acid molecule is not known or is not of importance. The term *sialylation* is used to designate the addition of a sialyl group to a sugar sequence. It is also used if the structure of sialic acid, e.g., N-acetylneuraminic acid, is known and if the structure is of biological importance, e.g., for antigenicity. Previous abbreviations of N-acetylneuraminic acid were NANA or NA. It has been recommended to introduce the term *Neu5Ac* to indicate the acetylation at C-5 [8]. Another designation indicating the acetylation of the amino group at C-5 is Neu*N*Ac. Although NeuAc was the most common abbreviation for N-acetylneuraminic acid for several years, Neu*N*Ac is now the prevailing abbreviation and therefore is used in this chapter.

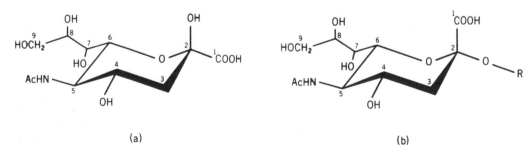

OH
OH
9 HOCH2
8
7
6
2
1 COOH
O
HO
4
AcHN
3
5
OH
(a)
OH
1 COOH
9 HOCH2
8
7
6
2
O
O
R
HO
4
AcHN
3
5
OH
(b)

Figure 2 1 C conformation of N-acetylneuraminic acid. β configuration is shown in (a) and α configuration in (b).

C. Sialidase: Specificity and Terminology

Sialidase, E. C. 3.2.1.18, is an exoglycosidase that cleaves terminal sialic residues. It is an acylneuraminylhydrolase hydrolyzing α2,3–, α2,6–, and α2,8-ketosidic bonds linking NeuNAc and other (but not all) sialic acids to glycoconjugates of glycoproteins, glycolipids, or oligosaccharides. Sialidase splits terminal linkages between NeuNAc and galactose, N-acetyl-glucosamine, N-acetylgalactosamine, NeuNAc and N-glycolylneuraminic acid.

Producers of sialidase are myxoviruses and many bacteria. Several sialidases are commercially available; e.g., from *Vibrio cholerae, Clostridium perfringens,* or *Arthrobacter ureafaciens*. Some preferential activities toward distinct ketosidic bonds, e.g., α2,3 linkage of NeuNAc, have been described particularly within myxovirus sialidases (9). Sialidases, however, do not specifically cleave certain ketosidic linkages, although quantitative differences can be observed. The enzyme from *Clostridium perfringens* hydrolyzes α2,3 bonds most rapidly, whereas the *Arthrobacter* sialidase prefers α2,6 linkages.

The term *sialidase* has now been substituted for the term *neuraminidase* because the designation neuraminidase implies enzymatic hydrolysis of neuraminic acid (see Fig. 1), which is not a naturally occurring substance (this is N-acylneuraminic acid) and is not a substrate for sialidase.

An earlier abbreviation for sialidase was RDE (receptor-destroying enzyme), since sialidase destroys the receptors (acceptors) for certain infectious agents; e.g., myxoviruses (10). Receptor-destroying enzyme is a historical name not based on the substrate specificity of the enzyme; therefore, name and its abbreviation should be avoided.

II. SIALIC ACID IN GLYCOPHORIN ALLOANTIGENS

A. MN Antigens

The structural differences between M and N antigens are based on amino acid exchanges in positions 1 and 5 of the amino terminus of glycophorin A (GP A) (11,12), as shown in Figure 3. The amino terminus includes three O-glycosidically linked oligo(tetra)saccharides (O-glycans) at amino acid residues 2, 3, and 4 (Fig. 3). They are identical in M and N GP A molecules. The complex terminal GP A region contains up to six NeuNAc groups. Its molecular weight is approximately 4,000 d (13) and seems to be too large to represent a single antigenic determinant. It should be expected that M and N determinants are centered primarily around amino acid residues at positions 1 or 5 encompassing adjacent peptide and/or carbohydrate structures. In this situation, sequences not specific for M and N antigens would contribute to the construction of M- and

```
              *    *    *
M      1H2N-Ser-Ser-Thr-Thr-5Gly-Val-Ala-Met-

              *    *    *
N      1H2N-Leu-Ser-Thr-Thr-5Glu-Val-Ala-Met-


*      O glycan attached:

          NeuNAcα2
                   \6
       NeuNAcα2-3Galβ1-3GalNAc-Ser/Thr
```

Figure 3 Aminoterminals (positions 1–8) of M- and N-specific glycophorin A.

N-specific structures. These structures are the peptide sequences of positions 2 and 3 or 6 and above and/or the O-glycans at the amino acid residues of positions 2, 3, and/or 4.

Two possible effects of these common structures are to be considered. On one side, they may be responsible for the cross-reactivity of many anti-M and anti-N, and on the other hand, they may also account for the generation of the specific epitope structure. As judged by the structure of the terminal GP A pentapeptide with three O-glycans, each possessing two NeuNAc groups, the O-glycans, and especially sialic acids, could play a major part in these effects. A simple tool to study the role of sialic acid is the use of sialidase-treated antigen material for antibody binding and immunization.

First reports on destroying MN antigens by sialidase treatment of RBCs date from 1958 (4,5). Judd et al. (14) tested several anti-M and anti-N sera for agglutination of sialidase-treated RBCs. Several failed to agglutinate the treated RBCs, but several, however, agglutinated the treated RBCs, as well as untreated RBCs. Lisowska and Kordowicz (15) immunized rabbits with sialidase-treated RBCs yielding anti-M and anti-N reacting exclusively with sialidase-treated RBCs. Pedersen et al. (16) demonstrated the reaction of anti-M and anti-N with synthesized M- and N-specific carbohydrate-free octapeptide, respectively. The data document that NeuNAc is not a prerequisite for M and N determinants, but it is necessary for antibody binding in several cases.

In these studies, polyclonal antibodies were used that are not suited to define distinct epitopes. Monoclonal antibodies to M and N antigens produced in the last years allowed to localize distinct epitopes on the complex GP A amino-terminus and to obtain a clearer picture of the contribution of sialic acid to certain epitopes. The data are summarized in Table 1. Confirming earlier results, antibodies were found that do not require NeuNAc for binding. Most antibodies, however, require NeuNAc. In principle, two main groups of NeuNAc-dependent epitopes can be distinguished.

1. NeuNAc influences the peptide, creating the epitope.
2. The peptide influences the sialylated O-glycan, creating the epitope.

Table 1 Suggested Epitopes Recognized by Monoclonal M and N Antibodies

Example	Ref. no.	Designation	Spec.	NeuNAc	peptide resid.[a]	Cross-reaction[b]
1	17	8A2	N	+	1	+
2		6A7	M	+	5	−
3		9A3	M	+	1	−
4	18	LM110/140	M	+		+
		110/149	M			
5		BS38	M	−	6–8	(+)
6		BS44	M	(+)	5	−
7	19	E3	M	−		+
8		G8	M	+		+
9	20	A09,AH7,B010	M,N,N	+		−,−,+
10	21	425/2B	M	(+)	5	+
11	22	M2A1	M	+	1	−
12	23	2/23	N	+		+
13	24	NN 3,4,5	N	+	1	+
14	25	N61	N	+	1	+
15		N92	N	−	1+5	+

Main structure of epitope

[a]Deduced, e.g., from results with Henshaw and M^c variants exhibiting amino acid variations in positions 1 and 5.
[b]Tentative data because of different techniques used for antigen determination. Reaction of anti-N with "N" antigen on glycophorin B not excluded in all cases.

It is important to distinguish the groups because epitopes of group 1 can or cannot contain NeuNAc, whereas the sialylated O-glycan is always part of the epitopes of group 2. Without going into details (and referring to the original papers), the epitopes listed in Table 1 can be attributed more or less to one of the two groups. A pH-dependent M epitope that belongs possibly to both groups has been described (21); at pH 7, the O-glycan(s) are predominant, whereas the amino acid in position 5 contributes predominantly to the epitope at pH 8.3.

In the first international workshop on monoclonal antibodies against human RBC and related antigens, 31 monoclonal antibodies against glycophorins were tested by several groups (26–29). The findings on MN antigens expanded and confirmed the findings discussed above.

The O-glycans contain two sialyl groups; i.e., NeuNAcα linked 2–3 to galactose and NeuNAcα linked 2–6 to N-acetylgalactosamine of the Galβ1-3 GalNAc core disaccharide. In experiments to restore MN antigen activity by resialylation of desialylated RBCs, Sadler et al. (30) used sialyltransferases capable of linking NeuNAcα2-3 to galactose and NeuNAcα2-6 to galactosamine, respectively. Either one of the two sialyltransferases could restore the MN antigens, although some antibodies appeared to require selectively the product of only one of the enzymes. Thus, one anti-M required the NeuNAcα2-3 Gal but not the NeuNAcα2-6 GalNAc structure, a second anti-M required the product of either enzyme alone, and a third anti-M preferred the product of both enzymes together. Polyclonal antibodies were used for this study. Monoclonal antibodies could probably define still more precisely the effect of distinct NeuNAc residues for anti-M and anti-N binding.

Using rabbit anti-M, -N sera, Ebert et al. [31] studied the effect of chemical modifications of glycophorin-bound NeuNAc on M and N antigens. They showed that periodate/borohydride treatment of glycophorins, which shortens the sidechain of NeuNAc, abolishes NeuNAc-dependent M and N antigens. The finding demonstrates that NeuNAc itself, and not (only) its electric charge, contributes to the constitution of M and N epitopes. Although this effect has been confirmed by other groups, it can not be excluded that certain M and N epitopes require only the charge effect of NeuNAc.

The significance of O-glycans for certain epitopes is not necessarily restricted to sialic acid(s). One monoclonal anti-N reacted to the same degree with untreated and desialylated N-GPA but did not react with the de-O-glycosylated antigen [25]. Dahr has shown (unpublished results) that rabbit anti-M, -N sera reacting with NeuNAc-independent M and N antigens did not react with Tn RBCs, indicating that galactosyl groups are required for binding of these antibodies.

The data discussed were obtained from results with animal antibodies, including hybridoma monoclonal antibodies and human alloantibodies. Autoanti-M and autoanti-N were not included in immunochemical studies on M and N epitopes. In view of the immunogenicity of autoantigens, it would be interesting to know the structures inducing autoanti-M and autoanti-N.

In this connection, autoantibodies against Pr^M (and Pr^N) determinants should be mentioned. The determinants are the O-glycans with immunodominant NeuNAc not only of the amino terminus of GP A but also of the whole extracellular domain of glycophorins A and B. They are, however, optimally expressed only if they are attached to the terminal M (and N) specific pentapeptide backbone (see Sect. III.A.1 on Pr antigens).

In conclusion, the contribution of NeuNAc to M and N antigens varies markedly. NeuNAc may be not involved in epitopes. It may simply facilitate antibody binding with the peptide epitope or influence the peptide epitope to adopt the definite (tertiary) structure either by participating in the epitope or not. It may be part of an O-glycan epitope depending on the peptide backbone. In an extreme case, it may be the immunodominant component of an O-glycan epitope not dependent on, but influenced by, the peptide backbone for full expression.

B. En^a Antigens

En^a antigens are found on GP A. They have been subdivided into En^{a}TS (trypsin-sensitive), En^{a}FS (ficin-sensitive), and En^{a}FR (ficin-resistant) antigens (32). They are a heterogeneous group of antigens recognized by alloantibodies from individuals lacking GP A or possessing GP variants. En^a autoantibodies also are known.

From the localization of protease-sensitive sites on GP A, it should be expected that En^{a}TS antigens are located on the amino terminal GP A portion reaching to residue 39 but excluding the sequence of positions 1–26 that is shared by GP A and GP B. En^{a}FS antigens that are trypsin-resistant but ficin sensitive should be located on the GP A portion of residues approximately 40–56. En^{a}FR antigens should be found on the membrane near the region of residues 57–72 (approximately). The latter sequence is not glycosylated. Possible effects of Neu$N$Ac on En^a determinants should be limited to En^{a}TS and En^{a}FS antigens.

Like anti-M and anti-N, several anti-En^{a}TS and anti-En^{a}FS require Neu$N$Ac for binding, whereas several do not. A detailed study on these antigens has been presented by Dahr et al. (33). One of three En^{a}TS determinants required Neu$N$Ac, probably of the O-glycan at threonine at position 33. Most of En^{a}FS determinants (5/6) required Neu$N$Ac of the O-glycan attached to threonine at position 50.

The role of Neu$N$Ac for antibody binding is not clear. Probably a spectrum of possibilities exists, as discussed in the Section II.A on MN determinants. Neu$N$Ac could facilitate antibody binding without belonging to the En^a epitope. It could influence a peptide epitope with or without participating in the epitope. It could be part of a glycan epitope oriented by the peptide backbone. Furthermore, Neu$N$Ac residues differently linked to the disaccharide core structure of O-glycans could have different effects on epitopes. The O-glycans with the structures 1, 2, and 3 of Figure 4 are found in a ratio of 8:3:1 on GP A (34). The monosialoglycans of structures 2 and 3 are predominantly found on more internal regions of GP A, where En^{a}TS and En^{a}Fs determinants are also located.

Interestingly, desialylation of GP A had always the same effect on En^{a}TS and En^{a}FS determinants as had deglycosylation (33). In no case had the core disaccharide structure maintained the effect after Neu$N$Ac had been removed from the O-glycan(s). The finding underlines the essential role of Neu$N$Ac for carbohydrate-dependent En^a antigens.

C. Gerbich Antigens

In 1982, Daniels (35) reported that several human anti-Ge2 and anti-Ge3 failed to react with sialidase-treated RBCs. The two major high-frequency antigens Ge2 and Ge3 could be attributed to the minor RBC membrane sialoglycoproteins GP D and GP C. Ge2 determinants are located on a tryptic glycopeptide of GP D. Ge3 determinants are found on GP C in proximity to the

(1)
$$NeuNAc\alpha2 \diagdown_{6}$$
$$^{3}GalNAc\text{-}Ser/Thr$$
$$NeuNAc\alpha2\text{-}3Gal\beta1 \diagup$$

(2) $NeuNAc\alpha2\text{-}3Gal\beta1\text{-}3GalNAc\text{-}Ser/Thr$

(3)
$$NeuNAc\alpha2 \diagdown_{6}$$
$$Gal\beta1\text{-}3GalNAc\text{-}Ser/Thr$$

Figure 4 Sialo-O-glycans of glycophorins.

tryptic cleavage site (position 48) and on a similar region of GP D (36). All anti-Ge2 studied (36,37) required NeuNAc of O-glycan(s) for binding. Some anti-Ge3 required epitopes depending on NeuNAc of O-glycans at serine in position 42, whereas others did not require NeuNAc for binding (36,37), although the NeuNAc free disaccharide might be necessary also in these cases (36).

Various murine monoclonal antibodies recognizing GP C ("Ge-related") determinants have been prepared (reviewed in refs. 38–40). All seven antibodies studied in detail required O-glycans for binding. Four recognized determinants comprising the amino terminal amino acids together with the sialyl groups of the glycans at positions 3 and/or 4. One required the O-glycan at position 15, although sialidase treatment did not prevent antibody binding. Two required NeuNAc of O-glycans at a not definitely defined peptide sequence also of the amino-terminal region of GP C.

As outlined in the Section II.A MN antigens, the role of NeuNAc to effect antibody binding also may vary markedly in Ge antigens. It could range from facilitating antibody binding without contributing to the epitope to being an essential component of a Ge epitope.

D. MNSs-Related Antigens

There are numerous variants of MNSs antigens (satellite antigens) (41). They are characterized by complex interrelationships with each other and the MN and Ss antigens, respectively. They are expressed on GP A and/or GP B. These MNSs-related antigens can be based on amino acid variations and/or on variations in the degree and type of glycosylation. Because it is beyond the scope of this section to discuss the numerous MNSs related antigens, only one recent paper [42] on Tm, Sj, M_1, Can, Sext, and Hu antigens is mentioned that illustrates, on a biochemical basis, the complex interrelations which may exist between peptide and O-glycan structures to create the majority of these antigens. It is apparent that the contribution of NeuNAc to MNSs satellite antigens varies to that degree which has been discussed for MN and other glycophorin alloantigens.

The glycophorin alloantigens MN, En^a, and Ge share several characteristics:

1. Peptide structures are a prerequisite for the antigens.
2. The peptide structures are confined to certain glycophorins.
3. The antigens are heterogeneous, i.e., different determinants are designated by the same name, e.g., En^{a}TS, or the antigens are based on complex structures that may present several biochemical and antigenic variations, e.g., the amino-terminal region (positions 1–5) of GP A.
4. NeuNAc (and O-glycans) may or may not be required for antibody binding.
5. Most antibodies recognizing the antigens are alloantibodies.

In all these respects, the antigens differ from Pr and related antigens described in the next section.

III. SIALOAUTOANTIGENS

A. Glycophorin Sialoautoantigens

1. Pr Antigens

In 1969, we described two examples of autoantibodies that recognized antigens that were destroyed on RBCs by sialidase (6). Because the antigens also were inactivated by *proteases*, they were termed Pr antigens (43) (formerly called HD (6) or Sp_1 (44)).

The autoantibodies recognizing Pr antigens belong to one of the two major groups of human autoantibodies against RBCs, the so-called cold agglutinins (CAs). Cold agglutinins are fascinating antibodies because their heterogeneity is highly restricted. Postinfection CAs are oligoclonal antibodies. Cold agglutinins persistently occurring in chronic CA disease represent a monoclonal B lymphocyte proliferation and are invariably monoclonal antibodies (45). Concerning the antigens they recognize, CAs are the best investigated naturally occurring monoclonal antibodies in humans. All decisive findings on Pr antigens were obtained using monoclonal anti-Pr CAs.

a. Pr Antigen and Determinant.   Anti-Pr CAs do not react with protease-treated RBCs and most do not react with sialidase-treated RBCs (46). These anti-Pr CAs are termed anti-Pr$_1$, anti-Pr$_2$, and so forth (Table 2). Occasionally, anti-Pr CAs are found that react with sialidase-treated RBCs but fail to react with protease-treated RBCs. They are called anti-Pr$_a$ (Table 2) (46).

Because Pr$_1$ and other Pr antigens are protease and sialidase sensitive, it was suggested that they represent sialoglycoproteins or glycophorins in the RBC membrane. All 36 anti-Pr from our collection studied for reactivity with the glycophorin mixture obtained by phenol/saline extraction of RBC ghosts were reactive (46). The isolated GP A is also Pr active (47). The rare genetic variant RBCs with the En(a–) phenotype selectively lack GP A and are only weakly agglutinated by anti-Pr (48). Because of the weak reaction of En(a–) RBCs with anti-Pr, at least one other GP must carry Pr determinants. In addition to GP A, GP B is Pr active (49). The rare individuals homozygous for the M^k gene lack GP A and GP B on their RBCs (50) and their RBCs are not agglutinated by anti-Pr (48). Because absorption/elution studies with M^kM^k RBCs were not performed, it is not excluded (but probable) that the minor glycophorins GP C and GP D also carry Pr determinants.

From these data, it is apparent that Pr determinants are structures shared by (all) glycophorins. Since Pr$_1$ and other Pr determinants are sialoantigens, these structures are the di/mono-sialo-tetra/tri-saccharides or O-glycans O-glycosidically linked to serine or threonine of the peptide backbone of glycophorins. Accordingly, after splitting off the O-glycans from the peptide backbone glycophorins are Pr$_{1-3}$ inactive (51), and one anti-Pr$_2$ reacted with the isolated O-glycans (51). Furthermore, all fragments of glycophorins carrying O-glycans are Pr$_{1-3}$ active (49). Therefore, Pr$_{1-3}$ determinants do not depend on interactions of the O-glycans with distinct peptide core sequences but are pure carbohydrate determinants. Despite these clear data and the significant contribution of NeuNAc to the Pr$_{1-3}$ determinants, it is not clear whether the NeuNAcα2-3Gal . . . or the NeuNAcα2-6GalNAc . . . structure or both components of O-glycans are responsible for Pr$_{1-3}$ determinants. Sialidases selectively splitting one of the two NeuNAc bindings are not available. Another approach to resolve this question would be desialylation and resialylation of RBCs and glycophorins with specific sialyltransferases. These studies are in progress.

b. Pr$_1$, Pr$_2$, Pr$_3$ Subspecificities.   Pr$_1$, Pr$_2$, and Pr$_3$ antigens are inactivated by sialidase. To study the role of NeuNAc for the determinants, we modified NeuNAc residues on glycophorins chemically and tested the derivatives for Pr antigenicity. Periodate-oxidized (31,52) and carbodiimide-treated (53) GPs were used (Fig. 5). Periodate oxidation shortens the trihydroxyside chain of NeuNAc, creating a C7 NeuNAc derivative (54). Carbodiimide may cause a N-acyl-urea derivative of NeuNAc, which is formed by rearrangement from O-acyl-urea derivative of NeuNAc after reaction with the carboxy group of NeuNAc (55). The results with modified glycophorins were surprising. Not only inactivation or nonalteration but also marked increase of antigenicity of distinct Pr antigens was observed. Pr antigens that are inactivated by both procedures are termed Pr$_1$. Pr$_2$ antigenicity is increased 100- to 200-fold by oxidation and is abolished by carbodiimide treatment. Pr$_3$ antigenicity is increased 100- to 200-fold by carbodiimide treatment and is abolished by oxidation. In the Pr$_1$ group, Pr antigens are included that are not (completely) inactivated by carbodiimide treatment but are activated neither by carbodiimide treatment nor by oxidation (46). All O-glycan–carrying fragments of GP A are activated in terms of Pr$_2$ and Pr$_3$ antigenicity by

Table 2 Serological and Biochemical Characterization of Pr Antigen Subspecificities and Sa Antigen

Antigen	Expression on RBCs human adult/newborn			Expression on glycophorins			Expression on RBCs of dog			Reaction with	
	untr.	pap.	sialid.	untr.	oxid.	carb.	untr.	pap.	sialid.	NeuNAc	NeuNAcα2-3lactose
Pr_{1h}	+	−	−	+	−	−/+	−			−	−
Pr_{1d}	+	−	−	+	−	−/+	+	−/+	−	−	−
Pr_2	+	−	−	+	←	−	←	←	−	−	−
Pr_{3h}	+	−	−	+	−	←	−	−/+	−	−	−
Pr_{3d}	+	−	−	+	−	←	+	−	−	−	−
Pr^M	+*	−	−	+**	+	+	+	−	−	−	−
Pr_a	+	−	+	+	↑/−	↑/−	+	+	−	−	−
Sa	+	→	−	+	−	−				−	+

Abbreviations: untr., untreated; pap., papain treated; sialid., sialidase treated; oxid., oxidized; carb., carbodiimide treated; +, present; −, not present/no reaction; /or; ↑, enhanced ↓, decreased; *, preferential expression on M RBC's; **, preferential expression on (the aminoterminal fragment of) glycophorin A.

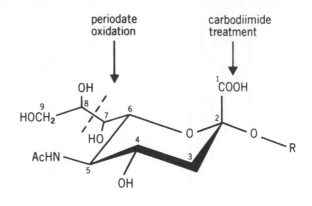

Pr₁ :	inactiv.	inactiv./not altered
Pr_1 :	inactiv.	inactiv./not altered
Pr_2 :	activated	inactiv.
Pr_3 :	inactiv.	activated

Figure 5 Chemical modifications of NeuNAc and their influences on Pr_1, Pr_2, Pr_3 antigenicities.

periodate and carbodiimide treatment, respectively (49). No effect is observed after previous desialylation of GP A (49). The effects cannot be prevented by previous modifications of the peptide backbone (49). The data confirm that NeuNAc is the immunodominant component of Pr_1, Pr_2, and Pr_3 antigens (and does not interfere with neighboring structures, e.g., by electrostatic interactions, thus creating the actual Pr determinant by conformational changes). They further confirm that Pr determinants are O-glycans not dependent on interactions with the peptide backbone. The only exception is the Pr^M antigen described below.

By these results, a definite biochemically based subspecification of Pr antigens could be introduced. It should be mentioned that Pr_2 and Pr_3 antigens are the only known natural antigens that can be increased by chemical modification of their immunodominant component; i.e., NeuNAc.

c. Pr_{1h}/Pr_{1d}, Pr_{3h}/Pr_{3d} Subclassification.   Among anti-Pr_1 and anti-Pr_3 CAs, several examples are found that agglutinate exclusively human RBCs. The antigens are termed Pr_{1h} (56) and Pr_{3h} (h for human) (46). Other examples are found that also react with animal RBCs, including RBCs of the dog. These antigens are termed Pr_{1d} (56) and Pr_{3d} (d for dog) (46) antigens (see Table 2). Among more than 60 anti-Pr samples studied in this laboratory, only one example did not fit into the Pr_h/Pr_d subclassification because it reacted with RBCs of several species but failed to react with RBCs of the dog (57).

Pr_2 antigens that would be limited to human RBCs are not known. The use of RBCs of the dog for Pr subclassification has the advantage that these cells show a characteristic reaction pattern with anti-Pr_2 (see Table 2). Contrasting Pr_{1d} and Pr_{3d} antigens, Pr_2 antigens are stronger expressed on dog compared to human RBCs, and proteases do not destroy them on dog RBCs (56).

d. Pr^M (and Pr^N) Antigen.   We have found a human monoclonal CA, termed anti-Pr^M (58), that agglutinates RBCs independently of their MN blood groups at lower temperatures like anti-Pr. But at higher temperatures, the antibody reacts preferentially with M positive RBCs, thus resembling anti-M. The antibody does not react with sialidase-treated RBCs. The slight reaction of anti-Pr^M with N-positive cells at 25°C could be markedly increased in low ionic strength medium, whereas the reaction with M positive RBCs could be enhanced only scarcely. The finding supports the suggestion that anti-Pr^M recognizes sialoantigens present on M and N RBCs with a different degree of affinity. Anti-Pr^M reacts with GP A, GP B, GP C, and their fragments (58). It reacts, however, best with GP A from M RBCs and its amino terminal fragment. It does not react with GP A from M RBCs after sialidase treatment or alkaline borohydride degradation that removes O-glycans from the peptide backbone by β-elimination (58).

It is apparent that anti-Pr^M recognizes O-glycans with immunodominant NeuNAc on glycophorins but binds best with the O-glycans attached to the M-specific peptide backbone of GP A. As had been discussed in the section on MN antigens, the Pr^M determinants are obviously O-glycans influenced by, but not completely dependent on, peptide backbone interference.

A murine monoclonal antibody with a specificity like anti-Pr^M has been described (59). A human CA that looks like an analogue to anti-Pr^M has been reported (60). It reacts preferentially with N RBCs at higher temperatures and could be termed anti-Pr^N.

  e. Pr$_a$ Antigen.   Despite their resistance to sialidase-treatment, Pr$_a$ antigens will be reviewed with NeuNAc-dependent glycophorin antigens. Two of the three anti-Pr$_a$ of our collection were tested for reaction with modified glycophorins (46). One anti-Pr$_a$ reacted strongly with periodate-oxidized and carbodiimide-treated glycophorins, but the other did not. Because oxidation and carbodiimide treatment should alter exclusively sialyl groups, the results are evidently incompatible with the serological results, which seem to exclude NeuNAc as a component of Pr$_a$ antigens. Possibly, anti-Pr$_a$ CAs recognize sialidase-insensitive NeuNAc molecules on glycophorins.

2. Sa Antigen

We have found a human monoclonal CA, anti-Sa (47), that shows a reaction pattern with human RBCs similar to, but not identical with, anti-Pr$_{1-3}$. The autoantibody recognizes an antigen, termed Sa (for sialic acid) that is completely inactivated by sialidase like Pr$_{1-3}$ but is only partially destroyed by papain, contrasting the completely protease-sensitive Pr$_{1-3}$ antigens (see Table 2). A second example of anti-Sa has been described (61). We have studied a third example (kindly provided by Dr. Pereira, Barcelona, Spain).

  Glycophorins and isolated GP A carry Sa determinants (47). The data of Dahr et al. (49) show that the more internal regions of GP A are Sa active, thereby contrasting Pr$_{1-3}$ activity. These regions are known to carry incompletely sialylated O-glycans (see structures 2 and 3 in Fig. 4) preferentially with the structure NeuNAcα2-3Galβ1-3GalNAc (34). We have shown that anti-Sa is inhibited by sialyllactose and that the isomer NeuNAcα2-3Galβ1-4Glc is responsible for anti-Sa binding (47). These data are consistent with the conclusion that Sa determinants are (predominantly) the NeuNAcα2-3Gal . . . structure found on the more internal regions of glycophorins and on NeuNAcα2-3lactose.

  The serological and biochemical data on Pr and Sa antigens are summarized in Table 2.

3. Broader Reactivity of Anti-Pr2 and Anti-Sa

Because anti-Sa also reacts with protease-treated human RBCs (47), and because anti-Pr$_2$ reacts very strongly with protease-treated RBCs of the dog (56), it can be assumed that both antibodies recognize antigens not limited to glycophorins. Tsai et al. (62) have shown that an anti-Pr$_2$ reacts with the short-chain ganglioside G$_{M3}$ and with sialylneolactotetraosylceramide with the terminal NeuNAcα2-3Gal sequence (Table 3). Our reference anti-Pr$_2$ reacts also with G$_{M3}$ and type 2 chain-based gangliosides of the neolacto series (63). In addition, this antibody reacts with sialoglycolipids of the ganglio series (63). This is in accordance with earlier immunocytochemical studies that have shown strong anti-Pr$_2$ binding to brain tissues of several mammalian species (64). The anti-Pr$_2$ recognizes NeuNAcα2-3Gal, NeuNAcα2-6Gal, and NeuNAcα2-8NeuNAc structures. It shows a specificity for N-acetyl- rather than N-glycolylsialic acid. Because anti-Pr$_2$ does not agglutinate protease-treated human RBCs, it is doubtful whether gangliosides contribute to the reaction of this antibody with human red cells. Probably it reacts

Table 3 Designations and Structures of G_{M3} and Neolacto Series (type 2) Chain Glycolipids and Sialoglycolipids (Gangliosides)

Designation	Sugar sequence
Sialyllactosylceramide (G_{M3})	NeuNAcα2-Galβ1-4Glc-Cer
Neolactotetraosylceramide (PG)	Galβ1-4GlcNAcβ1-3Galβ1-4Glc-Cer
Sialylneolactotetraosylceramide (SPG)	NeuNAcα2-3Galβ1-4GlcNAcβ1-3Galβ1-4Glc-Cer
Neolactohexaosylceramide, linear	[Galβ1-4GlcNAc]$_2$β1-3Galβ1-4Glc-Cer
Neolactohexaosylceramide, biantennary	Galβ1-4GlcNAcβ1 $\qquad\qquad\searrow^{3}$ $\qquad\qquad\qquad$Galβ1-4Glc-Cer $\qquad\qquad\nearrow^{6}$ Galβ1-4GlcNAcβ1
Sialylneolactohexaosylceramide, linear	NeuNAcα2-3[Galβ1-4GlcNAc]$_2$β1-3Galβ1-4Glc-Cer
Sialylneolactohexaosylceramide, biantennary	NeuNAcα2-3 Galβ1-4GlcNAcβ1 $\qquad\qquad\qquad\searrow^{3}$ $\qquad\qquad\qquad\qquad$Galβ1-4Glc-Cer $\qquad\qquad\qquad\nearrow^{6}$ (NeuNAcα2-3)Galβ1-4GlcNAcβ1
Sialylneolactooctaosylceramide, linear	NeuNAcα2-3[Galβ1-4GlcNAc]$_3$β1-3Galβ1-4Glc-Cer
Sialylneolactooctaosylceramide, biantennary	NeuNAcα2-3 Galβ1-4GlcNAcβ1 $\qquad\qquad\qquad\searrow^{3}$ $\qquad\qquad\qquad\qquad$Galβ1-4GlcNAcβ1-3Galβ1-4Glc-Cer $\qquad\qquad\qquad\nearrow^{6}$ (NeuNAcα2-3)Galβ1-4GlcNAcβ1

with gangliosides on RBCs of the dog. Binding of our reference anti-Pr_1 and anti-Pr_3 with the various gangliosides was not observed (63), indicating that Pr_1 and Pr_3 determinants could be limited to glycophorins.

Sa antigens are also gangliosides (63), thus resembling Pr_2 antigens. However, Sa and Pr_2 differ. Pr_2 antigens are represented by gangliosides of the neolacto and ganglio series, whereas Sa antigens are restricted to that of the neolacto series. Like anti-Pr_2, anti-Sa showed a specificity for N-acetyl- rather than N-glycolyl sialic acid presented by polylactosamine chains of neolacto gangliosides (63).

Pr_{1h}, Pr_{1d}, Pr_2, Pr_{3h}, Pr_{3d}, Pr^M, (Pr^N), Pr_a, and Sa antigens represent a main group of autoantigens recognized by cold agglutinins. The determinants are O-glycans of glycophorins, perhaps with the exception of Pr_a determinants. Nevertheless, in some instances (Pr_2, Sa), the antibodies recognize structures not limited to O-glycans of glycophorins. The extreme example is anti-Pr_2, which shows the broadest spectrum of reactivity with sialyl groups. A comparison of these glycophorin autoantigens with the glycophorin alloantigens MN, En^a, and Ge permits us to ascertain some general differences.

1. Peptide structures, which are essential for the alloantigens, are not involved in the autoantigens. The only exception is the Pr^M antigen. In this respect, $Pr^{M/N}$ is a connection link between M/N and Pr antigens.
2. In contrast to the alloantigens, the autoantigens are not confined to distinct glycophorins.
3. Contrasting the heterogeneity and/or complexity of the alloantigens, the autoantigen determinants are simple carbohydrates that can be surveyed easily. Owing to the monoclonality of cold agglutinins, several epitopes could, however, be defined on the O-glycans.
4. NeuNAc is required for the epitopes and is, perhaps with the exception of Pra, the immunodominant component of all autoantigens, whereas the role of NeuNAc for alloantigens varies considerably.
5. It is highly improbable that alloantibodies against Pr and Sa antigens would exist because RBCs lacking all glycophorins (and their O-glycans) are not known.

B. Sia-l1, Sia-b1, Sia-lb1 Autoantigens

1. Characteristics of Differentiation Sialoautoantigens

In 1981, we found an antibody belonging to the cold-reactive autoantibodies (CAs) like anti-Pr that recognizes the first NeuNAc-dependent developmentally regulated or differentiation antigen on the RBC surface, termed Fl (65). The detection was the starting point for the definition of several developmentally regulated sialoautoantigens that have been recently integrated into the Sia-l, -b, -lb antigen complex (66).

The expression of these sialoautoantigens compared with that of Ii antigens, which are also developmentally regulated, on untreated and enzyme-treated RBCs is shown in Table 4. The antigens share several characteristics.

1. The antigens are differentiation antigens. Sia-b1 (formerly Fl) is fully expressed only on adult RBCs. Sia-l1 (formerly Vo) is fully expressed only on newborn RBCs. As an exception, Sia-lb1 (formerly Gd) is expressed on adult and newborn RBCs in equal strength.
2. The antigens are present on the rare adult RBCs with the i phenotype (i adult RBCs) in equal strength as on newborn (i cord) RBCs. It can, therefore, be concluded that the structures responsible for Ii and Sia-l, -b, -lb antigens are related.
3. The antigens are inactivated by sialidase treatment of RBCs, indicating that NeuNAc, not involved in Ii antigenic determinants, serves as immunodominant component.

Table 4 Expression of Sia-b1, Sia-l1, Sia-lb1 Antigens Compared to Ii Antigens on Human Untreated and Enzyme-Treated Red Blood Cells

Antigen	Previous designation	Human RBCs									i Adult	O_h
		Adult				Newborn						
		untr.	pap.	sial.	endo.	untr.	pap.	sial.	pap./sial.	endo.	untr.	untr.
I		+	←	←	→	→					→	+
Sia-b1	Fl	+	+	–	+	→	←	←	←		→	→
i		→				+	←	+	–	–	+	+*
Sia-l1	Vo	→	+		+	+	+	–	–	–	+	+*
Sia-lb1	Gd	+	+	–	+	+				+	+	+

Abbreviations: untr., untreated; pap., papain treated; sial., sialidase treated; endo., endo-β-galactosidase treated; pap./sial., sialidase treated after papainization; +, optimal reaction with untreated RBCs; ↑, reaction (slightly) increased; ↓, reaction markedly decreased; –, no reaction; *, expressed as on adult RBCs.

4. The antigens are protease resistant and may be represented by gangliosides or protease-resistant glycoproteins of the RBC membrane.

Developmentally regulated glycoconjugates of the RBC membrane are the sugar chains of the neolacto series or type 2 chains; i.e., is [Galβ1-4GlcNAcβ1-3]n chains. The chains of fetal and newborn RBCs are linear, and those of adult RBCs are branched and are generated by adding a lactosamine unit in β1-6 linkage to the penultimate galactose of the linear sequence (Table 5). The linear chains are known to be the i antigens; the branched to be the I antigens (67,68). In accordance with the serological results, it is now clear that the developmentally regulated sialoautoantigens of the Sia-1, -b, -lb series are sialylated linear and/or branched type 2 chains. The names of the antigens have been deduced from their structural features. Antigens represented by *sia*lylated *l*inear chains are termed Sia-l1, antigens represented by *sia*lylated *b*ranched chains are called Sia-b1, and antigens expressed on both *sia*lylated *l*inear and *b*ranched chains are named Sia-lb1.

a. Sia-b1 Antigen.   Sia-b1 antigens are fully expressed only on adult RBCs (see Table 3). They are glycoproteins and glycolipids (gangliosides). I-active glycoproteins from papainized RBCs (69) are Sia-b1 active (70). They lose Sia-b1 activity after sialidase treatment that does not alter (but even increases) I antigenicity (70). Kannagi et al. (71) demonstrated the fucoganglioside with structure 4 in Table 5 to be Sia-b1 active. The basic structure of the Sia-b1 ganglioside is the branched neolactooctaosylceramide known to be I antigen active. Uemura et al. (63) also found a preferential reaction of anti–Sia-b1 with gangliosides with branched neolacto basic sequences in a chromatogram binding assay.

Table 5   Unsubstituted and Sialylated Type 2 Chains Generating Ii and Sia-l1, Sia-b1, Sia-lb1 Antigens, Respectively

Structure No.	Determinant	Type 2 chain[a]
1	i	Galβ1-4GlcNAcβ1-3Galβ1-4GlcNAcβ1-3Galβ1-4GlcNAc/Glc-
2	Sia-l1	Neu$N$Acα2-3Galβ1-4GlcNAcβ1-3Galβ1-4GlcNAcβ1-3Galβ1-4GlcNAc/Glc-
3	I	Galβ1-4GlcNAcβ1$\diagdown$ $\qquad\qquad\qquad$ 3 $\qquad\qquad\qquad\qquad$ Galβ1-4GlcNAcβ1-3Galβ1-4GlcNAc/Glc- $\qquad\qquad\qquad\diagup$ 6 Galβ1-4GlcNAcβ1$\diagup$
4	Sia-b1	Neu$N$Acα2-3Galβ1-4GlcNAcβ1$\diagdown$ $\qquad\qquad\qquad$ 3 $\qquad\qquad\qquad\qquad$ Galβ1-4GlcNAcβ1-3Galβ1-4GlcNAc/Glc- $\qquad\qquad\qquad\diagup$ 6 Fucα1-2Galβ1-4GlcNAcβ1$\diagup$
5	Sia-lb1	Neu$N$Acα2-3Galβ1-4GlcNAcβ1$\diagdown$ $\qquad\qquad\qquad$ 3 $\qquad\qquad\qquad\qquad$ Galβ1-4GlcNAcβ1-3Galβ1-4GlcNAc/Glc- $\qquad\qquad\qquad\diagup$ 6 (Neu$N$Acα2-3)Galβ1-4GlcNAcβ1$\diagup$
(2)		Neu$N$Acα2-3Galβ1-4GlcNAcβ1-3Galβ1-4GlcNAcβ1-3Galβ1-4GlcNAc/Glc-

[a]For designations see Table 3.

The structure of the Sia-b1 determinant is remarkable. It is

NeuNAcα2-3Galβ1-4GlcNAcβ1\
                          \
                           3
                            Galβ1-4GlcNAcβ1-3Galβ1-4Glc-Cer
                           /
                          6
    Fucα1-2Galβ1-4GlcNAcβ1
         ↑
         R = OH
         R = GalNAcα1-3
         R = Galα1-3

1. The fucosylated 1–6 branch represents a H determinant. It can be converted into blood group A substance by adding GalNAcα1-3 and blood group B substance by adding Galα1-3 to Gal, as indicated, without losing Sia-b1 activity, thus explaining the ABO blood group–independent Sia-b1 expression on RBCs.

2. Among the several glycolipids isolated from human RBC membrane, the only (strongly) Sia-b1 active ganglioside is the fucoganglioside (71). In particular, the nonfucosylated ganglioside is Sia-b1 inactive. The Sia-b1 determinant is a biantennary structure because both branches are required for Sia-b1 antigenicity. This biantennary determinant is unique because it requires different branches compared with the I determinant requiring two identical branches (structure 3 in Table 5). The Sia-b1 determinant is the first example demonstrating the construction of an epitope by two branches with different terminal sugars. It contributes to the possibilities that exist to generate numerous carbohydrate antigens from a limited number of single sugars used to build up carbohydrate antigens (and receptors). However, because the nonfucosylated ganglioside was from bovine RBCs having predominantly N-glycolylneuraminic acid, and because N-acetylneuraminic acid is essential for Sia-b1 antigenicity, the nonreactivity of this ganglioside with anti–Sia-b1 could be due to the lack of N-acetylneuraminic acid. But we have shown that O_h RBCs have a strongly reduced reactivity with anti–Sia-b1 (72) (see Table 4), indicating that fucosyl groups like NeuNAc are essential for optimal Sia-b1 antigen expression. In other words, the Sia-b1 determinant has two different immunodominant components. Nevertheless, two alternate explanations can be discussed. First, the actual Sia-b1 epitope could be one branch that is held in an appropriate conformation by interaction with the other branch. Second, the failure of fucosylation in O_h cells could result in sialylation of the 1–6 branch, thereby blocking the Sia-b1 epitope. Further studies are necessary to identify this interesting epitope definitely.

3. Sialylation (and fucosylation) of the neolactooctaosylceramide not only creates Sia-b1 antigenicity but also cancels I antigen activity. Although the antigens are related biochemically, they are entirely different immunologically.

All data on the Sia-b1 antigen mentioned above were obtained with the anti–Sia-b1 Fl (65). It is a monoclonal IgM-κ CA and is the only monoclonal anti–Sia-b1 known. After it could be defined, we have reinvestigated several CAs originally specified as anti-I by absorption studies with sialidase-treated RBCs but did not find a further example. However, by these experiments we found that several sera of patients suffering from recent *Mycoplasma pneumoniae* infections contained a mixture of anti-I and anti–Sia-b1 (73,74). These postinfection (polyclonal or oligoclonal) anti–Sia-b1 examples meet the serological criteria for anti–Sia-b1. But the Sia-b1 antigens recognized by the postinfection CAs differ from the monoclonal anti–Sia-b1 Fl in two respects (72). First, they are fully expressed on O_h cells, indicating that fucosyl groups are not required for these Sia-b1 determinants. Second, they are partially destroyed by endo-β-galactosidase-treatment of RBCs, whereas the Sia-b1 determinant recognized by the monoclonal anti–Sia-b1 Fl is not affected on the RBC membrane by the enzyme. As will be discussed later, the data are consistent with the postinfection nature of the antibodies recognizing these Sia-b1 antigens. (To avoid confusion, they are not considered in Table 4.)

b. Sia-l1 Antigen. A monoclonal IgM-λCA, originally termed anti-Vo, recognizes a NeuNAc-dependent antigen fully expressed only on newborn RBCs (75) (see Table 4). The corresponding antigen, now termed Sia-l1 (66,72), is fully accessible for antibody binding only after protease treatment of RBCs, and it is also accessible for the enzyme sialidase only after protease treatment. Biochemical data on the Sia-l1 determinant with isolated RBC membrane gangliosides (or protease-resistant RBC membrane glycoproteins) are not available. The serological findings could, however, be decisively supplemented by experiments with the enzyme endo-β-galactosidase. This enzyme of *Bacteroides fragilis,* like that of *Escherichia freundii,* hydrolyses internal β-galactosidic bonds of lacto-N-glycosyl oligosaccharides with the common sequence GlcNAcβ1-3Galβ1-4GlcNAc/Glc (76). Hydrolysis is limited to linear sequences. Branch point sequences are resistant to hydrolysis (77). The enzyme acts on the RBC surface (78). Endo-β-galctosidase treatment of newborn RBCs abolishes completely Sia-l1 antigens (66).

Based on the results with enzyme-treated RBCs and the fact that Sia-l1 antigens are strongly expressed on newborn and on adult RBCs with the i phenotype, a conclusive characterization of the Sia-l1 determinant is possible. Sialidase inactivates the Sia-l1 determinant, indicating that Sia-l1 is a sialoautoantigen with immunodominant NeuNAc. Endo-β-galactosidase from *B. fragilis* also inactivates the Sia-l1 antigen. Endo-β-galactosidase cleaves type 2 GlcNAcβ1-3Galβ1-4GlcNAc/Glc sequences much more effectively than type 1 GlcNAcβ1-3Galβ1-3GlcNAc/Glc sequences (76). Since the Sia-l1 antigen is strongly expressed only on RBCs abundantly equipped with linear type 2 chains, i.e., i cord and i adult RBCs, it is apparent that the Sia-l1 determinant is represented by sialylated linear type 2 chains (structure 2 in Table 5).

In biochemical terms, Sia-l1 resembles i as Sia-b1 resembles I. The expression of Sia-l1 on the human RBC is complementary to Sia-b1 like the expression of i and I. We have studied a family with three members of the i phenotype (unpublished observations). The three members had high Sia-l1 RBC levels (and strongly reduced Sia-b1 and I levels). Although it is clear that Sia-l1 determinants are sialylated linear type 2 chains, nothing is known about the length of the chains required for Sia-l1 determinants. Because the determinants are optimally accessible for the Sia-l1 antibody only on protease-treated RBCs, relatively short chains might account for Sia-l1 antigenicity. We have reinvestigated 42 examples of anti-i sera for possible anti–Sia-l1 CAs. Neither anti–Sia-l1 alone nor anti–Sia-l1 coexisting with anti-i was found (unpublished data). The situation contrasts that of postinfection anti-I sera that frequently contain coexisting anti–Sia-b1 and anti-I CAs.

c. Sia-lb1,2 Antigens. In 1977, we found two monoclonal IgM-κ CAs (79) recognizing antigens that were previously named Gd (for glycolipid dependent) and are now termed Sia-lb1 (66). Further anti–Sia-lb1 examples are known (80,81). As shown in Table 4, Sia-lb1 antigens are expressed on human adult and newborn RBCs in equal strength. They are protease resistant and are destroyed by sialidase treatment of RBCs. It was suggested that the antigens belong to the group of type 2 (neolacto series) sialoautoantigens discussed in this section. Unlike Sia-b1 and Sia-l1 antigens, the Sia-lb1 antigen is not developmentally regulated. It should, therefore, be represented by sialylated linear and branched type 2 chains. This assumption turned out to be true. Sia-lb1 antigens are gangliosides. Glycophorins do not carry Sia-lb1 determinants (47). Anti–Sia-lb1 CAs react with sialylated type 2 chains of gangliosides of the neolacto series and show a preference for longer sequences. Sialylneolactohexaosylceramide was 10-fold more active than sialylneolactotetraosylceramide (82). Using a thin-layer chromatogram binding assay, Uemura et al. (63) also demonstrated Sia-lb1 antigenicity of various neolacto series–based gangliosides, including linear and branched sialylneolactotetra/hexa/octa/deca/dodecaosyl-ceramides (see Table 3). Interestingly, G_{M3} with the short-chain Neu$N$Acα2-3Galβ1-4Glc-Cer was also active. It can be easily explained by this reaction profile of anti–Sia-lb1 with linear as well as with branched sialo-type 2 chains that Sia-lb1 antigens are not developmentally regulated but are expressed equally well on adult RBCs possessing predominantly branched chains and on newborn RBCs presenting predominantly linear chains (see Table 5).

The reaction pattern of the Sia-lb1 antibody could be due to the recognition of large domains of type 2 chains, including the branch point of branched chains. Alternatively, it could be due to short parts of the sequences common for branched and linear chains. In this case, the short sequence Neu$N$Acα2-3Galβ1-4GlcNAc or an even shorter sequence would be the Sia-lb1 epitope. We have shown that anti–Sia-lb1 can be weakly but definitely inhibited by sialyllactose, Neu$N$Acα2-3Galβ1-Glc (83). Because the 2–6 isomer is inactive (70), the isomer Neu$N$Acα2-6Galβ1-4Glc is responsible for Sia-lb1 activity, which could be confirmed by commercially available Neu$N$Acα2-3lactose (unpublished data). Neu$N$Ac and lactose alone are Sia-lb1 inactive. The data were confirmed by Kundu et al. (82), who showed that Neu$N$Acα2-6 isomers of Sia-lb1–active Neu$N$Acα2-3 gangliosides are also Sia-lb1 inactive, as are neolactoglycolipids without Neu$N$Ac. Because sialyllactose is Sia-lb1 active, it was possible to study related oligosaccharides for Sia-lb1 activity. The disaccharide Neu$N$Acα2-3Glc (1.2–5.6 diisopropylidene) inhibits one of the original anti–Sia-lb1 (Kn) but fails to inhibit the other (Hei). Another anti–Sia-lb1 (MAT; see ref. 80) is weakly inhibited (84). Anti–Sia-lb1 Kn does not require the subterminal Gal, contrasting the anti–Sia-lb1 Hei. The role of the subterminal Glc (1.2–5.6 diisopropylidene) for the Sia-lb1 determinant Kn was studied by inhibition experiments with several Neu$N$Ac monosaccharide derivatives (84). As shown in Figure 6, 2αmethylC9Neu$N$Ac is Sia-lb1 active (84). Therefore, a subterminal sugar is not required for this Sia-lb1 epitope, but only α-configuration of the monosaccharide Neu$N$Ac is required that is already induced by methylation of C2 of Neu$N$Ac (structure 2 in Fig. 6). Because of the clear-cut biochemical distinction between the Sia-lb1 determinants Kn and Hei, we have introduced the designations Sia-lb1 for Kn and Sia-lb2 for Hei; formerly termed Gd1 and Gd2, respectively (84). The Sia-lb1, Sia-lb2 minimum structures are:

Sia-lb1: Neu$N$Acα2-R
Sia-lb2: Neu$N$Acα2-3Galβ1 . . .

Because the monosaccharide 2αmethylC9Neu$N$Ac is Sia-lb1 active, modifications of the monosaccharide could be studied for effects on Sia-lb1 antigenicity. As can be seen in Figure 6, 2βmethylC9Neu$N$Ac (structure 3 in Fig. 6) is Sia-lb1 inactive, shortening of the trihydroxys-ide chain (structure 4 in Fig. 6) reduces Sia-lb1 antigenicity, and alterations of the carboxy group eliminating the electrostatic potential (structures 5 and 6 in Fig. 6) abolish Sia-lb1 antigenicity. Not only the intact carboxy group and the complete trihydroxyside chain are essential for optimal Sia-lb1 antigenicity, but the hydroxy group at C4 and the N-acetyl group at C5 (Brossmer and Roelcke, to be published) are necessary as well. The significance of the N-acetyl group has been demonstrated by Uemura et al. (63), who showed that neolacto gangliosides with N-glycolylNeu$N$Acα2-3 are Sia-lb1 inactive.

The Sia-lb1 minimum structure is remarkable. It is restricted to the immunodominant monosaccharide. Thus, all prominent groups of Neu$N$Ac essential for Sia-lb1 antigenicity can be identified (Fig. 7). Because the monosaccharide Neu$N$Ac is Sia-lb1 active and the short sequence Neu$N$Acα2-3Galβ1(-4Glc) is Sia-lb2 active, it can be assumed that the short-chain domain (before the branch point of branched type 2 chains) common for linear and branched

Structure No	Designation	NeuAc Structure	Antigenicity
1	βNeuNAc	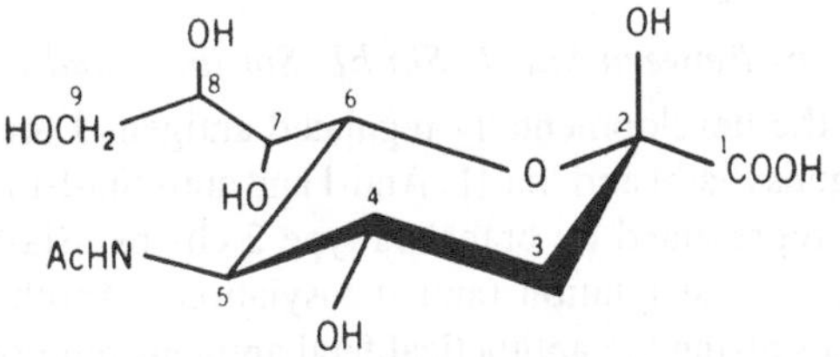	Sia-lb1 −
2	2αmethylC9NeuNAc	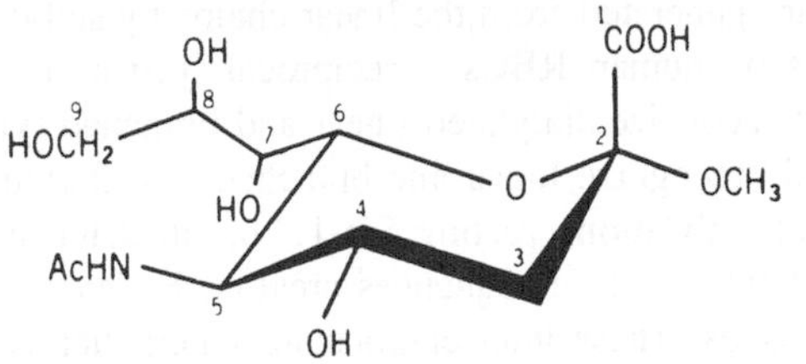	Sia-lb1 +
3	2βmethylC9NeuNAc	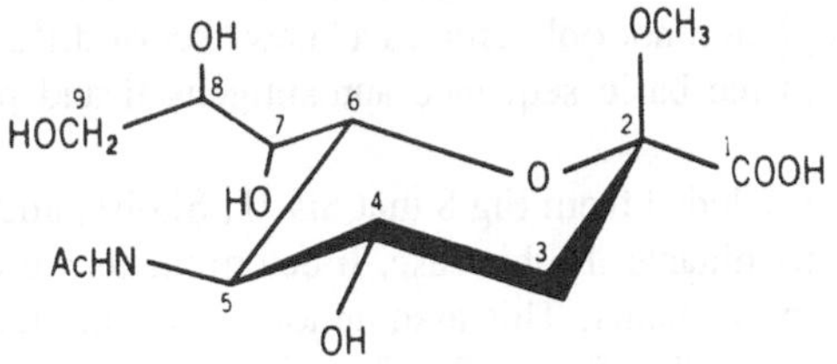	Sia-lb1 −
4	2αmethylC7NeuNAc	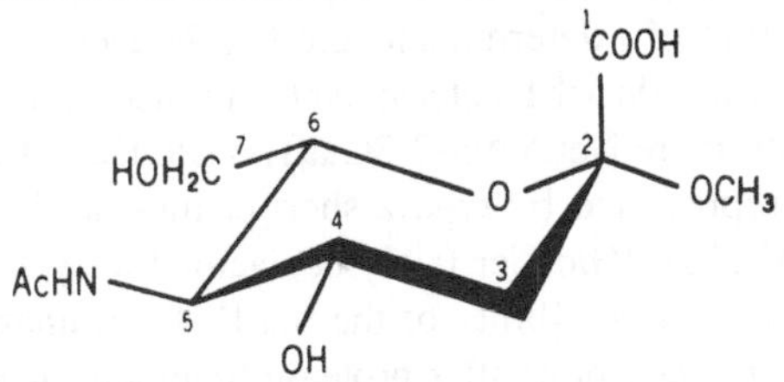	Sia-lb1(+)
5	2αmethylC9NeuNAc alcohol C1	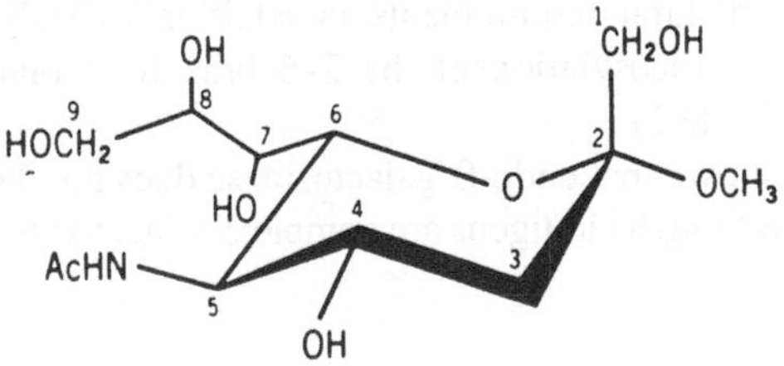	Sia-lb1 −
6	2αmethylC9NeuNAc methyl ester	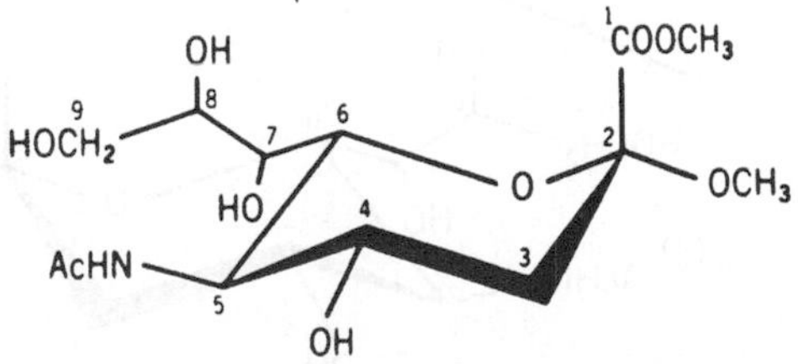	Sia-lb1 −

Figure 6 N-acetylneuraminic acid monosaccharide derivatives and their Sia-lb1 antigenicity.

type 2 sequences account for the reactivity of Sia-lb1 and Sia-lb2 antibodies with linear as well as with branched type 2 chains.

2. *Interrelations Between Sia-l1, Sia-b1, Sia-lb1,2 and Ii and H, AB Antigens*

In addition to the developmentally regulated antigens I and i, there exist the developmentally regulated antigens Sia-bl and Sia-l1. Anti-I and anti–Sia-b1 are a pair of antibodies that recognize adult antigens represented by branched type 2 chains. Sia-b1 determinants are generated from branched chains by sialylation (and fucosylation). Another pair of antibodies are anti-i and anti–Sia-l1 recognizing the antithetical fetal antigens represented by linear type 2 chains. Sia-l1 determinants are generated from the linear chains by sialylation. The expression of Sia-b1 and Sia-l1 antigens on human RBCs is reciprocal, just as is the expression of I and i antigens. Anti–Sia-lb1,2 recognize sialylated linear and branched type 2 chains. A pendant to anti–Sia-lb1,2 that would recognize linear and branched type 2 chains without sialylation is missing. It is apparent that sialylation creating Sia-1, -b, -lb determinants is an alternative pathway for fucosylation of type 2 basic sequences creating H determinants that can be converted into A and B blood groups. These interrelations are schematically shown in Figure 8. Because of the significance of differentiation antigens, e.g., as tumor-associated antigens, it is important to realize that sialylation not only creates a "new" set of differentiation sialoautoantigens but also masks (partially) the basic sequence autoantigens Ii and prevents the generation of A and B blood groups.

It could be concluded from Fig 8 that Sia-l1, Sia-b1, and Sia-lb1 determinants are generated from i and I determinants. In this case, Ii determinants were structures that have been left after sialylation of type 2 chains. This assumption is too simple.

1. A critical length of type 2 sequences is required to represent Ii determinants. The minimum structure of i determinants are two N-acetyllactosamine units (reviewed in refs. 67 and 68). In contrast, Sia-lb1 determinants are also represented by short-chain gangliosides as G_{M3} with the structure NeuNAcα2-3Galβ1-4Glc-Cer. It is not known whether Sia-l1 determinants are also represented by type 2 short-chain–based gangliosides like NeuNAcα2-3Galβ1-4Glc-NAcβ1-3Galβ1-4Glc-Cer (sialylneolactotetraosylceramide). As discussed, this could be concluded from the accessibility of the Sia-l1 determinant to the Sia-l1 antibody Fl as well as to the enzyme sialidase only after protease treatment of RBCs.

2. Further structural requirements in addition to sialylation are met with the Sia-b1 Fl determinant; i.e., fucosylation of the 2–6 branch of biantennary type 2 sequences (71,72) (structure 4 in Table 5).

3. We have shown that endo-β-galactosidase does not destroy Sia-b1 Fl and Sia-lb1 antigens on RBCs (66), although i antigens are completely inactivated and I antigens are strongly reduced

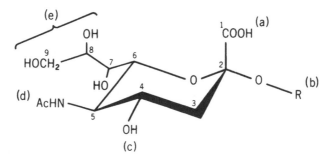

Figure 7 Role of C-1–C-9 of N-acetylneuraminic acid for Sia-lb1 antigenicity. Essential are (a) electric charge; (b) induction of α configuration; (c) intact hydroxyl group; (d) N-acetyl-group rather than N-glycolyl-group; (e) unshortened trihydroxyside chain.

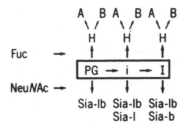

Figure 8 Interrelations between Ii, ABH and Sia-11, -b1, -lb1 antigens.

by the enzyme on RBCs (78). Scudder et al. (77) have shown that terminal sialylation (NeuNAcα2-3) of type 2 chains does not hamper (but even increases) the susceptibility of type 2 chains to endo-β-galactosidase. It is, therefore, not the susceptibility to the enzyme but obviously the accessibility for the enzyme on the RBC membrane that discriminates between Ii and Sia-b1 Fl/Sia-lb1 antigens. This finding points out differences between Ii and the sialoantigens resulting in a different availability for the corresponding antibodies on the RBC surface.

A significant exception are the Sia-b1 antigens recognized by postinfection CAs. Contrasting the Sia-b1 Fl determinant, they do not need fucosyl groups for full expression, as demonstrated by their reactivity with O$_h$ RBCs (72). Contrasting the Sia-b1 Fl determinant again, they are decreased like I determinants on RBCs by endo-β-galactosidase (72). It can be assumed that these Sia-b1 determinants are, in fact, sialylated I determinants. This assumption is in accordance with conceptions on the etiology of postinfection CAs that have been discussed recently in the literature (72) and are discussed below.

C. Sialoautoantigens Not Yet Attributed to Autoantigen Complexes

1. Li Antigen

A cold agglutinin of our collection recognizes an antigen, termed Li, that is inactivated by sialidase on RBCs but resembles the i antigen in all serological respects (85). It is fully expressed only on newborn and i adult RBCs. The Li antigen differs from the Sia-11 antigen, which is also a fetal sialoautoantigen recognized by CAs (75), since it is accessible for sialidase on intact cell surface, whereas the Sia-11 antigen is accessible for sialidase only after protease treatment of RBCs. All data would be consistent with the assumption that the Li antigen is represented by sialylated linear type 2 chains. Surprisingly, Li determinants are not destroyed by endo-β-galactosidase treatment of RBCs (66), contrasting the complete inactivation of i and Sia-11 antigens by the enzyme. The Li antigen has, therefore, not yet been included into the Sia-11, Sia-b1, Sia-lb1 series of sialoautoantigens.

2. Lud Antigen

In 1981, we found a CA recognizing an antigen termed Lud (86). Further examples are known (87,88). The Lud antigen is fully expressed only on adult RBCs and is, therefore, developmentally regulated. Lud antigenicity is abolished by sialidase on RBCs. In this respect, Lud determinants resemble Sia-b1 determinants. Contrasting Sia-b1 antigens, Lud antigens are fully expressed on adult RBCs with the i phenotype, thus obviously excluding type 2 chains to be responsible for Lud determinants. The Lud antigen is the only known developmentally regulated sialoautoantigen not based on type 2 chains. Accordingly, the glycoprotein obtained from papainized RBCs with I and Sia-b1 antigenicity (69) is Lud inactive (89), just as various type 2 chain–based gangliosides (63). The Lud antigen is partially destroyed by proteases on RBCs, thus resembling the Sa antigen. Glycophorins, however, do not express Lud determinants (unpublished data). Immunoblotting results described by Kajii et al. (88) suggest that Lud determinants are found on a 43,000d-RBC membrane glycoprotein.

Pennington and Feizi (90) studied the CA character and the specificity of type XIV pneumococcus antisera. The antisera react like anti-Lud with I, i cord, and i adult RBCs, but they do not require NeuNAc for reaction. The authors speculated that these antibodies could recognize a developmentally regulated increase of unsubstituted type 1 chain sequences, Galβ1-3GlcNAcβ1-3, which are the basic structures of Lewis antigens. It could be further speculated that anti-Lud recognizes sialylated type 1 chains.

3. Ju Antigen

Göttsche et al. (91) described a CA termed anti-Ju that reacts with untreated, protease- and sialidase-treated adult and newborn RBCs in equal strength at 0°C but shows a preferential reaction with untreated RBCs at higher temperatures. The antibody is not inhibited by sialyllactose. We have shown (unpublished data) that the antibody is not inhibited by native and modified glycophorins and isolated glycophorin A but is inhibited by the glycoprotein from papainized RBCs with I and Sia-b1 antigenicity (69). It is uncertain whether the CA recognizes (sialylated) type 2 chains on the glycoprotein and on the RBC membrane.

D. Immunobiologic Relevance of Sialoautoantigens

Contrasting the situation of alloantibody induction, the mechanisms of autoantibody induction are only poorly understood. As will be outlined briefly, the definition of sialoautoantigens contributes substantially to studies on the generation of cold-reactive autoantibodies against red cells (CAs).

1. Association Between Cold Agglutinin Specificities and Structures

a. Variable H and L Chain Regions of Cold Agglutinins.   Because CAs in chronic lymphoproliferative processes are monoclonal antibodies, structural analyses of variable regions of CA H and L chains could be performed. Most anti-I CAs have $V_\kappa III$ L chains and belong to the V_H IV gene family (reviewed in refs. 92 and 93). They express a H chain–associated cross-reactive idiotype codified by the V_H 4-21 germline gene (94–96). Anti-i CAs share the $V_H 4$ preference but do not show preference for $V_\kappa III$ (94).

Variable region data on anti-Pr CAs are limited but informative. Anti-Pr L and H chains belong to other subgroups than anti-I chains. The L chains belong predominantly to the $V_\kappa IV$ subgroup that was only detected by sequence analyses of anti-Pr CAs (97). Four of five anti-Pr κ chains are $V_\kappa IV$ (97–99) and one is $V_\kappa III$ (100). Anti-Pr CAs possess $V_H I$ (100), $V_H II$, and $V_H III$ (97,98) subgroups. Cross-reacting idiotypes among anti-Pr not related to anti-I have been known since 1974 (101); their structures are, however, to be identified.

The data on variable region characteristics of anti-Pr supplement data on anti-Ii. They document a restricted use of H and/or L chain V genes in cold agglutinins dependent on their specificities.

b. Cold Agglutinin Isotypes.   Isotypes, represented by the constant regions of H and L chains, are genetically independent from V_H and V_L regions and are involved neither in antigen-binding sites nor in frame work residues nor in idiotypes but nevertheless show preferences for distinct CA specificities (reviewed in ref. 89). Most strikingly, all rare IgA CAs have specificity for the glycophorin sialoautoantigens Pr and Sa (101a). This apparent restriction of the H chain isotype α to the anti–Pr/-Sa specificity is unexplained. A conclusive explanation of monoclonal CA generation must include an explanation of this peculiar association.

2. Interrelations Between Cold Agglutinin Specificities and Infectious Agents

Certain infectious agents induce CAs with certain specificities. Best known is the induction of anti-I by *Mycoplasma pneumoniae* and of anti-i by the Epstein-Barr virus (reviewed in ref. 89). More recently, we have identified viruses capable of inducing CAs with anti-Pr specificity; i.e., the rubella virus (102,103) and varicella virus (104). Because certain infectious agents induce CAs with distinct specificities, the infectious agent must be responsible for CA specificity. An earlier concept has proposed cross-reactive antigens on the agent and on the red cells. Modern concepts based on experimental data propose that antigens corresponding to CAs are the receptors (acceptors) for the agents rendering them autoimmunogenic by binding. Loomes et al. (105) have demonstrated an interaction of *Mycoplasma pneumoniae* with RBC type 2 chains ("Ii antigen type") provided that type 2 chains are sialylated; i.e., Sia-l1, Sia-b1, and Sia-lb1 antigens. We have shown that sera from patients with recent *Mycoplasma pneumoniae* infections frequently contain mixtures of anti-I plus anti–Sia-b1 autoantibodies (73). Another mechanism of autoantibody induction would be that CAs are anti-idiotypic antibodies against the antibodies to the agent that recognize the ligand for the receptor on the infectious agent (106). In all instances, NeuNAc contributes essentially to the specificity of oligoclonal CAs induced by *Mycoplasma pneumoniae* and obviously also by rubella and varicella viruses. It is either the immunodominant component of a cross-reactive antigen, or it is an essential component of the receptor for the infectious agent, or the binding site of an anti-idiotype is similar to its structure.

ACKNOWLEDGMENT

I am grateful to Hildegard Hack for arranging, correcting, and improving the manuscript. I thank Prof. Dr. W. Dahr for his comments on glycophorin alloantigens.

REFERENCES

1. Hübener G. Untersuchungen über Isoagglutination mit besonderer Berücksichtigung scheinbarer Abweichungen vom Gruppenschema. Z Immun Forsch 1926; 45:223.
2. Thomsen O. Ein vermehrungsfähiges Agens als Veränderer des isoagglutinatorischen Verhaltens der roten Blutkörperchen, eine bisher unbekannte Quelle der Fehlbestimmung. Z Immun Forsch 1927; 52:85.
3. Friedenreich V. The Thomsen hemagglutination phenomenon production of a specific receptor quality in red cell corpuscles by bacterial activity. Doctoral dissertation, Levin University Munksgaard, Copenhagen, 1930.
4. Mäkelä O, Cantell K. Destruction of M and N blood group receptors of human red cells by influenza viruses. Ann Med Exp Biol. Fenniae 1958; 36:366.
5. Springer GF, Ansell NJ. Inactivation of human erythrocyte agglutinogens M and N by influenza viruses and receptor-destroying enzymes. Proc Natl Acad Sci USA 1958; 44:182.
6. Roelcke D. A new serological specificity in cold antibodies of high titer: Anti-HD, Vox Sang 1969; 16:76.
7. Haverkamp J, van Halbeck H, Dorland L, Vliegenthart JFG, Pfeil R, Schauer R. High-resolution ^{1}H-NMR spectroscopy of free and glycosidically linked O-acetylated sialic acids. Eur J Biochem 1982; 122:305.
8. Fifth International Symposium on Glycoconjugates. Kiel, Germany, 1979.
9. Drzeniek R. Substrate specificity of neuraminidases. Histochem J, 1973; 5:271.
10. Burnet FM, Stone D. The receptor destroying enzyme of V. cholerae. Aust J Exp Biol Med Sci 1947; 25:227.
11. Dahr W, Uhlenbruck G, Janssen E, Schmalisch R. Different N-terminal amino acids in the MN-glycoprotein from MM and NN erythrocytes. Hum Genet 1977; 35:335.

12. Wasniowska K, Drzeniek R, Lisowska E. The amino acids of M and N blood group glycopeptides are different. Biochem Biophys Res Commun 1977; 76:385.

13. Anstee DJ. The structure of the MN and Ss blood group antigens. Biotest Bull 1983; 4:318.

14. Judd WJ, Issitt PD, Pavone PG, Anderson J, Aminoff D. Antibodies that define NANA-independent MN-system antigens. Transfusion 1979; 19:12.

15. Lisowska E, Kordowicz M. Specific antibodies for desialized M and N blood group antigens. Vox Sang 1977; 33:164.

16. Pedersen JT, Kaplan H, Wedeck L, Murphy RB, LoBue J, Pincus MR. Octapeptide segments from the amino terminus of glycophorin A contain the antigenic determinants of the M and N blood group systems. J Lab Clin Med 1990; 116:527.

17. Bigbee WL, Vanderlaan M, Fong SSN, Jensen RH. Monoclonal antibodies specific for the M- and N-forms of human glycophorin A. Mol Immunol 1983; 20:1353.

18. Fraser RH, Inglis G, Mackie A, Munro AC, Allan EK, Mitchell R, Sonneborn HH, Uthemann H. Mouse monoclonal antibodies reacting with M blood group-related antigens. Transfusion 1985; 25:261.

19. Nichols ME, Rosenfield RE, Rubinstein P. Two blood group M epitopes disclosed by monoclonal antibodies. Vox Sang 1985; 49:138.

20. Rubocki R, Milgrom F. Reaction of murine monoclonal antibodies to blood group MN antigens. Vox Sang 1986; 51:217.

21. Lisowska E, Messeter L, Duk M, Czerwinski M, Lundblad A. A monoclonal antiglycophorin A antibody recognizing the blood group M determinant: studies on the subspecificity. Mol Immunol 1987; 24:605.

22. Jaskiewicz E, Moulds JJ, Kraemer K, Goldstein AS, Lisowska E. Characterization of the epitope recognized by a monoclonal antibody highly specific for blood group M antigen. Transfusion 1990; 30:230.

23. Fletcher A, Harbour C. An interesting monoclonal anti-N produced following immunization with human group O, NN erythrocytes. J Immunol Genet 1984; 11:121.

24. Bigbee WL, Langlois RG, Vanderlaan M, Jensen RH. Binding specificities of eight monoclonal antibodies to human glycophorin A—studies with $M^{c}M$, and $M^{k}En(UK)$ variant human erythrocytes and M- and MN^{v}-type chimpanzee erythrocytes. J Immunol 1984; 133:3149.

25. Wasniowska K, Duk M, Steuden I, Czerwinski M, Wiedlocha A, Lisowska E. Two monoclonal antibodies recognizing different epitopes of blood group N antigen. Arch Immunol Ther Exp Warsz 1988; 36:623.

26. Lisowska E, Wasniowska K, Jaskiewicz E, Czerwinski M, Steuden I. Monoclonal antibodies against glycophorins. Rev Fr Transfu Immunohématol 1988; 31:261.

27. Zelinski T, Coghlan G, Belcher E, Philipps S, Kaita H, Lewis M. Preliminary serological studies on 31 samples of monoclonal antibodies directed against red cell glycophorins. Rev Fr Transfu Immunohématol 1988; 31:273.

28. Tippett P, Green CA. Monoclonal anti-glycophorin antibodies. Rev Fr Transfu Immunohématol 1988; 31:281.

29. Fraser RH, Murphy MT, Inglis G, Mitchell R. Characterization of antiglycophorin monoclonal antibodies. Rev Fr Transfu Immunohématol 1988; 31:289.

30. Sadler JE, Paulson JC, Hill RL. The role of sialic acid in the expression of human MN blood group antigens. J Biol Chem 1979; 254:2112.

31. Ebert W, Metz J, Roelcke D. Modifications of N-actetylneuraminic acid and their influence on the antigen activity of erythrocyte glycoproteins. Eur J Biochem 1972; 27:470.

32. Issitt PD, Daniels G, Tippett P. Proposed new terminology for En^{a}. Transfusion 1981; 21:473.

33. Dahr W, Müller T, Moulds J, Baumeister G, Issitt PD, Wilkinson S, Garratty G. High frequency antigens of human erythrocyte membrane sialoglycoproteins. I. En^{a} receptors in the glycosylated domain of the MN sialoglycoprotein. Biol Chem Hoppe-Seyler 1985; 366:41.

34. Lisowska E, Duk M, Dahr W. Comparison of alkali-labile oligosaccharide chains of M and N blood-group glycopeptides from human erythrocyte membrane. Carbohydrate Res 1980; 79:103.

35. Daniels GL. Studies on Gerbich negative phenotypes and Gerbich antibodies (abstr). Transfusion 1982; 22:405.

36. Dahr W, Kiedrowski S. Blanchard D, Hermand P, Moulds J, Cartron J. High frequency antigens

of human erythrocyte membrane sialoglycoproteins. V. Characterization of the Gerbich blood group antigens: Ge2 and Ge3. Biol Chem Hoppe-Seyler 1987; 368:1375.

37. Dahr W, Moulds J, Baumeister G, Moulds M, Kiedrowski S, Hummel M. Altered membrane sialoglycoproteins in human erythrocytes lacking the Gerbich blood group antigens. Biol Chem Hoppe-Seyler 1985; 366:201.

38. Dahr W, Blanchard D, Kiedrowski S, Poschmann A, Cartron J, Moulds J. High frequency antigens of human erythrocyte membrane sialoglycoproteins. VI. Monoclonal antibodies reacting with the N-terminal domain of glycophorin C. Biol Chem Hoppe-Seyler 1989; 370:849.

39. Dahr W. Immunochemistry of sialoglycoproteins in human red blood cell membranes. In: Vengelen-Tylev, Judd WJ, eds. Recent Advances in Blood Group Biochemistry. Arlington, VA: American Association of Blood Banks, 1986:23.

40. Reid ME. Hybrid sialoglycoproteins, Gerbich, Webb and Cad blood group determinants. In: Vengelen-Tyler V, Judd WJ, eds. Recent Advances in Blood Group Biochemistry. Arlington, VA: American Association of Blood Bands, 1986:67.

41. Issitt PD. The MN Blood Group System. Cincinnati, OH, Montgomery Scientific Publications, 1981.

42. Dahr W, Knuppertz G, Beyreuther K, Moulds J, Moulds M, Wilkinson S, Capon C, Fournet B, Issitt PD. Studies on the structures of the Tm, Sj, M_1, Can, Sext and Hu blood group antigens. *Biol Chem Hoppe-Seyler* 1991; 372:573.

43. Roelcke D, Uhlenbruck G. Letter to the Editor. Vox Sang 1970; 18:478.

44. Marsh WL, Jenkins WJ. Anti-Sp_1: the recognition of a new cold auto-antibody, Vox Sang 1968; 15:177.

45. Roelcke D. Cold agglutination. Antibodies and antigens. Clin Immunol Immunopathol 1974; 2:266.

46. Roelcke D, Kreft H. Characterization of various anti-Pr cold agglutinins. Transfusion 1984; 24:210.

47. Roelcke D, Pruzanski W, Ebert W, Römer W, Fischer E, Lenhard V, Rauterberg E. A new human monoclonal cold agglutinin Sa recognizing terminal N-acetylneuraminyl groups on the cell surface. Blood 1980; 55:677.

48. Anstee DJ. Blood group MNSs-active sialoglycoproteins of the human erythrocyte membrane. In: Sandler SG, Nusbacher J, Schanfield MS, eds. Immunobiology of the Erythrocytes, Proceedings of the 11th American Red Cross Scientific Symposium. New York: Liss, 1980:67–98.

49. Dahr W, Lichthardt D, Roelcke D. Studies on the receptor sites of the monoclonal anti-Pr and -Sa cold agglutinins. Protides Biol Fluids 1981; 29:365.

50. Tokunaga E, Sasakawa S, Tamaka K, Kawamata H, Giles CM, Ikin EW, Poole J. Anstee DJ, Mawby W, Tanner MJA. Two apparently healthy Japanese individuals of type M^kM^k have erythrocytes which lack both the blood group MN and Ss-active sialoglycoproteins. J Immunogenet 1979; 6:383.

51. Ebert W, Fey J, Gärtner C, Geisen HP, Rautenberg U, Roelcke D, Weicker H. Isolation and partial characterization of the Pr autoantigen determinants. Mol Immunol 1979; 16:413.

52. Lisowska E, Roelcke D. Differentiation of anti-Pr_1- and anti-Pr_2-sera with periodate-oxidized erythrocyte glycoproteins. Blut 1973; 26:339.

53. Roelcke D, Ebert W, Geisen HP. Anti-Pr_3: serological and immunochemical identification of a new anti-Pr subspecificity. Vox Sang 1976; 30:122.

54. Suttajit M, Winzler RJ. Effect of modification of N-acetylneuraminic acid on the binding of glycoproteins to influenza virus and on susceptibility to cleavage by neraminidase. J Biol Chem 1971; 246:3398.

55. Hoare DG, Koshland DE. A method for the quantitative modification and estimation of carboxylic acid groups in proteins. J Biol Chem 1967; 242:2447.

56. Roelcke D. Serological studies on the Pr_1/Pr_2 antigens using dog erythrocytes. Differentiation of Pr_2 from Pr_1 and detection of a Pr_1 heterogeneity: Pr_{1h}/Pr_{1d} Vox Sang 1973; 24:354.

57. Roelcke D, Ebert W, Feizi T. Studies on the specificities of two IgM lambda cold agglutinins. Immunology 1974; 27:879.

58. Roelcke D, Dahr W, Kalden JR. A human monoclonal IgMκ cold agglutinin recognizing oligosaccharides with immunodominant sialyl groups preferentially at the blood group M-specific peptide backbone of glycophorins: anti-Pr^M. Vox Sang 1986; 51:207.

59. Ochiai Y, Furthmayr H, Marcus DM. Diverse specificities of five monoclonal antibodies reactive with glycophorin A of human erythrocytes. J Immunol 1983 131:864.

60. Hinz CF Jr, Boyer JT. Dysgammaglobulinemia in the adult manifested as autoimmune hemolytic anemia. N Engl J Med 1963; 269:1329.
61. Suzuki S, Miura H, Hirakawa S, Sunada M, Amano T, Nishiya K, Ota Z, Roelcke D. A monoclonal IgM/κ cold agglutinin bearing a new anti-Sa subspecificity, Acta Haematol Japonica 1985; 48:1074.
62. Tsai CM, Zopf DA, Yu RK, Wistar R Jr, Ginsburg V. A Waldenström macroglobulin that is both a cold agglutinin and a cryoglobulin because it binds N-acetylneuraminosyl residues. Proc Natl Acad Sci USA 1977; 74:4591.
63. Uemura K, Roelcke D, Nagai Y, Feizi T. The reactivities of human erythrocyte autoantibodies anti-Pr_2, anti-Gd, -Fl and -Sa with gangliosides in a chromatogram binding assay. Biochem J 1984; 219:865.
64. Römer W, Seelig HP, Lenhard V, Roelcke D. The distribution of I/i, Pr and Gd antigens in mammalian tissues. Invest Cell Pathol 1979; 2:157.
65. Roelcke D. A further cold agglutinin, Fl, recognizing a N-acetylneuraminic acid-determined antigen. Vox Sang 1981; 41:98.
66. Roelcke D, Hengge U, Kirschfink M. Neolacto(type-2 chain)-sialoautoantigens recognized by human cold agglutinins. Vox Sang 1990; 59:235.
67. Feizi T. The blood group Ii system: a carbohydrate antigen system defined by naturally monoclonal or oligoclonal autoantibodies of man. Immunol Commun 1981; 10:127.
68. Hakomori S. Blood group ABH and Ii antigens of human erythrocytes: chemistry, polymorphism and their developmental change. Semin Hematol 1981; 18:39.
69. Ebert W, Roelcke D, Weicker H. The I antigen of human red cell membrane. Eur J Biochem 1975; 53:505.
70. Roelcke D, Brossmer R, Ebert W. Anti-Pr, -Gd and related cold agglutinins. Human monoclonal antibodies against neuraminyl groups. Protides Biol Fluids 1981; 29:619.
71. Kannagi R, Roelcke D, Peterson KA, Okada Y, Levery SB, Hakomori S. Characterization of an epitope (determinant) structure in a developmentally regulated glycolipid antigen defined by a cold agglutinin Fl, recognition of α-sialosyl and α-L-fucosyl groups in a branched structure. Carbohydrate Res 1983; 120:143.
72. Roelcke D, Kreft H, Northoff H, Gallasch E. Sia-b1 and I antigens recognized by Mycoplasma pneumoniae-induced cold agglutinins. Transfusion 1991; 31:627.
73. König AL, Kather H, Roelcke D. Autoimmune hemolytic anemia by coexisting anti-I and anti-Fl cold agglutinins. Blut 1984; 49:363.
74. Roelcke D, Weber MT. Simultaneous occurrence of anti-Fl and anti-I cold agglutinins in a patient's serum. Vox Sang 1984; 47:122.
75. Roelcke D, Kreft H, Pfister AM. Cold agglutinin Vo. An IgMλ monoclonal human antibody recognizing a sialic acid determined antigen fully expressed on newborn erythrocytes. Vox Sang 1984; 47:236.
76. Scudder P, Uemura K, Dolby J, Fukuda MN, Feizi T. Isolation and characterization of endo-β-galactosidase from Bacteroides fragilis. Biochem J 1983; 213:485.
77. Scudder P, Hanfland P, Uemura K, Feizi T. Endo-β-galactosidase of Bacteroides fragilis and Escherichia freundii hydrolyze linear but not branched oligosaccharide domains of glycolipids of the neolacto series. J Biol Chem 1984; 259:6586.
78. Fukuda MN, Fukuda M, Hakomori S. Cell surface modification by endo-β-galactosidase. J Biol Chem 1979; 254:5458.
79. Roelcke D, Riesen W, Geisen HP, Ebert W. Serological identification of the new cold agglutinin specificity anti-Gd. Vox Sang 1977; 33:304.
80. Weber RJ, Clem LW. The molecular mechanism of cryoprecipitation and cold agglutination of an IgMλ Waldenström macroglobulin with anti-Gd specificity: sedimentation analysis and localization of interacting sites. J Immunol 1981; 127:300.
81. Staub CA. Cold reacting antibodies recognizing antigens dependent on N-acetylneuraminic acid. Transfusion 1985; 25:414.
82. Kundu SK, Marcus DM, Roelcke D. Glycosphingolipid receptors for anti-Gd and anti-p cold agglutinins. Immunol Lett 1982; 4:263.
83. Roelcke D, Brossmer R, Riesen W. Inhibition of human anti-Gd cold agglutinins by siallyllactose. Scand J Immunol 1978; 8:179.

84. Roelcke D, Brossmer R. Different fine specificities of human monoclonal anti-Gd cold agglutinins. Protides Biol Fluids 1984; 31:1075.

85. Roelcke D. Li cold agglutinin: a further antibody recognizing sialic acid-dependent antigens fully expressed on newborn erythrocytes. Vox Sang 1985; 48:181.

86. Roelcke D. The Lud cold agglutinin: a further antibody recognizing N-acetylneuraminic acid-determined antigens not fully expressed at birth. Vox Sang 1981; 41:316.

87. Kaito K, Kajii E, Takayi S, Sakamoto S, Miura Y. Low titer cold agglutinin disease recognizing Lud or Lud-related antigen. Rinsho Ketsueki 1987; 28:451.

88. Kajii E, Ikemoto S, Miura Y. Localization of the Lud antigen by immunoblotting. Vox Sang 1988; 54:248.

89. Roelcke D. Cold agglutination. Transfu Med Rev 1989; 3:140.

90. Pennington J, Feizi T. Horse anti-type 14 pneumococcus sera behave as cold agglutinins recognizing developmentally regulated antigens apart from the Ii antigens on human erythrocytes. Vox Sang 1982; 43:253.

91. Göttsche B, Salama A, Müller-Eckhardt C. Autoimmune hemolytic anemia caused by a cold agglutinin with a new specificity (anti-Ju). Transfusion 1990; 30:261.

92. Silverman GJ, Dennis AC. Structural characterization of human monoclonal cold agglutinins: evidence for a distinct primary sequence defined V_H4 idiotype. Eur J Immunol 1990; 20:351.

93. Silverman GJ, Chen PP, Carson DA. Cold agglutinins: specificity, idiotypy and structural analysis. Chem Immunol 1990; 48:109.

94. Silberstein LE, Jefferies LC, Goldman J, Friedman D, Moore JS, Nowell PC, Roelcke D, Pruzanski W, Roudier J, Silverman GJ. Variable region gene analysis of pathologic human autoanibodies to the related i and I red blood cell antigens. Blood 1991; 76:2372.

95. Leoni J, Ghiso J, Goñi F, Frangione B. The primary structure of the Fab fragment of protein KAU, a monoclonal immunoglobulin M cold agglutinin. J Biol Chem 1991; 266:2836.

96. Pascual V, Victor K, Lelsz D, Spellerberg MB, Hamblin TJ, Thompson KM, Randen I, Natvig J, Capra JD, Stevenson FK. Nucleotide sequence analysis of the V regions of two IgM cold agglutinins: evidence that the V_H4-21 gene segment is responsible for the major cross reactive idiotype. J Immunol 1991; 146:4385.

97. Wang AC, Fudenberg HH, Wells JV, Roelcke D. A new subgroup of the kappa chain variable region associated with anti-Pr cold agglutinins. Nature 1973; 243:126.

98. Gergely J, Wang AC, Fudenberg HH. Chemical analyses of variable regions of heavy and light chains of cold agglutinins. Vox Sang 1973; 24:432.

99. Capra JD, Kehoe JM. Williams RC Jr, Feizi T, Kunkel HG. Light chain sequences of human IgM cold agglutinins. Proc Natl Acad Sci USA 1972; 69:40.

100. Silberstein LE, Litwin S, Carmack CE. Relationship of variable region genes expressed by a human B cell lymphoma secreting pathologic anti-Pr_2 erythrocyte autoantibodies. J Exp Med, 1989; 169:1631.

101. Feizi T, Kunkel HG, Roelcke D. Cross idiotypic specificity among cold agglutinins in relation to combining activity for blood group-related antigens. Clin Exp Immunol 1974; 18:283.

101a. Roelcke D, Hack H, Kreft H, Macdonald B, Pereira A, Habibi B. IgA cold agglutinins recognize Pr and Sa antigens expressed on glycophorins. Transfusion 1993 (in press).

102. Geisen HP, Roelcke D, Rehn K, Konrad G. Hochtitrige Kälteagglutinine der Spezifität Anti-Pr nach Rötelninfektion. Klin Wochenschr 1975; 53:767.

103. König A, Börner CH, Braun RW, Roelcke D. Cold agglutinins of anti-Pr_a specificity in rubella embryopathy (abstr). Immunobiology 1985; 170:46.

104. Northoff H, Martin A, Roelcke D. An IgG-κ monotypic anti-Pr_{1h} associated with fresh varicella infection. Eur J Haematol 1987; 38:85.

105. Loomes LM, Uemura K, Feizi T. Interaction of Mycoplasma pneumoniae with erythrocyte glycolipids of I and i antigen types. Infect Immun 1985; 47:15.

106. Plotz PH. Autoantibodies are anti-idiotype antibodies to antiviral antibodies. Lancet 1983; 2:824.

4

Erythrocyte Blood Group Antigens Associated with Phosphatidylinositol Glycan-Linked Proteins

MARILYN J. TELEN
Duke University Medical Center
Durham, North Carolina

I. INTRODUCTION

Early membrane biochemists divided membrane proteins into two classes: integral and peripheral. Integral membrane proteins are generally amphipathic and have one or more hydrophobic peptide segments of about 23 amino acids that span the lipid bilayer. Peripheral membrane proteins, on the other hand, are associated with the membrane but are completely external to the lipid bilayer. Prototypic peripheral membrane proteins are cytoskeletal proteins, such as spectrin and actin; such proteins remain attached to the plasma membrane when red blood cells are lysed owing to interactions with integral membrane proteins rather than with the lipid bilayer itself. However, more recently, investigators have realized that a number of proteins can be attached to the membrane via fatty acids that are linked to the protein and also insert into the membrane lipid bilayer. Fatty acids such as palmitate or myristate may be linked to one or more cysteine residues and, by inserting into the lipid bilayer, link the polypeptide to the membrane. A second mode of attachment involves a complex phosphatidylinositol-glycan (GPI) anchor attached to the C terminus of a protein (Fig. 1). A number of cell surface proteins are attached by this latter means, whereas several cytoskeletal proteins and cytoplasmic enzymes are attached to the membrane by cysteine-linked fatty acids.

II. PROTEINS WITH PHOSPHATIDYLINOSITOL-GLYCAN ANCHORS

Proteins with phosphatidylinositol-glycan anchors are found widely among animals and in most (if not all) human tissues (1,2). However, a protein may be GPI linked in one tissue and be expressed with a transmembrane domain in another tissue. Also, the structure of a protein's GPI anchor may vary somewhat from one tissue to another.

A. Structure and Synthesis of Phosphatidylinositol-Glycan Anchors

First well-described in trypanosomes, GPI anchors share a basic structure throughout phylogeny, although variations of the general structure are found among different species as well as among different tissues of the same animal (3–6). In this type of anchor, two fatty acids serve as anchoring lipids and are attached via a phosphate to inositol. In human erythrocytes, however, a third fatty acid (usually palmitate) is attached directly to the inositol (6). Attachment of the protein to the fatty acid anchor is via a tetrasaccharide linked by another phosphate group to ethanolamine. In humans, one such tetrasaccharide has been shown to consist of deacetylated N-glucosamine and three mannoses. The ethanolamine is joined to the carboxyl terminus of the

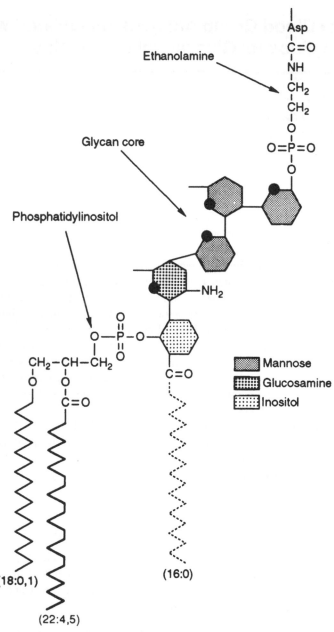

Figure 1 Schematic representation of a phosphatidylinositol-glycan anchor. The glycan core of the anchor is attached via inositol to two or three fatty acids. Two are always attached via phosphate to inositol, whereas a third fatty acid (usually palmitate [dotted line]) may be attached directly to inositol. At its other end, the glycan core is attached via phosphate to ethanolamine, which is in turn attached to the C terminal amino acid via an amide linkage. (From Telen MJ, Rosse WF: Baillieres Clin Haematol 1991; 4:849.)

protein via an amide bond. A second ethanolamine attached to the first mannose may also be present.

Although the process whereby the GPI anchor is synthesized and then attached to the protein is not fully known in detail, many of the steps have been identified (7). The anchor and the protein are initially made separately. The GPI anchor is synthesized in the endoplasmic reticulum, probably initially as a structure containing two fatty acids attached via phosphate to inositol. The other sugars are then added sequentially. N-acetylglucosamine is provided by UDP-N-acetylglucosamine, and the N-acetylglucosamine is deacetylated after its addition to phosphatidylinositol and before addition of the two mannoses. The latter is then followed by addition of phosphoethanolamine. Further modification of this anchor, including replacement of fatty acid or fatty alkyl groups and further glycosylation, may follow attachment of the phosphoethanolamine and even attachment of the anchor to its protein.

The GPI anchor is attached to its protein by a process that involves cleavage of a C terminal peptide from the immature protein and attachment of the GPI moiety to the new C terminus. The signal for this process is contained in the C terminal domain of GPI-linked proteins, but no two such proteins thus far identified share sequence homology in this area. Instead, the signal for GPI anchor attachment appears to reside in two characteristics of the mature protein (8,9). The protein must contain a hydrophobic domain near its C terminus. Then, for the cleavage and GPI anchor attachment to occur, there must also be a pair of small amino acids situated 10–12 residues N terminal to the hydrophobic domain.

B. An Enzyme that Specifically Cleaves Phosphatidylinositol-Glycan Anchors

GPI-anchored proteins can be distinguished from integral membrane proteins by their sensitivity to cleavage by phosphatidylinositol-specific phospholipase C (PI-PLC) and phosphatidylinositol-specific phospholipase D (10). PI-PLC, first well characterized in trypanosomes, can also be isolated from bacteria and mammals. It cleaves the fatty acids attached via the phosphate group from inositol. In those tissues in which a third fatty acid is not added directly to the inositol, this enzymatic action releases the protein from the cell membrane. However, in human erythrocytes, in which most GPI-linked proteins appear also to bear a palmitate directly attached to inositol (see Fig. 1), relatively little GPI-linked protein is released from the membrane by PI-PLC (6,11).

C. Phosphatidylinositol-Linked Proteins on Hematopoietic Cells

Differentiating and mature hematopoietic cells bear a large and ever-growing number of PI-anchored proteins on their surfaces (Table 1). Most of these proteins have been identified as GPI anchored by the finding that they can be removed from the cell by PI-PLC. In some cases, the presence of the anchor has also been demonstrated in biosynthetic experiments. It is interesting to note that some proteins are GPI anchored on erythrocytes, whereas they may be only partially GPI anchored on other cells (e.g., LFA-3) (12) or not GPI anchored at all in other tissues (e.g., acetylcholinesterase) (13). For acetylcholinesterase, for example, it has been shown that the peptide signal sequence for attachment of the GPI anchor is encoded by an exon used specifically in erythroid tissues (14).

Proteins with GPI anchors do not form a single functional class of proteins but rather subserve a variety of roles on the cell surface (see Table 1). Some, such as LFA-3 (CD57), are important to cell-cell interaction and signal transduction (15,16), whereas the type III Fc receptor (CD16) functions as a receptor for immune complexes (17). DAF (decay-accelerating factor) (CD55) and membrane inhibitor of reactive lysis (MIRL) (CD59) act to down-regulate the activation of autologous complement on cell surfaces (18). Other GPI-anchored proteins are enzymes, such as acetylcholinesterase, alkaline phosphatase, and alkaline phosphodiesterase I.

Table 1 Hematopoietic Cell Surface Proteins With
Phosphatidylinositol-Glycan Anchors

Complement regulatory proteins
  Decay accelerating factor (DAF, CD55)*
  Membrane inhibitor of reactive lysis (MIRL, CD59)*
  C8-binding protein (C8BP, HRF)*

Enzymes
  Alkaline phosphatase
  Acetylcholinesterase*
  Alkaline phosphodiesterase I
  5'-Ectonucleotidase (CD73)

Receptors and proteins that facilitate cell-cell interaction
  Lymphocyte function–associated antigen-3 (LFA-3, CD57)*
  Fc receptor III (FcR III, CD16)
  Folate-binding protein
  Neuronal cell adhesion molecule (N-CAM, CD56)

Proteins with other or unknown functions
  CD14
  CD48
  CD67
  JMH protein*
  Hy/Gy protein*

---

*Denotes proteins expressed by mature erythrocytes.

D. Paroxysmal Nocturnal Hemoglobinuria

Although absence of some GPI-linked proteins does not appear to be significantly detrimental
to circulating blood cells, others of these proteins are vital to normal cell survival and function.
This fact has been borne out by observations of patients with the acquired stem cell disease
paroxysmal nocturnal hemoglobinuria (PNH) (19). In PNH, circulating neutrophils, erythrocytes, and platelets derived from affected stem cell clones fail to express GPI-linked proteins.
In each patient, a variable proportion of cells are affected. The hallmark of PNH is hemolysis,
and this is due to the absence or marked underexpression of the complement regulatory proteins
DAF, C8 binding-protein, and MIRL. However, the absence of MIRL is the critical defect in
erythrocyte surface complement regulation (20). On platelets, MIRL may also be the critical
defect that leads to excessive thrombosis in patients with PNH (21). Investigators have shown
that PNH MIRL-deficient platelets, when exposed to complement components C5–C9,
demonstrate 10-fold excess alpha-granule secretion, microparticle formation, and factor Va
binding sites, all procoagulant processes. It is thus far not known if and how the lack of
GPI-linked proteins affects neutrophil function, although abnormal PNH neutrophils appear to
have a relatively normal life span (22).

E. Blood Group Antigens on PI-Linked Proteins

A number of blood group antigens have been shown to reside on GPI-linked proteins (Table
2) (23). Most such antigens so far identified have been found on erythrocytes, although the
NA1/NA2 polymorphism most often responsible for neonatal alloimmune neutropenia resides
on the neutrophil FcR III (24,25). NA1 and the FcR III protein were found to be GPI linked

Table 2 Blood Group Antigens on Proteins with Phosphatidylinositol Anchors

Blood group antigen or system	Protein involved in antigen expression
Cromer	Decay accelerating factor (DAF, CD55)
Cartwright (Yt)	Acetylcholinesterase
JMH	76 kD glycoprotein
Hy, Gy^a	47–58 kD glycoprotein
Dombrock	Possibly the same protein as Hy and Gy^a
Emm	Unknown

because they could be removed by PI-PLC and were also absent from PNH neutrophils (26). However, the erythrocyte antigens are only poorly cleaved from red cells by PI-PLC, presumably owing to direct attachment of a third fatty acid to inositol (6). In order to demonstrate what erythrocyte blood group antigens reside on PI-linked proteins, erythrocytes from patients with PNH were examined (23).

Earlier work by Chow and colleagues had demonstrated that normal and GPI-deficient PNH red cells could be separated by column chromatography dependent on the expression or absence of acetylcholinesterase (27). In this method, a suspension of washed red cells containing a mixture of normal and GPI-deficient cells is first incubated with murine monoclonal anti-acetylcholinesterase and then rabbit antimouse immunoglobulin G (IgG). The washed cells are then passed through a Sepharose 6MB-Staphylococcal Protein A column, to which only the antibody-coated cells adhere. Nonadherent GPI-deficient cells are then recovered in the effluent.

Cells obtained by this method were compared with complement-insensitive (and thus not GPI-deficient) cells from the same patients for expression of a variety of blood group antigens (23). Most blood group antigens tested were equally well expressed by both normal and PNH GPI-deficient erythrocytes. Those not expressed specifically by the GPI-deficient PNH cells were the Cromer blood group antigens, JMH, Holley/Gregory (Hy/Gy), Dombrock (Do^a and Do^b), Cartwright (Yt^a and Yt^b), and the high-incidence antigen Emm. The Cromer and Cartwright blood group antigens have now been shown to reside on known GPI-linked proteins (decay-accelerating factor and acetylcholinesterase, respectively), whereas the JMH and Hy/Gy antigens are partially characterized biochemically and appear at this writing to identify novel proteins. The Dombrock and Emm antigens remain biochemically uncharacterized.

III. DECAY-ACCELERATING FACTOR AND CROMER ANTIGENS

For many years, the defect(s) underlying the complement sensitivity of PNH erythrocytes was not understood, and cellular defenses against complement activation were unknown. However, in the early 1980s, largely through the work of Nicholson-Weller and her colleagues, the existence and role of decay accelerating factor became known (29,30). Demonstration that DAF was absent from PNH erythrocytes (31), as well other hematopoietic cells of PNH patients (32), led in turn to the understanding that PNH was associated with failure to express a number of proteins, all of which had in common that they were linked to the membrane via GPI anchors and some of which were complement-regulatory proteins (33).

A. Decay-Accelerating Factor Biochemistry and Genetics

Decay-accelerating factor is a glycoprotein that was first shown to destabilize the C3 convertase (C4bC2a) of the classic pathway of complement activation (34). It also has a similar effect on the C3 convertase of the alternative pathway (C3bBb).

As do all GPI-linked proteins investigated to date, DAF is organized so that its N terminus is distal from the membrane attachment site (Fig. 2) (35–37). Starting at the N terminus, DAF contains four homologous regions, most likely organized as loops held together by disulfide bonds. Each homologous region, also termed a short consensus repeat (SCR), is about 66 amino acids long and also shares homology with other complement-related proteins, including C2, factor B, factor H, complement receptors types 1 and 2, and C4-binding protein (38). Between the first and second SCRs is a single N-linked oligosaccharide. Potential sites for O-glycosylation also exist within the SCRs. The SCR region is linked to a 70–amino acid serine threonine–rich region that contains multiple sites for O-linked glycosylation and lacks sites for formation of disulfide bonds. This presumably more linearly arranged peptide domain may act as a stalk that serves to extend the SCR region, which is also the functional domain, into its appropriate milieu. Finally, the C terminus of the mature protein is produced by cleavage of a hydrophobic peptide domain encoded by the messenger ribonucleic acid (mRNA) and attachment of the glycolipid anchor to the enzymatically created C terminus.

Decay-accelerating factor is encoded by a gene within the regulation of complement activation (RCA) gene cluster on chromosome 1 (39,40). This gene cluster contains numerous genes encoding proteins that down-regulate the effects of complement activation, including complement receptors types 1 (CR1) and 2 (CR2), factor H, C4-binding protein (C4BP), membrane cofactor protein (MCP), and DAF (41,42). These genes have been partially mapped in relation to one another and are in the order: MCP-CR1-CR2-DAF-C4BP. Of these proteins, only DAF and CR1 are expressed on erythrocytes; CR1 is not GPI anchored and has recently been shown to bear the Knops/McCoy blood group antigens (43,44).

The organization of the DAF gene strongly suggests that the SCRs arose from a primordial

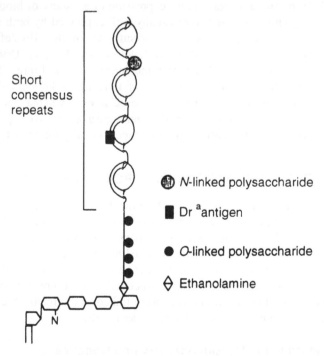

Figure 2   Organization of the decay accelerating factor (DAF) protein. The N terminal portion of DAF consists of four short consensus repeats, with one N-linked oligosaccharide situated between SCR1 and SCR2. The Dr[a] antigen is located within SCR 3. C-terminal to the SCRs is a serine/threonine–rich domain that is highly O-glycosylated. (From Telen MJ, Rosse WF: Baillieres Clin Haematol 4:849.)

gene (45), as SCRs 1, 2, and 4 are each encoded by a single exon. Short consenus repeat 3 is encoded by two exons, whereas a single exon encoding 5′ untranslated sequence and a signal peptide precedes the exon encoding SCR 1. The serine/threonine–rich region is encoded by three exons. One exon encodes an *Alu*-type sequence, but the corresponding RNA is found in only a minority of transcripts, and no protein domain corresponding to this exon has been demonstrated. Finally, the hydrophobic domain largely cleaved during attachment of the anchor is also encoded by a single exon that also contains 3′ untranslated sequence. The first 10 exons occur relatively close to one another, whereas exon 11, encoding the hydrophobic domain, is 20 kb away from exon 10, giving the total gene a size of about 40 kb. Three restriction fragment length polymorphisms (RFLPs) dependent on noncoding sequence have been described within the DAF gene region, whereas a fourth is related to the Dr(a+)/Dr(a–) polymorphism (see below).

B. Cromer Blood Group Antigens

The Cromer blood group comprises a group of antigens initially proposed to be related because they were all absent from the apparent null red cells of an individual denoted Inab (46). A number of high-frequency Cromer antigens have now been described (47). These include Cr^a, Tc^a, Dr^a, Es^a, WES^b, and UMC. Two low-frequency alleles of Tc^a—Tc^b and Tc^c—have been identified, and the rare WES^a allele has also been found. In addition, a second phenotype— Dr(a–)—has been shown to involve both absence of the Dr^a antigen as well as underexpression of all other high-frequency Cromer antigens. Finally, persons who fail to express all Cromer antigens (the Inab phenotype) make an antibody denoted anti-IFC that reacts with all cells not also of the Inab phenotype.

The first insights into the biochemistry of Cromer antigens were made by Spring and colleagues, who used murine monoclonal antibodies with IFC-like reactivity as well as human antibodies to demonstrated reactivity with an approximately 70-kd protein on Western (immuno) blots (48). This protein was then demonstrated to be DAF by a number of methods (28). Using biochemically rather than immunologically purified DAF, Telen and colleagues demonstrated that soluble DAF could inhibit the binding of human anti-Cr^a and anti-Tc^a to normal erythrocytes (28). They also demonstrated reactivity of these human antisera with purified DAF on immunoblots and showed that DAF-deficient PNH erythrocytes were also negative for all high-frequency Cromer antigens. Finally, they showed that rabbit polyclonal antibody to DAF did not bind to Inab erythrocytes, confirming these latter cells as Cromer-null.

C. The Inab Phenotype

The Inab phenotype has now been shown to arise from an inherited inability to express DAF protein (28,49,50). Persons with this phenotype, however, do not have hemolytic disease, although their erythrocytes exhibit increased complement sensitivity in several in vitro assays. Importantly, Inab cells are not PNH-like, in that they express other GPI-linked proteins normally (28). Among the GPI-linked proteins shown to be normally expressed on Inab cells are LFA-3, acetylcholinesterase, and CD59.

The existence of cells with the Inab phenotype has provided a unique opportunity to study the physiological role and importance of DAF (51,52). In the complement lysis sensitivity test of Rosse and Dacie (53), Inab cells are only about two times more sensitive to complement than are normal cells, whereas PNH cells are often at least 10 times more sensitive (51). However, other assays confirmed the difference between Inab and normal erythrocytes. When complement-fixing anti-I was used in varying dilutions, Inab cells were easily lysed at dilutions that caused no lysis of normal cells despite comparable levels of I expression (51). Also, the sucrose hemolysis test was weakly positive with Inab erythrocytes (51,52). Interestingly, however, the acidified serum lysis (Ham's) test was normal with Inab cells (51,52). The mechanism for the effect of DAF deficiency on Inab erythrocyte complement sensitivity was confirmed to be at the regulation of C3 convertase by direct measurement of C3 convertase activity in the alternative pathway (51). When nickel-stabilized C3 convertases were created with cobra venom factor, approximately the same amount of C3b was initially fixed to Inab and normal erythrocytes. However, over time, both PNH and Inab erythrocytes continued to allow fixation of additional C3b, whereas normal cells did not, indicating the defective ability to regulate this step of complement activation on Inab membranes. Inab cells differ from PNH cells, however, in that the regulation of the terminal complement components is normal owing to the presence of MIRL (CD59).

Thus far, the genetic basis for the Inab phenotype has been identified in only one individual, the original Inab (50). In this person, the DAF gene is grossly normal, as is mRNA from Epstein-Barr virus (EBV)–transformed lymphocytes. However, a single point mutation early in the gene causes a frameshift and premature termination of the gene product (D.M. Lublin, M.J. Telen, D.J. Anstee, and M.J.A. Tanner, unpublished data). A second individual with this phenotype is known not to have this mutation, but the genetic basis of the phenotype has not yet been established (D.M. Lublin and M.J. Telen, unpublished data). The sera of three Inab individuals have been looked at for expression of factor H and C4-binding protein, both of which were normal (M.J. Telen and W.F. Rosse, unpublished data). Thus, the Inab phenotype presumably arises from a variety of mutations, many or most of which do not involve large gene deletions. Also undetermined is the location of the IFC epitope recognized by antibodies made by Inab individuals.

D.   The Dr(a–) Phenotype

This unusual phenotype has thus far only been found in Jewish Israeli emigrants from the Bukhara region of Russia and in one other Eastern European. First described by Levene et al. (54,55), the proposita's cells were shown to react only weakly with anti-Cr^a, anti-Tc^a, and anti-IFC. In addition, the proposita produced an antibody that reacted with Cr(a–), Tc(a–) but not Inab erythrocytes and thus defined a new Dr^a antigen. This phenotype was later shown to be inherited.

The Dr(a–) phenotype has now been extensively investigated (56). Dr(a–) erythrocytes express about 40% of the normal amount of DAF, whereas other GPI-linked proteins are expressed normally on these cells. Immunoblots of Dr(a–) cell membrane proteins demonstrate reduced protein expression but normal or near-normal protein mobility, indicating that the DAF expressed in the Dr(a–) phenotype is largely normal biochemically. Complement lysis sensitivity testing is also normal.

Investigations at the genetic level have shown that the Dr(a–) phenotype is associated with a single point mutation in the second exon encoding SCR 3 (56). A C $\rightarrow$ T change results in a single amino acid substitution (^{165}serine to leucine), an event also likely to lead to reduced O-glycosylation in that region. This point mutation is also detectable as a TaqI RFLP when this region of genomic DNA is amplified by PCR techniques. Furthermore, transfectants containing DAF complementary deoxyribonucleic acid (cDNA) normal except for this point mutation fail to react with human anti-Dr^a, whereas transfectants expressing the "wild-type" cDNA do react with such antisera.

However, transfection of mammalian cells with Dr(a–)-type cDNA does not lead to lower levels of expression of DAF nor to abnormal synthesis and degradation kinetics (56). However, examination of EBV-transformed lymphocytes from Dr(a–) individuals shows the production of two mRNA species, one of which is not present in normal cells (D.M. Lublin and M.J. Telen, unpublished data). This second, predominant mRNA species contains a deletion apparently due to a missplicing event. This deletion, in turn, leads to a frame shift and premature stop codon. Thus, defective expression of DAF in Dr(a–) cells is due to expression of an aberrant transcript unable to be translated into a functional protein.

E. Other DAF/Cromer Polymorphisms

The most common polymorphisms of the Cromer blood group are the absence of Cr^a and Tc^a. Thus far, only the Cr(a–) phenotype has been investigated at the genetic level. This work (M.J. Telen and D.M. Lublin, unpublished data) has demonstrated that three unrelated individuals all have the same point mutation in the exon encoding SCR 4. Use of transfectants containing DAF cDNA in which various deletions have been made also map the Cr^a epitope to SCR 4.

IV. ACETYLCHOLINESTERASE AND CARTWRIGHT ANTIGENS

As mentioned above, acetylcholinesterase was the first protein found absent from PNH erythrocytes (57). When such erythrocytes were investigated for blood group antigen expression, Cartwright antigens were one group found to be lacking from PNH cells (23). However, investigation of the biochemical basis of Cartwright antigens has been hampered by the generally low titer and avidity of anti-Yt^a and lack of individuals with the Yt(a–b–) phenotype.

Two groups of investigators have now demonstrated that the Cartwright antigens reside on acetylcholinesterase (58,59). The first group to do so showed that anti-Yt^a and anti-Yt^b could be used to isolate acetylcholinesterase enzyme activity from lysates of erythrocyte membranes (58). Furthermore, proteins isolated with these antibodies showed identical migration in SDS-PAGE as did proteins isolated using monoclonal antibodies to acetylcholinesterase. The second group of investigators worked with cells from an individual who demonstrated an apparently transient Yt(a–b–) phenotype (59). During the time that he was Yt(a–b–), this individual's cells were markedly deficient in acetylcholinesterase activity and failed to bind numerous monoclonal antibodies to acetylcholinesterase. This group also showed that anti-Yt^a could immunoprecipitate a protein of the same size as acetylcholinesterase (59).

The location of the high-frequency Yt^a and low-frequency Yt^b epitopes has not yet been identified. Erythrocyte, muscle, and brain acetylcholinesterase share the same structure except for their modes of attachment to the membrane (60,61). Only the erythrocyte enzyme is GPI anchored. This anchor depends on use of a relatively small exon encoding the C terminus, including an appropriate hydrophobic domain (14). Studies to examine whether Yt antigens reside on muscle or brain acetylcholinesterase and search for a DNA polymorphism corresponding to the Yt^a/Yt^b blood group polymorphism should eventually elucidate the basis of the Yt blood group antigens.

V. THE JMH PROTEIN

The JMH antigen is another high-frequency antigen found to be missing from complement-sensitive PNH erythrocytes (23). First described in the 1970s (62), most antibodies to JMH are made by elderly individuals who themselves express a transient or acquired JMH-negative or JMH-weak phenotype. However, one family with an inherited JMH-negative phenotype as well as a family with an inherited JMH-weak phenotype have been described (63,64). In addition, several JMH-variant phenotypes have now been characterized serologically (65). Persons with these variant phenotypes have been found to produce antibodies to epitopes that are variably expressed by JMH-positive individuals. And finally, although the serology of the JMH system has been studied using erythrocytes, a monoclonal antibody with JMH-like reactivity has been produced by immunization of a mouse with a cells from a human T-cell line (66,67). Indeed,

JMH appears to be expressed at least weakly by peripheral blood lymphocytes as well as most human B- and T-lymphocyte cell lines.

Recently, investigators have used anti-JMH sera to identify a novel membrane protein and demonstrate it to be GPI linked (68). When JMH-negative red blood cells were examined for expression of known GPI-linked proteins, they were found to express DAF, acetylcholinesterase, LFA-3, and CD59 normally. These data suggested that the JMH antigen resided on a protein different from these well-characterized GPI-linked erythrocyte proteins.

Both human antisera to a polymorphic JMH epitope (Meged) as well as the monoclonal antibody H8, previously described as having JMH specificity, were used in immunoprecipitation and immunoblotting studies (68). Both techniques demonstrated that these antisera identified a protein of 76 kd found in human erythrocyte membranes. Interestingly, although the JMH antigen is destroyed by sulfhydryl-reducing reagents, electrophoresis of the isolated protein under reducing conditions produced no detectable shift in apparent molecular weight. This suggests that the JMH protein is a single-chain molecule that contains one or more disulfide bonds that contribute little to the physical dimensions of the protein. When JMH protein was isolated from a T-cell line, a similar protein of slightly lower apparent molecular weight (72–74 kd) was isolated.

In order to prove that the JMH protein was absent from PNH cells because it was GPI anchored, investigators have also directly demonstrated that the protein can be released from the membrane by cleavage using PI-PLC (68). However, as with acetylcholinesterase (6), only a small percentage of erythrocyte JMH protein was releasable with PI-PLC. Nevertheless, JMH protein could be isolated from the supernatant fluid of PI-PLC–treated erythrocytes. The released protein was similar in molecular weight to native, detergent-solubilized JMH protein, an observation similar to that made in the study of the GPI-linked Fc receptor CD16 (69), but unlike observations made in the study of DAF, LFA-3, and CD59 (70–73).

Also like FcR III (74), the JMH protein can be released largely intact via a protease (75). Although the protease responsible for this release has not been identified, its action has been shown to be inhibitable using a variety of protease inhibitors. The product of proteolytic release of JMH is a protein of 67 kd. However, unlike FcR III, no JMH protein has been detectable in serum (K.A. Bobolis and M.J. Telen, unpublished data). Thus, the physiological significance of this type of release via proteolysis is unclear; investigators have proposed such proteolysis as a possible mechanism for the acquired JMH-negative phenotype (75).

VI. THE HY/GY PROTEIN

The Hy and Gy^a erythrocyte blood group antigens have been associated with each other because of the high concordance of the Hy-negative and Gy(a–) phenotypes: Red cells that are Gy(a–) are nearly always Hy negative (76,77). The Hy and Gy^a antigens were also found to be absent from abnormal PNH erythrocytes, suggesting that they reside on phosphatidylinositol-linked proteins (23). Spring and Reid have now successfully used antisera to these antigens to identify immunoreactive proteins by Western blotting (78). Both types of antisera identified diffusely migrating proteins of approximately 46,750–57,550 d on antigen-positive cells. Membrane proteins from antigen-negative cells were appropriately nonreactive. Perhaps most interestingly, antigenic protein isolated via its reactivity with one type of antisera could be shown to be immunoreactive with the other sera by immunoblotting, implying that the Hy and Gy^a epitopes exist on the same protein species. The Hy/Gy^a protein appears to be a glycoprotein containing one or more N-linked oligosaccharides and was sensitive to digestion with a variety of proteases, including trypsin, chymotrypsin, and pronase. The protein identified with anti-Hy and anti-Gy^a appeared nonidentical to the similarly migrating GPI-linked protein LFA-3 (78).

VII. SUMMARY

Phosphatidylinositol-glycan linkage is a relatively recently described mechanism of anchoring surface membrane proteins. Thus far, a small number of erythrocyte blood group antigens have been identified as residing on proteins with GPI anchors. These antigens include those of the Cromer, Cartwright, JMH, Hy/Gy[a], and Dombrock blood group systems. In the first four of these blood groups, the protein bearing the antigens has been identified and at least partly characterized. Within the Cromer blood group, several of the phenotypes have been extensively investigated and their genetic bases delineated. Transfectants expressing different Cromer phenotypes have been shown to be useful in confirming antisera specificity. The use of blood group antisera to identify previously undescribed proteins is one of the other exciting aspects of research into GPI-anchored proteins.

ACKNOWLEDGMENTS

This work has been funded in part by grants RO1 HL35572 and RO1 HL44042 from the National Heart, Lung and Blood Institute, National Institutes of Health. M.J.T. is the recipient of Research Career Development Award KO4 HL02233 (NHLBI, NIH).

REFERENCES

1. Low MG, Saltiel AR. Structural and functional roles of glycosyl-phosphatidylinositol in membranes. Science 1988; 239:6740.
2. Cross GAM. Glycolipid anchoring of plasma membrane proteins. Ann Rev Cell Biol 1990; 6:1.
3. Ferguson MAJ, Homans SW, Dwek RA, Rademacher TW. Glycosyl-phosphatidylinositol moiety that anchors *Trypanosoma brucei* variant surface glycoprotein to the membrane. Science 1988; 239:753.
4. Homans SW, Ferguson MAJ, Dwek RA, Rademacher TW, Anand R, Williams AF. Complete structure of the glycosyl phosphatidylinositol membrane anchor of rat brain Thy-1 glycoprotein. Nature 1988; 333:269.
5. Roberts WL, Santikarn S, Reinhold VN, Rosenberry TL. Structural characterization of the glycoinositol phospholipid membrane anchor of human erythrocyte acetylcholinesterase by fast atom bombardment mass spectrometry. J Biol Chem 1988; 263:18776.
6. Roberts WL, Myher JJ, Kuksis A, Low MG, Rosenberry TL. Lipid analysis of the glycoinositol phospholipid membrane anchor of human erythrocyte acetylcholinesterase. Palmitoylation of inositol results in resistance to phosphatidylinositol-specific phospholipase C. J Biol Chem 1988; 263:18766.
7. Doering TL, Masterson WJ, Hart GW, Englund PT. Biosynthesis of glycosyl phosphatidylinositol membrane anchors. J Biol Chem 1990; 265:611.
8. Moran P, Caras IW. A nonfunctional sequence converted to a signal for glycophosphatidylinositol membrane anchor attachment. J Cell Biol 1991; 115:329.
9. Moran P, Caras IW. Fusion of sequence elements from non-anchored proteins to generate a fully functional signal for glycophosphatidylinositol membrane anchor attachment. J Cell Biol 1991; 115:1595.
10. Low MG, Stiernberg J, Waneck GL, Flavell RA, Kincade PW. Cell-specific heterogeneity in sensitivity of phosphatidylinositol-anchored membrane antigens to release by phospholipase C. J Immunol Methods 1988; 113:101.
11. Walter EI, Roberts WL, Rosenberry TL, Ratnoff WD, Medof ME. Structural basis for variations in the sensitivity of human decay accelerating factor to phosphatidylinositol-specific phospholipase C cleavage. J Immunol 1990; 144:1030.
12. Dustin ML, Selvaraj P, Mattaliano RJ, Springer TA. Anchoring mechanisms for LFA-3 cell adhesion glycoprotein at membrane surface. Nature 1987; 329:846.

13. Schumacher M, Maulet Y, Camp S, Taylor P. Multiple messenger RNA species give rise to the structural diversity in acetylcholinesterase. J Biol Chem 1988; 263:18979.

14. Li Y, Camp S, Rachinsky TL, Getman D, Taylor P. Gene structure of mammalian acetyl-cholinesterase: alternative exons dictate tissue-specific expression. J Biol Chem 1991; 266: 23083.

15. Krensky AM, Sanchez-Madrid F, Robbins E, Nagy JA, Springer TA, Burakoff SJ. The functional significance, distribution, and structure of LFA-1, LFA-2, and LFA-3: cell surface antigens associated with CTL-target interactions. J Immunol 1983; 131:611.

16. Springer TA, Dustin ML, Kishimoto TK, Marlin SD. The lymphocyte function-associated LFA-1, CD2, and LFA-3 molecules: cell adhesion receptors of the immune system. Ann Rec Immunol 1987; 5:223.

17. Selvaraj P, Rosse WF, Silber R, Springer TA. The major Fc receptor in blood has a phospha-tidylinositol anchor and is deficient in paroxysmal nocturnal hemoglobinuria. Nature 1988; 333:565.

18. Rosse WF. Phosphatidylinositol-linked proteins and paroxysmal nocturnal hemoglobinuria. Blood 1990; 75:1595.

19. Rosse WF. Paroxysmal nocturnal hemoglobinuria. In: Clinical Immunohematology: Basic Concepts and Clinical Applications. Oxford, England: Blackwell, 1990:593.

20. Holguin MH, Wilcox LA, Bernshaw NJ, Rosse WF, Parker CJ. Relationship between the membrane inhibitor of reactive lysis and the erythrocyte phenotypes of paroxysmal nocturnal hemoglobinuria. J Clin Invest 1989; 84:1487.

21. Wiedmer T, Hall SE, Ortel TL, Kane WH, Rosse WF, Sims PJ. Complement-induced vesiculation and exposure of membrane prothrombinase sites in PNH platelets. Blood 1991; 78(Suppl.):387a.

22. Brubaker L, Essig LJ, Mengel CE. Neutrophil life span in paroxysmal nocturnal hemoglobinuria. Blood 1977; 50:657.

23. Telen MJ, Rosse WF, Parker CJ, Moulds MK, Moulds JJ. Evidence that several high-frequency human blood group antigens reside on phosphatidylinositol-linked erythrocyte membrane proteins. Blood 1990; 75:1404.

24. Huizanga TWJ, Kleijer M, Tetteroo PAT, Roos D, Kr von dem Borne AEG. The biallelic neutrophil NA-antigen system is associated with a polymorphism in phosphoinositol-linked Fc receptor III (CD16). Blood 1989; 75:213.

25. Ory PA, Clark NR, Kwoh EE, Clarkson SB, Goldstein IM. Sequences of complementary DNAs that encode the NA1 and NA2 forms of Fc receptor III on human neutrophils. J Clin Invest 1989; 84:1688.

26. Selvaraj P, Rosse WF, Silber R, Springer TA. The major Fc receptor in blood has a phos-phatidylinositol anchor and is deficient in paroxysmal nocturnal hemoglobinuria. Nature 1988; 333:565.

27. Chow F-L, Hall SE, Rosse WF, Telen MJ. Separation of the acetylcholinesterase-deficient red cells in paroxysmal nocturnal hemoglobinuria. Blood 1986; 67:893.

28. Telen MJ, Hall SE, Green AM, Moulds JJ, Rosse WF. Identification of human erythrocyte blood group antigens on decay-accelerating factor (DAF) and an erythrocyte phenotype negative for DAF. J Exp Med 1988; 167:1993.

29. Nicholson-Weller A, Burge J, Austen KF. Purification from guinea pig erythrocyte stroma of a decay-accelerating factor for the classical C3 convertase, C4b,2a. J Immunol 1981; 127:2031.

30. Nicholson-Weller A, Burge J, Fearon DT, Weller PF, Austen KF. Isolation of a human erythrocyte membrane glycoprotein with decay-accelerating activity for C3 convertases of the complement system. J Immunol 1982; 129:184.

31. Nicholson-Weller A, March JP, Rosenfeld SI, Austen KF. Affected erythrocytes of patients with paroxysmal nocturnal hemoglobinuria are deficient in the complement regulatory protein decay accelerating factor. Proc Natl Acad Sci USA 1983; 80:5066.

32. Nicholson-Weller A, Spicer DB, Austen KF. Deficiency of the complement regulatory protein "decay accelerating factor," on membranes of granulocytes, monocytes, and platelets in paroxysmal nocturnal hemoglobinuria. N Engl J Med 1985; 312:1091.

33. Rosse WF. Phosphatidylinositol-linked proteins and paroxysmal nocturnal hemoglobinuria (PNH) red blood cells. Blood 1990; 75:1595.

34. Medof ME, Kinoshita T, Nussenzweig V. Inhibition of complement activation on the surface of cells after incorporation of decay-accelerating factor (DAF) into their membranes. J Exp Med 1984; 160:1558.

35. Davitz MA, Schlesinger D, Nussenzweig V. Isolation of decay accelerating factor (DAF) by a two-step procedure and determination of its N-terminal sequence. Journal of Immunolog Methods 1987;97:71.

36. Caras IW, Davitz MA, Rhee L, Weddell G, Martin DW Jr, Nussenzweig V. Cloning of decay-accelerating factor suggests novel use of splicing to generate two proteins. Nature 1987; 325:545.

37. Medof ME, Lublin DM, Holers VM, Ayers DJ, Getty RR, Leykam JF, Atkinson JP, Tykocinski ML. Cloning and characterization of cDNAs encoding the complete sequence of decay-accelerating factor of human complement. Proc Natl Acad Sci USA 1987; 84:2007.

38. Nicholson-Weller A, Zaia J, Raum MG, Coligan JE. Decay accelerating factor (DAF) peptide sequences share homology with a consensus sequence found in the superfamily of structurally related complement proteins and other proteins including haptoglobin, factor XIII, beta 2-glyco-protein I, and the IL-2 receptor. Immunol Lett 1987; 14:307.

39. Lublin DM, Lemons RS, Le Beau MM, Holers VM, Tykocinski ML, Medof ME, Atkinson JP. The gene encoding decay-accelerating factor (DAF) is located in the complement-regulatory locus on the long arm of chromosome 1. J Exp Med 1987; 165:1731.

40. Rey-Campos J, Rubinstein P, Rodriguez de Cordoba S. Decay-accelerating factor. Genetic polymorphism and linkage to the RCA (regulator of complement activation) gene cluster in humans. J Exp Med 1987; 166:246.

41. Rey-Campos J, Rubinstein P, Rodriguez de Cordoba S. A physical map of the human regulator of complement activation gene cluster linking the complement genes CR1, CR2, DAF, and C4BP. J Exp Med 1988; 167:664.

42. Carroll MC, Alicot EM, Katzman PJ, Klickstein LB, Smith JA, Fearon DT. Organization of the genes encoding complement receptors type 1 and 2, decay-accelerating factor, and C4-binding protein in the RCA locus on human chromosome 1. J Exp Med 1988; 167:1271.

43. Rao N, Ferguson DJ, Lee S-F, Telen MJ. Identification of human erythrocyte blood group antigens on the C3b/C4b receptor (CR1) J Immunol 1991; 146:3502.

44. Moulds JM, Nickells MW, Moulds JJ, Brown MC, Atkinson JP. The C3b/C4b receptor is recognized by the Knops/McCoy/Swain-Langley, and York blood group antisera. J Exp Med 1991; 173:1159.

45. Post TW, Arce MA, Liszewski MK, Thompson ES, Atkinson JP, Lublin DM. Structure of the gene for human complement protein decay accelerating factor. J Immunol 1990; 144:740.

46. Daniels GL, Tohyama H, Uchikawa M. A possible null phenotype in the Cromer-related blood group complex. Transfusion 1982; 22:362.

47. Daniels G. Cromer-related antigens—blood group determinants on decay-accelerating factor. Vox Sang 1989; 56:205.

48. Spring FA, Judson PA, Daniels GL, Parsons SF, Mallinson G, Anstee DJ. A human cell surface glycoprotein that carries Cromer-related blood group antigens on erythrocytes and is also expressed on leucocytes and platelets. Immunology 1987; 62:307.

49. Lin RC, Herman J, Henny L, Daniels GL. A family showing inheritance of the Inab phenotype. Transfusion 1988; 28:427.

50. Tate CG, Uchikawa M, Tanner MJ, Judson PA, Parsons SF, Mallinson G, Anstee DJ. Studies on the defect which causes absence of decay accelerating factor (DAF) from the peripheral blood cells of an individual with the Inab phenotype. Biochem J 1989; 261:489.

51. Telen MJ, Green AM. The Inab phenotype: characterization of the membrane protein and complement regulatory defect. Blood 1989; 74:437.

52. Merry AH, Rawlinson VI, Uchikawa M, Daha MR, Sim RB. Studies on the sensitivity to complement-mediated lysis of erythrocytes (Inab phenotype) with a deficiency of DAF (decay accelerating factor). Br J Haematol 1989; 73:248.

53. Rosse WF, Dacie JV. Immune lysis of normal human and paroxysmal nocturnal hemoglobinuria (PNH) red blood cells. I. The sensitivity of PNH red cells to lysis by complement and specific antibody. J Clin Invest 1966; 45:736.

54. Levene C, Harel N, Lavie G, Greenberg S, Laird-Fryer B, Daniels GL. A "new" phenotype confirming the relationship between Cr[a] and Tc[a]. Transfusion 1984; 24:13.

55. Levene C, Harel N, Kende G, Papo S, Bradford MF, Daniels GL. A second Dr(a–) proposita with anti-Dr[a] and a family with the Dr(a–) phenotype in two generations. Transfusion 1987; 27:64.

56. Lublin DM, Thompson ES, Green AM, Levene C, Telen MJ. Dr(a–) polymorphisms of decay accelerating factor: biochemical, functional and molecular characterization and production of allele-specific transfectants. J Clin Invest 1991; 87:1945.

57. Auditore JV, Hartmann RC, Flexner JM, Balchum OJ. The erythrocyte acetylcholinesterase enzyme in paroxysmal nocturnal hemoglobinuria. Arch Pathol 1960; 69:534.

58. Spring FA, Anstee DJ. Evidence that the Yt blood group antigens are located on human erythrocyte acetylcholinesterase (AChE) (abstr). Transfu Med 1(Suppl 2):42.

59. Telen MJ, Whitsett CF. Erythrocyte acetylcholinesterase bears the Cartwright blood group antigens. Clin Res. In press.

60. Schumacher M, Maulet Y, Camp S, Taylor P. Multiple messenger RNA species give rise to the structural diversity in acetylcholinesterase. J Biol Chem 1988; 263:18979.

61. Li Y, Camp S, Rachinsky TL, Getman D, Taylor P. Gene structure of mammalian acetyl-cholinesterase. Alternative exons dictate tissue-specific expression. J Biol Chem 1991; 266:23083.

62. Sabo B, Moulds JJ, McCreary J. Anti-JMH: another high-titer low-avidity antibody against a high frequency antigen (abstr). Transfusion 1978; 18:387.

63. Kollmar M, South SF, Tregallas WM. Evidence of a genetic mechanism for the production of the JMH-negative phenotype (abstr). Transfusion 1981; 21:612.

64. Bobolis KA, Moulds JJ, Lande WM, Telen MJ. Identification of a novel human erythrocyte phosphatidylinositol (PI)–linked protein with blood group activity (abstr). Blood (Suppl. 1), 76(Suppl 1):380a.

65. Moulds JJ, Levene C, Zimmerman S. Serological evidence for heterogeneity among antibodies compatible with JMH-negative red cells. Abstracts of the Joint Meeting of the 19th Congress of the International Society of Haematology and the 17th Congress of the International Society of Blood Transfusion (abstr). Budapest, 1982:287.

66. Daniels GL, Knowles RW. A monoclonal antibody to the high frequency antigen JMH. J Immunogenet 1982; 9:57.

67. Daniels GL, Knowles RW. Further analysis of the monoclonal antibody H8 demonstrating a JMH-related specificity. J Immunogenet 1983; 10:257.

68. Bobolis KA, Moulds JJ, Telen MJ. Isolation of the JMH antigen on a novel phosphatidylinositol-linked human membrane protein. Blood 1992; 79:1574.

69. Simmons D, Seed B. The Fc receptor of natural killer cells is a phospholipid-linked membrane protein. Nature 1988; 333:568.

70. Medof ME, Walter EI, Roberts WL, Haas R, Rosenberry TL. Decay accelerating factor of complement is anchored to cells by a C-terminal glycolipid. Biochemistry 1986; 25:6740.

71. Davitz MA, Low MG, Nussenzweig V. Release of decay-accelerating factor (DAF) from the cell membrane by phosphatidylinositol-specific phospholipase C (PIPLC). Selective modification of a complement regulatory protein. J Exp Med 1986; 163:1150.

72. Selvaraj P, Dustin ML, Silber R, Low MG, Springer TA. Deficiency of lymphocyte function-associated antigen 3 (LFA-3) in paroxysmal nocturnal hemoglobinuria: functional correlates and evidence for a phosphatidylinositol membrane anchor. J Exp Med 1982; 166:1011.

73. Holguin MH, Wilcox LA, Bernshaw NJ, Rosse WF, Parker CJ. Erythrocyte membrane inhibitor of reactive lysis: effects of phosphatidylinositol-specific phospholipase C on the isolated and cell-associated protein. Blood 1990; 75:284.

74. Huizinga TWJ, de Haas M, Kleijer M, Nuijens JH, Roos D, von dem Borne AEGKr. Soluble Fc receptor III in human plasma originates from release by neutrophils. J Clin Invest 1990; 86:416.

75. Bobolis KA, Telen MJ. Biochemical study of possible mechanisms of acquired loss of JMH antigen expression (abstr). Transfusion 1991; 31(Suppl):46S.

76. Issitt PD. Applied Blood Group Serology 3rd ed. Miami: Mongomery Scientific Publications, 1985:401.

77. Reid ME, Ellisor SS, Sabo B. Absorption and elution of anti-Hy from one of four Gy(a–) red blood cell samples. Transfusion 1982; 22:528.

78. Spring FA, Reid ME. Evidence that the human blood group antigens Gy^a and Hy are carried on a novel glycophosphatidylinositol-linked erythrocyte membrane glycoprotein. Vox Sang 1991; 60:53.

5

The Rh Blood Groups

PETER D. ISSITT
Duke University Medical Center
Durham, North Carolina

I. HISTORY AND INTRODUCTION

In 1939, Levine and Stetson (1) described a fatal case of hemolytic disease of the newborn (HDN). The woman who had been delivered of the stillborn fetus had a hemolytic transfusion reaction when she was subsequently transfused with blood from the infant's father. The report did not claim that the maternal antibody was responsible for the infant's death, nor was the antibody given a name. In 1940, Landsteiner and Wiener (2) described an antibody made in guinea pigs and rabbits in response to injections of red blood cells (RBCs) from rhesus monkeys. The anti-rh reacted visibly with the RBCs of some 85% of humans. In the same year, Wiener and Peters (3) reported that what appeared to be an antibody with the same specificity, when made in humans, caused hemolytic transfusion reactions. In 1941, Levine et al. (4–6) published a series of reports about HDN and correctly implicated the maternal antibody as the causative agent of RBC destruction. The antibodies studied by Levine and colleagues (1,4) appeared to have the same specificity as those raised in animals by Landsteiner and Wiener (2) and the examples from humans studied by Wiener and Peters (3). Although it is now known that the human antibodies were anti-Rh$_o$ (anti-D) and it is widely believed that the anti-rh made in animals were what was later (7) called anti-LW, there is no doubt that the reports cited above represent discovery of the human Rh blood group system. Although it has been pointed out (8) that as early as 1932, Buchbinder (9) was studying antibodies made in animals injected with rhesus monkey RBCs, examination of the report of that work suggests (at least to this author) that no clear differentiation was achieved between the species antibodies that would have been present in the animals' sera and anti-rh, if indeed that antibody was raised. Because Buchbinder was working in Landsteiner's laboratory, it seems reasonable to conclude that the 1940 report (2) described extension of the earlier studies.

II. Rh ANTIGENS AND PHENOTYPES

A. Rh Positive and Rh Negative Phenotypes

Since 1940, the study of the Rh blood group system has grown to the point that today it represents the most complex polymorphism of human red cell markers and one of the most complex of all human polymorphisms. As of December 1991, it was believed (10,11) that 46 different Rh antigens had been recognized at the serological level. However, as discussed later in this chapter, some of the names of these antigens may well describe groups of very similar but not identical antigens, whereas others may represent different epitopes of the same antigen. Table 1 lists the currently named Rh antigens; gives their names in the Fisher-Race CDE (12,13), Wiener Rh-Hr (14,15), and Rosenfield et al. (16) numerical terminologies; lists some names that do not truly fit any of these categories; and gives the incidence of each antigen in the American white population.

In spite of the enormous expansion of the Rh system, D or Rh_0, the first antigen found remains by far the most important in the system. This is because, as discussed in detail below, after A and B, D is very much more immunogenic than any other red cell blood group antigen. Thus, at the practical level in pretransfusion tests, the RBCs of all patients and donors are typed for D. Those individuals whose RBCs are found to carry the antigen are called Rh positive (Rh+), and those whose RBCs lack the antigen are called Rh negative (Rh–). In all normal circumstances, Rh– persons are transfused only with Rh– blood. Although nonimmunized Rh+ persons can receive either Rh+ or Rh– blood, the latter is normally only used in Rh– individuals. The division of persons into Rh+ and Rh– is not quite as simple as the above statements imply. Again as described below, some persons have a phenotype called D^u in which D is present, albeit in a weaker than usual form, whereas others have RBCs that carry some but not all epitopes of the D antigen. Such persons, who initially appear to be Rh+, are able to form alloimmune anti-D that is directed against the epitopes of D that their RBCs lack. Nevertheless, at the routine practical level, the overwhelming majority of persons can be classified as Rh+ or Rh– so that appropriate blood for transfusion can be selected.

In marked contrast to the situation with D, unless highly unusual circumstances prevail, there is no justification for selecting donor blood matched for any of the other 45 Rh antigens for transfusion to nonimmunized patients. This consideration relates to the low immunogenicity of all other Rh antigens when compared to D.

As already mentioned, and as will be apparent from Table 1, the Rh system is enormously complex at the serological level. Because this book is primarily concerned with the immunobiology of transfusion medicine, the serology of Rh will not be discussed in minute detail. Instead, in the following sections, certain Rh antigens will be grouped based on some common characteristics and some generalized observations will be made. Readers wishing to obtain more detailed information and references to the original findings described, are referred to a number of recent reviews (17–20).

B. Antigens C, c, E, and e

Soon after anti-D had been recognized, it became apparent that other antibodies defining antigens (C, c, E, and e) related to D are made in some humans following immunization by transfusion or pregnancy (6,21–24). It rapidly became clear that there is disequilibrium in the distribution of these antigens with regard to the Rh+ and Rh– states. For most practical purposes, C and c and E and e can be regarded as pairs of antithetical antigens (18,25). However, the incidence of C in Rh+ (D+) persons is approximately 70%, whereas in Rh– (D–) individuals, it is less than 1%. The E antigen has an incidence of around 30% in Rh+ persons; like C, it is found on the RBCs of less than 1% of Rh– individuals. This means, of course, that the overwhelming majority of Rh– persons have red cells that are c+ and e+. However, c and e also are found frequently on the RBCs of Rh+ persons. These findings are illustrated by the data described below and are summarized in Table 2. At the genetic level, control of Rh antigen production rests with a number of genes or gene complexes. Although the genes or gene complexes that produce C, D, and e, or c, D, and E, or c e without D are common, the others are rare in

Table 1 Rh Antigen Names in Different Terminologies and Antigen Frequencies

Numerical	CDE	Rh-Hr	Other	% Incidence (Whites)
Rh1	D	Rh_o		85
Rh2	C	rh'		70
Rh3	E	rh''		30
Rh4	c	hr'		80
Rh5	e	rh''		98
Rh6	ce or f	hr		64
Rh7	Ce	rh_i		70
Rh8	C^w	rh^{w1}		1
Rh9	C^x	rh^x		<1
Rh10	V or ce^s	hr^v		<1
Rh11	E^w	rh^{w2}		<1
Rh12	G	rh^G		85
Rh13		Rh^A		85
Rh14		Rh^B		85
Rh15		Rh^C		85
Rh16		Rh^D		85
Rh17		Hr_o		>99.9
Rh18		Hr or Hr^S		>99.9
Rh19		hr^S		98
Rh20	VS or e^s			>1
Rh21	C^G			70
Rh22	CE			<1
Rh23	D^w			<1
Rh24	E^T			30
Rh26	c-like			80
Rh27	cE			30
Rh28		hr^H		>1
Rh29		rh_m	Total RH	>99.9
Rh30	D^{Cor}		Go^a	<1
Rh31		hr^B		98
Rh32				<1
Rh33				<1
Rh34		Hr^B		>99.9
Rh35				<1
Rh36			Be^a	<1
Rh37			Evans	<1
Rh39	C-like			>99.9
Rh40			Tar	<1
Rh41	Ce-like			70
Rh42	Ce^s			<1
Rh43			Craw	<1
Rh44			Nou	>99.9
Rh45			Riv	<1
Rh46			Sec	>99.9
Rh47			Dav	>99.9
Rh48			JAL	<1

Table 2 The Eight "Standard" *Rh* Genes, Their Products, and Incidence

CDE Term	Rh-Hr Term	Shorthand Term	CcDEe Antigens Made	Percent incidence in			
				Whites	Blacks	American Indians	Orientals
CDe	*Rh¹*	*R¹*	C,D,e	42	17	44	70
cDE	*Rh²*	*R²*	c,D,E	14	11	34	21
cDe	*Rh⁰*	*R⁰*	c,D,e	4	44	2	3
CDE	*Rhᶻ*	*Rᶻ*	C,D,E	<1	<1	6	1
cde	*rh*	*r*	c,e	37	26	11	3
Cde	*rh'*	*r'*	C,e	2	2	2	2
cdE	*rh"*	*r"*	c,E	1	<1	1	<1
CdE	*rhʸ*	*rʸ*	C,E	<1	<1	<1	<1

the white population and, with the exception of the gene or gene complex that makes c, D, and e, also are rare in blacks. The early findings that inheritance of the *Rh* genes or gene complexes involves haplotypes that are almost invariably passed without change from parent to child prompted vigorous debate as to the probable genetic control of Rh antigen production. This, in turn, led to the introduction of two distinct terminologies. Fisher and Race (12,13) interpreted the early findings as indicating the existence of three sets of closely linked genes; i.e., *C* and *c*, *D* and *d*, and *E* and *e*. It was supposed that linkage was so close that crossing-over between the loci was an extraordinarily rare event but that very uncommon gene complexes such as *CDE* must originally have arisen by crossing-over between common genes complexes such as *CDe* and *cDE*. A different interpretation was made by Wiener et al. (14,15), who believed that a single *Rh* gene encodes production of an agglutinogen that is composed of a number of blood factors. For example, the presence of *Rh¹* was said to result in the production of Rh_1, a structure that included (at least) the Rh_o (D), rh' (C) and hr" (e) blood factors. It was supposed that the entire agglutinogen, any part thereof, and each blood factor could act as an immunogen. Table 2 lists the eight "standard" *Rh* genes (gene complexes), gives their names in three terminologies, lists the C, c, D, E, and e antigens that each encodes, and shows the incidence (26) of each in various population groups.

As discussed in more detail in a later section of this chapter, it now appears that the Fisher-Race and Wiener concepts were each partially correct. Current evidence (27) shows that more than one gene is involved in the control of Rh antigen production. However, unlike the original concept (12,13) of three genes, it now seems that two are involved. In Rh+ persons, one gene apparently encodes production of a D-bearing polypeptide, whereas a second either encodes one protein that carries the CcEe series of antigens or (perhaps via different control mechanisms) two proteins, one carrying the Cc and the other the Ee determinants. In Rh− persons, the gene encoding the D-bearing protein is apparently absent (and is not replaced by an allele), whereas the second gene (encoding CcEe or Cc and Ee polypeptides) is present. Although such findings partially favor the original Fisher-Race (12,13) postulate, the interaction of the Rh polypeptides at the phenotypic level suggests presence of a structure not totally unlike the agglutinogen of Wiener (14,15). These new findings also are totally consistent with the fact that during 50 years of serological study, no convincing evidence has ever emerged for the existence of a d antigen (or, hence, for a *d* gene). In spite of this, the designation d is often used (as below) at both the phenotypic and genetic levels. When used, *d* or d should be taken to indicate only the absence of *D* or D. Further, for the remainder of this discussion of the system at the practical level, the designation *Rh* gene should be taken to imply *Rh* gene, *Rh* gene complex, or *Rh* haplotype. It is now necessary to consider the haplotype in Rh+ persons as being genetic material that encodes D and Cc and Ee-bearing polypeptides. In Rh− people, the haplotype must be thought of as genetic material that encodes the Cc and Ee-bearing proteins.

C. Antigens f(ce,Rh6), rh$_i$(Ce,Rh7), cE(Rh27), CE(Rh22), G, and C^G

As work on the serology of Rh progressed, it became clear (28–32) that a number of antibodies exist that are similar to but not identical with those that define c, e, C, and E. As an example, anti-f (anti-ce, anti-Rh6) usually reacts only with RBCs that are c+, e+ and that come from an individual in whom the same gene encodes production of the two antigens; i.e., c and e are in *cis* position. That is to say, RBCs from an individual genetically *R^{1}r(CDe/cde)* are c+, e+, f+ because c and e are both encoded by the *r(cde)* gene. Red blood cells from an individual genetically *R^{1}R^2(CDe/cDE)* are c+, e+, f− because the genes that encode c and e are in *trans* position. In other words, the c is encoded by *R^2(cDE)* and the e by *R^1(CDe)* and, because those genes are on different chromosomes, no f is made. With the exception of some very rare *Rh* genes, some of which (33,34) make both C and c, whereas others (35–38) make no C, c, E, or e, or (39–42) no E or e, the same general rules apply to the production of rh$_i$(Ce,Rh7), cE(Rh27), and CE(Rh22). Table 3 lists the eight standard *Rh* genes in terms of their production of these antigens.

The antigen G differs from those described above in that it is almost always made by any gene that makes D (43) and, thus far, has always been seen to be made by any gene that makes C (18,43). Thus, all C+ RBCs are G+ and almost all D+, C− RBCs are G+, but the rare phenotypes C−, D+, G− (44–46) and C−, D−, G+ (43,47,48) have been found. The antigen C^G is regarded by some (49) as being a form of C that can be detected by eclectic sera that may or may not contain anti-C. However, an equally plausible explanation (34) is that C^G is the form of C made by genes that make C without e. Many examples of so-called anti-C are, in fact, composed largely of anti-rh$_i$. That portion of such antibodies that is not anti-rh$_i$ is considered by some workers to be anti-C and by others as the antibody that has been called anti-C^G. Table 3 also shows the usual production of G and C^G by the eight "standard" *Rh* genes but, as mentioned above, rare exceptions exist.

D. Rh Antigens of Very High Incidence

Thus far, this account has considered only the eight genes listed in Tables 2 and 3. There are, however, a series of much rarer genes whose actions differ from those already described. The genes *cD−*, *C^{w}D−* and *(C)D^{IV}−* encode what appear at the serological level to be exalted amounts of D (although, in fact, *(C)D^{IV}−* makes "partial" D; see below), normal amounts of G, and markedly reduced amounts of c, C^w, and C, respectively (39–42). Of much more importance

Table 3 Additional Products of the Eight "Standard" *Rh* Genes

Gene (Haplotype)	Product(s)
CDe	rh$_i$(Ce), G, C^G
cDE	cE(Rh27), G
cDe	f(ce), G
CDE	CE(Rh22), G, C^G
cde	f(ce)
Cde	rh$_i$(Ce), G, C^G
cdE	cE(Rh27)
CdE	CE(Rh22), G, C^G

in terms of alloimmunization, these and other (-D-, $\cdot D\cdot$, and so forth) *Rh deletion* genes (35–38) fail to encode production of a number of Rh antigens that are made by all other *Rh* genes regardless of their C or c, D or no D, and E or e production. Accordingly, when individuals homozygous for any *Rh deletion* gene are exposed (via transfusion or pregnancy) to RBCs from persons with "normal" *Rh* genes and antigens, they are at risk of becoming alloimmunized to an Rh antigen of very common occurrence. Although the *Rh deletion* genes are rare, individuals homozygous for any of them often become immunized because their rare phenotypes are not usually recognized before initial transfusions (Rh+ blood of patients and donors is not routinely typed beyond D). As a result, most of these individuals are recognized when their sera are found to react (in antibody screening tests during pregnancy or in tests before subsequent transfusions) with all RBCs that have "normal" Rh phenotypes. The antigens missing (35,50–52) from the RBCs of almost all *Rh deletion* homozygotes are Hr_o(Rh17), Hr(Hr^S or Rh18), and Hr^B(Rh34). Antibodies to these antigens can be identified from tests against the RBCs of other *Rh deletion* homozygotes and those of some even less frequent individuals whose RBCs carry some but not all the very common antigens involved (51–53). The antigens Rh44(Nou), Rh46(Sec), and Rh47(Dav) are missing from the RBCs of some but not all *Rh deletion* homozygotes (54–60). Again, differential reactivity of these antibodies with RBCs of ultrarare phenotypes can be used to establish specificity. In yet another extremely rare Rh phenotype, Rh_{null} (see below), in which no expression of Rh antigens is seen (61–63), another antigen of very high incidence is absent. Thus, in addition to antibodies to other Rh antigens mentioned in earlier sections and above, Rh_{null} persons can form allo–anti-Rh29. This antibody defines an antigen encoded by all *Rh* genes, including the *Rh deletion* genes, meaning that anti-Rh29 reacts (64) with all except the Rh_{null} RBCs of the antibody maker and others of the same extraordinarily rare phenotype. Another antigen present on all except Rh_{null} RBCs is Rh39. The antibody to this antigen has, thus far, been found (65) only as an autoantibody. Anti-Rh39 initially appears to have anti-C specificity but can be adsorbed to exhaustion by all C+ and C– RBCs with "standard" Rh antigens and by RBCs from persons homozygous for *Rh deletion* genes. Anti-Rh39 is not adsorbed by Rh_{null} RBCs. Rh antigens of very high incidence are of considerable academic and practical importance. At the academic level, study of the production and characteristics of these antigens has contributed significantly to current understandings of the Rh system. Although, for the sake of brevity, Hr_o, Hr, Rh29, and Hr^B have each been described as single entities, there are ample data that suggest that each name describes a group of closely similar but not identical antigens. As a single example, some anti-Hr_o antigens react preferentially with E+, e–, Hr_o+, some with E–, e+, Hr_o+ RBCs, and still others show no difference in reactivity against E+, e–, and E–, e+, RBCs that are Hr_o+. At the clinical level, antibodies to any of these very common antigens create an enormous problem in patients in need of transfusions.

E. Rh Antigens of Very Low Incidence

There are a number of Rh antigens that are found on the RBCs of less than 1% of random donors of most or all ethnic groups. Often such antigens appear (66,67) to be "markers" of certain rare *Rh* genes, and it is generally believed that each may represent the result of a single point mutation. In other words, it is supposed that a single nucleotide change can alter a codon in such a manner that a different to usual amino acid becomes incorporated into an Rh polypeptide. In some instances, the low-incidence marker antigen has been found (thus far at least) as the product of only one *Rh* gene. In other instances, several different *Rh* genes have been seen to encode the rare antigen. This latter finding does not exclude point mutation as an explanation for the appearance of these rare antigens. As discussed in detail below, different Rh polypeptides are known to contain large homologous regions. Thus, the same point mutation in two *Rh* genes, or one point mutation before one gene arose from the other, would explain production of the same rare antigen by different genes.

The presence of a rare Rh antigen is frequently associated with altered expressions of some more common Rh antigens. For example, the rare antigen Rh32 has, thus far, been seen (68) to be the product of a gene called $\overline{R}^N$. In addition to encoding Rh32, $\overline{R}^N$ appears (33) to make markedly weakened forms of C and e, an amount of rh_i (Ce) that can be detected (69) on the RBCs of some but not all persons who have inherited the gene, but a normal amount of D. In other words, $\overline{R}^N$ also can be described as *(C)D(e)R^{32}*, or a variant form of *CDe*, with the parentheses indicating reduced expression of the antigens encoded. It has been suggested (55,56,69) that at the phenotypic level, the presence of the rare antigen Rh32 causes steric rearrangement of the Rh polypeptide so that C, e, and rh_i, but not D, are in a spatial arrangement that makes approach and binding of their antibodies difficult. In other words, a single point mutation in an R^1 gene, leading to formation of the gene now called $\overline{R}^N$, might explain not only the appearance of the "new" antigen Rh32 but steric rearrangement (and hence all serological findings) of the other antigens encoded.

Table 4 lists the low-incidence Rh antigens that have been reported to date (December 1991) and shows the gene or genes with which each is usually associated. When the antigens C^w, C^x, and E^w were first recognized (70–72), it was supposed that C^w and C^x were the products of "new" alleles at the *Cc* locus or sublocus and that E^w represented the product of a third allele at the *Ee* locus or sublocus. However, more recent findings have caused reevaluation of such conclusions. First, although C^w and C^x initially appeared to be products of genes that also encoded C, it is now clear (82,83) that they also can be made by genes that make c but no C. Second, studies (for references, see Table 4) on the antigens Rh32, Rh33, Rh35, Be^a(Rh36), Evans(Rh37), Riv(Rh45), and JAL(Rh48) have not suggested close association with antigens in the Cc, D, or Ee series. Instead, these antigens have been considered to be products of unusual "whole" *Rh* genes, as suggested by the point mutation, amino acid substitution concept outlined above.

The low-incidence antigens D^w, Go^a, and Tar (Rh40) differ from those listed above in that they appear to be products of genes that "replace" part of the genetic material that normally

Table 4 Low-Incidence Rh Antigens and the Encoding Haplotypes Thus Far Recognized

Antigen	Encoding Haplotype(s)	Reference[a]
C^w	*CDe, Cde, cde* or *cDe*	70
C^x	*CDe, Cde, cde* or *cDe*	71
E^w	*cDE*	72
D^w	*cD^{Va}e, CD^{Va}e, cD^{Va}E*	73
Go^a	*cD^{IVa}e, cD^{IVa}E, (C)D^{IVa}-*	74
Rh32	$\overline{R}^N$, also written as *(C)D(e)R^{32}*	68
Rh33	*R^{oHar}*, also written as *c((D))(e)R^{33}, (C)D^{IVa}-*	75
Rh35	*(C)D(e)R^{35}*	76
Be^a	*(c)d(e)(f)*	25
Evans	*·D·*	37
Tar	*CDeR^{40}, -D-R^{40}*	77
Craw	*cde^{s}C^G*, also called *r'^{s}*	78
Riv	*(C)D^{IVa}-*	79
JAL	*(C)D(e)R^{48}, (c)D(e)R^{48}*	80, 81

[a]Additional information about many of these low-incidence antigens will be found in refs. 16, 18–20, 25, 26, 38, 55, 66, 67, 82, 83, 104, and 268.

encodes D in persons with "partial" D on their RBCs. The epitopes of D and the "partial" D situations are considered later in this chapter.

F. Variant Rh Antigens

In addition to Rh antigens of very high and very low incidence, some behave as variants of others. For example, among samples from American whites and blacks, those that carry the E antigen invariably react with another antibody (84), anti-E^T. That is to say, in such persons, there are two phenotypes E+, E^T+ and E-,E^T-. In Australian Aborigines, an additional phenotype, E+, E^T-, exists and is about equal in incidence to E+, E^T+. Individuals of the first phenotype can make allo–anti-E^T. The antigens hr^S and hr^B are present on almost all e+ RBCs. However, in South African Bantus and Cape Colored persons, in fewer American blacks and in very few American whites, the phenotypes e+, hr^S-, and e+, hr^B- are seen (18,51,52). The phenotype e-, hr^S+, or hr^B+ does not seem to exist. The antigens hr^S and hr^B are considered by some (85–87) to be "included within" (perhaps as epitopes) the antigens Hr_o and Rh34, respectively. The antigens Rh26 and Rh41 have somewhat similar relationships to c and rh_i respectively. The phenotypes c+, Rh:26 and c–, Rh:–26 are common, both c+, Rh:–26 and c–, Rh:26 have been seen (88). Genes in which C and e are in cis make rh_i and Rh41 and those that have C^w and e in cis make rh_i but not Rh41. Somewhat surprisingly, a gene called $r's$ (89), which is written by some (16,18,49,66) as cde^sC^G, encodes production of Rh41. The antigens listed as Rh^A, Rh^B, Rh^C, and Rh^D in Table 1 almost certainly represent epitopes of D and are discussed below in the section dealing with "partial" D.

G. Rh Antigens that Are Fairly Common in Blacks but Very Rare in Whites

The antigen V is found (90) on the RBCs of 20–25% of American blacks but is seldom seen in whites. The antigen is associated with an unusual form of e and is often found as a product of genes that have c and e^s in cis. The antigen VS, which also has been called e^s, has a similar incidence to V and often appears to be a product of the variant gene e^s when that gene is partnered by C and not c in cis (89). However, enough exceptions have been found to show that equating V with ce^s and VS with e^s represents oversimplification. The antigen hr^H has been studied (45) primarily among South African blacks and arguably may be present on some RBCs that type as V–, VS+. The antigen Rh42 might be though of as analogous to rh_i(Ce) when e^s replaces e; i.e., Ce^s (91). However, in view of what is stated above, equating Rh42 with Ce^s probably also represents oversimplification.

H. Antigens Previously Associated with the Rh System

At one time, the high-incidence antigens LW (now LW^a) and Duclos had Rh numbers, i.e., Rh25 and Rh38, respectively. It is now known that the genes that encode these antigens do not reside at the Rh locus. Thus, the association between these antigens and the Rh system is at the phenotypic level. RBCs that are D+ react more strongly with anti-LW^a (and anti-LW^b) than do RBCs that are D–, LW+. Indeed the initial confusion (7) between D and LW mentioned earlier arose in part because a weak example of anti-LW will give the visible serological reactions expected of anti-D. Differentiation between anti-D and anti-LW can be made in adsorption studies; although D–, LW+ RBCs may fail to react visibly with some anti-LW, they will adsorb such antibodies to exhaustion. Such cells will not adsorb anti-D. By the time that an antigen originally called Ne^a (92) was recognized as being LW^b (93), the antithetical partner to LW^a, the genetic independence of LW from Rh had been recognized, meaning that LW^b did not receive an Rh number.

It seems possible that the very common antigen Duclos (94) (previously Rh38) requires the presence of both Rh polypeptides and glycophorin B (the SsU-bearing sialoglycoprotein; see Chap. 2) for its expression (95). As might be expected, from their phenotypic associations with Rh, both LW and Duclos seem to have a biochemical relationship to the Rh polypeptides at the RBC membrane. Thus, the membrane structures that carry LW and Duclos are considered again later in this chapter.

I. The D^u Phenotype

In 1946, Stratton (96) described a phenotype, which he called D^u, in which the D antigen could be shown to be present only when in vitro tests more sensitive than those in routine use at that time were used. Over the years, through no fault of the original investigator, this phenotype has caused great confusion for both practicing physicians and blood bankers. There are a number of causes for this confusion. First, although RBCs of the D^u phenotype are D+, a minority of them come from individuals whose RBCs lack certain D epitopes, which means that such persons can produce anti-D (to the epitopes that their RBCs lack) if exposed to normal D+ red cells (i.e., all epitopes of D present). Second, because red cells of the D^u phenotype are D+, they can stimulate the production of anti-D if transfused into Rh– (D–) persons. These findings led to the introduction of a double standard by which potential transfusion recipients and pregnant women with the D^u phenotype were regarded as Rh–, whereas donors of that phenotype were called Rh+. Third, and adding considerably to the confusion outlined, definition of the D^u phenotype is very much technique dependent. Many blood samples typed as D^u in the 1940s and 1950s would type as D+ today because of the much more potent anti-D typing reagents now used. Fortunately, this change in in vitro determination of the D^u phenotype has been accompanied by the realizations that only a minority of D^u persons can form anti-D and that most D^u donors whose RBCs are immunogenic in D– recipients are now typed as D+. Thus, current thinking (97,98) is that the designation D^u should be replaced by the designation "weak D," that patients whose RBCs do not react in direct typing tests for D should be called Rh– without further testing being done (and should be transfused with Rh– blood), and that currently used D-typing tests on donors (often with monoclonal-based anti-D reagents) identify as Rh+ those persons whose RBCs might provoke production of anti-D if transfused into an Rh– recipient. Genetic backgrounds resulting in the D^u phenotype are discussed below.

J. D Variants

In the early 1950s, reports (99–101) appeared describing persons with D+ RBCs who had made alloimmune anti-D. Although uncommon, cases of this type have been studied in great detail over the years, and Tippett and her colleagues (102–106) have developed a comprehensive classification system. Two major types of tests were initially used (102–105). First, the D+ red cells of the antibody makers were tested with selected anti-D made by Rh– persons. Those anti-D were chosen because of their ability to characterize some D+ cells from which portions of D were missing. Second, cross tests were performed between the D+ RBCs of the antibody makers and the anti-D that they had made. At first the situation was said to indicate that the D antigen has a mosaic-like structure and that persons with a portion (or portions) of the mosaic missing were the ones who could form alloimmune anti-D to the portion (or portions) of D that their RBCs lacked. More recently, Tippett (104,105) has suggested that the situation is better described as one in which the individuals concerned have partial D on their RBCs. Early studies (102) divided persons of this type into six categories, I through VI, in which the RBCs and immune responses were similar in persons of the same category. Extension of those studies (103–105) excluded persons of category I from the scheme; subdivided those in categories III, IV, and V into three, two, and three subcategories, respectively, based on different reactions of their RBCs in cross tests with the anti-D; showed that although persons of category VI have similar RBCs, they can make two different specificity anti-D; and added category VII (Table 5).

A fascinating finding about these D variant RBCs is that some of them carry Rh antigens of low incidence that are thereby characteristic of a particular category or subcategory of partial D. Red blood cells of category IVa type as Go(a+), those of category IVb fail to react in direct tests with anti-Goᵃ, but at least some of them may carry a weak expression of the antigen as judged by adsorption/elution tests. The RBCs of other categories are Go(a–). Red blood cells of category Va are D^w+; those of other categories, including Vb and Vc are $D^w–$. Red blood cells of category VII are Tar+(Rh:40); those of other categories are Tar–(Rh:–40). One possible explanation for these findings is that the genetic material that would otherwise encode the epitopes of D missing in the partial D antigen is replaced. If the replacement material encodes a structure that is immunogenic, antibodies (i.e., to Goᵃ, D^w, and Tar) can be made. Lack of replacement antigens in other categories of partial D could represent nonimmunogenicity of the replacement product or deletion rather than replacement of the genetic material that would otherwise encode the missing epitopes of D.

Red blood cells that carry partial D are not often recognized from simple typing tests for D. That is to say, in many categories, the partial nature of the D antigen does not result in its giving a weaker than normal reaction. There are, of course, RBCs with partial D that give the reactions of the D^u phenotype as described above. However, because the anti-D made by persons with partial D on their RBCs often fail to react visibly with D^u variant (partial D^u) RBCs, such cells have not often been fully characterized. As described below, monoclonal antibodies to D are now being used further to investigate the partial D situation. No doubt some of these reagents will prove suitable to characterize blood with partial D^u. It should also be added that most RBCs of the D^u phenotype represent quantitative depression of expression of D and not the qualitative difference of partial D (see below).

In some instances, RBCs that carry partial D give enhanced reactions in routine typing tests with anti-D. The Go(a+) RBCs of category IVa often appear to carry more D than "normal" D+ RBCs. It is possible that steric rearrangement of the D-bearing polypeptide, occasioned by the presence of Goᵃ, results in a structure in which the epitopes of D that are present are more readily accessible to anti-D molecules than when Goᵃ is not present.

Serological studies (102–105) using D variant (partial D) RBCs and the anti-D made by persons with D variant RBCs clearly established the existence of the categories and subcategories described above. Once monoclonal (MAb) anti-D made by Epstein-Barr virus (EBV) transformation of human B cells and in hybridomas or heterohybridomas became available, they were

Table 5 Epitopes of D Present on (+) and Absent from (0) RBCs with Partial D Antigen, from Lomas et al. (106)

Partial D category	Epitopes						
	epD1	epD2	epD3	epD4	epD5	epD6	epD7
IIIa	+	+	+	+	+	+	+
IIIc	+	+	+	+	+	+	+
IVa	0	0	0	+	+	+	+
IVb	0	0	0	0	+	+	+
Va	0	+	+	+	0	+	+
Vc	0	0	0	0	+	+	+
VI	0	0	+	+	0	0	0
VII	+	+	+	+	+	+	+

used to confirm and extend these studies. Lomas et al. (106) demonstrated that among the partial D samples tested (some categories and subcategories were not available), the MAb to D defined six distinct epitopes; the existence of a seventh could be deduced from the results of earlier studies (107). The findings of these workers are illustrated in Table 5. That the seven epitopes of D thus far recognized to not completely explain the partial D situation is clear from a number of findings. First, RBCs of categories IIIa, IIIc, and VII carry all seven epitopes recognized, but these cells vary in terms of reactivity with anti-D made by persons with partial D on their RBCs. Second, the RBCs of categories IVb and Vc were shown to lack the same four epitopes and to carry the same three epitopes. Again, these RBCs give different results when tested with the anti-D made by D-variant individuals. Third, RBCs from categories II, IIIb, and Vb were not available for testing. These cells also differ from those tested when the anti-D made by individuals with partial D are used. In other words, although the results shown in Table 5 indicate the existence of seven different epitopes of D, still others must exist. Although these findings at first seem extraordinary in terms of complexity of a single Rh antigen, they fit well with other recent findings. As mentioned briefly earlier and as discussed in detail below, it is now known (27) that Rh+ people have two *Rh* genes, whereas Rh– persons have only one. Because the additional gene in Rh+ persons appears to encode a D-bearing polypeptide that is absent in Rh– people, it is not surprising that the polypeptide involved carries a large number of immunogenic epitopes. To conclude this section on partial D, it will be pointed out that the antigens Rh^A, Rh^B, Rh^C, and Rh^D, as listed in Table 1, are structures present on the RBCs of D+ persons who can form alloimmune anti-D. Because most of the informative studies have been performed using the category II to VII classifications, it is not known how Rh^A to Rh^D correlate with the categories. For this reason, the $Rh^{alphabet}$ terminology (108) is now seldom used.

K.   The Rh$_{null}$ and Rh$_{mod}$ Phenotypes and Other Suppressors of *Rh*

The phenotypes Rh$_{null}$ (61–63) and Rh$_{mod}$ (109,110) are extraordinarily rare but are of interest out of all proportion to their frequency. In the phenotype Rh$_{null}$, no Rh antigens can be detected on the RBCs by direct typing or in adsorption-elution studies. Family studies have shown that the phenotype can arise by either of (at least) two different genetic backgrounds. In the modifier or suppressor type (62), the Rh$_{null}$ individuals have *Rh* genes that in the probands fail to effect production of Rh antigens. When passed to their offspring, the *Rh* genes from this type of Rh$_{null}$ individual appear to function normally. Thus, in the mating Rh$_{null}$ by R^1R^2 producing one R^2r and one R^1R^1 child, it follows that the Rh$_{null}$ individual passed r to child 1 and R^1 to child 2. It has been supposed (62) that in this type of Rh$_{null}$ individual, genes at an unlinked locus effect suppression of expression of the *Rh* genes. It is said that in persons with normal Rh phenotypes, a gene called X^1r allows normal function of the *Rh* genes. In persons homozygous for X^0r, the rare allele of X^1r, *Rh* gene expression is blocked. Family studies have shown that the supposed X^1r and X^0r genes segregate independently of *Rh*. In spite of the names, X^1r and X^0r are not carried on the X chromosome. The mechanism by which X^0r in double dose prevents the expression of Rh antigens is not known.

In the amorph type (63) of Rh$_{null}$, it appears that the phenotype results from the inheritance of silent alleles at the *Rh* locus. This is exemplified by the apparent mating R^1R^1 by R^2R^2 producing apparent R^1R^1, R^2R^2 and actual Rh$_{null}$ offspring. Because in this mating parent 2 has apparently made no *Rh* contribution to child 1, parent 1 apparently no *Rh* contribution to child 2, and neither any *Rh* contribution to child 3, it is supposed (63) that the actual genotypes are $R^1\bar{r}$ by $R^2\bar{r}$ producing $R^1\bar{r}$, $R^2\bar{r}$ and $\bar{r}\bar{r}$, where $\bar{r}$ is a silent allele at the *Rh* locus.

The phenotype Rh$_{mod}$ is one in which expression of all or most Rh antigens is modified (109). In some persons of this phenotype, some Rh antigens give weak reactions in direct tests;

others can be shown to be present only by the use of adsorption-elution methods. In other persons with the phenotype (111), adsorption elution tests are necessary to demonstrate the presence of any Rh antigens. It is supposed (109) that the Rh_{mod} phenotype occurs in persons homozygous for a modifier gene that has been called X^Q. Although X^Q has been shown to segregate independently of the Rh locus and is assumed to be similar in action to X^0r, there is no direct evidence that X^Q and X^0r are allelles. However, based purely on serological observations, it is possible (18) that X^0r and X^Q are the same gene with different degrees of penetrance. Because the RBCs of Rh_{null} and Rh_{mod} persons do not enjoy normal in vivo life spans (112–115), these two phenotypes are considered again below in the section on function of the Rh polypeptides.

Over the years, other cases apparently involving suppression of Rh gene function have been reported (116,117). Family studies have often suggested that recessive genes at loci unlinked to Rh were responsible. Notably in these cases, not all Rh antigens in the affected individuals were suppressed to the same degree; suppression did not approach the level seen in the Rh_{mod} phenotype. In a highly unusual family, Kornstad (118) showed that 10 persons with Ol(a+) RBCs had suppression of Rh antigen expression, whereas their direct relatives (including siblings) with Ol(a–) red cells did not. Further, depression of C and E was marked, that of D less noticeable, whereas depression of c and e was not demonstrated. The Ol^a antigen is of very low incidence and Ol^a was shown to segregate independently of Rh. Because depression of Rh antigen expression was associated with the Ol(a+) phenotype, it appeared that the suppressor gene must be dominant in effect.

III. THE IMMUNOLOGY OF Rh

A. Immunogenicity of D in the Rh-Negative Phenotype

The reason that routine typing studies always include a test for the presence of D, with subsequent division of individuals into the Rh+ and Rh– phenotypes, is that if persons with D– RBCs are exposed to the D antigen, most of them will make anti-D. If Rh– individuals are transfused with 1 unit of Rh+ blood, there is a 70–80% chance that anti-D will be made (119,120). When the amount of D+ blood injected is less, the rate of immunization drops but is still considerable. In D– individuals given 25–40 ml of D+ RBCs, immunization to D occurs in between one third and one half (121,122). Even when the immunizing dose is much smaller, i.e., about 1 ml, immunization to D is still frequent. That is, about 25% of individuals make anti-D after a single injection, and almost 50% of them do so after a second injection (123–126).

Before the introduction of Rh immune globulin (RhIG), there was a high incidence of production of anti-D by Rh– women who bore Rh+ children. By pooling figures from several large series (127–130), it can be seen that among Rh– women who had two or more Rh+ pregnancies, between 15 and 22% eventually made anti-D. As discussed in detail in Chapter 20, the production of anti-D following the entry of fetal D+ RBCs into the maternal D– circulation can now be prevented if a sufficient amount of RhIG is injected at an appropriate time.

In spite of the very high immunogenicity of D, it is apparent (119,131–133) that some Rh– persons are incapable of making anti-D no matter how many times they are exposed to the D antigen. Although it was originally thought that as many as 25–30% of Rh– persons might be nonresponders to D, Mollison et al. (19) give reasons for supposing that the actual number is a little under 10% of Rh negatives. Although it can be presumed that the ability to respond to D is under genetic control, and although an early investigation (134) suggested that the HL-A3 antigen might be overrepresented among women immunized to D by pregnancy, other studies (135–137) have neither confirmed that association nor established any other. Mollison et al.

(19) point out that the lower the initial immunizing dose of D+ RBCs, the higher the apparent incidence of nonresponders to D. Further, if very small doses of immunoglobulin G (IgG) anti-D are given at the same time as the D+ RBCs, some poor responders are seen to make anti-D (126,138). In other words, it now appears that there is no sharp distinction between Rh–responders and nonresponders to D, but instead the ability seems to involve a sliding scale with perhaps only 7 or 8% of Rh– persons being complete nonresponders. As mentioned above, it has recently been shown (27) that at the genetic level, Rh+ and Rh– persons differ in that Rh+ persons have two *Rh* genes and Rh– persons only one. It will be fascinating to learn whether the inability of a minority of Rh– individuals to mount an immune response to D is related to the presence of the gene that in Rh+ persons encodes the D-bearing polypeptide, although that gene does not encode serologically detectable D antigen on the RBCs. Perhaps the true difference between the D+ and D– phenotypes will be better determined at the genomic level than at the serological level, and perhaps the difference will be totally correlated with the ability to mount an immune response to D.

Although Rh antigens, including D, are confined to RBCs, immunization to D can occur when Rh– patients are transfused with blood components from Rh+ donors, although those components are not given as a source of RBCs. For example, platelet concentrates contain some RBCs (even when the concentrates do not appear pink to the naked eye). In view of the small volume of RBCs needed to provoke alloimmunization to D (19), an Rh– patient given doses of platelets made from the blood of Rh+ donors is at risk of making anti-D (139). In those instances when an Rh– parous woman or a female child must be given platelets from an Rh+ donor or donors (e.g., need for HLA-matched platelets, shortage of concentrates made from Rh– blood), prevention of immunization to D can be accomplished by the use of RhIG. A useful rule of thumb is that one 250 to 300/μg dose of RhIG will prevent alloimmunization by a volume of RBCs up to about 15 ml and that a platelet concentrate that does not appear pink probably contains no more than 0.5 ml of RBCs. Some clinicians are reluctant to use RhIG in severely thrombocytopenic patients because of the danger that an intramuscular injection will cause bleeding into the tissue. Clearly, if RhIG for intravenous injection is available, its use is indicated. If such a product is not available, some clinicians elect to inject the intramuscular product immediately following infusion of the platelets, at a time when the patient's platelet count is likely to be at its highest. This author has heard anecdotal reports of RhIG prepared for intramuscular use being given intravenously. One dose of the RhIG is diluted in 100 ml of physiological saline and infused slowly, and the patient is closely watched for signs of any untoward reaction during the entire period of infusion. It must be added that the use of RhIG prepared for intramuscular use in this fashion violates licenced use of the product and that such use might well create liability for any serious consequences. Thus, the medical indication for such use should be documented in the patient's chart with risk-benefit considerations duly noted.

In terms of plasma transfusions, liquid stored plasma from Rh+ donors (that probably contains a few intact RBCs) has been seen to stimulate both primary (140,141) and secondary (141) responses to D in Rh– individuals. Frozen plasma and cryoprecipitate do not seem to have been incriminated as causative of primary immunization but can effect a secondary response, presumably because of the presence of RBC stroma (142).

In addition to the above rather obvious ways in which Rh– persons can be exposed to Rh+ RBCs, the production of anti-D has also followed exposure to such cells via renal transplantation (143), bone grafts (144,145), "therapeutic" injections of blood (146–148), blood exchange for "emotional gratification" (149,150), and the use of blood-contaminated syringes for the injection of illegal drugs (151,152).

There are a number of reasons for the importance of prevention of immunization to D. First, before the introduction of RhIG, among all cases of HDN that required treatment more extensive than simple phototherapy, some 93% involved Rh+ infants born to Rh– women immunized to D (153). Among cases in which in utero death of the fetus occurred following immune RBC destruction by the maternal antibody, close to 100% involved anti-D (153). The severity of anti-D HDN has not changed since the introduction of RhIG; the percentage of severe cases caused by anti-D has, of course, diminished. Second, development of anti-D by an Rh– individual means that subsequent transfusions must be with Rh– blood. As described below, Rh antibodies detected by conventional serological techniques are almost all clinically significant (i.e., capable of in vivo red cell destruction). Thus, although the production of anti-D in an Rh– person is not harmful per se, the consequences of its presence can be enormous. First, an Rh– female immunized to D by transfusion might never be able to bear a live child. Second, any Rh– person similarly immunized would be put at grave risk if later transfusions became essential and no Rh– blood was available. For these reasons, Rh– persons must be transfused with Rh– blood whenever possible. On those occasions when Rh– blood is in short supply and the deliberate use of Rh+ blood for an Rh– patient is unavoidable, the patient(s) to be exposed to the about 80% chance of forming anti-D must be chosen with some care. Candidates for such transfusion should be nonimmunized men or women beyond menopause in whom it is likely that only one series of transfusions will be required. If the patient is female, a careful history (i.e., concerning affected infants) must be taken to try to exclude the possibility that the woman was immunized to D by pregnancy but is no longer making serologically demonstrable anti-D (19). Although it is justifiable to use Rh+ blood for Rh– patients in times of acute shortage of Rh– units and in order to preserve the Rh– units for those who must receive them, i.e., women who may later become pregnant, any patient who has already made anti-D, such decisions should not become routine. It is far better to try to obtain more Rh– blood or to postpone some transfusions until Rh– blood is available than to use Rh+ blood for these patients in too cavalier a fashion.

B. Immunogenicity of D in the D^u and D-Variant Phenotypes

A problem that arises in considering the immunogenicity of D in this group of individuals is that recognition of the D^u phenotype does not indicate its cause and hence does not reveal whether or not the person can form alloimmune anti-D. When the weakening of D in the D^u phenotype is caused by the depressing effect of a C gene in *trans* to D (154), or by a D gene that encodes fewer than usual copies of its antigen (155,156), the D antigen present includes all epitopes of D (albeit in reduced amounts), meaning that the individual involved cannot make allo–anti-D. When the D^u phenotype represents absence of some D epitopes (101–105), the individual involved can form anti-D to the missing epitopes of that antigen. Although the majority of persons with the D^u phenotype are of one of the types who cannot form anti-D, there are no quick, easy, or reliable methods to establish that fact. The complexity of the situation is further compounded because most persons with partial D on their RBCs (the D variants who can form allo–anti-D) have RBCs that type as D+ (103–105). Thus, most individuals of this type are recognized only after they have formed the antibody.

The original solution to this problem was to call persons of the D^u phenotype Rh+ if they were donors and Rh– if they were patients. Fortunately, the need for this confusing solution has now largely disappeared (98). Currently used anti-D typing reagents and automated typing equipment (for donor samples) now comprise such sensitive test systems that many workers feel that most (or all) donor units that carry enough D to provoke production of anti-D in an Rh– individual are recognized as Rh+ and are labeled as such. Those few D^u samples with too little D to be detected are generally believed to be nonimmunogenic. In patients, it is felt that the initial test for D now identifies as Rh+ most persons who would previously have been called D^u. If the initial test for D is negative, no extension test for the D^u phenotype is needed;

instead the patient is called Rh–. Thus, a few patients with small amounts of D on their RBCs who might be able to form anti-D receive Rh– blood. The exercise of testing patients for the D^u phenotype so that they can be given Rh+ blood to preserve the Rh– blood supply, is now largely futile because most will initially type as D+. The currently used solution is a practical one that will occasionally backfire. There is, for example, no way of recognizing a patient with partial D on the RBCs when those cells type as D+. However, the practical solution's utility is greatly enhanced by the facts that D+ or D^u persons who can form allo–anti-D are quite rare, and that donor RBCs that fail to react in the initial test for D may not be capable of provoking production of anti-D in Rh– persons.

C.   Immunogenicity of Rh Antigens Other than D

That no Rh antigens even approached D in terms of immunogenicity became apparent from early studies in which volunteers were deliberately immunized with RBCs in attempts to provoke antibody production (157–160). It was found that repeated injections of RBCs carrying C, c, E, or e into volunteers whose RBCs lacked those antigens only seldom resulted in immunization. Such observations have been confirmed by transfusion therapy. Because Rh+ patients and donors are typed only for D, the transfusion of Rh+ blood into Rh+ patients results in many of the patients being exposed to Rh antigens that their RBCs lack. The total rate of alloimmunization to Rh antigens other than D via transfusion and pregnancy is probably less than 1% (161). Thus, although antibodies to virtually any Rh antigen can cause immune RBC destruction (and hence transfusion reactions and HDN), attempts to prevent their production by the provision of Rh phenotype–matched blood for transfusion are not cost effective.

Some workers elect, for special reasons, to try to prevent Rh alloimmunization in some circumstances. For example, patients with sickle cell anemia, who have D+, C–, E–, K–, RBCs are sometimes transfused with C–, E–, K–, blood even though they are not alloimmunized (162). The rationale is that on some occasions, alloimmunization is accompanied by the production of pathological autoantibodies. Because C, E, and K would be immunogenic in these patients, Rh (and K) matched units are used in an attempt to forestall alloimmunization and the possible development of autoimmune hemolytic anemia.

Problems associated with the production of antibodies to very common or very rare Rh antigens are addressed below in the section on the clinical relevance of Rh antibodies. Although this section has pointed out that alloimmunization to Rh antigens other than D is a relatively rare event (in view of the millions of transfusions given annually), it will be added that alloimmunization involving Rh is still somewhat more frequent than that involving other blood group systems. Several large surveys (161,163–165) on the detection of blood group antibodies have shown that if "naturally occurring" benign antibodies are excluded, about half the remaining (clinically significant) antibodies define an Rh antigen.

D.   Clinical Relevance of Rh Antibodies

The immune response to Rh antigens introduced on foreign RBCs seems to follow the most usual pattern seen in humans. That is to say, the first antibody made is IgM and there is then a switch to IgG. However, the switch from IgM to IgG production apparently occurs so early in many instances of Rh immunization, that the first antibody detected in serological tests may be IgG. Further, the IgM to IgG switch often seems to occur without the introduction of additional antigen. It is possible that with their fairly long in vivo life span, foreign RBCs supply both the primary and secondary immunizing stimuli. Late introduction of antigen-positive RBCs in an individual making potent Rh antibodies sometimes leads to the production of IgA and reappearance of IgM antibodies of the same specificity. Once any IgG Rh antibody detectable by conventional serological techniques is present, it is traditional to honor that antibody in all subsequent transfusions. This is because Rh antibodies of all specificities have caused immediate and/or delayed hemolytic transfusion reactions (18,19). It is likely that, as with IgG antibodies in other blood group systems, a few Rh antibodies might be benign in vivo. However, there is no reliable, rapid, or easy method to differentiate between pathological and benign forms, nor is there a method to determine which currently benign forms might become pathological because of a secondary immune response. Accordingly, prudence dictates that once an Rh antibody has been recognized in conventional tests antigen-negative blood be transfused.

Although IgG2 and IgG4 forms are seen (166,167), most Rh antibodies are IgG1 and/or IgG3 in nature (19,168–170). In Rh– women immunized to D by pregnancy, the antibody may be composed predominantly of one subclass; in volunteers deliberately injected with D+ RBCs, anti-D of more than one subclass are likely to be present (169,170). In spite of the regular occurrence of IgG1 and IgG3 Rh antibodies, only very rare examples have been seen to activate complement in vitro. Indeed, of thousands of examples tested, those with that property are invariably reported (171–173). As with IgG Rh antibodies, IgM forms fail to effect complement activation in vitro. From observations that in some cases (174–176) of hemolytic transfusion reactions caused by Rh antibodies hemoglobinemia and/or hemoglobinuria is seen, it has been speculated that some Rh antibodies may be able to activate complement in vivo with that ability not demonstrable in vitro. However, there is no direct evidence to support such speculation. Instead, it seems that most (or all) in vivo RBC destruction effected by these antibodies involves extravascular clearance mediated by tissue macrophages (see Chap. 16). In vivo RBC survival studies have shown (19) that within the variances effected by antibodies of different IgG subclasses, the rate and amount of in vivo RBC destruction caused by Rh antibodies is directly related to the amount of IgG that becomes RBC bound (see Chap. 16). The above considerations apply primarily to Rh antibodies whose production has been stimulated by the introduction of foreign RBCs via transfusion or pregnancy. Although most Rh antibodies fall into such a category, there are a few (described below) that do not and these may have somewhat different in vivo characteristics.

Rh antibodies directed against very common or very rare Rh antigens pose special problems. As already described, most Rh antibodies demonstrable in vitro by conventional serological techniques are clinically significant. Thus, when a patient is encountered in whom the antibody recognizes an antigen such as Hr, Hr_0 or Rh34, an acute problem in providing compatible blood exists. Indeed, because these antigens are so common, it is frequently necessary to use the services of one of the rare donor registries to obtain blood that will survive normally in vivo. The chief complication caused by an antibody to a rare Rh antigen is that it may cause HDN without the cause of that disease being apparent. As we (69) have pointed out, when an antibody to a rare antigen causes HDN severe enough to warrant some form of transfusion therapy, an Rh antibody should be a prime suspect. Most antibodies to rare Rh antigens have caused HDN (reviewed in ref. 69). In such cases, there is no difficulty in providing compatible blood; instead identification of the cause of HDN presents an intellectual challenge.

As described above, the majority of Rh antibodies are clearly RBC stimulated. However, there are some Rh antibodies found in the sera of persons who have never been pregnant, transfused, or exposed to foreign RBCs via any other route that are usually described as "naturally occurring." As this author has pointed out elsewhere (18), that term is probably self-contradictory because presumably the immune system must "see" an antigen in order to produce an antibody. Non-RBC–stimulated (naturally occurring) Rh antibodies may be IgM or IgG (or rarely mixtures of both); for unknown reasons two specificities, anti-E and anti-C^w, predominate. Relatively little work has been done to determine the clinical relevance of this subset of Rh antibodies. From the limited data available, it is clear that at least some of them do not destroy antigen-positive RBCs in vivo and that some of the antibody makers do not mount an immune response following exposure to those foreign RBCs (177). However, because it is usually easier to supply antigen-negative blood for patients with Rh antibodies demonstrable by conventional methods than to determine what caused antibody production in the first place, few attempts are made to differentiate between RBC and non-RBC–stimulated Rh antibodies at the level of practical transfusion.

The above section has several times mentioned Rh antibodies that are detectable by conventional methods. This is because there is a substantial subset of Rh antibodies detectable only by ultrasensitive methods. Good examples of such antibodies are those that react with protease (ficin, papain, bromelin)–modified RBCs but are not detectable in albumin or low ionic strength saline (LISS) to indirect antiglobulin test methods. Some antibodies in this subset are IgM, some IgG; some occur in persons who have been exposed to foreign RBCs, some are non-RBC stimulated. The existence of this subset of Rh antibodies has prompted some debate as to how the immunized patients should be handled. Some workers, usually practicing outside the United States, use enzyme-treated RBCs for pretransfusion antibody screening and identification tests. Patients with an antibody reactive solely in such tests are transfused only with antigen-negative blood. In other services, notably most of those in the United States, enzyme-modified RBCs are not routinely used in pretransfusion tests. In such services, patients with "enzyme-only" Rh antibodies must often receive antigen-positive blood because the antibody has not been detected. Failure to look for these antibodies does not seem to be of any consequence to the patients; the incidences of immediate and delayed transfusion reactions and posttransfusion alloimmunization seem the same in services honoring or not testing for the enzyme-only Rh antibodies. Because comparison of such incidences provides only a crude measure of the significance of these antibodies, we undertook a large retrospective study involving 10,000 recently transfused patients (178). We found that the overwhelming majority of patients with an enzyme-only Rh antibody in the serum before transfusion, who had by chance received antigen-positive blood, fared as well in terms of transfusion outcome as those who had, by chance, received only antigen-negative blood. Further, in these patients, secondary immune responses after transfusion were rare (4 of 33 patients) and were not correlated with the transfusion of antigen-positive blood. We concluded that based on the enormous increase in workload that results when enzyme-modified RBCs are used in pretransfusion tests (cold-reactive antibodies enhanced, enzyme-only autoagglutinins found), the benefits obtained (we would have prevented one delayed hemolytic transfusion reaction in 10,000 patients) do not justify such use. Although we cannot prove the point, we (18,178) suspect that the noticeable paucity of secondary immune responses in patients transfused with antigen-positive blood indicates that most enzyme-only Rh antibodies are in fact directed against other antigens (that may have nothing to do with human RBCs) and simply have the ability to cross-react with Rh antigens. We believe that reintroduction of the original (unknown) immunogen would be necessary to prompt a secondary immune response.

From our finding (178) that about half the enzyme only antibodies are also detectable by polyethylene glycol (PEG) and Polybrene methods, it became clear that when those techniques are used as a routine, some patients are given antigen-negative blood when, in fact, such selected units are not necessary. However, unlike the use of enzyme-premodified RBCs, PEG and Polybrene methods do not result in the detection of large numbers of other clinically irrelevant antibodies. In other words, the "price paid" (unnecessary use of a few antigen-negative units) is justified by the increased sensitivity of PEG and Polybrene methods in detecting antibodies that are of clinical significance.

E. Rh Autoantibodies

Although "warm" autoantibody-induced hemolytic anemia (WAIHA) is described in detail in Chapter 18, no account of the Rh blood group system would be complete without mention of the role of Rh autoantibodies in that condition. The first association of Rh with WAIHA appears to be the 1953 report of Weiner et al. (179) of a case in which the causative autoantibody had anti-e specificity; Wiener and Gordon (180) simultaneously and independently forecast that autoantibodies to "core" Rh antigens would be found in exactly such circumstances. If easily recognizable Rh antibodies (i.e., those directed against D, C, E, c, e, G, rh_i, and so forth) are considered, only about 3–4% of patients with WAIHA are seen immediately to have Rh autoantibodies (181). In other words, 96–97% of the autoantibodies react with all RBCs with "normal" Rh phenotypes. However, in 1963, Weiner and Vos (182) showed that if the causative autoantibodies are tested against Rh deletion (e.g., -D-/-D-, C^WD-/C^WD-) and Rh_{null} RBCs, a closer relationship to Rh is seen. Table 6 shows the reaction patterns of three major specificity autoantibodies that cause WAIHA. The designation anti-nl indicates an antibody that reacts with all RBCs with a normal (hence nl) Rh phenotype but fails to react with those that are partially deleted (e.g., -D-/-D-) or fully deleted (Rh_{null}). Anti-pdl reacts with all cells with normal and partially deleted (hence pdl) Rh phenotypes but not with fully deleted cells. Anti-dl reacts with all RBCs, including those that are fully deleted (hence dl), and may have no association with the Rh system. The bottom portion of Table 6 lists a number of alloantibodies that have, at least ostensibly, the same specificities as anti-dl and anti-pdl. These alloantibodies result from immunization to antigens (many but not all in the Rh system) lacking from the patient's RBCs; for example, anti-Hr_0 in the serum of an immunized -D- homozygote and anti-Rh29 in the serum of an immunized Rh_{null}. The alloantibodies listed under anti-dl in Table 6 represent some actual specificities found among antibodies initially characterized as anti-dl.

If anti-nl and anti-pdl are considered to be Rh antibodies, some 50% of all warm-reactive autoantibodies are associated with the Rh system. We (181) studied 150 individuals with a positive DAT and warm-reactive autoantibody in the serum and/or an eluate made from the RBCs. Of the 150 individuals, 87 had WAIHA, 33 had formed autoantibodies while being treated with alpha-methyldopa, and 30 were hematologically normal (for additional information on the latter two groups, see below). We identified a total of 311 autoantibodies among the 150 patients; in all, 157 (50.5%) of them were in the Rh system. As in other similar studies (183–187), Rh specificity of the autoantibodies was not always immediately apparent. For example, a serum or eluate that at first appears to contain anti-dl can sometimes be shown to contain anti-pdl and/or anti-nl following adsorption with Rh_{null} and/or -D-/-D- RBCs. Further adsorption of the anti-nl component with R_2R_2 RBCs may then reveal the presence of auto–anti-e. Although we (181) found only four cases with "simple" specificity Rh antibodies

Table 6 Reactions of Autoantibodies to nl, pdl, and dl and Some Ostensibly Similar Alloantibodies

Test Red Cells	Antibody Reactions		
	Anti-nl	Anti-pdl	Anti-dl
Normal Rh phenotype	+	+	+
Rh-deletion	0	+	+
Rh_{null}	0	0	+
	Some examples of ostensibly similar alloantibodies		
	Anti-Hr	Anti-Rh29	Anti-Wr[b]
	Anti-Hr_0	Anti-Rh39	Anti-En[a]
	Anti-Rh34	Anti-LW[ab]	Anti-Kp[b]
		Anti-U	Anti-K13

(three with auto–anti-e, one with auto–anti-c and anti-E) as the only autoantibody present, we found another 56 such antibodies during the adsorption studies.

To add to the complexity of Rh autoantibodies, it is now known that some with apparently simple specificities are not what they initially appear to be (188–191). For example, an antibody that initially appears to have anti-E specificity but can be recovered by elution from the patient's E– RBCs may actually have anti-Hr or anti-Hr_0 specificity. Identification of the real specificity of such autoantibodies is accomplished in adsorption-elution studies. The antibody described above, which initially appears to be anti-E, will be seen to have anti-Hr/Hr_0 specificity when shown to be adsorbed to exhaustion (and recovered by elution) from E+ and E– but not -D-/-D- RBCs. The presence of an autoantibody mimicking an alloantibody is often initially suspected when the serology appears wrong; i.e., an apparent specificity recovered by elution from antigen-negative RBCs (188,189). However, it should be remembered that a sizable proportion of antibodies initially recognized as being autoimmune in nature (i.e., eluted from antigen-positive RBCs) also mimic specificities they do not truly possess (190).

As mentioned above, not all Rh autoantibodies are pathological. Patients who form autoantibodies while being treated with alpha-methyldopa often have a strongly positive direct antiglobulin test (DAT) but no increase in the rate of in vivo RBC destruction; many of the autoantibodies involved have Rh specificity (181,187,192–194). A subset of individuals who have neither WAIHA nor drug-induced antibody production also exists in which the DAT is strongly positive but there are no in vivo sequelae; again Rh autoantibodies are seen (181,187,195). These two groups of individuals provide a graphic reminder that although the DAT may indicate autoantibody production, a positive test is not diagnostic of WAIHA.

IV. BIOCHEMISTRY OF THE Rh PROTEINS

A. Early Findings

Because of its considerable importance at the practical level and its intellectual challenge at the serological and genetic levels, the Rh system was an early target for biochemical study. In spite of the considerable efforts of many prominent investigators, relatively little was learned about the biochemistry of the system in the first 40 years after its discovery. Early attempts to isolate and characterize the Rh antigens or the membrane structures that carry them were thwarted by a variety of problems.

First, Rh antigens seem to be confined to the RBCs of humans and a few higher primates. Although it now appears (see below) that homologues of human Rh antigen-bearing membrane structures are present on the RBCs of some other animals (196), Rh antigens cannot be detected on those cells. Further, although there have been occasional claims to the contrary, most workers agree that human leukocytes, platelets, and tissue cells lack Rh antigens. Soluble forms of the antigens, analogous to those of the ABO, *Hh*, Ii, Lewis, P, Sd, and so forth systems, that so facilitated biochemical studies do not exist.

Second, Rh antigens are present on RBCs in only about one tenth of the number of copies of antigens of the ABO and MN systems (197–199). Thus, large amounts of RBCs yield only small amounts of isolated Rh-associated structures.

Third, it seems likely that older biochemical isolation procedures were harsh enough that they caused denaturation of the Rh antigens during isolation and/or the techniques available to study the isolates were insufficiently sensitive to identify Rh-containing material.

Fourth, it is now known (see below) that for Rh antigen activity to be expressed, rather critical in situ configurations of membrane components are essential. In other words, when the components presumed to be involved in Rh antigen structure are extracted from the membrane, the Rh antigens do not retain the steric arrangement that permits them to complex with antibodies. Indeed this problem continues to hinder progress in this area. In spite of the considerable advances described in the next section, the evidence that it is the Rh polypeptides that have been isolated is indirect in that, as yet, no isolate capable of complexing with an Rh antibody has been obtained (200).

Despite the problems listed above, some progress was made. Green (201) showed that the D activity of isolated RBC membranes could be destroyed by treatment with butanol and restored by the addition of phosphatidylcholine. Hughes-Jones et al. (202) showed that phopholipase A_2 caused partial denaturation of D; an effect that could be blocked if anti-D was allowed to bind to the D+ RBCs before the membrane preparations were made. These and other (203) findings suggested that the Rh antigens were associated in some way with membrane lipoproteins. Even at this early stage, it seemed probable (202) that the Rh antigens were carried on protein structures and that the lipids served to orient the proteins in a manner that allowed recognition of the antigens by antibodies. Another important early observation by Green (204) was that the reactivities of the Rh antigens D and C were dependent on the presence of a thiol group at or near the outer surface of the RBC membrane.

B. Nonglycosylated Rh Proteins

In 1982, two reports (205,206) appeared from workers who independently, but simultaneously, succeeded in the initial isolation of what are now known collectively as the Rh polypeptides. Moore et al. (205) radiolabeled intact RBCs, bound Rh antibodies to the cells, then used staphylococcal protein A to isolate immune complexes from membrane preparations made from the RBCs. At first, a labeled protein with a molecular weight of about 28.5 kd was isolated. By using antibodies to c, D, and E and R_2R_2 RBCs and by modifying the methods used to characterize the isolated proteins, these workers (205,207) then showed that at least two polypeptides had been obtained. One appeared to have been precipitated by anti-D and the other by anti-c and anti-E. However, even at this early stage, these investigators (207) suspected that anti-c and anti-E might have precipitated different polypeptides of closely similar molecular weights and that the differences between the proteins could not be resolved by the methods used. Gahmberg (206) also using a method that involved radiolabeling and immunoprecipitation with anti-D, isolated a previously unrecognized polypeptide with a molecular weight described as being between 28 and 33 kd. There was no doubt that the protein isolated by Moore et al. (205) and Gahmberg (206), using anti-D, was the same one. In both studies, it was shown that the isolated proteins were highly unusual in that they were not glycosylated. Following these initial breakthrough studies, other investigators isolated the same proteins and information about them rapidly accumulated (198,199,208–210).

Ridgwell et al. (211) used the earlier observation of Green (204) on the need for a thiol group for certain Rh antigen activity and showed the Rh$_{null}$ RBCs lack two thiol group–containing proteins that are present on RBCs of all normal Rh phenotypes. One of these proteins, with a molecular weight of 32 kd could be precipitated by anti-D and undoubtedly was the same as the protein isolated by Moore et al. (205) and Gahmberg (206) using that same antibody. By this time, Moore and Green (212) had shown that the protein that they had isolated with anti-D had a molecular weight of 31.9 kd. The second protein present on normal cells but missing from those of the Rh$_{null}$ phenotype had a molecular weight of 34 kd and could be precipitated (211) by a monoclonal antibody, R6A, that in serological tests reacts with all except Rh$_{null}$ RBCs (213). This 34-kd protein corresponded to the 33.1-kd protein (or proteins) immunoprecipitated by anti-c and anti-E (214).

The Paris workers (198,199,208,210,215,216) then used a series of potent monoclonal Rh antibodies (to D, c, E, and G) made by EBV transformation of human B cells (217) in a series of critical experiments. Using competitive immunoassays and flow cytometric studies with two separate labels, these workers showed that on intact RBCs one polypeptide appears to carry D and G, a second c, and a third E. These studies supported the earlier suggestion of Moore and Green (207,212) that anti-c and anti-E precipitate different proteins of the same molecular size. The monoclonal antibodies were then used to isolate the Rh polypeptides and peptide mapping studies were undertaken (208,215). When the isolates were digested with trypsin or chymotrypsin, three distinct but similar blotting patterns were seen. When V-8 proteinase was used, few differences in the blots were noted. These findings were taken to indicate that the D, c, and E proteins are distinct but are very closely related as shown by their large areas of homology. In amino acid composition studies (210) on the peptide precipitated by anti-D, a high proportion of hydrophobic amino acids was seen, a finding that correlates well with earlier suggestions (201–204) that the Rh proteins are largely embedded within the RBC membrane. The presence of cysteine (in the form of cysteic acid) correlated with the earlier observation (204) on the need for thiol groups for antigen integrity.

A considerable disadvantage in using immunoprecipitation methods to isolate the Rh polypeptides is that only small amounts of finishing material are obtained for further study. This problem was addressed by the Baltimore workers (196,218,219), who devised a nonimmunological method for isolation of the proteins. The yield when this method is used is almost 10 times greater than that obtained by immunoprecipitation, and many of the investigations described in the section on the function of the Rh polypeptides were made possible when greater yields of the proteins were obtained. Peptide mapping and amino acid sequencing studies on the isolates made by Cartron et al. (208,210,215) and Agre et al. (218,219) showed that the same proteins had been isolated. The finding that the amino acid sequences of the D, c, and E polypeptides were the same from residue 1 to residue 21 (later extended to residue 41; see below) at the NH_2 terminal ends added support to the conclusion that the polypeptides are closely related. Still more evidence was provided by Suyama and Goldstein (220), who immunized a rabbit with a denatured isolate of D polypeptide and showed that the antibody made would also react with c and E polypeptides. Apparently the antibody was directed against a portion of the D polypeptide that is homologous with a portion of the Cc and Ee polypeptides. Although it is speculative, it is relatively easy to guess that human antibodies to Rh29 and Rh39 (see above) are somewhat like this rabbit antibody in terms of specificity. Antibodies to Hr_o, Hr, and Rh34 may differ in that they fail to react with Rh deletion (e.g., -D-/-D-, cD-/cD-) RBCs so they may detect a homologous portion of the Cc and Ee polypeptides that is not present on the D polypeptide. Suyama and Goldstein (221) also provided evidence for differences between the closely related Rh proteins. Digestion of intact RBCs with phospholipase A_2 followed by treatment of the digests with papain showed partial degradation of the D but not the Ċc or Ee polypeptides.

C.   Are the Rh Polypeptides Attached to the Cytoskeleton?

Soon after the Rh polypeptides were recognized, evidence emerged that was taken to indicate that the proteins are attached to the internal actin-spectrin skeleton of the RBC. Gahmberg and Karhi (222) and Ridgwell et al. (223) reported that when the Rh proteins were isolated using low concentrations (i.e., 1–5% vol/vol) of Triton X-100, 70–80% of the polypeptides remained attached to the insoluble cytoskeleton. Paradis et al. (224) showed that D antigen integrity was preserved by the cytoskeleton when membranes containing D to which anti-D had been bound were solubilized in nonionic detergents. It was speculated that the stomatocytic nature of Rh_{null} RBCs (see below) might relate to the absence of Rh polypeptide linkage to the cytoskeleton. However, more recent observations (200) have caused the assumption of direct linkage to be questioned, and it now seems possible that the earlier observations related to the relative insolubility of the Rh polypeptides in Triton X-100. Physical shaking of intact RBC membranes in 5% (wt/vol) Triton X-100 results in more than 70% of the Rh polypeptides being solubilized (198). When Triton X-100 was used to extract Rh polypeptides from whole RBC membranes and spectrin-depleted membrane vesicles, similar solubilities were seen, showing that the membrane skeleton is not a major constraint in solubilization of the Rh proteins (225). Thus, it currently appears that interaction between the Rh polypeptides and the membrane skeleton either does not exist or is relatively weak.

D. Homologues of Rh Proteins on the RBCs of Other Species

As mentioned earlier, the prime site of Rh antigens is on circulating human RBCs. Tests with human polyclonal antibodies failed to detect the Rh antigens on erythroid progenitor cells (226). More recent studies with monoclonal antibodies have suggested that the Rh antigens are present on some more mature progenitors but in lower site density than on mature RBCs (227). Some Old World monkeys have an antigen that resembles c and some New World monkeys have antigens that resemble c and D on their RBCs (228,229). Antigens in the Ee series have been found only on the RBCs of humans. When the RBCs of lower primates, cows, cats, and rats were studied using the nonimmunological method (218) for the isolation of Rh polypeptides, 32-kd proteins somewhat analogous to the human Rh polypeptides were found (196). However, when two-dimensional iodopeptide maps were prepared, little homology between the human and animal proteins was seen. In other words, although a similarly functional protein to the human Rh polypeptides may exist on the RBCs of various mammals, it is likely that there are differences in primary structure.

E. Rh Glycoproteins

In 1987, Moore and Green (212) reported that when immunoprecipitation is used to isolate the nonglycosylated Rh polypeptides from RBC membrane preparations, unique ABH antigen-bearing glycoproteins are coprecipitated. From the initial study, it was clear that immunoprecipitation was specific; mixtures of RBCs of different phenotypes were used to exclude nonspecific precipitation or de novo complex formation during the isolation procedure. Further, the glycoprotein of MW 45 to 100 kd that was immunoprecipitated with the 31.9-kd D polypeptide was shown to differ from the MW 35 to 60 kd glycoprotein coprecipitated with the 33.1-kd Cc and/or Ee polypeptide(s). As with the nonglycosylated Rh polypeptides described above, the isolated glycoproteins failed to cause inhibition of Rh antibodies, so that it is still not clear whether Rh antigens are carried on the polypeptides, on the glycoproteins, on both, or on neither (the antigens could represent interactions between the proteins). In spite of this, because immunoprecipitation was specific and because later findings (see below) confirmed the association of these structures with the Rh system, they are now called the Rh glycoproteins.

The Rh glycoproteins were then studied further by Avent et al. (214), who had earlier shown (213) that a monoclonal antibody R6A (that reacts serologically with all except Rh_{null} RBCs) also precipitates Rh-associated components from RBC membrane preparations. These workers used a terminology that is based on the specificity of the antibody effecting precipitation and the molecular size of the component obtained. Thus, D_{30} and D_{50} were precipitated by anti-D; D_{30} appears to correspond to the nonglycosylated D polypeptide described above, and D_{50} is the D glycoprotein (MW 45–100 kd). $R6A_{32}$ and $R6A_{45}$ were precipitated by monoclonal antibodies of the R6A type; both were described as being glycoproteins (214). Thus, it is not clear if $R6A_{32}$ corresponds to the nonglycosylated Cc and/or Ee polypeptide(s) described above. Although the presence of glycans on $R6A_{32}$ argues against identity of the two proteins, the finding (see below) that $R6A_{32}$, D_{30}, and the nonglycosylated D, Cc, and Ee polypeptides share an amino acid sequence (at least in terms of residues identified thus far) suggests that $R6A_{32}$ might be the same protein as that described as the Cc and/or Ee polypeptide. $R6A_{45}$ is a (presumably CcEe) glycoprotein (MW 35–52 kd). It has been shown (212) that im-munoprecipitation of these glycoproteins by Rh antibodies still occurs after glycosidase digestion, showing that Rh antigen structure is not (solely) the result of glycosylation. Although it was initially suspected that the Rh glycoproteins might be glycosylated versions of the nonglycosylated Rh polypeptides, this is not the case. Avent et al. (214) determined partial amino acid sequences of the components they had isolated. The D_{30} and $R6A_{32}$ sequences were the same and identical to that established by Cartron et al. (210) and Agre et al. (219) for the D polypeptide. The D_{50} and $R6A_{45}$ sequences were the same as each other but different from the smaller molecular weight proteins (214). Thus, it follows that D_{50} is not a glycosylated form of D_{30} and that $R6A_{45}$ is not a more heavily glycosylated form of $R6A_{32}$. Another suspicion that the glycosylated and nonglycosylated Rh proteins might be produced as a single protein then cleaved in a posttranslation change also seems to have been excluded. Based on the size of the proteins and what is known of the size of *Rh* genes (see below), it seems that the joined proteins would represent too large a product.

Although the amino acid sequencing studies of Avent et al. (214) showed that the smaller Rh proteins differ considerably from the Rh glycoproteins, it seems that some sort of ancestral relationship may exist. First, the putative N terminal membrane-spanning regions of the D_{30}, D_{50}, and $R6A_{45}$ proteins showed considerable homology (200,214). Second, when the D_{30} and D_{50} sequences were compared a number of "evolutionary homologous" pairs of residues were seen (200).

As mentioned earlier, the antigen Duclos (94) was recognized from the time of its discovery to have some sort of relationship (at least at the phenotypic level) to the Rh system. In studying monoclonal antibodies (called the 2D10 type) that have a specificity (230) that is either the same or very similar to anti-Duclos, von dem Borne et al. (231) showed that the antibodies react specifically with the $R6A_{45}$ and D_{50} glycoproteins. Different studies (232) have shown that the amino acids at positions 33–39 of glycophorin B(Ss SGP) are involved in the structure of the Duclos antigen. Thus, it seems that the Duclos determinant may represent a structure that involves interaction between glycophorin B and the Rh glycoproteins (2D10-reactive glycoproteins) in a manner analogous to the way in which Wr^b appears to involve glycophorin A (MN SGP) and protein band 3 (233).

F. The Rh Polypeptide In Situ

Two groups of workers (234,235) have succeeded in cloning an Rh complementary (cDNA); the results of the two studies were essentially identical. Although the evidence is somewhat indirect, it is believed that the cDNA identified represents the genetic material that encodes production of the nonglycosylated Cc and/or Ee polypeptide(s). The open reading frame of the Rh cDNA encodes 416 amino acids in the mature protein; the calculated molecular weight of the deduced protein is 45.5 kd. The finding that in sodium dodecylsulfate–polyacrylamine gel electrophoresis (SDS-PAGE) analysis, the polypeptide appears to have a molecular weight in the order of 30–32 kd is thought to be due to its high content of hydrophobic amino acid residues that have high affinity for SDS (236). A posttranslation change in the encoded protein is considered unlikely to explain a size difference because a tryptic digest of an isolated Rh polypeptide corresponds to a predicted seven amino acid sequence at the C terminal end of the predicted protein (237).

Examination of the amino acid sequence of the Rh polypeptide, as predicted from the Rh cDNA, strongly suggests (200,210,234) that most of the protein is situated within the RBC membrane bilayer. It appears that the protein may span the bilayer 13 times, with only small portions of the polypeptide outside the RBC. Although such a structure is highly reminiscent of a transporter protein, no such function has yet been unequivocally established for Rh. The

NH_2-terminus of the protein appears to be within the cytoplasm of the RBC, the C-terminus is thought to be outside the membrane and to include two related seven amino acid repeat sequences, with at least one tyrosine residue outside the cell (200). In terms of identity between the D, Cc, and Ee polypeptides, it is thought that polymorphisms begin at some point after residue 41 from the NH_2-terminus (235). Although it appears that an unblocked cysteine residue at position 284 and the external tyrosine at position 400 are outside the membrane, there is as yet no explanation for the enormous variety of different Rh immunogens (see section on Rh antigens and phenotypes above), particularly in view of the fact that most of the Rh protein is predicted to be embedded within the membrane bilayer. One of the most intriguing questions about Rh is why is D so immunogenic? The finding (discussed below) that Rh+ individuals have two *Rh* genes, whereas Rh– persons have only one, means that Rh+ RBCs will carry an Rh protein that Rh– persons lack. However, the data listed above suggest that rather than D being a simple highly immunogenic structure, it will be seen (eventually) to be an interaction product involving not only the D polypeptide but other structures (as discussed below).

As mentioned above, early studies (201–204) suggested a relationship between Rh antigens and RBC membrane lipids. Once the Rh polypeptides could be isolated, this relationship was examined more closely. de Vetten and Agre (238) showed that the Rh polypeptides are major fatty acylated membrane proteins. Further, acylation of the Rh proteins was predicted to occur exclusively at multiple sites close to the inner leaflet of the phospholipid bilayer. Once the amino acid sequence of the Rh polypeptide could be deduced, it became apparent that the acylation sites are cysteine residues at positions 11, 185, and 310, each of which is forecast to be at a point where the protein crosses the inner portion of the bilayer (238). The major membrane acylation role of Rh proteins is considered again in the section on possible functions of the Rh proteins.

G. Rh Cluster or Complex Models

Recognition of the Rh polypeptides and glycoproteins has not resulted in recognition of the structure of Rh antigens. Further to compound this situation, it seems that other membrane components whose production is not encoded by genes at the *Rh* locus, which is on chromosome 1, may interact with Rh proteins. Such a probability was clear from studies at the phenotypic level. Rh_{null} RBCs that lack all expression of Rh antigens are LW(a-b-) (93,239) and Fy:-5 (240) and have a marked depression of expression of U (112). This in spite of the fact that the LW antigens are encoded from a locus on chromosome 19 (241) and are carried on a distinct membrane glycoprotein (242–244). Although the *Fy* locus is also on chromosome 1 (245), it is distal to *Rh*, and although the glycoprotein that probably carries the Duffy system antigens (205,246) has some characteristics in common with $R6A_{45}$ and D_{50}, no clear relationship between the molecules has yet been established (247). Further, Rh_{null}, Fy:-5 RBCs can carry normal expressions of Fy^a or Fy^b or both (240). The U antigen is located on glycophorin B; the production of which is encoded from a locus on chromosome 4 (248). The depression of expression of U antigen on Rh_{null} RBCs is now known (249) to reflect the fact that such cells carry only some 30% of the number of copies of glycophorin B found on RBCs of normal Rh phenotypes. In addition, it is known that Rh_{null} RBCs lack other membrane components. The monoclonal antibody BRIC 125 defines a heavily glycosylated MW 47- to 52-kd glycoprotein; the antibody reacts poorly with Rh_{null} RBCs (213). A different monoclonal antibody, 1D8, defines a cell surface antigen encoded by a gene on chromosome 3; again, Rh_{null} cells fail to react with this antibody (250).

Findings such as these led Cartron (208) to propose an Rh cluster model. It is supposed that in the absence of Rh proteins, some other genetically independent components cannot properly be incorporated into the RBC membrane; a somewhat similar suggestion regarding association of other polypeptides with the Rh complex was made by Anstee (247). As yet, it is not clear what role the Rh cluster plays in the expression of Rh antigens. It is possible that in order for antibody recognition of Rh antigens to occur, some, many, or all the associated glycoproteins may be required for spatial orientation of the Rh antigens. If so, producing an Rh isolate capable of inhibiting antibody may require plucking the whole cluster from the membrane or producing transfectants by the incorporation of a series of unrelated genes (200). It also is possible that all that is needed for Rh antigen integrity is coexpression of the nonglycosylated and glycosylated Rh proteins. Agre et al. (218) showed that the nonimmunological method for isolation of Rh proteins does not result in an end product that includes the other glycoproteins, suggesting that the various components are only loosely associated at the membrane level.

It is clear that although the LW-, Duffy-, and U-bearing RBC membrane components may require the presence of the Rh proteins for full expression, the reverse is not true. LW(a-b-), Fy(a-b-), Fy:-3,-5, and S-s-U- RBCs all express Rh antigens normally (17–19).

V. FUNCTION OF THE Rh PROTEINS

Although much new information about the structure of the Rh proteins has recently been obtained, little is known about their function. It was hoped that studies on the Rh_{null} phenotype would reveal what roles the Rh proteins normally play. Indeed, it was seen that in Rh_{null} persons, many of the RBCs are stomatocytes and a few are spherocytes and that, as such, the RBCs show increased sensitivity to osmotic lysis (112,113). At the biochemical level Rh_{null} RBCs have increased adenosine triphosphatase (ATPase) activity (251), reduced cation and water contents, a relative deficiency of membrane cholesterol (252), and perturbation of membrane phospholipid distribution (253). At the clinical level, Rh_{null} persons present with a chronic hemolytic anemia that varies from being almost fully compensated in some to requiring splenectomy for correction in others (61,254). This variation is reflected by the in vivo survival time of autologous RBCs in different Rh_{null} persons; half-lives as short as 7 days (255) and as long as 18 days (256,257) have been reported. Similar physiological and clinical findings have been made in persons of the Rh_{mod} phenotype; indeed in such persons the need for splenectomy may be a little more common (109,110). Although all these observations suggest that the Rh proteins are necessary for RBC membrane integrity, they do not identify any clear or specific defects. Agre and Cartron (200) have suggested that the lack of severe clinical manifestations in the Rh_{null} and Rh_{mod} syndrome may reflect a fine-tuning mechanism for Rh in RBC membrane physiology. Additional evidence to suggest a functional role for Rh proteins was provided by the observations of the Baltimore workers (196) that although the nonhuman Rh homologues differed considerably in structure to the Rh proteins, they had retained their fatty acid acylation characteristic.

Phospholipids of the RBC membrane are known to be asymmetrically distributed with the membrane's outer leaflet being rich in phosphatidylcholine and the inner leaflet being rich in phosphatidylethanolamine and the sole site of phosphatidylserine (258–260). An ATP-dependent enzyme, often referred to as phosphatidylserine (PS) flippase, has been shown to regulate this asymmetry by the transfer of phosphatidylserine from the outer to the inner leaflet (261). In one laboratory, a PS flippase with a molecular size and many of the features of the Rh polypeptides was identified (262,263). Indeed in a later study, monoclonal Rh antibodies were shown to immunoprecipitate this PS flippase (264). However, the situation is not as straightforward as it might initially appear. First, the Rh protein may simply be attached to PS flippase in situ as part of the Rh cluster described above (200). Second, the PS flippase activity of Rh_{null} RBCs was found to be normal (265), although an entirely different form of the enzyme may exist (266) to account for this finding. Third, if the Rh polypeptides are noncatalytic subunits of PS flippase (264), presumably an analogue of the Rh polypeptide must exist within

Rh$_{null}$ RBCs. Although Moore and Green (212) described a component that would fit such a description, this author is not aware of its existence having been confirmed by others. Fourth, coating RBCs with Rh antibodies did not interfere with their membranes' PS flippase activity (265). Fifth, the deduced (from cDNA; see above) sequence of the Rh polypeptide is not characteristic of an ATPase. Although it remains possible that the Rh polypeptides play a role in PS flippase activity, much work will be needed to differentiate participation of the Rh polypeptides (if any) from that of the many other proteins with which they are apparently associated in the membrane. Because it is established that the Rh polypeptides are fatty acylated (238), perhaps their role is to maintain membrane lipid asymmetry once it has been established by other proteins (the author is not aware of any supporting evidence). That is, with palmitic acids covalently linked to cysteine residues (see above) on the inner edge of the membrane leaflet, perhaps the Rh proteins somehow ensure that phosphatidylserine remains in place. As mentioned above, Kuypers et al. (253) reported a perturbation of lipid organization in the membrane of Rh$_{null}$ RBCs.

Regardless of the function of the Rh polypeptides, it seems that the antigens play no role. In spite of the huge variation in *Rh* gene products in terms of recognizable antigens, it seems that any RBCs with readily detectable Rh antigens function normally no matter which antigens are present. Along similar lines, Hughes-Jones et al. (216) used flow cytometry to study individual RBCs from a donor of the R$_2$R$_2$ phenotype. Although there was considerable cell to cell variation in terms of number of copies of c, D, and E polypeptides carried, the total number of Rh proteins per cell was roughly the same. It has, of course, been known for some time (267,268) that if the antigens C, c, D, E, and e are considered, RBCs of "normal" Rh phenotypes carry roughly equal total numbers of sites. That is, the sum of C, D, and e antigens on R$_1$R$_1$ cells, c, D, and E antigens on R$_2$R$_2$ cells, and c and e antigens on rr cells is the order of 150,000 to 200,000 per cell. Studies designed to estimate the number of copies of Rh polypeptides per cell, using monoclonal antibodies for the measurements, have yielded similar results (197). Thus, it seems that as long as a certain amount of Rh protein per RBC is present, normal membrane function results. When the Rh proteins are either absent or present in grossly reduced amounts (or perhaps present in a nonfunctional form) as in the Rh$_{null}$ and Rh$_{mod}$ phenotypes, membrane integrity is compromised. All these data suggest, of course, that it is the basic Rh protein that is functional. This might also explain the huge polymorphism of Rh. If the *Rh* gene is ancient and subject to ready mutation, but if antigen variation does not affect protein function, the multiple variants (mutants) that have arisen over a long time period would provide neither selective advantage nor disadvantage, so all would propagate.

VI. GENETICS OF THE Rh SYSTEM

Theories about the genetic control of Rh antigen production have been debated so many times in so many different publications from the 1940s through the late 1980s that they need not be repeated here. Suffice it here to say that more than 50 years of speculation are coming to an end, finally to be replaced by scientific data. In 1991, Colin et al. (27) published the results of studies in which they used Southern blot analysis of genomic DNA from donors of different Rh phenotypes. Using an entire Rh cDNA probe and several exon-specific probes covering the cloned *Rh* gene, these workers showed that in the genome of Rh+ individuals there are two different but closely related *Rh* genes, whereas in the genome of Rh– persons there is only one. It was concluded that the gene present in both Rh+ and Rh– persons encodes production, probably via different mRNA transcripts (269) from the same gene, of the Cc and Ee polypeptides. The second gene present in Rh+ but not in Rh– persons encodes production of the D-containing Rh polypeptide. Somewhat surprisingly, the gene that normally encodes the Cc and Ee polypeptides was found (27) in the genome of a -D-/-D- person, although its products are not detectable on such RBCs. Lack of the *D* gene, or any allele thereof in Rh– persons, explains why no d antigen (and hence no anti-d) has ever been found. Although the explanation is highly satisfactory at the genetic level, it has not yet provided an explanation of the high immunogenicity of D in Rh– persons. In other words, although it can be deduced that Rh– persons lack an entire protein that is present in Rh+ RBCs, it is not yet known what makes that protein so immunogenic. Indeed, characterization of the *D* gene product and its difference from the Cc and Ee polypeptides will be necessary for such an explanation. Because the difference between Rh+ and Rh– involves the presence and absence, respectively, of a gene and a protein, perhaps Rh– persons can now be thought of as being D_{null}. It is well established that persons with null (or minus-minus) phenotypes in other blood group systems are readily susceptible to immunization when exposed to RBCs carrying normal expressions of antigens of those systems (18).

The practical demonstration of two *Rh* genes, one encoding the D-bearing polypeptide and the second encoding a CcEe or Cc and Ee-bearing polypeptide(s) was expertly and eloquently forecast on theoretical grounds by Tippett (270) 5 years before the confirmatory data emerged. As yet, there is no information regarding genetic control of production of the Rh glycoproteins described earlier in this chapter. The fact that two rather than one or three *Rh* genes appear to exist does not necessarily invalidate some earlier suggestions. For example, the presence of an antigen similar to c on the RBCs of some higher primates and the presence of antigens similar to c and D on the RBCs of others (228,229) is often taken to indicate that the "original" *Rh* gene may have been *c* and that *D* arose by gene duplication then modification. The close similarity of the two *Rh* genes identified by Colin et al. (27) certainly leaves such a theory entirely tenable. The often bewildering array of *Rh* genes (for a partial listing see Table 4) can still be explained by this author's suggestion (18,66,67) of ordered genes; i.e., genes in series with each being related to one of the "normal" ancestral genes in Table 2. The concept of different messenger RNA (mRNA) transcripts from genes in the *D* and *CcEe* series does not change such a proposal.

Even before the above findings about the *Rh* genes had been made, linkage studies (271) and observations in an individual with a gene deletion (272) had shown that the *Rh* locus is located on the short arm of chromosome 1; i.e., 1p3,4. In situ hybridization experiments then confirmed the localization to region 1p34.3–1p36.1 (273).

NOTE ADDED IN PROOF   Since this chapter was completed many additional findings about the Rh system have been made. Some of these findings alter some statements made in the chapter. Lomas et al. (letter to the Editor, Transfusion, in press 1993) have shown that the RBCs of partial D categories IVb and Vc are not different after all and have suggested that the designation for subcategory Vc be abolished. Le Van Kim et al. (Proc Natl Acad Sci 1992; 89:10925) have now cloned the *D* gene. Their study confirms that, as suspected, the *Rh* gene previously cloned (234,235) is the one that encodes the CcEe polypeptide(s). A forecast of the structure of the D polypeptide projects that it is of similar size and shape to the CcEe protein(s) but has different amino acids at 36 of its 417 positions. Surprisingly, less than 10 of the amino acid substitutions are forecast to be at or near the outer surface of the RBC membrane. The relationship (if any) between these amino acid substitutions and the epitopes of D described in the chapter is not yet known. Avent et al. (J Biol Chem 1992;267:15134) have presented additional evidence in support of their view that both the NH_2 and COOH terminals of the Rh polypeptides are located on the inner side of the RBC membrane. This model differs from the one of Cherif-Zahar et al. (234) described in the chapter in which the NH_2 terminus is forecast to be inside and the COOH terminus outside the RBC membrane. Ridgwell et al. (Biochem J 1992;287:223) have shown that production of the Rh glycoproteins is controlled from a locus on chromosome 6. This finding, together with those (271–273) that show that the nonglycosylated Rh polypeptides are encoded by genes at a locus on chromosome 1, clearly indicates that the nonglycosylated Rh polypeptides play a far larger role than do the Rh glycoproteins in Rh antigen structure and/or composition.

REFERENCES

1. Levine P, Stetson RE. An unusual case of intragroup agglutination. JAMA 1939; 113:126.
2. Landsteiner K, Wiener AS. An agglutinable factor in human blood recognized by immune sera for rhesus blood. Proc. Soc. Exp. Biol. NY 1940; 43:223.
3. Wiener AS, Peters HR. Hemolytic reactions following transfusions of blood of the homologous group, with three cases in which the same agglutinogen was responsible. Ann Intern Med 1940; 13:2306.
4. Levine P, Katzin EM, Burnham L. Isoimmunization in pregnancy, its possible bearing on the etiology of erythroblastosis fetalis. JAMA 1941; 116:825.
5. Levine P, Vogel P, Katzin EM, Burnham L. Pathogenesis of erythroblastosis fetalis: Statistical evidence. Science 1941; 94:371.
6. Levine P, Burnham L, Katzin EM, Vogel P. The role of isoimmunization in the pathogenesis of erythroblastosis fetalis. Am J Obstet Gynecol 1941; 42:925.
7. Levine P, Celano MJ, Wallace J, Sanger R. A human 'D-like' antibody. Nature 1963; 198:596.
8. Rosenfield RE. Who discovered Rh? Transfusion 1989; 29:355.
9. Buchbinder L. The blood grouping of Macacus rhesus: Including comparative studies of the antigenic structure of the erythrocytes of man and Macacus rhesus. J. Immunol 1933; 25:33.
10. Lewis M, Anstee DJ, Bird GWG, et al. Blood group terminology 1990. Vox Sang 1990; 58:152.
11. Lewis M, Anstee DJ, Bird GWG, et al. ISBT working party on terminology for red cell surface antigens: Los Angeles report. Vox Sang 1991; 61:158.
12. Fisher RA, cited by Race RR. An 'incomplete' antibody in human serum. Nature 1944; 153:771.
13. Fisher RA, Race RR. Rh gene frequences in Britain. Nature 1946; 157:48.
14. Wiener AS. Genetic theory of the Rh blood types. Proc. Soc. Exp. Biol. NY 1943; 54:316.
15. Wiener AS, Sonn EB. The Rh series of genes with special reference to nomenclature. Ann. NY. Acad. Sci 1946; 46:969.
16. Rosenfield RE, Allen FH Jr, Swisher SN, Kochwa S. A review of Rh serology and presentation of a new terminology. Transfusion 1962; 2:287.
17. Salmon C, Cartron JP, Rouger P. The Human Blood Groups. New York, Masson, 1984.
18. Issitt PD. Applied Blood Group Serology. 3rd ed. Miami, Montgomery Scientific, 1985.
19. Mollison PL, Engelfriet CP, Contreras M. Blood Transfusion in Clinical Medicine. 8th ed. Oxford, England, Blackwell Scientific, 1987.
20. Issitt PD. The Rh blood group system, 1988: Eight new antigens in nine years and some observations on the biochemistry and genetics of the system. Transf Med Rev 1989; 3:1.
21. Wiener AS. Hemolytic reactions following transfusion of blood of the homologous group. II. Arch. Pathol. 1941; 32:227.
22. Wiener AS, Sonn EB. Additional variants of the Rh type demonstrable with a special human anti-Rh serum. J. Immunol. 1943; 47:461.
23. Race RR, Taylor GL, Boorman KE, Dodd BE. Recognition of Rh genotypes in man. Nature 1943; 152:563.
24. Mourant AE. A new rhesus antibody. Nature 1945; 155:542.
25. Race RR, Sanger R. Blood Groups in Man. 6th ed. Oxford, England, Blackwell Scientific, 1975.
26. Walker RH, ed. Technical Manual. 10th ed. Arlington, VA, Am Assoc Blood Banks, 1990.
27. Colin Y, Cherif-Zahar B, Le Van Kim C, et al. Genetic basis of the Rh D-positive and Rh D-negative blood group polymorphism as determined by Southern analysis. Blood 1991; 78:2747.
28. Rosenfield RE, Vogel P, Gibbel N, et al. A 'new' Rh antibody, anti-f. Br Med J 1953; i:975.
29. Rosenfield RE, Haber GV. An Rh blood factor, rh$_i$ (Ce), and its relationship to hr (ce). Am J Hum Genet 1958; 10:474.
30. Gold ER, Gillespie EM, Tovey GH. A serum containing 8 antibodies. Vox Sang 1961; 6:157.
31. Keith P, Corcoran PA, Caspersen K, Allen FH Jr. A new antibody; anti-Rh(27) (cE) in the Rh blood-group system. Vox Sang 1965; 10:528.

32. Dunsford I. A new Rh antibody—anti-CE. Proc. 8th Cong. Europ. Soc. Haematol. Paper No. 491, Vienna, 1961.
33. Rosenfield RE, Haber GV, Schroeder R, Ballard R. Problems in Rh typing as revealed by a single Negro family. Am J Hum Genet 1960; 12:147.
34. Race RR, Sanger R. Wither Rh? International symposium on the immunology and biochemistry of human blood, Amsterdam 1959. Vox Sang 1961; 6:227.
35. Race RR, Sanger R, Selwyn JG. A probable deletion in a human Rh chromosome. Nature 1950; 166:520.
36. Race RR, Sanger R, Selwyn JG. A possible deletion in a human Rh chromosome: A serological and genetical study. Br J Exp Pathol 1951; 32:124.
37. Contreras M, Stebbing B, Blessing M, Gavin J. The Rh antigen Evans. Vox Sang 1978; 34:208.
38. Contreras M, Armitage S, Daniels GL, Tippett P. Homozygous •D•. Vox Sang 1979; 36:81.
39. Gunson HH, Donohoe WL. Multiple examples of the blood genotype $C^wD–/C^wD–$ in a Canadian family. Vox Sang 1957; 2:320.
40. Gunson HH, Donohue WL. The blood genotype $C^wD–/C^wD–$. Proc. 6th Cong. Int. Soc. Blood Transf., 1958:123.
41. Tate H, Cunningham C, McDade MG, et al. An Rh gene complex Dc-. Vox Sang 1960; 5:398.
42. Salmon C, Gerbal A, Liberge G, et al. Le complexe genique $D^{IV}(C)–$, (Fr). Rev Fr Transf 1969; 12:239.
43. Allen FH Jr, Tippett PA. A new Rh blood type which reveals the Rh antigen G. Vox Sang 1958; 3:321.
44. Stout TD, Moore BPL, Allen FH Jr, Corcoran PA. A new phenotype: D+, G– (Rh:1,–12). Vox Sang 1963; 8:262.
45. Shapiro M. Serology and genetics of a 'new' blood factor: hr^H. J Forens Med 1964; 11:52.
46. Zaino EC. A new Rh phenotype, Rh_orh, G-negative. Transfusion 1965; 5:320.
47. Tippett P. Serological Study of the Inheritance of Unusual Rh and Other Blood Group Phenotypes. PhD Thesis, University of London, London, England, 1963.
48. Case J. Quantitative variation in the G antigen of the Rh blood group system. Vox Sang 1973; 25:529.
49. Levine P, Rosenfield RE, White J. The first example of the Rh phenotype r^Gr^G. Am J Hum Genet 1961; 13:299.
50. Allen FH Jr, Corcoran PA. Evidence for a new blood group antigen of nearly universal occurrence (abstract), Proc. 11th Ann. Mtg. Am Assoc Blood Banks, Cincinnati, Ohio, 1958.
51. Shapiro M. Serology and genetics of a new blood factor: hr^S. J Forens Med 1960; 7:96.
52. Shapiro M, LeRoux M, Brink S. Serology and genetics of a new blood factor: hr^B. Haematologia 1972; 6:121.
53. Issitt PD, Gutgsell NS. Subdivisions of the Rh antigen, Hr_0 (abstract). Book of Abstracts, International Society of Blood Transfusion and the Am Assoc Blood Banks Joint Congress, Los Angeles, 1990:29.
54. Habibi B, Perrier P, Salmon C. Antigen Nou. A new high frequency Rh antigen. Blood Transf. Immunohematol 1981; 24:117.
55. Issitt PD, Gutgsell NS. Some new Rh antigens: Rh43 to Rh47. Immunohematology 1987; 3:1.
56. Issitt PD, Gutgsell NS, McDowell MA, Tregellas WM. Studies on anti-Rh46 (abstract). Blood 1987; 70(suppl 1):110a.
57. LePennec PY, Rouger P, Klein MT, et al. A serologic study of red cells and sera from 18 Rh:32,–46 ($\bar{R}^N/\bar{R}^N$) persons. Transfusion 1989; 29:798.
58. Daniels GL. Blood Group Antigens of High Frequency: a Serological and Genetical Study. PhD Thesis, University of London, London, England, 1980.
59. Daniels GL. An investigation of the immune response of homozygotes for the Rh haplotype -D- and related haplotypes. Blood Transf. Immunohematol 1982; 25:185.
60. Issitt PD. New Studies on the Serology and Genetics of the Rh Blood Group System. PhD Thesis, Columbia Pacific University, San Rafael, California 1987.
61. Vos GH, Vos D, Kirk RL, Sanger R. A sample of blood with no detectable Rh antigens. Lancet 1961; 1:14.
62. Levine P, Celano MJ, Falkowski F, et al. A second example of - - -/- - - blood, or Rh_{null}. Nature 1964; 204:892.

63. Ishimori T, Hasekura H. A case of a Japanese blood with no detectable Rh blood group antigen. Proc Jpn Acad 1966; 42:658.

64. Haber GV, Bastani A, Arpin PD, Rosenfield RE. Rh$_{null}$ and pregnancy complicated by maternal anti-"total Rh".I.Anti-Rh29(Rh) (abstract). Transfusion 1967; 7:389.

65. Issitt PD, Pavone BG, Shapiro M. Anti-Rh39- a 'new' specificity Rh system antibody. Transfusion 1979; 19:389.

66. Issitt PD. Serology and Genetics of the Rhesus Blood Group System. Cincinnati, OH, Montgomery Scientific, 1979.

67. Issitt PD. 'Ordered' genes of the Rh blood group system. Can J Med Technol 1978; 40:52.

68. Chown B, Allen FH Jr, Cleghorn TE, et al. Unpublished observations 1965 to 1968. Cited in: Race RR, Sanger R. Blood Groups in Man. 5th ed. Oxford, England, Blackwell Scientific, 1968.

69. Issitt PD, Gutgsell NS, Martin PA, Forguson JR. Hemolytic disease of the newborn caused by anti-Rh32 and demonstration that $\bar{R}^N$ encodes rh$_i$ (Ce, Rh7). Transfusion 1991; 31:63.

70. Callender ST, Race RR. A serological and genetical study of multiple antibodies formed in response to blood transfusion by a patient with lupus erythematosus diffusus. Ann Eugen 1946; 13:102.

71. Stratton F, Renton PH. Hemolytic disease of the newborn caused by a new Rh antibody, anti-C^X. Br Med J 1954; 1:962.

72. Greenwalt TJ, Sanger R. The Rh antigen E^W. Br J Haematol 1955; 1:52.

73. Chown B, Lewis M, Kaita H. A 'new' Rh antigen and antibody. Transfusion 1962; 2:150.

74. Lewis M, Chown B, Kaita H, et al. Blood group antigen Go^a and the Rh system. Transfusion 1967; 7:440.

75. Giles CM, Crossland JD, Haggas WK, Longster G. An Rh gene complex which results in a 'new' antigen detectable by a specific antibody, anti-Rh33. Vox Sang 1971; 21:289.

76. Giles CM, Skov F. The *CDe* rhesus gene complex; some considerations revealed by a study of a Danish family with an antigen of the Rhesus gene complex *(C)D(e)* defined by a 'new' antibody. Vox Sang 1971; 20:328.

77. Lewis M, Kaita H, Allderice PW, et al. Assignment of the red cell antigen Targett (Rh40) to the Rh blood group system. Am J Hum Genet 1978; 31:630.

78. Cobb ML. Crawford: Investigation of a new low frequency red cell antigen (abstract). Transfusion 1980; 20:631.

79. Delehanty C, Wilkinson SL, Issitt PD, et al. Riv: A new low incidence Rh antigen (abstract). Tranfusion 1983; 23:410.

80. Lomas C, Poole J, Salaru N, et al. A low-incidence red cell antigen JAL associated with two unusual Rh gene complexes. Vox Sang 1990; 59:39.

81. Poole J, Hustinx H, Gerber H, et al. The red cell antigen JAL in the Swiss population: Family studies showing that JAL is an Rh antigen (Rh48). Vox Sang 1990; 59:44.

82. Sachs HW, Reuter W, Tippett P, Gavin J. An Rh gene complex producing both C^W and c antigen. Vox Sang 1978; 35:272.

83. Sistonen P, Abdulle OA, Sahid M. Evidence for a 'new' Rh gene complex producing the rare C^X (Rh9) antigen in the Somali population of East Africa. Transfusion 1987; 27:66.

84. Vos GH, Kirk RL. A 'naturally-occurring' anti-E which distinguishes a variant of the E antigen in Australian aborigines. Vox Sang 1962; 7:22.

85. Moores PP. The Blood Groups of the Natal Negro People. MSc Thesis, University of Natal, Durban, Republic of South Africa, 1976.

86. Case J. Unpublished observations cited by Issitt PD. In: Serology and Genetics of the Rhesus Blood Group System. Cincinnati, OH, Montgomery Scientific, 1979.

87. Moores P, Smart E. Serology and genetics of the red blood cell factor Rh34. Vox Sang 1991; 61:122.

88. Huestis DW, Catino ML, Busch S. A 'new' Rh antibody (anti-Rh26) which detects a factor usually accompanying hr'. Transfusion 1964; 4:414.

89. Sanger R, Noades J, Tippett P, et al. An Rh antibody specific for V and R'^{s}. Nature 1960; 186:171.

90. DeNatale A, Cahan A, Jack JA, et al. V: a 'new' Rh antigen, common in Negros, rare in white people. JAMA 1955; 159:247.

91. Moulds JJ, Case J, Thornton S, et al. Anti-Ce^s: a previously undescribed Rh antibody (abstract). Transfusion 1980; 20:631.

92. Sistonen P, Nevanlinna HR, Virtaranta-Knowles K, et al. Ne^a, a new blood group antigen in Finland. Vox Sang 1981; 40:352.

93. Sistonen P, Tippett P. A 'new' allele giving further insight into the LW blood group system. Vox Sang 1982; 42:252.

94. Habibi B, Fouillade MT, Duedari N, et al. The antigen Duclos. Vox Sang 1978; 34:302.

95. Dahr W, Kruger J. Solubilization of various blood group antigens by Triton X-100. Proc. 10th Int. Cong. Soc. Foren. Haematogenet., 1983:141.

96. Stratton F. A new Rh allelomorph. Nature 1946; 158:25.

97. Moore BPL. Does knowledge of D^u status serve a useful purpose? Vox Sang 1984; 46(suppl):95.

98. Agre P, Davies DM, Issitt PD, et al. A proposal to standardize terminology for weak D antigen (letter). Transfusion 1992; 32:86.

99. Shapiro M. The ABO, MN, P and Rh blood group systems in the South African Bantu, Part 1. S Afr Med J 1951; 25:165.

100. Shapiro M. The ABO, MN, P and Rh blood group systems in the South African Bantu, Part 2. S Afr Med J 1951; 25:187.

101. Argall CI, Ball JM, Trentelman E. Presence of anti-D antibody in the serum of a D^u patient. J Lab Clin Med 1953; 41:895.

102. Tippett P, Sanger R. Observations on subdivisions of the Rh antigen D. Vox Sang 1962; 7:9.

103. Tippett P, Sanger R. Further observations on subdivisions of the Rh antigen D. Artzl Lab 1977; 23:476.

104. Tippett P. Rh blood group system: The D antigen and high and low frequency Rh antigens, In: Vengelen-Tyler V, Pierce S. eds. Blood Group Systems:Rh. Arlington, VA, Am Assoc Blood Banks, 1987:25.

105. Tippett, P. Sub-divisions of the Rh (D) antigen. Med Lab Sci 1988; 45:88.

106. Lomas C, Tippett P, Thompson KM, et al. Demonstration of seven epitopes on the Rh antigen D using human monoclonal anti-D antibodies and red cells from D categories. Vox Sang 1989; 57:261.

107. Gorick BD, Thompson KM, Melamed MD, et al. Three epitopes on the human Rh antigen D recognized by ^{125}I-labelled human monoclonal IgG antibodies. Vox Sang 1988; 55:165.

108. Wiener AS, Unger LJ. Further observations on the blood factors Rh^A, Rh^B, Rh^C and Rh^D. Transfusion 1962; 2:230.

109. Chown B, Lewis M, Kaita H, Lowen B. An unlinked modifier of Rh blood groups: Effects when heterozygous and when homozygous. Am J Hum Genet 1972; 24:623.

110. Mallory DM, Rosenfield RE, Wong KY, et al. Rh$_{mod}$, a second kindred (Craig). Vox Sang 1976; 30:430.

111. Stevenson MM, Anido V, Tanner AM, Swoyer J. Rh 'null' is not always null. Br Med J 1973; 1:417.

112. Schmidt PJ, Holland PV. Rh$_{null}$ disease. Proc. 12th Cong. Int. Soc. Blood Transf. 1969:145.

113. Sturgeon P. Hematological observations on the anemia associated with blood type Rh$_{null}$. Blood 1970; 36:310.

114. Saji H, Hosoi T. A Japanese Rh$_{mod}$ family: Serological and haematological observations. Vox Sang 1979; 37:296.

115. Schmidt PJ. Hereditary hemolytic anemias and the null blood types. Arch Intern Med 1979; 139:570.

116. Giles CM, Bevan B. Possible suppression of Rh antigens in only one generation of a family. Vox Sang 1964; 9:204.

117. Heiken A, Giles CM. Evidence of mutation within the rhesus blood group system. Nature 1967; 213:699.

118. Kornstad L. A rare blood group antigen, Ol^a (Oldeide), associated with weak Rh antigens. Vox Sang 1986; 50:235.

119. Pollack W, Ascari WQ, Crispen JF, et al. Studies on Rh prophylaxis. II. Rh immune prophylaxis after transfusion with Rh-positive blood. Transfusion 1971; 11:340.

120. Urbaniak SJ, Robertson AE. A successful program of immunizing Rh-negative male volunteers for anti-D production using frozen/thawed blood. Transfusion 1981; 21:64.

121. Davey MG, Campbell AL, James J. Some consequences of hyperimmunization to the Rhesus (D) blood group antigen in man (abstract). Proc. Austral. Soc. Immunol. 1963; Adelaide, December 1969.

122. Pollack W. Unpublished observations cited by Mollison PL. In: Blood Transfusion in Clinical Medicine. 5th ed. Oxford, England, Blackwell Scientific, 1972.
123. Mollison PL, Hughes-Jones NC, Lindsay M, Wesseley J. Suppression of primary immunization by passively-administered antibody. Experiments in volunteers. Vox Sang 1969; 16:421.
124. Woodrow JC, Clarke CA, Donohoe WTA, et al. Mechanism of Rh prophylaxis: An experimental study on specificity of immunosuppression. Br Med J 1975; 2:57.
125. Samson D, Mollison PL. Effect on primary immunization of delayed administration of anti-Rh. Immunology 1975; 28:349.
126. Contreras M, Mollison PL. Failure to augment primary Rh immunization using a small dose of 'passive' IgG anti-Rh. Br J Haematol 1981; 49:371.
127. Nevanlinna HR, Vainio T. The influence of mother-child ABO incompatibility on Rh immunization. Vox Sang 1956; 1:26.
128. Woodrow JC, Donohoe WTA. Rh-immunization by pregnancy: Results of a survey and their relevance to prophylactic therapy. Br Med J 1968; 4:139.
129. Ascari WQ, Levine P, Pollack W. Incidence of maternal Rh immunization by ABO compatible and incompatible pregnancies. Br Med J 1969; 1:399.
130. Woodrow JC. Rh immunization and its prevention. Ser Haematol 1970; 3:3.
131. Davey MG. Nonresponders and hyperresponders to Rh antigens. Proceedings of a Symposium Rh-antibody Mediated Immunosuppression. Ortho Diagnostics, Raritan, NJ, 1976:13.
132. Archer GT, Cooke BR, Mitchell K, Parry P. Hyperimmunization of blood donors for the production of anti-Rh(D) gamma globulin. Bibl Haematol 1971; 38(part II):877.
133. Pollack W, Ascari WQ, Kochesky RJ, et al. Studies on Rh prophylaxis. I. Relationship between doses of anti-Rh and size of antigenic stimulus. Transfusion 1971; 11:333.
134. Murray S, Dewar PJ, Lee E, et al. A study of HL-A types in Rh haemolytic disease of the newborn. Vox Sang 1976; 30:91.
135. Petrany GG, Ivanyi P, Hollan SR. Relations of HL-A and Rh systems to immune reactivity. Vox Sang 1974; 26:470.
136. Darke C, Street J, Sargeant C, Dyer PA. HLA-DR antigens and properdin factor B allotypes in responders and non-responders to the Rhesus-D antigen. Tissue Antigens 1983; 21:333.
137. Kruskall MS, Yunis EJ, Watson A, et al. Major histocompatibility complex markers and red cell antibodies to the Rh(D) antigen. Transfusion 1990; 30:15.
138. Contreras M, Mollison PL. Rh immunization facilitated by passively-administered anti-Rh? Br J Haematol 1983; 53:153.
139. Goldfinger D, McGinniss MH. Rh-incompatible platelet transfusions-risks and consequences of sensitizing immunosuppressed patients. N Engl J Med 1971; 284:942.
140. McBride JA, O'Hoski P, Blajchman MA, et al. Rhesus alloimmunization following intensive plasmapheresis (abstract). Transfusion 1978; 18:626.
141. Burnie KL, Barr RM, personal communication to Mollison PL, Engelfriet CP, Contreras M. In: Blood Transfusion in Clinical Medicine. 8th ed. Oxford, England: Blackwell Scientific, 1987.
142. Barclay GR, Greiss MA, Urbaniak SJ. Adverse effect of plasma exchange on anti-D production in rhesus immunization owing to removal of inhibitory factors. Br Med J 1980; 2:1569.
143. Kenwright MG, Sangster JM, Sachs JA. Development of Rh D antibodies after kidney transplantation. Br Med J 1976; 2:151.
144. Hill Z, Vacl J, Kalasova E, et al. Haemolytic disease of the newborn in a D^u positive mother. Vox Sang 1974; 27:92.
145. Johnson CA, Brown BA, Lasky LC. Rh immunization caused by osseous allograft (letter). N Engl J Med 1985; 312:121.
146. Thompson EF, Walsh RJ. Immunization against the Rh antigen by small amounts of blood. Med J Austr 1950; 1:440.
147. Bichler A, Hetzel H. An unusual case of sensitization against the Rh factor. Gebrutschilfe Frauenheilkd 1975; 35:640.
148. David MP, Milbauer B. Three instances of Rh immunization due to childhood heterohemotherapy. Clin Pediatr 1978; 17:924.
149. Aronsson S, Engelson G, Svenningsen NW. Rh-immunization after sworn 'brotherhood' (letter). Lancet 1965; 2:847.

150. Wong LK, Smith LH, Jensen HM. Hemolytic disease of the newborn following maternal self-injection of blood. Transfusion 1983; 23:348.

151. Vontver LA. Rh sensitization associated with drug use. JAMA 1973; 226:469.

152. McVerry BA, O'Connor MC, Price A, et al. Isoimmunization after narcotic addiction. Br Med J 1977; 1:1324.

153. Giblett ER. Blood group antibodies causing hemolytic disease of the newborn. Clin Obstet Gynecol 1964; 7:1044.

154. Ceppellini R, Dunn LC, Turri M. An interaction between alleles at the Rh locus in man which weakens the reactivity of the Rh_0 factor (D^u). Proc Natl Acad Sci 1955; 41:283.

155. Race RR, Sanger R, Lawler SD. Rh genes allelomorphic to D. Nature 1948; 162:292.

156. Stratton F, Renton PH. Rh genes allelomorphic to D. Nature 1948; 162:293.

157. Wiener AS. Further observations on isosensitization to the Rh blood factor. Proc Soc Exp Biol Med 1949; 70:576.

158. van Loghem JJ, Harkink H, van der Hart M. Production of the antibody anti-e by artificial immunization. Vox Sang (old series) 1953; 3:22.

159. Jones AR, Diamond LK, Allen FH Jr. A decade of progress in the Rh blood-group system. N Engl J Med 1954; 250:283.

160. Jones AR, Diamond LK, Allen FH Jr. A decade of progress in the Rh blood-group system. N Engl J Med 1954; 250:324.

161. Issitt PD. Clinical consequences and practical limitations of Rhesus negative blood transfusion. In: Rhesus Problems in Clinical Practice. Gröningen, The Netherlands: Red Cross Blood Bank, 1979:46.

162. Rosse WF, Gallagher D, Kinney TR, et al. Transfusion and alloimmunization in sickle cell disease. Blood 1990; 76:1431.

163. Kellner A. A new look at the crossmatch. Obstet Gynecol 1955; 5:499.

164. Levine P, Robinson E, Stroup M, et al. A summary of atypical antibodies, rare genotypes, and ABO hemolytic disease encountered in a one year survey. Blood 1956; 11:1097.

165. Sinclair M, Anderson C, Simpson S. Unpublished observations cited by Moore BPL, Humphreys P, Lovett-Moseley CA. In: Serological and Immunological Methods of the Canadian Red Cross Blood Transfusion Service. 7th ed. Toronto: Canadian Red Cross Society, 1972:147.

166. Frame M, Mollison PL, Terry WD. Anti-Rh activity of human gammaG4 proteins. Nature 1970; 225:641.

167. Abramson N, Schur PH. The IgG subclasses of red cell antibodies and relationship to monocyte binding. Blood 1972; 40:500.

168. Natvig JB, Kunkel HG. Genetic markers of human immunoglobulins: The Gm and Inv systems. Ser. Haematol 1968; 1:66.

169. Devey ME, Voak D. A critical study of the IgG subclasses of Rh anti-D antibodies formed in pregnancy and in immunized volunteers. Immunology 1974; 27:1073.

170. Engelfriet CP. Unpublished observations cited in Mollison PL, Engelfriet CP, Contreras M. Blood Transfusion in Clinical Medicine. 8th ed. Oxford, England: Blackwell Scientific, 1987.

171. Waller M, Lawler SD. A study of the properties of the rhesus antibody (Ri) diagnostic for rheumatoid factor and its application to Gm grouping. Vox Sang 1962; 7:591.

172. Ayland J, Horton MA, Tippett P, Waters AH. Complement binding anti-D made in a D^u variant woman. Vox Sang 1978; 34:40.

173. Kline WE, Sullivan CM, Pope M, Bowman RJ. An example of a naturally occurring anti-cE (Rh27) that binds complement. Vox Sang 1982; 43:335.

174. Roy RB, Lotto WN. Delayed hemolytic reaction caused by anti-c not detectable before transfusion. Transfusion 1962; 2:342.

175. Pickles MM, Jones MN, Egan J, et al. Delayed haemolytic transfusion reactions due to anti-C. Vox Sang 1978; 35:32.

176. Giblett ER. Unpublished observations cited in Mollison PL, Engelfriet CP, Contreras M. Blood Transfusion in Clinical Medicine. 8th ed. Oxford, England: Blackwell Scientific, 1987.

177. Contreras M, De Silva M, Teesdale P, Mollison PL. The effect of naturally occurring Rh antibodies on the survival of serologically incompatible red cells. Br J Haematol 1987; 65:475.

178. Issitt PD, Combs MR, Bredehoeft SJ, et al. Lack of clinical significance of "enzyme-only" red cell antibodies. Transfusion 1993; 33:284.

179. Weiner W, Battey DA, Cleghorn TE, et al. Serological findings in a case of haemolytic anaemia; with some general observations on the pathogenesis of the syndrome. Br Med J 1953; 2:125.

180. Wiener AS, Gordon EB. Quantitative test for antibody-globulin coating human blood cells and its practical applications. Am J Clin Pathol 1953; 23:429.

181. Issitt PD, Pavone BG, Goldfinger D, et al. Anti-Wr^b and other autoantibodies responsible for positive direct antiglobulin tests in 150 individuals. Br J Haematol 1976; 34:5.

182. Weiner W, Vos GH. Serology of acquired hemolytic anemias. Blood 1963; 22:606.

183. Vos GH, Petz L, Fudenberg HH. Specificity of acquired haemoloytic anaemia autoantibodies and their serological characteristics. Br J Haematol 1970; 19:57.

184. Vos GH, Petz LD, Fudenberg HH. Specificity and immunoglobulin characteristics of autoantibodies in acquired hemolytic anemia. J Immunol 1971; 106:1172.

185. Vos GH, Petz LD, Garratty G, Fudenberg HH. Autoantibodies in acquired hemolytic anemia with special reference to the LW system. Blood 1972; 42:445.

186. Marsh WL, Reid ME, Scott P. Autoantibodies of U blood group specificity in autoimmune haemolytic anaemia. Br J Haematol 1972; 22:625.

187. Petz LD, Garratty G. Acquired Immune Hemolytic Anemias. New York: Churchill Livingstone, 1980.

188. Issitt PD, Zellner DC, Rolih SD, Duckett JB. Autoantibodies mimicking alloantibodies. Transfusion 1977; 17:531.

189. Henry RA, Weber J, Pavone BG, Issitt PD. A "normal" individual with a positive direct antiglobulin test: Case complicated by pregnancy and unusual autoantibody specificity. Transfusion 1977; 17:539.

190. Issitt PD, Pavone BG. Critical re-examination of the specificity of auto-anti-Rh antibodies in patients with a positive direct antiglobulin test. Br J Haematol 1978; 38:63.

191. Weber J, Caceres VW, Pavone BG, Issitt PD. Allo-anti-C in a patient who had previously made an autoantibody mimicking anti-C. Transfusion 1979; 19:216.

192. Carstairs KC, Breckenridge A, Dollery CT, Worlledge SM. Incidence of a positive direct Coombs test in patients on alpha-methyldopa. Lancet 1966; 2:133.

193. Worlledge SM, Carstairs KC, Dacie JV. Autoimmune haemolytic anaemia associated with alpha-methyldopa therapy. Lancet 1966; 2:135.

194. Worlledge SM. Immune drug-induced haemolytic anaemias. Semin Hematol 1969; 6:181.

195. Weiner W. "Coombs-positive" "normal" people. Proceedings of the 10th Congress of the International Society of Blood Transfusion. Basel: Karger, 1965:35.

196. Saboori A, Denker BM, Agre P. Isolation of proteins related to the Rh polypeptides from non-human erythrocytes. J Clin Invest 1989; 83:187.

197. Merry AH, Thomson EE, Anstee DJ, Stratton F. The quantification of erythrocyte antigen sites with monoclonal antibodies. Immunology 1984; 51:793.

198. Bloy C, Blanchard D, Lambin P, et al. Human monoclonal antibody against Rh(D) antigen: Partial characterization of the Rh(D) polypeptide from human erythrocytes. Blood 1987; 69:1491.

199. Bloy C, Blanchard D, Lambin P, et al. Characterization of the C, c, E and G antigens of the Rh blood group system with human monoclonal antibodies. Mol Immunol 1988; 25:925.

200. Agre P, Cartron JP. Molecular biology of the Rh antigens. Blood 1991; 78:551.

201. Green FA. Phospholipid requirement for Rh antigen activity. J Biol Chem 1968; 243:5519.

202. Hughes-Jones NC, Green EJ, Hunt VA. Loss of Rh antigen activity following the action of phosphalipase A_2 on red cell stroma. Vox Sang 1975; 29:184.

203. Green FA. Erythrocyte membrane lipids and Rh antigen activity. J Biol Chem 1972; 247:881.

204. Green FA. Erythrocyte membrane sulfhydryl groups and Rh antigen activity. Immunochemistry 1967; 4:247.

205. Moore S, Woodrow CF, McClelland DBL. Isolation of membrane components associated with human red cell antigens Rh(D), (c), (E) and Fy^a. Nature 1982; 295:529.

206. Gahmberg CG. Molecular identification of the human Rh$_o$(D) antigen. FEBS Lett 1982; 140:93.

207. Moore S. Identification of red cell membrane components associated with Rhesus blood group antigen expression. In: Cartron JP, Rouger P, Salmon C, eds. Red Cell Membrane Glycoconjugates and Related Genetic Markers. Paris: Librairie Arnette, 1983:97.

208. Cartron JP. Recent advances in the biochemistry of blood group Rh antigens. In: Rouger P, Salmon

C, eds. Monoclonal Antibodies Against Human Red Blood Cell and Related Antigens. Paris: Librairie Arnette, 1987:69.

209. Krahmer M, Prohaska R. Characterization of human red cell Rh (Rhesus-) specific polypeptides by limited proteolysis. FEBS Lett 1987; 226:105.

210. Bloy C, Blanchard D, Dahr W, et al. Determination of the N-terminal sequence of human red cell Rh(D) polypeptide and demonstration that the Rh(D), (c) and (E) antigens are carried by distinct polypeptide chains. Blood 1988; 72:661.

211. Ridgwell K, Roberts SJ, Tanner MJA, Anstee DJ. Absence of two membrane proteins containing extracellular thiol groups in Rh$_{null}$ human erythrocytes. Biochem J 1983; 213:267.

212. Moore S, Green C. The identification of specific Rhesus-polypeptide blood-group-ABH-active-glycoprotein complexes in the human red-cell membrane. Biochem J 1987; 244:735.

213. Avent ND, Judson PA, Parsons SF, et al. Monoclonal antibodies that recognize different membrane proteins that are deficient in Rh$_{null}$ human erythrocytes. Biochem J 1988; 251:499.

214. Avent ND, Ridgwell K, Mawby WJ, et al. Protein-sequence studies on Rh-related polypeptides suggest the presence of at least two groups of proteins which associate in the human red-cell membrane. Biochem J 1988; 256:1043.

215. Blanchard D, Bloy C, Hermand P, et al. Two-dimensional iodopeptide mapping demonstrates that erythrocyte Rh D, c and E polypeptides are structurally homologous but nonidentical. Blood 1988; 72:1424.

216. Hughes-Jones NC, Bloy C, Gorick B, et al. Evidence that the c, D and E epitopes of the human Rh blood group system are on separate polypeptide molecules. Mol Immunol 1988; 25:931.

217. Goosens D, Champomier G, Rouger P, Salmon C. Human monoclonal antibodies against blood group antigens. J Immunol Methods 1987; 1:193.

218. Agre P, Saboori AM, Asimos A, Smith BL. Purification and partial characterization of the M$_r$ 30,000 integral membrane protein associated with the erythrocyte Rh(D) antigen. J Biol Chem 1987; 262:17497.

219. Saboori AM, Smith BL, Agre P. Polymorphism in the M$_r$ 32,000 Rh protein purified from Rh(D)-positive and negative erythrocytes. Proc Natl Acad Sci USA 1988; 85:4042.

220. Suyama K, Goldstein J. Antibody produced against isolated Rh(D) polypeptide reacts with other Rh-related antigens. Blood 1988; 72:1622.

221. Suyama K, Goldstein J. Enzymatic evidence for differences in the placement of Rh antigens within the red cell membrane. Blood 1990; 75:255.

222. Gahmberg CG, Karhi KK. Association of Rh$_o$(D) polypeptides with the membrane skeleton in Rh$_o$(D)-positive human red cells. J Immunol 1984; 133:334.

223. Ridgwell K, Tanner MJA, Anstee DJ. The Rhesus (D) polypeptide is linked to the human erythrocyte cytoskeleton. FEBS Lett 1984; 174:7.

224. Paradis G, Bazin R, Lemieux R. Protective effect of the membrane skeleton on the immunologic reactivity of the human red cell Rh$_o$(D) antigen. J Immunol 1986; 137:240.

225. Hartel-Schenk S, Agre P. Fatty acid acylation of human red cell membrane proteins and phospholipids (abstract). J Cell Biol 1990; 111:322a.

226. Rearden A, Chiu P. Lack of rhesus antigen expression on human committed erythroid progenitors. Blood 61:525.

227. Falkenburg JHF, Fibbe WE, van der Vaart-Duinkerken N. Human erythroid progenitor cells express Rhesus antigens. Blood 1985; 66:660.

228. Wiener AS, Moor-Jankowski J, Gordon EB. Blood groups of apes and monkeys: IV. The Rh-Hr blood types of anthropoid apes. Am J Hum Genet 1964; 16:246.

229. Wiener AS, Moor-Jankowski J, Gordon EB, Kratochvil CH. Individual differences in chimpanzee blood, demonstrable with adsorbed human anti-Rh$_o$ sera. Proc Natl Acad Sci USA 1966; 56:458.

230. Mallinson G, Anstee DJ, Avent ND, et al. Murine monoclonal antibody MB-2D10 recognizes Rh-related glycoproteins in the human red cell membrane. Transfusion 1990; 30:222.

231. von dem Borne AEG, Kr, Bos MJE, Lomas C, et al. Murine monoclonal antibodies against a unique determinant of erythrocytes related to Rh and U antigens. Br J Haematol 1990; 75:254.

232. Dahr W, Moulds JJ. High frequency antigens of human erythrocyte sialoglycoproteins. IV. Molecular properties of the U antigen. Hoppe Seyler Z Physiol Chemie 1987; 368:659.

233. Telen MJ, Chasis JA. Relationship of the human erythrocyte Wr^b antigen to an interaction between glycophorin A and band 3.Blood 1990; 76:842.
234. Cherif-Zahar B, Bloy C, Le Van Kim C, et al. Molecular cloning and protein structure of a human blood group Rh polypeptide. Proc Natl Acad Sci USA 1990; 87:6243.
235. Avent ND, Ridgwell K, Tanner MJA, Anstee DJ. cDNA cloning of a 30 kDA erythrocyte membrane protein associated with Rh (Rhesus)- blood-group-antigen expression. Biochem J 1990; 271:821.
236. Helenius A, Simons K. Solubilization of membranes by detergents. Biochim Biophys Acta 1975; 415:29.
237. Suyama K, Goldstein J, Aebersold R, Kent S. Regarding the size of Rh proteins (letter). Blood 1991; 77:411.
238. de Vetten MP, Agre P. The Rh polypeptide is a major fatty acid-acylated erythrocyte membrane protein. J Biol Chem 1988; 263:18193.
239. Levine P, Celano M, Vos GH, Morrison J. The first human blood, - - -/- - -, which lacks the 'D-like' antigen. Nature 1962; 194:304.
240. Colledge KI, Pezzulich M, Marsh WL. Anti-Fy5, an antibody disclosing a probable association between the Rhesus and Duffy blood group genes. Vox Sang 1973; 24:193.
241. Sistonen P. Linkage of the LW blood group locus with the complement C3 and Lutheran blood group loci. Ann Hum Genet 1984; 48:239.
242. Mallinson G, Martin PG, Anstee DJ, et al. Identification and partial characterization of the human erythrocyte membrane component(s) that express the antigens of the LW blood-group system. Biochem J 1986; 234:649.
243. Bloy C, Hermand P, Blanchard D, et al. Surface orientation and antigen properties of Rh and LW polypeptides of the human erythrocyte membrane. J Biol Chem 1990; 265:21482.
244. Bloy C, Hermand P, Cherif-Zahar B, et al. Comparative analysis by two-dimensional iodopeptide mapping of the RhD protein and LW glycoprotein. Blood 1990; 75:2245.
245. Donahue RP, Bias W, Renwick JH, McKusick VA. Probable assignment of the Duffy blood group locus to chromosome 1 in man. Proc Natl Acad Sci USA 1968; 61:949.
246. Hadley TJ, David PH, McGinniss MH, Miller LH. Identification of an erythrocyte component carrying the Duffy blood group Fy^a antigen. Science 1984; 223:597.
247. Anstee DJ. Blood group-active surface molecules of the human red blood cell. Vox Sang 1990; 58:1.
248. German J, Metaxas MN, Metaxas-Buhler M, Chaganti RSK. Further evaluation of a child with the M^k phenotype and a translocation affecting the long arms of chromosomes 2 and 4. Cytogenet Cell Genet 1979; 25:160.
249. Dahr W, Kordowicz M, Moulds J, et al. Characterization of the Ss sialoglycoprotein and its antigens in Rh$_{null}$ erythrocytes. Blut 1987; 54:13.
250. Miller YE, Daniels GL, Jones C, Palmer DK. Identification of a cell-surface antigen produced by a gene on human chromosome 3 (cen-q22) and not expressed by Rh$_{null}$ cells. Am J Hum Genet 1987; 41:1061.
251. Lauf PK, Joiner CH. Increased potassium transport and ouabain binding in human Rh$_{null}$ red blood cells. Blood 1976; 48:457.
252. Ballas S, Clark MR, Mohandas N, et al. Red cell membranes and cation deficiency in Rh null syndrome. Blood 1984; 63:1046.
253. Kuypers F, van Linde-Sibenius-Trip M, Roelofsen B, et al. Rh$_{null}$ human erythrocytes have an abnormal membrane phospholipid organisation. Biochem J 1984; 221:931.
254. Seidl S, Spielman W, Martin H. Two siblings with Rh$_{null}$ disease. Vox Sang 1972; 23:182.
255. Senhauser DA, Mitchell MW, Gault DB, Owens JH. Another example of phenotype Rh$_{null}$. Transfusion 1970; 10:89.
256. Polesky HF, Moulds JJ. Three Rh$_{null}$ siblings: Hematologic observations (abstract). Book of Abstracts. 25th Annual Meeting of the American Association of Blood Banks and 13th Congress of the International Society of Blood Transfusion, 1972:16.
257. Moulds JJ. Rh$_{nulls}$: amorphs and regulators. In Walker RH, ed. Recent Advances in Immunohematology. Chicago: Am Assoc Blood Banks, 1973:63.
258. Verkleji AJ, Zwaal RFA, Roelofsen B, et al. The asymmetric distribution of phospholipids in the human red blood cell membrane. Biochim Biophys Acta 1973; 323:187.

259. Gordesky SE, Marinetti GV. The asymmetric arrangement of phospholipids in the human erythrocyte membrane. Biochem Biophys Res Commun 1973; 50:1027.

260. Zwaal RFA, Roelofsen B, Comfurius P, van Deenen LLM. Organization of phospholipids in red blood cell membranes as detected by various purified phospholipases. Biochim Biophys Acta 1975; 406:83.

261. Zachowski A, Favre E, Cribier S, et al. Outside-inside translocation of aminophospholipids in the human erythrocyte membrane is mediated by a specific enzyme. Biochemistry 1986; 25:2585.

262. Schroit AJ, Madsen J, Ruoho AE. Radioiodinated, photoactivable phosphatidylcholine and phosphatidylserine: Transfer properties and differential photoreactive interaction with human erythrocyte membrane proteins. Biochemistry 1987; 26:1812.

263. Connor J, Schroit AJ. Transbilayer movement of phosphatidylserine in erythrocytes: Inhibition of transport and preferential labeling of a 31,000-dalton protein by sulfhydryl reactive reagents. Biochemistry 1988; 27:848.

264. Schroit AJ, Bloy C, Connor J, Cartron JP. Involvement of Rh blood group polypeptides in the maintenance of aminophospholipid asymmetry. Biochemistry 1990; 29:10303.

265. Smith RE, Daleke DL. Phosphatidylserine transport in Rh_{null} erythrocytes. Blood 1990; 76:1021.

266. Morrot G, Zachowski A, Devaux DF. Partial purification and characterization of the human erythrocyte Mg^{++} ATPase. A candidate aminophospholipid translocase. FEBS Lett 1990; 266:29.

267. Hughes-Jones NC, Gardner B, Lincoln PJ. Observations on the number of available c, D, e and E antigen sites on red cells. Vox Sang 1971; 21:210.

268. Skov F, Hughes-Jones NC. Observations on the number of available C antigen sites on red cells. Vox Sang 1977; 33:170.

269. Leff SE, Rosenfeld MG, Evans RM. Complex transcriptional units: diversity in gene expression by alternate RNA processing. Ann Rev Biochem 1986; 55:1091.

270. Tippett P. A speculative model for the Rh blood groups. Ann Hum Genet 1986; 50:241.

271. Ruddle F, Ricciuti F, McMorris FA, et al. Somatic cell genetic assignment of peptidase C and the Rh linkage group to chromosome A-1 in man. Science 1972; 176:1429.

272. Marsh WL, Chaganti RSK, Gardner FH, et al. Mapping human autosomes: Evidence supporting assignment of Rhesus to the short arm of chromosome No. 1. Science 1974; 183:966.

273. Cherif-Zahar B, Mattei MG, Le Van Kim C, et al. Localization of the human Rh blood group gene structure to chromosome region 1p34.3-1p36.1 by in situ hybridization. Hum Genet 1991; 86:398.

6

Platelet and Neutrophil Alloantigens: Their Nature and Role in Immune-Mediated Cytopenias

A. E. G. KR. VON DEM BORNE

University of Amsterdam
and Central Laboratory of the Netherlands Red Cross Blood Transfusion Service
Amsterdam, The Netherlands

S. SIMSEK, C. E. VAN DER SCHOOT, and R. GOLDSCHMEDING

Central Laboratory of the Netherlands Red Cross Blood Transfusion Service
Amsterdam, The Netherlands

I. INTRODUCTION

Platelet and neutrophil alloantigens are of great interest to the immunohematologist because of their involvement in a number of important immune-mediated diseases of the blood as well as in certain transfusion reactions.

In the past two decades, these antigens have been intensively studied. New methods to detect, measure, and characterize antigens and antibodies have been devised. This has led not only to the recognition of new antigen systems but also to new insights in the pathophysiology of immune-mediated disorders of the blood in which they are involved. Moreover, studies at the molecular level have added a new dimension to the field.

In this chapter various clinical and immunological aspects of platelet and neutrophil alloantigens are discussed, with an emphasis on their biochemical nature.

II. PLATELET ALLOANTIGENS

Different types of alloantigens are present on platelets. Some are shared with other blood cells and tissues. These are the glycoconjugate antigens of the blood group ABH, Le, I, and P systems and the highly polymorphous HLA class I (A, B, C) glycoprotein antigens. HLA class II (DP, DQ, DR) antigens are not expressed on platelets. Another set of so-called platelet-specific antigens has been considered to be unique for these cells. As is discussed later, many of these antigenic structures appear not to be as unique for platelets as previously thought.

The platelet-specific antigens or antigen systems described so far are listed in Table 1 together with the frequency of their occurrence. Many have been described under different names. Therefore, a new nomenclature of platelet alloantigens has been proposed (Table 2) (1). In this nomenclature, platelet-specific alloantigen systems are called HPA (from human platelet antigen). The different antigen systems are numbered chronologically in order of the date of publication of their descriptions. A high-frequency allele of a system is designated with the letter a and its low-frequency counterpart with the letter b. The older antigen systems Duzo and Pl^E are not included in the new nomenclature. This is because Duzo and Pl^{E2} antisera are

Table 1 Platelet-Specific Antigen Systems Described Currently

System	Antigens	Frequency (%)[a]	References
Duzo	Duzo^a	22.0	37
Zw=Pl^A	Zw^a=Pl^{A1}	97.9	32, 38, 137
	Zw^b=Pl^{A2}	26.5	
Ko=Sib	Ko^a=Sib^a	14.9	5, 138
	Ko^b	99.3	
Pl^E	Pl^{E1}	>99.94	139
	Pl^{E2}	5.0	
Bak=Lek	Bak^a=Lek^a	87.7	140–142
	Bak^b	64.1	
Pen=Yuk	Pen^a=Yuk^b	>99.9	143–145
	Yuk^a	<0.2	
Br=Hc=Zav	Br^a=Hc^a=Zav	20.6	146–149
Pl^T	Pl^{T1}	>98.1	150
Nak	Nak^a	96.00^b	151
Gov	Gov^a	78.1	152
	Gov^b	71.7	

^{a}In whites.
^{b}In Japanese (probably 100% in whites).

Table 2 A New Nomenclature of Platelet-Specific Alloantigens

System	Original name(s)	Antigens	Original name(s)
HPA-1	Zw, Pl^A	HPA-1a	Zw^a, Pl^{A1}
		HPA-1b	Zw^b, Pl^{A2}
HPA-2	Ko, Sib	HPA-2a	Ko^b
		HPA-2b	Ko^a, Sib^a
HPA-3	Bak, Lek	HPA-3a	Bak^a, Lek^a
		HPA-3b	Bak^b
HPA-4	Pen, Yuk	HPA-4a	Pen^a, Yuk^b
		HPA-4b	Pen^b, Yuk^a
HPA-5	Br, Hc, Zav	HPA-5a	Br^b, Zav^b
		HPA-5b	Br^a, Zav^a, Hc^a

not available anymore. Moreover, Pl^{E1} antiserum was probably from a patient with Bernard-Soulier syndrome immunized by blood transfusion; i.e., the serum may contain isoantibodies instead of alloantibodies (2). It has been decided that new antigens or antigen systems will only be included in this nomenclature if they are sufficiently well characterized in the workshops of the International Working Party on Platelet Serology of the ISBT and ISH.

It is noteworthy that all HPA systems described so far appear to be biallelic systems. In recently performed population studies, it was found that phenotype and genotype frequencies of some antigens may vary considerably between different ethnic groups (3–6). For example, HPA-1a (Zw^a) is ubiquitous in Japanese, Koreans, and blacks, whereas HPA-1b (Zw^b) is rare, HPA-4b (Yuk^a = Pen^b) is found in Japanese and Koreans, although quite infrequently. This antigen is rare or absent in whites (and has not yet been studied in blacks). South American Indians (Mapuches) also have (nearly) all HPA-1a (Zw^a) and have HPA-4b (Yuk^a) in a low frequency and HPA-5b (Br^a) in a lower frequency in comparison to whites (see Table 3).

The biallelic nature and the marked differences in gene frequency of some platelet antigens

Table 3 Phenotype Frequency (%) of Platelet Alloantigens in Different Populations

System	Antigens	Whites	Blacks	Japanese	Koreans	Indians
ZW=HPA-1	Zw^a=1a	97.9	99.6	>99.9	100	99.9
	Zw^b=1b	26.5	—	3.7	11.5	—
Ko=HPA-2	Ko^b=2a	99.3	—	—	—	—
	Ko^a=2b	14.9	—	25.4	—	—
Bak=HPA-3	Bak^a=3a	87.7	—	78.9	87.3	89.3
	Bak^b=3b	64.1	—	70.7	—	—
Pen=HPA-4	Pen^a=4a	>99.9	—	99.9	100	99.9
	Pen^b=4b	0.2	—	1.7	1.6	0.9
Br=HPA-5	Br^b=5a	99.2	—	—	—	—
	Br^a=5b	20.6	—	—	—	4.9

These figures represent means of frequencies published in the literature. Recent figures from a Dutch study (63) are 97.8 and 28.64% for HPA-1a and HPA-1b, 100 and 13.15% for HPA-2a and HPA-2b, 80.95%, and 69.8 for HPA-3a and HPA-3b, 100 and 0% for HPA-4a and HPA-4b, and 100 and 19.7% for HPA-5a and HPA-5b, respectively. Also, 100% of 200 donors typed in this study were Nak(a+).

in different ethnic groups suggest that single evolutionary events of quite recent date have been responsible for their occurrence.

A. Methods to Detect Platelet Antibodies and to Type and Characterize Platelet Antigens

Many different methods for antigen and antibody detection have been devised in the past decades. Those based on the direct detection of antibody binding have been found to be the most reliable and specific methods. Platelet immunofluorescence (7) has been adapted as standard method by the International Working Party. However, other methods such as solid-phase enzyme-linked immunosorbent assay (ELISA) and mixed agglutination or hemabsorption tests also appear to be useful and sufficiently reliable (8–10).

For research purposes, a number of other assays are in use. These are, for instance, the monoclonal antibody radioimmunoassay (MARIA) to quantify antibody binding and antigen amount on platelets (11,12), immunoprecipitation (after radiolabeling of platelet glycoproteins) and sodium dodedylsulfate–polyacrylamine gel electrophoresis (SDS-PAGE) (13), immunoblotting (14), and antibody binding to purified platelet glycoproteins (15).

Recently, a test based on monoclonal antibody immobilization of platelet antigens (MAIPA) has been devised (16). This method makes immunochemical characterization of platelet antigens on a more routine scale possible. It also appears to be the only method available at present that can be used to detect antibodies against and to type for antigens with a low expression level on platelets such as of the HPA-5 (Br) system. Platelets carry only a few thousand HPA-5 antigen molecules on their surface. Moreover, because it is a test performed on isolated glycoproteins, specificity analysis of a mixture of antibodies in a serum is much more easy to perform.

A problem with which platelet serologists are often confronted is whether certain platelet-reactive antibodies are directed against HLA class I antigens or platelet-specific antigens. Chloroquine stripping of platelets (to remove HLA class I molecules from the platelets) is then a helpful tool (17) but also MAIPA using the appropriate monoclonal antibodies for capture.

B.   Clinical Importance of Platelet Alloantigens

Platelet alloantigens play a crucial role in a number of different clinical situations. These are neonatal alloimmune thrombocytopenia, posttransfusion purpura, and refractoriness to platelet transfusion therapy. They may also be involved in febrile transfusion reactions.

1.   Neonatal Alloimmune Thrombocytopenia

Neonatal alloimmune thrombocytopenia (NAITP) is caused by alloimmunization of the mother against fetal platelet antigens. It is a rare but important disease. It occurs in the Western countries in about 1 of every 1,000–3,000 pregnancies (18,19) and may already affect the first born (in about 50%). This suggests that placental passage of platelets occurs during gestation. Typically, the newborn has a low platelet count at birth, which becomes even lower in the hours or days after birth. The count usually normalizes again within weeks. There is a purpuric bleeding type, and although bleeding may be mild or even absent at birth, it also can be severe. Much feared are visceral and intracranial bleeding. Intracranial bleeding may cause neurological damage (21%) and even death (7%). Sometimes intracranial bleeds occur already in utero, and may then cause intracerebral "holes," so-called porencephali (20).

Nowadays much effort is put into the intrauterine diagnosis and management of fetal alloimmune thrombocytopenia in which percutaneous umbilical blood sampling (PUBS) is an important tool (21). Treatment modalities are corticosteroids, intravenous gamma globulin, and transfusion of compatible platelets (obtained from typed donors or the mother) that are even given before birth by way of cord vein puncture if necessary (22–24). Cesarean section is often performed to make birth less traumatic (25). At present, intravenous gamma globulin is considered to be the treatment of first choice for the postnatal period. Different modalities of antenatal treatment are being evaluated.

For the diagnosis, blood counts and serological tests are necessary, including antibody detection and specificity analysis, antigen typing of the mother, father, and child, as well as HLA typing (see below). Prenatal monitoring is common policy in subsequent pregnancies in affected families. The recurrence rate of NAITP is high (90%) (19). Molecular genetics may find a place in the early identification of fetuses at risk (26,27).

2.   Posttransfusion Purpura

Posttransfusion purpura (PTP) is an acute and often severe thrombocytopenia purpura occurring approximately 1 week (5–8 days) after a blood transfusion. Its incidence is unknown, but many cases have been reported in the literature (2,28,29). The exact pathogenesis is unknown. Most patients are probably preimmunized against platelets, and most are women who have been pregnant. The provocative transfusion is often accompanied by a febrile reaction. Platelet-specific alloantibodies are detected in the patient's serum and are mostly anti–HPA-1a (anti–Zw[a]). Platelets obtained from the patient after recovery are unreactive with the alloantibodies. However, in the acute phase, immunoglobulin binding to the patients' platelets is detected and eluates from these platelets contain the alloantibodies (30,31). This suggests that either the alloantibodies produced in the acute phase cross-react with the antithetic antigen (so-called pseudospecificity) or that soluble or particle-bound antigen-antibody complexes are formed during the destruction of the donor's platelets, which bind specifically to the patient's platelets (32,33).

For the diagnosis, both blood counts and serological tests are necessary. The detection of severe thrombocytopenia and platelet-specific alloantibodies (notably of anti–HPA-1a) in the blood of a previously hematologically normal individual after a transfusion makes the existence of PTP likely.

Without therapy or with glucocorticoid therapy only, thrombocytopenia may persist for many weeks. The patient may suffer severe bleedings. Even intracranial haemorrhage may occur.

Plasma exchange may lead to dramatic improvement, presumably by removing antibodies, immune complexes, and/or transfused antigens. Also intravenous gamma globulin therapy appears to be successful. This may become the treatment of first choice. Compatible platelets are ineffective, presumably because they are destroyed as well (34). After recovery, PTP does not necessarily recur when patients are transfused again with incompatible blood, although the antibodies may persist (35).

3. Refractoriness to Platelet Transfusions

Platelet transfusion refractoriness (PTR) in pancytopenic patients is often due to non-immunologic causes. However, in a significant number of patients, alloimmunization against platelet alloantigens occurs and may be the cause of PTR. Alloimmune PTR has been reviewed in detail (36).

C. Platelet Alloantibody Specificity in Different Clinical Settings

The Duzo[a] antibodies were detected in the blood of a mother with a newborn suffering from neonatal alloimmune thrombocytopenia, whereas anti–HPA-1a (Zw[a]) antibodies were found for the first time in the blood of patients with posttransfusion purpura (37,38). Since these initial discoveries sera from such cases have been the main source for further studies. This has led to the identification of many new antibody specificities and antigens. Only recently, the study of platelet transfusion refractoriness also has contributed. The role of the different platelet antigen systems in specific clinical situations is summarized in Table 4. The diversity of antibody specificities involved in NAIT appears to be far greater than in PTP. In fact, with the possible exception of anti-Gov, the antibodies in PTP are all directed against antigens present on the glycoprotein IIb/IIIa complex of platelets. This intriguing association is still unexplained. A few cases have been reported in which alloantibodies against low-frequency and private (family) antigens were found to be responsible for NAIT (39–42). However, it should be stated that the antibody diversity in PTP and NAIT is more apparent than real. In whites, most (85–90%) clinically well-defined cases of PTP and NAITP are due to anti–HPA-1a alloantibodies (31,43).

Refractoriness to platelet transfusion is mostly due to alloantibodies directed against HLA class I antigens and sometimes anti A and/or anti B. That due to platelet-specific alloantibodies seems to be of rare occurrence. Refractoriness to platelet transfusion has been seen mostly in patients who have become refractory to transfusion of HLA-matched platelets (reviewed in ref. 36). In a large study, Kickler et al. (44) detected GPIIb/IIIa antibodies in the blood of 2% of patients with PTR. However, allospecificity of these antibodies was not studied.

D. Glycoprotein Localization of Platelet-Specific Antigens

With the help of techniques such as radioimmunoprecipitation, immunoblotting, and, more recently, monoclonal antibody capture immunoassays, most platelet-specific antigens have now

Table 4 Clinical Importance of Platelet Alloantigens

Clinical Situation	References
Neonatal alloimmune thrombocytopenia	
Duzo, HPA-1, HPA-2, HPA-3, HPA-4, HPA-5, Pl^E, Pl^T	37, 139–141, 143, 146, 150, 153–155
Posttransfusion purpura	
HPA-1, HPA-3, HPA-4, Gov	32, 38, 142, 152, 156–160
Transfusion refractoriness	
HLA-ABC, HLA-ABO, HPA-1, HPA-2, HPA-3, HPA-5, Nak, Gov	5, 36, 151, 152, 161

been localized on specific platelet membrane glycoproteins (GP) or glycoprotein complexes (Table 5) (reviewed in refs. 45–47). Many alloantigens appear to be localized on glycoproteins of the GP IIb/IIIa complex, notably HPA-1, HPA-3, HPA-, and HPA-4, and the recently discovered low-frequency or private antigens Sr^a, Va^a, Mo^a, and Gro^a (39–42). (discussed above).

HPA-2 (identical with Sib) (48) is present on GP Ibα, as in Pl^{E1} antigen, which, however, as mentioned is an isoantigen rather than an alloantigen. The not yet so well-defined alloantigen Pl^T may reside on GP V, a protein associated with GP Ibα, GP Ibβ, and GP IX in another complex (GP Ib/IX/V complex). HPA-5 is on the GP Ia/IIa complex (probably on GP Ia). The Gov system alloantigens were found to be located on a novel platelet glycoprotein of 175 kd.

Nak^a antigen, discovered in Japan with the serum of a patient with PTR appears to be located on GP IV. In fact, it has been shown that Nak^a-negative individuals have a deficiency of platelet GP IV (49). Thus, anti-Nak antibodies also are isoantibodies rather than alloantibodies. GP IV deficiency, which appears to occur rather frequently in the Japanese, is rare or absent in whites. We did not encounter any Nak^a-negative individuals while typing many hundreds of donor platelet samples with anti-Nak^a (unpublished data). So far, GP IV deficiency of platelets does not seem to have any clinical consequences.

In Table 5, the Cr-related antigens have been included. This family of red blood cell antigens (Cr^a, Tc^a, Tc^b, Tc^c, Dr^a, WES^a, WES^b, Es^a, UMC, and IFC) is located on the decay-accelerating factor (DAF or CD55 antigen) (reviewed in ref. 50). Decay-accelerating factor also is present on platelets (as well as on all white blood cells, endothelial cells, and most but not all tissue cells).

E. The Molecular Nature of Platelet-Specific Antigens

Studies on the molecular nature of platelet antigens have been a major issue lately. The Zw^a and Zw^b antigens (HPA-1a,b) are present on a small N terminal peptide fragment of 17–23 kd (140–190 amino acids) obtained by trypsin digestion of GP IIIa (51,52). The HPA-1 (Zw) antigens are destroyed by reduction (14), which shows that they are dependent on the tertiary structure of the protein with intact disulfide bridges. Newman et al. (53) used reverse transcriptase (RT) and the polymerase chain reaction (PCR) to study platelet RNA from donors with different HPA-1 (Zw) phenotypes. They found that a C → T substitution of base 196 of the GP IIIa DNA sequence forms the basis of HPA-1 (Zw) polymorphism. The C/T polymorphism leads to a unique NciI restriction enzyme cleavage site in HPA-1b (Zw^b) DNA.

Table 5 Glycoprotein Localization of Platelet Alloantigens

System	Original name(s)	Glycoprotein location	References
HPA-1	Zw, Pl^a	GP IIIa	52, 162
HPA-2	Ko, Sib	GPI bα	48
HPA-3	Bak, Lek	GP IIb	13, 52, 163
HPA-4	Pen, Yuk	GP IIIa	156, 164
HPA-5	Br, Hc, Zav	GP Ia	148, 149, 165
—	Pl^E	GP Ibα	166
—	Nak	GP IV	167
—	Pl^T	GP V	150
—	Gov	gp175	152
—	Cr related	gp75	50

The single base change results in a leucine/proline polymorphism at amino acid position 33 from the N terminal part of GP IIIa.

That the amino acid polymorphism alone is responsible for formation of the HPA-1 epitopes was shown by the production of allele-specific constructs of GP IIIa recombinant DNA. With these constructs, specific alloantigen expression could be induced in mammalian (COS-7) cells (54). However, 13-mer peptides straddling the HPA-1–specific amino acid polymorphism did not block HPA-1a or HPA-1b alloantibodies (55). This indicates that the amino acids leucine and proline are not part of the actual HPA-1 (Zw) epitopes but induce the epitopes in the folded GP IIIa chain at another site. The N terminal region of GP IIIa is particularly rich in cysteines (7 in the first 50 N terminal amino acids) and extensive disulfide pairing occurs around amino acid 33. This is an explanation for destruction by reduction of HPA-1 (Zw) antigens. The N terminal location of the HPA-1 (Zw) epitopes on GP IIIa also explains an older finding that anti–HPA-1A (Zw^a) antibodies inhibit platelet aggregation via the inhibition of fibrinogen binding (56). This part of the molecule is thought to be involved in the formation of a fibrinogen binding site.

The same methodology was applied by Newman and co-workers to study the nature of HPA-3 (Bak) polymorphism (57). Again, a single (T→G) base substitution is present, resulting in an isoleucine-serine polymorphism of residue 843 of the mature GP IIb heavy chain. Interestingly, this polymorphism is very close to the binding site of the monoclonal antibody PMI-1, a functionally important region of GP IIb regulated by divalent cation and ligand binding and involved in platelet adhesion to collagen (58). The base substitution in the case of HPA-3 polymorphism leads to a restriction site for the enzyme Fok 1 in the HPA-3 complementary DNA (cDNA). Also in this case, allele-specific transfection studies proved the direct role of the amino acid substitutions in allotype formation (54).

Anti–HPA-3b (Bak^a) alloantibodies may react with different epitopes. Some react with GP IIb only in its native configuration, whereas others also react with the denatured chain. Some of the latter fail to react after desialization of the denatured glycoprotein (59). This also indicates that anti–HPA-3 antibodies often do not recognize the primary sequence.

Recently, we elucidated the molecular nature of the HPA 2 = Ko polymorphism (60). The PCR was performed directly on genomic material (DNA). This was possible because GP Ibα is encoded by a single intron (exon free) gene. We found that the HPA-2a/b (Ko^b/Ko^a) polymorphism was due to a single C→T base substitution at position 434 of the DNA coding for the mature protein, leading to a threonine-methionine polymorphism at amino acid position 145. This is near the binding site of von Willebrand factor and explains why HPA-2 antibodies may interfere with the binding of this factor to platelets (48). The C/T polymorphism is reflected in a difference in restriction-enzyme recognition, an *Aha*2 site in the HPA-2b allele and a *SfaN*I site in the HPA-2a allele.

Finally, Wang et al. (61) showed that HPA-4 polymorphism (Pen=Yuk) is due to a single base substitution of base 526 of GP IIIa (G→A), leading to a arginine to glutamine change.

A summary of the data discussed above is given in Table 6 (reviewed in refs. 47 and 62). The molecular basis of the HPA-5 (Br) system is still under study.

It is noteworthy that all platelet specific alloantigens studied so far are the result of single base substitutions in membrane glycoprotein genes.

F. Molecular Genotyping of Platelet Alloantigens

Knowledge of the genetic basis of platelet-specific antigens makes molecular genotyping possible. The genomic organization of the DNA coding for the relevant glycoprotein chains is known. Thus, genotyping can be done directly on DNA obtained from whatever cell type or tissue is available. By PCR with suitable primers, a DNA fragment containing the relevant

Table 6 Amino Acid Substitutions Responsible for HPA Antigens

Platelet alloantigen	Amino acid position	Glycoprotein
	28 33 39	
HPA-1a (Zw^a)	D E A L P L G S P R C D	GP IIIa
HPA-1b (Zw^b)	. . . . . P	
	140 145 151	
HPA-2a (Ko^b)	P P G L L T P T P K L E	GP Ib
HPA-2b (Ko^a)	. . . . . M	
	838 843 849	
HPA-3a (Bak^a)	D W G L P I P S P S P I	GP IIb
HPA-3b (Bak^b)	. . . . . S	
	138 143 149	
HPA-4A (Yuk^b)	L A T Q M R K L T S N L	GP IIIa
HPA-4b (Yuk^a)	. . . . . Q	

mutation is amplified. This can then be analyzed with probes specific for the base sequence under study (so-called allele-specific oligonucleotides, ASOs) applied in dot blotting (27).

We studied 98 donors, serotyped for the HPA-1, HPA-2, and HPA-3 antigens with an adapted restriction enzyme method (allele-specific restriction enzyme analysis, ASRA). The DNA was obtained from peripheral blood mononuclear leukocytes. The primer combinations and enzymes were chosen in such a way that in all PCR products an "internal control" site (to check for efficiency of the enzyme) was present; i.e., a nonpolymorphous target site independent from the phenotype of the donor. In this way, an absolute concordance was found between serotyping and genotyping (63).

G. Platelet Specificity of So-Called Platelet-Specific Alloantigens

Many platelet alloantigens, previously considered as "platelet specific", have been found on other cells and tissues as well. Antigens of the HPA-1 (Zw) and HPA-4 (Pen=Yuk) system have been detected on endothelial cells, smooth muscle cells, and fibroblasts (64–66). Antigens of the HPA-5 (Br) system have been found on activated T lymphocytes and endothelial cells (67,68). HPA-2 (Ko) and HPA-3 (Bak) antigens, however, appear to be expressed on platelets only.

These findings are not unexpected. Many antigen-carrying glycoproteins of platelets are present in the surface membrane as heterodimeric or heterotrimeric complexes. The complexes have important functions as receptor molecules for ligand binding in platelet aggregation and adhesion. Similar or related receptors are present on other cells and involved in cell-cell or cell-matrix interactions in general. In fact, these glycoprotein complexes often belong to a large superfamily of adhesion molecules (integrins) (69). Integrins are heterodimers of a noncovalently linked α and β chain. The superfamily consists of at least three (sub)families: the VLA (very late antigens) family, the LFA (leukocyte function antigen) or leukocyte adhesion molecule (Leu-CAM) family, and the cytoadhesin family. Each family shares a common β chain (β_1, β_2, and β_3, respectively). The members of a family have different α chains and show different ligand binding specificity. The different family-specific β chains have homologous amino acid sequences, as have the different inter- and intrafamily α chains.

Platelet GP IIb and GP IIIa form a complex (also designated $\alpha^{IIb}\beta_3$), which belongs to the cytoadhesin family. Fibrinogen, fibronectin, von Willebrand factor (vWF), and vitronectin (S protein) are ligands for the GP IIb/IIIa complex. All these adhesive proteins share the short peptide stretch RGDS (arg-gly-asp-ser) involved in binding to the receptor (70). For instance, on endothelial cells, fibroblasts, smooth muscle cells, and osteoclasts (and in low amounts also on platelets), a related cytoadhesin is expressed, the vitronectin receptor (VNR). This receptor has the ability to bind vitronectin, fibrinogen, and vWF. The VNR (also designated $\alpha^v\beta_3$) has the same β_3 chain (GP IIIa) that, as discussed, carries HPA-1 (Zw) and HPA-4 (Yuk=Pen) antigens. However, the α chain (α^v) is different and does not to carry HPA-3 (Bak) antigens. Thus, HPA-3 antigens are truly unique for platelets. Patients with Glanzmann's disease have platelets deficient in the membrane GP IIb/IIIa complex $\alpha^{IIb}\beta_3$. Their endothelial cells may express the VNR or $\alpha^v\beta_3$ normally. Thus, endothelial cells (as well as smooth muscle cells) in patients with Glanzmann's disease are then expected to express HPA-1 (Zw) and HPA-4 (Pen) antigens normally. This was indeed found to be so for HPA-1 (66). However, patients with a combined deficiency of GP IIb/IIIa and VNR also have been seen (71). These patients do not seem to have a particularly severe form of the disease. In the first form of Glanzmann's disease, the genetic defect probably affects the GP IIb gene or its regulation; in the second form, it may affect the GP IIIa gene or its regulation (72).

Platelets express three members of the VLA family, i.e., VLA-2 ($\alpha_2\beta_1$) or GP Ia/IIa complex, VLA-5 ($\alpha_5\beta_1$) and VLA-6 ($\alpha_6\beta_1$), both known as GP Ic/IIa complex. These three VLA molecules are receptors for collagen, fibronectin, and laminin, respectively (73,74). The VLA family encompasses at least nine different members (VLA-1–9) that are expressed on nearly every cell of the body, albeit in a different composition (and with different ligand binding specificity). All cells that carry VLA-2 or GP Ia/IIa will, therefore, also carry HPA-5 (Br) antigens, including activated T cells and endothelial cells.

On platelets, GP Ib (itself a heterodimer of GP Ibα and GP Ibβ) is complexed to GP IX and GP V. The complex is a major vWF receptor of platelets. So far, it has been found to be a structure confined to platelets and megakaryocytes only. Thus, Pl^E, HPA-2 (Ko), and Pl^T antigens are probably unique for this cell lineage.

The broad tissue distribution of many platelet antigens is of more than basic interest. It suggests that antibodies directed against such antigens may not only attack and destroy platelets but other cells as well, including cells that form an integral part of vessel walls. More specifically, it is possible that purpura, which forms such a characteristic sign of immune-mediated thrombocytopenia, may also result from direct vessel wall damage by antibodies. Moreover, it is imaginable that an alloimmune response against these antigens may be elicited not only by blood transfusion, bone marrow transplantation, and pregnancy but also by organ transplantation. Conversely, it may be that graft rejection sometimes results from such an immune response.

H. Molecular Immunology of the Platelet-Specific Alloimmune Response

Originally, Reznikoff Etievant et al. (75,76) made the interesting and important observation that the anti–HPA-1a alloimmune response is linked to the HLA class I phenotypes HLA-A1, HLA-B8 and strongly linked to the HLA class II phenotype HLA-DR3. Subsequently, this was confirmed by others (77,78). We could show that it also was associated with the supertypic antigen DRw52, including DR3 and DRw6 (79). This observation has recently been extended in that it was demonstrated that it is the subtype HLA-DRw52a that is involved in the HPA-1a response (80,81). This subtype resides on the β3 chain of HLA class II DR molecules. In a collaborative study with platelet serology laboratories in Europe, we found that the HPA-1b alloimmune response is not associated with HLA-DRw52a, nor was any other HLA association encountered (82). This indicates that presentation of peptides containing the HPA-1a amino acid substitution (Leu-33) is facilitated by HLA-DRw52a molecules but not of peptides containing the HPA-1b substitution (Pro-33). Thus, the association of HLA-DRw52a and HPA-1a alloimmune response seems to be the result of immune enhancement. It may explain the fact that HPA-1b immunization occurs much less often and that HPA-1a immunization may also sometimes occur in HLA-DRw52a–negative individuals (81). Another example of such a HLA class II alloimmune-mediated immune enhancement may be HPA-5b alloimmune response, which appears to be associated with HLA-DRw6 (83).

III. NEUTROPHIL ALLOANTIGENS

Different types of antigens also are present on neutrophils. Common antigens shared with other blood cells and/or tissue cells are glycoconjugate antigens of the blood group I and P system and glycoprotein HLA class I (ABC) antigens. Blood group ABH and Le antigens are not present on neutrophils (84). They carry another type of complex sugars (unbranched and fucosylated in another way) different from those of red blood cells and platelets, which can not act as substrates for A, B, H, or Le transferases. These complex sugars are also present on monocytes (mainly in a sialated form). They react with murine monoclonal antibodies of the cluster CD15 that react with the Le^X structure or with sialyl-Le^X (85). HLA class II (DP, DQ, DR) are not present on neutrophils.

Neutrophils also carry antigens that have so far been detected only on these cells. These "neutrophil-specific antigens" are the antigens of the NA, NB, NC, ND, and NE system. The first three systems were all described by Lalezari and coworkers (86) in a series of classic studies with sera from mothers who gave birth to a neutropenic child. The last two systems were discovered with sera from patients with autoimmune neutropenia and are less well defined (87,88).

Finally, neutrophils express antigens that they share with other white blood cells (monocytes and lymphocytes). These antigens were defined in studies with selected sera from individuals alloimmunized by blood transfusion and/or pregnancy and are the 9 system, Ond^a=E27 and $Mart^a$ antigens (89–92). The 9 system antigens were later found to be identical with the antigens of the human monocyte system HMA-1 (93). In Table 7, the phenotype and gene frequencies of the different neutrophil-specific and leukocyte-associated antigen systems are shown. All appear to be biallelec systems as well. A possible exception is the NA system. In studies in various laboratories, a very strong association (P >0.001) has been found between positivity for the NA2 and the NC1 antigen. It might indicate the existence of a triallelic system with the alleles NA(2+)NC(1+), NA(1+)NC(1+), and NA(1+)NC(1–).

Table 7 Neutrophil-specific and Leukocyte-"Specific" Antigens

System	Antigen	Phenotype frequency	Gene frequency
		in %	
NA	NA1	46	0.38
	NA2	88	0.63
NB = 5?	NB1	97	0.83
	NB2	32	0.17
NC	NC1	91	0.72
ND	ND1	98.5	0.88
NE	NE1	23	0.12
9 = HMA	9^a = HMA1	69	0.44
	9^b = HMA2	81	0.56
Mart	$Mart^a$	99	0.91
Ond	Ond^a (E27)	>99	>0.91

Recently, it was demonstrated that the Japanese have a much higher frequency of the NA1 phenotype than Europeans and North Americans (±0.65 versus ±0.35) (Table 8) (94,95). The genetic basis of this difference is not yet clear. As discussed, divergent gene frequencies between Japanese and white people also have been found for platelet antigens. Of interest is that in Japan, the NA null phenotype (see below) also seems to be more frequent.

A. Methods to Detect Neutrophil Antibodies and to Type and Characterize Neutrophil Antigens

The tests most commonly used to detect neutrophil antibodies and to type and characterize neutrophil antigens are agglutination and immunofluorescence, but cytotoxicity and antibody-dependent cellular cytotoxicity are being applied as well (96,97). The neutrophil agglutination test (NAT) and the neutrophil immunofluorescence test (NIFT) are most suitable for routine use. Both have an acceptable sensitivity and specificity, although the NIFT scores higher in this respect. Both tests detect immunoglobulin (Ig) M and G antibodies (98). Agglutination with IgG antibodies is an active process that requires both F(ab) binding and Fc receptor binding. It is a kind of frustrated phagocytosis for which viable cells, energy, and an intact cell skeleton are necessary. As a consequence, agglutination is inhibited by a low temperature, metabolic inhibitors, and inhibitors of microfilament and/or micrutubule formation (99).

The neutrophil cytotoxic test (NCT) is not suitable for routine use. Only complement binding antibodies are detected in this assay. Moreover, aspecific positive test results may occur.

The antibody-dependent cellular cytotoxicity assay (100) is the most sensitive and specific test for neutrophil antibodies available. It measures lysis of ^{51}Cr-tagged neutrophils by killer lymphocytes on sensitization with antibodies. Because this is also an Fcγ receptor–dependent process only IgG antibodies (of the IgG1 and IgG3 subclass) are detected. Unfortunately, the test it is too complicated for routine use.

For scientific studies, methods such as immunoprecipitation, immunoblotting, and monoclonal antibody immobilization (MAINA) are used (92). The MAINA may gain a place in the routine laboratory.

B. Clinical Importance of Neutrophil Alloantigens

Antibodies against neutrophil antigens are involved in neonatal alloimmune neutropenia, autoimmune neutropenia, notably when occurring in infants, and in transfusion reactions.

1. Neonatal Alloimmune Neutropenia

Neonatal alloimmune neutropenia (NAIPN)[101] is a rare disease, occurring in less than 1 per 2,000 newborns. Nevertheless, it is an important disease. This is because it may lead to severe and sometimes (5%?) lethal infections in the newborn. However, it may also be an entirely asymptomatic disease. Infections associated with NAINP are often recurrent and caused by

Table 8 NA Genotype Frequencies in Different Populations

	NA1	NA2	NA null
Netherlands	0.374	0.625	0.001
France	0.332	0.640	0.028
United States	0.337	0.663	0.0
Japan	0.651	0.302	0.047

gram-positive bacteria (streptococci, staphylococci). The infections preferentially affect the skin and mucosal membranes of the airway tract (ENT, respiratory tract), but sepsis may also occur.

Detection of neutrophil specific alloantibodies in the blood of the mother is of great diagnostic value (sensitivity 96%). The blood of the newborn shows selective neutropenia and often compensatory monocytosis, whereas the bone marrow is normal or shows a maturation arrest of neutrophils. If untreated, alloimmune neutropenia may persist for 2–4 months. Treatment modalities are antibiotics (also given prophylactically), plasma exchange, and high-dose intravenous gamma globulin (reviewed in refs. 97 and 102).

2. Autoimmune Neutropenia of Infancy

Chronic idiopathic and secondary neutropenia is quite a rare hematological disorder.[103] Serological analysis of patients with this disease shows that often neutrophil-bound immunoglobulins are present and that the serum may contain neutrophil (auto)antibodies. In adults, these antibodies only rarely have antigen specificity. However, in primary autoimmune neutropenia of infancy, neutrophil autoantibodies of the IgG and/or IgM class with antigen specificity are found in about 50% of the cases. This disease is peculiar in that it occurs at a very early age (a few months to less than 2 years) without any apparent cause and spontaneously resolves with the disappearance of the antibodies in 6 months to 3 years.

Blood and bone marrow show the same abnormalities as found in NAINP patients. Infants with AIPN may also have recurrent infections. These infections are mostly of mild to moderate severity, and they usually affect the skin (boils, cellulitis), the middle ear (otitis media), the oropharynx and upper respiratory tract (stomatitis, tonsillitis, pharyngitis), and the digestive tract (gastroenteritis). Few affected children develop pneumonia. Sepsis occurs only rarely. Usually, infections can be managed with routine antibiotic therapy, but in severe cases, corticosteroids and high-dose intravenous IgG are therapeutical options (for more detailed information, see refs. 97 and 104–106).

3. Transfusion Reactions

In most cases, a transfusion reaction due to neutrophil-reactive alloantibodies is an uncomplicated febrile reaction. Treatment with an antipyretic drug is then an adequate measure. Leukocyte removal by filtration of the blood is usually an adequate preventive action. The responsible antibodies are regularly HLA antibodies but sometimes neutrophil-specific antibodies are involved (107). In some patients, a life-threatening acute respiratory distress syndrome may develop, which is also referred to as transfusion-induced acute lung injury (TRALI) (108).

C. Transfusion-Induced Acute Lung Injury

Transfusion-induced acute lung injury (TRALI) has always been considered to be a rare complication of transfusion. However, analysis of the causes of transfusion-associated deaths in the United States reported to the Food and Drug Administration from 1976 to 1985 (109) suggest that this is not an entirely correct view. Although hemolysis (acute, delayed) is the leading cause in 71.9% (184 of 256) of transfusion-associated deaths, TRALI is the second most common cause in 12.1% (31 of 256), which means that TRALI occurs more often than death due to bacterial contamination of blood or blood products (26 of 256, 10.2%) or anaphylaxis (8 of 256, 3.1%).

Transfusion-induced acute lung injury is an acutely occurring dramatic complication of transfusion therapy. It may develop within minutes after starting a transfusion. Signs are nausea and vomiting, a persistent cough with production of serosanguineous sputum, dyspnea, cyanosis, development of mental confusion, and even coma with progression to death. Symptoms are a noisy respiration, rales over the lungs, tachycardia, hypotension, hypoxia, and respiratory acidosis. A lung x-ray shows diffuse, mottled infiltrates. Treatment is difficult and consists of intensive respiratory and circulatory support, corticosteroids, and prophylactic antibiotics. Plasmapheresis may have a beneficial effect.

Transfusion-induced acute lung injury has occurred during the administration of leukocytes to individuals sensitized against leukocyte antigens. However, most cases of TRALI reported in the literature were due to alloantibody infusion; i.e., infusion of whole blood or plasma from donors containing alloantibodies reactive with the recipient's leukocytes. The condition is believed to result from an intravascular reaction between neutrophils (or leucocytes in general) and alloantibodies, leading to massive sequestration of these cells in the lung. Damage to the lung tissues may be caused by substances released from activated neutrophils such as neutral proteases and superoxides but perhaps also by various cytokines. Detailed studies are still necessary to obtain more exact information about the incidence of TRALI and the role of leukocyte antibodies in its pathogenesis.

D. Neutrophil Alloantibody Specificity in Different Clinical Settings

The neutrophil alloantibodies that are most commonly involved in NAINP are anti-NA1 and anti-NB1. Anti-NA2 and anti-NB2 are found less often, and anti-NC1 is rarely found. In many cases (40%), specificity is not clear (97,102).

As discussed, the autoantibodies only rarely show antigen-specificity in adults with AINP. Auto–anti-NA1, auto–anti-ND1, and auto–anti-NE1 have been found in a few cases. However, in primary AINP of infancy, neutrophil autoantibodies with antigen specificity are found in about 50% of the cases (mostly anti-NA1 and sometimes anti-NA2) (97,104,106).

Transfusion-induced acute lung injury has occurred after infusion of whole blood or plasma from donors containing neutrophil-specific antibodies (anti-NA1, anti-NA2, anti-NB1, anti-5[b]) and HLA class I antibodies (110–115). Recently, we observed a case in which TRALI occurred on infusion of a gamma globulin preparation containing high titers of both HLA class I and class II antibodies (116).

E. Glycoprotein Localization and Other Characteristics of Neutrophil Antigens

The study of the biochemical nature of neutrophil antigens also has made significant progress lately.

1. NB System Antigens

With the help of immunoprecipitation and immunoblotting, it was established that NB1 is present on a membrane glycoprotein of 56–62 kd under reducing conditions (M_r 49–55 kd nonreduced). It was shown that this glycoprotein is a glycosyl-phosphatidylinositol (GPI)–anchored N-glycosylated protein (see below). The allotypic NB1-epitope is also recognized by the mouse monoclonal antibody (1B5) (117–120). NB1 antigen staining of neutrophils varies greatly among different donors (range 0–100%) but is mostly constant in individual donors. Blood cells other than neutrophils do not stain (99,120). NB1 antigen is expressed not only on the plasma membrane but also intracellularly on the membranes of small vesicles and specific granules. Cross-linking of NB1 antigen on the plasma membrane resulted in internalization of the complex, whereas in vivo stimulation of neutrophils caused an increase in intensity of plasma membrane staining with anti-NB1 but only of those cells that were already positive prior to stimulation (118,120). The NB1 glycoprotein thus appears to identify a distinct subset of neutrophils. The function of the NB1 glycoprotein remains unclear but its behavior on cross-linking and stimulation suggests a possible role as receptor molecule.

2. NA System Antigens

Immunoprecipitation and immunoblot, and later also monoclonal antibody immobilization, failed to localize the important antigens of the NA system. However, by a different approach, this problem was solved. We produced two murine MAbs against the human neutrophil Fcγ receptor (FcGran1 and Gran11) (121). Later, these antibodies were clustered in the CD16 MAb cluster.

One antibody (FcGran1) was panreactive; i.e., it reacted with the neutrophils of all donors tested. The other antibody (FcGran11) reacted with only about 50% of the neutrophils of normal donors. Analysis with a panel of typed neutrophils showed that it was a murine anti-NA1.

In precipitation studies, the panreactive antibody reacted with the whole neutrophil FcRIII structure, a typical smearlike precipitate of 50–80 kd on SDS-PAGE. This broad smear is due to heavy but variable glycosylation of the molecule.

Monoclonal anti-NA1 FcGran11 precipitated only the lower half of the FcRIII smear, indicating that NA1-FcRIII has a faster electrophoretic mobility than NA2-FcRIII. This was confirmed when precipitations were performed with the neutrophils of different NA-typed donors. Thus, the NA allotypes of FcRIII also are reflected in electrophoretic mobility differences (122,123).

Neutrophils carry two types of FcR for IgG, FcRII and FcRIII. Other blood leukocytes that carry FcR for IgG are monocytes, with FcRI (the high-affinity Fc receptor) and FcRII, and natural killer (NK) cells with only FcRIII. However, NA antigens have only been detected on neutrophils (124). It indicated that FcRIII from neutrophils and NK cells are different structures; as was later confirmed in molecular genetic studies (125,126) (see below).

"NA null" Phenotype.   Neutrophils have the phenotype "null" or NA(1-2-) in two clinical situations: paroxysmal nocturnal hemoglobinuria and hereditary neutrophil FcRIII deficiency.

Paroxysmal nocturnal hemoglobinuria (PNH).   This is an acquired clonal defect of the bone marrow stem cell. In PNH, the red blood cells (and also other blood cells) are missing multiple membrane glycoproteins, including the important complement regulatory proteins decay accelerating factor (DAF), membrane inhibitor of reactive lysis (MIRL), and C8 binding protein. This makes these cells very sensitive to lysis by activated complement components. Because some complement activation always occurs in vivo, chronic intravascular hemolysis results, which in some patients for unknown reasons occurs most severely during the night.

Recently, it was found that the missing membrane proteins all belong to a new class of membrane glycoproteins, so-called phosphatidylinositol glycan (PIG)–linked proteins, which are anchored in the outer lipid layer of the cell membrane via PIG. Apparently, in PNH, a mutation has occurred in the hematopoietic stem cell that leads to defective anchoring of such proteins. The nature of the defect is not clear. The proteins are synthesized normally in blood precursor cells of patients with PNH.

When studying PNH neutrophils, we found that they do not express FcRIII and NA antigens, whereas PNH NK cells had normal expression of NA antigen–negative FcRIII (122,127,128). It has been established that the FcRIII of NK cells (and of macrophages) is a transmembrane and not a PIG-anchored molecule (see below).

Hereditary neutrophil FcRIII deficiency and neonatal isoimmune neutropenia.   In studying a case of neonatal neutropenia, we found that the cause was isoimmunization of the mother against neutrophil FcRIII of her child (129). The mother appeared to have a hereditary deficiency of this receptor. Clinically, this was a classic case of neonatal immune neutropenia. The affected baby (the third child of the family) recovered after intravenous gamma globulin treatment without any severe complications. The mother, who was healthy, had panreactive neutrophil antibodies in her blood not reacting with her own cells. Her neutrophils were typed as NA(1-2-) and lacked expression of FcRIII. The antibodies were isoantibodies directed against neutrophil FcRIII, which were strongly reactive in the immunoblot with the whole FcRIII smear. During this study, a healthy male blood donor was found to have the same abnormality. His neutrophils were unreactive with the mother's antibodies. He had not produced neutrophil antibodies himself. Hence, the isoantibodies in the mother were induced by immunization during pregnancy. The defective neutrophil FcRIII expression in these two individuals was studied in detail at the RNA/DNA level. In both, a deletion of the neutrophil FcRIIIB gene was found but not of the FcRIIIA gene (see below). Recently, another case of neonatal isoimmune neutropenia due to neutrophil FcRIII deficiency has been described (130). Also more healthy individuals and a patient with systemic lupus erythematosus and the defect have been discovered (131). Thus, hereditary neutrophil FcRIII deficiency does not seem to be an extremely rare genetic defect. Whether it will have any clinical effect, other than being a cause of neonatal immune neutropenia, has still to be studied.

Soluble NA Antigens in Plasma. In vitro, neutrophil FcRIII is released in a soluble form into the fluid phase on stimulation of neutrophils with various agonists. FcRIII is cleaved off, apparently by a latent membrane protease that becomes activated by the agonists. In vivo, soluble(s) FcRIII is also present in body fluids (127,132). We found it in plasma, in ascites, in lymph fluid in quite high amounts, and in traces in the urine.

Immunochemical studies have shown that most, if not all, sFcRIII in plasma stems from neutrophils. Plasma sFcRIII also carries the NA antigens. Its concentration is markedly decreased in the plasma of patients with PNH, and it is undetectable in plasma from individuals with neutrophil FcRIII deficiency. The level of sFcRIII in plasma is not markedly increased in patients with infectious or inflammatory disorders (132). Thus, it seems that the level of plasma sFcRIII is determined mainly by constitutive excretion from neutrophils. It could be that it is a good measure for the overall neutrophil mass in the body. Indeed, the level of sFcRIII is decreased in patients with neutropenia owing to cytostatic treatment and normalizes on recovery.

F. NC and ND Antigens

PNH neutrophils are not only NA1 and NA2 antigen negative but also NC1-, ND1- and NB1-antigen negative, indicating that all these antigens are on one or more PIG-linked membrane proteins. The PIG linkage of the NB1 antigen has already been discussed.

The PIG-linked structures can be removed by the enzyme GPI-PLC (glycophosphoinositol-specific phospholipase C). Indeed, neutrophils treated with the enzyme loose all the antigens mentioned. The strong association between NA2 and NC1, discussed previously, suggests that NC1 also is on the FcRIII of neutrophils. The absence of NC1 antigen from PNH and GPI-PLC–treated neutrophils is in agreement with this hypothesis.

The two neutrophil FcRIII–deficient individuals identified in our laboratory were both typed negative not only for NA1 and NA2 but also for NC1 and ND1 (and as expected positive for NB1). This again indicates that not only NA antigens but also NC and ND antigens are located on FcRIII.

G. Ond and Mart Antigens

The neutrophil antigens Ond[a] and Mart[a] also are expressed on other leukocytes; i.e., monocytes and lymphocytes. This suggests the presence of the antigenic epitope on a more common glycoprotein type. Likely candidates are leukocyte integrins; i.e., molecules of the Leu-CAM family.

To date, three members of this family have been identified: LFA-1, complement receptor 3 (CR3), and complement receptor 4 (CR4). They are detected by McABs of the cluster groups CD11 (α chain antibodies), including CD11a, CD11b, CD11c, and CD18 (β chain antibodies).

Definite localization of these alloantigens on Leu-CAM structures was achieved by applying immunoprecipitation and monoclonal antibody immobilization. It was further evidenced by immunofluorescence on cells from patients with hereditary leukocyte adhesion deficiency, who do not have Leu-CAM molecule expression.

Ond[a] antigen was located on the α^M chain (CD11b molecule) and Mart[a] antigen on the α^L chain (CD11a molecule) of the Leu-CAM family, respectively (92).

In 1987, Pischel et al. described an alloantiserum (E27) also reacting with a polymorphous structure on LFA-1 α chain (91). Serologically, E27 antigen and Ond[a] antigen were found to be identical.

As discussed previously, many platelet alloantigens (HPA-1, HPA-3, HPA-4, and HPA-5 system antigens) are located on integrin structures as well. Thus, the general message is that integrins tend to be polymorphic, which may lead to antigenicity and immune-mediated diseases.

H. The Molecular Nature of Neutrophil Antigens

So far, only the molecular nature of the NA system antigens has been elucidated. This was made possible by the finding mentioned above and by the cloning and sequencing of FcRIII cDNA (133–136).

From the cloning of FcRIII cDNA, it became again clear that there are two types of FcRIII: FcRIII-1 or FcRIIIB, a shorter structure of 233 amino acids, and FcRIII-2 or FcRIIIA, a somewhat longer structure of 254 amino acids. FcRIIIB is the neutrophil form, which becomes PIG linked possibly via a serine on position 234. FcRIIIA is the NK cell form, also expressed on macrophages, which is a transmembraneous structure. FcRIIIA and FcRIIIB are the products of two different genes, both present on chromosome 1 and very closely linked. The coding sequences are for more than 95% identical.

In the amino acid sequences of FcRIIIB and FcRIIIA from NA1 or NA2 donors, only very subtle differences have been found (Table 9). Some are specific for the FcRIII type, whereas others are probably related to the NA polymorphism and occur only in the FcRIIIB type. These are the amino acids arg-asn-asp-val (at positions 36-65-82-106) in NA1-FcRIII and ser-ser-asn-ile in NA2-FcRIII. The amino acid differences are all based on one nucleotide difference in the coding triplet. The ser and asn substitution in NA2-FcRIII (at positions 65–82) lead to two extra glycosylation sites. This explains the slower mobility of NA2-FcRIII compared to NA1-FcRIII-1 in SDS PAGE.

Thus, the molecular basis of the NA antigens differs from that of the platelet antigens in that multiple amino acid substitutions are found. The precise location of the NA epitopes on the FcRIII-1 molecule is not yet clear.

Table 9 Difference in Deduced Amino Acid Sequence of FcRIIIA and FcRIIIB Allo-Forms

FcRIII type	amino acid no.	Amino acid positions								
		36	65	82	106	147	158	176	203	234
NA1–FcRIIIB	233	arg	asn	asp	val	asp	his	val	ser[b]	—
NA2–FcRIIIB	233	ser	ser[a]	asn[a]	ile	asp	his	val	ser[b]	—
FcRIIIA	254	arg	ser[a]	asp	ile	gly	tyr	phe	phe	asp

[a]Extra glycosylation site underlined.
[b]PIG binding site?

IV. CONCLUSIONS

Much has been achieved in the fields of platelet and neutrophil immunology in the past decades. The insight in the various immune-mediated disorders of platelets and neutrophils and the nature of the antigens involved has markedly increased. Nevertheless, much has still to be learned.

It will be very important to obtain insight in how and why an immune response, leading to disease, is generated. The understanding of the process of presentation of antigens or antigenic peptides via HLA molecules and of selection and activation of T cells and B cells will be of great importance in this respect. We hope that our ongoing studies will allow disease-inducing immune reactions to be treated and prevented in a more rational way than is now possible.

REFERENCES

1. von dem Borne AEGKr, Decary F. Nomenclature of platelet-specific antigens. Transfusion 1990; 30:477.
2. Shulman NR, Jordan JV. Platelet Immunology. In: Colman RW, Hirsch J, Marder VJ, Salzman EW, eds. Hemostasis and Thrombosis. Basic Principles and Clinical Practice. 2nd ed. Philadelphia: Lippincott, 1987:452–529.
3. Ramsey G, Salamon DJ. Frequencly of PL^{A1} in Blacks. Transfusion 1986; 26:531–532.
4. Inostroza J, Kiefel V, Mueller Eckhardt C. Frequency of platelet-specific antigens Pl^{A1}, Bak^{a}, Yuk^{a}, Yuk^{b}, and Br^{a} in South American (Mapuches) Indians. Transfusion 1988; 28:586–587.
5. Saji H, Maruya E, Fujii H, et al. New platelet antigen, Sib^{a}, involved in platelet transfusion refractoriness in a Japanese man. Vox Sang 1989; 56:283–287.
6. Han KS, Cho HI, Kim SI. Frequency of platelet-specific antigens among Koreans determined by a simplified immunofluorescence test. Transfusion 1989; 29:708–710.
7. von dem Borne AEGKr, Verheugt FWA, Oosterhof F, et al. A simple immunofluorescence test for the detection of platelet antibodies. Br J Haematol 1978; 39:195–207.
8. Taaning E. Microplate enzyme immuno-assay for detection of platelet antibodies. Tissue Antigens 1985; 25:19–27.
9. Sintnicolaas K, van der Steuijt, KJ, van Putten WL, Bolhuis RL. A microplate ELISA for the detection of platelet alloantibodies: comparison with the platelet immunofluorescence test. Br J Haematol 1987; 66:363–367.
10. Rachel JM, Summers TC, Sinor LT, Plapp FV. Use of a solid phase red blood cell adherence method for pretransfusion platelet compatibility testing. Am J Clin Pathol 1988; 90:63–68.
11. Court WS, LoBuglio AF. Measurement of platelet surface-bound IgG by a monoclonal ^{125}-I-anti-IgG assay. Vox Sang 1986; 50:154–159.
12. Janson M, McFarland JG, Aster RH. Quantitative determination of platelet surface alloantigens using a monoclonal probe. Hum Immunol 1986; 15:251–262.
13. Mulder A, van Leeuwen EF, Veenboer GJM, Tetteroo PAT, von dem Borne AEGKr. Immunochemical characterization of platelet-specific alloantigens. Scand J Haematol 1984; 33:267–274.
14. Huisman JG. Immunoblotting: an emerging technique in immunohaematology. Vox Sang 1986; 50:129–136.
15. Collins J, Aster RH. Use of immobilized platelet membrane glycoproteins for the detection of platelet-specific alloantibodies in solid-phase ELISA. Vox Sang 1987; 53:157–161.
16. Kiefel V, Santoso S, Weisheit M, Mueller Eckhardt C. Monoclonal antibody-specific immobilization of platelet antigens (MAIPA): A new tool for the identification of platelet-reactive antibodies. Blood 1987; 70:1722–1726.
17. Nordhagen R, Flaathen ST. Chloroquine removal of HLA antigens from platelets for the platelet immunofluorescence test. Vox Sang 1985; 48:156–159.
18. Blanchette VS, Chen L, de Friedberg ZS, et al. Alloimmunization to the Pl^{A1} platelet antigen: Results of a prospective study. Br J Haematol 1990; 74:209–215.
19. Kaplan C, Daffos F, Forestier F, et al. Current trends in neonatal alloimmune thrombocytopenia: Diagnosis and therapy. In: Kaplan-Gouet C, Schlegel N, Salmon C, McGregor J, eds. Platelet immunology: Fundamental and clinical aspects. London: John Libbey, 1991:267–278.
20. Herman JH, Jumbelic MI, Ancona RJ, Kickler TS. In utero cerebral hemorrhage in alloimmune thrombocytopenia. Am J Pediatr Hematol Oncol 1986; 8:312–317.
21. Kaplan C, Daffos F, Forestier F, et al. Management of alloimmune thrombocytopenia: Antenatal diagnosis and in utero transfusion of maternal platelets. Blood 1988; 72:340–343.

22. Derycke M, Dreyfus M, Ropert JC, Tchernia G. Intravenous immunoglobulin for neonatal isoimmune thrombocytopenia. Arch Dis Child 1985; 60:667–669.

23. Suarez CR, Anderson C. High-dose intravenous gammaglobulin (IVG) in neonatal immune thrombocytopenia. Am J Hematol 1987; 26:247–253.

24. Ander MM, Fisch GR, Starobin SG, Aster RH. Use of "compatible" platelet transfusions in treatment of congenital isoimmune neonatal thrombocytopenic purpura. N Engl J Med 1969; 280:244.

25. Deaver JE, Leppert PC, Zaroulis CG. Neonatal alloimmune thrombocytopenic purpura. Am J Perinatol 1986; 3:127–131.

26. Kuijpers RWAM, Faber NM, Kanhai HHH, von dem Borne AEGKr. Typing of fetal platelet alloantigens when platelets are not available. Lancet 1990; 336:1319.

27. McFarland JG, Aster RH, Bussel JB, et al. Prenatal diagnosis of neonatal alloimmune thrombocytopenia using allele-specific oligonucleotide probes. Blood 1991; 78:2276–2282.

28. Mueller Eckhardt C. Post-transfusion purpura. Br J Haematol 1986; 64:419–424.

29. Aster RH. Post-transfusion purpura. In: Engelfriet CP, von dem Borne AEGKr, eds. Baillière's Clinical Immunology and Allergy. Vol 1/No. 2, Alloimmune and Autoimmune Cytopenias. London: Baillière Tindall, 1987:453–461.

30. Pegels JG, Bruynes ECE, Engelfriet CP, von dem Borne AEGKr. Post-transfusion purpura: A serological and immunochemical study. Br J Haematol 1981; 78:521–530.

31. von dem Borne AEGKr, van der Plas-van Dalen CM. Further observation on post-transfusion purpura. Br J Haematol 1985; 61:374–375.

32. Shulman NR, Aster RH, Leitner A, Hiller NC. Immunoreactions involving platelets. V. Posttransfusion purpura due to a complement fixing antibody against a genetically controlled platelet antigen. A proposed mechanism for thrombocytopenia and its relevance in "autoimmunity." J Clin Invest 1961; 40:1597–1620.

33. Berney SI, Metcalfe P, Wathen NC, Waters AH. Post-transfusion purpura responding to high-dose intravenous IgG: Further observation on pathogenesis. Br J Haematol 1985; 61:627.

34. Gerstner JB, Smith MJ, Davis KD. Post-transfusion purpura: Therapeutic failure of PI^{A1}-negative platelet transfusion. Am J Hematol 1979; 78:361.

35. Lau P, Sholtis CM, Aster RH. Post-transfusion purpura: An enigma of alloimmunization. Am J Hematol 1980; 9:331.

36. von dem Borne AEGKr, Ouwehand WH, Kuijpers RWAM. Theoretic and practical aspects of platelet crossmatching. Transf Med Rev 1990; 4:265–278.

37. Moulinier P. Iso-immunisation maternelle antiplaquettaire et purpura néonatal. Le système de group plaquettaire "duzo." (abstract). Proc 6th Congress Europ Soc Haemat, Copenhagen, 1957; 236:817–820.

38. van Loghem JJ, Dorfmeijer H, van der Hart M, Schreuder F. Serological and genetical studies on a platelet antigen (Zw). Vox Sang 1959; 4:161–169.

39. Kroll H, Kiefel V, Santoso S, Mueller Eckhardt S. Sr^a, a private platelet antigen on glycoprotein IIIa associated with neonatal alloimmune thrombocytopenia. Blood 1990; 76:2296–2302.

40. Kekomäki R, Raivio P, Kero P. A new low-frequency platelet alloantigen, Va^a, on glycoprotein IIbIIIa associated with neonatal alloimmune thrombocytopenia. Transf Med 1992; 2:27–33.

41. Kuijpers RWAM, Simsek S, Faber NM, et al. Single point mutation in glycoprotein IIIa gives rise to a new platelet specific alloantigen (Mo) involved in neonatal alloimmune thrombocytopenia. Blood 1993; 81:70–76.

42. Simsek S, Goldschmeding R, Kuijpers, RWAM, et al. A new private platelet alloantigen, Gro^a, localized on GPIIIa involved in neonatal alloimmune thrombocytopenia. 1992 (in preparation).

43. von dem Borne AEGKr, van Leeuwen EF, von Riesz LE, et al. Neonatal alloimmune thrombocytopenia: Detection and characterization of the responsible antibodies by the platelet immunofluorescence test. Blood 1981; 57:649–656.

44. Kickler TS, Kennedy SD, Braine HG. Alloimmunization to platelet-specific antigens on glycoproteins IIb-IIIa and Ib/IX in multiply transfused thrombocytopenic patients. Transfusion 1990; 30:622–625.

45. Kunicki TJ, Furihata K, Brull B, Nugent DJ. The immunogenicity of platelet membrane glycoproteins. Transf Med Rev 1987; 1:21–33.

46. von dem Borne AEGKr, Ouwehand WH. Immunology of platelet disorders. Baillieres Clin Haematol 1989; 2:749–781.

47. Newman PJ, Goldberger A. Molecular genetic aspects of human platelet antigen systems. Baillieres Clin Haematol 1991; 4:869–888.

48. Kuijpers RWAM, Ouwehand WH, Bleeker PMM, et al. Localization of the platelet-specific HPA-2 (Ko) alloantigens on the N-terminal globular fragment of platelet glycoprotein Iba. Blood 1992; 79:283–288.

49. Yamamoto N, Ikeda H, Tandon NN, et al. A platelet membrane glycoprotein (GP) deficiency in healthy blood donors: Nak(a-) platelets lack detectable GPIV (CD36). Blood 1990; 76:1698–1703.

50. Daniels G. Cromer-related antigens—Blood group determinants on decay-accelerating factor. Vox Sang 1989; 56:205–211.

51. Newman PJ, Martin LS, Knipp MA, Kahn RA. Studies on the nature of the human platelet alloantigen, Pl^{A1}: Localization to a 17,000-dalton polypeptide. Mol Immunol 1985; 22:719–729.

52. van der Schoot CE, Wester M, von dem Borne AEGKr, Huisman JG. Characterization of platelet-specific alloantigens by immunoblotting: Localization of Zw and Bak antigens. Br J Haematol 1986; 64:715–723.

53. Newman PJ, Derbes RS, Aster RH. The human platelet alloantigens. Pl^{a1} and Pl^{A2}, are associated with a leucine33/proline33 amino acid polymorphism in membrane glycoprotein IIIa, and are distinguishable by DNA typing. J Clin Invest 1989; 83:1778–1781.

54. Goldberger A, Kolodziej M, Poncz M, et al. Effect of single amino acid substitutions on the formation of the Pl^A and Bak alloantigenic epitopes. Blood 1991; 78:681–687.

55. Flug F, Espinola R, Liu L-X, et al. A 13-mer peptide straddling the leucine^{33}/proline^{33} polymorphism in glycoprotein IIIa does not define the PLA^1 epitope. Blood 1991; 77:1964–1969.

56. van Leeuwen EF, Leeksma OC, van Mourik JA, et al. Effect of the binding of anti-Zw^a antibodies on platelet function. Vox Sang 1984; 47:280–289.

57. Lyman S, Aster RH, Visentin GP, Newman PJ. Polymorphism of human platelet membrane glycoprotein IIb associated with the Bak^a/Bak^b alloantigen system. Blood 1990; 75:2343–2348.

58. Loftus JC, Plow EF, Frelinger AL, et al. Molecular cloning and chemical synthesis of a region of platelet glycoprotein IIb involved in adhesive function. Proc Natl Acad Sci USA 1987; 84:7114–7118.

59. Take H, Tomiyama Y, Shibata Y, et al. Demonstration of the heterogeneity of epitopes of the platelet-specific alloantigen, Bak^a. Br J Haematol 1990; 76:395–400.

60. Kuijpers RWAM, Faber NM, Cuypers HTM, van dem Borne AEGKr. The N-terminal globular domain of human platelet glycoprotein Iba has a methionine^{145}/threonine^{145} amino-acid polymorphism, which is associated with HPA-2 (ko) alloantigens. J Clin Invest 1992; 89:381–384.

61. Wang L, Juji T, Shibata Y, Kuwata S, Tokunaga K. Sequence variation of human platelet glycoprotein IIIa associated with the Yuk^a/Yuk^b alloantigen system. Proc Jpn Acad 1991; 67:102–106.

62. Newman PJ. Platelet GPIIb-IIIa: Molecular variations and alloantigens. Thromb Haemost 1991; 66:111–118.

63. Simsek S, Kuijpers RWAM, Faber NM, et al. Determination of human platelet antigen frequencies in the Dutch population by immunophenotyping and DNA (allele-specific restriction enzyme) analysis. Blood 1993; 81:835–840.

64. Leeksma OC, Giltay JC, Zandbergen Spaargaren J, et al. The platelet alloantigen Zw^a or Pl^{A1} is expressed by cultured endothelial cells. Br J Haematol 1987; 66:369–373.

65. Giltay JC, Leeksma OC, von dem Borne AEGKr, van Mourik JA. Alloantigenic composition of the endothelial vitronectin receptor. Blood 1988; 72:230–233.

66. Giltay JC, Brinkman HJ, van dem Borne AEGKr, van Mourik JA. Expression of the alloantigen Zw^a (or Pl^{A1}) on human vascular smooth muscle cells and foreskin fibroblasts: A study on normal individuals and a patient with Glanzmann's thrombasthenia. Blood 1989; 74:965–970.

67. Giltay JC, Brinkman HJ, Vlekke A, et al. The platelet glycoprotein Ia-IIa–associated Br-alloantigen system is expressed by cultured endothelial cells. Br J Haematol 1990; 75:557–560.

68. Santoso S, Kiefel V, Mueller Eckhardt C. Human platelet alloantigens Br^a/Br^b are expressed on the very late activation antigen 2 (VLA-2) of T lymphocytes. Hum Immunol 1989; 25:237–246.

69. Hynes RO. Integrins: A family of cell surface receptors. Cell 1987; 48:549–554.

70. Ginsberg MH, Loftus JC, Plow EF. Cytoadhesins, integrins and platelets. Thromb Haemost 1989; 59:1–6.
71. Coller BS, Cheresh DA, Asch E, Seligsohn U. Platelet vitronectin receptor expression differentiates Iraqi-Jewish from Arab patients with Glanzmann trombasthenia in Israel. Blood 1991; 77:75–83.
72. Newman PJ, Seligsohn U, Lyman S, Coller BS. The molecular genetic basis of Glanzmann thrombasthenia in the Irawi-Jewish and Arab populations in Israel. Proc Natl Acad Sci USA 1991; 88:3160–3164.
73. Sonnenberg A, Modderman PW, Hogervorst F. Laminin receptor on platelets is the integrin VLA-6. Nature 1988; 336:487–489.
74. Hemler ME. Adhesive protein receptors on hematopoietic cells. Immunol Today 1988; 9:109–113.
75. Reznikoff Etievant MF, Dangu C, Lobet R, HLA-B8 antigen and anti-Pl^{A1} alloimmunization. Tissue Antigens 1981; 18:66–68.
76. Reznikoff Etievant MF, Muller JY, Julien F, Patereau C. An immune response gene linked to HLA in man. Tissue Antigens 1983; 22:312–314.
77. Taaning E. HLA antigens and maternal antibodies in alloimmune neonatal thrombocytopenia. Tissue Antigens 1983; 21:351–359.
78. Mueller Eckhardt C, Mueller Eckhardt G, Willen Ohff H, et al. Immunogenicity of and immune response to the human platelet antigen Zw^a is strongly associated with HLA-B8 and DR3. Tissue Antigens 1985; 26:71–76.
79. de Waal LP, van Dalen CM, Engelfriet CP, von dem Borne AEGKr. Alloimmunization against the platelet-specific Zw^a antigen, resulting in neonatal alloimmune thrombocytopenia or posttransfusion purpura, is associated with the supertypic DRw52 antigen including DR3 and DRw6. Hum Immunol 1986; 17:45–53.
80. Valentin N, Vergracht A, Bignon JD, et al. HLA-DRw52a is involved in alloimmunization against PL-A1 antigen. Hum Immunol 1990; 27:73–79.
81. Decary F, L'Abbé D, Tremblay L, Chartrand P. The immune response to the HPA-1a antigen: Association with HLA-DRw52a. Transf Med 1991; 1:55–62.
82. Kuijpers RWAM, von dem Borne AEGKr, Kiefel V, et al. The leucine^{33}/proline^{33} substitution in human platelet glycoprotein IIIa determines the HLA-DRw52^a (DW24) association of the immune response against HPA-1a (Zw^a/Pl^{A1}) and HPA-1b (Zw^b/Pl^{A2}). Hum Immunol 1992; 34:253–256.
83. Mueller Eckhardt C, Kiefel V, Kroll H, Mueller Eckhardt G. HLA-DRw6, a new immune response marker for immunization against the platelet alloantigen Br^a. Vox Sang 1989; 57:90–91.
84. Dunstan RA, Simpson MB, Borowitz M. Absence of ABH antigens on neutrophils. Br J Haematol 1985; 60:651–657.
85. McMichael AJ et al. eds. Leukocyte Typing IV. White Cell Differentiation Antigens. Oxford, England: Oxford University Press, 1989:1–1182.
86. Lalezari P, Radel E. Neutrophil-specific antigens: Immunology and clinical significance. Semin Hematol 1974; 11:281–290.
87. Verheugt FWA, von dem Borne AEGKr, van Noord-Bokhorst JC, et al. ND1, a new granulocyte antigen. Vox Sang 1978; 35:13–17.
88. Claas FHJ, Langerak J, Sabbe LJM, van Rood JJ, NE1, a new neutrophil specific antigen. Tissue Antigens 1979; 13:129–134.
89. van Rood JJ, van Leeuwen A, Schippers AMJ. Leukocyte groups, the normal lymphocyte transfer test and homograft sensitivity. Histocompatibility Testing 1965; 37–50.
90. Kline WE, Press C, Clay ME, et al. Three sera defining a new granulocyte-monocyte–T-lymphocyte antigen. Vox Sang 1986; 50:181–186.
91. Pischel K, Marlin S, Springer TA, et al. Polymorphism of lymphocyte function-associated antigen-1 demonstrated by a lupus patient's alloantiserum. J Clin Invest 1987; 1607:1614.
92. van der Schoot CE, Daams M, Huiskes E, et al. Antigenic polymorphism of the Leu-CAM family recognized by human leukocyte alloantisera. Br J Haematol 1993 (accepted for publication).
93. Jager MJ, Claas FJH, Witvliet M, van Rood JJ. Correspondence of the monocyte antigen HMA-1 to the non-HLA antigen 9a. Immunogenetics 1986; 23:71–77.
94. Ohto H, Matsuo Y. Neutrophil-specific antigens and frequencies in Japanese. Transfusion 1989;
95. Bierling P, Poulet E, Fromont P, et al. Neutrophil-specific antigen and gene frequencies in the French population. Transfusion 1990; 30:848–849.

96. Engelfriet CP, Tetteroo PAT, van der Veen JPW, et al. Granulocyte-specific antigens and methods for their detection. In: Advances in Immunobiology: Blood Cell Antigens and Bone Marrow Transplantation. New York: Liss, 1984:121–154.

97. McCullough J, Clay ME, Press C, Kline WE. Granulocyte Serology. A Clinical and Laboratory Guide. Chicago: ASCP Press, 1988.

98. Verheugt FWA, von dem Borne AEGKr, Decary F, Engelfriet CP. The detection of granulocyte alloantibodies with an indirect immunofluorescence test. Br J Haematol 1977; 36:533–544.

99. Verheught FWA, von dem Borne AEGKr, van Noord-Bokhorst JC, van Elven EH. Serological, immunochemical and immunocytological properties of granulocyte antibodies. Vox Sang 1978; 35:294–303.

100. Logue GL, Kurlander R, Pepe P, et al. Antibody-dependent lymphocyte-mediated granulocyte cytotoxicity in man. Blood 1978; 51:97–108.

101. Lalezari P, Nussbaum M, Gelman S, Spaet TH. Neonatal neutropenia due to maternal isoimmunization. Blood 1960; 15:236–242.

102. Lalezari P. Alloimmune neonatal neutropenia. Alloimmune and Autoimmune Cytopenias. Baillieres Clin Immunol Allergy 1987; 1(2):443–452.

103. Lalezari P, Jiang AF, Yegen L, Santorineou M. Chronic autoimmune neutropenia due to anti-NA2 antibody. N Engl J Med 1975; 293:744–747.

104. Lalezari P, Khorshidi M, Petrosova M. Autoimmune neutropenia of infancy. J Pediatr 1986; 109:764–769.

105. Conway LT, Clay ME, Kline WE, et al. Natural history of primary autoimmune neutropenia in infancy. Pediatrics 1987; 79:728–733.

106. McCullough J, Clay ME, Thompson HW. Autoimmune granulocytopenia. Alloimmune and autoimmune cytopenias. Baillieres Clin Immunol Allergy 1987; 1(2):303–326.

107. de Rie MA, van der Plas-van Dalen CM, Engelfriet CP, van dem Borne AEGKr. The serology of febrile transfusion reactions. Vox Sang 1985; 49:126–134.

108. Popovsky MA, Abel MD, Moore SB. Transfusion-related acute lung injury associated with passive transfer of leukocyte antibodies. Am Rev Respir Dis 1983; 128:185–189.

109. Sazama K. Reports of 355 transfusion-associated deaths: 1976 through 1985. Transfusion 1990; 30:583–590.

110. Brittingham TE, Chaplin H. Febrile transfusion reactions caused by sensitivity to donor leukocytes and platelets. JAMA 1957; 165:819–825.

111. Andrews AT, Zmijewski CM, Bowman HS, Reihart JK. Transfusion reaction with pulmonary infiltrates associated with HL-A-specific leukocyte antibodies. Am J Clin Pathol 1976; 66:483–487.

112. Nordhagen R, Conradi M, Dromtorp SM. Pulmonary reaction associated with transfusion of plasma containing anti-5b. Vox Sang 1986; 51:102–107.

113. Yomtovian R, Kline WE, Press C, et al. Severe pulmonary hypersensitivity associated with passive transfusion of a neutrophil-specific antibody. Lancet 1984; 1:244–246.

114. Eastlund T, McGrath PC, Britten A, Propp R. Fatal pulmonary transfusion reaction to plasma containing donor HLA antibody. Vox Sang 1989; 57:63–66.

115. van Buren NL, Stroncek DF, Clay ME, et al. Transfusion-related acute lung injury caused by an NB2 granulocyte-specific antibody in a patient with thrombotic thrombocytopenic purpura. Transfusion 1990; 30:42–45.

116. Dooren MC, Kuijpers RWAM, Goldschmeding R, et al. Adult respiratory distress syndrome after administration of an experimental intravenous gammaglobulin concentrate with a high titre of monocyte reactive IgG antibodies. 1993, submitted for publication.

117. Clement LT, Lehmeyer JE, Gartland GL. Identification of neutrophil subpopulations with monoclonal antibodies. Blood 1983; 61:326–332.

118. Stroncek DF, Skubitz KM, McCullough JJ. Biochemical characterization of the neutrophil-specific antigen NB1. Blood 1990; 75:744–755.

119. Skubitz KM, Stroncek DF, Sun B. Neutrophil-specific antigen NB1 is anchored via a glycosyl-phosphatidylinositol linkage. J Leukocyte Biol 1991; 49:163–171.

120. Goldschmeding R, van Dalen CM, Faber N, et al. Further characterization of the NB1 antigen as a variably expressed 56-62 kD GPI-linked glycoprotein of plasma membranes and specific granules of neutrophils. Br J Haematol 1992; 81:336–345.

121. Werner WF, von dem Borne AEGKr, Bos MJE, et al. Localization of the human NA1 alloantigen on neutrophil Fc-gamma-receptors. In: Reinherz EL, Haynes BF, Nadler LM, Bernstein ID, eds. Leukocyte Typing II. Vol 3. Human Myeloid and Hematopoietic Cells. Berlin: Springer-Verlag, 1986:109–122.

122. Huizinga TWJ, Kleijer M, Tetteroo PAT, et al. Biallelic neutrophil NA-antigen system is associated with a polymorphism on the phospho-inositol-linked Fc gamma receptor III (CD16). Blood 1990; 75:213–217.

123. Ory PA, Goldstein IM, Kwoh EE, Clarkson SB. Characterization of polymorphic forms of Fc receptor III on human neutrophils. J Clin Invest 1989; 83:1676–1681.

124. Huizinga TWJ, Kleijer M, Ross D, von dem Borne AEGKr. Differences between FcRIII of human neutrophils and human K/NK lymphocytes in relation to the NA antigen system. In: Knapp W, Dörken B, Gilks WR, et al, eds. Leucocyte Typing IV. White Cell Differentiation Antigens. Oxford, England: Oxford University Press, 1989:582–585.

125. Huizinga TWJ, Roos D, von dem Borne AEGKr. Neutrophil Fc-gamma receptors: A two-way bridge in the immune system. Blood 1990; 75:1211–1214.

126. Huizinga TWJ, Roos D, von dem Borne AEGKr. Fc-gamma receptors: Mediators, targets and markers of disease. Mol Immunohaematol 1991; 4(4):889–902.

127. Huizinga TWJ, van der Schoot CE, Jost C, et al. The PI-linked receptor FcRIII is released on stimulation of neutrophils. Nature 1988; 333:667–669.

128. van der Schoot CE, Huizinga TWJ, van 't Veer-Korthof ET, et al. Deficiency of glycosyl-phosphatidylinositol-linked membrane glycoproteins of leukocytes in paroxysmal nocturnal hemoglobinuria, description of a new diagnostic cytofluorometric assay. Blood 1990; 76:1853–1859.

129. Huizinga TWJ, Kuijpers RWAM, Kleijer M, et al. Maternal genomic neutrophil FcRIII deficiency leading to neonatal isoimmune neutropenia. Blood 1990; 76:1927–1932.

130. Stroncek DF, Skubitz KM, Plachta LB, et al. Alloimmune neonatal neutropenia due to an antibody to the neutrophil Fc-gamma receptor III with maternal deficiency of CD16 antigen. Blood 1991; 77:1572–1580.

131. Clark MR, Lin L, Clarkson SB, et al. An abnormality of the gene that encoding neutrophil Fc receptor III in a patient with systemic lupus. J Clin Invest 1990; 86:341–346.

132. Huizinga TWJ, de Haas M, Kleijer M, et al. Soluble Fc gamma receptor III in human plasma originates from release by neutrophils. J Clin Invest 1990; 86:416–423.

133. Ravetch JV, Perussia BV. Alternative membrane forms of FcRII (CD16) on human natural killer cells and neutrophils. J Exp Med 1989; 170:481–489.

134. Peltz GA, Grundy HO, Lebo RV, et al. Human Fcgamma RIII: Cloning, expression, and identification of the chromosomal locus of two Fc receptors for IgG. Proc Natl Acad Sci USA 1989; 86:1013–1017.

135. Ory PA, Clark MR, Kwoh EE, et al. Sequences of complementary DNAs that encode the NA1 and NA2 forms of Fc receptor III on human neutrophils. J Clin Invest 1989; 84:1688–1691.

136. Trounstine ML, Peltz GA, Yssel H, et al. Reactivity of cloned, expressed human FcgammaRIII isoforms with monoclonal antibodies which distinguish cell-type–specific and allelic forms of FcgammaRIII. Int Immunol 1990; 2:303–310.

137. van der Weerdt CM, Veenhoven-von Riesz LE, et al. The Zw blood group system in platelets. Vox Sang 1963; 8:513–530.

138. van der Weerdt CM. The platelet agglutination test in platelet grouping. In: Histocompatibility Testing. Copenhagen: Munksgaard, 1965:161–165.

139. Shulman NR, Marder VJ, Hiller MC, Collier EM. Platelet and leukocyte isoantigens and their antibodies: Serologic, physiologic and clinical studies. In: Progress in Hematology. 4th ed. 1964:222–304.

140. von dem Borne AEGKr, von Riesz LE, Verheugt FWA, et al. Bak[a], a new platelet-specific antigen involved in neonatal alloimmune thrombocytopenia. Vox Sang 1980; 39:113–120.

141. Boizard B, Wautier JL, Lek[a], a new platelet antigen absent in Glanzmann's thrombasthenia. Vox Sang 1984; 46:47–54.

142. Kickler TS, Herman JH, Furihata K, et al. Identification of Bak[b], a new platelet-specific antigen associated with posttransfusion purpura. Blood 1988; 71:894–898.

143. Shibata Y, Matsuda I, Miyaji T, Ichikawa Y. Yuk^a, a new platelet antigen involved in two cases of neonatal alloimmune thrombocytopenia. Vox Sang 1986; 50:177–180.

144. Shibata Y, Miyaji T, Ichikawa Y, Matsuda I. A new platelet antigen system, Yuk^a/Yuk^b. Vox Sang 1986; 51:334–336.

145. Friedman JM, Aster RH. Neonatal alloimmune thrombocytopenic purpura and congenital porencephaly in two siblings associated with a "new" maternal antiplatelet antibody. Blood 1985; 65:1412–1415.

146. Kiefel V, Santoso S, Katzmann B, et al. A new platelet-specific alloantigen Br^a. Report of 4 cases with neonatal alloimmune thrombocytopenia. Vox Sang 1988; 54:101–106.

147. Kiefel V, Santoso S, Katzmann B, Mueller Eckhardt C. The Br^a/Br^b alloantigen system on human platelets. Blood 1989; 73:2219–2223.

148. Woods VL Jr, Pischel KD, Avery ED, Bluestein HG. Antigenic polymorphism of human very late activation protein-2 (platelet glycoprotein Ia-IIa). Platelet alloantigen Hc^a. J Clin Invest 1989; 83:978–985.

149. Smith JW, Kelton JG, Horsewood P, et al. Platelet specific alloantigens on the platelet glycoprotein Ia/IIa complex. Br J Haematol 1989; 72:534–538.

150. Beardsley DS, Ho JS, Moulton T. Pl^T; a new platelet specific antigen on glycoprotein V. Blood 1987; 70(suppl 1):347a.

151. Ikeda H, Mitani T, Ohnuma M, et al. A new platelet-specific antigen, Nak^a, involved in the refractoriness of HLA-matched platelet transfusion. Vox Sang 1989; 57:213–217.

152. Kelton JG, Smith JW, Horsewood P, et al. Gov$^{a/b}$ alloantigen system on human platelets. Blood 1990; 75:2172–2176.

153. Mueller Eckhardt C, Becker T, Weisheit M, et al. Neonatal alloimmune thrombocytopenia due to fetomaternal Zw^b incompatibility. Vox Sang 1986; 50:94–96.

154. Bizzaro N, Dianese G. Neonatal alloimmune amegakaryocytosis. Case report. Vox Sang 1988; 54:112–114.

155. McGrath K, Minchinton R, Cunningham I, Ayberk H. Platelet anti-Bak^b antibody associated with neonatal alloimmune thrombocytopenia. Vox Sang 1989; 57:182–184.

156. Furihata K, Nugent DJ, Bissonette A, et al. On the association of the platelet-specific alloantigen, Pen^a, with glycoprotein IIIa. Evidence for heterogeneity of glycoprotein IIIa. J Clin Invest 1987; 80:1624–1630.

157. Kiefel V, Santoso S, Glockner WM, et al. Post-transfusion purpura associated with an antibody against an allele of the Bak^a antigen. Vox Sang 1989; 56:93–97.

158. Keimowitz RM, Collins J, Davis K, Aster RH. Post-transfusion purpura associated with alloimmunization against the platelet-specific antigen, Bak^a. Am J Hematol 1986; 21:79–88.

159. Taaning E, Killmann SA, Morling N, et al. Post-transfusion purpura (PTP) due to anti-Zw^b (-Pl^{A2}): the significance of IgG3 antibodies in PTP. Br J Haematol 1986; 64:217–225.

160. Simon TL, Collins J, Kunicki TJ, et al. Posttransfusion purpura associated with alloantibody specific for the platelet antigen, Pen(a). Am J Hematol 1988; 29:38–40.

161. Langenscheidt F, Kiefel V, Santoso S, Mueller Eckhardt C. Platelet transfusion refractoriness associated with two rare platelet-specific alloantibodies (anti-Bak^a and anti-Pl^{A2}) and multiple HLA antibodies. Transfusion 1988; 28:597–600.

162. Kunicki TJ, Aster RH. Isolation and immunologic characterization of the human platelet alloantigen Pl^{A1}. Mol Immunol 1979; 16:353–360.

163. Kieffer N, Boizard B, Didry D, et al. Immunochemical characterization of the platelet-specific alloantigen Lek^a: A comparitive study with the Pl^{A1} alloantigen. Blood 1984; 64:1212–1219.

164. Santoso S, Shibata Y, Kiefel V, Mueller Eckhardt C. Identification of the Yuk^b allo-antigen on platelet glycoprotein IIIa. Vox Sang 1987; 53:48–51.

165. Santoso S, Kiefel V, Mueller Eckhardt C. Immunochemical characterization of the new platelet alloantigen system Br^a/Br^b. Br J Haematol 1989; 72:191–198.

166. Furihata K, Hunter J, Aster RH, et al. Human anti-Pl^{E1} antibody recognizes epitopes associated with the alpha subunit of platelet glycoprotein Ib. Br J Haematol 1988; 68:103–110.

167. Tomiyama Y, Take H, Ikeda H, et al. Identification of the platelet-specific alloantigen, Nak^a, on platelet membrane glycoprotein IV. Blood 1990; 75:684–687.

7

Cellular and Molecular Biology of Senescent Cell Antigen

MARGUERITE M. B. KAY
University of Arizona College of Medicine
Tucson, Arizona

I. INTRODUCTION

Senescent cell antigen (SCA), an aging antigen, was discovered in 1975 (1). It is a protein that appears on old cells and acts as a specific signal for the termination of that cell by initiating the binding of immunoglobulin G (IgG) autoantibody and subsequent removal by phagocytes (1–32). This appears to be a general physiological process for removing senescent and damaged cells in mammals and other vertebrates (4). Although the initial studies were cone using human red blood cells (RBCs) as a model, senescent cell antigen was discovered on cells besides RBCs in 1981 (4). It occurs on all cells examined (4). The aging antigen itself is generated by the degradation of an important structural and transport membrane molecule, protein band 3 (5). Besides its role in the removal of senescent and damaged cells, senescent cell antigen also appears to be involved in the removal of RBCs in clinical hemolytic anemias (7,18), sickle cell anemia (31,32), and the removal of malaria-infected RBCs (33,34). Oxidation generates senescent cell antigen in situ (6).

The presence of band 3–related molecules in nonerythroid tissues was first demonstrated in 1983 (35). A protein immunologically related to band 3 was demonstrated in such diverse cell types as isolated neurons, hepatocytes, squamous epithelial cells, alveolar (lung) cells, lymphocytes, neurons, and fibroblasts using an antibody to band 3 that reacts with the transmembrane anion transport domain of band 3 (35). The band 3–like protein in many of these cell types appeared to be a truncated version of the erythroid protein based on its molecular weight of approximately 60,000 estimated from its migration in polyacrylamide gels. We suggested that part of the cytoplasmic amino-terminus segment was missing from the band 3–like protein in these cell types, and that band 3 protein was modified to perform functions in different environments (15,16,35,36). Since then band 3 has been described in numerous cell types and tissues, including brain, fibroblasts, glial cells, kidney, placental syncytiotrophoblast, eye lens, hepatoma cells, and lymphoid cells (15,16,37–50). Band 3 is also present in nuclear (35), Golgi (52), and mitochondrial membranes (53) as well as in cell membranes. Band 3–like proteins in nucleated cells participate in band 3 antibody-induced cell surface patching and capping (35). A truncated version of band 3 that lacks the amino-terminus has also been described in kidney (48). Band 3 is present in the central nervous system, and differences have been described in band 3 between young and aging brain tissue (16). One autosomal recessive neurological disease, choreoacanthocytosis, is associated with band 3 abnormalities (17–19). The 150 residues of the carboxyl-terminus segement of band 3 appear to be altered (19). In brains from patients with Alzheimer's disease, antibodies to aged band 3 label the amyloid core of classic plaques and the microglial cells located in the middle of the plaque in tissue sections and an abnormal band 3 in immunoblots. Band 3 in nonerythroid tissues performs the same functions as it does in erythrocytes. Thus, senescent cell antigen generation from band 3 may be a generalized mechanism for cellular removal.

II. MECHANISM OF REMOVAL OF SENESCENT CELLS

The first hint that a "neo-antigen" appeared on senescent cells came from studies showing that IgG autoantibodies selectively bind to old human RBCs aged in situ (1,2) during investigations of the mechanism by which macrophages distinguish between senescent and other "self" cells.

A. RBCs as a Model

Human RBCs were used as a model for these studies because of the ready availability of these cells and the ease with which populations of different ages can be separated. In addition, RBCs do not synthesize proteins. Therefore, they provide information on cumulative protein aging and damage.

B. Hypothesis

It was hypothesized that Ig in normal human serum attaches to the surface of senescent RBCs until a critical level is reached that results in phagocytosis.

C. IgG Binds to Old but Not Young Cells

To test this hypothesis, RBCs separated by density centrifugation from freshly drawn blood were incubated with specific antibodies to human Igs conjugated to scanning immunoelectron microscopy markers. Old RBCs had IgG but no IgA or IgM on their surfaces as determined by scanning immunoelectron microscopy (1). Young RBCs did not have immunoglobulin on their surfaces. Incubation of old RBCs with autologous macrophages resulted in their phagocytosis regardless of whether incubations are performed in medium with serum, autologous Ig-depleted serum, or whole serum (1). Young RBCs are not phagocytized under any of these conditions. Thus, it appeared that the IgG attached in situ to senescent human RBCs and rendered them vulnerable to phagocytosis by macrophages. The presence of IgG autoantibodies on the surface of old cells indicated that a new antigen had appeared that is not present on other cells. This was the first indication that a "neo-antigen" appears on senescent cells.

D. Senescent Cell IgG Is an Autoantibody

Immunoglobulin G attached to senescent cells in situ was shown to be an autoantibody (2). The antibodies could be dissociated from senescent cells. The dissociated antibodies specifically reattached via the antigen binding (Fab) portion of the IgG molecule to homologous senescent but not to autologous or allogeneic mature or young cells (3). Fab binding was demonstrated by antigen-blockade studies, scanning immunoelectron microscopy, and ^{125}I-labeled protein A binding to the Fc region of IgG bound to senescent cells and vesicles (2,8,9,11). Thus, the antibody to the senescent cell antigen is an autoantibody and not a nonspecific or a cytophilic antibody (2). It exhibited specific immunological binding via the Fab region.

Other investigators have confirmed the presence of IgG on senescent, damaged, and stored RBCs (1–13,22–32; reviewed in refs. see 9,11, and 18). The amount of IgG on the surface of cells increases with storage.

Glass et al. (23) have found a 44% reduction in the mean life span of RBCs in old, specific pathogen–free (SPF) rats as compared with the life span in young rats, as determined by ^{59}Fe pulse labeling in vivo. The proportion of young cells circulating in the blood of old animals was increased. In old rats, young as well as old RBCs are heavily labeled with IgG, whereas predominantly old cells carried IgG in young rats. Extending their studies to humans, Glass, et al. (24) found a significant increase in reticulocytes in healthy elderly humans even though their hematocrits are the same as those of younger individuals. A significant increase in autologous IgG on lower middle-aged cells was consistently demonstrated in these elderly individuals. These findings suggest that young cells age prematurely in old individuals. Bartosz et al. (37) have found increased amounts of cell membrane–bound IgG on RBCs from patients with Down's syndrome and suggest that accelerated RBC aging occurs in these individuals. Accelerated aging of other cells and systems, including the immune system, has been reported in patients with Down's syndrome. Bosman et al. (57) have found that RBCs from patient's with Alzheimer's disease but not multi-infarct dementia show characteristics of accelerated aging.

The results of studies described above demonstrate that Ig was required to initiate phagocytosis of senescent and stored cells and that IgG attaches in situ to senescent human RBCs (1,2).

E. RBC Life Span Studies

These results are confirmed in vivo using mice that are bred and maintained in a maximum security barrier devoid of viruses, mycoplasma, and pathogenic bacteria; thus, excluding an exogenous source for the senescent cell antigen (3). Red blood cells are labeled in situ with ^{59}Fe that labels the newly synthesized hemoglobin in young cells. Red blood cells are separated on Percoll gradients, 1 or 40 days after radioactive iron injection, into young and old populations, and injected into separate groups of syngeneic mice. Kinetic studies revealed that <90% of the ^{59}Fe-labeled young RBCs are removed from the circulation within 45 days. In contrast, >90% of the ^{59}Fe-labeled old RBCs are removed within 20 days. The difference in the rate of removal of young and old RBCs was statistically significant ($P \leq 0.001$). Kinetic studies on density-separated spleen cell populations revealed that the radioactivity decreased in the RBC fraction concomitantly with an increase in radioactivity in the splenic macrophage fraction. The radioactivity was found to be inside macrophages (3).

Studies performed in vitro with mouse splenic macrophages and autologous young and old RBCs revealed that mouse macrophages phagocytized senescent but not young RBCs ($P \leq 0.001$). The phagocytosis of middle-aged RBCs (~23%) was intermediate between that of young RBCs (5%) and old RBCs (~50%). This suggested that the appearance of the senescent cell antigen and, thus, molecular aging of membranes was a cumulative process.

F. Cellular Removal in Other Vertebrates

Numerous investigators have confirmed the presence of IgG on old human cells using different methods. In addition, IgG binding to RBCs has been shown to be a mechanism of removal of old RBCs in SPF mice (3), conventionally housed mice (22), germ-free rats (23), cows (25), rabbits (28), and chickens (Bosman G, Harris E, and Kay MMB, unpublished data). Anion transport by old RBCs from chickens was consistent with band 3 aging (Bosman G, Harris E, and Kay MMB, unpublished data).

G. Role of Sialic Acid and Carbohydrate in Recognition and/or Removal of Senescent Cells

Other groups, extrapolating from the classic experiments of Ashwell and coworkers who showed that the lifetime of serum glycoproteins could be drastically shortened by removal of external carbohydrates, have suggested that binding and phagocytosis of old RBCs require the disappearance of terminal sialic acid residues and subsequent exposure of penultimate galactose residues.

In order to determine what role, if any, galactose has in the physiological removal of old RBCs, we tried to elute IgG from intact senescent RBCs, as well as from their membranes, with buffer containing galactose (55). Incubation of senescent RBCs with galactose did not inhibit their phagocytosis by macrophages, indicating that galactose did not displace senescent cell IgG. Incubation with galactose did not elute senescent cell IgG from the membranes of RBCs. In addition, absorption of senescent cell IgG with the carbohydrate portion of band 3 did not alter binding to band 3 in immunoblots. The fraction specifically eluted from affinity columns containing the carbohydrate portion of band 3 did not bind to erythrocyte membranes in immunoblots. These results suggest that the IgG binding specifically to senescent RBCs was not directed against galactose residues. In addition, our synthetic peptide studies described below show that carbohydrate is not required for senescent cell IgG binding because it binds to synthetic peptides that have no carbohydrate attached.

In summary, macrophages recognize old and damaged RBCs on the basis of binding of a specific IgG autoantibody to old cells. Immunoglobulin G is required for phagocytosis of old RBCs.

III. NEOANTIGEN APPEARS ON OLD CELLS

Binding of an IgG autoantibody to senescent RBCs through immunological mechanisms indicated that antigenic determinants recognized by these IgG autoantibodies appeared on the membrane surface as RBCs aged.

A. Isolation of Senescent Cell Antigen

As an approach to isolating and identifying this neoantigen, affinity columns are prepared with IgG isolated from old cells. Senescent cell antigen is isolated from sialoglycoprotein mixtures with affinity columns prepared with IgG eluted from senescent cells (4). Material specifically bound by the column is eluted with glycine-HCl buffer, pH 2.3. Both glycoprotein and protein stains of gels of the eluted material revealed a band migrating at a relative molecular weight of 62,000 in the component 4.5 region. These experiments suggested that the 62,000 M_r glycopeptide carried the antigenic determinants recognized by IgG obtained from freshly isolated senescent cells. The 62,000 M_r peptide, but not the remaining sialoglycoprotein mixture from which it is isolated, abolished the phagocytosis-inducing ability of IgG eluted from senescent RBCs in the erythrophagocytosis assay (4). This indicated that the 62,000 M_r peptide is the antigen that appeared on the membrane of cells as they aged.

B. Senescent Cell Antigen Is Present on Nucleated Cells

Examination of other somatic cells for the antigen that appears on senescent RBCs revealed its presence on lymphocytes, platelets, neutrophils, and cultured human adult liver cells and primary cultures of human embryonic kidney cells as determined by a phagocytosis inhibition assay (4) (Table 1). Senescent cell antigen is isolated from lymphocytes (4,56) with the senescent RBC IgG affinity column. Gel electrophoresis of the material obtained from the column revealed a

Table 1 Inhibition of the Phagocytosis-inducing Ability of IgG Autoantibody Eluted from Senescent RBCs by Previous Absorption with (A) Stored Platelets, Lymphocytes, or Neutrophils, and (B) Human Adult Liver Cells or Embryonic Kidney Cells

	Cell type used For absorption	Phagocytosis (%) (mean $\pm$ s.d.)
A	None	37 ± 4
	Platelets	2 ± 2
	Lymphocytes	0
	Neutrophils	0
B	None	38 ± 6
	Liver	0
	Kidney	7 ± 7

Source: From Ref. 4.

band migrating at a M_r of 62,000 at the same position as the antigen isolated from senescent RBCs (4). This finding confirmed the results obtained with the phagocytosis inhibition assay, indicating that the antigen that appeared on senescent RBCs also appeared on other somatic cells.

Appearance of the 62,000 M_r antigen on RBCs initiates binding of IgG autoantibodies in situ and phagocytosis of senescent cells by macrophages (1–4). The antigen is present on stored human lymphocytes, platelets, and neutrophils and on cultured liver and kidney cells. In addition, IgG autoantibodies in normal serum have been shown to bind to senescent RBCs in situ in humans (1,2), mice (3), rats (23), cows (25), rabbits (28), and chickens (Bosman G, Harris E, Kay MMB, unpublished data). Thus, the immunological mechanism for removing senescent and damaged RBCs appears to be a general physiological process for removing cells programmed for death in mammals and, possibly, other vertebrates (1,2,4).

C. Identification of Senescent Cell Antigen as a Band 3 Product

Since mature erythrocytes cannot synthesize proteins, senescent cell antigen is probably generated by modification of a preexisting protein of higher molecular weight (8,10,11). It is postulated that senescent cell antigen is a component of the 4.5 region that is derived from band 3 (8,10,11) based on both extraction and isolation conditions, relative molecular weight, and its characterization as a glycosylated peptide (4).

Experiments designed to test this hypothesis revealed that senescent cell antigen is immunologically related to band 3 and may represent a physiologically significant breakdown product of the parent molecule (8,10,11). Both band 3 senescent cell antigen abolished the phagocytosis-including ability of IgG eluted from senescent cells; whereas spectrin, bands 2.1 and 4.1, actin, glycophorin A, PAS staining bands 1–4, and desialylated PAS staining bands 1–4 did not. In addition, rabbit antibodies to both purified band 3 and senescent cell antigen and IgG eluted from senescent cells reacted with band 3 and its breakdown products, as determined by immunoautoradiography of RBC membranes, indicating that these molecules share common antigenic determinants not possessed by other RBC membrane components (8,10,11).

These results confirmed those obtained with the erythrophagocytosis assay by indicating that band 3 carries the antigenic determinants of senescent cell antigen. Thus, senescent cell antigen is immunologically related to band 3 and may be derived from it.

Senescent cell antigen is mapped along the band 3 molecule using topographically defined fragments of band 3. Both binding of IgG eluted from senescent RBCs ("senescent cell IgG") to defined proteolytic fragments of band 3 in immunoblots and two-dimensional peptide mapping of senescent cell antigen, band 3, and defined proteolytic fragments of band 3 are used to localize senescent cell antigen along the band 3 molecule (10). The data suggested that the antigenic determinants of senescent cell antigen that is recognized by physiological IgG autoantibodies reside on an external portion of a naturally occurring transmembrane fragment of band 3 that has lost an M_r 40,000 cytoplasmic (NH_2 terminal) segment and part of the anion transport region. A critical cell age-specific cleavage of a band 3 appears to occur in the transmembrane anion transport region of band 3.

IV. BAND 3 AGING

The demise of band 3, which is synonymous with generation of senescent cell antigen, occurs in two distinct steps. Structurally, band 3 undergoes an as yet uncharacterized initial change during cellular aging that triggers a series of events terminating the life of the cell. We have recently developed antibodies against aged band 3 that recognize this change because they bind to a distinct region of band 3 in old but not middle-aged or young cells (7). Following the change in intact band 3 with aging, band 3 undergoes degradation, presumably catalyzed by an enzyme (56). Preliminary experiments indicate that it is a calcium-dependent membrane-bound protease and suggest that the protease may be calpain. Cleavage of band 3 occurs in the transmembrane anion transport region (5–7,8,10,11,56). Fragments of band 3 are detected in membranes of old but not young cells by immunoblotting with antibodies to normal band 3. Following degradation, band 3 undergoes a change in tertiary structure (56), becoming senescent cell antigen. A physiological IgG autoantibody binds to senescent cell antigen and initiates cellular removal.

Since our previous studies indicated that senescent cell antigen is derived from band 3 by cleavage in the transmembrane anion transport region (5,8,9,56), we suspected that anion transport might be altered with cellular aging (6). If this suspicion proved to be correct, then we would have a functional assay for aging of band 3, the major anion transport protein of the RBC membrane.

Transport studies on age-separated rat RBCs indicated that anion transport decreased with age (6). The Michaelis constant (K_m) increased and the maximal velocity (V_{max}) decreased in old RBCs as compared with middle-aged RBCs in humans and rats (Table 2). These data provided us with another assay of cellular function to use to determine whether RBCs are "senescent." However, it is doubtful that the number of molecules of band 3 to which IgG is bound (100/cell) is adequate to account for the magnitude of change in anion transport. Therefore, we suspect that another as yet unidentified change precedes events initiating IgG binding and is responsible for the observed changes in anion transport.

The following functional changes in band 3 occur as RBCs age. These changes are decreased anion transport activity (increased K_m; decreased V_{max}), decreased number of high-affinity ankyrin binding sites, and binding of physiological IgG autoantibodies in situ (57). In addition, band 3 undergoes an as yet undefined change that results in binding of 980 antibodies to aged band 3 (7). These 980 antibodies recognize band 3 that has aged prior to its formation of senescent cell antigen. Degradation of band 3 generates senescent cell antigen.

V. MODELS FOR CELLULAR AGING

A. Oxidation and Vitamin E

We postulated that generation of senescent cell antigen may result from oxidation-induced cross-linking followed by proteolysis (6). As an approach to evaluating oxidation as a possible

Table 2 IgG Molecules per Cell and Glucose and Anion Transport Properties of Human Erythrocytes as a Function of Cellular Age[a]

	Middle age[b]	Old	Stored
IgG	7 ± 1	98 ± 7*	110 ± 8*
Molecules per cell			
Sulfate exchange			
K_m, mM sulfate	0.6 ± 0.1	1.1 ± 0.1*	1.5 ± 0.2*
V_{max}, molecules × 10–8/(108 cells/min) at 37°C	11.1 ± 0.6	6.5 ± 0.3*	6.2 ± 0.7*
Glucose influx[c]			
V_{max} mmol/ml cells/min at 4°C	12.8 ± 1.9	6.7 ± 1.7*	6.4 ± 1.0*
Glucose efflux			
K_m, mM glucose[d]	9.0 ± 1.2	22.1 ± 3.8*	20.5 ± 3.0*
V_{max}, mmol/mL cells/min at 4°C	19.9 ± 2.9	33.4 ± 3.5*	34.9 ± 4.3*
3-O-methylglucose[c]			
Influx			
V_{max}, molecules × (10-8/108 cells/min) at 37°C	12.7 ± 1.6	8.0 ± 1.5*	7.7 ± 0.6*
Efflux			
K_m, mmol/mL cells/min at 4°C	9.0 ± 1.9	21.3 ± 2.8*	16.8 ± 2.4*
V_{max}, molecules × (10-8/108 cells/min)	17.9 ± 2.0	28.1 ± 2.4*	29.5 ± 1.3*

[a]Cells were separated on Percoll gradients and the amount of cell-bound IgG was measured with ^{125}I protein A; anion transport was measured with a sulfate self-exchange assay; zero-trans efflux and infinite-trans influx of ^{14}C-glucose were measured as described in text. All values are the mean of at least three experiments; *$P < 0.01$ compared with fresh middle-aged cells.
[b]Middle-aged cells kept in Alsever's for 4 weeks at 4°C.
[c]There are no significant differences between the various cell types in K_m of glucose influx.
[d]There are no significant differences between D-glucose and 3-O-methylglucose ($P > 0.10$).
Source: From Ref. 51.

mechanism responsible for generation of senescent-cell antigen, we studied erythrocytes from vitamin E–deficient rats (6). The importance of vitamin E as an antioxidant, providing protection against free radical–induced membrane damage, has been well documented (6). Vitamin E is primarily localized in cellular membranes, and a major role of vitamin E is the termination of free radical chain reactions propagated by the polyunsaturated fatty acids of membrane phospholipids. Vitamin E–deficient RBCs are defective in their ability to scavenge free radicals. It is interesting that there is a correlation between life span and natural antioxidant levels in a variety of species and that the level of such antioxidants appears to correlate with metabolic activity of individual species. Specific biochemical alterations in the membrane of RBCs from vitamin E–deficient rhesus monkeys have been described (6). Furthermore, vitamin E deficiency represents a "physiological" method for rendering cells susceptible to free radical damage and may simulate conditions encountered in situ. We used vitamin E deficiency as a model for studying oxidation because studies show that, in mammals, vitamin E functions as an antioxidant and because vitamin E deficiency simulates conditions encountered in situ more closely than does chemical treatment of cells in vitro. Red blood cells from vitamin E–deficient rats behaved like old RBCs in the phagocytosis assay and in anion transport and glyceraldehyde-3-phosphate dehydrogenase activity. In addition, increased breakdown products of band 3 are observed in RBC membranes from vitamin E–deficient rats. Vitamin E–deficient rats developed a com- pensated hemolytic anemia as is observed in vitamin E–deficient humans.

Middle-aged RBCs from vitamin E–deficient rats behaved like old cells based on the phagocytosis assay, anion transport studies, and immunoblotting studies (6).

Immunoblotting studies revealed increased breakdown products of band 3 in cells from vitamin E–deficient rats as is observed in old cells (6). Thus, vitamin E deficiency leads to accelerated RBC aging, presumably through oxidation.

We have not observed high molecular weight complexes containing band 3 in membranes from vitamin E–deficient rats or old cells aged in situ except under conditions that precipitate IgG (unpublished observations).

Results of the experiments on vitamin E deficiency suggest that oxidation can cause aging of band 3. We suspect that this may be one of the mechanisms of cellular aging in situ. At this time, it appears that general cellular damage such as lysis (Kay MMB, unpublished data) and oxidation can result in the generation of senescent cell antigen. We suspect that many different cellular insults have a final common pathway that results in generation of senescent cell antigen.

B. Chemical Models

As part of our systematic ongoing studies of mechanisms of cellular and molecular aging, we developed a "chemical profile" of senescent human RBCs (57). This "RBC aging" panel allows us to assess functional RBC age independently of chronological age. The panel used to obtain this profile includes IgG binding, phagocytosis, enzyme activity, anion transport, ankyrin binding, and immunoblotting with antibodies to band 3.

As part of our ongoing studies on mechanisms of cellular aging, we searched for models of accelerated and decelerated cellular aging. We anticipated that such models would allow us to dissect molecular aging and provide insight into mechanisms. Initially, we investigated models for aging in vitro (57).

1. Free Radical–generating Systems

We subjected intact human RBCs to treatments that have been reported to result in changes in band 3 and/or to mimic aging in vitro. The validity of these treatments as model systems for erythrocyte aging is evaluated using a RBC aging panel that provides a biochemical profile of a senescent RBC (6,7,57). Treatments are assessed for their ability to induce the following changes in vitro that are observed in normal erythrocytes aged in vivo: (1) increased breakdown of band 3 as detected by immunoblotting; (2) decrease in anion transport efficiency as detected with a sulfate self-exchange assay; (3) decrease in total glyceraldehyde 3-phosphate dehydrogenase (G3PDH) activity with an increase in membrane-bound activity; and (4) increase in the binding of autologous IgG as detected with a protein A binding assay. Neither incubation with the free radical–generating xanthine oxidase/xanthine system nor treatment with malondialdehyde, an end product of free radical–initiated lipid (per)oxidation, results in age-specific changes (57). Loading of the cells with calcium and oxidation with iodate results in increased breakdown of band 3 but does not lead to increased binding of autologous IgG. Only RBCs that have been stored for 3–4 weeks show the same structural and functional changes as observed during aging in vivo (57).

2. Hemoglobin Cross-linking

Cross-linking of band 3 by hemoglobin has been suggested as a mechanism for generating senescent cell antigen. Results of experiments in which cells are treated with phenylhydrazine in order to cross-link band 3 revealed increased binding of autologous IgG. However, phenylhydrazine in the amounts used caused RBC lysis. Lysis by itself initiates IgG binding. For example, IgG binding by control RBC that are not exposed to phenylhydrazine and had 0% lysis as determined by the loss of RBCs after incubation in PBS + 10 mM glucose pH 7.4 for 1 hr at 37°C (5% hematocrit) is 18 ± 2 molecules IgG/cell (mean ± 1 SD). When the incubation is performed with 5 mM phenylhydrazine in the solution, 20% hemolysis is observed and IgG binding increased to 115 ± 7. At 10 mM phenylhydrazine, hemolysis increased to

50% and IgG binding is 129 ± 7. At 15 mM phenylhydrazine, hemolysis is 60% and IgG binding is 200 ± 34. Similar results are obtained with acridine orange at the concentrations employed to induce "cross-linking" of band 3. This supports our early finding that lysis can initiate IgG binding but does not provide any insight into the role of cross-linking in the generation of senescent cell antigen. Drs. Linss, Simon, Halbhuber and Neyer have shown independently that IgG binding in the induced Heinz body system is an artifact (presented at the XIIth International Symposium on the Structure and Function of Erythroid Cells, Berlin, 1989). Thus, it appears that hemichrome formation generates artifacts. The other problem with this suggested hypothesis for the generation of senescent cell antigen is that is limited to RBCs and can not explain the formation of senescent cell antigen in cells besides RBCs.

3. Hemoglobin Köln and G6PD Deficiency

We then began a search for "experiments of nature" that might provide insights into the process of normal cellular aging (12). Initially, we studied glucose-6-phosphate dehydrogenase deficiency (G6PD) and hemoglobin Köln as potential models (12). Membranes from both the G6PD-deficient and hemoglobin Köln cells that we studied have been reported to contain high molecular weight polymers (12). In addition, hemoglobin Köln cells contain hemoglobin precipitates. We used the RBC aging panel to compare the biochemical profile of glucose 6-phosphate dehydrogenase–deficient and hemoglobin Köln cells containing high molecular weight protein polymers or hemoglobin precipitates with that of normal senescent cells. However, accelerated cellular aging is not present as determined by a RBC aging panel, including lack of phagocytosis and IgG binding to young and middle-aged RBCs, normal ankyrin binding, normal anion transport, normal G3PDH activity, and no increase in band 3 breakdown products (12) (Table 3). We found no evidence in support of the concept that aggregation of band 3 plays a role in the mechanism for generating senescent cell antigen. Observations like these support the hypothesis that degradation of band 3, not aggregation, is a critical event in IgG binding and normal RBC aging.

VI. BAND 3 MUTATIONS/ALTERATIONS

We began a search for mutations and/or clinical alterations of erythrocyte band 3. Our search for band 3 protein alterations resulted in the discovery of the first band 3 alterations/mutations in any species. All three different alterations were discovered in humans (7,14,17,19). Anion and glucose transport of all three is summarized in Table 4. One mutation, high transport band 3 Texas, results from an addition of tyrosine-containing peptides in the transmembrane, anion transport region of band 3 (14). Cytochalasin B binding was slightly increased, but the increase

Table 3 Transport Properties of Glucose-6-Phosphate Dehydrogenase-deficient and Hemoglobin Köln-containing Erythrocytes[a]

Cell type	Anion transport		Glucose transport		
			influx		efflux
	K_m	V_{max}	V_{max}	K_m	V_{max}
Control	0.9 ± 0.1	14.0 ± 0.6	13.1 ± 1.0	9.0 ± 0.7	19.7 ± 1.5
Hemoglobin Köln	0.8 ± 0.1	12.7 ± 0.9	14.1 ± 1.4	10.2 ± 0.6	17.7 ± 0.5
G6PDMinn	0.7 ± 1.0	14.5 ± 0.4	13.5 ± 0.9	9.2 ± 1.2	17.2 ± 0.8

[a]Middle-aged erythrocytes were washed and assayed within 12 hr after the blood was collected.
Source: From Ref. 51.

Table 4 Anion and Glucose Transport by Middle-aged and Old RBCs from Normal Individuals and RBCs from Individuals with Band 3 Alterations

Cells	Anion		Glucose		
	K_m [b]	V_{max} [c]	K_m	V_{max} [d] efflux	influx
Middle-aged	0.9 ± 0.1	13.2 ± 1.4	8.9 ± 1.2	19.0 ± 2.9	12.8 ± 1.9
High transport weight					
Control	0.6 ± 0.1	11.1 ± 0.6	18.5 ± 2.5	9.2 ± 2.8	13.9 ± 3.4
Proband	0.5 ± 0.1	22.3 ± 1.0+	11.5 ± 2.6*	10.1 ± 0.3*	12.9 ± 1.0
Father	0.7 ± 0.1	15.8 ± 0.8*	7.4 ± 2.0	5.4 ± 2.4*	12.1 ± 2.0
Mother	0.7 ± 0.1	16.8 ± 1.0*	11.1 ± 2.1	5.7 ± 1.9*	12.1 ± 0.7
Sibling 1	0.6 ± 0.1	10.8 ± 0.9	10.4 ± 1.1	16.3 ± 1.9	13.6 ± 2.1
Sibling 2	0.7 ± 0.1	18.8 ± 1.1*	11.5 ± 1.8	6.6 ± 1.6*	10.9 ± 1.9
NEUROLOGICAL					
Control	0.7 ± 0.1	13.5 ± 0.7	ND	16.5 ± 0.6	10.1 ± 0.9
Propositi	0.9 ± 0.1	29.0 ± 1.0*	ND	8.2 ± 0.3	9.8 ± 1.2
Fast Aging					
Control	1.0 ± 0.1	12.4 ± 0.7		8.1 ± 1.1	13.2 ± 1.0
Proband	1.7 ± 0.2*	9.9 ± 1.0*	16.4 ± 0.4*	21.2 ± 0.7*	8.1 ± 1.1*
ABETALIPOPROTEINEMIA					
Proband	1.5 ± 0.2	5.8 ± 0.8*	17.1 ± 1.3*	25.9 ± 2.4*	8.6 ± 2.1

[a]Results are presented as the mean ± 1 SD; +$P \leq 0.001$ compared with control; *$p \leq 0.01$ compared with the control.
[b]K_m, exchange constant; i.e., the sulfate concentration (in millimoles) at which the transport rate is half the maximal value, as determined from a Lineweaver-Burk plot of the ascending branch of the rate curve.
[c]V_{max}, the maximal velocity in moles × $10^{-8}/10^8$ cells/min.
[d]μmol/ml cells/min; efflux, zero-trans-efflux.
Source: From Ref. 51.

was not statistically significant (Table 5) (51). It appears to be an autosomal recessive. This mutation is associated with acanthocyte ("thorny" cell) formation. However, RBC survival is normal in situ as determined by the reticulocyte count, and the RBCs do not exhibit accelerated aging as determined by the RBC aging panel (57).

A second band 3 alteration also exhibits acanthocytosis (17,19). This alteration is associated with ion and glucose transport abnormalities and neurological disease. The neurological disease is an autosomal recessive.

The third alteration of band 3 alteration is characterized by accelerated cellular aging as determined by a RBC aging panel and cellular removal. The propositus' reticulocyte count is approximately ~20%, indicating the destruction and replacement in situ of 20% of circulating erythrocytes daily and there is increased IgG binding to middle-aged cells. Both peripheral blood findings (e.g., the presence of nucleated erythrocytes and precursors of monocytes and lymphocytes) and bone marrow biopsy are consistent with a hemolytic anemia (7). The propositus had a low hematocrit and hemoglobin. The propositus was splenetomized to reduce RBC destruction. We gave this band 3 alteration the descriptive name "fast aging" band 3 because the propositus' young and middle-aged cells exhibit all the characteristics of old erythrocytes (e.g., increased IgG binding, decreased anion and altered glucose transport, and increased breakdown products of band 3 are observed on immunoblots). Aged band 3 antibodies, which do not bind to young or middle-aged cells, bind to a distinct region of a band 3 in immunoblots of membranes of middle-aged red cells and to intact middle-aged red cells as determined by immunoelectronmicroscopy. We suspect that "fast aging" band 3 is more susceptible to proteolysis than is normal band 3.

The data indicate that the band 3 alteration that results from an addition to band 3 does not alter the RBC life span or produce clinical disease. In contrast, band 3 alterations that are associated with band 3 aging and/or degradation are characterized by a shortened RBC life span and clinical diseases. We suspect that these latter alteration result from deletions or substitution in the band 3 gene.

The three band 3 mutations/alterations provide support for the hypothesis that the membrane-spanning domain of the anion transporter and glucose transporter(s) is functionally and structurally related. For example, high molecular weight band 3–containing cells exhibit changes in band 3 structure and function that are probably caused by a redundant segment in the anion transport region. Changes in other membrane proteins or lipids are not detected. The other parameter that is altered is V_{max} of glucose efflux. External modifications of band 3, probably at its cytoplasmic domain, that occur in G6PD-deficient cells or in cells containing unstable hemoglobin Köln have no effect on anion transport and do not affect glucose transport. At the present time, we cannot reconcile the sequence data of the available glucose transport proteins

Table 5 Binding of Cytochalasin B to High Transport Band 3 Texas Containing RBCs

Cell type	High affinity		Low affinity	
	B_{max}	Kd	B_{max}	Kd
Control	2.0 jj 0.2	0.22 jj 0.04	10.4 jj 0.6	5.4 jj 0.9
High transport band 3 Texas	2.5 jj 0.3	0.32 jj 0.07	9.1 jj 0.9	3.7 jj 0.9

B_{max}, maximal number of binding sites in $\mu M/1013$ cells; kd, dissociation constant in micromoles.
Source: From Ref. 51.

with the genetic, functional, cell biology, and immunological data that indicate a relationship between band 3 and glucose transport.

The results of the studies on aging in vivo indicate that IgG binding and anion transport are the two most sensitive screening assays for determining cellular age.

A band 3 mutation/alteration in Southeast Asian ovalocytosis has recently been reported (58). A deletion of band 3 amino acids 400–408 and a substitution of Glu-56 for Lys-56 was found in this alteration associated with rigid erythrocytes associated with resistance to invasion by several strains of malaria in vitro (58). Apparently, the Glu-56 for Lys-56 substitution is found in normal individuals and thus is a polymorphism. The ovaloytic individuals are reported to have reduced numbers of intracellular parasites in vivo (58). Because residues 400–408 are in the cytoplasmic segment of band 3, it would be interesting to know the mechanism by which a change in the cytoplasmic segment would interfere with invasion by a parasite at the cell surface.

VII. MOLECULAR BIOLOGY OF SENESCENT CELL ANTIGEN AND BAND 3

A. Aging Antigenic Site

We used synthetic peptides to identify antigenic sites recognized by the IgG that binds to old cells (18,20,21,59,60). Results indicate that crucial anion transport segments of the band 3 molecule carry the aging determinants and suggest that these may be the aging sites of the molecule. The purpose of this proposal is to further define and localize the antigenic sites in senescent cell antigen and the aging site(s) of the band 3 molecule.

We concluded from previous studies that senescent cell antigen is a degradation product of band 3 that includes most of the approximately 35,000-d carboxyl terminal segment and the approximately 17,000-d anion transport region (5). Both immunoblotting studies with IgG isolated from senescent cells and peptide mapping studies of senescent cell antigen indicated that senescent cell antigen lacks an approximately 40,000 molecular weight cytoplasmic segment that contains the amino-terminus and, possibly, additional peptides of band 3 (5–7). Peptide mapping studies and anion transport studies suggested that a cleavage of band 3 occurs in the anion transport region (5). Furthermore, breakdown products of band 3 are observed in the oldest cell fractions but not in young or middle-aged cell fractions, and anion transport in impaired in old cells (5–7).

Based on structural, biochemical, and immunological data (1–7), we deduced that cleavage of old band 3 occurred approximately a third of the way into the transmembrane anion transport region from the carboxyl-terminus end. Therefore, we synthesized peptides of RBC band 3 from the anion transport domain of the molecule. We "walked" the anion transport segment (18,20,21,59,60). By "walking" we mean the antigenic analysis of a series of synthetic overlapping peptides that encompass the entire polypeptide chain of the anion transport domain. The synthetic peptides are of uniform size and overlap their adjacent neighboring peptides by a predetermined number of residues in the overlap regions in order to optimize the feasibility of synthesis and to expect reasonable resolution of individual antigenic sites.

These studies focused on the 511 amino acid anion transport domain. Our results indicate that this domain carries both the SCA antigenic determinants (5–7,10–12,15,16,18) and the aging vulnerable site (5–7), whereas the 40,000-d cytoplasmic segment does not. Therefore, we focused on segments within the transport domain that are most likely to be hydrophilic and, therefore, exposed based on hydrophobicity/hydrophilicity scales, amino acid composition, and location along the molecule based on our model described by Kay et al. (20). We synthesized peptides that corresponded to external regions predicted by our model. The peptides with residue number are CYTO, 129–144: AGVANQLLDRFIFEDQ; 426–440, LLGEKTRNQMGVSEL; 515–531, FISRYTQEIFSFLISLI; 526–541, FLISLIFIYETFSKLI; 538–554, SKLIKIFQDHP-LQKTYN; 549–566, LQKTYNYNVLMVPKPQGP; 561–578, PKPQGPLPNTALLSLVLM;

573–591, LSLVLMAGTFFFAMMLRKF; ANION 2, 588–602, LRKFKNSSYFPGKLR; 597–614, FPGKLRRVIGDFGVPISI; 609–626, GVPISILIMVLVDFFIQD; 620–637, VDFFIQDTY-TQKLSVPD; GLYCOS, 630–648, QKLSVPDGFKVSNSSARGW; 645–659, ARGWVIHP-LGLRSEF; 684–704, ITTLIVSKPERKMVKGSGFHL; 752–769, IQEVKEQRISGLLVAVL; 776–793, MEPILSRIPLAVLFGIFL; 788–805, FGIFLYMGVTSLSGIQUL; 800–818, LSGI-QLFDRILLLFKPPKY; 813–818, FKPPKY; COOH, 812–827, LFKPPKYHPDVPYVKR; 812–830, LFKPPKYHPDVPYVKRVKT; 818–827, YHPDVPYVKR; 822–839, VPYVKRVK-TWRMHLFTGI; 869–879 + 881 + 883, LRRVLLPLIFRVL (the actual sequence in band 3 is LRRVLLPLIFRNVEL, but the N and E were not included in the peptide used for thes studies); 877–903, DADDAKATFDEEEGRDE; 902–910, DEYDEVAMP. As a control, we used a peptide from the cytoplasmic segment of band 3 within the region of the putative ankyrin binding site (61) (CYTO, 139–159). Peptides were synthesized based on the sequence data from the article by Tanner et al. (61). Peptides were analyzed by amino acid analysis and sequencing to determine purity.

The specific physiological autoantibody to the senescent cell antigen, senescent cell IgG (SCIgG), was isolated from old human RBCs, as described previously, using affinity chromatography (2,4). Immunoglobulin G eluted from senescent cells, rather than serum IgG, was used because normal serum contains antibodies to, e.g., spectrin and actin, 2.1 (8,9,11). Competitive inhibition studies were performed using synthetic peptides to absorb the IgG isolated from senescent RBCs. This is the same IgG that initiates phagocytosis in situ. The Fc portion of IgG is required for binding and phagocytosis of cells by macrophages (1,4,7). Fab fragments were not used because we were simulating the physiological situation. Intact dimeric, senescent cell IgG containing the Fc portion binds to senescent cell in situ and initiates their removal (1–7). Only IgG isolated from aged RBCs binds specifically to senescent cells. For example, IgG eluted from young control RBCs did not bind to senescent cells (2). Moreover, the specific binding capacity of the autoantibody was eliminated by absorption with purified senescent cell antigen (7). SCIgG (3 μg) is absorbed with synthetic peptides at the concentrations indicated or purified SCA, as a control, for 60 min at room temperature, and incubated with stored RBCs for 60 min at room temperature (1,2,4,7,15,16,20,21). Immunoglobulin G binding and inhibition were determined with a protein A binding assay. This biological assay measures the fate of RBCs in vitro and in vivo (1,3,62). Storage mimics normal aging in situ immunologically and biochemically (1–13,57). After incubation with absorbed IgG, cells are washed four times with 40–50 volumes of phosphate-buffered saline (PBS) containing 0.2% bovine serum albumin (BSA, fraction V, Sigma, St. Louis, MO) and 0.5% glucose. Washed cells are transferred to BSA-coated tubes (5×10^7 cells/50 μL) and incubated for 30 min at 37°C with ^{125}I-protein A (Amersham, Arlington Heights, IL, 30–38 mCi/mg, 10–15 ng/tube). Cells are then washed four times and transferred to new tubes before counting in a gamma scintillation counter (Beckman, Gamma 5,500). The number of RBC-bound IgG molecules is quantitated before and after absorption using equilibrium binding kinetics (7,31). Scatchard analysis is performed. Percent inhibition is calculated from the following formula: $100\{1^-(x^-b/\Gamma b]$, where x = molecules of IgG autoantibody bound per cell; T = total number of IgG antibody molecules bound in the absence of inhibitor; b = background protein A binding.

Results of these "walking" studies indicate that senescent cell IgG recognizes antigenic determinants that lie within the anion transport region 538–554 and putative transport site containing a cluster of lysines toward the carboxyl-terminus, 812–827 (Fig 1) (18–21,59,60). More recent studies indicate that that residues 812–830 are more potent inhibitors of SCIgG binding than 812–827 (inhibition: 812–830, 45 ± 6 ($P \leq 0.001$); 812–827, 32 ± 5 ($P \leq 0.01$). The peptide "CYTO" from the cytoplasmic domain does not inhibit. Immunoblotting studies demonstrate binding of senescent cell IgG to peptides ANION 1 and COOH but not to CYTO, the peptide from the cytoplasmic segment of band 3 containing the putative ankyrin binding site (61).

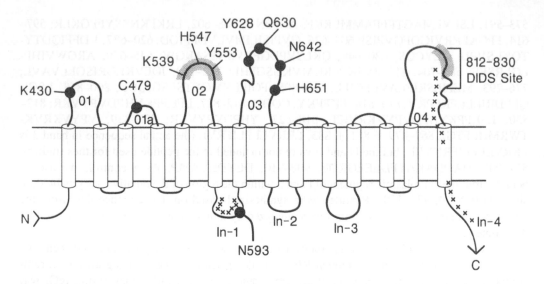

Figure 1 Model of membrane associated and external regions of anion transport protein band 3, approximate residues (R) 400–900 showing aging antigenic sites (///), anion transport sites (xxx), and DIDS binding site. K, lysine; C, cysteine; H, histidine; Y, tyrosine; N, asparagine; the number following a letter indicates residue number; In, inside the cell; O, outside of the cell; arrow C, carboxyl-terminus; arrow N, amino-terminus. The model was based upon application of the program PEPPLOT of the GCG package to identify membrane spanning nonpolar helices and intervening hydrophilic loops. The location of the hydrophilic loops as extracellular or intracellular was predicted on the basis of established chemical or biological markers, e.g., the demonstration that residues 814–829 contain a DIDS binding site accessible from the outside or external radioiodination of the tyrosine (Y) at position 553. Key residues are identified to facilitate their identification within the sequence. This is a two-dimensional representation that does not reflect three-dimensional associations of residues that are separated by long stretches of sequence. Results show, however, that close steric association must be maintained by external loops 02 and 04 and In-1 and In-4. The hydrophobicity plots indicate multiple turns/bends in the band 3 molecule in the region of the DIDS biding site. This is consistent with this site being in a pore. (From Ref. 63.)

These are the first studies using synthetic peptides to address mechanisms of aging. Results of our studies, to date, indicate that (1) an anion transport region of band 3 that appears to be extracellular carries active antigenic determinants of an aging antigen; (2) this transport site is located toward the carboxyl-terminal and overlaps or contains a stilbene disulfonate binding site; (3) a putative ankyrin binding region peptide is not involved in senescent cell antigen activity; and (4) synthetic peptides alone, without carbohydrate attached, abolish binding of senescent cell IgG to RBCs. Therefore, carbohydrate moieties are not required for the antigenicity or recognition of senescent cell antigen.

B. Active Aging Antigenic Amimo Acids

In order to define the aging antigenic site along the band 3 molecule and to determine the active antigenic residues, we tried substituting a neutral or positively charged amino acid for the positively charged lysine in pep-COOH peptide (LFKPPKYHPDVPYVKR) during synthesis. Sustitution of either neutral glycines (pep-COOH-G: LFGPPGYHPDVPYVGR) or positively charged arginines (pep-COOH-R: FRPPRYHPDVPYVRR) for lysine in pep-COOH reduced but did not abolish its activity in the competitive inhibition assay with senescent cell IgG (21). This suggests that (1) charge alone is not the critical determinant of antigenicity and (2) lysines contribute to the antigenicity of the aging antigen. Because we changed all three of the lysines in the synthetic peptide pep-COOH, we cannot determine at this time whether all lysines are critical or whether antigenicity depends on a specific lysine.

We have used synthetic peptides to locate a crucial aging antigen on band 3 and to create a synthetic senescent cell antigen. Results indicate that pep-ANION 1 (residues 538–554) and pep-COOH residues (812–827) may be the aging antigenic sites of the band 3 molecule and that lysine(s) is required for antigenicity. Generation of senescent cell antigen initiates IgG binding and removal of cells in situ. These results are consistent with the physiological data demonstrating that old erythrocytes have impaired anion transport (6,7,12,18,57) and the biochemical and immunological data indicating that band 3 undergoes degradation with loss of a cytoplasmic segment during the aging process (4–14,57).

C. Mapping of Aging Antigenic Sites in Relation to Anion Transport and Anion Transport Inhibitor Binding Site(s)

We have shown that senescent cell antigen contains pep-ANION 1 and pep-COOH (18–21). We suspected that senescent cell antigen is related to the anion transport site because peptide mapping studies and anion transport studies suggested that a cleavage of band 3 occurs in the anion transport region (5). Furthermore, breakdown products of band 3 are observed in the oldest cell fractions but not in young or middle-aged cell fractions (5,7). Fragments of the cytoplasmic segment of band 3 are detected with antipeptide antibodies in the cytoplasm of old RBCs and of RBCs with a band 3 alteration associated with accelerated aging (5,18). Anion transport is impaired in old cells (6,7,12,17,57) and band 3 mutations/alterations with damage to the transmembrane transport region result in accelerated aging and increased IgG binding (7). To clarify the relationship between senescent cell antigen and anion transport, we mapped the anion binding/transport properties of segments of band 3 using equimolar amounts of synthetic peptide and sulfate in a competitive inhibition assay (Figs. 2 and 3). Studies showed

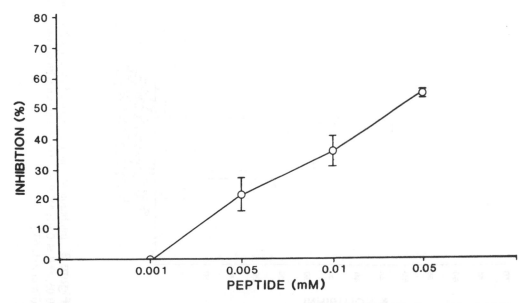

Figure 2 Inhibition of anion transport by varying concentrations of pep-COOH. Competitive inhibition studies were performed with pep-COOH as described in the text at the concentrations indicated on the graph. Influx buffer is 300 mM sucrose, 10 mM Tris-HEPES, pH 7.0. Sulfate concentration is 0.01 mM. (From Ref. 63.)

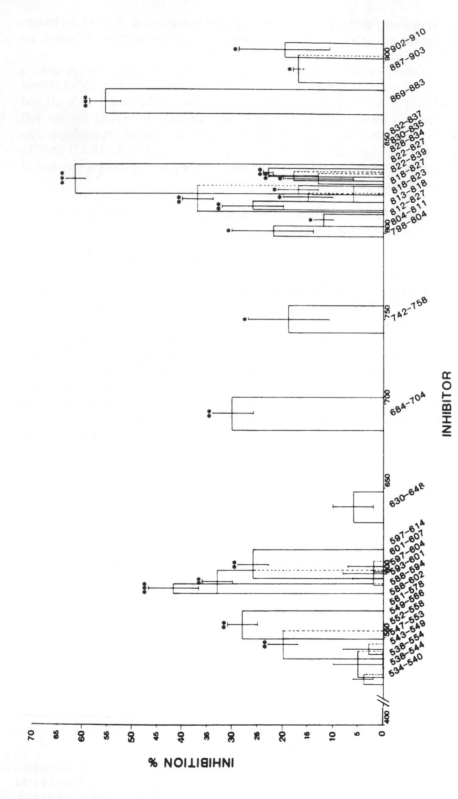

Figure 3 Inhibition of anion transported by band 3 synthetic peptides. Equimolar amounts of sulfate and band 3 peptides were used. *$P \leq$ 0.05; **$P \leq 0.01$; ***$P \leq 0.001$ compared with control without peptide. See Table 6 for amino acid sequences corresponding to residue number. (From Ref. 63.)

that the peptide was competing for the sulfate because increased amounts of sulfate overcame the inhibition (Hughes J, Haussler T, and Kay MMB, unpublished data).

1. Anion Binding/Transport Site

Peptides were tested in an anion transport inhibition assay to determine which ones are involved in anion binding/transport (63). Peptides inhibited transport in a dose-dependent manner (63). Peptide residues 588–594 (a seven amino acid peptide), 822–839, and 869–883 were the most active inhibitors of anion transport ($P \leq 0.001$ compared to control without peptide) (Fig. 3) (Table 6). The inhibitory activity of the last peptide, 869–883, could not be confirmed by testing adjacent peptides to the amino side because these regions are extremely hydrophobic. However, six to seven amino acid peptides from this region produced inhibition of transport (63) but to a lesser degree than 869–883. The component residues are probably additive. Peptide 869–879 + 881 + 883 seem to have special anion binding/transport properties, although both it and 869–883 produced significant inhibition ($P \leq 0.001$).

We performed synergy experiments with inhibitory peptides. Synergy was not observed inhibition: pep-COOH, 24 ± 5%, 822–827, 41 ± 7%; 869–879 + 881 + 883, 69 ± 3%; mixture of all three peptides, 41 ± 7%; or 588–594, 25 ± 4%; 822–839, 33 ± 5; 869–879 + 881 + 883, 70 ± 2; 597–614, 30 ± 6; mixture of all four peptides, 54 ± 3).

Anion transport has been attributed to residues 538–554 or, more recently, to a carboxyl segment of band 3, including pep-COOH, by investigators based on indirect evidence (64–66). Residues 538–554 include two important amino acids. The lysine at 538 (558 in the mouse) is a covalent binding site for the anion transport inhibitor, 4,4′-di-isothioayanato-stilbene-2,2′disulphonic acid (DIDS) (61) and the tyrosine at residue 553 is radioiodinated by extracellular lactoperoxidase (61). However, our present results indicate that the residues 538–554 are not anion binding, although segments carboxyl to them are. This agrees with the results of studies using mouse band 3 expressed in *Xenopus laevis* oocytes indicating that lysine 558 in the mouse sequence (539 on peptide 538–554 in the human sequence) is not involved in anion transport based on site-directed mutagenesis (67,68). These are two other lysines on peptide 538–554. Since the peptide does not inhibit anion transport, the other two lysines on peptide 538–554 at positions 542 and 551 do not function as anion binding sites. Because peptide 538–554 does not inhibit anion transport even though it has 3 lysines, anion transport binding must involve more than a mere positive charge. The configuration of the peptide is probably important. Results of the amino acid substitution studies support this interpretation.

2. Modification of Anion Transport/Binding Segments to Identify Active Amino Acids

Lysine has been implicated as an amino acid involved in anion transport based on DIDS inhibition studies (66). We decided to test this hypothesis by substituting a neutral or positively charged amino acid for the positively charged lysine or arginine in pep-COOH peptide. pep-COOH peptide was selected because (1) it is a highly conserved region of band 3 (18), (2) it is a crucial sequence in senescent cell antigen, and (3) it is an anion transport/binding peptide. Substitution of either neutral glycines (pep-COOH-G/K) or positively charged arginines (pep-COOH-R/K) for lysine in pep-COOH still resulted in significant inhibition, but the inhibition was significantly reduced compared with that of pep-COOH (Table 7). Because we changed all three of the lysines in the synthetic peptide pep-COOH, we can not determine at this time whether all lysines are critical or whether antigenicity depends on a specific lysine.

We then synthesized pep-COOH–related peptides in which glycines were substituted for arginines (pep-COOH G/R) and glycines were substituted for arginines and lysines (pep-COOH G/KR). Significant inhibition occurred with both altered peptides (Table 7), but only pep-COOH G/KR was significantly different than pep-COOH. No significant difference was observed between pep-COOH G/R and pep-COOH. Because all of the substituted peptides caused

Table 6 Inhibition of Anion Transport by Synthetic Peptides of Band 3 Protein[a]

Synthetic Peptide		Inhibition (%) of anion transport
residue	sequence	
426–440	LLGEKTRNQMGVSEL	20 ± 4**
534–540	YETFSKL	4 ± 2
538–544	SKLIKIF	0
538–554	SKLIKIFQDHPLQKTYN	5 ± 5
543–549	IFQDHPL	0
547–553	PLQKTY	0
552–558	TYNYNVL	3 ± 5
549–566	LQKTYNYNVLMVPKPQGP	20 ± 3**
561–578	PKPQGPLPNTALLSLVLM	28 ± 3**
588–602	LRKFKNSSYFPGKLR	33 ± 3**
588–594	LRKFKNS	42 ± 5***
593–601	NSSYFPGKL	2 ± 4
597–604	FPGKLRRV	2 ± 6
601–607	LRRVIGD	0
597–614	FPGKLRRVIGDFGVPISI	26 ± 3**
742–758	GKASTPGAAAQIQEVKE	19 ± 8**
798–804	TSLSGIQ	22 ± 8*
804–811	QLFDRILL	12 ± 2**
812–827	LFKPPKYHPDVPYVKR	37 ± 3**
813–818	FKPPKY	26 ± 6**
818–823	YHPDVP	15 ± 5*
818–827	YHPDVPYVKR	6 ± 5
822–827	VPYVKR	17 ± 4*
822–839	VPYVKRVKTWRMHLFTGI	61 ± 2***
827–835	RVKTWRMH	12 ± 4*
828–834	VKTWRMH	13 ± 7*
830–835	TWRMHL	18 ± 5**
865–870	LTVPLR	4 ± 4
869–875	LRRVLLP	11 ± 2**
875–881	PLIFRNV	11 ± 2**
879–884	RNVELQ	2 ± 3
869–883	LRRVLLPLIFRNVEL	33 ± 2***
869–879+881+883	LRRVLLPLIFRVL	77 ± 5***[b]
887–903	DADDAKATFDEEEGRDE	17 ± 1*
902–910	DEYDEVAMP	20 ± 9*

[a]Data are presented as the percentage inhibition of anion transport at 5 min ± S D. *$P \leq 0.05$, **$P \leq 0.01$, ***$P \leq 0.001$. We competed the peptides with sulfate to abolish transport. The sulfate concentration was 0.01 mM. Radioactive sulfate (0.018 μM) is added. The total peptide concentration used per sample was 0.01 mM. The position of these peptides and the inhibition they induce is graphed in Figure 2 so that anion binding sites can be more easily visualized.

[b]The N at residue 880 and   at residue 882 were omitted. They are not involved in binding because residues 879–884 containing these amino acids do not inhibit binding. Peptide 869–879+881+883 produced slight hemolysis of RBCs for unknown reasons. The degree of inhibition of transport might be responsible.

Source: From Ref. 63.

Table 7 Inhibition of Human RBC Anion Transport by Altered and Chicken pep-COOH Synthetic Peptides of Band 3 Protein[a]

Synthetic peptide		Inhibition (%) of	
residue	sequence	anion transport	
HUMAN 538–554	SKLIKIFQDHPLQKTYN	0	
CHICKEN 538–554	AKLVTILQAHPLQQSYD	0	
HUMAN pep-COOH	LFKPPKYHPKVPYVKR	31 jj 3***	
CHICKEN pep-COOH	LLMPPKYHPKEPYVTR	23 jj 2***	(*)
HUMAN pep-COOH-N6	FKPPKY	31 jj 5***	
CHICKEN-pep-COOH-N6	LMPPKY	30 jj 6***	[NS]
HUMAN pep-COOH-G/K	LFGPPGYHPDVPYVGR	17 jj 5**	(***)
HUMAN pep-COOH-R/K	LFRPPRYHPDVPYVRR	18 jj 8**	(*)
HUMAN pep-COOH-G/R	LFKPPKYHPDVPYVKG	27 jj 6**	(NS)
HUMAN pep-COOH-G/KR	LFGPPGYHPDVPYVGG	22 jj 6**	(*)

[a]Data are presented as the percentage inhibition $\pm$SD of anion influx by human erythrocytes. *$P \leq 0.05$; **$P \leq 0.01$; ***$P \leq 0.001$; NS, not significant compared with transport control without peptide if asterisk (*) is outside of parentheses; compared with human pep-COOH if asterisk (*) is within parenthesis; compared to human pep-pep-COOH-N6 if asterisk (*) is within brackets. P values calculated based on actual quantity of sulfate transported. From reference 63.
Source: From Ref. 63.

inhibition, it seems that the presence of lysine or arginine is not an absolute requirement for anion binding. Furthermore, it appears that another amino acid, perhaps glycine, can participate in anion binding.

Because the amino acid sequence of human and chicken pep-COOH and pep-COOH-N6 differs in several key amino acids, we synthesized peptides from the chicken sequence. Chicken pep-COOH has an M instead of K at a position corresponding to residue 814 of the human sequence, a K and E instead of a D and V at residue 821 and 822, and a T instead of K at residue 826. For example, substitution of a methionine (M) for a lysine (K) is significant because the former is nonpolar and the latter is a positively charged amino acid. Likewise, substitution of a negatively charged glutamic acid (E) for a nonpolar valine (V) or a positively charged lysine for a negatively charged aspartic acid (D) would be expected to alter tertiary configuration and binding properties. Thus, nature has performed "site-specific" mutagenesis for us.

Chicken pep-COOH inhibited anion transport, but the inhibition was significantly less than that of human pep-COOH ($P \leq 0.05$). Because chicken pep-COOH-N6 inhibited to the same degree as human pep-COOH-N6, the lysine at position 814 in the human sequence for which methionine is substituted in the chicken sequence is probably not critical for anion transport. This suggests that the change to a K and E instead of a D and V may be a significant change. A glutamic acid is implicated in transport (66,69). Neither human nor chicken pep-ANION 1, residues 538–554, inhibited transport.

Some investigators have suggested that lysines are not themselves part of the transport mechanism but are close to the transport site and that arginine is involved in anion transport (70,71). Residues 869–883 and 869–879 + 881 + 883, among the most potent inhibitors of anion transport, have arginines but no lysines. Other highly inhibitory peptides, residues 588–594 and 822–839, have lysines and arginines. Of the inhibitory peptides with $P \leq 0.01$, residues 804–811 and 830–835 have arginines and no lysines, and residues 549–566, 561–578, and 813–818 have lysines and no arginines. The substitution studies show that altered pep-COOH with glycines substituted for both lysine and arginine still inhibits anion transport, although the percent inhibition is reduced. Histidine and glutamine have also been implicated in anion transport (66). The peptide sequence recognized by stilbene disulphonate (SITS) anti-idiotypic antibodies overlaps a potent anion binding/transport peptide, 822–839, which is consistent with data indicating inhibition of transport by stilbene disulfonates. This site could also be adjacent to the other two potent inhibitory peptides in three-dimensional structure.

pep-COOH, a peptide from the carboxyl-terminus region, contains both hydrophobic and hydrophylic regions. The lysines found in this region comprise another binding site for the stilbene disulfonates based on data presented here and that of Jennings et al. (64). Our data suggest that this region has anion binding/transport capability as well. Residues 812–827 (pep-COOH) and 813–818 (N6, the six amino acids on the amino side of pep-COOH) are inhibitors of anion transport. Pep-COOH (residues 812–827) is part of senescent cell antigen (18,20,21,59,60). N6 is both an inhibitor of anion transport and of senescent cell IgG binding (IgG binding inhibition: 48 ± 1% at 10 μg) (19,54,58) even though it is only six amino acids long. However, COOH-N6 does contain a proline-proline bend tha may contribute to an anion pocket. It probably forms a loop in the membrane. These experiments suggest that at least part of a transport site is located on the same region of band 3 that generates senescent cell antigen.

3. Localization of SITS Binding Site on Band 3 Membrane Protein

Anti-idiotype antibodies recognize the receptor of the ligand against which the idiotype is prepared (63,72). This has provided an elegant method for preparing antibodies against membrane proteins without purifying them and for localizing active ligand binding sites on membrane receptors and proteins (63,72).

SITS is an inhibitor of anion transport. Anti-idiotypic antibodies to SITS react with band 3 and its breakdown products in erythrocyte membranes (58) and with band 3 peptide residues 788–805, 800–818, and strongest with 812–830 (Fig. 4A B) (58). Residues 812–827, three amino acids smaller that the peptide giving the strongest reaction, reacted as well as the other two peptides, 788–805 and 800–818, but weaker that 812–830. Anti-idiotypic antibodies did not react with residues 813–818, which are to the amino end of the peptide that reacts the strongest. In contrast, the antibodies reacted with peptide 818–827, which is toward the carboxyl end of the peptide giving the strongest reaction. This is consistent with the band 3 model that we have presented predicting that these residues are on external loop 04 (6,7). Reaction of anti-idiotypic antibodies with breakdown products of band 3 suggests that these breakdown products carry transport sites. This would indicate that these segments are not derived from the cytoplasmic segment of band 3.

In summary, our data indicate that residues 812–830 contain both a SITS binding site and an anion binding/transport site. Because the anti-idiotypic antibody does not react with residues 813–818, gives a weak reaction with residues 812–827, and a strong reaction with residues 812–830 and reacts weakly with 818–827, a crucial epitope probbly resides in the region of 828–830. Band 3 residues 788–805 and 800–818 may also be part of a SITS binding site. Data from chicken pep-COOH-N6 suggest that lysine 814 is not critical for anion transport. Data of Jennings et al. (64,73,75) indicate that one end of the dihydro derivative of DIDS, H_2DIDS, reacts covalently with a lysine that is between 70 and 168 residues from the C-terminus of band 3. This would be between residues 772 and 840 in the human sequence. Our data localizing the distilbene disulfonate binding site are consistent with this.

Results of this study, summarized in Figure 1, indicate that (1) regions with residues 588–594, 822–839, and 869–883 being the most active transport regions ($P \leq 0.001$); (2) residues 812–830 and, possibly, 788–805 and 800–818 are part of the stilbene disulfonate binding site; (3) residues 538–554, which have been reported to be a transport segment of band 3, do not bind anions; and (d) lysines themselves contribute to but are not required for anion binding and, thus, anion transport.

Results of these studies with synthetic peptides are consistent with the physiological data

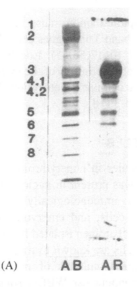

(A)   AB   AR

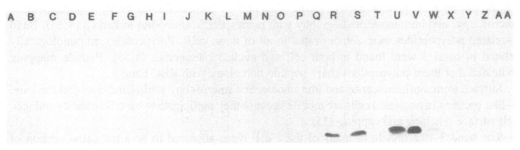

(B)

Figure 4 *A*, Antiidiotypic antibodies to SITS bind to band 3 and band 3 degradation products in RBC membranes. AB, amino black stain for proteins; AR, autoradiograph. (From Ref. 63.) *B*, "Walking" the band 3 molecule to localize the SITS binding site using anti-idiotypic antibody reactivity with synthetic peptides as determined by immunoblotting. Autoradiograph of immunoblot incubated with anti-idiotypic antibodies. Peptides were run on gradient gels with polyacrylamide concentrations of 12–26%. The peptides with residue number are (A) pep-CYTO, 129–144: AGVANQLLDRFIFEDQ; (B) 426–440, LLGEK-TRNQMGVSEL; (C) 515–531, FISRYTQEIFSFLISLI; (D) 526–541, FLISLIFIYETFSKLI; (E) 538–554, SKLIKIFQDHPLQKTYN; (F) 549–566, LQKTYNYNVLMVPKPQGP; (G) 561–578, PKPQGPLPNTAL-LSLVLM; (H) 573–591, LSLVLMAGTFFFAMMLRKF;(I) pep-ANION 2, 588–602, LRKFK-NSSYFPGKLR;(J) 597–614, FPGKLRRVIGDFGVPISI; (K) 609–626, GVPISILIMVLVDFFIQD; (L) 620–637, VDFFIQDTYTQKLSVPD; (M) pep-GLYCOS, 630–648, QKLSVPDGFKVSNSSARGW; (N) 645–659, ARGWVIHPLGRSEF; (O) 684–704, ITTLIVSKPERKMVKGSGFHL; (P) 752–769, IQEVKE-QRISGLLVAVL; (Q) 776–793, MEPILSRIPLAVLFGIFL; (R) 788–805, FGIFLYMGVTSLSGIQL; (S) 800–818, LSGIQLFDRILLLFKPPKY; (T) 813–818, FKPPKY; (U) pep-COOH, 812–827, LFKPPK-YHPDVPYVKR; (V) 812–830, LFKPPKYHPDVPYVKRVKT; (W) 818–827, YHPDVPYVKR; (X) 822–839, VPYVKRVKTWRMHLFTGI; (Y) 869–879 + 881 + 883, LRRVLLPLIFRVL (the actual sequence in band 3 is: LRRVLLPLIFRNVEL, but the N and E were not included in the peptide used for these studies); (Z) 887–903, DADDAKATFDEEEGRDE; (AA) 902–910, DEYDEVAMP. (From Ref. 63.)

demonstrating that old RBCs have impaired anion transport (6,7,34–37) and the biochemical and immunological data indicating that band 3 undergoes degradation with loss of a cytoplasmic segment during the aging process (4–7,10–12,56,57). Localization of the active site of SCA will facilitate the next logical step; namely, definition of the molecular changes occurring during aging that initiate molecular as well as cellular degeneration. Peptides ANION 1 and COOH are in highly conserved regions of band 3 (18).

VIII. BAND 3 IN NUCLEATED CELLS

The presence of band 3–related molecules in nonerythroid tissues was first demonstrated in 1983 (35). We suspected that band 3 was present in nucleated somatic cells as well as RBCs because senescent cell antigen, which is immunologically related to band 3 (8–10), is present on lymphocytes, platelets, adult liver cells, and embryonic kidney cells (4). Furthermore, antibodies prepared against senescent cell antigen isolated from white blood cells (WBCs) react with RBC band 3 (26,33); and other cells are known to transport anions.

As a test of this hypothesis, primary cultures of mouse neuroblastoma cells, human fibroblasts, lung cells, neutrophils, mononuclear WBCs, squamous epithelial (mouth) cells, lung squamous epithelial carcinoma, rhabdomyosarcoma, and rat hepatocytes were examined for the presence of immunoreactive forms of band 3 by immunofluorescence, immunoelectron microscopy, and immunoautoradiography with monospecific antibodies to band 3 (8,35). Band 3–related polypeptides were demonstrated in all of these cells. Polypeptides immunologically related to band 3 were found in both cell and nuclear membranes (8,35). Peptide mapping indicated that these polypeptides share peptide homology with RBC band 3.

Surface immunofluorescence and immunoelectron microscopy studies indicate that the band 3–like proteins in nucleated cells are mobile because they participate in band 3 antibody-induced cell surface patching and capping (35).

The band 3–like protein in many of these cell types appeared to be a truncated version of the erythroid protein based on its molecular weight of approximately 60,000 estimated from its migration in polyacrylamide gels. We suggested that part of the cytoplasmic amino-terminus segment was missing from the band 3–like protein in these cell types and that band 3 protein was modified to perform functions in different environments (35). Since then band 3 has been described in numerous cell types and tissues, including fibroblasts, hepatoma cells, and lymphoid cells (15,16,36,38–50).

Electron paramagnetic resonance spectroscopy (EPR) of cells incubated with spin-labeled (SL) SITS indicated that membranes of nucleated cells have an anion transporter that is accessible from the outside and behaves similar to RBC band 3 (Dalton L and Kay MMB, unpublished). Thus, polypeptides related to RBC senescent cell antigen (4,8–10) and RBC band 3 (35) have been demonstrated in nucleated cells, including brain (15,16,36,38–50).

A polyclonal antibody against the segment of band 3 containing senescent cell antigen was used to determine whether senescent cell antigen was altered by differentiation. In order to assess the amount of band 3 protein on living mitotic and differentiated cells, immunofluorescence was measured on a single-cell basis by flow cytometry. Differentiated N_{2AB-1} cells were shown to have more senescent cell antigen/band 3 protein on the cell surface on an individual cell basis (36). Because these cells do not change in size following differentiation, increased surface band 3 protein must be due to a change in density of this protein. These results were confirmed using immunoelectron microscopy. Preliminary studies on anion (sulfate) transport indicated that it increased following differentiation of N2AB-1 cells.

Examination of frozen brain sections from 10-year-old and 96-year-old individuals revealed labeling of fibrilary structures and processes with senescent cell antigen–band 3 antibodies in sections from old but not young brains (36).

Preliminary studies performed with Dr. R. T. of University of California, San Diego, show selective binding of band 3 antibodies to human cerebellum and cerebral cortex. Controls that consisted of preimmune serum incubated with brain tissue, liver, and myocardium were negative. In normal brains from elderly individuals, band 3 antibodies react with cortex neurons in layers III and IV, Purkinje cells and their dendrites extending into the molecular layer, and cerebellar dentate nucleus neurons. Aged band 3 (presenescent cell antigen) antibodies reacted with astrocytes in the white matter, a "mossy fiber" distribution in the cerebellum, and select Purkinje cells. Dentate neurons were strongly reactive, especially those containing lipofuscin, but the staining did not resemble that of lipofuscin. There was a moderately strong reaction with many, but not all, large neurons in the cerebrum. Aged band 3 antibodies recognize old band 3 before senescent cell antigen is formed. They bind to band 3 in old but not young middle-aged RBCs (7,17,19).

In brains from patients with Alzheimer's disease, aged band 3 antibodies labeled the amyloid core of classic plaques and the microglial cells located in the middle of the plaque. Adjacent neurons displayed a stronger and more widespread reaction than normals. In contrast, band 3 antibodies labeled the neuritic components of plaques, with some reaction noted in microglial cells, adjacent astrocytes, and neurons.

The anion exchange, band 3–related protein(s) in mammalian brain performs the same functions as that of erythroid band 3 (15,16). These functions are anion transport, ankyrin binding, and generation of senescent cell antigen. Structural similarity of brain and erythroid band 3 is suggested by the reaction of antibodies to synthetic peptides of erythroid band 3 with brain band 3, the inhibition of anion transport by the same inhibitors, and an equal degree of inhibition of brain and erythrocyet anion transport by synthetic peptides of erythroid band 3. One of these segments, COOH, contains antigenic determinants of SCA. These findings suggest that the transport domain of erythroid and neural band 3 is similar functionally and structurally and support the hypothesis that the immunological mechanism of maintaining homeostasis is a general physiological process for removing senescent and damaged cells in mammals and other vertebrates.

In summary, band 3 and senescent cell antigen are present in the central nervous system, and differences have been described in band 3 between young and aging brain tissue (15,16,36). This suggests that band 3 and senescent cell antigen may play a role in neurological health and disease.

ACKNOWLEDGMENTS

This work was supported by a Veterans Administration Merit Review, the International Foundation for Biomedical Aging Research, NIH grants AG08444, AG08574, and the Arizona Disease Control Commission.

REFERENCES

1. Kay MMB. Mechanism of removal of senescent cells by human macrophages *in situ*. Proc Natl Acad Sci 1975; 72:3521.
2. Kay MMB. Role of physiologic autoantibody in the removal of senescent human red cells. J Supramol Struct 1978; 9:555.
3. Bennett GD, Kay MMB. Homeostatic removal of senescent murine erythrocytes by splenic macrophages. Exp Hematol 1981; 9:297.
4. Kay MMB. Isolation of the phagocytosis inducing IgG-binding antigen on senescent somatic cells. Nature 1981; 289:491.
5. Kay MMB. Localization of senescent cell antigen on band 3. Proc Natl Acad Sci USA 1984; 81:5753.

6.   Kay MMB, Bosman GJCGM, Shapiro SS, et al. Oxidation as a possible mechanism of cellular aging: Vitamin E deficiency causes premature aging and IgG binding to erythrocytes. Proc Natl Acad Sci 1986; 83:2463.

7.   Kay MMB, Flowers N, Goodman J, Bosman GJCGM. Alteration in membrane protein band 3 associated with accelerated erythrocyte aging. Proc Natl Acad Sci 1989; 86:5834.

8.   Kay MMB, Sorensen K, Wong P, Bolton P. Antigenicity, storage & aging: Physiologic autoantibodies to cell membrane and serum proteins and the senescent cell antigen. Mol Cell Biochem 1982; 49:65.

9.   Kay MMB. Appearance of a terminal differentiation antigen on senescent and damaged cells and its implications for physiologic autoantibodies. Biomembranes 1983; 11:119–150.

10. Kay MMB, Goodman S, Sorensen K, et al. The senescent cell antigen is immunologically related to band 3. Proc Natl Acad Sci 1983; 80:1631.

11. Kay MMB. Senescent cell antigen: A red cell aging antigen. In: Garratty G, ed. Red Cell Antigens and Antibodies. Arlington, VA: American Association of Blood Banks, 1986:35.

12. Kay MMB, Bosman GJCGM, Johnson G, Beth A. Band 3 polymers and aggregates, and hemoglobin precipitates in red cell aging. Blood Cells 1988; 14:275.

13. Kay MMB. Immunologic techniques for analyzing red cell membrane proteins. In: Shohet S, Mohandas N, eds. Methods in Hematology: Red Cell Membranes. Churchill Livingston 1988:135.

14. Kay MMB, Bosman GJCGM, Lawrence C. Functional topography of band 3: A specific structural alteration linked to functional aberrations in human erythrocytes. Proc Natl Acad Sci USA 1988; 85:492.

15. Kay MMB, Hughes J, Zagon I, Lin F. Brain membrane protein band 3 performs the same functions as erythrocyte band 3. Proc Natl Acad Sci 1991; 88:2778.

16. Kay MMB. Aging of cell membrane molecules: Band 3 and senescent cell antigen in neural tissue. In: Beyreuther K, Schettler G, eds. Molecular Mechanisms of Aging, Berlin: Springer-Verlag 1990:110.

17. Kay MMB, Goodman J, Goodman S, Lawrence C. Membrane protein band 3 alteration associated with neurologic disease and tissue reactive antibodies. Clin Exp Immunogenet 1990; 7:181.

18. Kay MMB, Lin F, Bosman G, et al. Human erythrocyte aging: Cellular and Molecular biology. Trans Med Revs 1990; V:173.

19. Kay MMB, Goodman J, Lawrence C, Bosman G. Membrane channel protein abnormalities and autoantobodies in neurological disease. Brain Res Bull 1990; 24:105.

20. Kay MMB, Marchalonis JJ, Hughes J et al. Definition of a physiologic aging auto-antigen using synthetic peptides of membrane protein band 3: Localization of the active antigenic sites. Proc Natl Acad Sci 1990; 87:5734.

21. Kay MMB, Lin F. Molecular mapping of the active site of an aging antigen: Senescent cell antigen is located on an anion binding segment of band 3 membrane transport protein. Gerontology 1990; 36:293.

22. Singer JA, Jennings LK, Jackson C, et al. Erythrocyte homeostasis: Antibody-mediated recognition of the senescent state by macrophages. Proc Natl Acad Sci USA 83:5498.

23. Glass GA, Gershon H, Gershon D. The effect of donor and cell age on several characteristics of rat erythrocytes. Exp Hematol 1983; 11:987.

24. Glass GA, Gershon D, Gershon H. Some characteristics of the human erythrocyte as a function of donor and cell age. Exp Hematol 1985; 13:1122.

25. Bartosz G, Sosynski M, Wasilewski A. Aging of the erythrocyte XVII. Binding of autologous immunoglobin. Mech Aging Dev 1982; 20:223.

26. Bartosz G, Sosynski M, Kredziona J. Aging of the erythrocyte. VI. Accelerated red cell membrane aging in Down's syndrome. Cell Biol Int Rep 1982; 6:73.

27. Khansari N, Springer GF, Merler E, Fudenberg HH. Mechanisms for the removal of senescent human erythrocytes from circulation: Specificity of the membrane-bound immunoglobulin G. J Mech Aging Dev 1983; 21:49.

28. Khansari N, Fudenberg HH. Immune elimination of autologous senescent erythrocytes by Kupffer cells in vivo. Cell Immunol 1983; 80:426.

29. Walker WS, Singer JA, Morrison M, Jackson CW. Preferential phagocytosis of in vivo aged murine red blood cells by a macrophage-like cell line. Br J Haemat 1984; 58:259.

30. Lutz HU, Flepp R, Strigaro-Wipf G. Naturally occurring autoantibodies to exoplasmic and crytic regions of band 3 protein, the major integral membrane protein of human red blood cells. J Immunol 1984; 133:2610.

31. Petz LD, Yam P, Wilkinson L, et al. Increased IgG molecules bound to the surface of red blood cells of patients with sickle cell anemia. Blood 1984; 64:301.

32. Hebbel RP, Miller WJ. Phagocytosis of sickle erythrocytes. Immunologic and oxidative determinants of hemolytic anemia. Blood 1984; 64:733.

33. Okoye VC, Bennett V. Plasmodium falciparum malaria: Band 3 as a possible receptor during invasion of human erythrocytes. Science 1985; 227:169.

34. Friedman MJ, Fukuda M, Laine RA. Evidence for a malarial parasite interaction site on the major transmembrane protein of the human erythrocyte. Science 1985; 228:75.

35. Kay MMB, Tracey CM, Goodman JR, et al. Polypeptides immunologically related to erythrocyte band 3 are present in nucleated somatic cells. Proc Natl Acad Sci USA 1983; 80:6882.

36. Kay MMB, Bosman G, Notter M, Coleman P. Life and death of neurons: The role of senescent cell antigen. Ann NY Acad Sci 1988; 521:155.

37. Alper SL, Natale J, Gluck S et al. Subtypes of intercalated cells in rat kidney collecting duct defined by antibodies against erythroid band 3 and renal vacuolar H + ATPase. Proc Natl Acad Sci 1989; 86:5429.

38. Drenckhahn D, Zinke K, Schauer U, Identification of immunoreactive forms of human erythrocyte band 3 in nonerythroid cells. Eur J Cell Biol 1989; 34:144.

39. Drenckhahn D, Schulter K, Allen DP, Bennett V. Colocalization of band 3 with ankyrin and spectrin at the basal membrane of intercalated cells in the rat kidney. Science 1985; 230:1287.

40. Wolpaw EW, Martin DL. A membrane protein in LRM55 glial cells cross-reacts with antibody to the anion exchange carrier of human erythrocytes. Neurosci Lett 1986; 67:42.

41. Drenckhahn D, Merte C. Restriction of the human kidney band 3-like anion exchanger to specialized subdomains of the basolateral plasma membrane of intercalated cells. Eur J Cell Biol 1987; 45:107.

42. Hazen-Martin DJ, Pasternack G, Henningar RA, et al. Immunocytochemistry of band 3 protein in kidney and other tissues of control and cystic fibrosis patients. Pediatr Res 1987; 235.

43. Demuth DR, Showe LC, Ballantine M, et al. Cloning and structural characterization of a human non-erythroid band 3-like protein. Embo J 1986; 5:1205.

44. Alper SL, Kopito RR, Libresco SM, Lodish HF. Cloning and characterization of a murine band 3-related cDNA from kidney and from a lymphoid cell line. J Biol Chem 1988; 263:17092.

45. Vanderpuye OA, Kelley LK, Morrison MM, Smith CH. The apical and basel plasma membranes of the human placental syncytiotrophoblast contain different erythrocyte membrane protein isoforms. Evidence for placental forms of band 3 and spectrin. Biochim Biophys Acta 1988; 943:277.

46. Verlander JW, Madsen KM, Low PS, et al. Immunocytochemical localization of Band 3 protein in the rat collecting duct. Am J Physiol 1988; 255:F115.

47. Allen DP, Low PS, Dola A, Maisel H. Band 3 and ankyrin homologues are present in eye lens: Evidence for all major erythrocyte membrane components in same non-erythroid cell. Biochem Biophys Res Commun 1987; 149:266.

48. Brosius F, Alpert S, Garcia A, Lodish H. The major kidney band 3 gene transcript predicts an amino-terminal truncated band 3 polypeptide. J Biol Chem 1989; 264:7784.

49. Kudrycki KE, Shull GE. Primary structure of the rat kidney band 3 anion exchange protein deduced from a cDNA. J Biol Chem 1989; 264:8185.

50. Hazen-Martin DJ, Pasternack G, Spicer SS, Sens DA. Immunolocalization of band 3 protein in normal and cystic fibrosis skin. J Histochem Cytochem 1986; 34:823.

51. Bosman GJCGM, Kay MMB. Alterations of band 3 transport protein by cellular aging and disease: Erythroclyte band 3 and glucose transporter share a functional relationship. Biochem Cell Biol 1990; 68:1419.

52. Kellokumpu S, Neff L, Jamsa-Kellokumpu S, et al. A 115-kD polypeptide immunologically related to erythrocyte band 3 is present in Golgi membranes. Science 1988; 242:1308.

53. Schuster VL, Bonsib SM, Jennings ML. Two types of collecting duct mitochondria-rich (intercalated) cells: Lectin and band 3 cytochemistry. Am J Physiol 1986; 251:C347.

54. Bosman G, Bartholomeus I, DeMan C, et al. Alzheimer's Disease: Indications for disturbed erythrocyte aging. Neurobiol Aging 1991; 12: 13.

55.   Kay MMB, Bosman GJCGM. Naturally occurring human "antigalactosyl" IgG antibodies are heterophile antibodies recognizing blood group related substances. Exp Hematol 1985; 13:1103.

56.   Kay MMB. Aging of cell membrane molecules leads to appearance of an aging antigen and removal of senescent cells. Gerontology 1985; 31:215.

57.   Bosman GJCGM, Kay MMB. Erythrocyte aging: A comparison of model systems for stimulating cellular aging in vitro. Blood Cells 1988; 14:19.

58.   Jarolim P, Palek J, Amato D, et al. Deletion in erythrocyte band 3 gene in malaria-resistant Southeast Asian ovalocytosis. Proc Natl Acad Sci 1991; 88:11022.

59.   Kay MMB. Drosophilia to bacteriophage to erythrocyte: The erythrocyte as a model for molecular and membrane aging of terminally differentiated cells. Gerontology 1991; 37:5.

60.   Kay MMB, Marchalonis J. Synthetic aging antigen can be used to manipulate cellular lifespan. Life Sci 1991; 48:1603.

61.   Tanner MJA, Martin PG, High S. The complete amino acid sequence of the human erythrocyte membrane anion-transport protein deduced from the cDNA sequence. Biochem J 1988; 256:703.

62.   Branch DR, Gallagher MT, Mison AP, et al. In vitro determination of red cell alloantibody significance using an assay of monocyte-macrophage interaction with sensitized erythrocytes. Br J Haematol 1984; 56:19.

63.   Kay MMB. Molecular mapping of human band 3 anion transport regions using synthetic peptides. Fed Proc 1991; 5:109.

64.   Jennings ML, Anderson MP, Monaghan R. Monoclonal antibodies against human erythrocyte band 3 protein. Localization of proteolytic cleavage sites and stilbenedisulfonate-binding lysine residues. J Biol Chem 1986; 261:9002.

65.   Jennings ML, Monaghan R, Douglas SM, Nicknish JS. Functions of extracellular lysine residues in the human erythrocyte anion transport protein. J Gen Physiol 1985; 86:653.

66.   Jennings ML. Structure and function of the red blood cell anion transport protein. Annu Rev Biophys Biophys Chem 1989; 18:397.

67.   Bartel D, Hans H, Passow H. Identification by site directed mutagenesis of lysine 558 as a covalent attachment site of DIDS in mouse erythroid band 3. Biochem Biophys Acta 1989; 985:355.

68.   Garcia AM, Lodish HF. Lysine 539 of human band 3 is not essential for ion transport or inhibition of stilbene disulfonate. J Biol Chem 1989; 264:19607.

69.   Jennings ML, Anderson MP. Chemical modification and labeling of glutamate residues at the stilbenedisulfonate site of human red blood cell band 3 protein. J Biol Chem 1987; 262:1691.

70.   Bjerrum, PJ, Wieth JO, Minakami S. Selective phenylglyoxalation of functionally essential arginyl residues in the erythrocyte anion transport protein. J Gen Physiol 1983; 81:453.

71.   Zaki L. Anion transport in red blood cells and arginine specific reagents. (1) Effect of chloride and sulfate ions on phenylglyoxal sensitive sites in the red blood cell membrane. Biochem Biophys Res Commun 1983; 110:616.

72.   Kay MMB. Glucose transport protein is structurally and immunologically related to band 3 and senescent cell antigen. Proc Natl Acad Sci 1985; 82:1731.

II
Associations of Blood Groups with Disease

8

Do Blood Groups Have a Biological Role?

GEORGE GARRATTY
American Red Cross Blood Services
and University of California, Los Angeles
Los Angeles, California

I. INTRODUCTION

Some diseases are definitely associated with, or caused by, blood group antigen-antibody reactions (see below), but the medical literature is replete with unusual examples of associations of blood groups and disease. Many of these are pure statistical associations of ABO blood groups with certain diseases. Some of these associations have made some famous blood transfusion scientists suggest that such associations are part of the mythology of blood transfusion medicine (1–3). Examples of some early reports that led one to suspect that the associations were due to the misuse of statistics were reported by Prokop and Uhlenbruck (4). For example, in 1927, Warnowsky stated that "hangover" is more pronounced in persons of group A, and that members of group B defecate the most. In the same year, Bohmer found that there was an increased incidence of group B among criminals. In 1930, Suk found that persons of group O had the best teeth followed by those of group AB, whereas A and B persons were supposed to have the worst teeth. There were several papers correlating blood groups with personality traits. In fact, Schaer wrote a book on the subject in 1941; he found that group O individuals have less satisfactory strength of character and personality and group B individuals were impulsive. Other associations in the early literature have been made with homosexuality, lesbianism, platonism, sadism, and even flat feet.

Some of these rather unusual associations continue to appear in the literature. In 1972, Wood et al. (5) showed that the mosquito *Anopheles gambiae* (species A from Nkolmekok, Cameroons) was selective in its feeding habits, being influenced by the ABO blood group of its human host. In this study, the ABO status of the mosquito's meal was ascertained by extracting blood from the mosquito's gut and typing it! It was determined that the mosquitoes preferentially selected hosts of blood group O; a mean of 5.045 bites were found on O subjects compared to 3.276 on group A subjects! In 1973, another paper in the same highly respected journal, *Nature* (6), suggested that there may be an association between ABO blood groups and intelligence quotient (IQ). Individuals in group A_2 had the highest IQ, and both groups A_2 and O individuals had a higher IQ than the A_1 phenotype. In 1984, Golding et al. (7) reported that A blood groups are significantly more common among members of the higher socioeconomic groups; this led to some interesting correspondence in the same issue of *Nature*. As late as 1988, a book was published entitled *You Are Your Blood Type* (8), which was similar to Schaer's 1941 book (4) relating ABO blood type to personality traits.

My own interest in blood groups and disease became reactivated in the early 1970s, paralleling the developing field of tumor immunology and our increasing knowledge of the chemistry of blood group antigens. It was of interest that several of the basic concepts emerging from tumor immunology seemed to me perhaps to provide some rationale for the unusual statistical relationships between ABO blood groups and cancer. It has become obvious that some of the new so-called tumor antigens had been identified previously as blood group antigens and their chemical composition was already known by immunohematologists (see below).

Questions that are often not asked are: What are blood groups for? Do they have a biological role? Over 600 blood group antigens have been described and some of them (e.g., A, B, H, Le^a, Le^b, Le^Y, Le^x, I, i, P) are widely distributed. They are present on most circulating blood cells and present in many tissues (Table 1), some are also present in secretions (e.g., saliva, urine, semen, plasma). It is hard to believe that such a polymorphic system does not have a function. Blood groups are obviously not there to give us problems with artificial processes such as transfusion and transplantation! I believe that they do have a function and that the chemical moieties we call blood group antigens may play a biological role, sometimes related to the red blood cell (RBC) (e.g., structural) but often totally unrelated to their presence on RBCs. Some relationships of blood groups to disease, such as the relationships of blood group antigens to the immune destruction of circulating cells have been proven, but other relationships are just beginning to emerge. There is increasing literature on the relationship of certain RBC phenotypes, other than ABO, with disease, particularly hematological conditions, which suggest a structural function for some blood group antigens. There is also a current interest in defining

Table 1 Status of ABH Reactivity on Cells from Normal Organs

Organ	ABH Present	ABH Absent
Blood vessels	Endothelial cells	
Breast	Glands, ducts	
Bronchial tree	Respiratory epithelium	Serous glands, mucous glands
Colon, proximal	Surface epithelium glands	
Duodenum	Epithelium, Brunner's glands	
Endometrium	Epithelia (proliferative and secretory)	
Esophagus	Squamous epithelium	Basel cell layer of epithelium
Exocervix	Squamous epithelium	
Fallopian tube	Columnar epithelium	
Gallbladder	Columnar epithelium	
Kidney	Collecting tubules	Convoluted tubules
Larynx	Squamous epithelium, mucous glands	Serous glands
Liver	Kupffer cells	Hepatocytes
Pancreas	Exocrine glands	Islets
Pituitary	Colloid, pars intermedia	
Prostrate	Glands	
Skin	Stratum corneum	Cells of basal and malpighian layers
	Sweat glands	Sebaceous glands
Small intestine	Columnar epithelium	
Stomach	Columnar epithelium	
Tongue	Squamous epithelium	
Lower urinary system	Urinary bladder, ureter epithelium	
Vagina	Squamous epithelium, mucous glands	Basal layer of epithelium

bacterial and parasitic receptors, and some of these seem closely related to known blood group antigens. Finally, a thread of scientific rationale is beginning to emerge that might explain some of the unusual statistical associations of blood groups with cancer and coagulation (e.g., bleeding and thrombosis).

II. PROVEN RELATIONSHIPS OF BLOOD GROUPS WITH DISEASE

A. Hemolytic Disease of the Fetus/Newborn (HDF/N)

In 1905, Dienst clearly demonstrated that mothers could have an immune response to the baby's blood group antigens (9). It was suggested that susceptibility to pregnancy toxemia was partly dependent on the mother's blood group (9). In 1941, Levine et al. extended this observation by proving that HDF/N was due to a maternal antibody directed against the baby's Rh antigens (10). Since that time, antibodies to many blood group antigens have been shown to be capable of causing HDF/N (11,12) (see Chapter 20).

B. Autoimmune Hemolytic Anemia (AIHA)

In 1953 and 1954, several cases of AIHA were shown to be due to autoantibodies directed to the Rh blood group antigens e, c, C, and D (13–15). Since that time, many examples of these and other blood group antigens have been shown to be the targets for pathogenic autoantibodies (16) (see Chapter 18).

C. Hemolytic Transfusion Reactions

Hemolytic transfusion reactions have been recorded in the medical literature since the seventeenth century, but it was not until the discovery of ABO blood groups in 1900 that the cause was proven. Since that time, over 600 blood group antigens have been described as sometimes being present on the RBC (12); and antibodies to many of these antigens have been shown to be capable of causing shortened survival of transfused or fetal RBCs (11,12).

D. Graft Rejection and ABO Antibodies

Anti-A and anti-B appear to play a role in the rejection of ABO-incompatible solid organ (e.g., kidney) grafts (17–19). Although A and B antigens are present on early RBC precursors in the bone marrow, ABO incompatibility does not seem to be as important in bone marrow transplantation. Many successful bone marrow grafts have been achieved in the presence of major ABO incompatibility (20).

E. Early Abortion and P System Antibodies

Early abortion due to anti-P, anti-P_1, and anti-P^k in women of the rare p or P^k phenotypes have been described (21–28). The P antigen has been shown to be present in the placenta (28) and anti-PP_1P^k have been shown to be cytotoxic (24).

III. ASSOCIATION OF BLOOD GROUPS WITH MALIGNANCY

A. ABO/Lewis/Ii Blood Group Antigens

If one reviews the world literature on blood groups and disease, it is obvious that there is an increase of group A compared with group O in patients with cancer (29,30). Table 2 lists

Table 2 Statistically Significant Associations of ABO Blood Groups
with Disease

Disease	Comparison	Relative incidence[a]
Carcinoma		
Stomach	A:O	1.22
Colon and Rectum	A:O	1.11
Salivary Glands	A:O	1.64
Uterus	A:O	1.15
Cervix	A:O	1.13
Ovaries	A:O	1.28
Other Diseases		
Pernicious Anemia	A:O	1.25
Cholecystitis and Cholelithiasis	A:O	1.17
Rheumatic Disease	A:O	1.24
Duodenal Ulcer	O:A	1.35
Gastric Ulcer	O:A	1.17
Bleeding Ulcer	O:A	1.46

[a]Relative incidence, e.g., $A:O = \dfrac{\text{number of A patients} \times \text{number of O patients}}{\text{number of O patients} \times \text{number of A controls}}$

Source: Data mainly from Refs. 29 and 30.

some of the more significant associations. The first convincing study relating blood groups and disease showed a 20% increase of carcinoma of the stomach in group A as compared to group O (31). Since this observation, there have been over 150 separate sets of patients studied, more than 50,000 individuals, in different parts of the world; almost all these reports agree with the A/O relative incidence of about 1.2 in carcinoma of the stomach. Thus, the statistical data supporting a relationship of ABO blood groups to carcinoma of the stomach seem indisputable.

Other carcinomas of the gastrointestinal tract tend to show a raised A/O ratio, with the highest A/O relative incidence being 1.64 for salivary tumors (based on two series of 285 patients) (29,30). Carcinoma of the colon and rectum show an A/O ratio of 1.11 (based on 17 series of 7435 patients) (29,30). Carcinoma of other organs also generally shows an increased A/O ratio, but some of the series are not as large as those mentioned previously. One convincing association of a distinctly raised A/O ratio is carcinoma of the female genital tract. The A/O ratio in carcinoma of the ovary being 1.28 (17 series of 2326 patients), carcinoma of the uterus 1.15 (14 series of 2598 patients), and carcinoma of the cervix 1.33 (19 series of 11,927 patients) (29,30).

The risk of choriocarcinoma developing after a normal pregnancy or a hydatidiform mole is critically related to the ABO blood groups of the woman and her sexual partner. Women of group A whose sexual partners are men of group O seem to have the highest risk, whereas women of group A whose sexual partners are men of group A have the lowest risk. The relative risk of these two groups was found to be 10.4:1. Group AB patients tend to have rapidly progressive tumors that do not respond well to chemotherapy (32–34). Choriocarcinoma arising from the trophoblast of the placenta is a fetal tumor that invades the maternal host. It is distinguished from its host by the genetic constitution of the father. Evidence is conflicting for the presence of A antigen on human trophoblasts; some workers have detected A antigen on early, but not late, trophoblasts (35–37). It has been tentatively suggested that in some way an O trophoblast reacts to the foreign A antigen present in the mother.

1. Loss of ABH Antigens from Malignant Cells

Oh-Huti (38) seems to be the first to have described a loss of ABH antigens from malignant cells, and this was confirmed by Masamune et al. (39), Kawasaki (40), Kay and Wallace (41), Nairn et al. (42), and Davidsohn (43).

In a series of papers, Davisohn and his coworkers (reviewed in ref. 43) showed that isoantigens A, B, and H, present in epithelial cells of some normal tissues, could not be detected when carcinoma developed in these tissues. The specific red cell adherence test, a modification of Coombs' mixed cell agglutination test, was used for the detection of ABH antigens. The test was highly sensitive and specific. The age of paraffin-embedded tissues and hematoxylin-eosin stained slides did not affect the sensitivity of the test. The loss of the antigens was increasingly progressive from carcinoma in situ to anaplastic, invasive, and metastatic carcinoma and was interpreted as evidence of immunological dedifferentiation analogous to morphological dedifferentiation of anaplasia. Three hundred and fifty-five primary carcinomas of the uterine cervix, lung, pancreas, and stomach and 578 metastatic carcinomas of these organs were studied. With few exceptions, the loss of ABH antigens preceded the formation of distant metastases. The authors suggested that the test held promise: (1) in the diagnosis of early carcinoma in tissues that normally contain ABH antigens and in the prognosis of advanced carcinoma; and (2) to reduce the need for radical surgery in carcinoma in situ of the cervix. Since Davidsohn's studies (43), there have been hundreds of publications studying ABH antigens and many types of malignancy (44–49). In general, the results agree with, and extend, the earlier observations. Hakomori, in particular, has helped us considerably to understand the etiology of these changes (45–48).

The structure of the A, B, H, Lewis, and Ii antigens are discussed in detail in Chapter 1 and references 47, 49, and 50. In summary, A, B, H, Lewis, and Ii antigens are carbohydrate structures carried on glycoproteins (in secretions or on cells) or glycosphingolipids (a molecule of ceramide, which is a long-chain amino alcohol plus a long-chain fatty acid, inserted in the lipid bilayer, and a hydrophilic oligosaccharide chain projecting from the cell membrane). Their structures are based on four backbone sequences. The major two chains are Type 1 (containing Galβ→3GlcNac units) and Type 2 (containing Galβ→4GlcNAc units) to which L-fucose and, in some cases, N-acetyl-D-galactosamine or D-galactose are added as terminal sugars to produce the various blood group specificities. The Type 1 chain predominates over Type 2 in normal adult gastrointestinal epithelia, and the Type 1 chain is usually fucosylated (e.g., Le^a, Le^b, Le^c, Le^d). The majority of Type 1 chain H (le^d) in blood group A and B epithelia is converted to A and B. Type 2 chains are the major carriers of ABH on RBCs but are relatively minor components on normal epithelial cells. Fucosylated Type 2 chains yield Le^x and Le^y. More recently, Type 3 (repetitive globo sequences) chains were described to add to the complexity of the system. Some structures are linear (e.g., A^a, A^b, B_1, B_2, H_1, H_2, i), whereas others are branched (e.g., A^c, A^d, B_3, H_3, H_4, I). Some of the structures also have sialosylated versions (e.g., sialyl Le^a, sialyl Le^x).

The *A, B, H* genes are responsible for governing the synthesis of glycosyl transferases that are responsible for the blood group antigens. Other genes such as the *Lewis* and *Secretor* genes also play a role (50). Singhai and Hakomori (51) recently suggested that many of the carbohydrate changes associated with cancer take place at various stages of development and differentiation, and that the changes, associated with cancer, may result from activation or increased synthesis of different glycosyltransferases.

2. Appearance of "New" and "Illegitimate" ABH/Lewis/Ii Blood Group Antigens on Malignant Tissues

As a malignancy develops, the cells appear to lose normal antigens and new antigens appear (so-called tumor antigens). The "new" antigens may be represented by precursor substances of normal antigens or be "illegitimate" (incompatible) antigens; that is to say, antigens that are genetically dissimilar to the host. A similar pattern is observed with blood group antigens that are present on noncirculating cells (i.e., in tissue) (Table 3).

Watanabe and Hakomori (52) provided evidence that a genetic or epigenetic program for synthesizing blood group determinants and their carrier carbohydrate chains develops step-by-step during the process of ontogenesis, and that the program of synthesis is blocked or modified in the process of oncogenesis. Blood group ABH determinants in human RBCs are carried by four kinds of glycolipid carbohydrate chains differing in their structural complexity. They are A^a, A^b, A^c, and A^d for A variants and H_1, H_2, H_3, and H_4 for H variants. Based on the surface labeling of A variants, and on the reactivity of RBCs to antibodies directed against H_3 and against its degradation products, Watanabe and Hakomori (52) concluded that complex variants of A or H determinants (A^c and A^d/or H_3 and H_4) are absent or significantly low on fetal RBCs (80–150 days gestation) and on newborn RBCs, whereas these complex structures are fully developed on adult RBCs. In contrast, A determinants linked to simpler carbohydrate chains (A^a, A^b variants) are fully developed before birth and do not show significant change after birth. The precursor of blood group carbohydrate chains seems to be abundant on fetal or newborn RBCs. This assumption is based on the higher reactivity of fetal or newborn RBCs, with an antibody against the precursor N-acetyl-glucosaminyl $\beta1{\rightarrow}3$ galactosyl $\beta1{\rightarrow}4$ glycosylceramide, than the reactivity with adult RBCs. Reactions of glycolipids or gastrointestinal mucosa with antibodies directed against H_3 glycolipid and its degradation products were compared to that of gastrointestinal tumors. The reaction to $\beta GLcNAc1{\rightarrow}3$ $\beta Gal1{\rightarrow}4Glc$-ceramide, which is the precursor of all blood group glycolipids, was consistently higher in cases of tumor glycolipid than that of most normal glycolipid. Watanabe and Hakomori (52) suggested that this, as well as other evidence, supports a general concept that the process of ontogenesis of a blood group carbohydrate chain occurs as step-by-step elongation and arborization, and that blocking of such a development of a carbohydrate chain occurs in the process of oncogenesis (52).

In 1964, Hakomori and Jeanloz (53) isolated a glycolipid of unusual carbohydrate composition from a human adenocarcinoma; attempts to isolate a similar component from normal tissues were unsuccessful. In 1967, glycolipids extracted from different adenocarcinomas were shown to possess weak Le^b and H activity and moderate Le^a activity regardless of the Lewis type of the tissue donor (54). It is interesting to note that Hakomori has always detected both Le^a and Le^b in adenocarcinomas and glandular tissue but either Le^a or Le^b alone in parenchymatous organs or RBCs (52–54). Neither blood group A nor B activity was detected in glycolipid fractions from any adenocarcinomas even though some tumor donors were group A or B. In contrast, A and B activity was detected regularly in normal glandular tissue (52–54). Although the tumor glycolipid had no A activity there appeared to be a special relationship

Table 3 "New" and "Illegitimate" (Incompatible) Blood Group Antigens Appearing on Malignant Cells

---

"New" Antigens
   Type 1 chains (e.g., H type I, Le^c type)
   Type 2 chains (e.g., Ii type I, Le^x, Le^y)
"Illegitimate" (Incompatible) Antigens
   A and "A-like" in groups B and O patients
   Lewis antigens in Le(a–b–) patients
   P and P_1 antigens in gastric tissue of a patient with p phenotype
   P^k in a patient with Burkitt's lymphoma
   Forssman antigen in Forssman-negative tissue

---

between it and blood group substance A. Rabbit antisera against tumor glycolipid agglutinated type A red cells more readily than group B, AB, or O red cells. This and other experiments suggested that tumor glycolipid was a constituent of the surface of tumor cells, and that blood group A substance and group A red cells may contain a larger concentration of a hapten structure similar to, or identical with, the carbohydrate moiety of the tumor glycolipid than do substances or red cells of group B or O(H) (45). Hakomori et al. (45) suggested that it may be more difficult for the immunological system of the group A patient to recognize tumor cells, possessing "A-like" glycolipid, as foreign because of the latter's similarity to the host's own A substance and thus fail to reject them. This may possibly relate to the increase of group A compared with O in cancer patients. Other adenocarcinomas were found to have increased quantities of a ceramide pentasaccharide with Le^a structure and a ceramide hexasaccharide having Le^b activity (47,54). Increased levels of 2→3 sialyl Le^a and desialyl Le^a, both in the malignant cells and in the plasma, have been reported in colonic, pancreatic, and other cancers (51).

Since the original findings associating Lewis antigens with adenocarcinoma (53–55), there have been many papers elaborating on these findings. Many of these have appeared in the last decade and are appearing in increasing numbers in the last few years (56–82).

As mentioned above, Hakomori et al. (53) showed that a novel glycolipid with Le^a activity was isolated from a human adenocarcinoma and showed "A-like" activity. Over 60 years ago, Hirszfeld et al. (83) and Witebsky (84) had shown that an "A-like" antigen could be detected in cancer patients who were not group A. In 1970, Häkkinen and his coworkers (85,86) demonstrated clearly that A-like antigen could be detected in gastric juice and mucosa from group O and B patients with gastric cancer but was not detected in mucosa from patients with peptic ulcers. More recent studies suggest that the A-like antigen may be a true A antigen or an antigen cross-reacting with Forssman or Tn antigen (48,87–92) Glycolipids with clear A activity have been demonstrated in some cases of group O cancer patients (88,89,91). About 10–15% of group O or B patients with colonic cancer express mono- or di-fucosyl type 1 chain A antigen; A transferase activity was also detected in the A-expressing O tumors (91). Because of these findings, Hakomori (92) has suggested that the A transferase gene may not be a specific product of A individuals but may rather be suppressed in normal B or O tissues. The Forssman antigen is usually present on malignant cells independently from the A-like antigen (88,89). It seems that most of the A-like antigens appearing on malignant cells may be Tn (90) (see below).

Ørntoft et al. (79) reported in 1991 that Le(a-b-) individuals who did not have Le^a or Le^b in their saliva or α1→4 fucosyltransferase (the primary Lewis gene product) in saliva or normal tissues showed expression of Le^a, Le^b, and α1→4 fucosyltransferase in their tumors. Lacto-series Type 1 chain is a normal component of gastrointestinal cells. It appears that type 2 chain-based structures (e.g., Le^x, sialosyl Le^x, dimeric and trimeric Le^x) are major oncofetal antigens in human gastrointestinal colorectal and lung cancers (81). Large concentrations of Le^x antigen (fucosylated Type 2 chains, Galβ1→4 [Fuc α1→3]→GlcNAc), otherwise known as SSEA-1 (56), have been demonstrated in various tumors (59). Levels of another Type 2 antigen, Le^y (Fucα1→2Galβ1→4 [Fucα1→3] Glc-NAc) are significantly increased in colonic cancer (64). It appears that when malignant cells lose A and B antigens owing to blocked activity of A and B transferases, the Type 2 chain is fucosylated by enhanced α1→3 fucosyltransferase and accumulates Le^x hapten glycolipid. The Type 1 chain is fucosylated by enhanced α1→4 fucosyltransferase as well as α1→2 fucosyltransferase to accumulate both Le^a and Le^b hapten regardless of the Lewis status of the host (47,48).

An interesting recent finding was that the Le^x antigen might be a good marker for the Reed-Stenberg (RS) cell of Hodgkin's disease (HD). Ree et al. (80) used a monoclonal antibody specific for Le^x to study 103 cases of HD, in comparison with 57 cases of non-HD lymphoma, and 55 other diseases of the reticuloendothelial system. Reed-Sternberg cells stained selectively in 80 of 92 (87%) cases of HD, excluding 11 cases of lymphocyte predominance type. The authors found the method superior to staining results using Leu-M1. The Le^x staining also detected subcapsular clustering of Langerhans'-like cells in persistent generalized lymphadeno-pathy, which had not been described previously.

3.   Association of ABH/Lewis/Ii Antigens with Carcinoembryonic Antigen (CEA)

In 1965, Gold and Freedman (93) reported the presence of identical antigens on all malignant human tumors of the endodermally derived epithelium of the gastrointestinal tract, liver, and pancreas as well as in fetal gut, liver, or pancreas. No other adult or fetal tissues, benign or diseased, contained the antigens. The antigen was named carcinoembryonic antigen (CEA). More than 300 human tissues were studied for their ability to inhibit a tumor-specific antibody. Only digestive tract tumors did so. Two to 6-month-old fetal digestive tract organs gave reactions of identity in agar gels. All other adult or fetal tissues, normal or diseased, were negative. Since then, the original thesis that CEA is a single specific carcinofetal antigen has been vigorously disputed, and, indeed, CEA has now been shown to be present in a number of normal or tumor-free tissues. Gold et al. (94,95) showed that there was a degree of cross-reactivity between CEA and blood group A substance, and that anti-A combines with CEA. Simmons and Perlmann (96) suggested that CEAs were incomplete blood group substances of the ABO system. The incomplete ABO substance they described was very similar to that described for I specificity (96). They suggested that the genetic changes in oncogenesis include deletion or repression of the gene(s) controlling the transferase(s) for the terminal sequences of the ABO-active glycoproteins. Holburn et al. (97) produced evidence that A, B, and Lewis antigens share the same glycoprotein carrier molecule as CEA. No I or i activity was detected in the CEA preparations. In contrast, Cooper et al. (98) and Feizi et al. (99) reported that I and i antigenic sites were on different molecules than CEA in colon carcinoma extracts. Bloom et al. (100) found that sera from many patients with tumors showed demonstrable cytotoxic antibody activity against selected human tumor cells in culture. The antibody activity was not found to be specific for tumors but was shown to be directed against an antigen that is serologically related to blood group A. Direct cytotoxicity and absorption analyses, blocking tests, and erythrocyte adherence tests confirmed this conclusion. Antibody activity was found, as expected, frequently in sera from patients with blood groups O and B phenotypes and not in patients belonging to blood groups A or AB. The authors suggested that in view of the ubiquitous occurrence of blood group antibodies, their possible role in some human tumor serological studies should not be ignored. Magous (101) used a sandwich radioimmunoassay to demonstrate that blood group A antigens previously identified in CEA preparations were truly borne by the CEA molecule and not by a contaminating entity. Nichols et al. (102) studied the reactivities of eight purified preparations of CEA with monoclonal antibodies directed to tumor-associated carbohydrate determinants. All eight reacted with a monoclonal antibody (AH6) defining the Lewis (Le^y) blood group structure. A few preparations reacted also with an antibody defining the Le^x structure. Other authors (103) have also shown the presence of Le^x in one of the side chains of CEA. As mentioned previously, Le^y and Le^x have been detected in a wide variety of human cancers (47,48).

4.   Association of ABH/Lewis Antigens with Growth Factors and Adhesion Receptors

One of the most distinctive traits of malignant cells is the uncontrolled growth that occurs. Malignant cells fail to respect the territorial rules that confine normal cells to particular tissues (104). There have been some interesting associations of blood group antigens with cellular growth, wound healing, and more recently adhesion receptors.

There is an increase in blood group H antigen in HeLa cells and in cultured human epithelioid (primary amnion) cells (105,106) during mitosis. The expression of blood group A on primary amnion cells in culture also varies with growth conditions (105, 107), with the number of

A-positive cells being higher during rapid division (108). It was shown by clonal selection that antigen-negative cells gave rise to both positive and negative progeny (108). In 1971, Thomas (109) proposed a model for blood group B and H antigenic variation, during the division of mouse cells, that reacted with human anti-B and H antisera. He showed that (1) resting cells were B negative and H positive and gave rise to B+ and H– cells during exponential growth; (2) at mitosis, cells can proceed to a G_1 state that is B– and H+ or B+ and H–; (3) the B+ H– G_1 cells undergo synchronous division, whereas B– H+ G_1 cells are restricted to asynchronous growth; and (4) blood group B determinant is expressed on lymphocytes after treatment with phytohemagglutinin (PHA) and its appearance precedes DNA synthesis. Thus, the ability to express the α-galactosyl 1→ galactose moiety (B determinant) was a prerequisite for cell division. B and H expression were not thought to inhibit cell division but rather to provide an index of a cell committed to mitosis. Escape from growth inhibition was associated with the permanent expression of B at the cell surface. It was suggested that cells at mitosis can be diverted from a path of rapid proliferation to one of growth inhibition with arrest in a G_1 (or G_0) B– state.

Other interesting observations regarding ABO blood groups and cell growth concern loss of ABH antigens during wound healing (110). These studies suggest that there may be a correlation between loss of ABH antigens and certain cell processes such as mitosis and migration. Blood group B antigen was shown to be lost within hours from epithelial cells adjacent to healing wounds in the oral mucosa of monkeys (110). The region in which major cellular proliferation was occurring was outside the region of the B antigen deletion. This suggested that the cell surface changes were related primarily to control of cell movement rather than to control of proliferation. Cells participating in wound healing and malignant cells exhibit reduced contact-inhibition of movement (i.e., inhibition of locomotion of a cell in a direction taking it across another cell) (111). Thus, Mackenzie et al. (110) suggest that the altered (depressed) blood group antigen reactivity described earlier in some epithelial tumors may not be a tumor-specific change but rather reflect a common increased potential for cell mobility in both tumors and wounds.

All carbohydrate chains in glycoproteins or in glycolipids undergo rapid and dramatic changes during development and differentiation (112–114). Perhaps the most obvious developmentally regulated blood group antigens are I and i. The i antigen, prominent on fetal RBCs, diminishes after birth and during the first year of life, whereas the I antigen increases concomitantly. The Ii antigens are backbone structures (Type 2 chain) of ABH. They consist of repeating units of N-acetyllactosamine (Galβ1→4 GlcNAc). The i antigen is made up of unbranched oligosaccharides of three or four repeating N-acetyllactosamine units joined to each other by a β1→3 linkage (114). The corresponding branched structures found by β1→6 linkage of N-acetyl-lactosamine units to internal galactose residues of the repeating sequence express the I antigen (114). During the first year of life, there may be increased activity of a glycosyltransferase (branching enzyme) that transfers N-acetylglucosamine via a 1→6 linkage to a previously formed linear chain (114). Hakomori (112) has suggested that aberrant glycosylation in cancer cells may represent retrogenic expression of carbohydrate synthesis to a certain stage of embryogenesis and fetal development. He suggested that 10 types of chemical changes to glycolipids occur (Table 4). Types 1–5 are caused by incomplete synthesis of normally existing carbohydrate chains and accompanying precursor-accumulating types 6–10 are due to neosynthesis through activation of new glycosyltransferase that are characteristic of tumor cells and are absent, or present only in small quantities, in normal cells.

Feizi (113,114) has reviewed the use of monoclonal antibodies to demonstrate that the carbohydrate structures of glycoproteins and glycolipids are onco-developmental antigens. Table 5 lists some blood group related carbohydrate structures of glycoproteins and glycolipids recognized by monoclonal antibodies raised by immunizing mice with human tumor cells, tumor

Table 4 Chemotypes of Aberrant Glycosylation in Tumor Cells

In glycolipids
 Incomplete synthesis with or without precursor accumulation
  Type 1: Decrease or deletion of G_{M3}*, G_{D3}*: increase of LacCer, ClcCer
  Type 2: Decrease or deletion of G_{M1}*, G_T*, $G_{P1a/orb}$*: increase of G_{m3}*, G_{M2}*
  Type 3: Decrease or deletion of Gb_4*, Gb_5*, or other longer neutral glycosphingolipids
  Type 4: Accumulation of asialo core (Gg_4*, Gg_3*, nLc_4*) which is normally absent
  Type 5: Accumulation of G_{D3}* or G_{D2}*
 Neosynthesis (activation of a new addition of a glycosyl residue)
  Type 6: Neosynthesis of Gb_5 (Forssman) and other Forssman hapten
  Type 7: Neosynthesis of incompatible blood group antigen foreign to the host A like antigen in
       gastrointestinal tumors with blood group O or B host Pk antigen in Burkitt's lymphoma
       (irrespective of host blood group P status)
       P-like and P_1 antigen in the gastric cancer of the host with pp genotype
  Type 8: A linear chain elongation of Type 2 chain coupled with $\alpha 1 \rightarrow 3$ fucosylation at every GlcNAc
       residue
  Type 9: Enhanced synthesis of Le^x and its sialosylation
  Type 10: Enhanced synthesis of Le^a hapten and its sialosylation
In glycoproteins
 Increased branch: GlcNAc-mannosyl core structure of asparagine-linked oligosaccharide is increased
 Increased density: O-glycoside mucin-type oligosaccharide chain
 Changes in peripheral region: the same as incomplete synthesis or neosynthesis in glycolipids (types
   1–10)

---

*Ganglio-series gangliosides (see Ref 48 for structure).
Source: Data from Ref. 112.

Table 5 Blood Group–Related Carbohydrate Structures Recognized by Monoclonal Antibodies Raised by Immunizing Mice with Cells from Human Tissues

Designation of antigen	Immunogen
Type 1 based	
FC10.2	Embryonal carcinoma
A	Epidermal carcinoma
Le^a	Colon carcinoma
Le^b	Colon carcinoma
ALe^b	Epidermal carcinoma; Colon carcinoma
19.9 sialosyl-Le^a	Colon carcinoma
Type 2 based	
Lactosyl ceramide	Nonlymphoblastic leukaemia
H	Embryonal carcinoma
A	Epidermal carcinoma
B	Pancreatic carcinoma
SSEA-1 (Le^x)	Myelomonocytic leukaemia
C14 (Le^y)	Epidermial carcinoma; Colon carcinoma
ALe^y	Colon adenoma; Lung carcinoma; Gastric carcinoma; Embryonal carcinoma; Epidermal carcinoma
CSLEXI (Sialosyl-Le^x)	Gastric carcinoma
Type 3 based	
H	Breast carcinoma
SSEA-4	Embryonal carcinoma

Source: From Ref. 113.

cell lines, or their membranes (113). Feizi (113) points out that by using well-characterized monoclonal antibodies, the immunochemical approach is making it possible to monitor the normal developmental regulation of highly complex saccharide structures in whole cells as well as the derangement in their biosynthesis in tumor cells. For instance, hybridoma antibodies to single and repeating sequences of α1–3 fucosyl type 2 chains have shown that in certain fetal tissues (but not corresponding adult tissue) there is a predominance of these repeating units, and that they "reappear" as tumor-associated antigens in certain carcinomas (113).

Hakomori (81) recently reported that two selectins, endothelial leukocyte adhesion molecule 1 (ELAM-1) (expressed at the surface of activated endothelial cells) and GMP-140 (expressed at the surface of activated platelets or endothelial cells) would bind to the sialosyl-Le^x epitope. Berg et al. (115) also showed that a carbohydrate domain common to both sialyl Le^a and sialyl Le^x is recognized by ELAM-1. These selectins are expressed only after activation with lymphokines (transforming growth factor (TGF) beta or tumor necrosis factor (TNF) alpha). Metastatic deposits express more sialosyl-Le^x than primary colonic tumors (114). In a study of two colonic tumor cell lines, one showing high expression of sialosyl-Le^x (KM12-HX), adhered strongly to TNF-α–treated endothelial cells; whereas the other, showing no expression of sialosyl-Le^x (KM12-LX), did not adhere to such cells (81). Adhesion of KM12-HX cells to endothelial cells was inhibited by anti–ELAM-1. Sialosyl-Le^x expression in human tumors was inversely correlated with survival of patients with colonic cancer (81). Taken together, these findings suggested that cell adhesion events essential for progression of human colonic cancer involve expression of the tumor-associated antigen sialosyl-Le^x, which is recognized by selectins.

B. "Illegitimate" (Incompatible) P and Forssman Antigens on Malignant Cells

In 1951, Levine et al. (116) described the first example of anti-Tj^a (now known as anti-PP$_1$P^k), a clinically significant antibody that reacted with a new high-frequency red cell antigen. Most blood transfusion scientists are familiar with anti-Tj^a, but many do not know that the "T" stands for tumor. The antibody was found in a patient with gastric cancer (adenocarcinoma). The serum of the patient contained anti-Tj^a to a titer of 8. Her phenotype was Tj(a–) (now known as the p phenotype), which has a random incidence of about 1:150,000, but in the patient's family, the incidence was 1:4 because her parents were double first cousins; a younger sister was also of the p phenotype and therefore compatible with her sister. Because no other compatible donor could be found, the patient was given a trial injection of 25 ml of incompatible group O blood. This resulted in an immediate violent hemolytic reaction with hemoglobinuria. Several days later, when the patient was fully recovered, the anti-Tj^a rose to a titer of 512. Subtotal gastrectomy was then performed without benefit of transfusions. The excised tumor was lyophilized from the frozen state so that a fine white powder was available. Adsorption tests showed that 20 mg of the cancer tissue adsorbed 16–32 agglutinating units of the anti-Tj^a. Because of the inhibition by the tumor, it was postulated that the antibody was stimulated by antigens on the tumor, thus the antibody was named anti-Tj^a; the "T" standing for tumor and the "J" for the surname of the patient. The patient survived 22 years and died from a brain hemorrhage in 1973 at the age of 88; at no time was there any evidence of tumor recurrence and metastasis. This phenomenon was interpreted to mean that the incompatible blood transfusion had boosted the strength of the antibody that had caused the inhibition of tumor growth. The patient's sister, who was also of the rare p phenotype, but was not given incompatible P + blood, died of adenocarcinoma of the uterus in 1962 (117). In 1955, Sanger (118) showed that Tj^a was part of the P system; anti-Tj^a is now known as anti-PP$_1$P^k and the rare Tj(a–) individuals are of the p phenotype (12). Much is now known about the chemistry of the P system (119). The P antigen is globoside (globotetraosyl ceramide); the P^k antigen is globotriaosyl ceramide and is a precursor of P. Neither P^k nor P is a precursor of P_1. The P_1 determinant is formed from paragloboside (lactoneotetraosyl ceramide), the precursor of ABH, Lewis, and Ii. P_1 has a terminal galactose added to the paragloboside structure.

In 1987, Levine found some frozen tumor from his original patient with anti-Tj^a and had it examined by Hakomori. Hakomori's group found that the major glycolipid isolated from the tumor had the same mobility on thin-layer chromatography and antigenic reactivity as a new glycolipid of human RBCs that cross-reacts with antigloboside, and the structure was identified as GalNAcβ1→3Galβ1→4GlcNAcβ1→3Galβ1→4Glcβ1→1Cer (120). Although the purified glycolipid fraction displayed a clear inhibition of anti-P_1 agglutinins, only a minor component had the same mobility on thin-layer chromatography as P_1 glycolipid, which is a ceramide pentasaccharide susceptible to α-galactosidase. These results indicated that the tumor activated the synthesis of the globo-series glycolipid; it also showed an enhanced synthesis of the lacto-series glycolipid with the same terminal structure as globoside (120). The biochemical results supported the 1951 findings of a p individual having made "illegitimate" ("incompatible") P antigen on malignant cells.

Forssman antigen was first described in 1911 (121). Globoside (P antigen) has been found to be the biosynthetic precursor of Forssman glycolipid (122–124). Forssman antigen was found to be present in many animals, but until relatively recently humans were thought to be Forssman negative. Most human sera were known to contain naturally occurring Forssman antibodies that would react strongly (i.e., agglutinate and hemolyze) with Forssman-positive cells (e.g., sheep RBCs). It has also been known for many years that Forssman antigen cross-reacts with the A blood antigen, and later a cross-rection with P antigen was described (119,124). Hakomori (47) considered the possibility that the A-like antigen appearing in malignant tissue might be Forssman antigen. Forssman antigen was not detected in the gastrointestinal mucosa of most normal individuals, but it was detected in about 30% of the population studied (125). Tumors derived from Forssman-negative tissue contained Forssman antigen, whereas tumors from Forssman-positive tissue did not contain Forssman glycolipid (125). Other workers have also detected Forssman antigen in malignant tissue (126–129).

Young et al. (130) showed that the antibodies in normal human sera causing complement-dependent lysis of sheep RBCs are specific for the Forssman glycolipid structure (GalNAcα1→3GalNAcβ1→3GalNAcβ1→3Galα1→R). About 75% of random normal individuals appeared to have Forssman antibodies, reactive with sheep RBCs, in their sera (130). Most of their antibodies appeared to be immunoglobulin M (IgM), and their occurrence was independent of the ABO type of the serum donor. Sera from patients with cancer showed decreased Forssman antibody activity (130). Levine (131) confirmed these findings. Levine detected Forssman antibodies in 79% of normal sera compared with 32–39% of sera from cancer patients (131). The presence of Forssman antibodies in healthy individuals varied with the age. The highest incidence was >90% in the youngest age group (<19 years old) compared with 61% for the 50- to 80-year-old group. It was suggested that the decrease in Forssman antibody activity in cancer was due to the appearance of "illegitimate" Forssman antigen in the malignant tissue (131). Mori et al. (132) also reported that the sera of cancer patients contained less Forssman antibody than normal sera. Although Forssman antigen does appear as an "illegitimate" antigen in malignant tissue and can appear to be A-like, Hakomori now believes that this only accounts for 10–15% of the A-like antigens appearing in malignant tissue (48). Some "illegitimate" A antigens appear to be true A antigens, but the majority of them are probably Tn antigens (see below) that also cross-react with A antigens (90).

One further interesting finding concerning P blood group antigens and malignancy is that the antigen expressed on the tumor cells from Burkitt's lymphoma, irrespective of the cells having the Epstein-Barr virus (EBV) genome, has been identified as the P^k antigen—globotriaosylceramide (Galα1→4Galβ1→4Glcβ1→1Cer) (133,134).

C. T and Tn Antigens on Malignant Cells

In 1975, Springer et al. (135) showed that malignant cells, but not normal cells or benign tumors, had T antigen, a cryptantigen known to be present on human RBCs, and Tn antigen, a precursor of T, on their surface. They also showed that naturally occurring anti-T was severely depressed in the sera of many cancer patients (135,136). The T and Tn antigens were first described as blood group antigens that were acquired by RBCs in association with certain conditions. T and Tn antigens are not usually detected on the RBCs of healthy individuals. T antigen can appear as a transitory antigen on RBCs as a result of the action of bacterial sialidases (137,138); the acquisition of Tn by RBCs is a rare event and is often persistent; it is found usually in association with thrombocytopenia, leukopenia and/or hemolytic anemia, or leukemia (139–145). Tn expression on RBCs is thought to result from somatic mutation within stem cells of the bone marrow, resulting in lack of the $\alpha 3$-β-D-galactosyltransferase needed to convert Tn to T (146,147). Expression of T or Tn on RBCs was recognized because RBCs become polyagglutinable, when T and Tn are present, because almost all adult human sera (including some commercial blood-typing reagents) contain anti-T and anti-Tn (11,12). Anti-T and Tn, like anti-A and anti-B, are bacterial antibodies that cross-react with RBC antigens (148,149).

The plants *Arachis hypogea* (peanut) and *Salvia sclarea* contain lectins that react with T and Tn antigens, respectively (12). Unfortunately, the peanut lectin does not react specifically with the T antigen on malignant tissue (150). Two anti-T lectins that appear to be more specific are found in *Artocarpus intergrifolia* and *Amaranthus caudatus* (151,152). Several highly specific monoclonal antibodies to T and Tn have been produced; some of these were produced unintentionally by using malignant tissue (150).

Since 1975 Springer's group produced many paper confirming and extending their observations on the association of T and Tn antigens with malignancy (for complete details, see refs. 150,153,154,184,186. Many other authors have confirmed the presence of T and Tn on malignant cells (155–183,187–192).

It has been suggested that T and Tn are important for adhesion of cancer cells to their preferred target in metastasis; i.e., hepatocytes (154,180,193). The attachment of malignant cells (Esb T-lymphoma cells), which expressed T and Tn on their membranes, to hepatocytes was competitively inhibited by minute quantities of T and Tn antigen. Springer (154) suggested that T and Tn may be involved in specific cell-cell adhesions required for invasion and metastasis by cancer cells. It is of interest that T and Tn also appear to be differentiation antigens. Barr et al. (194) studied fetal tissue 45–117 days after ovulation for T and Tn reactivity. Most fetal tissues during normal morphogenesis appear to contain some T and Tn-specific structures during gestational days 45 through 117. Their highest density is in fetal epithelia and mesothelia. One monoclonal anti-T reacted with all elements of erythropoiesis but with none of the epithelia (i.e., hepatocytes and bile duct epithelia). The authors suggested that as ABH antigens appear around the third month of gestation, this probably is when T and Tn is no longer detectable in fetal tissue. This work would suggest that "illegitimate" T and Tn are examples of carcinoembryonic antigens.

D. Immune Response to T and Tn Antigens

As mentioned previously, anti-T and anti-Tn are detected in the sera of all healthy adults. They are usually not detected in fetal or cord sera; they appear in the serum at about the same time as anti-A and anti-B. Springer and Tegtmeyer (149) showed that White Leghorn chicks raised in a germ-free environment produced no anti-T nor anti-Tn. When one dose of live *Escherichia coli* O_{86} was given in the drinking water to germ-free chicks, the chicks produced both anti-T and anti-Tn. Control chicks raised under ordinary conditions produced anti-T and anti-Tn without being deliberately given *E. coli*. Killed *E. coli* O_{86} was also given to 13 adults and six diarrheic and five healthy human infants. All infants but one suffering from diarrhea showed a significant increase ($\geq$ fourfold) in anti-T/Tn; in some, these antibodies were elicited de novo. All four adults with intestinal lesions had a significant increase of anti-T/Tn subsequent to ingestion of killed *E. coli*, as did five of nine healthy adults but to a lesser extent. These findings seem to support that anti-T and anti-Tn, like anti-A and anti-B, are antibodies to bacterial antigens that cross-react with similar antigens on human RBCs.

Springer's group has used a series of tests for humoral and cellular responses to T and Tn in cancer (150).

1. Humoral Response

Anti-T agglutinin levels appear to remain remarkably constant from about 3 years of age through adulthood (137,195,196). The normal range for anti-T scores was found to be 20–25 (154). About 37% of 287 preoperative patients with breast, respiratory, or gastrointestinal tract carcinomas had severely depressed anti-T scores (<12). Anti-T scores were depressed in only 9% of 309 patients with benign disease and in 8.5% of 200 putatively healthy individuals ($p < 0.001$ for cancer patients versus patients without cancer). A substantial increase (>25%) in anti-T was observed 1–5 months following curative surgery for breast and lung cancer; the increases were not observed in patients having surgery not related to cancer (150,154,198,199). The response appeared to be specific as ABO and Forssman antibodies did not increase following cancer surgery. Thatcher et al. (199) showed that 55 patients with untreated, histologically proven, disseminated melanoma had depressed anti-T compared with 60 healthy individuals ($p < 0.0005$). Anti-T levels increased following one injection of *Corynebacterium parvum* but no increase was observed following a similar injection with bacillus Calmette-Guérin (BCG). Springer et al. (200) had previously shown that T and Tn were strongly expressed on *C. parvum* but not on BCG.

Solid-phase immunoassays (SPIA) more than doubled the sensitivity of cancer detection compared to hemagglutination assays (201,202). The SPIA for anti-T measures IgM anti-T as a proportion of total serum IgM. Springer et al. (150) applied this assay to study sera from 368 healthy individuals and preoperative patients; 216 of the patients had cancer. The SPIA detected cancer in 92.2% of 90 patients with lung cancer (100% of 19 patients with squamous cell lung cancer); 82.6% of patients with breast cancer; 81.8% of patients with cancer of the bladder; 94.7% of patients with pancreatic cancer (all five patients with pancreatitis were negative). Sera from patients with benign tumors of the lung yielded 6.3% positive reactions and benign tumors of the breast 15.4%. Only 7.5% of healthy controls yielded a positive test result.

2. Cellular Response

Sterile, pyrogen, and leukocyte-free T and Tn antigens were prepared from normal human RBCs and used for delayed-type skin hypersensitivity reactions (DTHRs) and in vitro cell-mediated immune response (CMIR) as measured by leukocyte migration inhibition (LMI) (150).

Delayed-type skin hypersensitivity reactions were observed following skin tests of 951 patients and controls (150). Only one of 127 healthy controls gave a positive reaction. Over 80% of the malignancies, most of which were adenocarcinomas, yielded a positive result (88.2%) of lung cancer, 83.4% of breast cancer, 88.5% of pancreatic cancer, 86.7% of colon cancer. 83.5% bladder cancer). Positive DTHRs were observed in less than 10% of patients with benign tumors of the lung, breast, pancreas, colon and genital tract. No positive DTHRs were observed in 45 patients with other benign tumors or diseases (150).

3. Detection of Preclinical Stages of Cancer

Perhaps the most dramatic results of the studies by Springer's group are the sensitivity of their T/Tn system assays for detecting early cancer. They have evaluated longitudinally 34 patients (32 with breast and lung cancer) who yielded repeatedly positive assays but were free of cancer according to biopsy and radiographic results at that time. As of May 1990, 32 of 34 (64.7%) of patients who showed positive results more than once developed biopsy-verified cancer within 3 months to 10 years of follow-up. The predictive value of Springer's assays for cancer appear to be 80% in 5 years for lung cancer and 8 years for breast cancer (150).

IV. ASSOCIATION OF BLOOD GROUPS WITH COAGULATION

A. Association of ABO Blood Groups with Bleeding

In 1954, Aird and Bentall (203) showed that group O individuals were 20% more likely to develop a peptic (gastric and duodenal) ulcer than those of group A. Duodenal ulceration is approximately 50% more likely to develop in nonsecretors of ABH blood group substances than in secretors. Taking the liability of the group least susceptible to duodenal ulcer as 1, the relative liability of O secretors has been estimated as 1.35, A and B nonsecretors as 1.6, and O nonsecretors as 2.5 (203,204). Langman and Doll (204) found that the low incidence of secretors among the patients with duodenal ulcer was associated with an increased tendency to need surgical intervention but not with bleeding. Thus, there appears to be a true association between ulceration and the absence of secretion.

It is not surprising that as large quantities of blood group substances (ABH) are found in the gastrointestinal mucosa, and failure to secrete these substances in the mucus is associated with peptic ulcer, a protective role has been suggested for ABH substances (206–210). A simple protective mechanism seems an unlikely explanation because the total amount of blood group substance is similar for nonsecretors and secretors (i.e., Lewis substance is present in nonsecretors) (208). Furthermore, a blood group effect on peptic ulcer can be shown in nonsecretors alone. There have been many studies to correlate ABH secretor status with gastric function (e.g., acid secretion) but the results are inconclusive (211–217). It is interesting to note that ABH antigens can be detected in most cells of the body regardless of the secretor status of the individual, but when the brush border of cells from duodenal ulcers is examined, ABH substances are detected only in cells from secretors (218). Glynn et al. (208) showed that the effect of the secretor status appears to be confined to the specificity of the blood group antigens in the superficial epithelium of both stomach and duodenum. Thus, in secretors, A and B substances were abundant in superficial mucosa but were replaced in nonsecretors by Le^a substance. In the deep layers, A and B substances were present in nonsecretors as well as in secretors. It has been suggested that foodstuffs may contain substances with anti-A and/or anti-B activity (e.g., lectins from the pea and bean family have powerful red cell activity in vitro), and that these may damage the duodenal mucosa in nonsecretors but be neutralized in secretors (219). Another suggestion has been that foodstuffs may contain substances closely resembling human A and B antigens, and that these may react with anti-A and/or anti-B (in the capillaries of the gastric mucosa membrane) of the host causing a local alteration in the tissues; e.g., on the marginal surface.

A decade after the original report by Aird and Bentall (203), Langman and Doll (205) and Merckas et al. (206) showed that the association of group O with ulcers was not the with the ulcer itself but with *bleeding* ulcers. The original study was performed on only hospitalized patients who tend to be admitted because their ulcers are bleeding. Thus, the bleeding tendency that brings the patient to the hospital may account for the excess of group O reported by Aird and Bentall (203).

B. Association of ABO Blood Groups with Clotting

In contrast to the above findings, there appears to be an association with group A, thrombosis, serum cholesterol level, and myocardial infarction. Mourant and coworkers (220) analyzed data from the world's literature and confirmed that patients with thromboembolic disease include a raised proportion who are of group A. This applied to women taking oral contraceptives, to pregnant and puerperal women, and to coronary thrombosis cases. There was a mean relative incidence of 1.27 among group A patients with coronary thrombosis (3,089 patients) and 1.41 for other cases of thromboembolic disease (847 patients). Among pregnant and puerperal women with thromboembolism (220 patients), the relative incidence of A was 1.85, whereas among women taking oral contraceptives, the relative incidence of A was 3.12 (146 patients). On the other hand, susceptibility to coronary insufficiency, as shown by angina pectoris or coronary occlusion, without evidence of infarction (1,577 patients) is little, if at all, affected by a person's blood group. It could be calculated that among 1,000,000 group O women practicing oral contraception for 20 years, the expected number of deaths due to the method of contraception will be 211, whereas among 1,000,000 group A women it will be about 680. Despite the small numbers on which the calculations were based, it seems that the death rate from thrombosis is at least twice as high in A women as in O women (220).

Many reports have appeared in the literature supporting these conclusions (221–235). For instance, a 5-year prospective study of 10,000 Israeli male government employees over 40 years of age was conducted as part of the Israeli Heart Disease Project: Subjects with blood groups A_1, B and A_1B had a higher incidence rate of myocardial infarction than those of group O (221). Kingsbury (233) showed an excess of group A over O in 1,222 patients with aortoiliac and femoropopliteal artherosclerosis. Separation of the patients according to the type and extent of their arterial disease assessed from arteriograms showed the excess of group A to be concentrated in those with an occlusion, whereas the proportion of blood group O increased with the degree of mural artheroma.

Various parameters of dynamic blood coagulation and thrombus formation have been associated with ABO blood groups, e.g., the viscosity of thrombus, which implies the degree of interference with blood flow, and the degree of thrombus degradation, which is thought to relate to the propensity of microemboli formation. It has been suggested that blood microrheology differs not only in various cardiovascular disease groups but also differs within each group depending on the ABO blood group of the patients. These differences might depend on the peculiarities of the cell surfaces and the plasma proteins, especially fibrinogen (or fibrinogenlike proteins), characteristic to certain ABO blood groups (238). It has been suggested that etiological pathways of cardiovascular diseases may differ in patients of different ABO blood groups owing to these differences in their blood rheology and plasma protein activities (236–241).

1. Association with Serum Cholesterol Levels

There have been several substantial studies agreeing that serum cholesterol levels are higher in group A (242–249). These studies consisted of mainly adults of Western European ethnic backgrounds. This association did not seem to hold for Asians (250–252), African–Americans (253), or children/neonates (252,253). It has been suggested that the ABO-cholesterol relationships may differ according to race (252), cholesterol level (253–255), or be secondary to a more direct effect on one of the cholesterol fractions, such as esterified cholesterol (251) or β-lipoprotein (247,255,256). Fox et al. (257) studied 656 white and black adolescent children to answer several questions:

1. Is the ABO blood group locus associated with serum lipid and lipoprotein levels, and if so, at what levels is this association discernable?
2. Do phenotypic variations at the ABO locus have a similar effect on the serum level of white and African-American children?
3. Is there a direct association between ABO phenotype and total serum cholesterol (TC), or is this mediated through one of the lipoprotein cholesterol (LPC) fractions?

The data provided definitive answers for the first two questions (257). Following appropriate adjustment of lipid values for concomitant variables, mean levels of ABO phenotypes were found to differ significantly in both races (A > B in whites, B > O in blacks). Differences between highest and lowest ranking phenotypic means amounted to approximately 8 mg/dl TC in both races. Slightly over 1% (white sample) or 2% (black sample) of the total variation of adjusted TC values was accounted for by ABO phenotype. Although the difference between B and O phenotypic means in blacks was not satistically significant when adjusted cholesterol values were $\log_{10}$ transformed, the transform had little effect on the results of F-tests for heterogeneity of means or r^2 estimates in either race. Analysis of phenotypic ratios at different percentile levels of lipid and lipoprotein distributions indicated that phenotypic ratios for black and white children ranking above the 85th percentile of their respective β-LPC distributions differed significantly from ratios prevailing in the remainder of the study population. Among children with high β-LPC levels O:non-O ratios were consistently reduced in all race-sex groups; concomitantly, A:non-A ratios were selectively increased in whites and B:non-B ratios increased in blacks. Although ratio changes in the TC and LP index distributions were concordant with those in the β-LPC distribution, the data strongly suggest that the most direct association between the ABO locus and serum lipids or lipoproteins is with the β-LPC fraction (257).

2. Association with Serum Alkaline Phosphatase

A fascinating association between blood groups and serum alkaline phosphatase has emerged. Human serum alkaline phosphatase can be separated by starch-gel electrophoresis into a fast-moving component, thought to be derived from liver or bone, and a slower-moving fraction, thought to be dervied from the small intestine. The fast-moving fraction is present in all sera, whereas the slower-moving isoenzyme originally was described to be present only in the serum of group B and O secretors and never in group A secretors or nonsecretors of any group (258–262). A more sensitive technique demonstrated small amounts of enzyme in 10–15% of group A secretors and a smaller number of nonsecretors.

Alkaline phosphatases are present in many human tissues, including bone, intestine, kidney, liver, placenta, and leukocytes. Their physiological function is unknown. However, their localization to membranes suggests that they may be involved in the active transport of substances across these membranes (263). Fat ingestion appears to stimulate the appearance of the enzyme, with protein and carbohydrate having no effect (264–266). It has been questioned whether the same genetic factors involved in the blood group secretor and isoenzyme relationship may influence fat handling in the intestine.

C. Hypothesis to Explain Associations of ABO Blood Groups with Coagulation

As previously mentioned, group O individuals tend to suffer with bleeding from ulcers more than group A individuals. Thus, on one hand, there is a tendency to thrombose in group A and, on the other, for group O to bleed. Mourant (220) makes the interesting point that an earlier paper (267) had described that group A individuals have a higher average level of antihemophilic globulin (factor VIII) present in their plasma than do group O individuals. He suggested that the difference in factor VIII in the plasma, even within the physiological range, may determine whether clinically detectable bleeding may ocur from a deep ulcer or, on the other hand, in an atheromatous blood vessel, whether clotting will ensure. Kingsbury (233) conjectured that the higher frequency of group O in the atherosclerotic patients with increased mural atheroma (as opposed to the lower ratio of group O in the occlusion group) could be due to a tendency of the group O patients to hemorrhage (rather than thrombose) into the arterial walls, thus sustaining more tissue damage. Several other workers had confirmed the association of group A with a higher factor VIII level (268–272). There have also been associations with other coagulation factors such as von Willebrand factor (vWF), factor V, and factor IX (271,273–278).

V. ASSOCIATION OF BLOOD GROUPS WITH BACTERIA/INFECTION

Many bacteria, particularly gram-negative organisms (e.g., *E. coli*) are known to have chemical moieties on their surface that resemble blood group antigens. Springer (148, 279) tested 282 bacterial strains, of which 137 showed A, B, or H(O) specificity. In vitro activity as high as that of the blood group glycoproteins from human secretions was encountered in about 20% of these active bacteria. Springer's classic experiments in chickens showed that the anti-B in White Leghorn chickens was produced as a result of exposure to *E. coli* (Fig 8–1). He showed that normally, Leghorn chicks produced anti-B by the age of 30 days, but if they were brought up under germ-free conditions, anti-B was not formed (280). In contrast, if the chicks then were deliberately fed *E. coli*, high titers of anti-B were produced (280). Most blood group workers believe that a similar mechanism must operate in humans for the production of the so-called "naturally occurring" anti-A and anti-B isoagglutinins and perhaps all so-called naturally occurring antibodies.

A. Do ABO Antibodies Play a Protective Role in Bacterial Infections?

Mourant (281) raised the question whether infecting organisms are the primary factors for the polymorphism of ABO blood groups. Vogel, et al. (282) suggested that the geographical distribution of the ABO blood types has been greatly influenced by the severe selection exercised by the pandemics, such as plague and smallpox. They suggested that if an infecting microbe possessed a particular blood group activity, the infection would be better contained by persons who had the antibody reactive with the specificity. Assuming that an infecting microbe possessed blood group A activity, then the naturally occurring anti-A possessed by individuals of group B and O might contribute to host defense mechanisms against this microbe.

Vogel et al. (282) claimed that *Pasteurella pestis* was rich in H antigen, and that patients of group O, because of their inability to produce anti-H, fared poorly in plague epidemics. In accord with this concept, the O gene is now very frequent in places where few or no plague

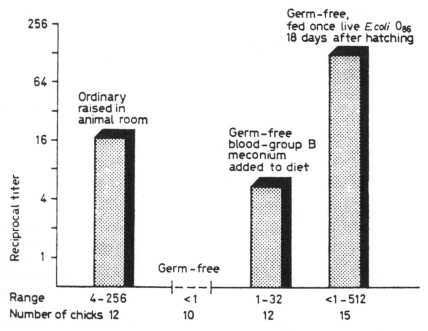

Figure 1 Production of anti-B by White Leghorn chickens. (From Ref. 280.)

epidemics have occurred, but its incidence is low in the ancient plague centers of Mongolia, the Orient (Turkey), and North Africa (lower Egypt). Vogel et al. (282) also showed the smallpox virus to possess an antigen similar to the A antigen, thus humoral resistance against smallpox may be more effective in patients of blood groups B and O who possess anti-A in their plasma. The Asian and African distribution of the A gene supports the theory of a selective disadvantage among individuals carrying this gene who are infected with smallpox virus. In areas with plague as well as smallpox, such as Mongolia, China, India, and parts of Russia, the relative frequency of the B gene is increased, possibly due to selection against the A as well as the O genes. Springer and Wiener disagreed with these conclusions, and the reader is referred to interesting communications from both sets of authors in the journal *Nature* (283). In 1985, Adalsteinsson (284) suggested that the low frequency of A and high frequency of O blood group genes in Iceland is the result of a selective disadvantage for group A during severe smallpox epidemics. He thought this was a much more likely explanation than the suggestion that the Icelandic population was more closely related to the Irish than Nordic peoples; a suggestion that was partly based on blood group distribution (285).

It has been suggested that blood group antibodies may play a protective role against bacteria. Springer (286) showed that hyperimmune anti-B sera retard the growth of *E. coli* O_{86} in the absence of complement, and Muschel (287) showed that in the presence of complement the bacterium is killed. Moody et al. (288) showed a decreased incidence of group O, as compared with group A, among patients infected with *Enterobacteriacae*. Robinson and coworkers (289) clearly demonstrated that there is an increased risk of gram-negative enteric infections, other than *Shigella*, to patients of blood groups B and AB when compared with individuals of blood group A and O. They showed that individuals of groups B and AB, regardless of ethnic background, have a 55% greater chance of developing an *E. coli* infection than patients of blood groups A and O. Among black and Puerto Rican patients, there was a 131% greater probability of *Salmonella* infections occurring in individuals of blood groups B and AB than A and O. Both *E. coli* and *Salmonella* have been shown by Springer to be rich in blood group B antigen; therefore they are perhaps able to survive better in individuals who lack anti-B (i.e., groups B and AB).

Wettels and Lichtman (290) compared the blood groups of 115 patients with *E. coli* septicemia with three control populations (138 patients with septicemia due to other organisms, 23,155 random hospitalized patients, and 40,038 normal blood donors). The relative incidence of B and AB (i.e., no anti-B) was significantly higher than A or O (i.e., possessing anti-B) in the group with *E. coli* septicemia. The conclusion was disputed by Sachs (291). In 1991, van Loon et al. (292) found no association of group O and *E. coli*–associated diarrhea in 510 rural Bangladeshis. Workers in the same institution (Matlab Hospital of the International Centre for Diarrhaeal Disease Research, Bangladesh) found a significant association of ABO blood groups and cholera (293). Patients with cholera were twice as likely to be of group O and one-ninth as likely to be group AB compared with community controls. Several other groups have reported similar associations (294–297).

Resistance to several other bacterial and viral infections have been associated with blood groups. An increased susceptibility to infection with *Neisseria gonorrhoeae* and blood group B has been noted in patients of different racial groups (298–300). Miller et al. (299) showed that *N. gonorrhoeae* could absorb anti-A and anti-B in vitro, which suggests the presence of A and B antigens on the gonococci. Anti-A and anti-B were shown not to be bactericidal for gonococci, but diferences were shown in the reactivity between gonococci and granulocytes and monocytes from donors of different ABO groups (301,302). Mandrell et al. (303) used a mouse monoclonal antibody to lipooligosaccharides of *N. gonorrhoeae* to define a similar structure on RBCs. This structure was type 1 (Galβ→4GlcNac) or n-acetyllactosamine. This structure is the terminal sequence in paragloboside, the precursor of A, B, H, I, i RBC antigens.

Two recent papers reported a possible association with acquired immune deficiency syndrome (AIDS). Adachi et al. (304) found that human T-cell lines infected with human immunodeficiency virus (HIV) and T cells from patients with AIDS expressed Le^y antigen, whereas normal T cells did not. Arendrup et al. (305) reported that carbohydrate epitopes on HIV may also be targets for monoclonal antibody (MAb)–mediated virus inhibition. They found that anti-A neutralized HIV produced by lymphocytes from group A donors but not from group B or O donors. The same workers had previously shown that a MAb, directed against blood group A antigen precipitated the major envelope glycoprotein gp 120 and that A-specific MAbs were able to inhibit cell-free HIV infection even though the A antigen is not normally expressed by the cells used for the production of HIV or as target cells for infection. Arendrup et al. (305) suggested that HIV infection of mononuclear cells from donors with blood group A appears to induce expression of host cell–encoded carbohydrate blood group A epitopes on HIV that can be targets for MAb-mediated viral neutralization. The authors (305) are currently trying to identify the possible A transferase mRNA in HIV-infected cells.

There have been other reports of associations of ABO group with many other infectious diseases. Table 6 lists the ones reviewed in 1989 by Berger et al. (306). The possible role of ABO blood group antibodies in protection against infection is very controversial, and the reader can obtain a great deal of information from several excellent reviews on the associations of bacteria with blood groups (148,307–309).

B. Blood Group Antibodies Other than Anti-A and Anti-B Associated with Infection

As mentioned previously, there is good evidence that so-called naturally occurring blood group antibodies are usually formed as an immune response to bacteria. Such antibodies are often predominately IgM and react optimally at colder temperatures. Relatively commonly encountered examples in healthy individuals, other than anti-A or anti-B, are anti-I, anti-M, anti-N, anti-P$_1$, anti-Le^a, anti-Le^b, anti-T, and anti-Tn. Rarer examples of seemingly naturally occurring

Table 6 Association of Blood Groups with Infectious Disease

Agent/Infection	Increased incidence of blood group antigen/antibody or secretor status
Bacterial	
Plague	O
Cholera	O
Leprosy	A,B (lepromatous form) O (tuberculoid form)
Yaws	M
Tuberculosis	O, B
Gonorrhoea	B
Streptococcus pneumoniae infection	B
Neisseria meningitidis infection	Nonsecretor
Haemophilus influenzae infection	Nonsecretor
Escherichia coli infection	B, AB
Viral	
Epstein-Barr Virus (EBV) infection	anti-i
Smallpox	A, AB
Mumps	O
Fungal	
Candida albicans	Nonsecretor

Source: Data from Ref. 306 (which contains all references to above associations).

antibodies in the Rh (especially anti-E) and Kell systems have been described. Sometimes "naturally occurring" autoantibodies, such as anti-I, can increase in titer and thermal range and cause autoimmune hemolytic anemia (AIHA) (Chapter 18). Other antibodies that usually occur as naturally occurring alloantibodies, such as anti-A, anti-B, anti-M, anti-N, anti-P_1, have been found sometimes as autoantibodies and sometimes they have been the cause of AIHA. Specificities of autoantibodies associated with AIHA are listed in Chapter XX and discussed in a comprehensive review by Garratty (16).

The occurrence of some blood group antibodies appear to be closely associated with certain diseases or infections. Approximately 50% of the cases of cold agglutinin syndrome (CAS) are secondary to *Mycoplasma pneumoniae* infection (310). These cases are associated with a hemolytic anemia caused by high-titer, high–thermal amplitude anti-I. The anti-I is often polyclonal in contrast to the monoclonal anti-I associated with chronic idiopathic CAS. This suggests that the condition may result from a stimulus to the naturally occurring anti-I. There are some data to support this conclusion but it is controversial whether CAS is purely due to an "I-like" antigen on *M. pneumoniae*. Two studies (from the same group) suggest that mycoplasma may alter the normal I antigen on RBCs causing it to become autogenic (311,312). In favor of this theory are the findings that it is difficult to adsorb anti-I with *M. pneumoniae* (313), and when rabbits are injected with mycoplasma alone, they do not make anti-I, but when injected with RBCs treated with mycoplasma, they produce anti-I (314).

In 1965, before any of the above work, Costea et al. (315) had reported that rabbits produced anti-I cold agglutinins when they were infected with *Listeria monocytogenes*, isolated from a patient with septicemia and CAS. Costea et al. (315) were able to adsorb anti-I with *L. monocytogenes*. In 1971, Costea et al. (316) injected rabbits and mice with live and killed *L. monocytogenes*, *M. pneumoniae*, and *Streptococcus* MG. In contrast to previous suggestions (311–314), Costea et al. (316) showed that modification of the RBC I antigen was not required for the induction of anti-I cold agglutinins. Killed organisms were as effective immunogens as live organisms. Rabbits produced anti-I cold agglutinins following immunization with all three organisms; maximum titers were similar. Adsorption of an immune serum with *M. pneumoniae* reduced its titer from 1024 to 20. Those that did not possess I antigens on their RBCs produced anti-I following challenge with (1) *M. pneumoniae* and (2) preincubation of live *M. pneumoniae* with human or rabbit RBCs having I antigen did not enhance the immune response. It is of interest to note that rabbit RBCs are richer in I antigen than human RBCs; thus they are probably not the ideal model to produce optimal amounts of anti-I. In a later paper, Costea et al. (317) produced support for their hypothesis that anti-I results from a direct stimulus of an I-like antigen on *M. pneumoniae*. They showed that the anti-I produced by rabbits and humans infected with *M. pneumoniae* could be inhibited by a crude lipopolysaccharide fraction isolated from the *M. pneumoniae*, *L. monocytogenes*, and *Streptococcus* MG (317). Lind (318) confirmed the findings of Costea et al. (316) that the anti-I induced by *M. pneumoniae*, *L. monocytogenes*, and *Streptococcus* MG could be adsorbed by the organism. Colhing and Brown (319) found anti-I was produced when rabbits were hyperimmunized with group C streptococcal vaccine.

Loomes et al. (320) showed that *M. pneumoniae* adheres to RBCs via receptors consisting of sialic acid α2-3 linked to long carbohydrate chains of Ii type, and they suggested that anti-I autoagglutinins are directed against the backbone on this receptor. Several experimental approaches led to this conclusion. First, oligosaccharides and glycoproteins containing sialic acid α2-3 linked to long-chain backbone structures of repeating N-acetyllactosamine (Galβ1→4GlcNAc) sequences of Ii antigen type were more potent inhibitors of *M. pneumoniae* binding than those with short carbohydrate chains. Second, glycophorin-deficient RBCs with normal levels of I antigen were shown to have normal *M. pneumoniae* binding. Third, the receptors on intact RBC membranes were shown to be susceptible to digestion with endo-β-galactosidase that specifically cleaves the linear domains of oligosaccharides of the Ii type.

Thus, it was deduced that minor sialyloligosaccharides, such as the long carbohydrate chains of bands 3 and 4.5 proteins rather than those of the major sialoglycoproteins (glycophorins) are the main receptors for this agent in intact RBC membranes. Such long carbohydrate chains also occur in minor Ii-active sialoglycolipids (gangliosides) of human RBC membranes and as major components of bovine RBC membranes.

In a later report, Loomes et al. (321) showed the inhibitory activity of a fraction of bovine RBCs containing long backbone structures of the I antigen type was 200 times greater than that of the short-chain gangliosides GM_3 and GT_{1b}. The binding of *M. pneumoniae* to I and i RBCs was similar, indicating the *M. pneumoniae* in its adhesive specificity may not distinguish between the branched carbohydrate I structures and the linear i structures (321). Loomes et al. (321) discussed the question: Why are autoantibodies to branched poly-N-acetyllactosamine (anti-I) rather than linear backbones produced following *M. pneumoniae* infection? *M. pneumoniae* infection usually occurs in children and young adults rather than neonates and the i type oligosaccharides of fetal erythrocytes are largely replaced by I structures during the first year of life. Moreover, the bronchial epithelium, which is the primary site of adhesion and infection by *M. pneumoniae,* produces sialoglycoproteins with branched carbohydrate backbones of the I antigen type. However, cells with the i type sequences are abundant in inflammatory tissues. For example, monocytes and lymphocytes are rich in sialylated sequences not only of I type but also of i type. Thus, massive amounts of immunogenic complexes may form in the inflamed respiratory tract containing the lipid-rich mycoplasma (a potential adjuvant) and I- and i-active host cells, including epithelium, lymphocytes, and accessory cells. It is intriguing that this infection ultimately results in the production of anti-I antibodies by B lymphocytes, which themselves express this antigen on their surface. Were it not for their cold-reactive properties, the anti-I antibodies would be suicidal for the B cells that produce them. Such autoablation may be the mechanism for selection against lymphocytes producing high-affinity (warm-reactive) anti-I antibodies and the survival of cells producing low-affinity (cold-reactive) antibodies (321). Further studies on the pathogenesis of the postinfective autoimmune disorder will be greatly facilitated by the knowledge of the adhesive specificity of *M. pneumoniae*.

In studying 192 sera containing cold autoagglutinis of anti-I specificity, König et al. (322) suggested that the sialylated structures described as a receptor for *M. pneumoniae* (320,321) are identical to the structures described for Fl and Gd. Fl and Gd have recently been renamed Sia-b1 (sialo-branched) and Sia/1b1,2 (sialo-linear and branched structures). Chapter 3 discusses the above in detail.

Anti-I^T is another cold autoagglutinin that was reported as a "naturally occurring" antibody but only in isolated populations (Melanesians [324]) and Yanomama indians in Venezuela (324). The occurrence of this antibody in isolated populations suggests that it may be there as a result of endemic infection. This hypothesis is supported by the transient nature of the antibody response in Venezuela (325). We described an interesting association of Hodgkin's disease with AIHA and anti-I^T in white Americans (326–327). In 1974, we reported finding an IgG auto anti-I^T in a 12-year-old white boy with Hodgkin's disease; no AIHA was obvious (326). In our 1974 study, four patients with warm antibody type AIHA associated with Hodgkin's disease were described (327). Three of the four had autoantibodies that demonstrated anti-I^T specificity. No further examples of auto-anti-I^T were found in 50 cases of Hodgkin's disease with no hemolytic anemia (47 cases had negative direct antiglobulin tests and 3 had positive direct antiglobulin tests but no hemolytic anemia). In addition, no further examples were found in 70 cases of warm-type AIHA either idiopathic or secondary to other diseases of the reticuloendothelial system (327). It should be noted that, as with the cold autoagglutinins showing anti-I^T specificity, the I^T specificity only becomes obvious when the eluates and/or serum were titrated against I adult, i cord, and i adult red cells and antiglobulin agglutination scores compared. In

1977, Freedman et al. (328) described a patient with AIHA with no history of Hodgkin's disease associated with an IgM complement-binding anti-I^T reacting optimally at 37C. Levine et al. (329) reported seven further cases of Hodgkin's disease associated with positive DATs due to IgG auto-anti-I^T. In 1990, we described an unusual case of cold agglutinin syndrome associated with anti-I^T (330).

Anti-i is not usually encountered in healthy individuals. It was first described in patients with diseases of the reticuloendothelial system (331,332) and can cause CAS (323). Later it was found to be detected in the sera of 70–90% of patients with infectious mononucleosis (333–335). McGinniss (336) made the suggestion that it would be most interesting to study the correlation of anti-i with antibodies to Epstein-Barr virus (EBV), especially in diseases such as Burkitt's lymphoma where high titer EBV antibodies are detected (337).

C. Miscellaneous Blood Groups Associated with Certain Organisms

McGinniss (336) discussed several rare associations of MN, K, and Jk^b with infections. Four children with bacterial infections associated with *Proteus mirabilis* in two cases and meningitis in two cases produced anti-M that was not detectable following resolution of the infection (338). An *E. coli* strain, causing pyelonephritis, would cause hemagglutination of only M + RBCs (339). It was suggested that this strain of *E. coli* recognized the NH_2 terminal amino acid sequence in glycophorin A, and that the M determinants may be present, as bacterial receptors, on uroepithelial cells, in addition to P determinants (see below).

Although "naturally" occurring anti-K are not common, most experienced immuno-hematologists have encountered at least one example of IgM agglutinating anti-K with no known antigenic stimulus. Examples of this phenomenon were first reported in 1963 (340). Tegoli et al. (341) and Kanal et al. (342) reported examples in patients with a mycobacterium infection. In 1978, Marsh et al. (343) and McGinniss et al. (344) reported cases associated with two other organisms. *E. coli*$_{0125}$:B15 and a D streptococcus *S. faecium* were shown to probably possess a "K-like" antigen on their membrane. Marsh et al. (343) showed that *E. coli* whole organisms inhibited an anti-A in their patient's (a 20-day-old baby) serum but not anti-K; disrupted organisms inhibited only the anti-K in the baby's serum. McGinniss et al. (344) showed that K– RBCs incubated in vitro with disrupted *S. faecium* became K+, but when incubated with whole organisms, the K type did not change. Another interesting finding was that *S. faecium* whole organisms would convert Jk(b–) RBCs to Jk(+) in vitro (336,344).

Although there have been no convincing further reports on the association of Jk^b with organisms, it is of interest that McGinniss et al. (345) also described an auto-anti-Jk^b found during a urinary tract infection due to *Proteus mirabilis*. When Jk(b–) RBCs were incubated in vitro with *P. mirabilis*, they reacted with some anti-Jk^b. McGinniss (336) also found that anti-Jk^b would react with Jk(b–) RBCs incubated in vitro with *Micrococcus* organisms.

It is of interest that Byrd et al. (346) showed a significant correlation between urinary tract infection with *S. faecalis* and renal graft failure, and that "K-like" and "Jk^b-like" antigens have been shown to be present on *S. faecium*. As far as I know, this relationship has not been pursued.

There have been several reports of human sera containing antibodies to various sugars. Bird et al. (347) found that 48% of the sera contained antibodies to the disaccharide melibiose. It was suggested that the melibiose antibodies might be stimulated by carbohydrate antigens on bacterial membranes.

D. Association of Blood Group Antigens and Bacterial Receptors

In the early 1980s, a series of papers were published showing that *E. coli* hemagglutinins reacted specifically with RBCs having P blood group antigens (348–353). Over 90% of *E. coli* isolated from 30 children with pyelonephritis showed mannose-resistant hemagglutination. The reactive target on human RBCs was found to be the P blood group antigen. The P glycolipids were shown to be the receptors for bacterial fimbriae (Fig 2). The P glycolipids are also present on uroepithelial cells and renal tissue where they mediate the adhesion of *E. coli* and their subsequent ascent to the kidney (351–358). This adhesion is necessary for the *E. coli* to resist the rinsing effect of urine and for efficient colonization (358).

Kaach et al. (359) immunized Rhesus monkeys with purified P fimbriae from *E. coli* during the last trimester of pregnancy. A delay in the onset of renal disease after bladder infection showed protection from passive immunization. This was associated with a high serum antibody titer. In addition to delayed onset of renal infection, a decreased number of immunized monkeys developed pyelonephritis. Cranberry juice is often recommended for treatment of urinary tract infections. It is of interest that cranberry (and blueberry) juice is thought to be effective because of its anti–*E. coli* adhesion properties (360–363). It would be of interest to see if there is any anti-P (lectin) activity in cranberry juice, thus competing with the *E. coli* fimbriae for the P receptor site.

Some other blood group antigens whose specificity is not determined by carbohydrates have been shown to be associated with the receptors for bacteria. Väisänen et al. (339) reported one strain of *E. coli* (018:K1:H7) associated with sepsis and meningitis of the newborn had hemagglutinating specificity associated with the MN sialoglycoprotein (SGP), glycophorin A. Their results suggested that the *E. coli* binds to the Neu-Acα2-Galβ1-3GalNAc sequence of the 0-linked saccharides of the MNSGP (glycophorin A). It is unfortunate that Parkinson et al. (364) termed their *E. coli* "S-fimbriated," which would imply that they were specific for the S blood group antigen that is found on glycophorin B not glycophorin A. Although no blood group associated was reported, Pieroni et al. (365) described a receptor on RBCs for an *E. coli* (078:H11) colonization factor antigen fimbriae. The receptor was identified as a sialoglycoprotein.

The specificity of about 20% of pyelonephritis-associated *E. coli* that are mannose-resistant hemagglutinins has not been identified and has been termed X. Nowicki et al. (366) used a systematic approach with RBCs of different phenotypes, including very rare types, to identify the receptor for an X hemagglutinin associated with the serotype 075 *E. coli*. The receptor was identified as the high-frequency Dr blood group antigen. The Dr antigen is a component of the

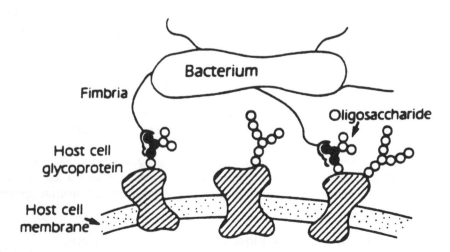

Figure 2   Fimbriae (pili) of *E. coli* attaching to oligosaccharides on host cell glycoproteins (e.g., P blood group antigen). (From Ref. 371.)

Cromer-related blood group complex (367) (Chapters 4 and 10). The molecule recognized by the Dr hemagglutinin is a chloramphenicol-like structure; tyrosine seems important to the specificity. Nowicki et al. (368,369) isolated the Dr hemagglutinin for a recombinant bacterial *E. coli* strain (BN406). A rabbit anti-Dr hemagglutinin was prepared and used by indirect immunofluorescence to study different tissues. The Dr antigen was expressed in different parts of the digestive, respiratory, urinary, and genital tracts and skin. Intense staining by Dr hemagglutinin was shown in colonic, bronchial, and endometrial glands. The strongest fluorescence was observed in the luminal domains of glands, but focal weak staining was also present in cell membranes. Renal tubular basement membrane and Bowman's capsule were strongly stained. P-fimbriated *E. coli* have been shown to adhere to glomeruli and to lumina of proximal and distal tubules but not to collecting ducts and peritubular sites. Dr hemagglutinin–positive strains shown adherence to Bowman's capsule and renal interstitium. The authors (368, 369) suggested that high density of the Dr-rich structures in the colon and urinary tract may permit *E. coli* to colonize the colon. Colonization of the lower urinary tract may occur due to attachment of *E. coli* to Dr-rich transitional epithelium in the ureter. High density of Dr in the Bowman's capsule may facilitate colonization of the glomerulus. It is of great interest that Dr^a is found on the same molecule as decay-accelerating factor (DAF) of the complement system (see Chapters 4 and 10). Nowicki et al. (370) have used the Dr hemagglutinin in a method for diagnosing paroxysmal nocturnal hemoglobinuria (PCH). Another interesting associated of Cromer-related antigens and disease is that two of only four known individuals whose RBCs lack all Cromer-related antigens (the Inab phenotype) and another individual who had anti-IFC but whose RBCs were never confirmed as being of the Inab phenotype had protein-losing enteropathy (367).

Rosenstein et al. (371) described a new type of adhesive specificity, revealed by oligosaccharide probes, in *E. coli* from patients with urinary tract infection. This adhesive specificity was unrelated to the presence of fimbriae. The new oligosaccharide receptor was affected by the presence of blood group genetic markers. It involved the dissacharide sequence linked to the membrane-associated lipid moiety of the host-cell glycolipids. It was proposed that this type of adhesive specificity may have had an important role in the invasion of damaged epithelial membranes where the saccharide-lipid function may be exposed. When the lactose-containing sequence is modified by additional monosaccharides (including the blood group monosaccharides), binding of *E. coli* is greatly impaired. It was predicted that the *Secretor* gene and the genes that code for blood group enzymes, or for other glycosyltransferases whose levels change in epithelial cells during differentiation, proliferation, and maturation, would strongly influence binding and hence susceptibility to invasion. It was pointed out that an association has already been suggested between nonsecretion of blood group B and AB antigens and susceptibility to recurrent urinary tract infections (322). Blackwell et al. (373) showed that although anti-B is known to be bactericidal for some serotypes of *E. coli* associated with urinary tract infection, it is not responsible for the association of groups B and AB with recurrent urinary tract infections. Lomberg et al. (374) reported that the ability of bacteria to bind to epithelial cells is increased in nonsecretors of ABH as compared with secretors. They suggested that products of the *Secretor* gene may shield the receptors. Sheinfeld et al. (375) found an increased frequency of Le(a+b–) and Le (a–b–) nonsecretors in 49 white women with recurrent urinary tract infections. In contrast to the recurrent urinary tract infection data, Lurie et al. (376) could find no association of ABO, Lewis, and P with recurrent pelvic inflammatory disease.

Some strains of *Haemophilus influenzae* also have fimbriae and cause in vitro hemagglutination (377). The degree of hemagglutination was found to correlate with adherence to buccal epithelial cells (377). The receptor for the fimbriae of *H. influenzae* has been found to be the AnWj blood group antigen (378,379). Red blood cells from the rare individuals of the Lu(a–b–)

dominant phenotype lack or have very weak AnWj and *H. influenzae* adherence receptor. The receptor molecule on the surfaces of the epithelial cell and the RBC are different, but the binding sites for the fimbriae are similar (380).

E. Association of Blood Group Antigens and Parasitic Infections

1. Association with Malaria

In 1975, Miller et al. (381) showed an association between malaria and Duffy blood group antigens. Red blood cells lacking Fy^a and Fy^b [Fy(a–b–)] were shown to be resistant to invasion by a monkey malaria, *Plasmodium knowlesi*. *Plasmodium knowlesi* is genetically related to the human malaria *P. vivax*. It has been known since the 1930s that many black people are resistant to infection by *P. vivax*. It had also been known that about 70% of the American black population and nearly 100% of the West African black population are Fy(a–b–). Epidemiological studies in endemic areas showed that *P. vivax* infections do not occur in individuals who are Fy(a–b–). *Plasmodium vivax* does not occur in West Africa where nearly 100% of the population is Fy(a–b–). Studies using *P. vivax* in volunteers demonstrated that the resistance in black people correlated with the Fy(a–b–) phenotype (382). Recently, a short-term in vitro culture system for *P. vivax* has been developed, and it has been shown that these parasites, like *P. knowlesi*, cannot invade Fy(a–b–) erythrocytes (383). It is important to note that Fy^a and Fy^b epitopes per se do not appear to constitute the actual binding site recognized by the parasite for the following reasons: (1) *P. knowlesi* parasites invade Fy(a+b–) and Fy(a–b+) human erythrocytes equally well; and (2) erythrocytes of rhesus and Kra monkeys, which express Fy^b, can still be invaded after Fy^b is removed by chymotrypsin. It is likely that the actual binding site recognized by *P. knowlesi* and *P. vivax* is on the same protein as the Fy^a and Fy^b determinants (384). It is of interest that *P. vivax* requires two ligands for invasion. One ligand may be associated with Duffy antigens and the other may be expressed on reticulocytes but not on mature RBCs (385). The Duffy associated ligand may be one designated Fy^6 (383).

The ligand for *P. falciparum* is different from that of *P. vivax*. *Plasmodium falciparum* invades Fy(a–b–) RBCs equally to Fy(a+) and Fy(b+) RBCs. Miller et al. (386) tested RBCs of various null phenotypes and found that none resisted invasion by *P. falciparum* to the extent noted with Fy(a–b–) and *P. vivax*. Red blood cells of the En(a–) phenotype, neuraminidase-treated RBCs of common phenotype, showed a 50% reduction in invasion by *P. falciparum*. Subsequent studies in other laboratories using different strains of *P. falciparum* showed a 95% reduction in invasion with neuraminidase-treated RBCs (387,388). Pavsol et al. (389) and Cartron et al. (390) showed that En(a–), Tn, Cad, and Wr(b–) RBCs resisted invasion. In contrast to Miller et al. (386), Pavsol et al. (389) and Facer et al. (391) found that S–s–U– and S–s–U+ RBCs showed considerable resistance to invasion by *P. falciparum;* trypsinized S–s– and En(a–) RBCs were almost completely resistant to invasion. All the phenotypes that showed resistance to invasion by *P. falciparum* had abnormalities of glycophorin A or B. Pavsol et al. (389) suggested that the initial attachment of the merozoite surface coat to the red cell may reflect a lectin-ligand like interaction in which the parasite binds in a specific manner to a cluster of oligosaccharides present on glycophorin A or B (or both). Once attachment has occurred and the apical end of the merozoite with a specialized organelles has oriented to the membrane, further specific conformational alterations may occur that trigger the process of red cell deformation and parasite entry. They suggested that possibly the Wr^b determinant on glycophorin A (and possibly a homologous portion of glycophorin B) located close to the membrane acts as the trigger. Later studies (392–395) revealed that the results obtained with Wr(b–) RBCs were inaccurate owing to the age of the Wr(b–) RBCs used by Pavsol et al. (389); fresh Wr(b–) RBCs were found to be fully susceptible to invasion by *P. falciparum* (392–395).

The above results suggest that as glycophorin A–deficient En(a–) RBCs are resistant to invasion, that glycophorin A is an important ligand. Glycophorin B also appears to play a role as glycophorin B–deficient RBCs (S–s–U–) are less susceptible to invasion. Trypsin-treated RBCs are also resistant to invasion; trypsin treatment cleaves glycophorins A and C, whereas glycophorin B remains unchanged. Although trypsin-treated En(a–) RBCs are more resistant to invasion than untreated En(a–) RBCs (391), which would suggest that glycophorin C may also be invaded, recent studies showed that neuraminidase-treated RBCs of the rare Gerbich null RBCs of the Leach type, which lack glycophorin C, are invaded by *P. falciparum* comparably to normal neuraminidase-treated RBCs (394). Sialic acid is required for all strains of *P. falciparum* to bind to human RBCs. Hadley et al. (396) showed that M^kM^k RBCs, which lack glycophorin A and B, showed resistance to invasion by some strains of *P. falciparum* but was invaded by other strains. The 7G8 strain invaded M^kM^k erythrocytes and neuraminidase-treated normal erythrocytes with >50% the efficiency of normal erythrocytes. In contrast, the Camp strain invaded M^kM^k erythrocytes at 20% of control and neuraminidase-treated normal erythrocytes at only 1.8% of control. Invasion of M^kM^k erythrocytes by 7G8 parasites was unaffected by treatment with neuraminidase but was markedly reduced by treatment with trypsin. In contrast, invasion of M^kM^k cells by Camp parasites was markedly reduced by neuraminidase but was unaffected by trypsin. The authors concluded that the 7G8 and Camp strains differ in ligand requirements for invasion and that 7G8 requires a trypsin-sensitive ligand distinct from glycophorins A and B. The data suggest that the ligand on glycophorin is primarily the sialic acid and possible other sugars and may not require the peptide backbone. Furthermore, the receptor heterogeneity includes differing requirements for sialic acid, and the requirement for a trypsin-sensitive ligand distinct from glycophorins A and B.

Several *P. falciparum* merozoite antigens involved in the invasion process have been isolated (397–399). One of these, a major *P. falciparum* merozoite antigen Pf200, has the property of binding to sialic acid. Genes for RBC-binding proteins for *P. knowlesi* (400). *Plasmodium vivax* (401) and *P. falciparum* (402–404) have also been cloned and sequenced. Hadley (384) suggested two hypotheses:

Hypothesis 1: There is a proven receptor heterogeneity among *P. falciparum* parasites. Parasites that depend heavily on sialic acid for invasion also depend heavily on the presence of glycophorin A; parasites that are less dependent on sialic acid are less dependent on glycophorin A.

Hypothesis 2: The importance of glycophorin A resides in the fact that it provides sialic acid for a sialic acid–dependent site rather than a peptide domain for parasite binding.

2. Association with Parasites Other than Malaria

In 1957, Cameron and Staveley showed that the fluid from granuloma, formed in response to infection with *Echinococcus* tapeworm, contained a substance that would inhibit anti-P_1 and anti-P (405,406). Hydatid cyst fluid provided a rich source of P substance for studies on the chemistry of P blood group system antigens. Prokop and Schlesinger reported that extracts from the worms *Lumbricus terrestris* (407) and *Ascaris suum* (408) inhibited anti-P_1. Devan et al. (409) suggested that liver flukes may also possess P_1 antigen.

There are three reports showing an increase of group A compared with group O in patients with giardiasis *(Giardia lamblia)* (410–412). One study did not agree with this association (413). Leishmanial parasites have been shown to react with anti-B, anti-M, anti-N, and anti-T (414–416). Greenblatt et al. (416) suggested that *Leishmania* parasites may utilize a system of camouflage or mimicry of host blood group antigens to evade host defense mechanisms.

VI. ASSOCIATION OF DISEASE WITH DECREASES AND INCREASES OF RBC ANTIGENS, ACQUIRED RBC ANTIGENS, AND "NULL" PHENOTYPES

A. Diseases Associated with Decreases in Blood Group Antigens on RBCs

1. Decreased ABH Antigens on RBCs

Modifications of blood group antigens by disease was first noted in the course of acute leukemia (417). Numerous reports exist of weakened A, B, H, and I RBC antigens in leukemia (418,419). A patient may start with a normal A_1 antigen, which during the course of the disease may begin to react more weakly with anti-A serum, eventually perhaps appearing like A_3; finally, the RBCs may not agglutinate at all but can be shown to absorb anti-A, which has been termed A_g. If the patient is a secretor, then A substance will be present in the saliva, thus the reactions are similar to those seen in the genetically weak A termed A_m. The A antigen has been shown to weaken also in preleukemia, aplastic anemia, and refractory anemia (Fig 3) (418–422). It was suggested that the antigenic abnormalities may be of enzymatic origin. ABH antigens were reported to be depressed in about 20% of group O patients with acute leukemia (418,421,423).

It is of interest to note that sometimes only some of the RBCs are affected, suggesting an abnormal clone of cells (418,424,425). Renton et al. (426) described a fascinating example of this. A group A_1B leukemic patient lost all A_1 antigenic activity. Renton et al. were able to separate AB, A, B. and O cells from the patient's blood. The proportions were as follows: 20% O, 12% A, 42% B, and 20% AB. It was thought that the O cells were produced as the result of two independent processes (i.e., loss of A and B), suggesting that the alteration was at a

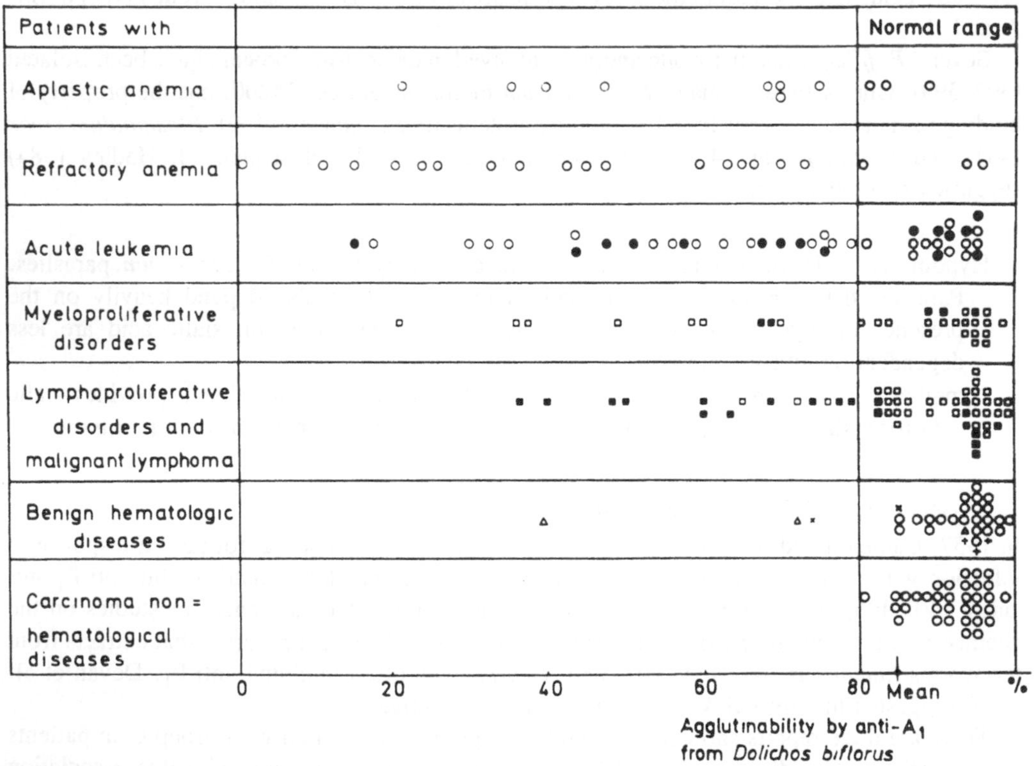

Figure 3 Reactions of group A RBCs, from patients with various hematological conditions, with anti-A_1. The mean agglutination scores and normal range are in the box on the right side of the figure. Any scores on the left side of this box indicate reduced A antigen status of RBCs. (From Ref. 422.)

chromosomal level. Renton et al. (426) and others (427) have shown that normal RBCs transfused into such patients retain an intact A antigen, whereas the patients' own cells continue to undergo modification. Depressions of ABH antigens have been noted in pregnancy (428) and on rare occasions in normal individuals (particularly the aged). Salmon (421) describes a case of an elderly woman (70 years when first seen) who was hematologically normal, with a dual population of RBCs, 50% of the hematopoietic tissue being unable to produce A_1 antigen. These RBCs were shown also to have a deficiency of the RBC enzyme adenylate kinase 1 (AK1). It is known that the *AK1* locus is close to the *ABO* locus on the long arm of chromosome 9 at 9q34. It was suggested that in one clone of cells in these individuals, the portion of chromosome 9 carrying *ABO* and *AK1* is affected (418,421). A patient with erythroleukemia with weakened A antigens and AK1 deficiency has also been described (429).

Salmon's group (421) demonstrated that the N-acetylgalactosaminyl transferase activity in a leukemic male patient, with depressed A antigen, was significantly less active than the product of the same gene in his daughter. The same was noted in another family of a leukemic patient (421). Thus, the antigenic modification in leukemia appeared to be related to a defect in the direct product of the gene rather than a membrane defect. Salmon believes there are striking differences between the antigenic modifications associated with disease (e.g., leukemia) and those appearing in normal individuals (e.g., the elderly). In normal individuals, the modifications seem to affect only one clone of cells, with only the blood group antigens (ABH) usually being affected, whereas in the leukemic or preleukemic states, modifications are multiple, polyclonal, and independent. The patients with leukemia or refractory anemia demonstrated depressions in RBC enzymes and immunoglobulin genetic markers (420–422). Kuhns et al. (439) confirmed the depression of transferase activity in leukemia, but found that the effect was mainly on the H-transferase. The serum level of H-transferase was correlated with the course of the disease in 54 patients with acute myeloid leukemia (AML), whereas the serum level of A-transferase was often unchanged. In almost all patients with AML, the serum A-transferase level was normal or low-normal range before treatment, whereas the serum level of H-transferase was uniformly low (430). During remission, H-transferase activity increased and fell again during relapse. In four of eight group A patients, A-transferase activity increased during remission but remained unchanged in the other four patients. These findings were confirmed by Koscielak et al. (431), who added the interesting findings that platelets are a rich source of at least one α-L-fucosyltransferase. The authors suggested the presence of platelets would influence transferase assay results and may explain some of the discrepancies in the literature.

Crookston (419) discussed the possible etiology of the blood group changes associated with leukemia and emphasized that only about 20–30% of the A- and B-transferases present in serum comes from hemopoietic tissue, whereas the H-transferase in serum appears to be derived entirely from hemopoietic tissue (the latter was disputed by Yoshida et al. [430]). If these assumptions, are true, then in patients whose RBC ABH antigens are weakened, one might expect this change to correlate with the level of H-transferase but not with the level of A- or B-transferase in the serum (419). The cause of a specific deficiency of the α-2-fucosyltransferase (H-transferase) in acute myeloid leukemia is unknown. The low level is not related to anemia but may be related to a deficiency of the enzyme in leukocytes; leukemic leukocytes are known to have a low level of H-enzyme (430).

Crookston (419) also discusses the interesting facts that the locus for the *A* and *B* genes is on chromosome 9 (at position 9q34). In chronic myeloid leukemia (CML), there is commonly a reciprocal translocation between a segment of the long arm of chromosome 9 and a segment of the long arm of chromosome 22. After the translocation, chromosome 22 is smaller but it now carries an oncogene (in 9q34). This chromosome is found in 96% of patients with typical chronic myeloid leukemia (CML). If ABO was involved in the 9; 22 translocation, one would expect to find weakened A and B antigens more often in CML, but the phenomenon is much more common in AML. In AML, a consistent chromosome translocation is from the long arm of 21 to the long arm to chromosome 8 (419); so far, neither of these chromosomes has been shown to carry a locus for blood group genes. Yoshida et al. (432) described a preleukemic patient whose RBC B antigens were severely depressed prior to treatment. The plasma and bone marrow H-transferase activity was not severely depressed; however, B-transferase activity was drastically reduced in the patient's bone marrow. The amount of H on the patient's RBCs was comparable to a group O. The authors suggested that the diminished B antigen was caused mainly by the blockage of conversion of H substance to B substance. The viral oncogene c-abl, linked to the ABO locus at q34 of chromosome 9, may occasionally suppress the expression of A and B enzymes and antigens. Atkinson et al. (433) described a group A patient with myelomonocytic leukemia who lost his RBC A antigens. The membranes were incubated with uridine diphosphate (UDP)-N-acetyl-D-^{14}C galactosamine in plasma from the patient and controls with group A and O RBCs. Red blood cell membranes from the patient behaved normally in that they incorporated the terminal carbohydrate responsible for blood group A activity. Scanning electron microscopy showed that the patient's RBCs had striking morphological changes, with marked crenation and numerous knisocytes and dacryocytes. It was concluded that loss of the A antigen in this patient was not due to an abnormality of the enzyme required to convert H substance to A substance. It was postulated that weakening of the A antigen in some patients with leukemia may be related to a steric modification associated with abnormal RBC morphology. It is of great interest that this depression of ABH antigens on RBCs appears to predict a leukemic state just as loss of ABH on tissue appear to predict metastases (see above). Several cases of depressed antigens being noted before clinically active leukemia was detected have been recorded (434,435).

2. Decreased RBC Antigens Other than ABH Associated with Leukemia and Other Malignant Blood Disorders

It is rare to encounter depressed antigens other than ABH associated with leukemia but some have been described. Depressed Rh antigens and Rh mosaicism have been reported associated with leukemia (436–439), myeloid metaplasia (440), myelofibrosis (441,442), and polycythemia (443,444). It is interesting to note that only depressions of D, C, and E have been described; so far, c and e antigens appear to be unaffected in this group of diseases, all of which may represent an abnormal clone of stem cells.

As the gene for Rh is located on chromosome 1, the loss of Rh antigens has often been associated with chromosome abnormalities. Marsh et al. (442) described a patient with myelofibrosis whose RBCs lost D antigen and who had deletion of chromosome 1. Bracey et al. (438) described a patient with CML whose RBCs had depressed D and C antigens. At the time when the patient's bone marrow revealed 100% Philadelphia (Ph^1)–positive chromosomes, the blood group antigens were normal. When 25% of the cells where Ph^1 negative, only 27% of the RBCs expressed D antigen. When the Ph^1-negative RBCs rose to 75%, the D antigen was present in 75% of the RBCs. This suggested that normalization of previously altered RBC antigens may reflect resurgence of normal stem cell lines. Cooper et al. (440) reported a male patient with myeloid metaplasia who lost RBC D antigens and who had an anomaly involving chromosomes 1 and 13 in 100% of the cells. An interesting finding in this patient was anti–D + C in the serum when the patient had never been transfused. Abnormalities of chromosome 1 do not explain all the Rh depressions, as some patients have been described with depressed Rh antigens and normal chromosome 1 (438,445).

Depressions of some blood group antigens associated with leukemia other than ABH and Rh have been described. Those include M, N. Le^a, Le^b, and I (446–451). Some patients have shown a depression of several antigens (448).

3. Miscellaneous Diseases Associated with Depressed RBC Antigens

Booth et al. (452) reported that many antigens, including I^T, I^F, CW, D, C, e, S, s, U, Kp^b, Jk^a, Jk^b, Xg^a, Wr^b, Sc1, Di^b, and En^a, were depressed in Melanesians with recessively inherited ovalocytosis. About 15% of Melanesians from the coastal areas of Papua, New Guinea, have ovalocytosis and depressed antigens.

There have now been many reports of a variety of blood group antigens becoming depressed in cases of autoimmune hemolytic anemia. The antigens include those of the Rh, Kell, Duffy, and Kidd systems, LW, Ge, AnWj, En^a, Co, and Sc1 (references for each of these are listed in the review by Garratty [452]). The depression usually occurs when antibody to the respective antigen is present in the serum. Thus, as the antibody can appear to be an alloantibody, it is often termed a mimicking antibody. When the antibody weakens, the antigen appears again on the patients's RBCs. It is unknown what causes this phenomenon. It is possible that viruses may depress RBC antigens enough that autoantibodies of the mimicking type are produced; they may sensitize RBCs with the most antigen, leading to their premature destruction, leaving only RBCs with depressed or absent antigens in the circulation.

4. Decreased Blood Group Antigens on Leukocytes

ABH antigens are present on normal lymphocytes but are absent or depressed on the lymphocytes of patients with chronic lymphatic leukemia (CLL) (453). The i antigen on lymphocytes, unlike RBCs, is detectable throughout adult life (454). In a series of papers, Shumak et al. (455–457) showed that the amount of i antigen on lymphocytes can aid in the differential diagnosis of leukemia (Table 7). They showed that i antigen is markedly decreased on the lymphocytes of patients with CLL. The authors suggested that this was useful in differentiating CLL from lymphocytosis due to other causes (e.g., malignancy or infection) where i antigen status is normal. They also showed that blast cells can be classified as myeloid or lymphoid according to their i status (456). Lymphoid blast cells had normal amounts of i antigen, but the amount of i antigen on myeloid blast cells was greatly decreased. One interesting finding was that the

Table 7 Reactions of Lymphocytes and Blast Cells with Anti-i: An Aid in the Diagnosis of Leukemia

Cells	Reaction[a] with anti-i (Den.)
Lymphocytes	
reactive lymphocytosis[b]	Normal
classic CLL	Decreased
early or morphologically atypical CLL	Decreased
lymphosarcoma-cell leukemia	Normal
Blast Cells	
classic AML (M2)[c]	Decreased
classic ALL	Normal
CML blast-cell crisis	Decreased or normal
acute undifferentiated leukemia	
myeloid (M1)	Decreased
lymphoid	Normal

[a]Compared with reaction of normal lymphocytes
[b]Lymphocytosis due to solid tumor or infection
CLL = chronic lymphoid leukemia
AML = acute myeloid leukemia
ALL = acute lymphoid leukemia
[c]FAB classification of acute leukemia
Source: Modified from Ref. 491.

source of anti-i was important for these differential diagnoses; the anti-i associated with infectious mononucleosis was found to be unsuitable (455,456).

The i antigen is also detected on granulocytes and macrophages during adult life (458). O'Hara et al. (45974) studied i antigen on myeloid progenitors of human bone marrow cultured in vitro. Colony-forming units-erythroid (CFU-E) were found to be relatively rich in i antigen, but the amount of i antigen varied considerably from person to person. The variation in antigen expression on these cells distinguishes them qualitatively from i_{cord} RBCs and circulating lymphocytes, which express i antigen on all cells, and from circulating granulocytes and macrophages, the majority of which express i antigen, although none are in cell cycle. Thomas (475) has shown that anti-i reacts with cultured lymphocytes that are in the S or G_2 phase of the cell cycle but not with cells in the G_1 or G_0 phase. Thus, O'Hara et al. (459) suggested that the i antigen is restricted to those marrow progenitor cells that are cycling, and that this raises the possibility that i may have a role in the progression of cells through the cell cycle.

B. Disease Associated with Increases of Blood Group Antigens on RBCs

The i antigen is the only blood group antigen that is found commonly to be increased on RBCs associated with certain hematological conditions (419,460–4652). Table 8 lists conditions that have been shown to be sometimes associated with increased i antigen. By far the most impressive increase is that associated with the most common form of dyserythropoietic anemia, HEMPAS (hereditary erythroblastic multinuclearity with a positive acidified-serum test) (463). Red blood cells from patients with HEMPAS react as strongly with anti-i as i_{cord} RBCs. In contrast to the rare i_{adult} RBCs, HEMPAS RBCs react normally, or even give stronger reactions than normal, with anti-I. There is no correlation with the expression of i and fetal hemoglobin (461,464,465). Hillman and Giblett (464) bled volunteers of up to 3,500 ml of blood and showed that the i antigen increased on their RBCs but ABH antigens were unchanged. They suggested that the increase in i was related to the shortened marrow transit time. This is an interesting hypothesis because it assumed that young RBCs in the bone marrow have more i than mature RBCs. Although at that time, everyone agreed that fetal RBCs had more i than adult RBCs, and that after 18 months of age most of the circulating RBCs have very little i present, there were no data showing that the same applied to maturing RBCs in the marrow. More recently, several studies have suggested that i is present in greater quantities on RBC precursors and younger

Table 8 Hematological Conditions Where i Antigen Is
Usually or Sometimes Increased

Usually Increased
    congential dyserythropoietic anemia type 2 (HEMPAS)
    thalassemia
    acute leukemia
    paroxysmal nocturnal hemoglobinuria
    myeloproliferative disorders
    aplastic anemia
    refractory anemia
Sometimes Increased
    sickle cell anemia
    congenital spherocytosis
    autoimmune hemolytic anemia

Source: Data from Refs. 460–463.

RBCs in the bone marrow (467,468). Nevertheless, two studies disagreed with the marrow transit time hypothesis (464,469). Cooper et al. (469) found that RBCs of 13 of 15 patients with sideroblastic anemia and 7 of 8 patients with megaloblastic anemia had increased i and I on their RBCs. They were unable to correlate the increased i with a decreased marrow transit time; the authors considered disordered erythropoiesis to be a more likely explanation. Similarly, Maniatis and Bertkes (464) did not agree that the increase in i in sickle cell anemia was associated with marrow transit time; these authors suggested that the i increase may reflect on alteration of the cell membrane.

It has been suggested that the i antigen is increased on the RBCs of children with congenital hypoplastic anemia and not on RBCs from patients with transient erythroblastopenia (469). Determination of RBC i status is often used in the differential diagnosis of this condition. I have never been impressed with the data that supports these claims.

One other blood group antigen, the Bg antigen, has been shown to increase in strength when associated with certain hematological conditions. Morton et al. (471,472) showed that Bg, which is an HLA-related RBC antigen (473,474) is increased in many hematological conditions. Bg antigens are thought to be remnants of HLA antigens on RBCs. A considerable increase of Bg on RBCs was noted in infectious mononucleosis (471) and hematological diseases of the lymphoid system (e.g., chronic lymphatic leukemia) (472). Twenty-nine percent of normal donor RBCs reacted with anti-Bg^a (HLA-B7), but 77% of RBCs from CLL reacted, and 42–48% of RBCs from AML, CML, lymphoma, myeloma, and hemolytic anemia (reticulocytes >30%) reacted. With anti-Bg^b (HLA-B17), only 12% of normal donors reacted, but 50% of RBCs from CLL and 52% of RBCs from lymphomas and myelomas reacted (472).

C. Diseases that Are Associated with Acquired RBC Antigens

Some antigens have been described that appear to be acquired by the RBCs of the patient during an illness. The antigens may be cryptantigens that are normally "hidden" or covered" on RBCs of healthy individuals (476). The antigens are most often acquired transiently and disappear when the illness (e.g., infection) resolves; a few acquired antigens appear to be persistent. The antigens are often detected because they cause the RBCs to become poly-agglutinable; that is to say, the RBCs will react with most sera from adults. This is because the reactive sera contain naturally occurring antibodies to the acquired antigens. This subject has been reviewed comprehensively in the literature and will only be summarized and updated in this chapter. The reader should refer to the excellent reviews by Beck (476), Levine et al. (477), and Judd (478).

1. Acquired B Antigens

There have been many papers on this subject. Since it was first reported in 1959, conclusions that have been drawn are (1) most cases are associated with diseases of the intestine (e.g., cancer of the colon); (2) usually only group A individuals acquire the B antigen; (3) the anti-B present in the serum of the group A individual acquiring the B antigen does not react with any acquired B antigens; and (4) there appear to be two mechanisms that may cause the phenomenon, but the most common mechanism is probably deacetylation of the A structure by bacterial enzymes. Gerbal et al. (479) suggested that a bacterial deacetylase could convert the terminal sugar N-acetylgalactosamine of the A antigen into galactosamine that may cross-react with anti-B. This can be reproduced in vitro with the deacetylase produced by Clostridium tertium. Later Gerbal et al. (480) supported their hypothesis by showing that the acquired B could be abolished by reacetylation induced by mild treatment of the RBCs in vitro with acetic anhydride. There is some evidence to suggest that sometimes the acquired B might be caused by adsorption of a B-like substance from E. coli$_{O86}$ and Proteus vulgaris onto group A and O RBCs.

2. *Acquired Antigens (T, Tn, Th, Tx, VA) Associated with Polyagglutinable RBCs*

The structure of T and Tn is well defined but, Th, Tx, and VA are not so well defined. They are all present as cryptantigens', that is to say, none of them are usually available for reaction with their respective antibodies on the RBCs of healthy individuals. It has been known for years that bacterial (e.g., *Clostridium perfringens, Vibrio cholerae*) or viral (e.g., influenza) neuraminidases can cleave the terminal N-acetyl-neuraminic acid (NeuAc) from RBC membrane sialoglycoproteins (SGPs), exposing B-linked D-galactose, which is the immunospecific sugar for T specificity (137,138,476,478). This can be shown readily in vitro, and sometimes T appears on RBCs in vivo. The T structure will react with anti-T present in most sera from adults and will react with several lectins (e.g., *Arachis hypogae* [peanut], *Vicia cretica, Glycine soja*]). The reactions with *G. soja* reflect the reduced level of sialic acid; this is also reflected by the finding that T-transformed RBCs do not aggregate in hexadimethrine bromide (Polybrene). Tn, the precursor of T, is formed when galactose is removed from the T structure.

Acquired T Antigen. As mentioned previously, in vivo T-transformed RBCs are most commonly encountered in patients with febrile infections. Rawlinson and Stratton (481) detected only one case in 10,000 random hospital patients, but Buskila et al. (482) detected T-transformed RBCs in 55% of a selected group of 238 patients with malignancies and sepsis. Lenz et al. (482) studied 53 adult surgical intensive care unit patients with septicemia. When using *A. hypogoea* and *G. soja* by direct antiglobulin tests (as used by Buskila et al. [482]), 4% of the patients were found to have T-transformed RBCs, but when an antiglobulin test utilizing rabbit anti–*A. hypogoea* was used in addition, 32% of the patients had reactive RBCs. Serum neuraminidase and serum hemoglobin were found to be elevated in 71% of the patients with T-transformed RBCs and 19 and 14%, respectively, of patients with no T transformation. The authors concluded that T transformation of RBCs may be a significant factor in the hemolytic anemia associated with severe infection. Adams et al. (484) studied T transformation in 108 patients with AIDS; 7% of patients with AIDS and 3% of patients without AIDS had T-transformed RBCs. The authors suggested that T transformation should be considered in the differential diagnosis of the hemolytic anemia associated with AIDS.

A very interesting association of T transformation with hemolytic uremic anemia (HUS) has been noted (476,477). In a series of 24 children exhibiting T transformation of their RBCs, Porschmann and Fischer (484) found that 7 had HUS. Klein et al. (486) and Seger et al. (485) described four cases of HUS associated with T-transformed RBCs and pneumonococcal pneumonia. Klein et al. (458) demonstrated T antigen on the RBCs and renal glomeruli of both their patients. It was suggested that pneumoccal neuraminidase might have caused the T transformation. Hamilton et al. (488) also described a case of fatal HUS associated with T-transformed RBCs. The authors suggested that the acute hemolysis was due to renal microangiopathy, probably the result of T-transformation of renal endothelial cells.

Acquired Tn Antigen. One of the most interesting forms of RBC polyagglutination is that associated with the appearance of Tn on the RBCs and platelets. Such patients often have an associated thrombocytopenia and less commonly a hemolytic anemia (139–145, 476–478). Tn transformation of RBCs, in contrast to T, Tk, Th, and Tx transformation, appears to be unassociated with bacterial infection. Tn is the immediate precursor of T. It appears that the appearance of Tn is due to a deficiency of a galactosyl transferase that prevents Tn from being made into T (146,147,489). The transferase deficiency is thought to be the result of genetic dysfunction in a mutant hemopoietic stem cell (490,492). Only some of the RBCs have Tn on them; this can vary from 5 to 95%. Thus, some aspects of the Tn syndrome are similar to paroxysmal nocturnal hemoglobinuria. Tn RBCs are agglutinated specifically by adult sera containing anti-Tn and *Salvia sclarea;* they will also cross-react with lectins that detect A structures that are similar to Tn (e.g., *Dolichos biflorus* and *Helix promatia*). Because the RBCs have decreased sialic acid they also react with *Glycine soja* and do not aggregate normally in Polybrene.

Tn RBCs have usually been detected in patients with a hematological problem but have sometimes been found in seemingly healthy blood donors and in newborns (476). Perhaps one of the most interesting findings is the presence of Tn RBCs in leukemia and the possibility of using Tn antigen as a marker for preleukemia (140–145). We reported a patient with thrombocytopenia of unknown cause who was admitted for splenectomy and found to have Tn RBCs (143). Two years later, the patient was diagnosed as acute myelomonocytic leukemia; Tn RBCs were no longer demonstrable. In 1983, Tiji et al. (497) reported a patient with Tn-RBCs and "ringed" sideroblasts who was successfully treated for pancytopenia. Following treatment, Tn was no longer detectable on the RBCs. In a Letter to the Editor of the journal *Blood* in 1979, Tiji (494) reported that 1 year following the disappearances of Tn RBCs, the patient relapsed and was diagnosed as having acute myeloid leukemia.

Acquired Tk, Th, Tx and VA Antigens.   The appearance of Tk, Th, Tx, and VA on RBCs is less common than the appearance of T and Tn. The appearance of Tk on RBCs appears to be associated with infectious agents (e.g., *Bacteroides fragilis, Serratia marscescens, Aspergillus niger, Candida albicans*). These organisms produce endo- and exo-β-galactosidases that can expose the Tk cryptantigen. These enzymes can also weaken ABH/li/P_1 activity. Tk can be detected by naturally occurring anti-T^k in adult sera or the lectins of *Griffonia simplicifolia* (previously called *Bandeiraea simplicifolia*) and *Vicia hyranica* that contains easily separable anti-T and -T^k. T^k RBCs have no decrease in sialic acid thus are not agglutinated by *G. soja* and aggregate normally in Polybrene.

As Th RBCs are agglutinated by *V. hypoaea, V. cretica,* and *Medicago disciformis* but not by *G. soja* or *G. simplicifolia*, it has been suggested that Th is a weak or intermediate form of T. Sondag-Thull et al. (495) induced Th transformation of RBCs in vitro using a neuraminidase from *Corynebacterium aquaticum*. Other neuraminidases would cause Th but not T transformation if used under very mild conditions of hydrolysis. Release of <20 $\mu g/10^{10}$ RBCs yield T. Herman et al. (496,497) made the fascinating observation that Th-transformed RBCs were present in five of seven (71%) children with congenital hypoplastic anemia. All three children with Diamond-Blackfan syndrome reacted with *A. hypogaea*, but RBCs of one of the three still reacted with ficin-treated RBCs, suggesting T or Tx rather than Th transformation. Th RBCs were present in three of four children with Fanconi's anemia; the Th RBCs were no longer detectable following bone marrow transplant in one child. Th RBCs were not detected in any of three children with undefined bone marrow function (including transient erythroblastopenia of childhood). None of the Th RBCs were detectable with the anti-Tn in adult human sera (i.e., no polyagglutination was noted). Another interesting finding was that 13.5% of RBCs from 74 random cord bloods were found to have Th RBCs present compared with 0% in 20 healthy children, 1.5% in 132 healthy adults, and 1.8% in a group of 96 children with hypoproliferative and congenital hemolytic anemias (it is interesting to note that 15.4% of these 96 children with hematological problems appeared to have T-transformed RBCs). Herman et al. (496) suggested that the Th transformation may be caused by expression of a fetal RBC antigen that is usually lost after infancy. This antigen may reappear in congenital hypoplasia. As they found no difference in i antigen, HbF, or MCV in any of the three groups with hypoplastic anemia, the authors suggested that Th is a RBC developmental marker that is more specific for congenital hypoplastic anemia than i antigen expression or other fetal RBC characteristics. To support this concept and to contrast it with the theory that Th is a weak form of T, Herman et al. (497) used ^{125}I-labeled *A. hypogaea* by Western blotting and [^{3}H]sialic acid with a purified sialyltransferase to show that the Th determinant on the RBCs of patients Fanconi's anemia was qualitatively different than T.

Table 9 Abnormalities Associated with Depressed or Lack of Common Blood Group Antigens

Phenotype	Abnormality
Rh_{mod}/Rh_{null}	Stomatocytosis of RBCs; hemolytic anemia
McLeod	Acanthocytosis of RBCs; muscle abnormalities
Lu_{null}(InLu type)	Acanthocytosis of RBCs; suppressed CD44
Ge_{null}(Leach type)	Elliptocytosis
Cr_{null}(Inab type)	Protein-losing enteropathy; RBCs have increased sensitivity to complement-mediated lysis

Tx RBCs were first described in children with pneumococcal infections (498). Tx-converting enzymes were shown to be present in the supernatants of pneumococcal cultures (477). Tx RBCs react with *A. hypogaea* but not *V. cretica* or *M. disciformis* in contrast to T and Th RBCs that react strongly with all three lectins.

A rare form of polyagglutination was described in a patient with chronic hemolytic anemia and termed VA (V = Vienna) (13, 14). VA RBCs react with most adult sera but do not react with *A. hypogaea* or *D. biflorus*; the RBCs showed a stippled appearance with *Helix pomatia* and have decreased H antigen. VA is protease resistant. Because of the decreased H activity, it has been suggested that an α-fucosidase of microbial origin could be responsible for VA-RBCs.

D. Diseases Associated with a Lack of Common RBC Antigens

In some systems, phenotypes exist where some common antigens are missign from the RBCs; this is often genetic due to racial differences (e.g., the Fy[a–b–] phenotype is rarely encountered in whites but is found in 68% of American blacks and in almost all blacks in some parts of Africa). Sometimes phenotypes with severe depressions of RBC antigens are encountered (e.g., Rh_{mod}, McLeod). For many of the blood group systems, rare null phenotypes have been described; that is to say, none of the antigens in this system are expressed on the RBCs.

Perhaps the first report of one of these phenotypes being related to disease, and suggesting that blood group antigens may play a role in the integrity of the RBC membrane, was the reported association of stomatocytosis and hemolytic anemia associated with the Rh_{null} phenotype (501,502). Since that time, there have been increasing numbers of reports of associations of hematological abnormalities, reflecting abnormalities in membrane structure, with both of the groups above, but especially with the null phenotypes (503). Table 9 summarizes some of these findings. All of these are discussed in Chapters 4, 5, and 9 and are not discussed in this chapter.

REFERENCES

1. Manuila A. Blood groups and disease—hard facts and delusions. JAMA 1958; 167:2047.
2. Wiener AS. Modern blood group mythology. J Forensic Med, 1960; 7:166.
3. Wiener AS. Blood groups and disease. Am J Hum Genet 1970; 22:476.
4. Prokop O, Uhlenbruck G. Human Blood and Serum Groups. London, Maclaren, 1969:690.
5. Wood CS, Hattison GA, Dore C, Weiner JS. Selective feeding of *Anopheles gambiae* according to ABO blood group status. Nature 1972; 239:165.
6. Gibson JR, Harrison GA, Clarke VA, Hiorns RW. IQ and ABO blood groups. Nature 1973; 246:498.
7. Golding J, Hicks P, Butler NR. Blood group and socio-economic class. Nature 1984; 309:396.
8. Nomi T, Besher A. You Are Your Blood Type. New York, Pocket Books, 1988.
9. Dienst A. Das Eklampsiegift. Zbl Gynäk 1905; 29:353.

10. Levine P, Katzin EM, Burnham L. Isoimmunisation in pregnancy. Its possible bearing on the etiology of erythroblastosis foetalis. JAMA 1941; 116:825.

11. Mollison PL, Engelfriet CP, Contreras M. Blood Transfusion in Clinical Medicine. 8th ed. Oxford, Blackwell Scientific, 1987.

12. Issitt PD. Applied Blood Group Serology. 3rd ed. Miami, Montgomery Scientific, 1985.

13. Weiner W, Battey DA, Cleghorn TE, et al. Serological findings in a case of haemolytic anaemia. Br Med J 1953; 2:125.

14. Hollander L. Specificity of antibodies in acquired haemolytic anaemia, Experientia 1953; 9:468.

15. Dacie JV, Cutbush M. Specificity of auto-antibodies in acquired haemolytic anaemia. J Clin Pathol 1954; 7:18.

16. Garratty G. Target antigens for red-cell-bound autoantibodies. In: Nance SJ, ed. Clinical and Basic Science Aspects of Immunohematology. Arlington, VA, American Association of Blood Banks, 1991:33.

17. Szulman SE. The histological distribution of the blood group substances A and B in man. J Exp Med 1960; 11:785.

18. Starzl TE, Marchioro TL, Holmes JH, et al. Renal homografts in patients with major donor-recipient blood group incompatibilities. Surgery 1964; 55:195.

19. Thorpe SJ, Hunt B, Yacoub M. Expression of ABH blood group antigens in human heart tissue and its relevance to cardiac transplantation. Transplantation 1991; 51:1290.

20. Petz LD. Immunohematologic problems associated with bone marrow transplantation. Trans Med Rev 1987; 1:85.

21. Race RR, Sanger R. Blood Groups in Man. 6th ed. Oxford, England, Blackwell, 1975;139.

22. Levine P. Biological and clinical significance of differences between RBC membrane (Rh) and non-membrane (ABH, MN, P) antigenic sites: illegitimate ABO, M-N (T), P (Tj^a) antigens in malignancy. Rev Fr Transfus Immunohematol 1976; 19:213.

23. Levine P. Comments on hemolytic disease of newborn due to anti-PP$_1$P^k (anti-Tj^a). Transfusion 1977; 17:573.

24. Lopez M, Cartron J, Cartron JP, et al. Cytotoxicity of anti-PP$_1$P^k antibodies and possible relationship with early abortions of p mothers. Clin Immunol Immunopathol 1983; 28:296.

25. Cantin G, Lyonnais J. Anti-PP$_1$P^k and early abortion. Transfusion 1983; 23:350.

26. Yoshida H, Ito K, Emi N, Kanzaki H, Matsuura S. A new therapeutic antibody removal method using antigen-positive red cells. II. Application to a P-incompatible pregnant woman. Vox Sang 1984; 47:216.

27. Shirey RS, Ness PM, Kickler TS, et al. The association of anti-P and early abortion. Transfusion 1987; 27:189.

28. Hansson GC, Wazniowska K, Rock JA, et al. The glycosphingolipid composition of the placenta of a blood group P fetus delivered by a blood group P$_1$^{k} woman and analysis of the anti-globoside antibodies found in maternal serum. Arch Biochem Biophys 1988; 260:168.

29. Vogel F, Druger J. Statistische Beziehung zwischen den ABO-Blutgruppen und Krankheiten mit Ausnahme der Infektionskrankheiten. Blut 1968; 16:351.

30. Vogel F. ABO blood groups and disease. Am J Hum Genet 1970; 22:464.

31. Aird I, Bentall HH, Roberts JAF. A relationship between cancer of stomach and the ABO blood groups. Br Med J 1953; 1:799.

32. Bagshawe KD, Rawlins G. ABO blood-groups in trophoblastic neoplasia. Lancet 1971; i:553.

33. Dawood MY, Teoh ES, Ratnam SS. ABO blood group in trophoblastic disease. J Obstet Gynaecol Br Commonw 1971; 78:918.

34. Morgensen B, Kissmeyer-Nielsen F. Current data on HL-A and ABO typing in gestational choriocarcinoma and invasive mole. Transplant Proc 1971; 3:1267.

35. Gross SJ. Human blood group A substance in human endometrium and trophoblast localized by chromatographed rabbit antiserum. Am J Obstet Gynecol 1956; 95:1149.

36. Szulman AE. The A, B and H blood-group antigens in human placenta. N Engl J Med 1972; 286:1028.

37. Loke YW. Blood group A antigen on human trophoblast cells. Nature 1973; 245:329.

38. Oh-Huti K. Polysaccharides and glycidamin in tissue of gastric cancer. Tohoku J Exp Med 1949: 51:297.

39. Masamune H, Yosizawa Z, Masukawa A. Comparison of group carbohydrate of gastric cancer with corresponding carbohydrate of gastric mucosa. Tohoku J Exp Med 1953; 58:381.

40. Kawasaki H. Molisch positive mucopolisaccharides of gastric cancers as compared with corresponding components of gastric mucosae. Tohoku J Exp Med 1958; 68:119.

41. Kay HEM, Wallace DM. A and B antigens of tumors arising from urinary epithelium. J Natl Cancer Inst 1961; 26:1349.

42. Nairn RC, Fothergill JE, McEntegart MG, Richmond HG. Loss of gastro-intestinal-specific antigen in neoplasia. Br Med J 1962; i:1791.

43. Davidsohn, I. Early immunologic diagnosis and prognosis of carcinoma. Am J Clin Pathol 1972; 57:715.

44. Coon JS, Weinstein RS. Blood group-related antigens as markers of malignant potential and heterogeneity in human carcinomas. Hum Pathol 1986; 17:1089.

45. Hakomori S. Fucolipids and blood group lipids in normal and tumor tissue. Prog Biochem Pharmacol 1975; 10:167.

46. Hakomori S, Young WW Jr. Tumor-associated glycolipid antigens and modified blood group antigens. Scand J Immunol 6(Suppl):97.

47. Hakomori S. Philip Levine Award Lecture: Blood group glycolipid antigens and their modifications as human cancer antigens. Am J Clin Pathol 1984; 82:635.

48. Hakomori S. Aberrant glycosylation in tumors and tumor-associated carbohydrate antigens. Adv Canc Res 1989; 52:257.

49. Lloyd KO. Blood group antigens as markers for normal differentiation and malignant change in human tissue. Am J Clin Pathol 1987; 87:129.

50. Watkins WM. Biochemistry and genetics of the ABO, Lewis, and P blood group system. Adv Hum Genet 1980; 10:1.

51. Singhai A, Hakomori S., Molecular changes in carbohydrate antigens associated with cancer. BioEssays 1990; 12:223.

52. Watanabe K, Hakomori S. Status of blood group carbohydrate chains in ontogenesis and in oncogenesis. J Exp Med 1976; 144:644.

53. Hakomori S, Jeanloz W. Isolation of glycolipid containing fucose, galactose, glucose, and glucosamine from human cancerous tissue. J Biol Chem 1964; 239:PC3606.

54. Hakomori S, Koschielak J, Bloch KJ, Jeanloz RW. Immunologic relationship between blood group substances and a fucose-containing glycolipid of human adenocarcinoma. J Immunol 1967; 98:3.

55. Hakomori S, Andrews H. Sphingoglycolipids with Le^b-activity, and the co-presence of Le^a- and Le^b-glycolipids in human tumor tissue. Biochim Biophys Acta 1970; 202:225.

56. Solter D, Knowles B. B. Monoclonal antibody defining a stage-specific mouse embryonic antigen (SSEA-1). Proc Natl Acad Sci USA 1978; 75:5565.

57. Koprowski H, Brockhaus M, Blaszczyk, et al: Lewis blood-type may affect the incidence of gastrointestinal cancer. Lancet 1982; 1:1332.

58. Wang S, Huang TW, Hakomori S. Immunohistochemistry of two glycolipid tissue antigens in human gastric carcinoma. Cancer 1983; 52:2072.

59. Fukushi Y, Hakomori S, Nudelman E, Cochran N. Novel fucolipids accumulating in human adenocarcinoma: II. Selective isolation of hybridoma antibodies that differentially recognize mono-, di-, and trifucosylated type 2 chain. J Biol Chem 1984; 259:4681.

60. Blaszcyk M, Hansson GC, Karlsson K, et al. Lewis blood group antigens defined by monoclonal anti-colon carcinoma antibodies. Arch Biochem Biophys 1984; 233:161.

61. Iguro T, Wakisaka A, Terasaki PI, et al. Sialylated Lewis[x] antigen detected in the sera of cancer patients. Lancet 1984; 2:817.

62. Limas C, Lange PH. Lewis antigens in normal and neoplastic urothelium. Am J Pathol 1985; 121:176.

63. Limas C. Detection of urothelial Lewis antigens with monoclonal antibodies. 1986; Am J Pathol 1986; 125:515.

64. Abe K, Hakomori S, Ohshiba S. Differential expression of difucosyl type 2 chain (Le^y) defined by monoclonal antibody AH6 in different locations of colonic epithelia, various histological types of colonic polyps, and adenocarcinomas. Cancer Res 1986; 46:2639.

65. Cooper HS, Marshall C, Ruggerio F, Steplewski Z. Hyperplastic polyps of the colon and rectum. Lab Invest 1987; 57:421.

66. Law KL, Smith DF. III^{6}NeuAcLc$_4$Cer in human SW116 colorectal carcinoma cells: A possible oncofetal antigen that is not dependent on Lewis gene expression. Arch Biochem Biophys 1987; 258:315.

67. Itai S, Arii S, Tobe R, et al. Significance of 2-3 and 2–6 sialylation of Lewis A antigen in pancreas cancer. Cancer 1988; 61:775.

68. Young WW Jr, Mills SE, Lippert MG, et al. Deletion of antigens of the Lewis a/b blood group family in human prostatic carcinoma. Am J Pathol 1988; 131:578.

69. Torrado J, Blasco E, Cosme A, et al. Expression of type 1 and type 2 blood group-related antigens in normal and neoplastic gastric mucosa. Am J Clin Pathol 1989; 91:249.

70. Uemura K, Hattori H, Ono K, et al. Expression of Forssman glycolipid and blood group-related antigens A, Le(x), and Le(y) in human gastric cancer and in fetal tissues. Jpn J Exp Med 1989; 59:239.

71. Jovanovic R, Jagirdar J, Thung SN, Paronetto F. Blood-group–related antigen Lewis^x and Lewis^y in the differential diagnosis of cholangiocarcinoma and hepatocellular carcinoma. Arch Pathol Lab Med 1989; 113:139.

72. Hall JB, Chou ST, Louis CJ. The expression of Lewis antigens in neoplasms of the gastrointestinal tract. Pathology 1989; 21:239.

73. Makovitzky J, Schwenk J. Comparative study on the expression of the blood group antigens Le a, Le b, Le x, Le y and the carbohydrate antigens CA 19-9 and CA-50 in chronic pancreatitis and pancreatic carcinoma. Acta Histochemica 1990; 40(Suppl):143.

74. Torrado J, Blasco E, Gutierrez-Hoyos A, et al. Lewis system alterations in gastric carcinogenesis. Cancer 1990; 66:1769.

75. Stroud MR, Levery SB, Nudelman ED, et al. Extended type 1 chain glycosphingolipids: Dimeric Le^a (III^{4}V^{4}Fuc$_2$Lc$_6$) as human tumor-associated antigen. J Biol Chem 1991; 266:8439.

76. Itai S, Nishikata J, Yoneda T, et al. Tissue distribution of 2-3 and 2-6 sialyl Lewis A antigens and significance of the ratio of two antigens for the differential diagnosis of malignant and benign disorders of the digestive tract. Cancer 1991; 67:1576.

77. Langkilde, NC, Wolfe H, Ørntoft TF. Lewis antigen expression in benign and malignant tissues from RBC Le(a–b–) cancer patients. Br J Haematol 1991; 79:493.

78. Limas C. Quantitative interrelations of Lewis antigens in normal mucosa and transitional cell bladder carcinomas. J Clin Pathol 1991; 44:983.

79. Ørntoft TF, Holmes EH, Johnson P, et al. Differential tissue expression of the Lewis blood group antigens: Enzymatic immunohistologic, and immunochemical evidence for Lewis a and b antigen expression in Le(a–b–) individuals. Blood 1991; 77:1389.

80. Ree HJ, Teplitz C Khan S. The Lewis X antigen. A new paraffin section marker for Reed-Sternberg cells. Cancer 1991; 67:1338.

81. Hakomori S. Possible functions of tumor-associated carbohydrate antigens. Curr Opin Immunol 1991; 3:646.

82. Inoue M, Fujita M, Nakazawa A, et al. Sialyl-Tn, sialyl-Lewis Xi, CA 19-9, Ca 125, carcinoembryonic antigen, and tissue polypeptide antigen in differentiating ovarian cancer from benign tumors. Obstet Gynecol 1992; 79:434.

83. Hirszfeld L, Halber W, Laskowski J. Untersuchungen über die serologischen Eigenschaften der Gewebe. II: Uber serologische Eigenschaften der Neubildungen. Z Immunitatsforsch 1929; 64:61.

84. Witebsky E. Zur serologischen Spezifitat des Cardinomgewebes. Klin Wochenschr 1930; 9:58.

85. Häkkinen I, Virtanen S. The blood group activity of human gastric sulphoglycoproteins in patients with gastric cancer and normal controls. Clin Exp Immunol 1967; 2:669.

86. Häkkinen I. A-like blood group antigen in gastric cancer cells of patients in blood groups O or B. J Natl Cancer Inst 1970; 44:1183.

87. Breimer ME. Adaptation of mass spectrometry for the analysis of tumor antigens as applied to blood group glycolipids of a human gastric carcinoma. Cancer Res 1980; 40:897.

88. Hattori H, Uemura K, Taketomi T. Glycolipids of gastric cancer. The presence of blood group A–active glycolipids in cancer tissues from blood group O patients. Biochim Biophys Acta 1981; 666:361.

89. Yokota M, Warner G, Hakomori S. Blood group A–like glycolipid and a novel Forssman antigen in the hepatocarcinoma of a blood group O individual. Cancer Res 1981; 41:4185.

90. Hirohashi S, Clausen H, Yamada T, et al. Blood group A cross-reacting epitope defined by monoclonal antibodies NCC-LU-35 and -81 expressed in cancer of blood group O or B individuals: Its identification as Tn antigen. Proc Natl Acad Sci USA 1985; 82:7.

91. Clausen H, Hakomori S, Graem N, Dabelsteen E. Incompatible A antigen expressed in tumors of blood group O individuals: Immunochemical, immunohistologic, and enzymatic characterization. J Immunol 1986; 136:326.

92. Hakomori S, Clausen H, Levery SB. A new series of blood group A and H antigens expressed in human erythrocytes and the incompatible A antigens in tumours of blood group O and B individuals. Biochem Soc Trans 1987; 15:593.

93. Gold P, Freedman SO. Demonstration of tumor-specific antigens in human colonic carcinoma by immunological tolerance and absorption techniques. J Exp Med 1965; 121:439.

94. Gold JM, Freedman SO, Gold P. Human anti-CEA antibodies detected by radioimmuno-electrophoresis. Nature 1972; 234:60.

95. Gold JM, Gold P. The blood group A-like site on carcinoembryonic antigen. Cancer Res 1973; 33:2821.

96. Simmons AR, Perlmann P. Carcinoembryonic antigen and blood group substances. Cancer Res 1973; 33:313.

97. Holburn AM, Mach JP, MacDonald D, Newlands M. Studies of the association of the A, B and Lewis blood group antigens with carcinoembryonic antigen (CEA). Immunology; 1974; 26:831.

98. Cooper AG, Brown MC, Kirch ME, Rule AH. Relationship of carcinoembryonic antigen to blood substances A and i: Evidence that the antigenic sites are on different molecules. J Immunol 1974; 113:1246.

99. Feizi T, Tuberville C, Westwood JH. Blood-group precursors and cancer-related antigens, Lancet 1975; 2:391.

100. Bloom ET, Fahey JL, Peterson IA, et al. Anti-tumor activity in human serum: antibodies detecting blood-group-A–like antigen on the surface of tumor cells in culture. Int J Cancer 1973; 12:21.

101. Magous R, Lecou C Bali J. Evidences for the association of blood group determinants with the carcinoembryonic antigen molecule. Molec Immunol 1980; 17:1039.

102. Nichols EJ, Kannagi R, Hakomori S, et al. Carbohydrate determinants associated with car-cinoembryonic antigen (CEA). J Immunol 1985; 135:1911.

103. Chandrasekaran EV, Davila M, Nixon DW, et al. Isolation and structures of the oligosaccharide units of carcinoembryonic antigen. J Biol Chem 1983; 258:6213.

104. Liotta LA. Cancer cell invasion and metastasis. Sci Am 1992; 266:54.

105. Kuhns W J, Bramson S. Variable behaviour of blood group H on HeLa cell populations synchronized with thymidine. Nature 1968; 219:938.

106. Kuhns WJ, Pann C. Relationship of phenotypic expression of blood group H to changes in growth kinetics of cultured primary and transformed epitheloid cells. Am J Pathol 1973; 73:789.

107. Dawson A, Franks D. Factors affecting the expression of blood group antigen A in cultured cells. Exp Cell Res 1967; 47:377.

108. Franks D, Dawson A. Variations in the expression of blood group antigen A in clonal culture of rabbit cells. Exp Cell Res 1966; 42:543.

109. Thomas DB. Cyclic expression of blood group determinants in murine cells and their relationship to growth control. Nature 1971; 233:317.

110. MacKenzie IC, Dabelsteen E, Zimmerman K. The relationship between expression of epithelial B-like blood group antigen, cell movement and cell proliferation. Acta Pathol Microbiol Scand 1977; 85:49.

111. Abercrombie M. Behaviour of cells toward one another. Adv Biol Skin 1964; 5:95.

112. Hakomori S. Aberrant glycosylation in cancer cell membranes as focused on glycolipids: Overview and perspectives. Cancer Res 1985; 45:2405.

113. Feizi T. Carbohydrate antigens in human cancer. Cancer Surv 1985; 4:245.

114. Feizi T. Demonstration by monoclonal antibodies that carbohydrate structures of glycoproteins and glycolipids are onco-developmental antigens. Nature 1985; 314:53.

115. Berg EL, Robinson MK, Mansson O, et al. A carbohydrate domain common to both sialyl Le(a) and sialyl Le(X) is recognized by the endothelial cell leukocyte adhesion molecule ELAM-1. J Biol Chem 1991; 266:14869.

116. Levine P, Bobbitt OB, Waller RK, Kuhmichel A. Isoimmunization by a new blood factor in tumor cells. Proc Soc Exp Biol (NY) 1951; 77:403.
117. Levine P. Blood group and tissue genetic markers in familial adenocarcinoma: Potential specific immunotherapy. Semin Oncol 1978; 5:25.
118. Sanger R. An association between the P and Jay systems of blood groups. Nature 1955; 176:1163.
119. Marcus DM, Kundu SK, Suzuki A. The P blood group system: Recent progress in immunochemistry and genetics. Semin Hematol 1981; 18:63.
120. Kannagi R, Levine P, Watanabe K, Hakomori S. Recent studies of glycolipid and glycoprotein profiles and characterization of the major glycolipid antigen in gastric cancer of a patient of blood group genotype pp (Tj^{a-}) first studied in 1951. Cancer Res 1982; 42:5249.
121. Forssman J. Die Herstellung hochwertiger spezifisher Schafhämolysine ohne Verwendung von Schafblut: Ein Beitrag zur Lehre von heterologer Antikörperbildung. Biochem Z 1911; 37:78.
122. Siddiqui B, Hakomori S. A revised structure for Forssman hapten glycolipid. J Biol Chem 1971; 246:5766.
123. Stellner K, Hakomori S, Warner GA. Enzymic conversion of "H$_1$-glycolipid" and deficiency of these enzyme activities in adenocarcinoma. Biochem Biophys Res Commun 1973; 55:439.
124. Karol RA, Kundu SK, Marcus DM. Immunochemical relationship between Forssman and globoside glycolipid antigens. Immunol Commun 1981; 10:237.
125. Hakomori S, Wang SM, Young WW Jr. Isoantigenic expression of Forssman glycolipid in human gastric and colonic mucosa: Its possible identity with "A like" antigen in human cancer. Proc Natl Acad Sci USA 1977; 74:3023.
126. Yoda Y, Ishibashi T, Makita A. Isolation, characterization, and biosynthesis of Forssman antigen in human lung and lung carcinoma. J Biochem (Tokyo) 1980; 88:1887.
127. Taniguchi N, Yokosawa N, Narita M, et al. Expression of Forssman antigen synthesis and degradation in human lung cancer. J Natl Cancer Inst 1981; 67:577.
128. Mori E, Mori T, Sanai Y, Nagai T. Radioimmun-thin-layer chromatographic detection of Forssman antigen in human carcinoma cell lines. Biochem Biophys Res Commun 1982; 108:926.
129. Mori T, Sudo T, Kano K. Expression of heterophile Forssman antigens in cultured malignant cell lines. J Natl Cancer Inst 1983; 70:811.
130. Young WW Jr, Hakomori S, Levine P. Characterization of anti-Forssman (anti-Fs) antibodies in human sera: their specificity and possible changes in patients with cancer. J Immunol 1979; 123:92.
131. Levine P. Self-nonself concept for cancer and diseases previously known as "autoimmune" diseases. Proc Natl Acad Sci USA 1978; 75:5697.
132. Mori T, Fuji G, Kawamura A, Jr, et al. Forssman antibody levels in sera of cancer patients. Immunol Commun 1982; 11:217.
133. Wiels J, Fellous M, Tursz T. Monoclonal antibody against a Burkitt lymphoma associated antigen. Proc Natl Acad Sci USA 1981; 78:6485.
134. Nudelman E, Kannagi R, Hakomori S, et al. A glycolipid antigen associated with Burkitt lymphoma defined by a monoclonal antibody. Science 1983; 220:509.
135. Springer GF, Desai PR, and Banatwala I. Blood group MN antigens and precursors in normal and malignant breast glandular tissue. J Natl Cancer Inst 1975; 54:335.
136. Springer GF, Desai PR, Scanlon EF. Blood group MN precursors as human breast carcinoma-associated antigens and "naturally" occurring human cytotoxins against them. Cancer 1976; 37:169.
137. Friedenreich V. The Thomsen hemagglutination phenomenon. Copenhagen, Levin and Munksgaard, 1930.
138. Springer GF, Ansell NJ. Inactivation of human erythrocyte agglutinogens M and N by influenza viruses and receptor-destroying enzyme. Proc Natl Acad Sci USA 1958; 44:182.
139. Moreau R, Dausset J, Bernard J, Moullec J. Anemie hemolytique acquise avec polyagglutinabilite des hematies par un nouveau facteur present dans le serum humain normal (anti-Tn). Bull Soc Med Hop Paris, 73:569.
140. Bird GWG, Wingham J, Pippard MJ, et al. Erythrocyte membrane modification in malignant diseases of myeloid and lymphoreticular tissues. I. Tn-polyagglutination in acute myelomonocytic leukaemia, Br J Haematol 1976; 33:289.
141. Beck ML, Hicklin BL, Pierce SR. Observations on leucocytes and platelets in six cases of Tn-polyagglutination. Med Lab Sci 1977; 34:325.

142. Bird GWG, Wingham J, Richardson SGN. Myelofibrosis, autoimmune haemolytic anaemia, and Tn-polyagglutinability, Haematologica 1985; 18:99.

143. Ness PM, Garratty G, Morel PA, Perkins HA. Tn polyagglutination preceding acute leukemia. Blood 1979; 54:30.

144. Baldwin ML, Barrasso C, Ridolfi RL. Tn-polyagglutinability associated with acute myelomonocytic leukemia. Am J Clin Pathol 1979; 72:1024.

145. Roxby DJ, Morley AA, Burpee M. Detection of the Tn antigen in leukaemia using monoclonal anti-Tn antibody and immunohistochemistry. Br J Haematol 1987; 67:153.

146. Cartron J-P, Andreu G, Cartron J, et al. Demonstration of T-transferase deficiency in Tn-poly-agglutinable blood samples. Eur J Biochem 1978; 92:111.

147. Cartron J-P, Andreu G, Cartron J, et al. Selective deficiency of 3-β-D-galactosyltransferase (T-transferase) in Tn-polyagglutinable erythrocytes, Lancet 1978; 1:856.

148. Springer GF. Blood-group and Forssman antigenic determinants shared between microbes and mammalian cells. Prog Allergy 1971; 15:9.

149. Springer GF, Tegtmeyer H. Origin of anti-Thomsen-Friedenrich (T) and Tn agglutinins in man and in White Leghorn chicks. Br J Haematol 1981; 47:453.

150. Springer GF, Desai PR, Wise W, et al. Pancarcinoma T and Tn epitopes. Autoimmunogens and diagnostic markers that reveal incipient carcinomas and help establish prognosis. In: Herberman RB, Mercer DW, eds. Immunodiagnosis of Cancer. 2nd ed. New York: Marcel Dekker 1990:p. 587.

151. Sastry MVK, Banarjee P, Patanjali SR, Swamy MJ et al. Analysis of saccharide binding to *Artocarpus integrifolia* lectin reveal specific recognition of T-antigen (β-D-Gal(1→3)D-GalNAc). J Biol Chem 1986; 261:11726.

152. Rinderle SJ, Goldstein IJ, Matta KL, Ratcliffe RM. Isolation and characterization of amaranthin, a lectin present in the seeds of *Amaranthus caudatus*, that recognizes the T-(or cryptic T)-antigen. J Biol Chem 1989; 264:16123.

153. Springer GF, Desai PR, Murthy MS, et al. Precursors of the blood group MN antigens as human carcinoma-associated antigens. Transfusion 1979; 19:233.

154. Springer GF. T and Tn, general carcinoma autoantigens. Science 1984; 224:1198.

155. Weinstein RS, Schwartz D, Coon JS. Blood group autoantigens and ploidy as prognostic factors in urinary bladder carcinoma. Fenoglio-Preiser CM, Weinstein RS, Kaufmann N, eds. New Concepts in Neoplasia as Applied to Diagnostic Pathology (Intl Acad Pathology Monograph. Vol. 27). Baltimore: Williams & Wilkins, 1986:255.

156. Seitz RC, Fischer K, Stegner HE, Poschmann A. Detection of metastatic breast carcinoma cells by immunofluorescent demonstration of Thomsen-Friedenreich antigen. Cancer 1984; 54:830.

157. Ghazizadeh M, Kagawa S, Izumi K, Kurokawa K. Immunohistochemical localization of T antigen–like substance in benign hyperplasia and adenocarcinoma of the prostate. J Urol 1984; 132:1127.

158. Ohoka H, Shinomiya H, Yokoyama M, et al. Thomsen-Friedenreich antigen in bladder tumors as detected by specific antibody: a possible marker of recurrence. Urol Res 1985; 13:47.

159. Howard DR, Taylor CR. An antitumor antibody in normal human serum: reaction of anti-T with breast carcinoma cells. Oncology 1980; 37:142.

160. Clausen H, Stroud M, Parker J, et al. Springer, GF, and Hakomori, S-I. (1988). Monoclonal antibodies directed to the blood group A associated structure, galactosyl-A:Specificity and relation to the Thomsen-Friedenreich antigen. Mol Immunol 1988; 25:199.

161. Springer GF, Murthy MS, Desai PR, Scanlon EF. Breast cancer patient's cell-mediated immune response to Thomsen-Friedenreich (T) antigen. Cancer 1980; 45:2949.

162. Codington JF, Yamazaki T, van den Eijnden DH, et al. Unequivocal evidence for a β-D-config-uration of the galactose residue in the disaccharide chain of epiglycanin, the major glycoprotein of the TA3-Ha tumor cell. FEBS Lett 1979; 99:70.

163. Kjeldsen T, Clausen H, Hirohashi S, et al. Preparation and characterization of monoclonal antibodies directed to the tumor-associated O-linked Sialosyl-2→α-N-acetylgalactosaminyl (Sialosyl-Tn) epitope, Cancer Res 1988; 48:2214.

164. Stein R, Chen S, Grossman W, Goldenberg DM. A human lung carcinoma monoclonal antibody specific for the Thomsen-Friedenreich antigen. Cancer Res 1989; 49:32.

165. Altavilla G, Lanza G Jr, Rossi S, Cavazzini L. Morphologic changes, mucin secretion, carcinoembryonic antigen (CEA) and peanut lectin reactivity in colonic mucosa of patients at high risk for colorectal cancer. Tumori 1984; 70:539.

166. Ørntoft TF, Mors NPO, Eriksen G, et al. Comparative immunoperoxidase demonstration of T-antigens in human colorectal carcinomas and morphologically abnormal mucosa. Cancer Res 1985; 45:447.

167. Yuan M, Itzkowitz SH, Boland CR, et al. Comparison of T-antigen expression in normal, premalignant, and malignant human colonic tissue using lectin and antibody immunohistochemistry. Cancer Res 1986; 46:4841.

168. Nishiyama T, Matsumoto Y, Watanabe H, et al. Detection of Tn antigen with *Vicia villosa* agglutinin in urinary bladder cancer: Its relevance to the patient's clinical course. J Natl Cancer Inst 1987; 78:1113.

169. Kellokumpu I, Kellokumpu S, Andersson LC. Identification of glycoproteins expressing tumour-associated PNA-binding sites in colorectal carcinomas by SDS-GEL electrophoresis and PNA-labelling. Br J Cancer 1987; 55:361.

170. Kjeldsen T, Hakomori S, Springer GF, et al. Coexpression of sialosyl-Tn (NeuAcα2→6GalNacα→O-Ser/Thr) and Tn (GalNAcα→O-Ser/Thr) blood group antigens on Tn erythrocytes. Vox Sang 1989; 57:81.

171. Roxby DJ, Skinner JM, Morley AA, et al. Expression of a Tn-like epitope by carcinoma cells. Br J Cancer 1987; 56:734.

172. Böcker W, Kalubert A, Bahnsen J, et al. Peanut lectin histochemistry of 120 mammary carcinomas and its relation to tumor type, grading, staging, and receptor status. Virchows Arch (Pathol Anat) 1984; 403:149.

173. Howard DR, Taylor CR. A method for distinguishing benign from malignant breast lesions utilizing antibody present in normal human sera. Cancer 1979; 43:2279.

174. Yokoyama M, Ohoka H, Oda H, et al. Thomsen-Friedenreich antigen in bladder cancer tissues detected by monoclonal antibody. Acta Urol Jpn 1988; 34:255.

175. Blasco E, Torrado J, Belloso L, et al. T-antigen. A prognostic indicator of high recurrence index in transitional carcinoma of the bladder. Cancer 1988; 61:1091.

176. Cooper HS, Reuter VE. Peanut lectin-binding sites in polyps of the colon and rectum. Adenomas, hyperplastic polyps, and adenomas with in situ carcinoma. Lab Invest 1983; 49:655.

177. Ghazizadeh M, Kagawa S, Kurokawa K. Immunohistochemical studies of human renal cell carcinomas for ABO(H) blood group antigens, T antigen-like substance and carcinoembyronic antigen. J Urol 1985; 133:762.

178. Itzkowitz SH, Yuan M, Montgomery CK, et al. Expression of Tn, sialosyl-Tn, and T antigens in human colon cancer. Cancer Res 1989; 49:197.

179. Ghazizadeh M, Oguro T, Sasaki Y, et al. Immunohistochemical and ultrastructural localization of T antigen in ovarian tumors. Am J Clin Pathol 1990; 93:315.

180. Schlepper-Schäfer J, Springer GF. Carcinoma autoantigens T and Tn and their cleavage products interact with Gal/GalNAc-specific receptors on rat Kupffer cells and hepatocytes. Biochim Biophys Acta, 1989; 89:266.

181. Holt S, Wilkinson A, Suresh MR, et al. Radiolabelled peanut lectin for the scintigraphic detection of cancer. Cancer Lett. 1984; 25:55.

182. Laurent JC, Noël P, Faucon M. Expression of a cryptic cell surface antigen in primary cell cultures from human breast cancer. Biomedicine 1978; 29:260.

183. Boland CR, Montgomery CK, Kim YS. Alterations in human colonic mucin occurring with cellular differentiation and malignant transformation. Proc Natl Acad Sci USA 1982; 79:2051.

184. Springer GF, Desai PR, Banatwala I. Blood group MN antigens and precursors in normal and malignant human breast glandular tissues. J Natl Cancer Inst 1975; 54:335.

185. Springer GF. Tn epitope (N-acetyl-d-galatcosamineα-O-serine/threonine) density in primary breast carcinoma: a functional predictor of aggressiveness. Mol Immunol 1989; 26:1.

186. Springer GF, Taylor CR, Howard DR, et al. Tn, a carcinoma-associated antigen, reacts with anti-Tn of normal human sera. Cancer 1985; 55:561.

187. Coon JS, Weinstein RS, Summers JL. Blood group precursor T-antigen expression in human urinary bladder carcinoma. Am J Clin Pathol 1982; 77:692.

188. Ghazizadeh M, Oguro T, Sasaki Y, et al. Immunohistochemical and ultrastructural localization of T antigen in ovarian tumors. Am J Clin Pathol 1990; 93:315.

189. Kjeldsen T, Clausen H, Hirohashi S, et al. Preparation and characterization of monoclonal antibodies directed to the tumor-associated O-linked sialosyl-2-6α-N-acetylgalatcosaminyl (sialosyl-Tn) epitope, Cancer Res 1988; 48:2214.

190. Itzkowitz SH, Yuan M, Montgomery CK, et al. Expression of Tn, sialosyl-Tn, and T antigens in human colon cancer. Cancer Res 1989; 49:197.

191. Itzkowitz SH, Bloom EJ, Kokal WA, et al. Sialosyl-Tn. Cancer 1990; 66:1960.

192. Inoue M, Ton S, Ogawa H, Tanizawa O. Expression of Tn and sialyl-Tn antigens in tumor tissues of the ovary. Am J Clin Pathol 1991; 96:711.

193. Springer GF, Cheingsong-Popov R, Schirrmacher V, et al. Proposed molecular basis of murine tumor cell-hepatocyte interaction. J Biol Chem 1983; 258:5702.

194. Barr N, Taylor CR, Young T, Springer GF. Are pancarcinoma T and Tn differentiation antigens? Cancer 1989; 64:834.

195. Lind PE, McArthur NR. The distribution of "T" agglutinins in human sera. Aust J Exp Biol Med Sci 1947; 25:247.

196. Schneider AW, Fischer K, Stegner HE, Poschmann A. Automatic determination of anti-T antibodies in patients with breast carcinoma and controls. Tumor Diagn Ther 1986; 7:78.

197. Springer GF, Desai PR, Scanlon EF. Blood group MN precursors as human breast carcinoma-associated antigens and "naturally" occurring human cytotoxins against them. Cancer 1976; 37:169.

198. Springer GF, Murthy SM, Desai PR, et al. Patients' immune response to breast and lung carcinoma-associated Thomsen-Friedenreich specificity. Klin Wochenschr 1982; 60:121.

199. Thatcher N, Hashmi K, Chang J, et al. Anti-T antibody in malignant melanoma patients. Cancer 1980; 46:1378.

200. Springer GF, Desai PR, Murthy MS, Tegtmeyer H, Scanlon EF. Human carcinoma-associated precursor antigens of the blood group MN system and the host's immune responses to them. Ishizaka K, Kallós P, Waksman BH, de Weck Al, eds. Progress in Allergy. Vol 26. Basel: Karger, 1979:42.

201. Springer GF, Desai PR. Detection of lung- and breast carcinoma by quantitating serum anti-T IgM levels with a sensitive, solid-phase immunoassay, Naturwissenschaften 1982; 69:346.

202. Desai PR, Springer GF. Carcinoma detection by quantitation and interrelation of serum anti-T IgM and total IgM. Protides Biol Fluids Proc 1984; 31:421.

203. Aird I, Bentall HH, Mehigan JA, Roberts JAF. The blood group in relation to peptic ulceration and carcinoma of colon, rectum, breast, and bronchus: An association between the ABO groups and peptic ulceration. Br Med J 1954; 2:315.

204. Clark CA, Cowan WK, Edwards JW, et al. The relationship of the ABO blood groups to duodenal and gastric ulceration. Br Med J 1955; 2:643.

205. Langman MJS, Doll R. ABO blood group and secretor status in relation to clinical characteristics of peptic ulcer. Gut 1965; 6:270.

206. Merikas G, Christakopoulos P, Petropoulos E. Distribution of ABO blood groups in patients with ulcer disease. Its relationship to gastroduodenal bleeding. Am J Dig Dis 1966; 11:790.

207. Clarke CA, Edwards JW, Haddock DRW, et al. ABO groups and secretor character in duodenal ulcer. Population and sibship studies. Br Med J 1956; 2:725.

208. Glynn LE, Holborow EJ, Johnson GD. The distribution of blood group substances in human gastric and duodenal mucosa, Lancet 1957; 2:1083.

209. Szulman AE. The histological distribution of blood group substances A and B in man. J Exp Med 1960; 111:785.

210. Szulman AE. The histological distribution of blood group substances in man as disclosed by immunofluorescence: 2. The H antigen and its relation to A and B antigen. J Exp Med 1962; 115:977.

211. Sievers ML. Hereditary aspects of gastric secretory function. Am J Med 1959; 27:246.

212. Koster KH, Sindrup E, Seele V. ABO blood groups and gastric acidity. Lancet 1955; 2:52.

213. Niederman JC, Gilbert EC, Spiro HM. The relationship between blood pepsin level, ABO blood group and secretor status. Ann Intern Med 1962; 56:564.

214. Hanley WB. Hereditary aspects of duodenal ulceration: Serum pepsinogen level in relation to ABO blood groups and salivary ABH-secretor status. Br Med J 1964; 1:936.

215. Denborough MA. ABO blood group, secretor status and gastric secretion. Aust Ann Med 1966; 15:314.
216. Brown DAP, Melrose AS, Wallace J. The blood groups in peptic ulceration. Br Med J 1956; 2:135.
217. Ventzke LE, Grossman MI. Response to patients with duodenal ulcer to augmented histamine test as related to blood groups and to secretor status. Gastroenterology 1962; 42:292.
218. Selsnick F. A Study of ABH Blood Group Substances on Duodenal Mucosal Cells. ChM Thesis, Liverpool, England: Liverpool University, 1959.
219. Cain JA. Possible significances of secretor. Lancet 1957; 1:212.
220. Mourant AE, Kopec AC, Domainiewska-Sobczak K. Blood-groups and blood-clotting, Lancet 1971; 1:223.
221. Medalie JH, Levene C, Papier C, et al. Blood groups, myocardial infarction and angina pectoris among 10,000 adult males. N Engl J Med 1971; 285:1348.
222. Gertler MM, White PD. Coronary Heart Disease in Young Adults: A Multidisciplinary Study. Cambridge, MA: Harvard University Press, 1954.
223. Allan TM, Dawson AA. ABO blood groups and ischaemic heart disease in men. Br Heart J 1968; 30:377.
224. Nefzger MD, Hrubee Z, Chalmers TC. Venous thromboembolism and blood-group. Lancet 1969; 1:887.
225. Denborough MA. Blood groups and ischaemic heart disease. Br Med J 1962; 2:927.
226. Bronte-Stewart B, Botha MC, Krut LH. ABO blood groups in relation to ischaemic heart disease. Br Med J 1962; 1:1646.
227. Havlik RJ, Feinleib M, Garrison RJ, Kannel WB. Blood-groups and coronary heart-disease. Lancet 1969; 2:269.
228. Jick H, Slone D, Westerhold B, et al. Venous thromboembolic disease and ABO blood type: A cooperative study. Lancet 1969; 1:539.
229. Talbot S, Wakley EJ, Ryrie D, Langman MJS. ABO blood-groups and venous thromboembolic disease. Lancet 1970; 1:1257.
230. Dick W, Schneider W, Brockmüller K, Mayer W. Interrelationships of thromboembolic diseases and blood-group distribution. Thromb Diath Haemorrh 1963; 9:472.
231. Weiss NS. ABO blood type and arteriosclerosis obliterans. Am J Hum Genet 1972; 24:65.
232. Morris T, Bouhoutsos J. ABO blood groups in occlusive and ectatic arterial disease. Br J Surg 60:892.
233. Kingsbury KJ. Relation of ABO blood groups to atherosclerosis. Lancet 1971; 1:199.
234. George VT, Elston RC, Amos CI, Ward LJ, Berenson GS. Association between polymorphic blood markers and risk factors for cardiovascular disease in a large pedigree. Genet Epidemiol 1987; 4:267.
235. Whincup PH, Cook DG, Phillips AN, Shaper AG. ABO blood group and ischaemic heart disease in British men. Br Med J 1990; 300:1679.
236. Dintenfass L. Formation, consistency and degradation of artificial thrombi in severe renal failure. Thromb Diath Haemorrh 1968; 20:267.
237. Dintenfass L. The role of ABO blood groups in dynamic coagulation and thrombus formation in vascular disease. Haematologia 1971; 5:205.
238. Dintenfass L. The role of ABO blood groups in blood rheology of cardiovascular disorders. Angiology 1973; 24:442.
239. Dintenfass L, Forges CD, McNicol GP. Viscosity of blood in patients with myocardial infarction, haemophilia and thyroid diseases. Effect of fibrinogen, albumin and globulin. Biorheology 1972; 9:150.
240. Dintenfass L. ESR and aggregation of red cells after addition of fructose or glucose: Effect of ABO blood groups. Med J Aust 1972; 2:425.
241. Ionescu DA, Ghitescu M, Marcu I, Xenakis A. Erythrocyte rheology in acute cerebral thrombosis. Effects of ABO blood groups. Blut 1979; 39:351.
242. Oliver MF, Geizerova H, Cumming RA, Heady, JA. Serum cholesterol and ABO and Rhesus blood groups. Lancet 1969; 2:605.
243. Langman MJS, Elwood PC, Foote J, Ryrie DR. ABO and Lewis blood groups and serum cholesterol, Lancet, 1969; 2:607.

244. Flat G. Serum-cholesterin, ABO-glutgruppen and Häemoblobintyp, Humangenetik 1970; 10:318.
245. Beckman L, Olivecrona T, Hernell O. Serum lipids and their relationship to blood groups and serum alkaline phosphatase isozymes. Hum Hered 1970; 20:569.
246. Morton NE. Genetic markers in atherosclerosis: A review. J Med Gener 1976; 13:81.
247. Garrison RJ, Havlik RJ, Harris RB, et al. ABO blood group and cardiovascular disease. The Framingham Study. Atherosclerosis 1976; 25:311.
248. Sing CF, Orr JD. Analysis of genetic and environmental sources of variation in serum cholesterol in Tecumseh, Michigan. III. Identification of genetic effects using 12 polymorphic genetic blood marker systems. Am J Hum Genet 1976; 28:453.
249. Polychronopoulou A, Georgiadis E, Kalandidi A, et al. Serum cholesterol, triglycerides and phospholipids, and ABO and Rhesus (RH₀D) antigen among young Greeks. Hum Biol 1977; 49:605.
250. Srivastava BK, Sinha AS. Observations on serum cholesterol and lipid phosphorus levels in relation to ABO blood groups. J Indian Med Assoc 1966; 47:261.
251. Banerjee B, Saha N. Blood-groups and serum-cholesterol. Lancet 1969; 2:961.
252. Saha N, Banerjee B. Blood-groups and serum-cholesterol. Lancet 1971; 1:969.
253. Hames CG, Greenberg BG. A comparative study of serum cholesterol levels in school children and their possible relation to atherogenesis. Am J Public Health 1961; 51:374.
254. Mayo O, Wiesenfeld SL, Stamatoyannopoulos G, Fraser GR. Genetical influences on serum-cholesterol level. Lancet 1971; 2:554.
255. Ledvina M, Kellen J. Die Beziehungen der β-Lipoproteine des Serums zu den Blutgruppen. Folia Haematol (Leipz) 1962; 79:382.
256. Polychronopoulou A, Miras CJ, Trichopoulos D. Lipoprotein types, serum cholesterol, and ABO blood groups. Br J Prev Sco Med 1974; 28:60.
257. Fox MH, Webber LS, Srinivasan SR, et al. ABO blood group associations with cardiovascular risk factor variables. I. Serum lipids and lipoproteins. The Bogalusa Heart Study. Hum Biol 1981; 53:411.
258. Arfors KE, Beckman L, Lundin LG. Genetic variations of human serum phosphatases. Acta Genet 1963; 13:89.
259. Arfors KE, Beckman L, Lundin LG. Further studies on the association between human serum phosphatases and blood groups. Acta Genet 1963; 13:366.
260. Beckman L. Associations between human serum alkaline phosphatases and blood groups. Acta Genet 1964; 14:286.
261. Bamford KF, Harris H, Luffman JE, et al. Serum-alkaline-phosphatase and the ABO blood groups. Lancet 1965; 1:530.
262. Shreffer DG. Genetic studies of blood group-associated variations in human serum alkaline phosphatase. Am J Genet 1965; 17:71.
263. Kaplan MM. Current concepts: Alkaline phosphatase. N Engl J Med 1972; 286:200.
264. Langman MJS, Leuthold E. Robson EB, Harris J, Luffman JE, Harris H. Influence of diet on the intestinal component of serum alkaline phosphatase in people of different ABO blood groups and secretor status. Nature 1966; 212:41.
265. Inglis NI, Krant MJ, Fishman WH. Influence of a fat enriched meal on human serum (L-phenyl-alanine-sensitive) 'intestinal' alkaline phosphatase. Proc Soc Exp Biol Med 1967; 124:699.
266. Kleerekoper M, Horne M, Cornish CJ, Posen S. Serum alkaline phosphatase after fat ingestion: An immunological study. Clin Sci 1970; 38:339.
267. Preston AE, Barr A. The plasma concentration of factor VIII in the normal population. II. The effects of age, sex and blood group. Br J Haematol 1964; 10:238.
268. Jeremic M, Weisert O, Gedde-Dahl TW. Factor VII (AHG) levels in 1016 regular blood donors. Scand J Clin Lab Invest 1976; 36:461.
269. McCallum CJ, Peake IR, Newcombe RG, Bloom AL. Factor VIII levels and blood group antigens. Thromb Haemostas 1983; 50:757.
270. Mohanty D, Ghosh K, Marwaha N, et al. Major blood group antigens—a determinant of Factor VIII levels in blood? Thromb Haemostas 1984; 51:414.
271. Ørstavik KH, Magnus P, Reisner H, et al. Factor VIII and Factor IX in a twin population. Evidence for a major effect of ABO locus on factor VIII level. Am J Hum Genet 1985; 37:89.

272. McLellan DS, Knight SR, Aronstam A. The relationship between coagulation factor VIII and ABO blood group status. Med Lab Sci 1988; 45:131.

273. Gedde-Dahl TW, Jeremic M, Weisert O. Factor V (proaccelerin) concentration in 1016 blood donors, Scand J Clin Lab Invest 1975; 35:25.

274. Mazurier C, Samor B, Mannessier L, et al. Blood group A and B activity associated with factor VIII–von Willebrand factor, Blood Trans Immunohaematol 1981; XXIV:3.

275. Gill JC, Endres-Brooks J, Bauer PJ, et al. The effect of ABO blood group on the diagnosis of von Willebrand disease, Blood 1987; 69:1691.

276. Korsnan-Bengtsen K, Wilhelmsen L, Nilson LÅ, Tibblin G. Blood coagulation and fibrinolysis in relation to ABO, Rh, MN and Duffy blood groups in a random population sample of men aged 54 years. Thromb Res 1972; 1:549.

277. Fagerhol M, Abildgaard U, Kornstad L. Antithrombin III concentration and ABO blood groups. Lancet 1971; 2:664.

278. Stormorken H, Erikssen J. Plasma antithrombin III and factor VIII antigen in relation to angiographic findings, angina and blood groups in middle-aged men. Thromb Haemost 1977; 38:874.

279. Springer GF, Williamson P, Brandes WC. Blood group activity of gram-negative bacteria. J Exp Med 1961; 113:1077.

280. Springer GF, Horton RE, Forbes M. Origin of anti-human blood group B agglutinins in white leghorn chicks. J Exp Med 1959; 110:221.

281. Mourant AE. The Distribution of the Human Blood Groups, Oxford, England: Blackwell Scientific, 1964.

282. Vogel F, Pettenkofer HJ, Helmbold W. Uber die Populationsgenetik der ABO-Blugruppen. 2. Mitteilung. Genhaüfigkeit und epidemische Erkrankunge. Acta Genet Statis Med 1960; 10:267.

283. Springer GF, Wiener AS. Alleged causes of the present-day world distributions of the human ABO blood groups. Nature 1962; 193:444.

284. Adalsteinsson S. Possible changes in the frequency of the human ABO blood groups in Iceland due to smallpox epidemics selection. Ann Hum Genet 1985; 49:275.

285. Bjarnason O, Bjarnason V, Edwards JH, et al. The blood groups of Icelanders. Ann Hum Genet 1973; 36:425.

286. Springer GF, Ansell N, Brandes W, Norris RF. Relation of blood group specific substances from bacilli and a higher plant to hemagglutinin formation. Proc 6th Congr Int Soc Blood Transf, Bibl Haematol Vol. 7, Basel: Karger, 1958:190,

287. Muschel LH, Osawa E. Human blood group substances B and *Escherichia coli* O_{86}. Proc Soc Exp Biol Med 1959; 101:614.

288. Moody MP, Young VM, Faber JE. Relationship of blood group antigens of the *Enterobacteriacea* to infections in humans. Proc Interscience Conf Antimicrob Agents and Chemotherapy, Washington DC, Am Soc Microbiol. Antimicrobiol Agents Chemother 1969; 424.

289. Robinson MG, Folchin D, Halpern C. Enteric bacterial agents and the ABO blood groups. Am J Hum Genet 1971; 23:135.

290. Wittels EG, Lichtman HC. Blood group incidence and *Escherichia coli* bacterial sepsis. Transfusion 1986; 26:533.

291. Sachs V. ABO blood groups and *Escherichia coli* sepsis. Transfusion 1987; 27:504.

292. van Loon FPL, Clemens JD, Sack DA, et al. ABO blood groups and the risk of diarrhea due to enterotoxigenic *Escherichia coli*. J Infect Dis 1991; 163:1243.

293. Glass RI, Holmgren J, Haley CE, et al. Predisposition for cholera of individuals with O blood group. Am J Epidemiol 1985; 121:791.

294. Barua D, Paquio AS. ABO blood groups and cholera. Ann Hum Biol 1977; 4:489.

295. Chaudhuri A. Cholera and blood-groups. Lancet 1977; 2:404.

296. Levine MM, Nalin DR, Rennels MB, et al. Genetic susceptibility to cholera. Ann Hum Biol 1979; 6:359.

297. Clemens JD, Sack DA, Harris JR, et al. ABO blood groups and cholera: New observations on specificity of risk and modification of vaccine efficacy. J Infect Dis 1989; 159:770.

298. Foster MT, Labrum AH. Relation of infection with *Neisseria gonorrhoeae* to blood groups. J Infect Dis 1976; 133:329.

299. Miler JJ, Novotney P, Walker PD, et al. *Neisseria gonorrhoeae* and ABO isohaemagglutinins. Infect Immun 1977; 15:713.

300. Kinane DF, Blackwell CC, Winstanley FP, Weir DM. Blood group secretor status and susceptibility to infection by *Neisseria gonorrhoeae*. Br J Vener Dis 1983; 59:44.

301. Kinane DF, Blackwell CC, Weir DM et al. ABO blood groups and susceptibility to gonococcal infection. III. Role of isohaemagglutinins in increased association of *Neisseria gonorrhoeae* to monocytes from blood group B individuals. J Clin Lab Immunol 1983, 12:83.

302. Blackwell CC, Kowolik M, Winstanley FP, et al. ABO blood group and susceptibility to gonococcal infection. I. Factors affecting phagocytosis of *Neisseria gonorrhoeae*. J Clin Lab Immunol 1983; 10:173.

303. Mandrell RE, Griffiss JM, Macher BA. Lipooligosaccharides (Los) of *Neisseria gonorrhoeae* and *Neisseria meningitidis* have components that are immunochemically similar to precursors of human blood group antigens. J Exp Med 1988; 168:107.

304. Adachi M, Hayami M, Kashiwagi N, et al. Expression of Le^y antigen in human immunodeficiency virus-infected human T cell lines and in peripheral lymphocytes of patients with acquired immune deficiency syndrome (AIDS) and AIDS-related complex (ARC). J Exp Med 1988; 167:323.

305. Arendrup M, Hansen J-ES, Clausen H, et al. Antibody to histo-blood group A antigen neutralizes HIV produced by lymphocytes from blood group A donors but not from blood group B or O donors. AIDS 1991; 5:441.

306. Berger SA, Young NA, Edberg SC. Relationship between infectious diseases and human blood type. Eur J Clin Microbiol Infect Dis 1989; 8:681.

307. Gershowitz H, Neel JV. The blood group polymorphisms: Why are they there? In: Aminoff D, ed. Blood and Tissue Antigens. New York: Academic Press, 1970:33.

308. Muschel LH. Blood groups, disease and selection. Bacteriol Rev 1966; 30:427.

309. Springer G.F. Importance of human red cell surface structures in reactions between man and microbes. In: Aminoff D, ed. Blood and Tissue Antigens. New York: Academic Press, 1970:265.

310. Garratty G, Petz LD. Acquired Immune Hemolytic Anemias. New York: Churchill Livingstone, 1980.

311. Schmidt PJ, Barile MF, McGinniss MH. *Mycoplasma* (pleuropneumonia-like organisms) and blood group I: Associations with neoplastic disease. Nature 1965; 205:371.

312. Smith CB, McGinniss MH, Schmidt PJ. Changes in erythrocyte I agglutinogen and anti-I agglutinins during *Mycoplasma pneumoniae* infection in man. J Immunol 1967; 99:333.

313. Feizi T, Taylor-Robinson D. Cold agglutinin anti-I and *Mycoplasma pneumoniae*. Immunology 1967; 13:405.

314. Feizi T, Taylor-Robinson D. Production of cold agglutinins in rabbits immunized with human erythrocytes treated with *Mycoplasma pneumoniae*. Nature 1969; 222:1253.

315. Costea N, Yakulis VJ, Heller P. Experimental production of cold agglutinins in rabbits. Blood 1965; 26:323.

316. Costea N, Yakulis VJ, Heller P. The mechanism of induction of cold agglutinins by *Mycoplasma pneumoniae*. J Immunol 1970; 106:598.

317. Costea N, Yakulis VJ, Heller P. Inhibition of cold agglutinins (anti-I) by *M. pneumoniae* antigens. Proc Soc Exp Biol Med 1972; 139:476.

318. Lind K. Production of cold agglutinins in rabbits induced by *Mycoplasma pneumoniae*, *Listeria monocytogenes*, or *Streptococcus MG*. Acta Path Microbiol Scand Section B 1973; 81:487.

319. Colling RG, Brown JC. The appearance of IgM and IgG cold agglutinins in rabbits hyperimmunized with group C streptococcal vaccine. J Immunol 1979; 122:202.

320. Loomes LM, Uemura K, Childs RA, et al. Erythrocyte receptors for *Mycoplasma pneumoniae* are sialylated oligosaccharides of li antigen type, Nature 1984; 307:560.

321. Loomes LM, Uemura K, Feizi T. Interaction of *Mycoplasma pneumoniae* with erythrocyte glycolipids of I and i antigen types. Infect Immun 1985; 47:15.

322. König AL, Kreft H, Hengge U, et al. Coexisting anti-I and anti-FI/Gd cold agglutinins in infections by *Mycoplasma pneumoniae*. Vox Sang 1988; 55:176.

323. Roelcke D, Kreft H, Northoff H, Gallasch E. Sia-b1 and I antigens recognized by *Mycoplasma pneumoniae*–induced human cold agglutinins. Transfusion 1991; 31:627.

324. Booth PB, Jenkins WJ, Marsh WL. Anti-I^T: A new antibody of the I blood group system occurring in certain Melanesian sera. Br J Haematol 1966; 12:341.
325. Layrisse Z, Layrisse M. High incidence cold autoagglutinins of anti-I^T specificity. Vox Sang 1968; 14:369.
326. Garratty G, Haffleigh B, Dalziel J, et al. An IgG anti-I^T detected in a Caucasian American. Transfusion 1972; 12:325.
327. Garratty G, Petz LD, Wallerstein RO, Autoimmune hemolytic anemia in Hodgkin's disease associated witn anti-I^T. Transfusion 1974; 14:226.
328. Freedman J, Newlands M, Johnson CA. Warm IgM anti-I^T causing autoimmune haemolytic anaemia. Vox Sang 1977; 32:135.
329. Levine AM, Thornton P, Forman SJ, et al. Positive Coombs test in Hodgkin's disease: Significance and implications. Blood 1980; 55:607.
330. Postoway N, Capon S, Smith L, et al. Cold agglutinin syndrome caused by anti-I^T. In: International Society of Blood Transfusion/American Association of Blood Banks Joint Congress, Book of Abstracts, 1990:85.
331. Marsh WL, Jenkins WJ. Anti-i: A new cold antibody. Nature 1960; 188:753.
332. Pitney WR, Thomas HN, Wells JV. Cold hemagglutinins associated with splenomegaly in New Guinea. Vox Sang 1968; 14:438.
333. Jenkins WJ, Koster HG, Marsh WL, Carter RL. Infectious mononucleosis: An unexpected source of anti-i. Br J Haematol 1965; 11:480.
334. Rosenfield RE, Schmidt PJ, Calvo RC, McGinnis MH. Anti-i: A frequent cold agglutinin in infectious mononucleosis. Vox Sang 1965; 10:631.
335. Capra JD, Dowling P, Cook S, Kunkel HG. An incomplete cold reactive γG antibody with i specificity in infectious mononucleosis. Vox Sang 1969; 16:10.
336. McGinniss MH. The ubiquitous nature of human blood group antigens as evidenced by bacterial, viral and parasitic infections. In: Garratty G, ed. Blood Group Antigens and Disease. Arlington, VA: American Association of Blood Banks, 1983:25.
337. Henle G, Henle W, Diehl V. Relation of Burkitt's tumor-associated Herpes-type virus to infectious mononucleosis. Proc Natl Acad Sci USA 1968: 59:94.
338. Kao YS, Frank S, DeJongh DS. Anti-M in children with acute bacterial infections. Transfusion 1978; 18:320.
339. Väisänen V, Korhonen TK, Jokinen M, et al. Blood group M specific haemagglutinin in pyelonephritogenic Escherichia coli, Lancet 1982; 1:1192.
340. Morgan P, Bossom EL. "Naturally occurring" anti-Kell (K1): Two examples. Transfusion 1963; 5:397.
341. Tegoli J, Sausais L, Issitt PD. Another example of a "naturally-occurring" anti-K1. Vox Sang 1967; 12:305.
342. Kanel GC, Davis I, Bowman JE. "Naturally-occurring" anti-K1: Possible association with Mycobacterium infection. Transfusion 1978; 18:472.
343. Marsh WL, Nichols ME, Oyen R, et al. Naturally occurring anti-Kell stimulated by E coli enterocolitis in a 20 day old child. Transfusion 1978; 18:149.
344. McGinniss MH, MacLowry JD, Holland PV. Acquisition of Kell-like antigen by Kell negative red cells. Transfusion 1978; 18:624.
345. McGinniss MH, Leiberman R, Holland PV. The Jk^b red cell antigen and gram-negative organisms. Transfusion 1979; 19:663.
346. Byrd LH, Cheigh JS, Stenzel KH, et al. Association between Streptococcus faecalis urinary infections and graft rejection in kidney transplants. Lancet 1978; 2:1167.
347. Bird GWG, Roy TCF. Human serum antibodies to melibiose and other carbohydrates. Vox Sang 1980; 38:169.
348. Källenius G, Möllby R, Svenson SB, et al. The P^k antigen as a receptor for the haemagglutinin of pyelonephritic Escherichia coli. FEMS Microbiol Lett 1980; 7:297.
349. Väisänen V, Elo J, Tallgren LG, et al. Mannose-resistant haemagglutination and P antigen recognition are characteristic of Escherichia coli causing primary pyelonephritis. Lancet 1981; 2:1366.
350. Källenius G, Möllby R, Svenson SB, et al. Occurrence of P-fimbriated Escherichia coli in urinary tract infections. Lancet 1981; 2:1369.

351. Korhonen TK, Väisänen V, Saxén H, et al. P-antigen-recognizing fimbriae from human uropathogenic *Escherichia coli* strains. Infect Immun 1982; 37:286.

352. Lomberg H, Hanson LÅ, Jacobsson B, et al. Correlation of P blood group, vesicoureteral reflux, and bacterial attachment in patients with recurrent pyelonephritis. N Engl J Med 1983; 308:1189.

353. Gander RM, Thomas VL, Forland M. Mannose-resistant hemagglutination and P receptor recognition of uropathogenic *Escherichia coli* isolated from adult patients. J Infect Dis 1985; 151:508.

354. Martenson E. On the neutral glycolipids of human kidney. Acta Chem Scand 1963; 17:2356.

355. Makita A, Yamakawa T. Biochemistry of organ glycolipids. III. The structures of human kidney cerebroside sulfuric ester, ceramide dihexoside and ceramide trihexoside. J Biochem 1964; 55:365.

356. Leffler H, Svanborg CE. Chemical identification of glycosphingolipid receptor for *Escherichia coli* attaching to human urinary tract epithelial cells and agglutinating human erythrocytes. FEMS Microbiol Lett 1980; 8:127.

357. Sussman M, Parry SH, Rooke DM, Lee MJS. Bacterial adherence and the urinary tract. Lancet 1982; 1:1352.

358. Editorial. What makes microbes stick? Lancet, 1988; 2:1343.

359. Kaack MB, Roberts JA, Baskin G, Patterson GM. Maternal immunization with P Fimbriae for the prevention of neonatal pyelonephritis. Infect Immun 1988; 56:1.

360. Sobota AE. Inhibition of bacterial adherence by cranberry juice: Potential use for the treatment of urinary tract infection. J Urol 1984; 131:1013.

361. Schmidt DR, Sobota AE. An examination of the anti-adherence activity of cranberry juice on urinary and nonurinary bacterial isolates. Microbios 1988; 55:173.

362. Zafriri D, Ofek I, Adar R, Pocino M, Sharon N. Inhibitory activity of cranberry juice on adherence of type 1 and type P fimbriated *Escherichia coli* to eucaryotic cells. Antimicrob Agents Chemother 1989; 33:92.

363. Ofek I, Goldhar J, Zafriri D, et al. Anti–*Escherichia coli* adhesin activity of cranberry and blueberry juices. N Engl J Med 1991; 324:1599.

364. Parkkinen J, Rogers GN, Korhonen T, et al. Identification of O-linked sialyloligosaccharides of glycophorin A as the erythrocyte receptors for S-fimbriated *Escherichia coli*. Infect Immun 1986; 54:37.

365. Pieroni P, Worobec EA, Paranchych W, Armstrong GD. Identification of a human erythrocyte receptor for colonization factor antigen I pili expressed by H10407 enterotoxigenic *Escherichia coli*. Infect Immun 1988; 56: 1334.

366. Nowicki B, Moulds J, Hull R, Hull S. A hemagglutinin of uropathogenic *Escherichia coli* recognizes the Dr blood group antigen. Infect Immun 1988; 56:1057.

367. Daniels G. Cromer-related antigens—blood group determinants on decay-accelerating factor. Vox Sang 1989; 56:205.

368. Nowicki B, Truong L, Moulds J, Hull R. Presence of the Dr receptor in normal human tissues and its possible role in the pathogenesis of ascending urinary tract infection. Am J Clin Pathol 1988; 133:1.

369. Nowicki B, Holthöfer H, Saraneva T, et al. Location of adhesion sites for P-fimbriated and 075X-positive *Escherichia coli* in the human kidney. Microb Pathog 1986; 1:169.

370. Nowicki B, Hull R, Moulds J. Use of the Dr hemagglutinin of uropathogenic *Escherichia coli* to differentiate normal from abnormal red cells in paroxysmal nocturnal hemoglobinuria. N Engl J Med 1988; 319:1289.

371. Rosenstein IJ, Stoll MS, Mizuochi T, et al. New type of adhesive specificity revealed by oligosaccharide probes in *Escherichia coli* from patients with urinary tract infection. Lancet 1988; 1327.

372. Kinane DF, Blackwell CC, Brettle RP, et al. ABO blood group, secretor state, and susceptibility to recurrent urinary tract infection in women. Br Med J 1982; 285:7.

373. Blackwell CC, Andrew S, May SJ, et al. ABO blood group and susceptibility to urinary tract infection: no evidence for involvement of isohaemagglutinins. J Clin Lab Immunol 1984; 15:191.

374. Lomberg H, Cedergren B, Leffler H, et al. Influence of blood groups on the availability of receptors for attachment of uropathogenic *Escherichia coli*. Infect Immun 1986; 51:919.

375. Sheinfeld J, Schaeffer AJ, Cordon-Cardo C, et al. Association of the Lewis blood-group phenotype with recurrent urinary tract infections in women. N Engl J Med 1989; 320:773.

376. Lurie S, Sigler E, Fenakel K. The ABO, Lewis or P blood group phenotypes are not associated with recurrent pelvic inflammatory disease. Gynecol Obstet Invest 1991; 31:158.

377. Pichichero ME, Loeb M, Anderson P, Smith DH. Do pili play a role in pathogenicity of haemophilus influenzae type B? Lancet 1982; 1:960.

378. van Alphen L, Poole J, Overbeek J. The Anton blood group antigen is the erythrocyte receptor for *Haemophilus influenzae*. FEMS Mibrobiol Lett 1986; 37:69.

379. Poole J, van Alphen L. *Haemophilus influenzae* receptor and the AnWj antigen. Transfusion 1988; 28:289.

380. van ALphen L, Levene C, Geelen-van den Broek L, et al. Combined inheritance of epithelial and erythrocyte receptors for *Haemophilus influenzae*. Infect Immun 1990; 58:3807.

381. Miller LH, Mason SJ, Dvorak JA, et al. Erythrocyte receptors for (*Plasmodium knowlesi*) malaria: Duffy blood group determinants. Science 1975; 189:561.

382. Miller LH, Mason SJ, Clyde DF, McGinniss MH. The resistance factor to *Plasmodium vivax* in blacks. N Engl J Med 1976; 295:302.

383. Barnwell JW, Nichols ME, Rubinstein P. In vitro evaluation of the role of the Duffy blood group in erythrocyte invasion by *Plasmodium vivax*. J Exp Med 1989; 169:1795.

384. Hadley TJ, Miller LH, Haynes JD. Recognition of red cells by malaria parasites: The role of erythrocyte-binding proteins. Trans Med Rev 1991; 5:108.

385. Hadley TJ, McGinniss MH, Klotz FW, Miller LH. Blood group antigens and invasion of erythrocytes by malaria parasites. In: Garratty, ed. Antigens and Antibodies Arlington, VA: American Association of Blood Banks, 1986:17.

386. Miller LH, Haynes JD, McAuliffe FM, et al. Evidence for differences in erythrocyte surface receptors for the malarial parasites, *Plasmodium falciparum* and *Plasmodium knowlesi*. J Exp Med 1977; 146:277.

387. Perkins ME. Inhibitory effects of erythrocyte membrane proteins on the in vitro invasion of the human malarial parasite (*Plasmodium falciparum*) into its host cell. J Cell Biol 1981; 90:563.

388. Breuer WV, Ginsburg H Cabantchik ZI. An assay of malaria parasite invasion into human erythrocytes. The effects of chemical and enzymatic modification of erythrocyte membrane components. Biochem Biophys Acta 1983; 755:263.

389. Pasvol G, Jungery M, Weatherall DJ, et al. Glycophorin as a possible receptor for plasmodium falciparum. Lancet 1982; 1:947.

390. Cartron JP, Prou O, Lulier PM, Soulier JP. Susceptibility to invasion by *Plasmodium falciparum* of some human erythrocytes carrying rare blood group antigens. Br J Haematol 1983; 55:639.

391. Facer CA. Erythrocyte sialoglycoproteins and *Plasmodium falciparum* invasion. Transac Roy Soc Trop Med Hyg 1983; 77:524.

392. Hermentin P, Enders B, Neunziger G, et al. Wr(a+b–) red blood cells are fully susceptible to invasion by plasmodium falciparum. Lancet 1984; 2:466.

393. Cartron JP, Tounkara A, Prou O, et al. Wr^b antigen not required for invasion of human erythrocytes by plasmodium falciparum. Lancet 1984; 2:466.

394. Facer CA, Mitchell GH. Wr^b negative erythrocytes are susceptible to invasion by malaria parasites. Lancet 1984; 2:758.

395. Hermentin P, David PH, Miller LH, et al. Wright (a+b–) human erythrocytes and *Plasmodium falciparum* malaria. Blut 1985; 50:75.

396. Hadley TJ, Klotz FW, Pasvol G., et al. Falciparum malaria parasites invade erythrocytes that lack glycophorin A and B (M^kM^k). J Clin Invest 1987; 80:1190.

397. Perkins ME. Stage-dependent processing and localization of a a *Plasmodium falciparum* protein of 130,000 molecular weight. Exp Parasitol 1988; 65:61.

398. Camus D, Hadley TJ. A *Plasmodium flaciparum* antigen that binds to host erythrocytes and merozoites. Science 1985; 230:553.

399. Perkins ME, Rocco LJ. Sialic acid-dependent binding of *Plasmodium falciparum* merozoite surface antigen, Pf200, to human erythrocytes. J Immunol 1988; 141:3190.

400. Ravetch JV, Kochan J, Perkins M. Isolation of the gene for a glycophorin-binding protein implicated in erythrocyte invasion by a malaria parasite. Science 1985; 227–1593.

401. Fang X, Kaslow DC, Adams JH, et al. Cloning of the *Plasmodium vivax* Duffy receptor. Mol Biochem Parasitol 44:125.

402. Orlandi PA, Sim BKL, Chulay JD, et al. Characterization of the 175-kilodalton erythrocyte binding antigen of *Plasmodium falciparum*. Mol Biochem Parasitol 1990; 40:285.

403. Sim BKL, Orlandi PA, Haynes JD, et al. Primary structure of the 175 K *Plasmodium falciparum* erythrocyte binding antigen and identification of a peptide which elicits antibodies that inhibit malaria merozoite invasion. J Cell Biol 1990; 111:1877.

404. Orlandi PA, Sim BKL, Chaulay JD, et al. Characterization of the 175-kilodalton erythrocyte binding antigen of *Plasmodium falciparum*. Mol Biochem Parasitol 1990; 40:285.

405. Cameron GL, Staveley JM. Blood group P substance in hydatid cyst fluids. Nature 1957; 179:147.

406. Staveley JM, Cameron GL. The inhibiting action of hydatid cyst fluid on anti-Tj^a sera. Vox Sang 1958; 3:114.

407. Prokop O, Schlesigner D. Über das vorkommen von P$_1$-blutgruppensubstanz oder einer P$_1$-like substany bei lumbricus terrestris. Z Immun Forsch 1965; 129:344.

408. Prokop O, Schlesigner, D. Über das vorkommen von P$_1$ blutgruppensubstanz bei *Ascaris suum*. Dtsh Gesd Wes 1965; 20:1584.

409. Bevan B, Hammond W, Clarke RI. Anti-P$_1$ associated with liver fluke infection. Vox Sang 1970; 18;188.

410. Barnes GL, Kay R. Blood-groups in giardiasis. Lancet 1977; 1:808.

411. Zisman, M. (1977). Blood-group A and giardiasis. Lancet 1977; 2:1285.

412. Sotto A, Cabrera S, Castro J, et al. Blood groups in recurrent giardiasis. Lancet 1983; 2:1312.

413. Jokipii L, Jokippi A. Is predisposition to giardiasis associated with the blood groups? Am J Trop Med 1980; 29:5.

414. Pardoe GI, Jaquet H, Hahn R, et al. The immunochemistry of surface antigens of *Leishmania enrietti*. Behring Inst Mitt 1975; 58:30.

415. Decker-Jackson JE, Honigberg BM. Glycoproteins released by *Leishmania donovani*. Immunological relationships with host and bacterial antigens and preliminary biochemical analysis. J Protozool 1978; 25:515.

416. Greenblatt CL, Kark JD, Schnur LF, Slutzky GM. Do Leishmania serotypes mimic human blood group antigens? Lancet 1981; 1:505.

417. van Loghem JJ, Dorfmeier H, van der Hart M. Two antigens with abnormal serologic properties. Vox Sang 1957; 2:16.

418. Salmon C. A tentative approach to variations in ABH and associated erythrocyte antigens. Ser Haematol 1969; II:3.

419. Crookston MC. Anomalous ABO, H and Ii phenotypes in disease. In: Garratty G, ed. Blood Group Antigens and Disease. Arlington, VA: American Association of Blood Banks, 1983:67.

420. Dreyfus B, Sultan C, Rochant H, et al. Anomalies of blood group antigens and erythrocyte enzymes in two types of chronic refractory anaemia. Br J Haematol 1969; 16:303.

421. Salmon C. Blood groups changes in preleukemic states. Blood Cells 1976; 2:211.

422. Rochant H, Tonthat H, Henri A, et al. Abnormal distribution of erythrocytes A$_1$ antigens in preleukemia as demonstrated by an immunoflourescence technique. Blood Cells 1976; 2:237.

423. Saichua S, Chiewsilp P. Red cell ABH antigens in leukaemias and lymphomas. Vox Sang 1978; 35:154.

424. Salmon CH, Andre R, Dreyfus B. Arguments en faveur de mutations somatiques du gene de groupe sanguin A, au cours de certaines leucemies aigues. Proc 7th Congr Europ Soc Haematol 1959; 2:1171.

425. Salmon CH, Andre R, Dreyfus B. Double population de globules, differant seulement par l'antigene de groupe ABO, observe chez un malade leucemique, Rev Hematol 1958; 13:148.

426. Renton PH, Stratton F, Gunson HH, Hancock JA. Red cells of all four ABO groups in a case of leukemia. Br Med J 1962; i:294.

427. Salmon CH, Andre R, Philippon J. Agglutinabilite normale des hematies A$_1$ transfusees a trois malades leucemiques de phenotype A modifie. Rev Franc Etudes Clin Biol 1961; 6:792.

428. Tilley CA, Crookston MC, Crookston JH, et al. Human blood-group A- and H-specified glycosyltransferase levels in the sear of newborn infants and their mothers. Vox Sang 1978; 34:8.

429. Kahn A, Vroclans M, Hakim J, Boivin P. Differences in the two red cell populations in erythroleukaemia. Lancet 1971; 2:933.

430. Kuhns WJ, Oliver RTD, Watkins WM, Greenwell P. Leukemia-induced alterations of serum glycosyltransferase enzymes. Cancer Res 1980; 40:268.

431. Koscielak J, Pacuszka T, Miller-Podraza H, Zdziechowska H. Activities of fucosyltransferases in sera of leukaemic patients: Platelet origin of serum α-6-L-fucosyltransferase. Biochem Soc Transac 1987; 15:603.

432. Yoshida A, Kumazaki T, Davé V, et al. Suppressed expression of blood group B antigen and blood group galactosyltransferase in a preleukemic subject. Blood 1985; 66:990.

433. Atkinson JB, Tanley PC, Wallas CH. Loss of blood group A in acute leukemia. Transfusion 1987; 27:45.

434. Lopez M, Bonnet-Gajdos M, Reviron M, et al. An acute leukaemia augured before clinical signs by blood group antigen abnormalities and low levels of A and H blood group transferase activities in erythrocytes. Br J Haematol 1986; 63:535.

435. Benson K. Decreased ABH blood group antigen expression associated with preleukemic conditions and acute leukemia: Loss of detectable B, then A antigens in a group AB patient progressing from a myelodysplastic syndrome to leukemia. Immunohematology 1991; 7:89.

436. Tovey GH, Lockyer JW, Tierney RBH. Changes in Rh grouping reactions in a case of leukaemia. Vox Sang 1961; 6:628.

437. Garner RJ, Rembe AM, Landells M. Loss of Rh₀(D) antigen. Transfusion 1980; 20:619.

438. Bracey AW, McGinniss MH, Levine RM, Whang-Peng J. Rh mosaicism and aberrant MNSs antigen expression in a patient with chronic myelogenous leukemia. Am J Clin Pathol 1983; 79:397.

439. Májsky A. Some cases of leukemia with modifications of the D (Rho) receptor. Neoplasma 1967; 14:335.

440. Cooper B, Tishler PV, Atkins L, Breg WR. Loss of Rh antigen associated with acquired Rh antibodies and chromosome translocation in a patient with myeloid metaplasia. Blood 1979; 54:642.

441. van Brockstaele DR, Berneman ZN, Muyelle L, et al. Flow cytometric analysis of erythrocytic D antigen density profile. Vox Sang 1986; 51:40.

442. Marsh WL, Chaganti RSK, Gardner FH, et al. Mapping human autosomes: evidence supporting assignment of rhesus to the short arm of chromosome no. 1. Science 1974; 183:966.

443. Levan A, Nichols WW, Hall B. Mixture of Rh positive and Rh negative erythrocytes and chromosomal abnormalities in a case of polycythemia. Hereditas 52:89.

444. Callender ST, Kay HEM, Lawler SD, et al. Two populations of Rh groups together with chromosomally abnormal cell lines in the bone marrow. Br Med J 1971; 1:131.

445. Marsh WL, Johnson CL, DiNapoli J, et al. Two cases of acquired in vivo change in red cell Rh type. Transfusion 1980; 20:619.

446. Kassulke JT, Hallgren HM, Yunis EJ. Studies of red cell isoantigens on peripheral leukocytes from normal and leukemic individuals. Am J Pathol 1969; 56:333.

447. Gold ER, Tovey GH, Benney WE, Lewis FJW. Changes in the group A antigen in a case of leukemia. Nature 1959; 183:892.

448. Kolins J, Holland PV, McGinniss MH. Multiple red cell antigen loss in acute granulocytic leukemia. Cancer 1978; 42:2248.

449. Ayres M, Salzano FM, Ludwig OK. Blood group changes in leukemia. J Med Genet 1966; 3:180.

450. McGinniss MH, Schmidt PJ, Carbone PP. Close association of I blood group and disease. Nature 1964; 202:606.

451. McGinniss MH, Kirkham WR, Schmidt PJ Modified expression of the ABO, I, and H antigens in acute myelogenous leukemia. Transfusion 1964; 4:310.

452. Garratty G. Target antigens for red cell-bound autoantibodies. In: Nance SJ, ed. Clinical and Serological Aspects of Immunohematology. Arlington, VA: American Association of Blood Banks, 1991:33.

453. Brody JI, Beizer LH. Alteration of blood group antigens in leukemic lymphocytes. J Clin Invest 1965; 44:1582.

454. Shumak KH, Rachkewich RA, Crookston MC, Crookston JH. Antigens of the li system on lymphocytes. Nature New Biol 1971; 231:148.

455. Shumak KH, Beldotti LE, Rachkewich RA. Diagnosis of haematological disease using anti-i. I. Disorders with lymphocytosis. Br J Haematol 1979; 41:399.
456. Shumak KH, Rachkewich RA Beldotti LE. Diagnosis of haematological disease using anti-i. II. Distinction between acute myeloblastic and acute lymphoblastic leukaemia. Br J Haematol 1979; 41:407.
457. Shumak KH, Baker MA, Taub RN, et al. Myeloblastic and lymphoblastic markers in acute undifferentiated leukemia and chronic myelogenous leukemia in blast crisis. Cancer Res 1980; 40:4048.
458. Pruzanski W, Farid N, Keystone E, Armstrong M. The influence of homogeneous cold agglutinins on polymorphonuclear and mononuclear phagocytes. Clin Immunol Immunopathol 1975; 4:277.
459. O'Hara CJ, Shumak KH. Price GB. The i antigen on human myeloid progenitors. Clin Immunol Immunopathol 1978; 10:420.
460. Issitt PD. I blood group system and its relationship to disease. J Med Lab Technol 1968; 25:1.
461. Giblett ER, Crookston MC. Agglutinability of red cells by anti-i in patients with thalassaemia major and other haematological disorders. Nature 1964; 201:1138.
462. Rochant PH, Tonthat H, Man NM, et al. Étude quantitative des antigènes érythrocytaires I et i en pathologie. Nouv Rev Fr d'Hematol 1973; 13:307.
463. Crookston JH, Crookston MC, Burnie KL, et al. Hereditary erythroblastic multinuclearity associated with a positive acidified-serum test: A type of congenital dyserythropoietic anaemia. Br J Haematol 17:11.
464. Maniatis A, Bertles JF. Erythrocyte I-i antigens: Distribution in normal and sickle erythrocytes and relationship of i antigenicity to hemoglobin F cell content. In: Kruckeberg WC, et al, eds. Erythrocyte Membranes: Recent Clinical and Experimental Advances. New York: Liss, 1978:159.
465. Papayannopoulu T, Chen P, Maniatis A, Stamatoyannopoulos G. Simultaneous assessment of i-antigenic expression and fetal hemoglobin in single red cells by immunofluorescence. Blood 1980; 55:221.
466. Hillman RS, Giblett ER. Red cell membrane alteration associated with "marrow stress." J Clin Invest 1965; 44:1730.
467. Vainchenker W, Testa U, Rochant H, et al. Cellular regulation of i and I antigen expressions in human erythroblasts grown in vitro. Stem Cells 1981; 1:97.
468. Sieff C, Bicknell D, Caine G, et al. Changes in cell surface antigen expression during hemopoietic differentiation. Blood 1982; 60:703.
469. Cooper AG, Hoffbrand, AV, Worlledge SM. Increased agglutinability by anti-i of red cells in sideroblastic and megaloblastic anaemia. Br J Haematol 1968; 15:381.
470. Wang WC, Mentzer WC. Differentiation of transient erythroblastopenia of childhood from congenital hypoplastic anemia. J Pediatr 1976; 88:784.
471. Morton JA, Pickles MM, Darley JH. Increase in strength of red cell Bg[a] antigen following infectious mononucleosis. Vox Sang 1977; 32:26.
472. Morton JA, Pickles MM, Turner JE, Cullen PR. Changes in red cell Bg antigens in haematological disease. Immunol Commun 1980; 9:173.
473. Morton JA, Pickles MM, Sutton L. The correlation of the Bg[a] blood group with the HL-A7 leucocyte group; demonstration of antigenic sites on red cells and leucocytes. Vox Sang 1969; 17:536.
474. Morton JA, Pickles MM, Sutton L, Skov F. Identification of further antigens on red cells and lymphocytes. Association of Bg[b] with W17 (Te57) and Bg[c] with W28 (Dal5, Ba*). Vox Sang, 1971; 21:141.
475. Thomas DB. The i antigen complex: a new specificity unique to dividing human cells. Eur J Immunol, 1974; 4:819.
476. Beck ML. Blood group antigens acquired de novo. In: Blood Group Antigens and Disease. Arlington, VA: American Association of Blod Banks, 1983:45.
477. Levene C, Levene NA, Buskila D, Manny N. Red cell polyagglutination. Trans Med Rev 1988; 2:176.
478. Judd WJ. Polyagglutination. Immunohematology. 1992; 8:58.
479. Gerbal A, Maslet C, Salmon C. Immunological aspects of the acquired B antigen. Vox Sang 1975; 28:398.
480. Gerbal A, Ropars C, Gerbal R, et al. Acquired B antigen disappearance by in vitro acetylation associated with A₁ activity restoration. Vox Sang 1987; 31:64.

481. Rawlinson VI, Stratton F. Incidence of T activation in a hospital population. Vox Sang 1984; 46:306.

482. Buskila D, Levene C, Bird GWG, Levene NA. Polyagglutination in hospitalized patients: A prospective study. Vox Sang 1987; 52:99.

483. Lenz G, Goes U, Baron D, et al. Red blood cell T-activation and hemolysis in surgical intensive care patients with severe infections. Blut 1987; 54:89.

484. Adams M, Toy PTCY, Reid ME. Exposure of cryptantigens on red blood cell membranes in patients with acquired immune deficiency syndrome or AIDS-related complex. J Acquir Immune Defic Syndr 1989; 2:224.

485. Poschmann A, Fischer K. Hamolytisch-uramisches syndrome. Med Klin 1974; 69:1821.

486. Klein PJ, Bulla M, Newman R.A. et al. Thomsen-Friedenreich antigen in haemolytic-uraemic syndrome. Lancet 1977; 2:1024.

487. Seger R, Joller P, Baerlocher K, et al. Hemolytic-uremic syndrome associated with neuraminidase-producing microorganisms: Treatment by exchange transfusion. Helv Paediat Acta 1980; 35:359.

488. Hamilton DV, Black AJ, Darnborough J, Bird GWG. Haemolytic-uraemic syndrome and T-activation of red blood cells. Clin Lab Haematol 1983; 5:109.

489. Berger EG, Kozdrowski I. Permanent mixed-field polyagglutinable erythrocytes lack galacto-syltransferase activity. FEBS Lett 1978; 93:105.

490. Vainchenker W, Testa U, Deschamps JF, et al. Clonal expression of the Tn antigen in erythroid and granulocyte colonies and its application to determination of the clonality of the human megakaryocyte colony assay. J Clin Invest 1982; 69: 1081.

491. Brouet JC, Vainchenker W, Blanchard D, et al. The origin of human B and T cells from multipotent stem cells: A study of the Tn syndrome. Eur J Immunol 1983; 13:350.

492. Vainchenker W, Vinci G, Testa U, et al. Presence of the Tn antigen on hematopoietic progenitors from patients with the Tn syndrome. J Clin Invest 1985; 75:541.

493. Jiji RM, Jahn EFW, Bilenki LA. Tn-activation with acquired A-like antigens associated with pancytopenia and "ringed" sideroblasts. Transfusion 1973; 13:359.

494. Jiji RM. Letter to the Editor. Blood 1979; 54:1451.

495. Sondag-Thull D, Levene NA, Levene C, et al. Characterization of a neuraminidase from *Corynebacterium aquaticum* responsible for Th polyagglutination. Vox Sang 1989; 57:193.

496. Herman JH, Shirey RS, Smith B, et al. Th activation in congenital hypoplastic anemia. Transfusion 1987; 27:253.

497. Herman JH, Whiteheart W, Shirey RS, et al. Red cell Th activation: Biochemical studies. Br J Haematol 1987; 65:205.

498. Bird GWG, Wingham J. Tk: A new form of red cell polyagglutination. Br J Haematol 1987; 23:759.

499. Graninger W, Rameis H, Fischer K, et al. "VA": A new type of erythrocyte polyagglutination characterized by depressed H receptors and associated with hemolytic anemia. I. Serological and hematological observations. Vox Sang 1977; 32: 195.

500. Graninger W, Poschmann A, Fischer K, et al. "VA": A new type of erythrocyte polyagglutination characterized by depressed H receptors and associated with hemolytic anemia. II. Observations by immunofluorescence, electron microscopy, cell electrophoresis and biochemistry. Vox Sang 1977; 32:201.

501. Schmidt PJ. The hemolytic anemia of the Rh$_{null}$ blood group. In: Steane EA, ed. Cellular Antigens and Disease. Washington, DC: American Association of Blood Banks, 1977:31.

502. Vengelen-Tyler V. The Rh blood group system and its association with disease. In: Vengelen-Tyler V, Pierce S, eds. Blood Group Systems: Rh. Arlington, VA: American Association of Blood Banks, 1987:77.

503. Reid ME, Bird GWG. Associations between human red cell blood group antigens and disease. TransMed Rev 1990; 4:47.

9

Associations of Red Blood Cell Membrane Abnormalities with Blood Group Phenotype

MARION E. REID
The New York Blood Center
New York, New York

I. BLOOD GROUP ANTIGENS

Blood group antigens are polymorphic, inherited, structural characteristics that are located on proteins, glycoproteins or glycolipids on the outer surface of the red blood cell (RBC) membrane. For decades blood group antigens have been recognized to be clinically important in the immune destruction of RBCs in homologous blood transfusions, maternofetal blood group incompatibility, autoimmune hemolytic anemia, and organ transplantation.

The polymorphism of human blood groups has been exploited in the following ways: They have served as a valuable tool to monitor in vivo survival of transfused RBCs, originally by a differential hemagglutination technique and more recently by flow cytometry. By virtue of their relative ease of detection by hemagglutination and their generally straightforward mode of inheritance, blood group antigens have been used in anthropological, genetic and forensic investigations. Blood group antigen profiles have been used to predict inheritance of diseases that are encoded by genes in close proximity to the gene encoding the blood group antigen. The presence of certain antigens has been implicated in susceptibility or resistance to certain diseases.

The persistence of blood group structures in evolution suggests that blood group antigens are located on biologically important structures. Thus blood group antigens have been used as tools in the analysis of structure and function of RBC membrane components on which they are carried. These antigens also have been used as probes to study the complexities of genes that encode them. Information obtained by such studies has not only provided insight into the workings of the RBC but has served as a model for other cells. Many of the glycoproteins that are in the human RBC membrane are not restricted to the erythroid lineage but are present on other hemopoietic cells as well as cells from other tissues (1).

II. RED BLOOD CELL MEMBRANE

The RBC membrane consists of a lipid bilayer through which pass integral proteins. On the cytoplasmic aspect of the lipid bilayer is a membrane skeleton that interacts with the lipid bilayer to confer the dynamic, fluid properties of the RBC membrane. The RBC membrane skeleton consists of many interacting proteins and an absence, deficiency, or abnormality in a number of these proteins can result in hematological disease. For example, changes in protein 4·1 have caused hereditary elliptocytosis (HE); changes in spectrin have caused HE or hereditary spherocytosis (HS); changes in ankyrin or in protein 4·2 have caused HS; and a deficiency in band 7 has resulted in stomatocytosis (reviewed in ref. 2). As will be discussed below, the absence or presence of altered forms of critical transmembrane proteins can also induce RBC shape changes (see Table 1), possibly by upsetting the balance of skeletal protein interactions and/or by altering certain transport properties of the RBC membrane.

The major proteins of the RBC membrane were identified after separation of the components by electrophoresis on polyacrylamide gels in the presence of sodium dodecyl sulfate. Staining of the gels with Coomassie blue detects several proteins and staining with periodic acid Schiff's base detects the four major glycoproteins (reviewed in ref. 3). By using more sensitive techniques (immunoblotting and immunoprecipitation) with antibodies to blood group antigens (human polyclonal and human or murine monoclonal), numerous other glycoproteins have been identified. A summary of blood group antigens that have been assigned to a specific protein is shown in Table 2. Antigens carried on glycolipids are not included in Table 2. When a unique protein has been partially characterized, it can be studied in depth at protein and genetic levels. Once the structure of a protein has been established, the role it plays can often be predicted. Blood group antigens that are exclusively dependent upon carbohydrates, whether attached to glycoproteins or glycolipids (i.e., A, B, H, I, i, Le^a, Le^b, P, P^k, P$_1$, LKE, Sd^a, Cad, T, Tn, and Tk) and those that are on immunologically important membrane components in terms of complement regulation or bacterial receptors are discussed elsewhere within this book.

The purpose of this chapter is to review the association of demonstrable RBC membrane abnormalities and blood group phenotypes with disease. For situations where a disease causes an alteration in the RBC membrane and blood group antigen expression or where a disease inheritance pattern can be predicted through blood group antigen testing, see a recent review by Reid and Bird (19). This chapter concentrates on blood groups that have been associated with a compromised membrane in relation to the ability of the RBC membrane to maintain a normal morphology or function.

Table 1 RBC Shape Changes Induced by Absent or Altered Membrane Skeletal or Transmembrane Proteins

RBC Morphology	Skeletal Proteins	Transmembrane Proteins
Acanthocyte		Kx polypeptide
		Lutheran polypeptide
Elliptocyte	Protein 4·1	Glycophorin C and D
	Spectrin	Band 3
Ovalocyte		Band 3
Spherocyte	Spectrin	Band 3
	Ankyrin	
	Protein 4·2	
Stomatocyte	Band 7	Rh polypeptides

Table 2 Blood Group Antigens That Have Been Assigned to Specific RBC Membrane Proteins

Blood Group Antigen	RBC Membrane Component	Apparent Molar Mass (M_r)	Chromosome Location
ABH	Band 3 anion transport	90,000–110,000	9q 34
	Protein 4·5 glucose transporter	45,000–55,000	Transferase gene
M,N,En^a	Glycophorin A	43,000	4q28–q31
'N', S,s,U	Glycophorin B	25,000	4q28–q31
Numerous MNS-related antigens	Altered GPA, GPB, or hybrids of GPA and GPB		4q28–q31
Rh antigens	Complex of Rh polypeptides 2D10 type, CD47	30,000 45,000–100,000 47,000–52,000	1p36–p34
LW antigens	LW glycoprotein	40,000–47,000	19p13–p11
Fy antigens	Fy glycoprotein	35,500–90,000	1q22–q23
Lu antigens	Lutheran glycoprotein	78,000–85,000	19q12–q13
Kell antigens	Kell protein (metalloglycopeptidase)	93,000	7q33
Kx	Kx protein	37,000	Xp21.1
Ge2	Glycophorin D	30,000	2q14–q21
Ge3	Glycophorins C and D		2q14–q21
Ge4	Glycophorin C	40,000	2q14–q21
Wb, Dh^a, An^a, Ls^a	Altered forms of GPC, GPD or both		2q14–q21
Ok^a	Ok^a glycoprotein	35,000–69,000	19p13.2–pter
In antigens	CD44	80,000	11p13
Sc antigens	Scianna protein	68,000	1p32–p32
Cromer-related antigens	DAF (CD55)	70,000	1q32
Gy^a, Hy; Jo^a, Do^a, Do^b	Gregory glycoprotein	47,000–56,000	
Yt antigens	Acetylcholinesterase	72,000 (reduced)	7q22
JMH	JMH protein	76,000	
Chido; Rodgers	C4	Multiple bands	6p21.3
McCoy, Knops, Sl^a, Yk^a	CRI (CD35)	160,000–250,000	1
Xg^a	Xg^a glycoprotein	22,000–25,000; 26,500–29,000	Xp22–pter
Pt^a	Pt^a protein	31,600	

Data from Refs. 1 and 4–18.

III.   DISEASES ASSOCIATED WITH RBC SHAPE CHANGES AND BLOOD GROUP PHENOTYPES

A.   Hereditary Acanthocytosis

1. McLeod Phenotype

Red blood cells with the McLeod phenotype react weakly with Kell system antibodies, lack the common Kx antigen, are acanthocytic, and have a reduced in vivo survival (20). McLeod phenotype RBCs lack Kx protein and have a marked deficiency of Kell protein (21). The altered properties of McLeod phenotype RBCs are unlikely to be a consequence of their reduced level of Kell protein because Ko RBCs which totally lack this protein, are apparently normal. Ko RBCs have about twice the amount of Kx protein as do RBCs of common Kell type. Red blood cells with common Kell phenotypes possess Kell protein and low levels of Kx antigen in the approximate proportion of 10:1 (21). The relationship between Kell and Kx proteins in the RBC membrane is not known. Kell protein has an apparent M_r of 93,000 and is encoded by a gene on chromosome 7 (22), whereas Kx protein has an apparent M_r of 37,00 and is encoded by a gene on the X chromosome (23). Because of its X-linked inheritance, all known individuals of McLeod type have been males. The Kx protein appears to be required for normal expression of Kell protein and, thus, Kell antigens, and it may be required for maintenance of normal RBC morphology. Marsh and Redman (24) point out that if Kx protein in involved in maintaining a normal RBC morphology, then the small amount of Kx protein in RBCs with common Kell phenotypes may do so through a catalytic rather than a structural function.

Red blood cells with the McLeod phenotype have an apparently normal complement of glycolytic enzymes and nonglycolytic enzymes and adenosine triphosphate (ATP), membrane skeletal proteins, and membrane lipids, and a normal phospholipid:cholesterol ratio (25–28). In contrast, RBCs with an acquired form of acanthocytosis associated with liver disease have an altered phospholipid:cholesterol ratio (29). Those with the McLeod phenotype have an enhanced exchange rate of membrane phosphatidylcholine with an exogenous source (28) and exhibit a selective increased phosphorylation of β spectrin and band 3 (25). They have a decreased surface area and potassium content, an increased density, and are more rigid than RBCs with common Kell phenotype (30). The acanthocytic morphology of McLeod RBCs can be corrected in vitro by expanding the inner lipid bilayer leaflet with chloropromazine (31). This suggests that the characteristic membrane abnormality may be due to derangement of the lipid bilayer. It is of interest to note that other lesions in vertical RBC membrane protein interactions (e.g., β spectrin:ankyrin:band 3) are associated with destabilization of the lipid bilayer (32). Correction of the acanthocytic morphology of McLeod RBCs does not affect the expression of Kell-related antigens.

Other abnormalities found in individuals with the McLeod phenotype are now believed to be a consequence of changes to the adjacent areas of the X chromosome and not due to the absence of the Kx antigen. Individuals with the McLeod phenotype have late onset of muscular dystrophy, increased serum creatinine phosphokinase of the MM isoenzyme, increased carbonic anhydrase III, cardiomegally, and frequently neurological changes (33,34). Because the genes encoding Duchenne muscular dystrophy, Kx, and chronic granulomatosis disease are all located on the X chromosome in the Xp21 region (23,35,36), a deletion could affect one or more of them. Thus, an absence of Kx protein from the RBC membrane probably causes acanthocytosis, whereas the clinical syndrome associated with the McLeod phenotype is probably due to alteration of a gene(s) in close proximity to the XK gene.

2. Dominant Type Lu(a–b–) Phenotype

Inheritance of the *In(Lu)* gene, which gives rise to the dominant type of Lu(a–b–), has been associated with abnormal RBC morphology (37), whereas no abnormal RBC morphology or function has been associated with either the recessive type or the X-linked type of Lu(a–b–). Red blood cells from some individuals with the dominant type of Lu(a–b–) phenotype are acanthocytic or poikilocytic but appear to have a normal in vivo survival (37).

Fresh RBCs with the dominant type Lu(a–b–) phenotype have a normal osmotic fragility and electrolyte balance, but after incubation at 37°C for 24 hours, they have a significant resistance to osmotic lysis, a loss of K^+, and a slight gain of Na^+ as compared with RBCs of common Lutheran type. Red blood cells with this phenotype have a decreased expression of the concanavalin A receptor that has been attributed to abnormal glycosylation of band 3 (37).

In addition to a marked suppression of blood group antigens in the Lutheran system (38), RBCs with the dominant type Lu(a–b–) phenotype have suppressed P₁ and Au[a] antigens (39). Suppression of the Au[a] antigen is hardly surprising because it is now known to be a Lutheran antigen (40). These RBCs also have a weakened expression of Cs[a], Yk[a], Kn[a], McC[a], and Sl[a] antigens (41), all of which, except Cs[a], are carried on the C3b/C4b receptor (14,15). Red blood cells with the dominant type of Lu(a–b–) phenotype also have a weak expression of MER2 (42), Anwj (43–45), and In[b] (46) antigens. Because In[b] is located on CD44, a portion of which appears to be attached to the RBC membrane skeleton, it has been suggested that the association of CD44 with the Lutheran glycoprotein may contribute to the maintenance of a normal morphology in RBCs with common Lutheran antigens, and that a disruption of this association may lead to the altered morphology in RBCs with the dominant type of Lu(a–b–) phenotype (46). The role of CD44 in the RBCs membrane is unknown, but in lymphocytes, it is involved in mediating lymphocyte-endothelial cell interactions and in lymphocyte homing (1,4,47). These blood group antigens may be suppressed by the *In(Lu)* gene directly as a result of reduced levels of the glycoproteins or their abnormal glycosylation. Alternatively, the antigens could be suppressed indirectly by changes in conformation of membrane components as a consequence of reduced levels of glycoprotein or abnormal glycosylation of unrelated structures (48).

B. Hereditary Elliptocytosis

1. Leach Phenotype

Red blood cells from the nine individuals known to have the Leach phenotype lack Gerbich blood group antigens and a proportion of their RBCs are elliptocytic (49–53). These RBCs lack glycophorin C and glycophorin D (49,54) and have altered membrane mechanical properties. In ektocytometric analysis, the mechanical stability of these RBCs (which is a measure of membrane structural integrity) was 50% of normal, and their deformability was 40% of normal (55). Some individuals with the Leach phenotype have experienced long-standing anemia (52), whereas others maintain a low-normal hematocrit and high-normal reticulocyte count (50). On close examination of the ektocytometric plots, it is apparent that Leach phenotype RBCs have a slightly increased osmotic fragility (unpublished observation). Red blood cells from the original Leach donor had a slightly increased osmotic fragility as determined by the standard test and a normal composition and organization of membrane phospholipids (28). Red blood cells with the two other Gerbich-negative phenotypes (Gerbich and Yus) also lack glycophorin C and glycophorin D (54) but possess altered forms of these glycophorins that functionally substitute for their normal counterparts in maintaining normal RBC morphology, membrane mechanical stability, and deformability (56). Red blood cells with the Leach phenotype have a normal complement of membrane skeletal proteins, suggesting that the membrane mechanical and morphological abnormalities ascribed to these RBCs are primarily due to the glycophorin deficiency and not to any of the skeletal protein alterations previously described (55). It has been suggested that the ability of glycophorin C and glycophorin D to maintain the normal RBC shape and membrane mechanical properties may be modulated through their interaction with components of the membrane skeleton (55); namely, protein 4·1 (reviewed in refs 57 and 58).

Leach phenotype RBCs have a weak expression of Kell blood group antigens (reviewed in refs. 4 and 57). Gerbich negative phenotype RBCs also exhibit this property, thereby eliminating Kell protein as a candidate for the cause of the abnormal RBC properties associated with the Leach phenotype. These results do, however, suggest that an interaction with at least some of the amino acids encoded by exon 3 of the glycophorin C gene are required for the normal expression of Kell blood group antigens (4,57).

2. RBCs with a Protein 4·1 Deficiency

Red blood cells that lack protein 4·1 are elliptocytic and have approximately 10% of the normal content of glycophorin C (reviewed in ref. 57). These RBCs have a weak expression of Gerbich antigens and indeed by direct testing have been typed as Ge negative (P. Walker, personal communication, May 1986).

C.   Hereditary Ovalocytosis

The oval, rigid RBCs from individuals with hereditary ovalocytosis or stomatocytic HE who are found predominantly in Southeast Asia have a weakened expression of the following blood group antigens: I, LW^a, D, C, e, S, s, U, Kp^b, Jk^a, Xg^a, Scl, and En^a (59). The reason for the weakened expression of this diverse collection of antigens has yet to be determined; however, three independent groups of workers have shown that these RBCs have a point mutation (Lys^{56} → Glu) and a deletion of amino acid residues 400–408 from band 3 (60–62). Amino acid residues 400–408 of normal band 3 occur at the junction of the cytoplasmic and first transmembrane domains of band 3. Presumably, deletion of these amino acid residues induces the dramatic rigidity of RBCs from Southeast Asians with hereditary ovalocytosis. The physical rigidity of these RBCs may render them less agglutinable than normal RBCs or the altered band 3 may affect its interaction with other transmembrane components and thereby cause a weak expression of the antigens mentioned above.

D.   Hereditary Stomatocytosis

1. Rh_{null} and Rh_{mod} Phenotypes

Red blood cells with the Rh_{null} phenotype are known to lack Rh blood group system antigens and several polypeptides (4,63,64). Those with the Rh_{mod} phenotype have a weak expression of Rh antigens and traces of some polypeptides (64). Red blood cells with both phenotypes are stomatocytic and have a reduced in vivo survival (63,64). The hemolytic anemia in individuals with either phenotype varies in severity, and such patients may require splenectomy to control their anemia (64).

Red blood cells with the Rh_{null} phenotype have an increased K^+ and Na^+ permeability (65,66) and an increased number of Na^+K^+ pumps as compared to those with common Rh phenotypes (67). Rh_{null} RBCs have a normal membrane skeletal protein composition and lipid composition (64) but an altered phospholipid organization in that twice the normal amount of phosphatidylethanolamine is in the outer lipid leaflet and the transbilayer movement of phosphatidylcholine is faster than in normal control RBCs (68). Because some of the polypeptides that are absent from Rh_{null} RBCs interact with the membrane skeleton (reviewed in ref. 4), this is another example of where a change in vertical RBC membrane protein interactions causes alterations in the lipid bilayer, and this suggests that the multiple polypeptides that form the

Rh complex play a significant role in maintaining the phospholipid symmetry of the normal RBC membrane. It has been appreciated for some time that expression of the D antigen requires an interaction with phospholipid (69,70), and recently it has been suggested that the Rh complex of polypeptides may maintain the normal phospholipid asymmetry through covalent bonds to fatty acid side chains (71).

Red blood cells with Rh_{null} phenotype lack several polypeptides, which probably form a complex in the membrane (reviewed in ref. 4). These polypeptides include the Rh polypeptides (with apparent M_r of 30,000 and 45,000–100,000), LW polypeptide, BRIC 125 polypeptide, Fy glycoprotein, and glycophorin B. Several of these polypeptides have N-glycans attached to them, and it has been suggested that the complex may have a receptor or adhesive function (4). The cation abnormalities described above imply that Rh_{null} RBCs have an impaired transport function that may be a consequence of the absence of some or all of the polypeptides that form the "Rh complex." The actual number of polypeptides in the complex is unknown, as is the manner in which they interact.

IV. RBC MEMBRANE FUNCTION ABNORMALITIES AND BLOOD GROUP PHENOTYPES

A. Urea Transport and the Jk(a–b–) Phenotype

Red blood cells with the Jk(a–b–) phenotype are resistant to lysis when suspended in 2 M urea (72). Numerous investigations have been carried out in an attempt to isolate the protein on which the Jk antigens are carried and to determine the nature of the defect in Jk(a–b–) RBCs (reviewed in ref. 73). Because the most probable mechanism for hemolysis involves the entry of water as a result of the influx of urea, the resistance to lysis that is exhibited by Jk(a–b–) RBCs suggests they lack proteins that transport urea and/or water. Jk(a–b–) RBCs have a 1,000-fold reduction in their rate of urea transport and lack the kinetic characteristics associated with mediated transport, implying that in these RBCs urea and thiourea move across the lipid bilayer by simple passive diffusion (74). The permeability of chloride, water, and ethylene glycol are the same in Jk(a–b–) and control RBCs (74). Collectively, these results imply that Jk blood group antigens are carried on a protein that forms a channel through the lipid bilayer of the RBC membrane for the active transport of urea.

A glycoprotein (CHIP28) that is abundant in RBCs and renal tubules has recently been cloned (75). Because CHIP28 shares homology with major intrinsic protein (MIP), which forms channels that are permeable in water (75), one wonders if these proteins are altered in Jk(a–b–) RBCs.

A brief report has suggested that Jk antigens may be carried on a protein with an apparent M_r of 45,000 (76); however, this protein has not been isolated from RBC membranes. Recent attempts to clone the gene that encodes the Jk antigens suggests that the resultant protein would be more likely to have an apparent M_r of 77,000 (77–79). These studies have proven that the Jk^a antigenic determinant is protein and not carbohydrate because the expressing bacteria used do not glycosylate proteins. These studies also indicate that the Jk protein has a predicted sequence that is consistent with a transmembrane protein with its C-terminal domain oriented to the external face of the membrane. The N-terminal domain has six α-helices consisting of 20–25 amino acids each, and the last 12 amino acid residues at the C-terminus contain four residues of cysteine (79).

Until recently, no pathological findings have been associated with the Jk(a–b–) phenotype. However, it is now known that individuals with the Jk(a–b–) phenotype have a moderate decrease in their ability to maximally concentrate urine (80). It has been postulated that a lack of facilitated urea transport in the medulla impairs urea recycling in the kidney so that urine cannot be maximally concentrated. It has also been suggested that the erythrocyte urea transporter and the kidney urea transporter may be encoded by a single gene (80).

B. Malarial Parasite Invasion of RBCs

Successful invasion of RBCs by malarial parasites is a receptor-mediated process and requires at least two ligand sites: one for attachment and one for junction formation. If RBCs have an altered membrane that lacks one of these ligands, RBCs resist invasion by the *Plasmodium* parasite and, to varying degrees, protect the host from malaria.

1. Plasmodium vivax and Plasmodium knowlesi

Plasmodium vivax is one of four species that cause human malaria. Because it is extremely difficult to culture in vitro, *P. knowlesi* has been used in vitro to study the process by which the parasite invades human RBCs. Red blood cells with the Fy(a–b–) phenotype resist invasion by *P. knowlesi*, whereas Fy(a+b-), Fy(a+b+), and Fy(a–b+) RBCs are invaded equally. Invasion of Fy(a+b–) and Fy(a–b+) RBCs is blocked by anti-Fy^a and anti-Fy^b, respectively. *Plasmodium knowlesi* merozoites attach to Fy(a–b–) RBCs as well as they do to Fy(a+) or Fy(b+), indicating that Fy(a–b–) RBCs possess the ligand for attachment but lack the ligand for junction formation (reviewed in ref. 81). Presumably the glycoprotein that carries the Duffy blood group antigens is involved in the mechanism by which *P. knowlesi* and *P. vivax* invade the human RBC.

2. Plasmodium falciparum

Plasmodium falciparum uses different RBC ligands for invasion than *P. vivax* or *P. knowlesi*. To varying degrees, *P. falciparum* invades RBCs with membrane alterations that involve changes in sialic acid. Thus, RBCs that are deficient in glycophorins A, B, or C or that have the Tn or Cad 1 blood group antigens are resistant to varying degrees to invasion by *P. falciparum*. Red blood cells treated with sialidase or trypsin have a marked reduction in invasion by *P. falciparum*, but the exact ligands involved in attachment and junction formation have not been determined. Clearly, there is heterogeneity in receptors for *P. falciparum* and that at least two receptors are required (reviewed in ref. 81). The *P. falciparum* merozoite protein that binds to RBCs has been well characterized (82).

The RBCs from Southeast Asian individuals with hereditary ovalocytosis resist invasion by *P. knowlesi* and *P. falciparum* (83–85). This may be due to a physical barrier induced by the extremely rigid membranes of these RBCs and/or to the specific band 3 alteration (59–62). The degree of resistance to invasion by RBCs from different Southeast Asian individuals with ovalocytosis correlates with the extent of their decreased deformability as determined by an ektacytometer (85). This finding, together with the knowledge that when antibodies bind to glycophorin A, they decrease RBC membrane deformability (86), highlights the difficulty of using antibodies as probes for identifying the domain(s) of glycophorin A that may be involved in malaria invasion.

V.   DISEASES ASSOCIATED WITH OTHER RBC MEMBRANE PROTEINS AND BLOOD GROUP PHENOTYPES

A. Paroxysmal Nocturnal Hemoglobinuria

The RBCs from patients with paroxysmal nocturnal hemoglobinuria (PNH) lack, to a varying degree, glycosylphosphatidylinositol (GPI)–anchored proteins. Many of these proteins carry blood group antigens; i.e., Cromer-related antigens (4,87), Gy^a and Hy antigens (11,87), Yt^a antigen (12), JMH antigen (18,87), and Do^a and Do^b antigens (87). Some of the proteins lacking from RBCs from patients with PNH are involved in regulating the activity of complement, and their absence renders these RBCs susceptible to hemolysis (88). Because this subject is described in detail elsewhere in this book, it is not expanded here.

Individuals whose RBCs selectively lack the GPI-linked Gy^a glycoprotein have no known pathological abnormalities. Gy(a–) RBCs have recently been shown to lack Do^a and Do^b antigens (88). The four examples of Gy(a–) RBCs had the previously undescribed Do(a–b–) phenotype. It is probable that Dombrock antigens reside on the same RBC membrane glycoprotein as Gy^a and Hy (88). In contrast, as described below, individuals whose RBCs selectively lack either decay-accelerating factor (DAF), which carries Cromer-related antigens (Inab phenotype); the protein that carries JMH antigens; or acetylcholinesterase (AChE), which carries Cartwright blood group antigens exhibit pathological changes.

B. Intestinal Disorders

Individuals with Inab phenotype RBCs are rare. Of the four proposita described, three have had intestinal disorders (90–91). The reason for this has not been determined, but it has been suggested that an absence of DAF from cells that do not possess substitutes for complement regulation may result in increased in situ complement activation. This could lead to cell damage and release of anaphylatoxins and arachidonic acid derivatives, thereby promoting a complex inflammatory mechanism involving a progression of degenerative changes (91).

C. Congenital Dyserythropoietic Hemolytic Anemia

The RBCs from two brothers with congenital dyserythropoietic hemolytic anemia have a specific marked reduction in the expression of JMH antigens (18,92). The GPI-linked JMH protein in RBCs from these patients was present in less than half the normal amount but was qualitatively normal. The mechanism leading to the reduced amount of JMH protein in these RBCs is unknown but is apparently different from that which causes the acquired loss of JMH antigens (18).

D. Erythroleukemia and Acute Myeloid Leukemia

The enzyme acetylcholinesterase (AChE) has recently been shown to carry Yt^a and Yt^b blood group antigens (12,93,94). Expression of multiple forms of AChE in various tissues is the result of alternative splicing of mRNA and post-translational modification. Multiple peptides have been identified which contain identical catalytic domains but different C termini (95). Acetylcholinesterase is an essential component of cholinergic neutrotransmission but its function on RBCs is unknown. In the RBC membrane, AChE is attached via a GPI anchor, where it exists predominantly as a dimer (reviewed in ref. 96). It is increased in RBCs from patients with HS, pernicious anemia, some hemolytic disorders, and after acute blood loss (95), but this may be a nonspecific effect as a result of the presence of an increased number of young RBCs in the patients. Acetylcholinesterase is decreased on RBCs from patients with PNH, alloimmune and autoimmune hemolysis, erythroleukemia, and acute myeloid leukemia (96). A hereditary deficiency of RBC AChE has been reported (97,98) but no pathological abnormalities were detected in these patients.

The gene encoding AChE is located at 7q22 (99,100) in a cluster of genes whose products are expressed on hematopoietic tissues (100). The *AChE* gene is located in the same region in which frequent chromosome 7 deletions occur in leukemias of myeloid cells precursors, in acute nonlymphocytic leukemia, myelodysplastic syndromes, and megakaryoblastic leukemia (100). This would account for the reduced expression of AChE in RBCs from these patients and is reminiscent of the weakened expression of A and B blood group antigens in some patients with chronic myeloid leukemia. This has been shown to be due to the translocation of the long arm of chromosome 9 to chromosome 22. Such a translocation can result in a reduction of *A* gene–*B* gene–specific transferases because these genes are located on the long arm of chromosome 9 (19). Presumably rearrangement of a chromosome in the vicinity of a gene encoding a blood group antigen could potentially affect the expression of the antigen and induce a malignancy. The chromosome locations of some blood group antigens are shown in Table 2.

E. Systemic Lupus Erythematosus

1. Chido-Negative, Rodgers-Negative Phenotype

A deficiency of C4A and C4B has been described in numerous patients with SLE. The importance of this association in determining disease susceptibility was reported in a study of families of 29 patients with SLE (101) and a study of 189 patients with SLE from three distinct populations (102). These studies revealed that complete or partial deficiency of C4A is a genetic determinant of this disease (102). Because Chido and Rodgers blood group antigens are carried on different components of C4 (13,103), patients with SLE often type as Chido negative and/or Rodgers negative. The association of these blood group antigens and C4 is described in detail elsewhere in this book.

2. McCoy-, Knops-, Sl^a-, or Yk^a-Negative RBCs

The RBCs from patients with SLE often lose the complement receptor type 1 (CRI) (104,105) and thus type McCoy-negative, Knops-negative, Sl(a–), or Yk(a–). As has been described elsewhere in this book, CRI carries McCoy, Knops, Sl^a, and Yk^a blood group antigens (14,15).

VI. CONCLUSION

In this chapter, several examples have been described where the absence of a membrane skeleton protein or transmembrane protein has induced an alteration in the expression of other proteins or in the arrangement of bilayer lipids. Numerous examples exist where more than one protein is required for blood group antigen expression (e.g., Fy5, Wr^b) or where the presence of a blood group antigen reduces the expression of other antigens on the same protein (e.g., the presence of Kp^a sometimes causes a weak expression of other Kell system antigens and the presence of Dr^a causes a dramatically weakened expression of other Cromer-related antigens). Further, RBCs deficient in glycophorin A (En[a–] and MkMk) have an increased glycosylation of band 3 whereas RBCs with an increased number of glycophorin molecules (St(a+) and Dantu+) have a decreased glycosylation of band 3 (reviewed in ref. 4). This implies a functional interaction of RBC membrane proteins and the way in which they are glycosylated. Knowledge about individual proteins carrying blood group antigens in the RBC membrane has advanced greatly in the last few years, but there is still much to learn about interaction of different components and their effect on the normal functioning of the RBC.

REFERENCES

1. Anstee DJ, Spring FA. Red cell membrane glycoproteins with a broad tissue distribution. Transf Med Rev 1989; 3:13.

2. Zail S. Clinical disorders of the red cell membrane skeleton. CRC Oncol Hematol 1986; 5:379.

3. Darnell J, Lodish H, Baltimore D. Molecular Cell Biology. 2nd ed. New York: WH Freeman, 1990:506.

4. Anstee DJ. Blood group-active surface molecules of the human red blood cell. Vox Sang 1990; 58:1.

5. Tippett PA, Reid ME, Poole J, et al. The Miltenberger subsystem: Is it obsolescent? Transf Med Rev 1992; 6:170.

6. Redman CM, Avellino G, Pfeffer SR, et al. Kell blood group antigens are part of a 93,000 dalton red cell protein. J Biol Chem 1986; 261:9521.

7. Lee S, Zambas ED, Marsh WL, Redman CM. Molecular cloning and primary structure of Kell blood group protein. Proc Natl Acad Sci USA 1991; 88:6353.

8. Spring FA. Immunochemical characterisation of the low-incidence antigen, Dh[a]. Vox Sang 1991; 61:65.

9. Daniels GL, Khalid G, Cedergren B. The low frequency red cell antigen An[a] is located on glycophorin D. Proceedings International Society of Blood Transfusion and American Association of Blood Banks Joint Congress. Los Angeles, Nov 10–15, 1990:194.

10. Spring FA, Herron R, Rowe G. An erythrocyte glycoprotein of apparent Mr 60,000 expresses the Sc1 and Sc2 antigens. Vox Sang 1990; 58:122.

11. Spring FA, Reid ME. Evidence that the human blood group antigens Gy[a] and Hy are carried on a novel glycosylphosphatidylinositol-linked erythrocyte membrane glycoprotein. Vox Sang 1991; 60:53.

12. Spring FA, Anstee DJ. Evidence that the Yt blood group antigens are located on human erythrocyte acetylcholinesterase (AChE). Transf Med 1991; 1(Suppl 2):42.

13. O'Neill GL, Yang SY, Tegoli J, et al. Chido and Rodgers blood groups are distinct antigenic components of human complement C4. Nature L 1978; 273:668.

14. Moulds JM, Nickells MW, Moulds JJ, et al. The C3b/C4b receptor is recognized by the Knops, McCoy, Swain-Langley and York blood group antisera. J Exp Med 1991; 173:1159.

15. Rao N, Ferguson DJ, Lee S-F, Telen MJ. Identification of human erythrocyte blood group antigens on the C3b/C4b receptor. J Immunol 1991; 146:3502.

16. Herron R, Smith GA. Identification and immunocharacterization of the human erythrocyte membrane glycoproteins that carry the Xg[a] antigen. Vox Sang 1989; 262:369.

17. Herron R, Smith GA, Young D, Smith DS. Partial characterization of the human erythrocyte antigen Pt[a]. Vox Sang 1989; 56:112.

18. Bobolis KA, Telen MJ. Biochemical study of possible mechanisms of acquired loss of JMH antigen expression. Transfusion 1991; 31(Suppl):46S.

19. Reid ME, Bird GWG. Associations between human red cell blood group antigens and disease. Transf Med Rev 1990; 4:47.

20. Wimer BM, Marsh WL, Taswell HF, Galey WR. Haematological changes associated with the McLeod phenotype of the Kell blood group system. Br J Haematol 1977; 36:219.

21. Redman CM, Marsh WL, Scarborough A, et al. Biochemical studies on McLeod phenotype red cells and isolation of Kx antigen. Br J Haematol 1988; 68:131.

22. Zelinski T, Coghlan G, Myal Y, et al. Genetic linkage between the Kell blood group system and prolactin-inducible protein loci provisional assignment to chromosome 7. Ann Hum Genet 1991; 55:137.

23. Bertelson CJ, Pogo AO, Chaudhuri A, et al. Localization of the McLeod locus (Xk) within Xp21 by deletion analysis. Am J Hum Genet 1988; 42:703.

24. Marsh WL, Redman CM. Recent developments in the Kell blood group system. Transf Med Rev 1987; 1:4.

25. Tang LL, Redman CM, Williams D, Marsh WL. Biochemical studies on McLeod phenotype erythrocytes. Vox Sang 1981; 40:17.

26. Galey WR, Evan AP, Van Nice PS, et al. Morphology and physiology of the McLeod erythrocyte.

1. Scanning electron microscopy and electrolyte water transport properties. Vox Sang 1978; 34:152.

27. Symmans WA, Shepherd CS, Marsh WL, et al. Hereditary acanthocytosis associated with the McLeod phenotype of the Kell blood-group system. Br J Haematol 1979; 42:575.

28. Kuypers FA, Van Linde-Sibenius-Trip M, Roelofsen B, et al. The phospholipid organization in the membranes of McLeod and Leach phenotype erythrocytes. Fed Eur Biochem Soc 1985; 184:20.

29. Cooper RA, Dilog-Puray M, Lardo P, Greenberg MS. An analysis of lipoproteins, bile acids and red cells membranes associated with target cells and spur cells in patients with liver disease. J Clin Invest 1972; 51:3182.

30. Ballas SK, Bator SM, Aubuchon JP, et al. Abnormal membrane physical properties of red cells in McLeod syndrome. Transfusion 1990; 30:722.

31. Khodadad JK, Weinstein RS, Steck TL. Correction of the acanthocytic shape of McLeod red blood cells with chlorphromazine. J Cell Biol 1986; 103:63a (abstr).

32. Pakek J. Disorders of red cell membrane skeleton: An overview. In: Kruckeberg WC, Eaton JW, Aster J, Bewer GJ (eds): Erythrocyte Membranes 3: Recent Clinical and Experimental Advances. New York: Alan R Liss, 1984:177.

33. Marsh WL, Marsh NJ, Moore A, et al. Elevated serum creatinine phosphokinase in subjects with McLeod syndrome. Vox Sang 1981; 40:403.

34. Swash M, Schwartz MS, Carter ND, et al. Benign X-linked myopathy with acanthocytes (McLeod syndrome). Its relationship to X-linked muscular dystrophy. Brain 1983; 106:717.

35. Franke U, Ochs HD, de Martinville B, et al. Minor Xp21 chromosome deletion in a male associated with expression of Duchenne muscular dystrophy, chronic granulomatous disease, retinitis pigmentosa, and McLeod Syndrome. Am J Hum Genet 1985; 37:250.

36. Mikusick VA. Mendelian Inheritance in Man. Catalogs of Autosomal Dominant, Autosomal Recessive, and X-linked Phenotypes. 7th ed. Baltimore: The Johns Hopkins University Press, 1986.

37. Udden MM, Umeda M, Hirano Y, Marcus DM. New abnormalities in the morphology, cell surface receptors, and electrolyte metabolism of In(Lu) erythrocytes. Blood 1987; 69:52.

38. Crawford MN, Greenwalt TJ, Sasaki T, et al. The phenotype Lu(a–b–) together with unconventional Kidd groups in one family. Transfusion 1961; 1:228.

39. Crawford MN, Tippett P, Sanger R. The antigens Au[a], i, and P[1] of the cells of the dominant type of Lu(a–b–). Vox Sang 1974; 26:283.

40. Daniels GL, LePennee PY, Rouger P, et al. The red cell antigens Au[a] and Au[b] belong to the Lutheran system. Vox Sang 1991; 60:191.

41. Daniels GL, Shaw MA, Lomas CG, et al. The effect of In(Lu) on some high-frequency antigens. Transfusion 1986; 26:171.

42. Tippett P. Contribution of monoclonal antibodies to understanding one new and some old blood group systems. In: Garratty (ed): Red Cell Antigens and Antibodies. Arlington, VA: American Association of Blood Banks, 1986:84.

43. Daniels G. The Lutheran blood group system: Monoclonal antibodies, biochemistry and the effect of In(Lu). In: Pierce SR, Macpherson CR (eds): Blood Group Systems: Duffy, Kidd and Lutheran. Arlington, VA: American Association of Blood Banks, 1988:133.

44. Marsh WL, Brown PJ, DiNapoli J, et al. Anti-Wj: an autoantibody that defines a high-incidence antigen modified by the In(Lu) gene. Transfusion 1983; 23:128.

45. Poole J, Giles C. Anton and Wj, are they related? Transfusion 1985; 25:443 (letter).

46. Spring FA, Dalchau R, Daniels GL, et al. The In[a] and In[b] blood group antigens are located on a glycoprotein of 80,00 MW (the CDw44 glycoprotein) whose expression is influenced by the In(Lu) gene. Immunology 1988; 64:37.

47. Jalkanen ST, Bargatze RF, Herron R, Butcher EC. A lymphoid cell surface glycoprotein involved in endothelial cell recognition and lymphocyte homing in man. Eur J Immunol 1986; 16:1195.

48. Shaw MA, Tippett P. Proposed new notation for In(Lu) modifying gene—Another view. Transfusion 1985; 25:170.

49. Anstee DJ, Parsons SF, Ridgwell K, et al. Two individuals with elliptocytic red cells apparently lack three minor red cell membrane sialoglycoproteins. Biochem J 1984; 218:615.

50. Daniels GL, Shaw M-A, Judson PA, et al. A family demonstrating inheritance of the Leach phenotype: A Gerbich negative phenotype associated with elliptocytosis. Vox Sang 1986; 50:117.

51. Reid ME, Martynewycz M-A, Wolford FE, et al. Leach type Ge– red cells and elliptocytosis. Transfusion 1987; 27:213 (letter).

52. Rountree J, Chen J, Moulds MK, et al. A second family demonstrated inheritance of the Leach phenotype. Transfusion 1989; 29(Suppl):15S.

53. McShane K, Chung A. A novel human alloantibody in the Gerbich system. Vox Sang 1989; 57:205.

54. Reid ME, Anstee DJ, Tanner MJA, et al. Structural relationship between human erythrocyte sialoglycoproteins β and γ and abnormal sialoglycoproteins found in certain rare human erythrocyte variants lacking the Gerbich blood group antigen(s). Biochem J 1987; 244:123.

55. Reid ME, Chasis JA, Mohandas N. Identification of a functional role for human erythrocyte sialoglycoproteins β and α. Blood 1987; 69:1068.

56. Reid ME, Anstee DJ, Jensen RH, Mohandas N. Normal membrane function of abnormal related erythrocyte sialoglycoproteins. Br J Haematol 1987; 67:467.

57. Reid ME. Biochemistry and molecular cloning analysis of human red cell sialoglycoproteins that carry Gerbich blood group antigens. In: Unger P, Laird-Fryer B (eds): Blood Group Systems: MN and Gerbich. Arlington, VA: American Association of Blood Banks, 1989:73.

58. Reid ME, Takakuwa Y, Conboy J, et al. Glycophorin C content of human erythrocyte membrane is regulated by protein 4•1. Blood 1990; 75:2229.

59. Booth PB, Serjeantson S, Woodfield DG, Amato D. Selective depression of blood group antigens associated with hereditary ovalocytosis among Melanesians. Vox Sang 1977; 32:99.

60. Tanner MJA, Burce L, Martin PG, et al. Melanesian hereditary ovalocytes have a deletion in red cell band 3. Blood 1991; 78:2785 (letter).

61. Jarolim P, Palek J, Amato D, et al. Deletion in erythrocyte band 3 gene in malarial-resistant Southeast Asian ovalocytes. Blood 1991; 78(Suppl 1):252a (abstr).

62. Chasis J, Knowles D, Winardi R, et al. Conformational changes in cytoplasmic domains of band 3 and glycophorin A affect red cell membrane properties. Blood 1991; 78(Suppl 1):252a (abstr).

63. Schmidt PJ, Vos GH. Multiple phenotype abnormalities associated with Rhnull (——/——). Vox Sang 1967; 13:18.

64. Nash R, Shojania AM. Hematological aspect of Rh deficiency syndrome: A case report and a review of the literature. Am J Hematol 1987; 24:267.

65. Lauf PK, Joiner CH. Increased potassium transport and ouabain binding in human Rhnull red blood cells. Blood 1976; 48:457.

66. Ballas SK, Clark MR, Mohandas N, et al. Red cell membrane and cation deficiency in Rhnull syndrome. Blood 1984; 63:1046.

67. Lauf PK. Membrane transport changes in Rhnull erythrocytes. In: Steane EA (ed): Cellular Antigens and Disease. Washington, DC: American Association of Blood Banks, 1977:41.

68. Kuypers F, Van Linde-Sibenius-Trip M, Roelofsen B, et al. Rh$_{null}$ human erythrocytes have an abnormal membrane phospholipid organisation. Biochem J 1984; 221:931.

69. Green FA. Phospholipid requirement of Rh antigenic activity. J Biol Chem 1968; 243:5519.

70. Hughes-Jones NC, Green EJ, Hunt VAM. Loss or Rh antigen activity following the action of phospholipase A$_2$ on red cell stroma. Vox Sang 1975; 29:184.

71. Vetten M-P, Agre P. The Rh polypeptide is a major fatty acid-acetylated erythrocyte membrane protein. J Biol Chem 1989; 263:18193.

72. Heaton DC, McLoughlin K. Jk(a–b–) red blood cells resist urea lysis. Transfusion 1982; 22:70.

73. Edwards-Moulds J. The Kidd blood group systems: Drug-related antibodies and biochemistry. In: Pierce SR, Macpherson CR (eds): Blood Group Systems: Duffy, Kidd and Lutheran. Arlington, VA: American Association of Blood Banks, 1988:73.

74. Fröhlich O, Macey RI, Edwards-Moulds J, et al. Urea transport deficiency in Jk(a–b–) erythrocytes. Am J Physiol 1991; 260:C778.

75. Preston GM, Agre P. Cloning the cDNA of red cell Mr 28kDa integral membrane protein: A probable volume-regulatory channel. Blood 1991; 78(Suppl 1):364a.

76. Sinor LT, Eastwood KL, Plapp FV. Dot-blot purification of the Kidd blood group antigen. Med Lab Sci 1987; 44:294.

77. Gargus JJ, Brunner-Jackson B, Malone L. Cloning the human gene encoding a putative urea transport mechanism. FASEB J 1988; 2:A300.

78. Allen JR, Mikas M, Malone L, et al. Inborn error in human urea transport: Analysis of the cDNA encoding the putative transporter. Am J Hum Genet 1988; 43:A1.

79. Gargus JJ, Steele E, Feng Y, et al. Expression studies of human urea transporter cDNA. Biophys J 1991; 59:330a.

80. Sands JM, Gargus JJ, Fröhlich O, et al. Importance of carrier-mediated urea transport to urine concentrating ability in patients with Jk(a–b–) blood type. Nephrology 1992; (in press).

81. Hadley TJ, Miller LH, Haynes JD. Recognition of red cells by malaria parasites: The role of erythrocyte-binding proteins. Transf Med Rev 1991; 5:108.

82. Kochan J, Perkins M, Ravetch JV. A tandemly repeated sequence determines the binding domain for an erythrocyte receptor binding protein of P. falciparum. Cell 1986; 44:689.

83. Kidson C, Lamont G, Saul A, Nurse GT. Ovalocytic erythrocyte from Melanesians are resistant to invasion by malaria parasites in culture. Proc Natl Acad Sci USA 1981; 78:5829.

84. Hadley T, Saul A, Lamont G, et al. Resistance of Melanesian elliptocytes (ovalocytes) to invasion by *Plasmodium knowlesi* and *Plasmodium falciparum* malaria parasites in vitro. J Clin Invest 1983; 71:780.

85. Mohandas N, Lie-Injo LE, Friedman M, Mak JW. Rigid membranes of Melayan ovalocytes: A likely genetic barrier against malaria. Blood 1984; 63:1385.

86. Chasis JA, Reid ME, Jensen RH, Mohandas N. Signal transduction of glycophorin A: Role of extracellular and cytoplasmic domains in a modulatable process. J Cell Biol 1988; 107:1351.

87. Telen MJ, Rosse WF, Parker CJ, Moulds MK, Moulds JJ. Evidence that several high frequency human blood group antigens reside on phosphatidylinositol-linked erythrocyte membrane proteins. Blood 1990; 75:1404.

88. Banks JA, Parker N, Poole J. Evidence to show that Dombrock (Do) antigens reside on Gy^a/Hy glycoprotein. Transf Med 1992; 2(suppl 1):68.

89. Rosse W. Abnormal sensitivity to complement due to abnormalities of the cell membrane. In: Nance SJ (ed): Clinical and Basic Science Aspects of Immunohematology. Arlington, VA: American Association of Blood Banks, 1991:13.

90. Daniels G. Cromer-related antigens-blood group determinants on decay-accelerating factor. Vox Sang 1989; 56:205.

91. Reid ME, Mallinson G, Sim RM, et al. Biochemical studies on red blood cells from a patient with the Inab phenotype (decay-accelerating factor deficiency). Blood 1991; 78:3291.

92. Bobolis KA, Lande WM, Telen MJ. Markedly weakened expression of JMH in a kindred with congenital hemolytic anemia. Transfusion 1991; 31(Suppl):46S.

93. Telen MJ, Whitsett CF. Erythrocyte acetylcholinesterase bears the Cartwright blood group antigens. Clin Res 1992; 40:170A.

94. Spring FA, Gardner B, Anstee DJ. Evidence that the antigens of the Yt blood group system are located on human erythrocyte acetylcholinesterase. Blood 1992; 80: 2136–2141.

95. Taylor P. The cholinesterases. J Biol Chem 1991; 266:4025.

96. Lawson AA, Barr RD. Acetylcholinesterase in red blood cells. Am J Hematol 1987; 26:101.

97. Johns RJ. Familial reduction in red-cell cholinesterase. N Engl J Med 1962; 267:1344.

98. Shinohara K, Tanaka KR. Hereditary deficiency of erythrocyte acetylcholinesterase. Am J Hematol 1979; 7:313.

99. Zelinski T, White L, Coghlan G, Philipps S. Assignment of the YT blood group locus to chromosome 7q. Genomics 1991; 11:165.

100. Getman DK, Eubanks JH, Camp S, et al. The human gene encoding acetylcholinesterase is located on the long arm of chromosome 7. Am J Hum Genet 1992; 51:170.

101. Fielder AHL, Walport MJ, Batchelor JR, et al. Family study of the major histocompatibility complex in patients with systemic lupus erythematosus: Importance of null alleles of C4A and C4B in determining disease susceptibility. Br Med J 1983; 286:425.

102. Dunckley H, Gatenby PA, Hawkins B, et al. Deficiency of C4A is a genetic determinant of systemic lupus erythematosus in three ethnic groups. J Immunogenet 1987; 14:209.

103. Giles CM. Antigenic determinants of human C4, Rodgers and Chido. Exp Clin Immunogenet 1988; 5:99.
104. Walport M, Ng YC, Lachmann PJ. Erythrocytes transfused into patients with SLE and haemolytic anaemia lose complement receptor type 1 from their cell surface. Clin Exp Immunol 1987; 69:501.
105. Walport MJ, Lachmann PJ. Erythrocyte complement receptor type 1, immune complexes and the rheumatic diseases. Arthritis Rhemat 1988; 31:153.

10

Association of Blood Group Antigens with Immunologically Important Proteins

JOANN M. MOULDS
University of Texas Medical School
Houston, Texas

I. INTRODUCTION

Following the discovery and serological classification of the human blood groups, studies regarding their function and biological significance became one of the more fascinating areas of research. As we have seen from previous chapters, blood group antigens have been associated with malignancy, hematological abnormalities, and parasitic invasion of red blood cells (RBCs). It is difficult to believe, however, that the sole purpose of some proteins carrying blood group antigens is to act as receptors for infection. More likely, these proteins have other yet undefined functions. The purpose of this chapter is to describe some of the immunologically important proteins that express blood group polymorphisms, and to study their role not only in transfusion medicine but also disease associations and biological functions.

II. RECEPTORS FOR ADHESION MOLECULES

A. Indian Blood Group

In order to clarify the confusing array of names for the same protein and provide a common reference point, a new nomenclature was adopted termed cluster differentiation (CD) (1). The CD antigens represent a wide range of proteins with different biological functions, a number of which have now been shown to carry blood group antigens. The first to be discussed here is CD44, which carries the Indian blood group antigens.

1. Serology

The identification of the first Indian antibodies is in itself an intriguing story. Commercial firms in Bombay utilized a donor for stimulation of anti-D in their hyperimmunized donors. Unknown to them, the donor's RBCs were positive for a new low-frequency antigen later named In^a (2,3). These immunizations resulted in a total of 41 donors who produced anti-In^a often in combination with anti-D. Using absorbed antisera, Badakere et al. (3,4) found the antigen in 51 of 1749 (2.9%) Bombay blood donors or patients, 59 of 557 (10.6%) Iranians, and 29 of 246 (11.8%)

Arabs but none in Thai, Indonesians, or Chinese. Thus, they suggested that the probable epicenter of the antigen might be the Middle East rather than India.

In 1963, an antibody to a high-frequency antigen (Salis) was found in a transfused patient from Pakistan (5). Later, two additional examples were identified in antenatal samples. All three antibody producers were In^a positive, and family studies demonstrated the antithetical relationship between the Salis antibody and anti-In^a. Although population tests were never reported using anti-In^b, the calculated gene frequencies for In^a and In^b are 0.037 and 0.963, respectively.

The Indian blood group system is similar to Lewis in that the antigens become greatly depressed during pregnancy and are very weak at birth (6). Using an indirect immunoradiometric assay, the mean number of In^a sites per RBC was estimated as 74,000 for normal adults, 28,000 for pregnant women, and 20,000 in newborn infants (7). This suggests that even though these are immune antibodies, they may not cause significant hemolytic disease of the newborn (HDN). Indeed, Bhatia et al. (6) did not find any cases of neonatal jaundice in any of the In(a+) infants they studied. Anti-In^a may, however, cause transfusion reactions as antigen-positive RBCs were cleared from circulation within 20 minutes in antibody producers.

2. Biochemistry/Molecular Genetics

Because blood group antigens are not restricted to RBCs, they provide a mechanism for the investigation of protein structure and function on a broad range of cells and tissues. In their studies of RBC membranes, Spring et al. (8) located the Indian blood group antigens on an RBC protein of 80–85 kd. They were able to show that In^b was also expressed on granulocytes and lymphocytes. The glycoprotein appeared to be the same as that reported by Dalchau et al. (9), Telen et al. (10), and Letarte et al. (11) and was assigned the number CD44.

Some interesting observations regarding an 80-kd protein (now known to be CD44) and the InLu phenotype were made by several groups in the early 1980s. Using various monoclonal antibodies stimulated by T cells, investigators (10–13) found that CD44 was suppressed on InLu RBCs but not on those from the recessive type of Lu(a–b–). Anstee et al. (14) found that the number of CD44 sites was reduced by 21–61% of normal on these cells. Udden et al. (15) later found that the *InLu* RBC had morphological abnormalities and a defect in electrolyte metabolism.

The CD44 protein is first synthesized as a 37-kd molecule and then is glycosylated to the 80-kd form. It contains 248 amino acids in the extracellular domain, a 21 amino acid transmembrane region, and a 72 amino acid cytoplasmic domain (16). The molecule contains several disulfide bonds and is rich in o-linked carbohydrate. It has been speculated that the InLu phenotype results from the lack of a carbohydrate transferase that is needed to produce the carbohydrate antigens CD44 (In^a and In^b) as well as P_1, i, Lu^a, and Lu^b.

The gene for CD44 has been cloned and mapped to the short arm of chromosome 11 at p13 (15,17). The alleles for *In^a* and *In^b* have not been investigated at the molecular level but probably represent a single amino acid substitution. Recently, size variants of CD44 have been studied at both the protein and gene levels (18). The myelomonocytic cell line KG1a expresses CD44+ proteins that are 85, 115, and 130 kd. Both of the larger forms have an additional serine-threonine–rich insert that may allow further glycosylation or sulfation and contribute to the tissue specificity of CD44.

3. Function/Disease

The migration of peripheral lymphocytes from the blood stream into lymphoid tissue and inflammation sites is dependent on their adhesion to vascular endothelium. Many cell surface glycoproteins play a role in this interaction including CD44.

Initially CD44 was named lymphocyte-homing receptor because it demonstrated tissue specificity. Although this homing ability is crucial in the immune response, it also can be detrimental. Because CD44 recognizes hyaluronate and possibly other cell adhesion molecules (19), it could serve as a tool for invasion by cancer cells. In a study using nude mice, Sun et al. (20) found that clones expressing the 80-kd form of CD44 had greatly enhanced tumorigenicity and metastatic potential. Indeed, some human studies have shown a better prognosis among patients with non-Hodgkin's lymphoma that have CD44-negative lymphocytes (21). Monoclonal antibodies to CD44 may be a potential treatment for these and other types of cancer.

Recently, CD44 was found to play a role in inflammatory synovitis. Patients with rheumatoid arthritis (RA) or osteoarthritis had higher levels of CD44 in their joint fluid than did controls (22). Thus, new therapeutic modalities for RA might include ways to inhibit interactions of membrane CD44.

What began as the identification of an antibody to a new low-frequency antigen has now expanded into other areas. The investigation of the alternative allele, i.e., *In*^{a}, may be of importance in the worldwide study of epidemiology as well as anthropology. Certainly, the suppression of CD44 in the In(Lu) phenotype needs further investigation and may yield important clues for the study of cancer.

III. RECEPTORS FOR BACTERIA

A. Anton/Wj and *Haemophilus*

1. Serology

Initially Anton was considered to be one of the "para-Lutheran" antigens and was given the designation Lu15. However, Poole and Giles (23) reported that two samples of the recessive Lu(a–b–) phenotype reacted as strongly with several Anton antisera as did those having normal Lutheran phenotypes. In addition, the Anton determinant was affected differently by proteolytic enzymes; thus, they suggested that Anton was separate from the Lutheran blood group system.

Anti-Wj was first reported as an autoantibody (24) that reacted with all RBCs tested except Lu(a–b–) RBCs of the In(Lu) type and cord RBC. Other examples of auto-anti-Wj have been found, some of which occur concomitantly with the loss of the RBC antigen (25,26). In the transient Wj- case reported by Mannessier et al. (26), the RBCs were also nonreactive with a monoclonal anti-Wj as well as anti-Anton. This fact and the similar reactivity with cord cells, enzyme-treated RBCs, and the In(Lu) cells provided convincing evidence that anti-Anton and anti-Wj were recognizing the same determinant.

2. Biochemistry/Molecular Genetics

The fact that An/Wj is lacking on RBCs having the dominant Lu(a–b–) phenotype suggests that this antigen might also be part of the paragloboside series. As a receptor for *Haemophilus* (see below), the binding site has not been identified but is probably a disaccharide unit involving galactose. Otherwise, there is no known biochemical or gene structure information available for An/Wj.

3. Function/Disease

Most bacteria that are pathogenic for humans adhere to the surface of host cells (particularly epithelial layers) where they can localize and colonize. This is accomplished through the attachment of bacterial fimbriae (hairlike structures) to host receptor molecules. Some bacteria have demonstrated blood group specificity of their adhesins; e.g., P and Dr^a antigens for strains of *Escherichia coli* (27). In 1986, van Alphen et al. (28) found that the Anton antigen was the RBC receptor for fimbriated strains of *Haemophilus influenzae*. In a later study using RBCs from newborns, these authors found that the epithelial receptor was similar to but different from

An/Wj (29). Thus, although the relevance of this antigen to bacterial infection has been questioned, it points out the diversity of functions associated with blood groups.

B. P and *Escherichia*

1. Serology

The P blood group was identified by Landsteiner and Levine (30) after a deliberate search to find new blood group factors. These investigators inoculated rabbits with human RBCs and tested the rabbit sera for reactivity; thus anti-P_1 was discovered. Since these initial experiments, a number of antibodies have been added, including anti-p, anti-P, anti-P^k, anti-Tj^a, and anti-Luke. Anti-Luke (LKE) is nonreactive with all p and P^k RBCs (31) but also shows an association with ABO. Other "compound antibodies" require specific Ii antigens to be present in combination with P antigens; e.g., anti-IP_1, anti-iP_1, and anti-iP (32,33).

Most of these antibodies are cold reactive and thus are of little significance in transfusion. There have been some reports (34) of increased frequency of abortion in women who have naturally occurring anti-Tj^a. The Donath-Landsteiner (D-L) hemolysin, which has been associated with paroxysmal cold hemoglobinuria (PCH), has been shown to have P specificity.

2. Biochemistry/Molecular Genetics

Because of their widespread distribution, the P blood group antigens have been the focus of considerable investigation. Much is known regarding the biochemical structures of these antigens but little is understood about the genes or their probable products; i.e., glycosyltransferases.

P system antigens are formed by the addition of carbohydrates to the fatty acid chain of sphingolipids. The pathway shown for the formation of the P blood group antigens (Fig 1) is also involved in the formation of the ABH and Ii antigens. P^k, or ceramide trihexoside (CTH), is the precursor for P (globoside). Paragloboside is the precursor for the P_1 and p (sialosylparagloboside) antigens and the type II precursor for the ABH antigens.

Although much has been learned about the P blood group antigens at the protein level, this knowledge has not helped clarify the genetic background. There are several hypotheses for the formation of the various antigens, and the interested reader is referred to other references (35,36) for more detail. Perhaps when these genes have been cloned, we will have a better understanding of the genetic background.

3. Function/Disease

Unlike some of the proteins to be discussed later, the glycosphingolipids carrying the P blood group antigens have no known specific function other than they constitute part of the cell membrane. Thus, the increased expression of some of these antigens, e.g., P^k in Burkitt cell tumors (B lymphocytes), is intriguing (37,38). The potential usefulness of the P system antigens as tumor markers or even targets for immunotherapy deserve investigation. Indeed, a woman with gastric carcinoma (39) and a potent anti-$P + P_1 + P^k$ (Tj^a) has been reported. It was postulated that her antibody was cytotoxic to the tumor cells and this resulted in her prolonged survival rate.

Because of its wide antigenic distribution, many of the P system antibodies result from the immune response to other organisms. The D-L antibody discussed previously is thought to be such a response. Many examples of PCH in children are preceded by a flulike illness or respiratory infection (40). In adults, this antibody may appear transiently associated with syphilis. It is possible that both the virus and spirochete carry a P-like carbohydrate structure that stimulates the autoantibody production.

High-titer anti-P_1 has been found in pigeon breeders, patients with hydatid cyst disease (*Echinococcus granulosus*), and patients harboring the liver fluke *Fasciola hepatica* (41).

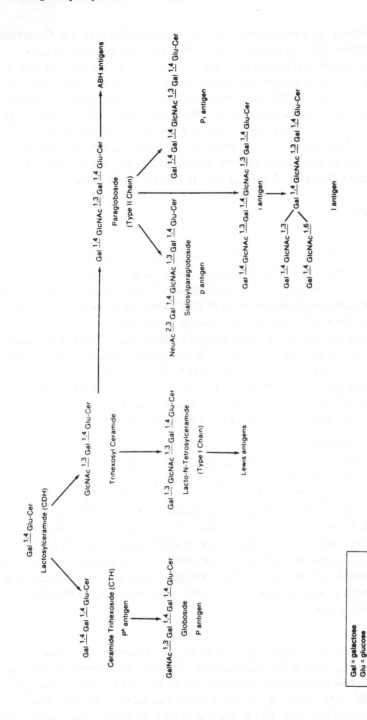

Figure 1 Biochemical pathway for the formation of the I and P blood group antigens.

Hydatid cyst fluid and pigeon egg albumin have been shown to be a rich source of P_1 substance. Thus, one might expect these patients to have a potent immune response to P_1 antigen.

Bacterial adhesion to human epithelial cells of the urinary tract is an important step in the establishment of urinary tract infections and childhood diarrhea. Strains of *Escherichia coli* that cause pyelonephritis attach to Gal(1,4)Gal structures found as part of the membrane globosides (42,43). This carbohydrate structure occurs as part of the P^k, P, and P_1 blood group antigens. One study (43) showed that girls whose RBC typed as P_1 positive had an increased risk for recurring pyelonephritis. The presence of the fimbriae that cause attachment appears to be inducible and is due to a 92-kb plasmid found in the infectious strains (44). Screening for these diseases using RBC with high-density P_1 antigen may be a useful clinical test.

C. I and *Mycoplasma*

1. Serology

For many years the term *nonspecific cold agglutinin* was used to describe the autoantibody now called anti-I. In 1956, Wiener et al. (45) found five donors who lacked the corresponding antigen; thus, they named the antigen "I" for "individuality." The strength of the I antigen showed variability among adult blood donors but cord RBCs almost always typed as I negative. The rare I negative adult donor often had allo anti-I in the serum (46).

As with the P blood group system, I and i antibodies have been found that require the presence of other blood group antigens for reactivity. Some examples include anti-IA, anti-IB, anti-IH, anti-H(i), anti-O(i), anti-iH, anti-IP$_1$, and anti-ILe^{bh}. In addition to these, other I antibodies have been serologically defined that appear to recognize a heterogeneous group of epitopes; e.g., anti-I^T, anti-I^D, and anti-I^F (47,48). The association of some of these antibodies with hemolytic anemia made the investigation of this blood group a fruitful area of research.

2. Biochemistry/Molecular Genetics

The serological study of the I/i antigens has proved a useful basis for the biochemical analysis of these blood group antigens. It is now known that I/i are "precursor" structures for H and eventually the A and B antigens. The i antigen is an unbranched, linear structure, whereas I results from repeated branching of this chain by the addition of Gal(1,4)GlcNAc residues (see Fig 1). These carbohydrates are mostly carried on band 3 of the RBC membrane (49). More details regarding these structures and their relationship to ABH can be found in Chapter 1.

Because there is not a single sugar that can be identified with I or i specificity, one cannot be sure that there is a single gene for each of these antigens. This may be a worthy area for investigation by molecular geneticists who may be able to more clearly define the genetic background of the I blood group system.

3. Function/Disease

The specific purpose for the glycosphingolipids carrying I/i antigens is not known, but the antigens show an interesting association with bacteria. Early in the history of blood group serology, it was noted that horse antiserum to *Pneumococcus* type XIV was able to agglutinate human RBCs of all ABO types (50). After considerable biochemical investigation, it was confirmed that these antibodies recognized terminal Gal(1,4) units. The pneumococcal polysaccharide coat was a linear polymer containing short side chains of Gal(1,4) linked to GlcNac. Thus, the horse antiserum was thought to be cross-reacting with the human I blood group antigen (51).

Another aspect of the immune response and the I blood group regards the increased frequency of anti-I following *Mycoplasma pneumoniae* infection. Naturally occurring anti-I antibodies will increase in titer and thermal range following infection. Loomes et al. (52,53) postulated that these autoantibodies occurred as a result of the interaction of the I antigen with the

Mycoplasma and presentation of this "self"-antigen to the immune system. They later showed that *M. pneumoniae* could bind to both I and i antigens on the RBC. The bacteria recognized the structure NeuAc(2,3)Gal(1,4)GlcNAc and thus had a specificity similar to the cold autoantibody named Gd (54). Recently, Roelcke et al. (54) found coexisting anti-I and anti–Sia-b1 (Gd) in the sera of patients with recent *Mycoplasma* infections.

IV. COMPLEMENT PROTEINS

A. Cromer and Decay-Accelerating Factor

The next protein to be discussed, which bears blood group antigens, is one that crosses many disciplines. Decay-accelerating factor (CD55) is a complementary-regulatory protein that carries the Cromer blood group antigens and acts as a bacterial receptor. Thus, it could have been placed in the previous section but is listed under complement proteins as this is its major function.

1. Serology

The first case of what is now known as anti-Cr[a] was found in a Go[a]-positive woman and originally thought to be anti-Go[b] (55). The Cromer blood group first began to take form in 1975 when Stroup and McCreary (56) described four black individuals who had produced antibodies to a public antigen. Two of these cases had identical specificity to the first case (surname Cromer). Because the new evidence did not support the proposition that Cromer serum contained anti-Go[b], the antibodies were renamed anti-Cr[a].

In 1981, Daniels et al. (57) reported the null phenotype for the Cromer system in a Japanese patient (Inab). Because the patient had a protein-losing enteropathy and ileocecal tumor, it was unknown at that time whether this phenotype was inherited or was due to the disease process. Another example of the null phenotype was found in 1983 in a patient (surname Freiberger) who had Crohn's disease and an antibody to a high-frequency antigen (58). The antibody was later named anti-IFC for Inab-Freiberger-Cromer (59). Finally, in 1987, a family was reported demonstrating inheritance of the Inab phenotype (60).

At the same time that the Cromer-Inab relationship was being explored, another Cromer-related group was defined. Anti-Tc[a], an antibody to a high-frequency antigen, was nonreactive with the original Inab RBCs (61,62). Two low-frequency alleles have been reported (60,63), Tc[b] and Tc[c]. The corresponding antigen is detected in approximately 5% of blacks.

Levene et al. (64) described a new phenotype that further substantiated the relationship between Cromer and Tc[a]. The RBCs of an Israeli woman exhibited weakened expression of the Cr[a], Tc[a] and IFC antigens. Her serum contained an antibody to a high-frequency antigen that was distinct from anti-IFC and thus named anti-Dr[a]. Further studies have confirmed the genetic inheritance of this factor (65).

Other antigens have been included in the Cromer blood group system because of their lack of reactivity with the Inab RBCs. These include the high-frequency antigens WES[b] and Es[a] (66,67). The antithetical antigen to WES[b], WES[a], has been found as a low-incidence antigen in the Finnish population occurring with a frequency of 0.56% (68,69).

2. Biochemistry/Molecular Genetics

The Cromer-related antibodies were originally grouped together because of their lack of reactivity with Inab RBCs and because the antigens they defined were similarly destroyed by some enzymes. This complex, however, was elevated to blood group status when it was found that these antigens resided on a 70-kd protein known as decay-accelerating factor (DAF, CD55) (68,70).

The gene for DAF has been mapped to chromosome 1q32 and is part of a group known as

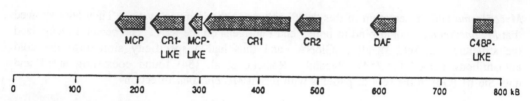

Figure 2 The regulators of complement activation (RCA) complex genes on chromosomes 1q32.

the regulators of complement activation (RCA) complex (71,72). Other genes (Fig 2) that are closely linked include complement receptors one and two (*CR1* and *CR2*), C4-binding protein (*C4bp*), membrane cofactor protein (*MCP*), factor H, and factor XIIIb (73,74). Additional partially duplicated sequences have also been found in this region and are called MCP-like, CR1-like, and so on (75).

Both the cDNA and the gene for DAF have been cloned (76,77). The *DAF* gene is approximately 35 kb in length and demonstrates three restriction fragment length polymorphisms (RFLPs) using the enzymes *Hin*dIII and *Bam*HI (78). How these various RFLPs relate to the known blood group polymorphisms is unknown at this time. Sequence analyses of DNA from cells of the original Inab phenotype demonstrate a single nucleotide mutation in codon 53 (79). This results in a stop codon, which explains the lack of DAF and consequently all Cromer blood group antigens on the Inab RBCs.

3. Function/Disease

The broad distribution of DAF on RBCs, leukocytes, platelets, epithelial cells, for example, suggests that its function is of major physiological significance (80,81). The primary purpose of DAF is to downregulate complement activation by preventing the formation of C3 and C5 convertases and dissociate preformed convertases. This goal is achieved through the interaction of several membrane proteins and serum cofactors (Table 1). The ability of DAF to bind both C3b and C4b makes it doubly important because it can function in the regulation of both the classic and alternative pathways. Thus, DAF can not only protect host tissue from antibody-dependent inflammation but can also deflect low-level complement activation away from the self-tissue. This basic premise has lead to investigations of the potential utility of DAF to prevent complement-mediated tissue injury in xenotransplants (82).

One might presume that the depression or complete lack of DAF on the RBC might be quite injurious. Several such examples have been identified: the Dr(a−) phenotype, the pathological condition of paroxysmal nocturnal hemoglobinuria (PNH), and the Inab phenotype. One should note that the DAF-negative status of PNH RBCs is an acquired defect, whereas the Inab phenotype is a genetic defect.

Table 1 Proteins Regulating Complement Activation

Pathway	Dissociation of C4b/C3b	Cleavage of C4b/C3b
Classical		
Membrane	DAF, CR1	CR1, MCP
Serum	C4bp	C4bp, factor I
Alternative	C3bBb	
Membrane	DAF, CR1	
Serum	Factor H	

Individuals with the Inab phenotype are extremely rare and this fact has limited this area of research. Unlike patients with PNH, these individuals do not have episodes of in vivo hemolysis. Their RBCs, however, do show an increased sensitivity to complement-mediated lysis in vitro (83,84). Telen et al. (83) showed that RBCs from two Inab individuals had normal levels of other GPI-linked proteins.

Although persons with the Inab phenotype do not demonstrate any hematological abnormalities, it is interesting to note that the first three examples had protein-losing enteropathies or Crohn's disease. The current consensus is that an autoimmune process is the underlying cause of such inflammatory bowel diseases (85). Immune complex formation and complement activation are important in disease pathogenesis. Therefore, the lack of the complement-regulatory protein DAF may be more than coincidence in these individuals. However, studies of patients with Crohn's disease or ulcerative colitis have not yielded any further examples of this phenotype (86).

It was postulated that the GPI anchor of DAF allowed for rapid lateral mobility in the membrane, making it more effective in the dissociation of C3 convertases. However, Lublin and Coyne (87) showed that mutant DAF molecules having a transmembrane region functioned as well as wild-type DAF. Other research suggests that the DAF GPI anchor may be linked to protein tyrosine kinases and may be involved in T-cell signaling and activation (88–90). Although the Cromer blood group polymorphism does not appear to compromise DAF's function as a regulatory protein (D. Lublin, personal communication, September, 1991), its possible role in cell signaling simply has not been studied.

A number of organisms, including parasites, bacteria, and viruses, can utilize membrane proteins to initiate infection. Decay-accelerating factor is yet another example of a blood group protein acting as a bacterial receptor. In 1988, Nowicki et al. (27) reported that the Dr^a antigen (carried on DAF) was the receptor recognized by the 075X adhesion of *E. coli*. The bacteria did not agglutinate Dr(a–) or IFC-negative RBCs. The Dr(a–) phenotype has recently been shown to be due to a C to T change in nucleotide 649 (91). This results in an amino acid change from serine to threonine and the creation of a *Taq*I RFLP. Because of the abundance of Dr(a+) DAF in the colon and urinary tract, it has been suggested that this molecule may play a role in the colonization of *E. coli* and urinary tract infection (92).

There is one final point to note regarding the role of DAF and the immune response to parasitic infection. Some parasites, such as *Schistosoma mansoni*, can absorb DAF molecules from the host, thus resisting destruction by the alternative pathway of complement (93). Other parasites may produce DAF-like molecules on their cell surface. *Trypanosoma cruzi* produces a 160-kd protein that is very homologous to human DAF at the protein and DNA levels (93,94). Vaccine development to produce anti–"DAF-like" antibodies is currently under investigation. It is unknown whether this may result in the appearance of Cromer complex antibodies in immunized individuals, but it must be considered as a possibility.

The identification of the Cromer blood group antigens on DAF has already enhanced the studies of this molecule both at the functional and molecular levels. The presence of specific negative phenotypes, e.g., Dr(a–) in Jews or Cr(a–) in blacks, in conjunction with the disease associations, suggests that these may be more than just random mutations. Clearly there is a broad range of research to pursue in this area.

B. Knops/McCoy/York and CR1

1. Serology

In 1965, the sera from three unrelated patients (Copeland, Stirling, Wainwright) were reported to have an antibody of similar specificity (95). The antibody was named anti-Cs^a after the first two producers. Ten years later, a new antigen, York (Yk^a), was reported (96). The York serum was originally thought to be anti-Cs[a] until the RBCs of the donor (surname York) were found to be Cs(a+). This same study found that 12 of 1,246 white donors were both Cs(a–) and Yk(a–). Thus, these two antigens appeared to be phenotypically related. They became part of a collection of antibodies known as "high-titer, low-avidity" (HTLA) antibodies.

During this time period, another group of antibodies with HTLA characteristics was being investigated. The first of these to be named was the Knops-Helgeson (Kn[a]) antigen (97). The RBCs from the donor Helgeson were found to be compatible and thought to be negative for the high-incidence antigen Kn[a]. In 1980, an antibody to the corresponding low-incidence antigen was found in a serum (Hall) and given the name Kn[b] (98).

Molthan and Moulds (99) first noted the relationship between Knops and a new high-incidence antigen McCoy (McC[a]). They found that 53% of McC(a–) samples were also Kn(a–), including the Helgeson RBCs. Anti-McC[a] appeared to be more common among black patients. Through studies of black individuals who had antiglobulin-reactive antibodies, other McCoy specificities were found. Swain-Langley (Sl[a]), or McC[c], was reported in simultaneous abstracts in 1980 (100,101). Since then, a series of McCoy antibodies has been named (102,103) that are based on their lack of reactivity with the Helgeson cells.

In 1991, two groups of researchers independently found that the Knops, McCoy, and York antigens were located on complement receptor 1 (CR1) (104,105). Studies using sensitive radioimmunoprecipitation techniques showed that the RBCs from Helgeson, the putative Knops-McCoy null phenotype, carried at least McC[a] and Yk[a] (146). The lack of serological reactivity appeared to be due to low numbers of CR1 protein per RBC (106).

2. Biochemistry/Molecular Genetics

The most common form of CR1 is a glycoprotein containing >2,000 amino acids: a 41–amino acid signal peptide, a 1930–amino acid extracellular domain, a 25–amino acid transmembrane region, and a 45-amino acid cytoplasmic tail (107). Similar to DAF, this protein is composed of short consensus repeats (SCRs) but contains many more SCRs; 4 versus 30, respectively (108). The SCRs contain 60–70 amino acids that show high homology. Disulfide bonding among the four internal cysteines gives the molecule a looped structure.

In 1980, Fearon et al. (109), using pooled donor RBCs, purified CR1 and estimated its molecular weight to be 200,000. Subsequent studies by other investigators (110,111) led to the discovery of a size polymorphism for this receptor. Four codominantly inherited allelic size variants have been identified with molecular weights of 190(C), 220(A), 250(B), and 280(D) kd on SDS-PAGE (sodium dodecylsulfate–polyacrylamide gel electrophoresis) under reducing conditions (112). There do not appear to be any functional differences between these different molecular weight variants (110–113).

In addition to the size polymorphism, a quantitative polymorphism of CR1 has been described. Although the number of CR1 molecules on most cells appears to vary little from person to person, RBC expression is quite variable. This appears to be regulated by a cis-acting regulatory element and may represent a further polymorphism of the promoter region of the *CR1* gene (75,114). Using RFLP analyses, Wilson et al. (115) and Wong et al. (116) found several polymorphisms, one of which correlated with high and low expression of RBC CR1. The *L* allele (low) correlated with a 6.9-kb genomic *Hind*III fragment, whereas the *H* allele (high) showed a 7.4-kb fragment.

There is evidence to suggest that CR1 copy number may affect the Knops, McCoy, and York reactivity in hemagglutination assays (106). Many false-negative reactions are obtained when the RBCs have low expression of CR1. Some investigators have suggested that low copy number may play a role in the deposition of immune complexes in blood vessel walls leading to inflammatory damage (117). Acquired deficiencies of CR1 can occur in some malignant tumors (118), acquired immune deficiency syndrome (AIDS) (119), systemic lupus erythematosus (120), and other autoimmune diseases (121). These facts make serological typing of the CR1-related blood group antigens very unreliable in a patient population.

The *CR1* gene has been mapped to chromosome one (see Fig 2) and is part of the RCA complex (122). The *CR1* gene is rather large; e.g., the *B* allele covers 160 kb (114). Studies of this gene suggest that the CR1 size variants were generated by a duplication or deletion of a highly homologous unit generated by unequal crossover rather than by alternative splicing of the mRNA (75,114,123,124).

3. Function/Disease

Activation of the complement system via the classic or alternative pathways results in the formation of C3 convertases. Cleavage of C3 leads to several important biological activities. Control of the pivotal C3 component is accomplished by both fluid-phase and cell-bound regulators (see Table 1). In the plasma, factor H and C4bp act as cofactors for the serine protease factor I. The RBC membrane control proteins are DAF (CD55) and CR1 (CD35). Considerable interest has arisen regarding the use of these regulatory proteins to control damage by complement in xenotransplantation (82,125), myocardial infarction (126), and autoimmune disease (127).

CR1, also known as the immune adherence or C3b/C4b receptor, plays an important role in the processing of immune complexes. Erythrocyte CR1 binds immune complexes and transports them to the liver and spleen where they can be removed from the circulation. The distribution of CR1 on B lymphocytes, monocytes, granulocytes, some T cells, glomerular podocytes, and follicular dendritic cell suggests that CR1 plays multiple roles in the immune response (109). Cross-linking of CR1 leads to the activation of B lymphocytes and secretion of interleukin-1 by monocytes (128). Furthermore, complement receptors, CR1 and CR3, appear to influence T-cell responses (129).

Some pathogens have developed the ability to disassemble C3 convertase and protect themselves from destruction by the complement system. *Trypanosoma cruzi*, herpes simplex virus, and Epstein-Barr virus have all produced proteins homologous to human CR1 (93). Other pathogens such as *Babesia rodhaini*, *Legionella pneumophilia*, and *Mycobacterium leprae*, allow themselves to be coated with C3b so that they may bind to CR1 and initiate infection of the host cell. One might speculate that the protein polymorphisms, now recognized by blood group antibodies, may have been a host response to differentiate self-CR1 from pathogen CR1!

C. Rodgers/Chido and C4

1. Serology

In a short report published in 1967, Harris et al. (130) described three patients who had antibodies to a high-frequency antigen and named the antibody anti-Chido after one of the early antibody producers. Chido antibodies could not be inhibited by saliva, urine, or hydatid cyst fluid. However, Middleton and Crookston (131) found that plasma contained "Chido substance" and described a test, i.e., plasma inhibition, to differentiate positive from negative donors. Using this method, they typed 639 random donors in Toronto and found that 11 (1.7%) were Chido negative.

Longster and Giles (132) first described anti-Rodgers and noted its similarity to anti-Chido. The Rodgers serum contained an enzyme-reactive anti-E and a second antibody that gave positive reactions ranging from very weak to 4+. Plasma from donors, thought to be Rg(a+) by RBC typing, could inhibit the Rg^a antibody. Negative donor plasma would not inhibit the antibody; however, a certain portion of the samples tested were found to inhibit anti-Rg^a partially. By testing random donors using the plasma inhibition test, these investigators found 3.1% to be Rg^a negative and 2.6% to be Rg partial inhibitors.

Some blood group serologists believed that Rodgers and Chido might represent remnants of HLA antigens on the RBC. This led to the investigation of the HLA phenotypes of Chido- or Rodgers-negative individuals. Middleton et al. (133) studied 15 families and found that HLA-B12 and Bw5 (B5) occurred more frequently among Chido-negative subjects. They calculated the odds in favor of linkage between Chido and HLA to be 1,450,000 to 1. The Rodgers antigens also appeared to be linked to HLA; Rg(a–) individuals were found in a higher frequency among HLA-B8 (134) and possibly Bw40 persons (135). In a large study of 19 families, no Rg negative, Ch negative individuals were found and close linkage between these genes was confirmed.

The association between Rg-Ch and HLA became clear when the fourth component of complement, C4, was reported to carry these blood group antigens (136,137). Individuals having only the fast-moving bands of C4 (C4A) usually had the HLA type B12, Bw35, B5, or B18 and were Chido negative. Those persons with only the slow bands (C4B) were almost exclusively HLA-B8 positive and Rodgers negative (137).

To date, nine antigenic determinants on the C4 molecule have been defined (Fig 3). Approximately 82% of a random white population are positive for the high-frequency antigens Rg1,2 and Ch1,2,3 (138). Ch4 is detected on all C4B allotypes and probably represents the C4B isotype (139). Ch6 is present on most C4B proteins and is frequently absent when Ch3 is missing. It may also be detected on some C4A proteins that type as Rg1-2 (140). All these new antigens are of high frequency. Only one low-frequency antigen (WH) has been described that appears to detect a conformational epitope requiring Ch6 and Rg1 in the rare cis conformation (140).

As always, rare exceptions to these observations have been found (141). The only C4A allotype that has neither Rg1 nor Rg2 is C4A1 (142). The C4A1 allotype carries Ch1-2,3, in its place; this phenomenon is referred to as "reversed antigenicity." Another unusual allotype that may carry reversed antigens is C4B5. This C4B/Rg+ allotype shows linkage to C4A4 along with HLA-B60, B35, or B18 (143,144). Although these individuals do not express Ch1, Ch2, or Ch3, they do carry Ch4 on their C4B molecule (139).

2. Biochemistry

C4 is synthesized by hepatocytes and macrophages (145) as a single protein of 1722 amino acids known as pro-C4. Pro-C4 undergoes posttranslational cleavage by a plasminlike protease

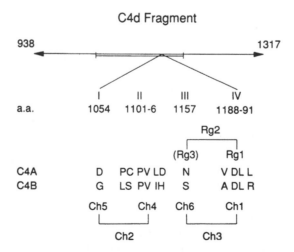

Figure 3   Structural model for C4. (Adapted from Refs. 139 and 163.)

at two arginyl-rich regions to produce three polypeptide chains joined together by disulfide bonds (Fig 4) (146). The molecular weight of the processed C4 molecule is approximately 200 kd.

The α-chain has a molecular weight of 94–96 kd, carries three complex oligosaccharides (containing mannose fucose, glucosamine, and sialic acid), and one sulfated site (147). The β-chain is 72–77 kd in size and has a single high-mannose oligosaccharide of the Man_2 $GlcNAc_2$ type. The smallest chain, γ, is not glycosylated and weighs only 32–35 kd.

Two mature forms (isotypes) of C4 exist known as C4A and C4B. In addition to these two major isotypes of C4, at least 13 C4A and 16 C4B allotypes have been described based on their electrophoretic mobility (148). Rodgers antigens are strongly associated with most of the C4A allotypes, whereas Chido determinants are found on C4B. The lack of either C4A or C4B protein has been given the abbreviation "Q0" meaning "quantity naught."

3. Molecular Genetics

The major histocompatibility complex (MHC) in humans is a highly polymorphic region encompassing 2 centimorgans (cM) (3800 kb) in length on the short arm of chromosome 6. The class III region, which spans 1100 kb between class I and class II, includes the genes from the complement proteins C2, C4, and factor B as well as the genes for 21-hydroxylase (21-OH), heat-shock protein (HSP70), and tumor necrosis factor (TNF) (149). The two C4 loci are separated by 10 kb and both are flanked by a 21-OH gene located 3 kb from the 3' end of the C4 gene (150,151).

Despite the large size of the MHC, there is a paucity of crossover events occurring either within or around the class III genes. Therefore, the C4 genes have a tendency to be inherited along with factor B and C2 as a single haplotype known as a "complotype." Certain complotypes may be further extended to include HLA-B or DR genes as an inherited unit. This is referred to as an "extended haplotype" (152,153). These closely linked loci are inherited at a frequency significantly greater than would be expected from their individual frequencies and are in linkage disequilibrium.

Four separate genetic events can result in an apparent C4 null status (Rodgers or Chido negative): deletion, duplication, conversion, or an amorphic (nonfunctional) allele. An example of an extended haplotype carrying a deleted gene is HLA-B8, DR3, C4A*Q0. This is due to a 28-kb deletion that removes both the C4A and 21-OHA genes (154). Unequal crossover with subsequent gene deletion explains approximately 60% of the apparent C4 null genes (149). The duplicated C4A*3, *2, B*Q0 allotype, which is associated with the Rg pi serological phenotype,

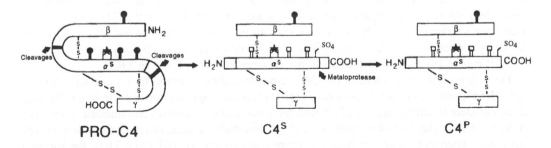

PRO-C4   C4S   C4P

- ♦ = High mannose type oligosaccharide
- ♦ = Biantennary complex type oligosacchraide
- ★ = Thiolester bond
- SO₄ = Sulfate

Figure 4 Post-translational processing of the C4 molecule (From Ref. 147.)

is frequently found with *HLA-B35, DR1* (155). Using the enzymes *Nla*IV and *Eco*O 109 for RFLP analysis of the *C4* genes, Yu and Campbell (156) found that in the extended haplotype *HLA-B44, DR6, C4B*Q0*, the *C4B* gene had been converted to a *C4A* gene. Other situations exist where the gene is present but not expressed. This may be due to defects in transcription, translation, or post-translational processing.

The *C4* genes can differ in their size; the *C4A* gene is almost always long (22 kb), whereas *C4B* genes may be short (16 kb) or long (22 kb) (157,158). This is due to the presence or absence of a 6.5-kb intron located 2.5 kb from the 5' end of the gene (158,159). Most *C4B*Q0* genes are 22 kb in size and thus are more homologous with the *C4A* gene. Schendel et al. (160) suggested that the *C4B* long genes are twice as frequent as the shorter version. Aside from the variable presence of this intron, the *C4A* and *C4B* genes are 99% homologous (146).

In order to compare the genes for *C4A* and *C4B* more completely, the genes were cloned and sequenced. Only 14 differences were found out of 4,600 nucleotides compared; 12 of these were in the C4d region and 1 each in the β and γ chains (150,155). The C4A protein had the sequence PCPVLD at positions 1101–1106, whereas C4B had LSPVIH, which was thought to be the isotypic site (161). The change of D to H at position 1106 accounts for the switch in functional activity, whereas the substitution of C for S at position 1102 affects hemolytic activity and immunoglobulin (IgG) binding (162). It is this region that is solely responsible for modulation of the thioester bond. The change of P to L at position 1101 results in different mobilities of the α chains on SDS-PAGE.

The Rodgers and Chido blood group antigens have also been located using cloning techniques and the rare allotypes C4A1 and C4B5 (156). The structural model (see Fig 3), as proposed by Yu and modified by Giles, accounts for all known Rodgers and Chido antigens (139,163). According to this model, most C4A allotypes are Rg1,2 and Ch-1-2-3; most C4B allotypes are Rg-1-2 and have at least Ch1. Expression of Rg1 is determined by VDLL and Ch1 by ADLR at positions 1188–1191. Yu and Campbell (156) have developed RFLPs using a C4d-specific probe to characterize these antigens. A *C4A* gene is recognized by 276- and 191-bp *Nla*IV fragments and (if Rg1 is expressed) a 565 bp *Eco*O 109 fragment. A *C4B* gene shows a single 467-bp *Nla*IV fragment with a 458-bp EcoO 109 fragment present for Ch1.

4. Function

A major function of the complement cascade is to assist the immune response by promoting phagocytosis or lysing foreign cells. The classic pathway begins with the activation of C1, which is the major interface with the humoral response. C1s then activates C4 by cleaving 77 amino acids from the N terminus of the α chain (164). This small polypeptide of ~9 kd, designated C4a, diffuses into the fluid phase. One molecule of C1 can cleave multiple C4 molecules resulting in an amplification of the cascade. The remainder of the C4 molecule, C4b, undergoes a conformational change that exposes an internal thioester site and allows it to bind the target surface. Once C4b is bound, it can either produce an active C3 convertase by binding C2 or it can be inactivated by factor I in the presence of C4bp, CR1, or MCP.

There is no difference between the C4 isotypes regarding cleavage by C1s, inactivation by factor I, or assembly of the C3 convertase (165). There does appear, however, to be a difference in the covalent binding reactions of C4 with the surface of erythrocytes and immune aggregates in vitro (166). The thioester bond of C4A preferentially transacylates onto amino groups (proteins), whereas C4B prefers hydoxyl groups (carbohydrates) (165,167). Thus, the apparent hemolytic differences between C4A and C4B are not due to an impairment of C4A function but rather the target surface; i.e., RBC, which are rich in sialic acid and can bind more C4B. C4A is more effective than C4B at solubilizing immune complexes and inhibiting immune precipitation (168). C4A is also more effective in binding immune complexes to RBCs cells and is two to two and a half times more efficient in binding to IgG. On an evolutionary level, the ability of the C4 isotypes to bind to different types of invading targets would be desirable and may explain their simultaneous presence.

The role of complement in antibody response was highly controversial when first postulated. Animals deficient in C4 failed to develop immunological memory, suggesting that both C4 and C3 were necessary for the immune response (169). Recent studies by Finco et al. (170) showed that C4-deficient guinea pigs reconstituted with human C4A and immunized with bacteriophage had titers five times higher than those reconstituted only with C4B. Additionally, the animals lacking C4B had no secondary response. In human studies, blood donors with *C4B*Q0* genes had higher titers to cytomegalovirus (CMV) than those without C4 null genes (171,172). It is unclear at this time whether the lack of C4B protein or the increased levels of C4A (171) are responsible for the increased antibody response.

5. Disease

Because of the known HLA association with various diseases, the *C4* genes became a target for investigation. Low levels of C4 have been suggested to be inherited predisposing factors for diseases such as insulin-dependent diabetes (173) and autoimmune chronic active hepatitis (174). Some specific C4 allotypes (175,176) have been associated with various diseases (Table 2). Other diseases show an association with an extended MHC haplotype such as HLA B44, DR4, C4B3 with rheumatoid arthritis and HLA B17, C4A6 with psoriasis (177,178).

Processing of immune complexes is important in the pathogenesis of autoimmune diseases. Therefore, it was postulated that lack of either C4A or C4B might play a role in these diseases. *C4A* null genes (*C4A*Q0*, *Rg*) have been implicated in a number of autoimmune diseases, including Graves' disease, systemic sclerosis, rheumatoid arthritis, Sjögren's syndrome, and juvenile dermatomyositis (179,180). A high frequency of *C4A*Q0* has also been found in cases of IgA nephropathy and subacute sclerosing panencephalitis (82,149).

Table 2 C4 Genes Associated with Various Diseases

Disease	C4A Loci	C4B Loci	References
Psoriasis	*6	–	177
Subacute sclerosing panencephalitis (SSPE)	*Q0	–	199
Juvenile dermatomyositis	*Q0	–	180
Graves' disease	*Q0	–	179
Systemic lupus erythematosus	*Q0	–	190
Sjögren's syndrome	*Q0	–	200
Systemic sclerosis (scleroderma)	*Q0	*Q0	201,202
IgA nephropathy	*Q0	*Q0	181,203
Rheumatoid arthritis	*Q0	*2.9	204
		*3	178
		*5	205
Felty's syndrome	–	*Q0	182,183
Scleroderma	–	*Q0	202
AIDS	–	*Q0	185
AIDS-related complex	–	*Q0	186,206
Bacterial meningitis	–	*Q0	184
Schizophrenia	–	*Q0	207
Autism	–	*Q0	208
Paracoccidioidomycosis	–	*Q0	196
Glomerulonephritis	–	*2.9	176
Parkinson's disease	–	*2	209
Alzheimer's dementia	–	*2	209
Biliary cirrhosis	–	*2	175

Interestingly, some of the same diseases listed previously are also associated with *C4B* null genes (*C4B*Q0, Ch*); e.g., IgA nephropathy (181) and rheumatoid arthritis (182,183). The complete lack of C4B protein (Chido negative) results in increased susceptibility to bacterial meningitis in children (184). The influence of *C4B*Q0* on human immunodeficiency (HIV) infection may be of interest to blood bankers. The presence of these null genes seems to effect the progression of AIDS-related complex (ARC) to AIDS (185,186).

C4 null genes have become of even greater importance in the study of systemic lupus erythematosus (SLE), which is a chronic multisystem inflammatory illness that appears to result from a disturbance in immune regulation owing to genetic, hormonal, and environmental factors (187). Fielder et al. (188) reported the increased presence of *C4* null genes along with HLA-DR3 in patients with SLE but was unable to distinguish the relative contribution of each as risk factors. Other studies (189,190) reached similar conclusions regarding the increased frequency of *C4A*Q0* in patients with SLE. Carroll (154) found that a *C4A/21-OHA* gene deletion occurred with the HLA haplotype HLA-B8, DR3. Later studies on DNA using C4-specific probes found that the *C4* gene deletion occurred frequently in the lupus population and could be used as a genetic marker in this disease.

Goldstein et al. (190) noted that *C4A*Q0* genes occurred in both white and black patients with SLE; however, in blacks, the null gene did not always occur with the HLA A1, B8, DR3 phenotype. Other workers (191) also found an increase of *C4A* nulls but concluded that it was a relatively weak risk factor in blacks. Additional work using RFLP analysis has shown that the *C4A* gene deletion is a significant risk factor (RR = 4). It appears to travel with HLA-B44 and DR2 in blacks as well as the known HLA-B8, DR3 haplotype (192). In fact, the *C4A*Q0* allele appears to be the only risk factor that crosses racial boundaries, having been found in Chinese, Japanese, whites, blacks, and Mexican-Americans (193,194).

Even stronger evidence for the role of *C4A* null alleles is the fact that of 18 published cases of total C4 deficiency, all but 4 have SLE (195,196). The lack of both C4A and C4B may be related to other immune response problems. Several reports have noted abnormalities in Ig memory, failure to switch from IgM to IgG during secondary immune response, and marked impairment in the opsonization of microbes.

Several totally C4-deficient patients have been studied at the DNA level (190,197,198) using both C4 and 21-OH probes. Three of these patients showed normal intact genes. Two other C4-deficient individuals had large deletions of their *C4B/21-OHA* genes, which often occurs with HLA-B35, Cw4. The lack of any C4 protein in the plasma was apparently due to nonfunctional genes at the remaining loci. Clearly, there are many intriguing questions yet to be answered regarding the association of the Rodgers/Chido blood group and autoimmune disease.

V. SUMMARY

Initially the identification of blood group polymorphisms was of interest only to those involved with transfusion medicine. Changes in blood groups relative to disease evoked investigations into the biochemical structures of these epitopes. As we have seen in this chapter, interest in blood group polymorphisms now extends beyond the field of serology into immunology, bacteriology, rheumatology, and other fields. Advances in these fields will surely affect the practice of transfusion medicine in the future.

REFERENCES

1. Cobbold S, Hale G, Waldmann H. Non-lineage, LFA-1 family, and leucocyte common antigens: New and previously defined clusters. McMichael AJ, ed. Leukocyte Typing III: White Cell Differentiation Antigens. London: Oxford University Press, 1987:788.

2. Badakere SS, Joshi SR, Bhatia HM, et al. Evidence for a new blood group antigen in the Indian population (a preliminary report). Indian J Med Res 1973; 4:563.
3. Badakere SS, Parab BB, Bhatia HM. Further observations on the In[a] antigen in Indian populations. Vox Sang 1974; 26:400.
4. Badakere SS, Vasantha K, Bhatia HM, et al. High frequency of In[a] antigen among Iranians and Arabs. Hum Hered 1980; 30:262.
5. Giles CM. Antithetical relationship of anti-In[a] with the Salis antibody. Vox Sang 1975; 29:73.
6. Bhatia HM, Badakere SS, Mokashi SA, Parab BB. Studies on the blood group antigen In[a]. Immunol Commun 1980; 9:203.
7. Dumasia AN, Gupte S. Quantitation of In[a] blood group antigens. Indian J Med Res 1990; 92:50.
8. Spring FA, Dalchau R, Daniels GL, et al. The In[a] and In[b] blood group antigens are located on a glycoprotein of 80,000 mw (the CDw44 glycoprotein) whose expression is influenced by the *In(Lu)* gene. Immunology 1988; 64:37.
9. Dalchau R, Kirkley J, Fabre JW. Monoclonal antibody to a human brain-granulocyte–T-lymphocyte antigen probably homologous to the W3/13 antigen of the rat. Eur J Immunol 1980; 10:745.
10. Telen MJ, Palker TJ, Haynes BF. Human erythrocyte antigens: II. The *In(Lu)* gene regulates expression of an antigen on an 80-kilodalton protein of human erythrocytes. Blood 1984; 64:599.
11. Letarte M, Iturbe S, Quackenbush EJ. A glycoprotein of molecular weight 85,000 on human cells of B-lineage: Detection with a family of monoclonal antibodies. Mol Immunol 1985; 22:113.
12. Knowles RW, Bai Y, Lomas C, et al. Two monoclonal antibodies detecting high frequency antigens absent from red cells of the dominant Lu(a–b–) Lu:-3. J Immunogenet 1982; 9:353.
13. Telen MJ, Eisenbarth GS, Haynes BF. Human erythrocyte antigens. Regulation of expression of a novel erythrocyte surface antigen by the inhibitor Lutheran *In(Lu)* gene. J Clin Invest 1983; 71:1878.
14. Anstee DJ, Gardner B, Spring FA, et al. New monoclonal antibodies in CD44 and CD58: Their use to quantify CD44 and CD58 on normal human erythrocytes and to compare the distribution of CD44 and CD58 in human tissues. Immunology 1991; 74:197.
15. Udden MM, Umeda M, Hirano Y, Marcus DM. New abnormalities in the morphology, cell surface receptors, and electrolyte metabolism of *In(Lu)* erythrocytes. Blood 1987; 69:52.
16. Haynes BF, Telen MJ, Hale LP, Denning SM. CD44– a molecule involved in leukocyte adherence and T-cell activation. Immunol Today 1989; 10:423.
17. Goodfellow PN, Banting G, Wiles MV, et al. The gene, MIC4, which controls expression of the antigen defined by monoclonal antibody F10.44.2, is on human chromosome 11. Eur J Immunol 1982; 12:659.
18. Dougherty GJ, Lansdorp PM, Cooper DL, Humphries RK. Molecular cloning of CD44R1 and CD44R2, two novel isoforms of the human CD44 lymphocyte "homing" receptor expressed by hemopoietic cells. J Exp Med 1991; 174:1.
19. Miyake K, Underhill CB, Lesley J, Kincade PW. Hyaluronate can function as a cell adhesion molecule and CD44 particpates in hyaluronate recognition. J Exp Med 1990; 172:69.
20. Sy MS, Guo YJ, Stamenkovic I. Distinct effects of two CD44 isoforms on tumor growth in vivo. J Exp Med 1991; 174:859.
21. Jalkanen S, Joensuu H, Soderstrom KO, Klemi P. Lymphocyte homing and clinical behavior of non-Hodgkin's lymphoma. J Clin Invest 1991; 87:1835.
22. Haynes BF, Hale LP, Patton KL, et al. Measurement of an adhesion molecule as an indicator of inflammatory disease activity. Arthritis Rheum 1991; 34:1434.
23. Poole J, Giles CM. Observations on the Anton antigen and antibody. Vox Sang 1982; 43:220.
24. Marsh WL, Brown PJ, DiNapoli J, et al. An autoantibody that defines a high incidence antigen modified by the *In(Lu)* gene. Transfusion 1983; 23:128.
25. Harris T, Marsh WL. A Wj-negative patient with anti-Wj (letter). Transfusion 1986; 26:117.
26. Mannessier L, Rouger P, Johnson CL, et al. Acquired loss of red-cell Wj antigens in a patient with Hodgkin's Disease. Vox Sang 1986; 50:240.
27. Nowicki B, Moulds J, Hull R, Hull S. A hemagglutinin of uropathogenic *Escherichia coli* recognizes the Dr blood group antigen. Infect Immun 1988; 56:1057.
28. vanAlphen L, Poole J, Overbeeke M. The Anton blood group antigen is the receptor for *Haemophilus influenzae*. FEMS Microbiol Lett 1986; 37:69.

29. vanAlphen L, Poole J, Geelen L, Zanen HC. The erythrocyte and epithelial cell receptors for *Haemphilus influenzae* are expressed independently. Infect Immun 1987; 40:2355.

30. Landsteiner K, Levine P. Further observations on individual differences of human blood. Proc Soc Exp Biol Med 1927; 24:941.

31. Tippett P, Sanger R, Race RR. An agglutinin associated with the P and ABO blood group systems. Vox Sang 1965; 10:269.

32. Allen FH Jr, Marsh WL, Jensen L, Fink J. Anti-IP: An antibody defining another product of interaction between the genes of the I and P blood group systems. Vox Sang 1974; 27:422.

33. Booth PB. Anti-I[T]P₁: An antibody showing a further association between the I and P blood groups systems. Vox Sang 1970; 19:85.

34. Levene C, Sela R, Rudolphson Y, et al. Hemolytic disease of the newborn due to anti-PP₁P[k] (anti-Tj[a]). Transfusion 1977; 79:569.

35. Moulds MK. Serology of P, I, Sd[a], Rx and Pr. In Moulds JM, Woods LL (eds): Blood Groups: P, I, Sd[a] and Pr. Arlington, VA: American Association of Blood Banks, 1991:113.

36. Marcus DM. The Ii and P blood group systems. In: Litivin SD (ed): Human Immunogenetics. Basic Principles and Clinical Relevance. New York: Marcel Dekker 1989:701.

37. Wiels J, Fellous M, Tursz T. Monoclonal antibody against a Burkitt lymphoma-associated antigen. Proc Natl Acad Sci USA 1981; 78:6485.

38. Nudelman E, Kannagi R, Hakomori S, et al. A glycolipid antigen associated with Burkitt lymphoma defined by a monoclonal antibody. Science 1983; 220:509.

39. Issitt PD. The P blood group system. In: Issitt PD (ed): Applied Blood Group Serology. Miami: Montgomery Scientific Publications, 1985:203.

40. Levine P, Celano MJ, Falkowski F. The specificity of the antibody in paroxysmal cold hemoglobinuria (PCH). Transfusion 1963; 3:278.

41. Ben-Ismail R, Rouger P, Carme B. Comparative automated assay of anti-P₁ antibodies in acute hepatic distomiasis (fascioliasis) and in hydatidosis. Vox Sang 1980; 38:165.

42. Leffler H, Svanborg-Eden C. Glycolipid receptors for uropathogenic *Escherichia coli* on human erythrocytes and uroepithelial cells. Infect Immun 1981; 34:920.

43. Lomberg L, Hanson LA, Jacobsson B, et al. Correlation of P blood group, vesicoureteral reflux, and bacterial attachment in patients with recurrent pyelonephritis. N Engl J Med 1983; 308:1189.

44. Giron JA, Ho ASY, Schoolnik GK. An inducible bundle-forming pilus of enteropathogenic *Escherichia coli*. Science 1991; 254:710.

45. Wiener AS, Unger LJ, Cohen L, Feldman J. Type-specific cold auto-antibodies as a cause of acquired hemolytic anemia and hemolytic transfusion reactions: Biologic test with bovine red cells. Ann Intern Med 1956; 44:221.

46. Jenkins WJ, Marsh WL, Noades J. The I antigen and antibody. Vox Sang 1960; 5:97.

47. Booth PB, Jenkins WJ, Marsh WL. Anti-I[T]: A new antibody of the I blood-group system occurring in certain Melanesian sera. Br J Haematol 1966; 12:341.

48. Marsh WL, Nichols ME, Reid ME. The definition of two I antigen components. Vox Sang 1971; 20:209.

49. Hakomori S. Blood group ABH and Ii antigens of human erythrocytes: Chemistry, polymorphism, and their developmental change. Semin Hematol 1981; 18:39.

50. Finland M, Curen EC. Agglutinins for human erythrocytes in type XIV anti-pneumococci horse serums. Science 1938; 87:417.

51. Feizi T. The blood group Ii system: a carbohydrate antigen system defined by naturally monoclonal or oligoclonal autoantibodies of man. Immunol Comm 1981, 10:127.

52. Loomes LM, Uemura K, Childs RA, et al. Erythrocyte receptors for *Mycoplasma pneumoniae* are sialyated oligosaccharides of Ii antigen type. Nature 1984; 307:560.

53. Loomes LM, Uemura K, Feizi T. Interaction of *Mycoplasma pneumoniae* with erythrocyte glycolipids of I and i antigen types. Infect Immun 1985; 47:15.

54. Roelcke D, Kreft H, Northoff H, Gallasch E. Sia-b1 and I antigens recognized by *Mycoplasma pneumoniae*-induced human cold agglutinins. Transfusion 1991; 31:627.

55. McCormick EE, Francis BJ, Belb AG. A new antibody apparently defining an allele of Go[a]. Transfusion 1965; 5:369.

56. Stroup M, McCreary J. Cr[a], another high frequency blood group factor. Transfusion 1975; 15:522.

57. Daniels GL, Tohyama H, Uchikawa M. A possible null phenotype in the Cromer blood group complex. Transfusion 1982; 22:362.

58. Walthers L, Salem M, Tessel J, et al. The Inab phenotype: Another example found. Transfusion 1983; 23:423.

59. Daniels GL, Walthers L. Anti-IFC, an antibody made by Inab phenotype individuals (letter). Transfusion 1986; 26:117.

60. Lin RC, Herman J, Henry L, Daniels GL. The Inab phenotype: The first family to demonstrate inheritance (abstr). Transfusion 1987; 27:515.

61. Laird-Fryer B, Dukes CV, Lawson J, et al. Tc[a]: A high frequency blood group antigen. Transfusion 1983; 23:124.

62. Gorman MI, Glidden HM, Behzad O. Another example of anti-Tc[a] (abstr). Transfusion 1981; 21:579.

63. Lacey PA, Block UT, Laird-Fryer BJ, et al. Anti-Tc[b], an antibody that defines a red cell antigen antithetical to Tc[a]. Transfusion 1985; 25:373.

64. Levene C, Harel N, Lavie G, et al. A "new" phenotype confirming a relationship between Cr[a] and Tc[a]. Transfusion 1984; 24:13.

65. Levene C, Harel N, Kende G, et al. A second Dr(a–) proposita with anti-Dr[a] and a family with the Dr(a–) phenotype in two generations. Transfusion 1987; 27:64.

66. Daniels GL, Green CA, Darr FW, et al. A "new" Cromer-related high frequency antigen probably antithetical to WES. Vox Sang 1987; 53:235.

67. Tregellas WM. Description of a new blood group antigen, Es[a]. Abstracts Int Soc Blood Transfusion 1984:163.

68. Spring FA, Judson PA, Daniels GL, et al. A human cell-surface glycoprotein that carries Cromer-related blood group antigens on erythrocytes and is also expressed on leucocytes and platelets. Immunology 1987; 62:307.

69. Sistonen P, Nevanlinna HR, Virtaranta-Knowles K, et al. WES, a new infrequent blood group antigen in Finns. Vox Sang 1987; 52:111.

70. Telen MJ, Hall SE, Green AM, et al. Identification of human erythrocyte blood group antigens on decay-accelerating factor (DAF) and an erythrocyte phenotype negative for DAF. J Exp Med 1988; 167:1993.

71. Lublin DM, Lemons RS, LeBeau MM, et al. The gene encoding decay-accelerating factor (DAF) is located in the complement-regulatory locus on the long arm of chromosome 1. J Exp Med 1987; 165:1731.

72. Rey-Campos J, Rubinstein P, Rodriguez de Cordoba S. Decay-accelerating factor: Genetic polymorphism and linkage to the RCA (regulator of complement activation) gene cluster in humans. J Exp Med 1987; 166:246.

73. Rey-Campos J, Rubinstein P, Rodriquez de Cordoba S. A physical map of the human regulator of complement activation gene cluster linking the complement genes CR1, CR2, DAF, and C4BP. J Exp Med 1988; 167:664.

74. Lublin DM, Liszewski KM, Post TW, et al. Molecular cloning and chromosomal localization of human membrane cofactor protein (MCP). J Exp Med 1988; 168:181.

75. Hourcade D, Holers VM, Atkinson JP. The regulators of complement activation (RCA) gene cluster. Adv Immunol 1989; 45:381.

76. Caras IW, Davitz MA, Rhee L, et al. Cloning of decay-accelerating factor suggests novel use of splicing to generate two proteins. Nature 1987; 325:545.

77. Post TW, Arce MA, Liszewski KM, et al. Structure of the gene for human complement protein decay accelerating factor. J Immunol 1990; 144:740.

78. Stafford HA, Tykocinski ML, Lublin DM, et al. Normal polymorphic variations and transcription of the decay accelerating factor gene in paroxysmal nocturnal hemoglobinuria cells. Proc Natl Acad Sci USA 1988; 85:88.

79. Mallinson G, Tanner MJA, Thompson ES, et al. Sequence analysis of decay-accelerating factor cDNA and gene in original propositus of decay-accelerating-factor-negative Inab phenotype (abstr). Complement Inflamm 1991; 8:189.

80. Nicholson-Weller A, March JP, Rosen CE, et al. Surface membrane expression of human blood

leukocytes and platelets of decay-accelerating factor, a regulatory protein of the complement system. Blood 1985; 65:1237.

81. Kinoshita T, Medof EM, Silber R, Nussenzweig V. Distribution of decay-accelerating factor in the peripheral blood of normal individuals and patients with paroxysmal nocturnal hemoglobinuria. J Exp Med 1985; 162:75.

82. Dalmasso AP, Vercellotti GM, Platt JL, Bach FH. Inhibition of complement-mediated cell cytotoxicity by decay-accelerating factor. Potential for prevention of xenograft hyperacute rejection. Transplantation 1991; 52:530.

83. Telen MJ, Green AM. The Inab phenotype: Characterization of the membrane protein and complement regulatory defect. Blood 1989; 74:437.

84. Tate CG, Uchikawa M, Tanner MJ, et al. Studies on the defect which causes absence of decay accelerating factor (DAF) from the peripheral blood cells of an individual with the Inab phenotype. Biochem J 1989; 261:489.

85. Morgan BP. Complement in other diseases. In Morgan BP (ed): Complement; Clinical Aspects and Relevance to Disease. San Diego: Academic Press, 1990:184.

86. Daniels GL. Cromer-related antigens-blood group determinants on decay-accelerating factor (review). Vox Sang 1989; 56:205.

87. Lublin DM, Coyne KE. Phospholipid-anchored and transmembrane versions of either decay-accelerating factor or membrane cofactor protein show equal efficiency in protection from complement-mediated cell damage. J Exp Med 1991; 174:35.

88. Davis LS, Patel SS, Atkinson JP, Lipsky PE. Decay-accelerating factor functions as a signal transducing molecule for human T cells. J Immunol 1988; 141:2246.

89. Fujita T, Shibuya K, Abe T. Activation of human monocytes through decay-accelerating factor (abstr). Complement Inflamm 1989; 8:152.

90. Stefanova I, Horejsi V, Ansotegui IJ, et al. GPI-anchored cell-surface molecules complexed to protein tyrosine kinases. Science 1991; 254:1016.

91. Lublin DM, Thompson ES, Green AM, et al. Dr(a–) polymorphism of decay accelerating factor. Biochemical, functional, and molecular characterization and production of allele-specific transfectants. J Clin Invest 1991; 87:1945.

92. Nowicki B, Truong L, Moulds J, Hull R. Presence of the Dr receptor in normal human tissues and its possible role in the pathogenesis of ascending urinary tract infection. Am J Pathol 1988; 133:1.

93. Cooper NR. Complement evasion strategies of microorganisms. Immunol Today 1991; 12:327.

94. Norris KA, Bradt BM, Cooper NR. Inhibition of alternative complement pathway activation by a 160-kDa binding protein of *Trypansoma cruzi* (abstr). Complement Inflamm 1991; 8:200.

95. Giles CM, Huth MC, Wilson TE, et al. Three examples of a new antibody anti-Cs[a], which reacts with 98% of red cell samples. Vox Sang 1965; 10:405.

96. Molthan L, Giles CM. A new antigen, Yk[a], and its relationship to Cs[a] (Cost). Vox Sang 1975; 29:145.

97. Helgeson M, Swanson J, Polesky HF. Knops-Helgeson (Kn[a]), a high frequency erythrocyte antigen. Transfusion 1970; 10:737.

98. Mallan MT, Grimm W, Hindley L, et al. The Hall serum: detecting Kn[b], the antithetical allele to Kn[a] (abstr). Transfusion 1980; 20:630.

99. Molthan L, Moulds J. A new antigen, McC[a] (McCoy), and its relationship to Kn[a] (Knops). Transfusion 1978; 18:566.

100. Lacey P, Laird-Fryer B, Block U, et al. A new high incidence blood group factor, Sl[a]; and its hypothetical allele. Transfusion 1980; 20:632.

101. Molthan L. The new McCoy antigens, McC[c] and McC[d] (abstr). Transfusion 1980; 20:622.

102. Molthan L. Expansion of the York, Cost, McCoy, Knops blood group system: The new McCoy antigens McC[c] and McC[d]. Med Lab Sci 1983; 40:113.

103. Molthan L. The status of the McCoy/Knops antigens. Med Lab Sci 1983; 40:59.

104. Moulds JM, Nickells MW, Moulds JJ, et al. The C3b/C4b receptor is recognized by the Knops, McCoy, Swain-Langley, and York blood group sera. J Exp Med 1991; 173:1159.

105. Rao N, Ferguson DJ, Lee SF, Telen MJ. Identification of human erythrocyte blood group antigens on the C3b/C4b receptor. J Immunol 1991; 146:3501.

106. Moulds JM, Moulds JJ, Brown MC, Atkinson JP. Antiglobulin testing for CR1-related

(Knops/McCoy/Swain-Langley/York) blood group antigens: Negative and weak reactions are caused by variable expression of CR1. Vox Sang 1992; 62:230.

107. Ahearn JM, Fearon DT. Structure and function of the complement receptor, CR1(CD35) and CR2(CD21). Adv Immunol 1989; 46:183.

108. Hourcade D, Post TW, Holers VM, et al. Polymorphism of the regulators of complement activation gene cluster. Complement Inflamm 1990; 7:302.

109. Fearon D. Identification of the membrane glycoprotein that is the C3b receptor of the human erythrocyte polymorphonuclear leukocyte, B lymphocyte, and monocyte. J Exp Med 1980; 152:20.

110. Wong WW, Wilson JG, Fearon D. Genetic regulation of a structural polymorphism of human C3b receptor. J Clin Invest 1983; 72:685.

111. Dykman TR, Hatch JA, Aqua MF, Atkinson JP. Polymorphism of the C3b/C4b receptor (CR1): characterization of a fourth allele. J Immunol 1985; 134:1787.

112. Van Dyne S, Holers VM, Lublin DM, Atkinson JP. The polymorphism of the C3b/C4b receptor in the normal population and in patients with systemic lupus erythematosus. Clin Exp Immunol 1987; 68:570.

113. Dykman TR, Cole JL, Iida K, Atkinson JP. Polymorphism of human erythrocyte C3b/C4b receptor. Proc Natl Acad Sci USA 1983; 80:1698.

114. Wong WW, Cahill JM, Rosen MD, et al. Structure of the human CR1 gene. Molecular basis of the structural and quantitative polymorphisms and identification of a new CR1-like allele. J Exp Med 1989; 169:847.

115. Wilson JG, Murphy EE, Wong WW, et al. Identification of a restriction fragment polymorphism by a CR1 cDNA that correlates with the number of CR1 on erythrocytes. J Exp Med 1986; 164:50.

116. Wong WW, Kennedy CA, Bonaccio ET, et al. Analysis of multiple restriction fragment length polymorphisms of the gene for the human complement receptor type 1. Duplication of genomic sequences occurs in association with a high molecular mass receptor allotype. J Exp Med 1986; 164:1531.

117. Ng YC, Schifferli JA, Walport MJ. Immune complexes and erythrocyte CR1 (complement receptor 1): effect of CR1 numbers on binding and release reactions. Clin Exp Immunol 1988; 71:481.

118. Currie MS, Vala M, Pisetsky DS, Greenberg CS, Crawford J, Cohen HJ. Correlation between erythrocyte CR1 reduction and other blood proteinase markers in patients with malignant and inflammatory disorders. Blood 1990; 75:1699.

119. Tausk FA, McCutchaan JA, Spechko P, Schreiber RD, Gigli, I. Altered erythrocyte C3b receptor expression, immune complexes, and complement activation in homosexual men in varying groups for acquired deficiency syndrome. J Clin Invest 1986; 78:977.

120. Iida K, Mornaghi R, Nussenzweig V. Complement receptor (CR1) deficiency in erythrocytes from patients with systemic lupus erythematosus. J Exp Med 1982; 155:1427.

121. Walport MJ, Lachmann PJ. Erythrocyte complement receptor 1, immune complexes, and the rheumatic diseases. Arthritis Rheum 1988; 31:153.

122. Rodriguez de Cordoba S, Lublin DM, Rubinstein P, Atkinson JP. Human genes for three components that regulate the activation of C4 are tightly linked. J Exp Med 1985; 161:1189.

123. Hourcade D, Miesner DR, Bee C, Zeldes W, Atkinson JP. Duplication and divergence of the amino-terminal coding region of the complement receptor 1 (CR1) gene. An example of concerted (horizontal) evolution within a gene. J Biol Chem 1990; 265:974.

124. Holers VM, Chaplin DD, LeyKam JF, et al. Human complement C3b/C4b receptor (CR1) mRNA polymorphism that correlates with the CR1 allelic molecular weight polymorphism. Proc Natl Acad Sci USA 1987; 84:2459.

125. Pruitt SK, Baldwinn WM III, Marsh HC Jr, et al. The effect of soluble complement receptor type 1 on hyperacute xenograft rejection. Transplantation 1992; 52:868.

126. Weisman HF, Bartwow T, Leppo MK, et al. Soluble human complement receptor type 1: In vivo inhibitor of complement suppressing post-ischemic myocardial inflammation and necrosis. Science 1990; 249:146.

127. Fearon DT. Anti-inflammatory and immunosuppressive effects of recombinant soluble complement receptors. Clin Exp Immunol 1991; 86:43.

128. Bacle F, Haeffner-Cavaillon N, Laude M, et al. Induction of IL-1 release through stimulation of

the C3b/C4b complement receptor type one (CR1,CD35) on human monocytes. J Immunol 1991; 144:147.

129. Betz M, Filsinger S. Modulation of T cell functions through CR1 and CR3. Complement Inflamm 1991; 8:128.

130. Harris JP, Tegoli J, Swanson J, et al. A nebulous antibody responsible for cross-matching difficulties (Chido). Vox Sang 1967; 12:140.

131. Middleton J, Crookston MC. Chido substance in plasma. Vox Sang 1972; 23:256.

132. Longster G, Giles CM. A new antibody specificity, anti-Rg^a, reacting with a red cell and serum antigen. Vox Sang 1976; 30:175.

133. Middleton J, Crookston MC, Falk JA, et al. Linkage of Chido and HL-A. Tissue Antigens 1974; 4:366.

134. James J, Stiles P, Boyce F, Wright J. The HL-A type of Rg(a–) individuals. Vox Sang 1976; 30:214.

135. Giles CM, Gedde-Dahl T Jr, Robson EB, et al. Rg^a (Rodgers) and the HLA region: Linkage and associations. Tissue Antigens 1976; 8:143.

136. Tilley CA, Romans DG, Crookston MC. Localisation of Chido and Rodgers determinants to the C4d fragment of human complement. Nature 1991; 276:713.

137. O'Neill G, Yang SY, Tegoli J, et al. Chido and Rodgers blood groups are distinct antigenic components of human complement C4. Nature 1978; 273:668.

138. Giles CM. Antigenic determinants of human C4, Rodgers and Chido. Exp Clin Immunogenet 1988; 5:99.

139. Giles CM, Uring-Lambert B, Goetz J, et al. Antigenic determinants expressed by human C4 allotypes; A study of 325 families provides evidence for the structural antigenic model. Immunogenetics 1988; 27:442.

140. Giles CM, Jones JW. A new antigenic determinant for C4 of relatively low frequency. Immunogenetics 1987; 26:392.

141. Boksch W, Braum M, Brenden M, et al. C4A proteins with C4B antigenic epitopes (abstr). Immunobiology 1986; 173:451.

142. Rittner C, Giles CM, Roos MH, et al. Genetics of human C4 polymorphism: Detection and segregation of rare and duplicated haplotypes. Immunogenetics 1984; 19:321.

143. Roos MH, Giles CM, Demant P, et al. Rodgers (Rg) and Chido (Ch) determinants of two C4B5 subtypes, one of which contains Rg and Ch determinants. J Immunol 1984; 133:2634.

144. Hing SN, Giles CM, Fielder AHL, Batchelor JR. HLA haplotypes with C4B5; evidence for further allelic heterogeneity. Immunogenetics 1986; 23:151.

145. Colten HR. Genetics and synthesis of components of the complement system. In: Ross GD (ed): Immunobiology of the Complement System. An Introduction for Research and Clinical Medicine. New York: Academic Press, 1986:174.

146. Belt KT, Carroll MC, Porter RR. The structural basis of the multiple forms of human complement component C4. Cell 1984; 36:907.

147. Chan AC, Atkinson JP. Oligosaccharide structure of human C4. J Immunol 1985; 134:1790.

148. Mauff G, Alper CA, Dawkins RL, et al. C4 nomenclature statement (1990). Complement Inflamm 1991; 7:261.

149. Robinson MA, Carroll MC, Johnson AH, et al. Localization of C4 genes within the HLA complex by molecular genotyping. Immunogenetics 1985; 21:143.

150. Carroll MC, Belt KT, Palsdotirr A, Yu CY. Molecular genetics of the fourth component of human complement and steroid 21-hydroxylase. Immunol Rev 1985; 87:39.

151. Campbell RD, Carroll MC, Porter RR. The molecular genetics of components of complement. Adv Immunol 1986; 38:203.

152. Awdeh ZL, Raum D, Yunis EJ, Alper CA. Extended HLA/complement allele haplotypes: Evidence for T/t-like complex in man. Proc Natl Acad Sci USA 1983; 80:259.

153. Carroll MC, Campbell RD, Bently DR, Porter RR. A molecular map of the major histocompatibility complex III region linking complement genes C4, C2 and factor B. Nature 1984; 307:237.

154. Carroll MC, Palsdotirr A, Belt KT, Porter RR. Deletion of complement C4 and 21-hydroxylase genes in the HLA class III region. EMBO J 1985; 4:2547.

155. Bruun-Peterson G, Lamm, LU, Jacobson BK, Kristensen T. Genetics of complement C4. Two homoduplication haplotypes C4SC4S and C4FC4F in a family. Hum Genet 1982; 61:36.

156. Yu CY, Campbell RD. Definitive RFLPs to distinguish between the human complement C4A/C4B isotypes and the major Rodgers/Chido determinants: Application to the study of C4 null alleles. Immunogenetics 1987; 25:383.

157. Schneider PM, Carroll MC, Alper CA, et al. Polymorphism of the human complement C4 and steroid 21-hydroxylase genes. Restriction fragment length polymorphism revealing structural deletion, homoduplications and size variants. J Clin Invest 1986; 78:650.

158. Palsdotirr A, Arnason A, Fossdad R, et al. Heterogeneity of human C4 gene size. Immunogenetics 1987; 25:299.

159. Hellman U, Eggertson G, Lundwall A, et al. Primary sequence difference between Chido and Rodgers variants of tryptic C4d on the human complement system. FEBS Lett 1984; 170:254.

160. Schendel DJ, O'Neill GJ, Wank R. MHC-linked class III genes. Analysis of C4 gene frequencies, complotypes, and associations with distinct HLA haplotypes in German Caucasians. Immunogenetics 1984; 20:23.

161. Yu CY, Belt KT, Giles CM, Campbell RD, Porter RR. Structural basis of the polymorphism of human complement components C4A and C4B: gene size, reactivity and antigenicity. EMBO J 1986; 5:2873.

162. Carroll MC, Fathallah DM, Bergamaschini L, et al. Substitution of a single amino acid (aspartic acid for histidine) converts the functional activity of human complement C4B to C4A. Proc Natl Acad Sci USA 1990; 87:6868.

163. Yu CY, Campbell RD, Porter RR. A structural model for the location of the Rodgers and the Chido antigenic determinants and their correlation with the human complement component C4A/C4B isotypes. Immunogenetics 1988; 27:399.

164. Hughes-Jones NC. The classical pathway. In: Ross GD (ed): Immunobiology of the Complement System. An Introduction for Research and Clinical Medicine. New York: Academic Press, 1986:21.

165. Law SKA, Dodds AW, Porter RR. A comparison of the properties of two classes of C4A and C4B of the human complement component C4. EMBO J 1984; 3:1819.

166. Schifferli JA, Paccaud JP. Two isotypes of human C4, C4A and C4B have different structure and function. Complement Inflamm 1989; 6:19.

167. Isenman DE, Young JR. The molecular basis of the difference in immune hemolytic activity of the Chido and Rodgers isotype of human complement component C4. J Immunol 1984; 132:3019.

168. Paul L, Skanes VM, Mayden J, et al. C4-mediated inhibition of immune precipitation and differences in inhibitory action of genetic variants C4A3 and C4B1. Complement 1988; 5:110.

169. Morgan BP. The biological effects of complement activation. In: Morgan BP (ed): Complement, Clinical Aspects and Relevance to Disease. New York: Academic Press, 1990:53.

170. Finco O, Li S, Cuccia MC, Carroll MC. Regulation of the immune response by polymorphism of human C4 (abstr). Complement Inflamm 1991; 8:149.

171. Moulds JM, deJongh R. Influence of C4B null genes on cytomegalovirus antibody titers from healthy blood donors. Transfusion 1992; 32:145.

172. Partanen J, Koskimies S, Soininen R. High Anti-CMV antibody titer in healthy blood donors is associated with homozygous C4B deficiency. Proceedings of the 2nd European Meeting Complement in Human Disease, 1988:189.

173. Vergani D, Johnston C, B-Abdullah N, Barnett AH. Low serum C4 concentrations: an inherited predisposition to insulin dependent diabetes? Br Med J 1983; 286:926.

174. Vergani D, Larcher VF, Davies ET, et al. Genetically determined low C4: a predisposing factor to autoimmune chronic active hepatitis. Lancet 1985; 2:294.

175. Briggs DC, Donaldson PT, Hayes P, et al. A major histocompatibility complex class III allotype (C4B2) associated with primary biliary cirrhosis (PBC). Tissue Antigens 1987; 29:141.

176. Wank R, O'Neill GJ, Held E, et al. Rare variant of complement C4 is seen in high frequency in patients with primary glomerulonephritis. Lancet 1984; 1:872.

177. Wyatt RJ, Wang C, Hudson EC, et al. Complement phenotypes in patients with psoriasis. Hum Hered 1989; 39:327.

178. Fielder AHL, Ollier W, Lord DK, et al. HLA class III haplotypes in multicase rheumatoid arthritis families. Hum Immunol 1989; 25:75.

179. Ratanachaiyavong S, Demaine AG, Campbell RD, and McGregore AM. Heat shock protein 70

(HSP70) and complement C4 genotypes in patients with hyperthyroid Grave's disease. Clin Exp Immunol 1991; 84:48.

180. Robb SA, Fielder AHL, Saunders CEL. C4 complement allotypes in juvenile dermatomyositis. Hum Immunol 1988; 22:31.

181. Welch TR, Beischel LS, Choi EM. Molecular genetics of C4B deficiency in IgA nephropathy. Hum Immunol 1989; 26:353.

182. Hillarby MC, Strachan T, Grennan DM. Molecular characterisation of C4 null alleles found in Felty's syndrome. Ann Rheum Dis 1990; 49:763.

183. Thomson W, Sanders PA, Davis M, et al. Complement C4B-null alleles in Felty's syndrome. Arthritis Rheum 1988; 31:984.

184. Rowe PC, McLean RH, Wood RA, et al. Association of homozygous C4B deficiency with bacterial meningitis. J Infect Dis 1989; 160:448.

185. Cameron PU, Cobain TJ, Zhang WJ, et al. Influence of C4 null genes on infection with human immunodeficiency virus. Br Med J 1988: 296:1627.

186. Plum G, Siebel E, Bendick C, et al. Major histocompatibility complex class I to III allotypes in patients with AIDS-related complex/Walter-Reed 5, desseminated Kaposi's sarcoma and in normal controls. Vox Sang 1990; 59(Supp 1):15.

187. Schumacher HR (ed). Systemic lupus erythematosus pathology and pathogenesis. In: Primer on the Rheumatic Diseases. Atlanta: Arthritis Foundation, 1988:96.

188. Fielder AHL, Walport MJ, Batchelor JR, et al. Family study of the major histocompatibility complex in patients with systemic lupus erythematosus: importance of null alleles of C4A and C4B in determining disease susceptibility. Br J Med 1983; 286:425.

189. Kemp ME, Atkinson JP, Skanes VM, et al. Deletion of C4A genes in patients with systemic lupus erythematosus. Arthritis Rheum 1987; 30:1015.

190. Goldstein R, Arnett FC, McLean RH, et al. Molecular heterogeneity of complement component C4-null and 21-hydroxylase genes in systemic lupus erythematosus. Arthritis Rheum 1988; 31:736.

191. Wilson WA, Perez MC, Michalski JP, Armatis PE. Cardiolipin antibodies and null alleles of C4 in black Americans with systemic lupus erythematosus. J Rheum 1988; 15:1768.

192. Olsen ML, Goldstein R, Arnett FC, et al. C4A gene deletion and HLA associations in black Americans with systemic lupus erythematosus. Immunogenetics 1989; 30:27.

193. Dunckley H, Gatenby PA, Hawkins B, et al. Deficiency of C4A is a genetic determinant of systemic lupus erythematosus in three ethnic groups. J Immunogenet 1987; 14:209.

194. Kumar A, Kumar P, Schur PH. DR3 and non-DR3 associated complement component C4A deficiency in systemic lupus erythematosus. Clin Immunol Immunopathol 1991; 60:55.

195. Hauptmann G, Goetz J, Uring-Lambert B, Grosshans E. Component deficiencies 2: The fourth component. Progr Allergy 1986; 39:239.

196. deMassias IJT, Reis A, Brenden M, et al. Association of major histocompatibility complex class III complement components C2, BF, and C4 with Brazilian paracoccidioidomycosis. Complement Inflamm 1991; 8:288.

197. Uring-Lambert B, Mascart-Lemone F, Tongio MM, et al. Molecular basis of complete C4 deficiency. A study of three patients. Hum Immunol 1989; 24:125.

198. Uring-Lambert B, Vegnaduzzi-Lamouche N, Carroll MC, et al. Heterogeneity in the structural basis of the human complement C4A null allele (C4A*Q0) as revealed by Hind III restriction fragment length polymorphism analysis. Fed Eur Biochem 1987; 217:65.

199. Rittner C, Meier EMM, Stradman B, et al. Partial C4 deficiency in subacute sclerosing panencephalitis. Immunogenetics 1984; 20:407.

200. Moriuchi J, Ichikawa Y, Tayaka M, et al. Association of the complement allele C4AQ0 with primary Sjögren's syndrome in Japanese patients. Arthritis Rheum 1991; 34:224.

201. Briggs DC, Welsh K, Pereira RS, Black CM. A strong association between null alleles at the C4A locus in the major histocompatibility complex and systemic sclerosis. Arthritis Rheum 1986; 29:1274.

202. Mollenhauer E, Schmidt R, Heinrich, M, Rittner C. Scleroderma: Possible significance of silent alleles at the C4B locus. Arthritis Rheum 1984; 27:711.

203. Wyatt RJ, Julian BA, Woodford SY, et al. C4A deficiency and poor prognosis in patients with IgA nephropathy. Clin Nephrol 1991; 36:1.

204. O'Neill GJ, Nerl CW, Kay PH, et al. Complement C4 is a marker for adult rheumatoid arthritis. Lancet 1982; 2:214.

205. Takeuchi F, Mimori A, Matsuta K, et al. Association of complement alleles C4AQ0 and C4B5 with rheumatoid arthritis in Japanese patients. Arthritis Rheum 1989; 32:691.

206. Cameron PU, Mallal SA, French MAH, Dawkins RL. Major histocompatibility complex genes influence the outcome of HIV infection. Ancestral haplotypes with C4 null alleles explain diverse HLA associations. Hum Immunol 1990; 29:282.

207. Rudduck E, Beckman L, Franzen G, et al. Complement factor C4 in schizophrenia. Hum Hered 1985; 35:223.

208. Warren RP, Singh VK, Cole P, et al. Increased frequency of the null allele at the complement C4B locus in autism. Clin Exp Immunol 1991; 83:438.

209. Nerl C, Mayeux R, O'Neill GJ. HLA-linked complement markers in Alzheimer's and Parkinson's disease: C4 variant (C4B2) a possible marker for senile dementia of the Alzheimer type. Neurology 1984; 34:310.

11

Use of Hematopoietic Cells and Markers for the Detection and Quantitation of Human In Vivo Somatic Mutation

STEPHEN G. GRANT and RONALD H. JENSEN
University of California, San Francisco
San Francisco, California

I. INTRODUCTION

In general, the elucidation of the biochemistry and genetics of blood cells and blood cell markers has been in advance of other physiological systems for two practical reasons: accessibility and medical importance. A blood sample is relatively easy to obtain, and analysis of its components can be diagnostic of many types of disease states. The use of hematopoietic cells and cell-specific markers to study human in vivo somatic mutation is a logical extension of this concept. In the last few years we have begun to realize the significance of stable genetic alterations in somatic cells as important contributors to such ailments as cancer and aging. Direct detection and measurement of the processes that collectively can be termed somatic segregation may become an important prognostic tool in the clinical evaluation of affected individuals and, further, may point the way toward a better understanding and treatment of such degenerative states.

II. GENETIC DESIGN OF GENOTOXICITY ASSAYS

In designing a system to detect human in vivo somatic mutation, the tissue to be used should be fairly accessible to allow collection of a large, representative, population of cells (each representing at least one mitotic event), and the assay should be applicable to as large a segment of the population as possible. The first point takes into account the assumption that events that stably alter the genetic material are relatively rare; so to obtain a reasonable estimate of frequency or rate, a large number of potential events must be sampled. The second point is important because of the inherent genetic diversity of the human population; because suitable assayable genotypes cannot be produced by breeding or engineering, one must design the putative assay to be applicable to as large a segment of the human population as possible without regard for race or geographical distribution.

In order to create a sensitive genetic assay for somatic cells, one wishes to be able to detect single genetic events. In diploid mammals, there are three possible ways of detecting such events: dominant mutations, hemizygous loci, and heterozygous loci. Direct detection of a dominant mutation circumvents the problem of a diploid genotype; however, it severely limits the type of mutation one can detect. Dominant mutations must almost always produce very specific changes in the regulation of a gene or the ultrastructure of a gene product to be detectable. At the morphological level, the mutation must result in an obvious phenotype that can have occurred by only one mechanism to avoid the problem of overlapping gene effects and phenocopies. Although such phenotypic dominant mutations have been studied in a number of mammalian systems, their utilization for in vivo human somatic mutations is rare.

The detection of mutation in lower eukaryotes and prokaryotes is simplified by their monozygous genotype, such that all loci are hemizygous. In mammals, a large portion of the X chromosome is similarly hemizygous: in males, owing to the nonhomologous structures of the X and Y sex chromosomes and in females owing to the phenomenon of X chromosome inactivation (1). Thus, a single somatic event at the single functional allele of an X-linked locus can result in a mutant phenotype even if the mutant phenotype would be recessive had it occurred at an autosomal, diploid locus. Such a system is ideal for detecting classic mutational events; that is, events affecting only a single gene. However, such mutational events are not the only, nor indeed the most important, contributors to human somatic variation.

Since the greatest part of the mammalian genome is autosomal and diploid, an assay utilizing such a locus will be more representative of the actual scale of genetic variation, and the range of mechanisms by which such variation occurs, than an assay using an X-linked gene. Besides the dominant mutation assay mentioned earlier, there is a second method of circumventing the problem of diploidy to detect mutations at a single allele. If the locus in question is heterozygous, and the two alleles and/or their allelic products can be easily and unambiguously distinguished, then mutation at either allele can be detected while the allelic homologue remains unaffected. Indeed, the proper expression of the homologous allele can be used to screen against phenocopies. This type of assay can be utilized when the two alleles are codominant or alternatively to detect the reexpression of a recessive allele or phenotype upon the mutation of the corresponding dominant homologue. The range of possible mechanisms of variation and the expected results of these events are shown graphically in Figure 1.

This diploid heterozygous type of mutation assay, like the other two types, has been utilized extensively in somatic cell culture (2). Originally it was thought that this type of assay would detect essentially the same types of events as the dominant and hemizygous types of assays. Now it is clear, however, that the presence of a homologous chromosome can affect the frequency and mechanisms of variation at a dizygous locus in ways the other two types of assays cannot detect. Since the range of mutations that can be detected at a diploid locus involves any event that results in the absence or aberrant expression of one allele, all the events detected by an assay at a hemizygous locus should also be detected by the diploid heterozygous assay. At a diploid locus, however, there may be additional types of allowable mechanisms because any chromosomal or regulatory event that affects expression of only one allele can also result in the "mutant" phenotype. This would include gross chromosome deletion or loss, events that would have substantial deleterious effects upon the viability of the cell were they to occur at a hemizygous locus. A subtler effect is that of allelic inactivation; for example, by de novo DNA methylation that can affect a single gene or a variable region of a chromosome.

Finally, two chromosomal mechanisms that result in no gross changes in the structure or quantity of the genetic material have been detected in cultured somatic cells (2,3). The first involves the loss or substantial deletion of one copy of the chromosome carrying the gene of interest, with an associated duplication of the remaining homologue. These two events could occur simultaneously through an aberrant chromosome disjunction (although this would presuppose some interaction of the two homologues at mitosis) or sequentially by two nondisjunction events, although no molecular mechanism has yet been demonstrated experimentally for this sequence. A second chromosomal event involves a mitotic recombination between homologous chromosomes (strongly implicating some association between chromosomal homologues), followed by a fortuitous segregation of chromatids at mitosis. Note that although the

Allele Loss Mechanisms

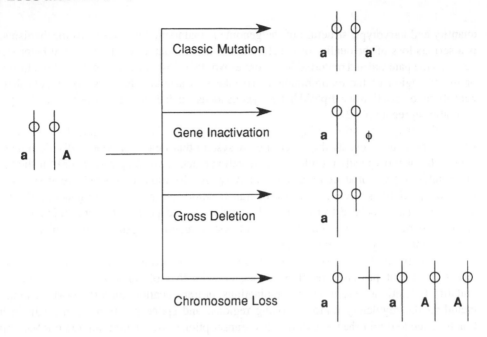

Allele Loss and Duplication Mechanisms

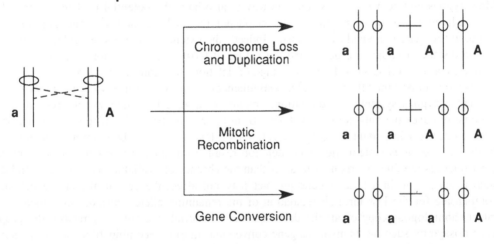

Figure 1   Potential mechanisms of allele loss and loss and duplication at some putative locus, A, heterozygous for the wild-type allele and a recessive genetic marker, a. In the upper figure, four mechanisms of loss of the remaining wild-type A allele are described. These include (1) mutation at the A allele resulting in loss of activity (see text for further elaboration); (2) inactivation of the A allele by a clonally inheritable event such as DNA methylation; (3) deletion of an entire region of the chromosome, including the A allele; or (4) loss of the entire chromosome carrying the A allele. The latter event is shown as occurring via nondisjunction during mitosis, with the simultaneous generation of a daughter cell trisomic for the chromosome of genotype A/A/a. In the lower figure, three potential mechanisms leading to homozygosity for the a allele are described, including (1) chromosome loss and duplication, which may occur via two successive nondisjunctional events or by a single aberrant disjunction in which paired chromatids segregate into daughter cells leading to the generation of both types of homozygous daughter cells, as shown; (2) a mitotic recombination event between the centromere and the A locus would lead to the indicated daughter cells 50% of the time depending on chromosomal segregation at mitosis; and (3) a putative gene conversion event in which the DNA from one chromatid is replicated using information from the homologous chromosome, with the result that one allele, in this case the A allele, is not replicated. (From Ref. 34.)

quantity and karyotypic structure of the genome is maintained by these two mechanisms, there is a serious loss of the quality of genetic information in that all of the potential heterozygosity between the paternal and maternal homologues would be lost either along the entire chromosome or in the region of the recombination. To take into account the range of events that could contribute to variation at a diploid heterozygous locus, such events have been collectively termed "somatic segregation" (2,3).

Another way of descriminating these three study designs is by examining the potential "target size" of the genetic events they measure. A system that detects a genetically dominant event does so by phenotypically monitoring or selecting (such as for drug resistance) for the presence of an altered gene product or a novel activity. At the molecular level, very specific point mutations, deletions, recombinations, or translocations are necessary to generate the required alteration, and associated transcriptional, translation, and posttranslational regulatory regions of the gene must be unaffected. This type of system requires a gain of function and, therefore, operates under very strict constraints.

Alternately, both monozygous and heterozygous detection systems deal with essentially recessive phenotypes and are often associated with loss of function events. Random point mutations, deletions, insertions, recombinations, or translocations almost anywhere in the gene, including the regulatory regions, coding regions, and splice junctions, can result in loss of function due to diminished or extinguished transcription or translation, altered mRNA or protein processing or stability, altered protein targeting, conformation, or activity. Thus, these systems detect a wider range of the same types of gene-specific events that occur in dominant systems. Monozygous and hemizygous systems, however, also have the potential to detect events that affect a larger region of the genome. Since the phenotypes are based on loss of function, deletion of the entire gene is a viable mechanism. Indeed, the extent of the possible deletion depends on the distance to adjoining genes and the nature of those genes. Deletion of all or part of a gene critical for cell survival limits the range of deletions that can be recovered.

There are important differences in the consequences of such deletion between the monozygous and heterozygous systems. By definition, deletion of a gene in a monozygous region of the genome removes the only copy of that gene from the cell irretrievably. If the gene function is even moderately important for cell survival, such a loss is likely to be extremely deleterious. In the heterozygous system, however, deletion results in a reduction in gene dosage and the consequences are due to a reduction rather than the absence of available gene product. Indeed, such a loss, even in a critical gene product may not affect the cell at all, or the cell may compensate for the loss through regulation of the remaining allele. Indeed, since there is an intact, homologous copy of all the deleted genetic material, the cell may restore the proper gene dosage by such mechanisms as gene conversion, mitotic recombination, or chromosome missegregation depending on the extent of the deletion. This results in the qualitative loss of heterozygosity mentioned above. In effect, the range of events that can be detected in such a system include almost any size deletion up to and including the complete loss of the chromosome carrying the gene of interest.

In this chapter, we describe four different assays for performing somatic cell mutation analysis on humans using hematopoietic cells. One of these assays analyzes for effects on an X-linked locus, hypoxanthine phosphoribosyltransferase, whereas the other three assays analyze for codominant effects occurring at diploid loci; the hemoglobin β-chain gene, the glycophorin A gene, or the *HLA-A* gene of the major histocompatibility locus.

III. ERYTHROCYTE ASSAYS

The erythrocyte is an excellent target for a mutagenesis assay primarily because of its abundance. From in vitro studies, we expect the frequency of mutations to be approximately 10^{-6}; since there are more than 10^9 red blood cells (RBCs) per milliliter of peripheral blood, analysis of 10^8 cells is feasible. Thus, the frequency of mutation is not a limitation on the accuracy of an assay based on RBC markers. On the other hand, RBCs have several major disadvantages. Despite a great deal of excellent scientific investigation, basic parameters of RBC metabolism, such as the number and turnover of stem cell populations, the persistence of intermediate phenotypes, and the significance of nucleated precursors in the peripheral circulation, are not clearly understood. These uncertainties make it virtually impossible to convert the frequency of variant erythrocytes measured in peripheral blood samples into a segregation rate in erythroid stem cells. A second major disadvantage of RBCs is their lack of genetic material, which precludes any attempt to discern the underlying genetic mechanisms responsible for variant phenotypes.

A. Hemoglobin

This in vivo mutation assay involves the generation of unique mutant β-chain hemoglobins in normal individuals. Owing to their medical significance, genetic variants of the hemoglobin gene and proteins were among the first human mutants to be isolated and characterized, with the result that methods of detecting such aberrant products were developed for diagnostic purposes. It was also important that such variants were known to be natural products of mutation during meiosis and were viable at the cellular level if not the organismal level. If indeed mitotic and meiotic mutations are similar, then the presence of rare cells expressing variant hemoglobins should be detectable in normal individuals at a frequency representative of the frequency of the underlying mutational events in the erythroid stem cells. Further, mutant hemoglobins could be selected based on their mutational mechanism of generation. Mutant hemoglobins that result from single base mutations can thus be targeted exclusively, allowing for the detection of variants caused by a single genetic event.

The first such assays were designed to detect two well-known hemoglobin variants, hemoglobin S and hemoglobin C (4,5). Since the mutations responsible for these aberrant proteins do not strongly affect the expression of the gene, the mutant allele is expressed codominantly with the remaining wild-type allele. The mutant protein can then be detected unambiguously with antiserum that differentiates between the normal and variant forms of the protein. Thus, the assay is essentially taking advantage of the presence of an altered protein to distinguish the progeny of a stem cell carrying a mutated allele from unaltered cells and to distinguish the normal and mutant allelic products in a single cell. In initial studies, populations of peripheral blood erythrocytes were labeled with fluorescently conjugated antibodies specific to the mutant hemoglobin S and C proteins. By scanning slides by fluorescence microscopy and counting the number of labeled versus unlabeled cells, a mutation frequency of approximately 10^{-8} was determined for each of these mutant alleles. Thus, such mutations did indeed occur somatically but at much lower frequency than originally predicted.

In common with in vitro dominant mutation assays, the in vivo hemoglobin assay is limited by the very specific types of events it can detect. Instead of a whole gamut of different mutations, only a single, specific base change can create the mutagenic endpoint it is designed to detect. This assay is therefore not properly assessing mutation at the β-globin locus in general but only at a single base pair at a time. Therefore, one should not be surprised that the mutation frequency measured by this type of assay is much lower than the 10^{-6} predicted for whole gene mutations (6,7).

Owing to the extreme rarity of such events, attempts were made to increase the cellular analysis rate for the hemoglobin assay significantly. The first method utilized flow cytometric detection and quantitation of variant erythrocytes (8–10). Although hemoglobin is the most abundant protein in the erythrocyte, it is an internal protein, so that the RBCs had to be partially permeabilized prior to labeling to allow the antibody access to the protein. This was not a significant problem in preparations of erythrocytes on microscope slides but caused difficulties for labeling in suspension. To improve the consistency and specificity of labeling, monoclonal antibodies against variant proteins were isolated and used for analysis (11). Ultimately, although the flow analysis confirmed the frequencies previously determined by manual microscopic analysis, the assay remained impractical for two reasons. Owing to the low frequency of variant events, the increased speed of analysis afforded by flow cytometric technology at the time was not enough to allow practical analysis of more than a few samples. Also, because of the low frequency of events, the detection system was working at the threshold of its capability necessitating flow sorting and manual microscopic confirmation of putative variant cells. More recently, the process of image analysis has been used to automate the detection of variant erythrocytes carrying mutant hemoglobins on microscope slide preparations (12,13). This computerized process, although still expensive and time consuming, offers the possibility that optical and mechanical improvements will yet render the hemoglobin assay practical and applicable.

The human β-globin gene has been well characterized at the molecular level. It is part of a cluster of six related genes and pseudogenes on chromosome 11, and it consists of three exons and two introns spanning less than 2 kilobases (kb) (14). As far as target size is concerned, however, the organization of the gene is unimportant because the assay screens directly for new mutations with specific amino acid replacements. To date, the assay has been performed with antibodies against three different variant hemoglobins, hemoglobins S and C, as described above, as well as hemoglobin$_{San Jose}$ (15), that require not only a mutation at a specific base in the coding sequence but a specific change at that base. Thus, the target size for this assay consists of a single base, and even then only one of three possible base changes are detectable. Recently, the assay has been extended to a second type of mutant by utilizing antibodies against an inherited abnormal hemoglobin, hemoglobin$_{Leiden}$, a variant that requires the in-frame deletion of one codon from the coding sequence (15).

A nonmechanical method of improving the hemoglobin assay that has been suggested involves the simultaneous screening of slides with antibodies to many of the more than 300 known hemoglobin variants (16). Not only would this significantly increase the frequency of positive events (an expected 10^{-8} per variant added) but it would also increase the ability of the assay to represent properly a larger range of mutagenic events occurring at the hemoglobin locus. A preliminary version of such an assay has been described in which antibodies against three different hereditary hemoglobin variants were used simultaneously and resulted in the expected threefold increase in mutation frequency (15).

Indeed, with modern genetic techniques it is no longer necessary for known genetic variants to exist in order to serve as a template for a possible somatic mutant. Gene cloning, expression vectors, site-specific mutagenesis, and in vitro translation would allow virtually any hemoglobin variant to be produced in quantities sufficient for the production of polyclonal or monoclonal antibodies. Thus, by mixing and matching the "cocktail" of detecting antibodies, an overview of mutation at the hemoglobin locus might be accomplished.

Ultimately, however, the molecular basis of the hemoglobin assay will always severely limit its applicability. Since a variant protein product must be expressed, all mutations causing loss of expression are invisible to the assay; likewise, all base changes that do not cause a change in the amino acid structure of the protein. Also, undoubtably there are amino acid substitutions that do not create a conformational change significant enough to create a distinguishable epitope. In the end, one saving grace of the hemoglobin assay is that the molecular nature of the mutagenic endpoint can be determined unambiguously without the need for analysis of genetic material, which is not present in erythrocytes.

B. Glycophorin A

Another assay that measures in vivo effects on RBCs involves phenotypic analysis of cell surface antigens on a cell by cell basis and enumeration of the frequency of variant cells that occur as a result of in vivo allele loss at the glycophorin A *(GPA)* locus in erythroid precursor cells in the bone marrow (9,10,17,18). The *GPA* gene codes for the most abundant RBC surface sialoglycoprotein at approximately 500,000 copies per cell. This gene occurs in two major allelic forms, M and N, that are expressed codominantly on RBCs in peripheral blood and are responsible for the MN blood group. Thus, people who are heterozygous at the *GPA* locus express an equal amount of each allelic form on RBCs. These two alleles occur at approximately equal frequency in most human populations; approximately half are therefore heterozygous at the *GPA* locus (19).

The population genetics of the *GPA* locus are important because the somatic cell mutation assay based on this gene is applicable only to $GPA^{M/N}$ heterozygotes. This heterozygous allele loss assay in its most improved version (20) uses two-color fluorescence labeling with two different monoclonal antibodies, each of which specifically recognizes one of the two allelic forms of the GPA protein (M and N). The assay is specifically designed to detect rare variant RBCs that have lost normal expression of one of the two *GPA* alleles. It can detect two distinctly different variant cell types. One variant cell type, the N/Ø variant, has a hemizygous phenotype. Such cells might arise by single base changes (causing transcriptional or translational inactivation or altering the protein product so that it is no longer recognized by the N-specific antibody), deletion or inactivation of the GPA^M allele, or loss of the chromosome carrying that allele in erythroid precursor cells. The other variant cell type detected is a homozygous N/N variant that has not only lost expression of the GPA^M allele but also expresses the GPA^N allele at twice the heterozygous level. These homozygous variant cells might be generated by chromosomal loss and duplication, gene conversion, or mitotic recombination in erythroid precursor cells. Thus, the *GPA* assay is potentially sensitive to all mechanisms of somatic segregation (as represented in Fig. 1) not merely classical mutations. An important feature of the *GPA* assay is that it requires normal expression of the GPA^N homologue; thus guaranteeing that all variant cells are capable of expressing this cell surface antigen. Because of this built-in safeguard, RBCs that have epigenetically lost the capability to retain any cell surface GPA (e.g., by membrane defects, carbohydrate metabolism defects, or by cellular degeneration) are not included as false positives (phenocopies) in the enumeration of variant cells, and the only mutations scored are *GPA* allele specific (17,18). The data obtained by performing this assay are the frequencies of N/Ø and N/N variant cell types for each sample analyzed. Such variant cell frequencies provide a measure of the sum of all the different types of gene-loss somatic cell mutations that have occurred at the *GPA* locus in the bone marrow of that individual. If, for example, an individual was exposed to ionizing radiation, one would predict that the frequency of such variant cells would be higher than in individuals who were not exposed. Because two exceedingly different kinds of variant cells are enumerated, different kinds of genotoxicity should be distinguishable. Thus, one might expect that radiation exposure would result in DNA damage that leads to deletions of chromosomes or subchromosomal deletions affecting specific genes. These would yield hemizygous variant cell types, and the assay would show a high frequency of hemizygous (N/Ø) variant cells with a near-normal frequency of homozygous (N/N) variant cells. However, if a particular chemical exposure leads to increases in somatic cell recombinations, one would expect to see an increased frequency of N/N variant cell types in the *GPA* genotoxicity assay with a near-normal frequency of N/Ø variant cells.

The human *GPA* gene has been localized to chromosome 4, closely linked to genes coding for two other, closely related erythrocyte membrane proteins: glycophorins B and E. In addition to defining the amino acid sequence of the mature GPA protein, the *GPA* coding region contains information for a leader peptide sequence as well as an extensive 3' untranslated region. The gene extends over 40 kb and is organized into seven exons, with the first two exons separated by an intron of over 30 kb (19). Since this is an expression loss assay, mutation throughout this entire region might be involved in producing the required variant phenotypes.

The improved version of the *GPA* assay allows it to be performed on commercially available single-beam flow cytometers such as the Becton Dickinson FACScan System, using their conventional Consort 30 software package (20). With this system, cells can be processed at a rate of 4,000 cells/sec, so that analysis of 5 million cells can be completed in 30 min. Because of the stability of the Becton Dickinson FACscan cytometer and its capacity to rapidly analyze many cells, the reproducibility of this improved assay for measuring such rare events as somatic segregation is excellent.

Since it is very easy to use, the *GPA* assay has become the most widely applied human in vivo somatic segregation assay. Average background variant frequencies in peripheral blood samples from normal populations are on the order of 10^{-5}, although the distribution of frequencies is considerably skewed to higher values, such that median levels are typically somewhat lower. We have identified at least two sources of this skewing. The first is a small age effect on the two endpoints, resulting in a 0.6 variants/year increase in frequency in NØ variant cells and a considerably larger increase of 3.6 variants/year in the N/N endpoint (21,22). There are also a variable number of individuals in normal populations that for no apparent reason manifest significantly higher variant frequencies for either endpoint. Again, this effect is more apparent with the homozygous than with the hemizygous class of variant, and the incidence of these "outlier" individuals increases with age in an exponential manner (23,24).

The *GPA* assay has been used extensively as a biodosimeter for exposure to ionizing radiation. Results from studies of survivors of the atomic bombing of Hiroshima (25–28) demonstrate the ability of the assay to detect persistent mutagenic effects. Even with no allowance made for the presence of the expected outliers in this elderly population (as described above), there is a significant positive response for the N/Ø variant frequency versus the estimated radiation dose of these individuals. Quantitatively consistent results have been reported in other accidentally exposed individuals, such as the survivors of the Goiania, Brazil, cesium source incident (29) and victims of the Chernobyl nuclear power plant accident (30,31). *GPA* variant frequency, in concert with other sensitive biodosimetric assays, has also been used to confirm lifetime radiation dose due to occupational exposure (32). Conversely, *GPA* variant frequency was not detectably altered by localized radiotherapy for solid tumours (33), although significantly elevated levels of homozygous variants were observed in preliminary experiments with patients treated with pelvic irradiation for benign gynecological disorders (34). It is clear that the specific intensity, extent, and geometry of radiation exposure is key to its mutagenic effect on erythroid bone marrow.

A biphasic response of the *GPA* assay was observed upon longitudinal study of patients undergoing chemotherapy (34–36). Large initial increases in variant cell frequencies were associated with induction of mutation in the dividing and differentiating erythrocyte precursor cells, whereas persistent effects suggested involvement of the stem cells. Different agents caused different levels of initial response and persistence. Much more subtle effects were detectable in populations environmentally exposed to chemical mutagens, such as smokers (37,38), styrene workers (38,39), and pesticide applicators (40).

Finally, significant elevations in *GPA* variant frequency have been demonstrated in individuals suffering from diseases of DNA repair and metabolism. Ten-, 50-, and 100-fold increases in hemizygous variant frequency were associated with the cancer-prone syndromes ataxia telagiectasia, Fanconi's anemia, and Bloom's syndrome, respectively (41–44). A concurrent 100-fold increase in homozygous variants was also observed in the patients with Bloom's syndrome (42–43). Increased levels of spontaneous *GPA* N/Ø variants have also been documented in the rare chromosome instability disease Nijmegan breakage syndrome and in Werner's syndrome, which is associated with premature aging (45).

As with the hemoglobin-based assay, the *GPA* assay has several drawbacks. First, it can be applied only to individuals who are heterozygous at the glycophorin A locus, such that only 50% of the human population can be analyzed. Also, the GPA antigen is expressed only on mature erythroid cells, and since peripheral blood erythrocytes do not carry DNA, the genetic changes that result in cellular phenotype changes cannot be assessed directly. Nevertheless, as demonstrated above, it is convenient and sensitive enough to be used for monitoring relatively large populations for mutagenic effects resulting either from lifestyle or from susceptibility factors.

IV. LYMPHOCYTE ASSAYS

Lymphocytes are significantly less abundant than RBCs in peripheral blood; however, they have several features that make up for this seeming disadvantage. First, some types of lymphocytes, particularly primary T lymphocytes, can be grown in cell culture. A related feature is their relative ease of immortalization by a number of agents to produce established cell lines. In addition, lymphocytes in peripheral blood retain their genetic material, so that although it may be more difficult to identify a mutant of this cell type, genotypic analysis can be performed with such a mutant once it is isolated. Lymphocytes share some disadvantages with erythrocytes: their kinetics of development are equally unknown and their differentiation is much more complex than erythroid cells. It is known that after release from the bone marrow, T lymphocytes are sequestered in the thymus and undergo further differentiation and multiplication. This phenomenon has been shown to lead to clonal amplification of mutated cells and result in a high frequency of mutant cells as a result of cellular stimulation rather than cellular mutagenesis. Genetic methods have been devised to assess the independence of mutations based on the novel rearrangement of the T-cell receptor locus during maturation in the thymus; thus assuring that clonal expansion of single bone marrow cell mutants can be detected if not precluded (46). These complexities with analysis prevent T lymphocyte–based assays from being applied easily to large populations.

A. Major Histocompatibility Locus

The human class I histocompatibility locus consists of a family of closely linked autosomal genes mapped to chromosome 6. This *HLA* gene family, part of the immunoglobin gene superfamily, consists of six genes encoding polypeptide subunits that form noncovalently linked heterodimers with the β_2-microglobulin polypeptide. The *HLA-A*, *-B*, and *-C* genes are expressed at the cell surface on a majority of cell types, including peripheral blood lymphocytes, although *HLA-C* expression is significantly lower than *HLA-A* and *HLA-B*. These genes are highly polymorphic, with at least 20 common alleles of the *HLA-A* gene identified in the human population and 40 for *HLA-B* (47). The molecular biology of the locus has also been well characterized; the *HLA-A* gene spans approximately 4 kb and consists of a signal exon, three exons representing the three extracellular domains of the polypeptide, one exon encoding the transmembrane region, and three exons coding for the cytoplasmic domain, with a substantial 3′ untranslated region (48).

The *HLA* somatic mutagenesis assay is based on an immunologic selection procedure using allele-specific monoclonal antibodies to specifically bind allele-specific *HLA* surface antigens in cultured lymphocytes heterozygous for *HLA*; addition of complement is then used to select for variants with allele-loss phenotypes. In an identical manner to the *GPA* assay, two genetic classes of mutant cells can be isolated: hemizygous cells that can arise by inactivation, mutation, or deletion of one *HLA* allele or by rearrangement or missegregation of the copy of chromosome

6 carrying that allele; or homozygous cells that result from gene conversion, homologous recombination, or chromosome missegregation accompanied by duplication. Thus, like the *GPA* assay, the *HLA* assay can enumerate lymphocytes of variant phenotype arising from a spectrum of gene-specific as well as chromosomal mutational mechanisms.

Both the *HLA-A* and the *HLA-B* loci have been extensively studied as a target locus for somatic mutation in vitro. In early studies, human lymphoblastoid cell lines heterozygous for appropriate *HLA-A* and *HLA-B* alleles were identified or established and used as experimental systems. Putative mutant clones with *HLA* allele-loss phenotypes were then isolated using specific antisera or murine monoclonal antibodies for allelic antigens followed by complement killing of normally expressing cells. These studies demonstrated a spontaneous mutation frequency at this locus of 2–5 × 10^{-6}. By investigation of other linked *HLA* genes and the phosphoglucomutase-3 marker, they further showed that these cells lost expression of an HLA cell surface antigen as a result of mutation of a single *HLA* allele (49,50).

This in vitro system has also been used to study the effects of exposures to known mutagens on the *HLA* locus. In one study, treatment of these cultures with chemical mutagens produced up to 100-fold dose-dependent increases in the frequency of allele loss variants, and genetic analysis of variant clones revealed all of them to be single gene mutants (50). In contrast, a second study utilizing a cell line with a cytogenetically marked chromosome 6 demonstrated the loss of linked *HLA* alleles and the glyoxylase I gene, and in one case there was even cytological evidence for deletion of chromosomal material (51). Similar induction studies have been performed with ionizing radiation. Gamma radiation was effective in inducing variants, although unlike the spontaneous and chemical mutagen-induced mutants, the majority induced by irradiation were multiple gene-loss mutants, some of these extending to the *cis*-linked glyoxylase I locus (52). Again, in one case, a cytologically detectable chromosome deletion was shown (51). Similar results were observed after treatment with x-rays, with the recovery of approximately equal numbers of mutants losing expression of only the selected allele and variants losing expression of the entire *HLA* haplotype linked to the selected allele (53). A mouse model of this in vitro system has recently been reported (54).

HLA-A allele-loss has also been demonstrated in vivo, using HLA-A2– and HLA-A3–specific monoclonal antibodies and complement to isolate mutants preexisting in the circulating lymphocyte population (55). These antibodies were chosen because they are readily available and are specific for two of the most common *HLA-A* alleles. Variant cell frequencies (2–3 × 10^{-6}) were independent of the actual allele selected and increased with the age of the donor (56). Significantly, there was a dose-dependent increase in variant frequencies when these primary lymphocyte cultures were treated in vitro with either mitomycin C or x-rays (55). Molecular analysis, in conjunction with restriction enzymes that yield allele-specific *HLA-A* patterns (57), indicated that loss or rearrangement of DNA from the immunoselected allele occurred in 10–50% of spontaneous mutants (55,58), rising to 80% in x-ray– or mitomycin C–induced populations (55). The proportion of such mutants also missing the linked *HLA-B* allele, indicating the occurence of a large chromosomal alteration such as deletion, mitotic recombination, chromosome loss, or loss and duplication, was 30–40% in spontaneous variants. This proportion increased to 90% on treatment with mitomycin C and dropped to 15% in x-ray–treated populations (55). Further attempts to characterize the molecular mechanisms of mutation in spontaneous variants have involved quantitation of *HLA-A* band intensities and examination at linked polymorphic markers (58,59). Genetic characterization of 127 spontaneous mutants from 10 individuals revealed that mitotic recombination is responsible for up to 30% of *HLA-A* allele-loss mutants (58).

The *HLA* assay would appear to offer all the advantages of the *GPA* assay with the added ability to molecularly characterize isolated variants. The culture, selection, and cloning of lymphocytes, however, requires several weeks to determine variant frequencies (as opposed to minutes with *GPA*), with further molecular analysis currently requiring expansion of the clone preparatory to DNA isolation. The reagents and labor necessary for lymphocyte culture and selection cause the *HLA* assay to be much more expensive than the *GPA* assay, and the complement-based selection can be problematic. Since the assay is designed to detect a single event at a dizygous locus, the molecular analysis of variants is also complicated by the continued presence of the unaffected *HLA* homologue. Currently, this restricts such studies to the gross loss of the 3′ end of the *HLA-A2* allele, which can be identified by an allele-specific polymorphism (57). Indeed, the application of this assay has so far been restricted to loss of either the *A2* or *A3* alleles, whereas an increased repertoire of monoclonal antibodies would allow quantitation of allele loss mutants in all heterozygotes (80–90% of individuals, depending on the population [60]). The use of *HLA-B* alleles in vivo, as has been done in vitro (50–53), would further expand the potential application of this assay. Finally, emerging new technologies should aid in the development of more practically applicable versions of the *HLA* assay. Rather then cloning mutant lymphocytes after selection in culture, it should be possible to quantitate them directly using image analysis and/or isolate them quickly using flow cytometry. The problems associated with molecular analysis will be addressed with the development of a battery of polymerase chain reaction (PCR) procedures designed to distinguish alleles and easily identify the mechanism of mutation or segregation.

B. Hypoxanthine-Guanine Phosphoribosyltransferase

The hypoxanthine-guanine phosphoribosyltransferase gene *(HPRT)* codes for an enzyme of the purine scavenger or salvage pathway, which allows recycling of free purines and provides an alternative to the de novo synthesis of these nucleotides. *HPRT* is a constituitively expressed housekeeping enzyme present in all cell types, including lymphocytes. This gene is X-linked in mammals, making it structurally (in males) or functionally (in females) hemizygous, providing the basis for a mutational assay with single-hit kinetics that is applicable to almost the entire human population. Hereditary mutations at this locus are responsible for the human diseases Lesch-Nyhan syndrome and gouty arthritis. *HPRT* activity has been used extensively to manipulate cells in culture using simple methods of selecting either for or against enzyme expression. By poisoning de novo purine biosynthesis (with azaserine or folate inhibitors such as aminopterin), cells can be made to rely solely on the salvage pathway and, therefore, functional *HPRT* for viability. Alternately, *HPRT* will convert the purine analogues 6-thioguanine and 8-azaguanine into toxic nucleotides, so that media containing toxic concentrations of these compounds can be used to select for loss of *HPRT* expression. The *HPRT* gene has been cloned and characterized in a number of mammals, including humans. The human *HPRT* gene spans 44 kb and includes nine exons; it is not part of a linked gene family as are the other target loci under consideration. The *HPRT* assay as applied to a normal individual is an expression-loss assay, and there is a large amount of accumulated information on both hereditary mutations at this locus and on mutations and reversions in cell culture (61).

The *HPRT* assay was the first in vivo somatic mutation system to be practically applicable, and it is now performed in many laboratories throughout the world. Thus, there is a considerable amount of accumulated data that can only be briefly summarized in the context of this chapter. In addition, there is a wealth of molecular data derived from this system, and there is comparable information from in vitro human and animal studies and in vivo animal studies to which we refer the reader to recent reviews (61,62).

There are two versions of the *HPRT* assay used for the measurement of human in vivo mutation. The first method involves the direct microscopic detection of lymphocytes that continue to incorporate labeled pyrimidines (either [^{3}H]thymidine or 5-bromodeoxyuridine) in the presence of cytotoxic levels of purine analogues and thus are *HPRT* deficient (63,64). The second method is more quantitative in that *HPRT* mutations are detected as primary human T-lymphocyte clones in culture following selection in medium containing toxic concentrations of purine analogues. This second method (called the *HPRT* clonogenic assay) also has the advantage of allowing recovery of viable mutant clones for further analysis. An in vivo model of this assay has been described and applied in the mouse allowing manipulation of the system in situ (65).

Variant and mutant frequencies from normal individuals are similar as measured by the two versions of the in vivo *HPRT* assay, ranging from 1.9–9.5 × 10^{-6} (66,67). A slight increase in frequency (similar to that seen in the hemizygous class of *GPA* variants) with age has been documented (13,68–70), and newborn mutation frequencies are significantly (~10-fold) lower than those of the adult (71,72).

When used as a biodosimeter, the *HPRT* assay has shown significantly increased mutation frequencies in Hiroshima atomic bomb survivors (27,73,74) and in others exposed to ionizing radiation either medically (75–78), occupationally (66,79), or accidently (80). Similar results were found in individuals undergoing medical chemical therapy (including cancer chemotherapy) with a regimen that included cyclophosphamide, a known mutagen (67,81), and in workers occupationally exposed to the same compound (82). The *HPRT* assay also has proven to be sensitive to genetic predisposition, registering high mutation frequencies in individuals homozygous for the DNA repair deficiencies xeroderma pigmentosum, Cockayne's syndrome, and ataxia telangiectasia (13,83,84).

As mentioned earlier, a major advantage of lymphocyte-based assays is the ability to isolate and culture mutants for further analysis. Given the fact that *HPRT* and associated X-linked genes are hemizygous in mammalian somatic cells, the first question to be asked was whether "chromosomal" events, such as chromosome loss, translocation, or cytogenetically detectable deletion, contribute significantly to variation at this locus. Several studies have demonstrated that such karyotypic alteration is rare among in vivo T-lymphocyte mutants, and in these studies no chromosomal aberrations could be detected at Xq27, where the *HPRT* gene is located (85–87). A similar result has been demonstrated for spontaneous HPRT mutation in a cultured rodent fibroblast system (88). Germ cell mutations recovered from patients with the Lesch-Nyhan syndrome also show no evidence for cytogenetically detectable chromosomal changes (89). These results are in stark contrast to results in an artificially constructed diploid *HPRT* somatic system, where chromosome loss or gross deletion accounted for all observed *HPRT* segregation (2,3,90). Thus, it is clear that the unique behavior of this gene located hemizygously on the X chromosome limits the types of mutation one can recover at the *HPRT* locus.

Nevertheless, detailed molecular analysis has displayed a large spectrum of changes at this locus (for a thorough review, see ref. 62). Beginning with Southern analysis to identify gene rearrangements (91–93), for example, it has been shown that 15% of the mutations occurring in *HPRT*-deficient clones isolated from normal adults are the result of deletions, rearrangements, and duplications that are large enough to be detected by restriction fragment length polymorphisms (greater than a few kilobases) (94). Other powerful molecular methods that have been used to characterize the spectrum of mutations in the *HPRT* locus include PCR amplification and sequencing (95), HOT (hydroxylamine–osmium tetroxide) analysis (96), denaturing gradient gel electrophoresis (97), and pulse-field gel electrophoresis (98). In general, these techniques allow the display of many different kinds of fine structural changes, including base substitutions, small deletions or insertions, frameshifts, and splice-site alterations, all of which result in a loss of expression of this housekeeping gene (99).

At the other extreme, relatively large deletions are detected in mutant clones from individuals exposed to ionizing radiation. At present, the only radiation-exposed individuals who have been studied for molecular defects at the *HPRT* locus are patients who were treated with radioimmunotherapy (78,100,101). Results in these studies indicate that deletions occur much more frequently in these patients after radioimmunotherapy (20% of mutants pretherapy versus 40% of mutants posttherapy). In addition, radioimmunotherapy increases the proportion of large deletion mutations. Of the deletions that occur, the fraction that eliminate the entire 44-kb *HPRT* gene increases from 15% in pretreatment samples to 43% in posttreatment samples. Some clones isolated posttreatment contained X chromosome deletions estimated to be as large as 21 Mb, including the *HPRT* gene (98).

Another intriguing observation is that in blood from the human fetus, the proportion of mutants that are deletions at the *HPRT* locus is exceedingly high (85% of all mutants) even though, as we previously mentioned, the total *HPRT* mutation frequency is one tenth that of adults. Subsequent molecular analysis of mutant clones from fetal blood shows a characteristic pattern of deletion for half of these mutants, in which the region that includes exon 2 and exon 3 of the *HPRT* gene is deleted (102). By detailed characterization, it has been shown that these deletions occurred via illegitimate recombination events promoted by the VDJ recombinase activity that acts in T-cell receptor gene rearrangement and B-cell immunoglobulin gene rearrangement (103). This unique pattern in fetal blood may be due to high activity of the recombinase in the rapidly developing thymus cells in the fetus and induction of subsequent erroneous recombination.

The advantage that detailed molecular analyses can be performed using mutants isolated from the *HPRT* clonogenic assay serves as a balance to the disadvantages that this assay displays. Since it requires cell growth, samples must be treated with great care prior to performing the assay to retain cellular viability, and once the assay is begun, a large amount of time, labor, and cell culture material must be expended. Thus, it is not particularly suited to prospective analysis of large populations or to producing rapid results for subsequent treatment of patients. A second disadvantage is the hemizygosity of the locus due to its X chromosome linkage, as has been previously discussed. Selection at the *HPRT* locus will clearly result in different types of stable mutations than those typically found in autosomal loci, so that the mutation frequency and spectrum probably do not represent that found in genes that are responsible for subsequent pathological changes. Therefore, using this assay alone as a basis for projecting risk may be suspect. The fact that the radiation dose-response for *HPRT* mutations in atomic bomb survivors is very small (73,74) indicates that the mutant cells have a limited lifetime and that the assay may not serve as a long-time biodosimeter. Finally, there is evidence that the HPRT-deficient phenotype is actually selected against in vivo precluding the accu- mulation of variants and an accurate assessment of total genetic damage (104).

V. MULTI-ENDPOINT ANALYSIS

In reviewing research progress on the development of in vivo somatic mutation assays, we have seen that each assay described suffers some flaws and that different assays often complement one another. It appears, therefore, that the optimum strategy for performing human in vivo somatic mutation analysis would be multi-endpoint analysis using more than one of these procedures on each individual. Table 1 gives a brief overview of the advantages and disadvantages of the four assays that have been described.

One might use these overall characteristics to choose a particular combination of assays for a particular population to be analyzed. For example, we are now attempting to analyze the population effects of the accident at the Chernobyl, Ukraine, nuclear reactor in 1986. Since the population exposed to significant amounts of ionizing radiation appears to number greater than 300,000 people, we have chosen to use the easily applied *GPA* assay to characterize specific subpopulations to identify those who appear to have received the most biologically significant doses. Those subpopulations that appear to be most heavily exposed will subsequently be analyzed more completely using the *HPRT* assay, including detailed molecular genotyping to identify any radiation-specific effects in the X chromosome and the *HLA* assay to analyze for

Table 1 Overview of Current in Vivo Somatic Mutation Assays

Locus	Cell Type	Advantages	Disadvantages	Prospects
Hb β-chain	Red blood cells	Can potentially assay entire population Autosomal locus, codominant expression Screen for specific mutations Molecularly defined phenotypes Long-term persistence (probable for certain mutations) Can be performed on small blood sample Samples can be stored indefinately after slide preparation	Expensive/labor intensive Requirement for expression limits mechanisms Presently, limited mutation sampling Genotypic analysis not possible Requires 4 months for full expression May be selected against in vivo (probable for certain mutations) Cannot address issues of variant clonality	Simultaneous selection for multiple mutants Improved technology, automated image analysis
GPA	Red blood cells	Inexpensive, rapid, easily performed Autosomal locus, codominant expression Assays wide range of mechanisms Proven long-term persistence Can be performed on small blood sample	Can assay only 50% of population Genotypic analysis not possible Requires 4 months for full expression Requires fresh blood Cannot address issues of variant clonality	Extension to reticulocytes, bone marrow Improved technology, automation, faster flow rate Sample freezing after fixation In vitro, in vivo model systems
HLA	T lymphocytes	Can potentially assay major fraction of population Autosomal locus, codominant expression	Expensive/labor intensive Presently, limited population sampling T-cell differentiation is complex	Adaptation to flow cytometry, image analysis Development of large array of allele-specific antibodies

	Advantages	Disadvantages	Future directions
	Assays wide range of mechanisms Variants can be recovered for molecular analysis Long-term persistence (probable for certain mutations) Samples, variants can be frozen for later analysis In vitro model systems (human, mouse) Can unambiguously establish clonality with T-cell receptor (TCR) locus Panel of polymorphic probes to analyze recombination	Requires large blood sample May be selected against in vivo (probable for certain mutations)	In vivo model systems (mouse, rat) Establishment of a multiplex PCR panel Determination of "molecular spectra"
HPRT T lymphocytes	Can assay entire population Variants can be recovered for molecular analysis Samples, variants can be frozen for later analysis Extensive in vitro, in vivo meiotic, somatic data Can unambiguously establish clonality with TCR locus Multiplex PCR panel for molecular analysis	X-linked, hemizygous locus Expensive/labor intensive Evidence of limited range of mechanisms T-cell differentiation is complex Requires large blood sample Evidence for in vivo selection against variants	Adaptation to image analysis, flow cytometry Panel of linked polymorphic probes to analyze deletion Determination of "molecular spectra"

autosomal effects of radiation in this population. Since radiation damage has been well characterized in both in vivo and in vitro systems as causing deletions and translocations, the hemoglobin assay would not appear to be as useful in this study.

This plan illustrates the presumption that the results of any one blood cell–based mutation assay cannot completely represent all the types of mutagenic events that occur in vivo (105). As seen in Section IV, there is a clear difference in the pattern of molecular events contributing to the two lymphocyte-based assays. Although this gross difference can be attributed to the X-linked and autosomal localizations of the genes involved, there are likely to be more subtle differences between different X-linked and autosomal systems owing to such vaguaries as distance of the gene from the centromere, the presence of fragile sites (as well as other, as yet unknown, aspects of chromosomal architecture), or the degree of association with critical genes. If, as is indicated by in vitro studies, mutation frequency and mechanism is associated with mitotic cell cycling, the mutation frequency in blood cell–based assays will be affected by the kinetics of cell turnover and maturation and may not be representative of mutation in other cell types. In addition, the target genes themselves are likely to have a unique pattern of mutation susceptible and resistant sequences, such as CG-rich HTF islands, that are not representative of all genes in the genome. For all these reasons, it is important that in vivo mutation be measured using a number of different assays or endpoints in different tissues, with the results of each contributing to a better understanding of the mutagenic state of an individual.

Despite the greater depth of molecular data available from the lymphocyte assays, their relative expense and labor intensity precludes them from widespread application. There are ongoing efforts to improve the ease of application of these assays. For example, the radiolabeling version of the *HPRT* assay might be automated through an image analysis system (106) or by flow cytometry (107). Since the *HLA* assay uses cell surface markers, it might also lend itself to flow cytometry in an assay similar to the *GPA* flow assay. Attempts are also underway to allow a limited amount of molecular data to be recovered from mutants isolated via the *GPA* assay by specifically analyzing the reticulocyte fraction, which retains mRNA, or circulating nucleated normoblasts using fluorescence-activated cell sorting to isolate phenotypic variants (108). Even as these assays begin to overlap in terms of convenience and depth of analysis, new approaches are being proposed, such as utilizing the antigens defining the ABO blood group as a heterozygous RBC system (109–111) and extending the *HPRT* assay to B lymphocytes (122). Ideally, one would like to analyze an individual with a gamut of fast, inexpensive assays designed to cover a representative amount of the genome both karyotypically and at the level of the nucleotide sequence. The results of such a comprehensive analysis would have significant consequences for the possible medical outcome of mutagenic exposure of an individual and could be used diagnostically to determine the level of risk and urgency of treatment.

Several comprehensive comparative studies of the various currently available biodosimetry assays are underway; several limited comparisons of such techniques have already been completed. In an earlier review of this subject (105), we compared the results of the four assays, as reported by various laboratories in separate studies, when applied to normal individuals, individuals exposed to ionizing radiation or genotoxic chemicals, or individuals manifesting DNA repair/cancer-prone syndromes. Given the known characteristics of these assays (as described in detail in Secs. III and IV), the variant frequencies as measured by the four assays were consistent: The frequency of specific hemoglobin variant erythrocytes (10^{-8}) was several orders of magnitude lower than that of *HPRT*-deficient lymphocytes and hemizygous NØ variant RBCs (10^{-6}), whereas the frequency of *HLA* allele-loss in lymphocytes was equivalent to the sum of both hemizygous and homozygous variant erythrocytes at the *GPA* locus. Chemical mutagen effects were also very similar; however, as mentioned earlier, the magnitude of persistent response to ionizing radiation in atomic bomb survivors was quite different between the *HPRT* and *GPA* assays.

Perhaps more revealing are those studies in which two or more biodosimetric assays were applied to the same population at the same time. In the most comprehensive studies thus far, frequencies of *HPRT*-deficient lymphocytes, *GPA* variant RBCs, and chromosomal aberrations (as estimated by conventional staining, banding, and chromosome-specific fluorescent in situ hybridization) were established for a population of atomic bomb survivors selected for the level of confidence of their exposure estimates (27,28). Significantly, the assays correlated better with each other than they did with dose (although all three assays showed significant dose dependence). These results may simply indicate problems with dosage estimates; or they may reflect individual differences in susceptibility to DNA damage by ionizing radiation that affect all three assays in a similar manner. The correlation of assay results was not perfect; however, further evidence that the results of these assays are complementary not merely redundant.

VI. APPLICATION AND SIGNIFICANCE

To varying degrees all four biodosimetry assays under consideration have been validated by demonstrating appropriate responses to known genotoxic exposures and/or molecular analysis of isolated variant cells. Depending on their relative sensitivities, these assays should therefore be useful in establishing the level of inherent genetic damage sustained by an individual up to the time of sampling; if the health effects of such damage could be established, these assays could then be applied medically to anticipate the development of disease states associated with somatic variation. In this section, we attempt to elucidate the importance of somatic DNA damage for the health and survival of an individual and to suggest instances in which the currently available genotoxicity assays might be used to screen and monitor the human population to predict and characterize the level and mechanisms of somatic DNA damage and its medical consequences.

A. Somatic Mutation and Human Disease

Somatic cell culture and the field of somatic cell genetics were pursued because they offered the possibility of a model system for the study of genetic mechanisms in higher eukaryotes. From the beginning, however, there was considerable debate over whether such in vitro systems accurately modeled genetic processes in somatic cells in the body. A major source of contention was the perceived karyotypic instability of such cells in culture and the karyotypic evolution of established cell lines. It was widely believed that such processes did not go on in situ, or if they did, they were not important because the types of events that occurred, chromosome loss, duplication, deletion, and translocation, caused significant loss of genetic material and therefore monozygosity for the genes in the affected region. Based on the meiotic effects of such monozygosity, these events were thought to have drastically deleterious if not lethal effects upon the viability of the cell, at the very least affecting its ability to compete with unaffected neighbors. Somehow the culture conditons, or the transformed nature of such cells, were thought to allow them to survive in vitro, whereas they would not in situ, or indeed were thought to induce such events, making their study largely artefactual. The segregation (in this case meaning loss) of chromosomes from somatic cell hybrids was widely utilized for gene mapping studies, and eventually it was recognized that at least some types of somatic cell variation were analagous to classic meiotic mutation mechanisms, but there was no thought of the implications or significance of such mechanisms occuring in vivo (113).

At the same time, it was widely accepted that somatic mutation played some role in two very important physiological processes: aging and oncogenesis. It is only relatively recently, with the advent of molecular biotechnology, that strong associations have been established between somatic variation and these processes, and that somatic events mechanistically distinct from those involved in the hereditary processes of germ cell mutation have been implicated and appreciated. It is now clear that somatic mutational and segregational mechanisms are instrinsic to not only aging and oncogenesis but also to other types of human disease, such as Alzheimer's syndrome and atherosclerosis (114, 115). Besides the in vivo applications of somatic mutation and segregation assays discussed in Sections III and IV, the greatest amount of information on the occurrence and significance of these events has come from studies of carcinogenesis.

It is now generally accepted that all cancer has a genetic basis and that the steps in multistage carcinogenesis represent discrete genetic events. Two genetic mechanisms have been characterized. In the first, a normal cellular gene, often involved either directly or indirectly with regulation of cell growth, is "activated" by a mutational mechanism to become an "oncogene." This activation event most often results in the overexpression, unregulated expression, or inappropriate expression of the gene product causing an uncontrolled stimulation of cell growth. This event can occur by a variety of mechanisms, including base mutation, deletion, insertion, and translocation but is highly constrained because it must retain expression of the gene and the functionality of the gene product. The particular changes necessary for activation vary with each "proto-oncogene," but in each case, the situation is very similar to that revealed with the hemoglobin assay, where a specific conformational change must be produced in an expressed gene product. Activated oncogenes are thought to act in a dominant manner because mutation of both copies of autosomal loci are not necessary for progression of oncogenesis. Oncogenes have been implicated directly with cancer in studies of viral oncogenesis, in various in vitro systems, and in transgenic mouse studies, although it has not yet been determined unequivocally whether cancer in situ can be caused by activation of a single oncogene (116,117).

The second mutational mechanism implicated in oncogenesis involves the loss of expression of one of a second set of genes, the tumor suppressor genes. These genes are also known as recessive oncogenes because expression of both copies of autosomal genes of this type must be lost before their oncogenic potential is manifested. Some examples of tumor suppressor gene products have been shown to interact directly with the products of oncogenes and/or cellular proto-oncogenes, presumably regulating them, leading to their designation as antioncogenes, although it is clear that not all tumor suppressor genes act in this manner. An example of a cancer involving loss of a single tumor suppressor gene has been identified, retinoblastoma (118). Retinoblastoma was distinguished by its distinct patterns of onset and presentation: either early onset with multiple, bilateral tumors or relatively later onset with often a single malignant focus. These patterns were found to correspond to the number of genetic events necessary to cause cancer; the early-onset cases were often associated with familial occurrence. It was speculated, and later proven, that such families carried a germinal mutation in one copy of the putative retinoblastoma locus. Although carried in all somatic cells, this predisposing genotype acted as a recessive on the cellular level producing no phenotypic alteration until a second, somatic event occurred, usually in the retina, causing loss of expression of the remaining functional allele. The frequency of this secondary event was so high, however, that it was a virtual certainty to occur, causing retinoblastoma predisposition to appear as a dominant disease on the organismal level. The late-onset pattern is associated with a normal germinal genotype, with both steps in the oncogenic pathway occurring as somatic events.

Both of the genetic events associated with recessive oncogenesis involve loss of function. Thus, any mechanism that affects the functionality of the gene product, the expression of the gene, or indeed removes the gene from the genome is a potential candidate. The range of such mechanisms is much less limited than those discussed above for the activation of proto-oncogenes; it encompasses all local or gene-specific mutational events such as occur at the *HPRT* gene but also all the segregational mechanisms that contribute to allele loss at the *GPA* and *HLA* loci. Indeed, the types of mutations responsible for activating proto-oncogenes are also likely to be similar to the mutations that inactivate these marker loci making these assays excellent model systems for the events that occur in both genetic mechanisms of oncogenesis (2,117). In terms of modeling events necessary for oncogenesis, however, the distinction between events causing activation of proto-oncogenes and inactivation of tumor suppressor genes may be completely arbitrary because, other than in retinoblastoma, all known cancers appear to require a series of events involving both types of cancer genes to occur before a tumor develops (119).

B. Risk Analysis

Owing to their mechanistic modeling of the types of molecular events important for somatic disease and cancer the results of in vivo somatic genotoxicity assays may provide valuable information for risk estimations specific for each individual. A high frequency of variant cell types as measured by any one of the four current assays is indicative of a higher than normal amount of DNA damage, which if representative of the whole genome, would suggest that the individual might have a correspondingly higher than normal chance of developing cancer and other somatic diseases. It should be stressed at this point, however, that the target loci for the current assays have been chosen such that the resultant allele-loss phenotypes do not have significant deleterious effects on cell survival (except perhaps in the case of HPRT deficiency) and that disease states, especially cancer, do not rely directly on mutational or segregational events at these target loci.

There are two obvious ways that biological dosimetric assays can contribute to human health and preventive medicine. The first involves elucidating, quantitating, and, in some cases, characterizing the effects of background, environmental, accidental, medical, and occupational exposures on the frequency and mechanisms of human somatic mutation and subsequent medical consequences. All of the currently available assays have been utilized in pilot studies of this type to varying degrees and have demonstrated different sensitivities. Thus, depending on the type of exposure, the above biodosimetric assays, and others still to be developed, will be important in determining the genotoxic risk to individuals and populations. For example, a particularly important application of in vivo biodosimetric assays will be to assess the amount of persistent genetic damage caused by current cancer therapy regimens to determine the contribution of such treatments to the induction of secondary tumors (34).

It is important to remember, however, that the target tissues for all four current assays are all hematopoietic, such that they are useful for noninvasive screening but may not be representative of genotoxic damage occurring in the tissue at risk. These considerations are important in exposure measurements because different tissues may be exposed to different effective doses of potential mutagens or may respond differently to similar doses than the bone marrow, thymus, or circulating T lymphocytes. In the case of whole-body exposure, it may be possible that the relationships between genetic damage in these marker tissues and other tissues can be determined in vivo, especially with the use of model systems. In the case of partial body exposures, there can be no replacement for biodosimetric assays applicable directly to the cell type(s) at risk.

The second manner in which in vivo bioassays of genotoxicity are applicable to human health is in determining the genetic predisposition of an individual or a population to specific genotoxic events, both spontaneous and induced. The *GPA* and *HPRT* assays have both demonstrated increased frequencies of variants in individuals with cancer-prone syndromes; indeed the *GPA* assay has been proposed as a simple means of confirming preclinical diagnosis of Fanconi's anemia (44). These studies, and the consistent increases in variant frequencies with age seen in the *GPA, HLA,* and *HPRT* assays, suggest that they may be capable of detecting much more subtle differences in the normal human population that might have important consequences for human longevity and disease susceptibility. An important potential application of these assays might, therefore, be the monitoring of individuals scheduled to undergo medical therapy with genotoxic agents, both before and throughout treatment, in order to design and revise the protocol according to the individual response of each patient to that particular regimen (120).

Ultimately, the applicability of the current assays, and biodosimetric assays in general, will have to be evaluated independently for each disease. Besides the cell type effects discussed with respect to exposure above, there are also considerations related to the discussion of target size given in Section II. For any particular disease the relative genetic context (chromosome, linked genes) of the causative or predisposing gene, and of the assayed locus, will determine how well the assay predicts health outcomes (e.g., there has been a report of a tumor suppressor gene important in hepatocarcinoma localized to chromosome 4, where the *GPA* gene is located [121]). Individuals may also have chromosome-specific abnormalities, such as translocations and fragile sites that differentially affect disease and marker loci. Since different oncogenes are implicated in different cancers, and the somatic diseases thus far elucidated are also cell type specific, there may be also be differential cell type effects with respect to mutation and segregation frequency owing to different cell cycle kinetics, metabolism, and regulation. Despite these caveats, the only viable means of determining how the current array of bioassays may be clinically and epidemiologically useful will be to apply them and evaluate the results.

VII. CONCLUSIONS

The progress made in measuring somatic mutations in vivo during the last 10 years is remarkable. Technical difficulties in measuring such rare events in human specimens have been gigantic, and somatic genetics has been enough different from germinal genetics that interpreting results has not been an easy task. The fact that the analyses described in this chapter are now being tested in the field for applications to human biodosimetry and risk analysis indicates that these exceedingly large problems have nearly been solved. We expect that a combination of these analytical procedures will begin to be used routinely during the next 10 years and will have a significant effect on determining effects on individuals of exposures to toxic chemicals and/or radiation.

We also believe that the most meaningful and useful somatic cell mutation analyses have not yet been devised. The fact remains that the analyses that have been developed to date are ones that showed feasibility, not necessarily powerful applicability. At the present time, there certainly are different kinds of somatic mutation assays being devised that measure mutational damage to DNA directly within cells or tissues. These should be much easier to interpret than the ones that we now have in hand. In addition, more specificity toward the tissues at risk to mutagenic damage and the tissues at risk to develop cancer will become usable. Finally, the intense research efforts being put into understanding the molecular nature of induction of carcinogenesis and progression to metastaces of tumors will certainly give important information that should lead to new methods for determining the risk of cancer in individuals. Undoubtedly, the somatic mutation and cancer risk assays of the next generation will entail analysis of oncogenes and tumor suppressor genes in tissues at risk in individuals. We look forward to such developments in the context of health maintenance services in that extremely early determination of molecular events that may lead to pathological conditions can be eliminated or repaired long before any physiological consequences have occurred.

ACKNOWLEDGMENTS

The authors wish to thank Drs. William L. Bigbee, Richard G. Langlois, and Elbert W. Branscomb for their insightful contributions to our thinking and their determined experimental efforts in this research. This work was performed under the auspices of the US Department of

Energy at Lawrence Livermore National Laboratory under contract number W-7405-ENG-48, with additional support from NIH grant CA 48518 and the US-USSR Joint Coordinating Committee for Nuclear Reactor Safety.

REFERENCES

1. Grant SG, Chapman VM. Mechanisms of X-chromosome regulation. Ann Rev Genet 1988; 22:199.
2. Worton RG, Grant SG. Segregation-like events in Chinese hamster cells. In: Gottesman MM, ed. Molecular Cell Genetics. New York: Wiley 1985:831.
3. Grant SG, Campbell CE, Duff C, et al. Gene inactivation as a mechanism for the expression of recessive phenotypes. Am J Hum Genet 1989; 45:619.
4. Papayannopoulou T, McGuire TC, Lim G, et al. Identification of haemoglobin S in red cells and normoblasts, using fluorescent anti-Hb S antibodies. Br J Haematol 1976; 34:25.
5. Papayannopoulou T, Lim G, McGuire TC, et al. Use of fluorescent antibodies for the identification of haemoglobin C in erythrocytes. Am J Haematol 1977; 34:25.
6. Stamatoyannopoulos G. Possibilities for demonstrating point mutations in somatic cells, as illustrated by studies of mutant haemoglobin. In: Berg K, ed. Genetic Damage in Man Caused by Environmental Agents. New York: Academic Press 1979:49.
7. Stamatoyannopoulos G, Nute P, Lindsley D, et al. Somatic-cell mutation monitoring system based on human hemoglobin mutants. In: Ansari AA, De Serres FJ, eds. Single-Cell Mutation Monitoring Systems: Methodologies and Applications. New York: Plenum Press, Top Chem Mutagen 1984; 1:1.
8. Bigbee WL, Branscomb EW, Weintraub HB, et al. Cell sorter immunofluorescence detection of human erythrocytes labeled in suspension with antibodies specific for Haemoglobins S and C. J Immunol Methods 1981; 45:117.
9. Bigbee WL, Branscomb EW. Use of fluorescence-activated cell sorter for screening mutant cells. In: Ansari AA, De Serres FJ, eds. Single-Cell Mutation Monitoring Systems: Methodologies and Applications. New York: Plenum Press, Top Chem Mutagen 1984; 2:37.
10. Jensen RH, Bigbee WL, Branscomb EW. Somatic mutations detected by immunofluorescence and flow cytometry. In: Eisert WG, Mendelsohn ML, eds. Biological Dosimetry: Cytometric Approaches to Mammalian Systems. Berlin: Springer-Verlag 1984:161.
11. Jensen RH, Vanderlaan J, Grabske RJ, et al. Monoclonal antibodies specific for sickle cell hemoglobin. Hemoglobin 1985; 9:349.
12. Verwoerd NP, Bernini LF, Bonnet J, et al. Somatic cell mutations in humans detected by image analysis of immunofluorescently stained erythrocytes. In: Burger G, Ploem JS, Goettler K, eds. Clinical Cytometry and Histometry. San Diego: Academic Press 1987:465.
13. Tates AD, Bernini LF, Natarajan AT, et al. Detection of somatic mutants in man: HPRT mutations in lymphocytes and hemoglobin mutations in erythrocytes. Mutat Res 1989; 213:73.
14. Karlsson S, Nienhuis AW. Developmental regulation of human globin genes. Ann Rev Biochem 1985; 54:1071.
15. Bernini LF, Natarajan AT, Schreuder-Rotteveel AHM. et al. Assay for somatic mutation of human hemoglobins. Prog Clin Biol Res 1990; 340C:57.
16. Weatherall DJ, Clegg JB, Higgs DR, Wood, WG. The hemoglobinopathies. In: Scriver CR, Beaudet A, Sly W, Valle D, eds. The Metabolic Basis of Inherited Disease. 6th ed. New York: McGraw Hill 1989:2281.
17. Langlois RG, Bigbee WL, Jensen RH. Flow cytometric characterization of normal and variant cells with monoclonal antibodies specific for glycophorin A. J Immunol 1985; 134:4009.
18. Langlois RG, Bigbee WL, Jensen RH. Measurements of the frequency of human erythrocytes with gene expression loss phenotypes at the glycophorin A locus. Hum Genet 1986; 74:353.
19. Cartron J–P, Colin Y, Kudo S, Fukuda M. Molecular genetics of human erythrocyte sialoglycoproteins: Glycophorins A, B, C, and D. In: Harris JR, ed. Blood Cell Biochemistry. Vol 1; Erythroid Cells. New York: Plenum Press 1990:299.
20. Langlois RG, Nisbet BA, Bigbee WL, et al. An improved flow cytometric assay for somatic mutations at the glycophorin A locus in humans. Cytometry 1990; 11:513.

21. Grant SG, Langlois RG, Jensen RH, Bigbee WL. Age-related increases in human autosomal somatic mutation occur primarily by an *in situ* dosage compensation mechanism. Genet Soc Can Bull 1990; 21(suppl):49.

22. Compton PJE, Smith MT, Grant SG, et al. Gene duplicating events increase with age in human blood cells. Proc Am Assoc Cancer Res 1991; 32:107.

23. Grant SG, Langlois RG, Jensen RH, Bigbee WL. Identification of individuals from normal populations with aberrantly high frequencies of somatic segregation. Environ Mol Mutagen 1991; 17(suppl 19):27.

24. Grant SG, Langlois RG, Jensen RH, Bigbee WL. Somatic mutation and segregation in normal individuals as determined using the *in vivo* GPA assay: Implications for oncogenesis and aging. Am J Hum Genet 1991; 49(suppl):448.

25. Langlois RG, Bigbee WL, Kyoizumi S, et al. Evidence for an increased frequency of somatic cell mutations at the glycophorin A locus in A-bomb survivors. Science 1987; 236:445.

26. Kyoizumi S, Nakamura N, Hakoda M, et al. Detection of somatic mutations at the glycophorin A locus in erythrocytes of atomic bomb survivors using a single beam flow sorter. Cancer Res 1989; 49:581.

27. Akiyama A, Kyoizumi S, Hirai Y, et al. Studies on chromosome aberrations and HPRT mutations in lymphocytes and GPA mutation in erythrocytes of Atomic bomb survivors. Prog Clin Biol Res 1990; 340C:69.

28. Langlois RG, Akiyama M, Kusonoki Y, et al. Analysis of somatic cell mutations at the glycophorin A locus in atomic bomb survivors: a comparative study of assay methods. Radiat Res (in press).

29. Straume T, Langlois RG, Lucas J, et al. Novel biodosimetry methods applied to victims of the Goiania accident. Health Phys 1991; 60:71.

30. Langlois RG, Bigbee WL, Jensen RH. The glycophorin A assay for somatic cell mutations in humans. Prog Clin Biol Res 1990; 340C:47.

31. Jensen RH, Bigbee WL, Langlois RG, et al. Laser-based flow cytometric analysis of genotoxicity of humans exposed to ionizing radiation during the Chernobyl accident. In: Akhmanov SA, Poroshina MY, eds. Laser Applications in Life Sciences, Part One: Laser Diagnostics of Biological Molecules and Living Cells - Linear and Nonlinear Methods. Bellingham, Massachusetts: Society of Photo-Optical Instrumentation Engineers, SPIE Proc 1991; 1403:372.

32. Straume T, Lucas JN, Tucker JD, et al. Biodosimetry for a radiation worker using multiple assays. Health Phys 1992; 62:122.

33. Mendelsohn ML. New approaches for biological monitoring of radiation workers. Health Phys 1990; 59:23.

34. Grant SG, Bigbee WL, Langlois RG, Jensen RH. Methods for the detection of mutational and segregational events: Relevance to the monitoring of survivors of childhood cancer. Curr Clin Oncol 1992; 2:133.

35. Bigbee WL, Wyrobek AW, Langlois RG, et al. The effect of chemotherapy on the *in vivo* frequency of glycophorin A "null" variant erythrocytes. Mutat Res 1990; 240:165.

36. Perera F, Bigbee W, O'Neill P, et al. Validation of biologic markers in chemotherapy patients. Proc Am Assoc Cancer Res 1991; 32:223.

37. Manchester DK, Grant SG, Langlois RG, et al. Occurrence of glycophorin A phenotypic variants in human umbilical cord blood. Am J Hum Genet 1990 47(suppl):A139.

38. Bigbee WL, Grant SG, Jensen RH, et al. Glycophorin A variant erythrocyte frequencies in Finnish reinforced plastics workers exposed to styrene. Environ Mol Mutagen 1991; 17(suppl):10.

39. Compton-Quintana PJE, Jensen RH, Bigbee WB, et al. Workers exposed to styrene studied with the glycophorin A human mutation assay. Environ Health Perspectives, 1993; 99:297.

40. Langlois RG, Garry VF, Bigbee WL, et al. Analysis of somatic cell mutations at the glycophorin A locus in workers occupationally exposed to agricultural pesticides and herbicides. Mutat Res (in press).

41. Bigbee WL, Langlois RG, Swift M, Jensen RH. Evidence for an elevated frequency of *in vivo* somatic cell mutations in ataxia telangiectasia, Am J Hum Genet 1989; 44:402.

42. Langlois RG, Bigbee WL, Jensen RH, German J. Evidence for increased *in vivo* mutation and somatic recombination in Bloom's syndrome. Proc Natl Acad Sci USA 1989; 86:670.

43. Kyoizumi S, Nakamura N, Takebe H, et al. Frequency of variant erythrocytes at the glycophorin-A locus in two Bloom's syndrome patients. Mutat Res 1989; 214:215.

44. Bigbee WL, Jensen RH, Grant SG, et al. Evidence for elevated *in vivo* somatic mutation at the glycophorin A locus in Fanconi anemia. Am J Hum Genet 1991; 49(suppl):446.

45. Grant SG, Langlois RG, Auerbach AD, et al. Analysis of human DNA metabolism/repair diseases with the *in vivo* glycophorin A somatic segregation assay: Application of an improved assay and extension to new syndromes. Environ Mol Mutagen 1992; 19(Suppl 20):20.

46. Nicklas JA, O'Neill JP, Albertini RJ. Use of T-cell receptor gene probes to quantify the *in vivo* hprt mutations in human T-lymphocytes. Mutat Res 1986; 173:65.

47. Bjorkman PJ, Parham P. Structure, function, and diversity of class I major histocompatability complex molecules. Ann Rev Biochem 1990; 59:253.

48. Malissen M, Malissen B, Jordan BR. Exon/intron structure and complete nucleotide sequence of an *HLA* gene. Proc Natl Acad Sci USA 1982; 79:893.

49. Pious D, Hawley P, Forrest G. Isolation and characterization of HL-A variants in cultured human lymphoid cells. Proc Natl Acad Sci USA 1973; 70:1397.

50. Pious D, Soderland C, Gladstone P. Induction of HLA mutations by chemical mutagens in cultured human lymphoid cells. Immunogenetics 1977; 4:437.

51. Gladstone P, Fueresz L, Pious D. Gene dosage and gene expression in the *HLA* region: Evidence from deletion variants. Proc Natl Acad Sci USA 1982; 79:1235.

52. Kavathas P, Bach FH, DeMars R. Gamma ray-induced loss of expression of HLA and glyoxalase I alleles in lymphoblastoid cells. Proc Natl Acad Sci USA 1980; 77:4251.

53. Nicklas JA, Miyachi Y, Taurog JD, et al. HLA loss variants of a B27$^+$ lymphoblastoid cell line: Genetic and cellular characterization. Hum Immunol 1984; 11:19.

54. Henson V, Palmer L, Banks S, et al. Loss of heterozygosity and mitotic linkage maps in the mouse. Proc Natl Acad Sci USA 1991; 88:6486.

55. Janatipour M, Trainor KJ, Kutlaca R, et al. Mutations in human lymphocytes studied by an HLA selection system. Mutat Res 1987; 198:221.

56. McCarron MA, Kutlaca A, Morley AA. The HLA-A mutation assay: Improved technique and normal results. Mutat Res 1989; 225:189.

57. Koller BH, Sidwell B, DeMars R, Orr HT. Isolation of *HLA* locus-specific DNA probes from the 3′untranslated region. Proc Natl Acad Sci USA 1984; 81:5175.

58. Morley AA, Grist SA, Turner DR, et al. Molecular nature of *in vivo* mutations in human cells at the autosomal HLA-A locus. Cancer Res 1990; 50:4584.

59. Turner DR, Grist SA, Janatipour M, Morley AA. Mutations in human lymphocytes commonly involve gene duplication and resemble those seen in cancer cells. Proc Natl Acad Sci USA 1988; 85:3189.

60. Allsopp CEM, Harding RM, Taylor C, et al. Interethnic genetic differentiation in Africa: HLA class I antigens in the Gambia. Am J Hum Genet 1992; 50:411.

61. Stout JT, Caskey CT. HPRT: Gene structure, expression, and mutation. Ann Rev Genet 1985; 19:127.

62. Albertini RJ, Nicklaus JA, O'Neill JP, Robison SH. In vivo somatic mutations in humans: Measurement and analysis. Ann Rev Genet 1990; 24:305.

63. Strauss GH, Albertini RJ. 6-Thioguanine resistant lymphocytes in human blood. In: Scott D, Bridges BA, Sobels FH, eds. Progress in Genetic Toxicology. Amsterdam: Elsevier, 1977:327.

64. Ostrosky-Wegman P, Montero RM, Cortinas de Nava C, et al. The use of bromodeoxyuridine labeling in the human lymphocyte HGPRT somatic mutation assay. Mutat Res 1988; 191:211.

65. Burkhart-Schultz K, Strout CL, Jones IM. Mouse model for somatic mutation at the HPRT gene: Molecular and cellular analyses. Prog Clin Biol Res 1990; 340C:5.

66. Messing K, Seifert AM, Bradley WEC. *In vivo* mutant frequency of technicians professionally exposed to ionizing radiation. In: Sorsa M, Norppa H, eds. Monitoring of Occupational Genotoxicants. New York: Liss, 1986:87.

67. Ammenhauser MM, Ward JB Jr, Whorton EB Jr, et al. Elevated frequencies of 6-thioguanine resistant lymphocytes in multiple sclerosis patients treated with cyclophosphamide: A prospective study. Mutat Res 1988; 204:509.

68. Trainor KJ, Wigmore DJ, Chrysostomou A, et al. Mutation frequency in human lymphocytes increases with age. Mech Ageing Dev 1984; 27:83.

69. Albertini RJ, Sullivan LS, Berman JK, et al. Mutagenicity monitoring in humans by autoradiographic assay for mutant T-lymphocytes. Mutat Res 1988; 204:481.

70. Cole J, Green MHL, James SE, et al. A further assessment of factors influencing measurements of thioguanine-resistant mutant frequency in circulating T-lymphocytes. Mutat Res 1988; 204:493.

71. Henderson L, Cole H, Cole J, et al. Detection of somatic mutations in man: Evaluation of the microtitre cloning assay for T-lymphocytes. Mutagenesis 1986; 1:195.

72. McGinniss MJ, Falta MT, Sullivan LS, Albertini RJ. *In vivo hprt* mutant frequencies in T-cells of normal human newborns. Mutat Res 1990; 240:117.

73. Hakoda M, Akiyama M, Kyoizumi S, et al. Increased somatic cell mutation frequency in atomic bomb survivors. Mutat Res 1988; 201:39.

74. Hakoda M, Akiyama M, Hirai Y et al. *In vivo* mutant T cell frequency in atomic bomb survivors carrying outlying values of chromosome aberration frequencies. Mutat Res 1988; 202:203.

75. Messing K, Bradley WEC. *In vivo* mutant frequency rises among breast cancer patients after exposure to high doses of γ-radiation. Mutat Res 1985; 152:107.

76. Seifert AM, Bradley WEC, Messing K. Exposure of nuclear medicine patients to ionizing radiation is associated with rises in HPRT-mutant frequency in peripheral T-lymphocytes. Mutat Res 1987; 191:57.

77. Ammenheuser MM, Ward JB, Au WW, Belli JA. A prospective study comparing 6-thioguanine-resistant variant frequencies with chromosome aberration frequencies in lymphocytes from radiotherapy and chemotherapy patients. Environ Mol Mutagen 1989; 14:9.

78. Nicklas JA, Falta MT, Hunter TC, et al. Molecular analyses of *in vivo hprt* mutations in human lymphocytes. V. Effects of total body irradiation secondary to radioimmunoglobulin therapy (RIT). Mutagenesis 1990; 5:461.

79. Messing K, Ferraris J, Bradley WEC, et al. Mutant frequency of radiotherapy technicians appears to be associated with a recent dose of ionizing radiation. Health Phys 1989; 57:537.

80. Ostrosky-Wegman P, Montero R, Gomez M, Cortinas de Nava C. 6-Thioguanine resistant T-lymphocyte determination as a possible indicator of radiation exposure. Environ Mutagen 1987; 9:81.

81. Dempsey JL, Seshadri RS, Morley AA. Increased mutation frequency following treatment with cancer chemotherapy. Cancer Res 1985; 45:2873.

82. Huttner E, Mergner W, Braun R, Schoneich J. Increased frequency of 6-thioguanine-resistant lymphocytes in peripheral blood of workers employed in cyclophosphamide production. Mutat Res 1990; 243:101.

83. Cole J, Green MHL, Stephens G, et al. HPRT somatic mutation data. Prog Clin Biol Res 1990; 340C:25.

84. Norris PG, Limb GA, Hamblin AS, et al. Immune function, mutant frequency, and cancer risk in the DNA repair defective genodermatoses xeroderma pigmentosum, Cockayne's syndrome, and trichothiodystrophy. J Invest Dermatol 1990; 94:94.

85. Muir P, Osborne Y, Morley AA, Turner DR. Karyotypic abnormality of the X chromosome is rare in mutant HPRT lymphocyte clones. Mutat Res 1988; 197:157.

86. Lambert B, Holmberg K, He S-H, Einhorn N. Karyotypes of human T-lymphocyte clones. IARC Sci Publ 1988; 89:469.

87. He SM, Holmberg K, Lambert B, Einhorn N. Hprt mutations and karyotype abnormalities in T-cell clones from healthy subjects and melphalan-treated ovarian cancer patients. Mutat Res 1989; 210:353.

88. Fuscoe JC, Fenwick RG, Ledbetter DH, Caskey CT. Deletion and amplification of the HGPRT locus in Chinese hamster cells. Mol Cell Biol 1983; 3:1086.

89. Yang TP, Patel PI, Chinault AL, et al. Molecular evidence for new mutation in the HPRT locus in Lesch-Nyhan syndrome. Nature 1984; 310:412.

90. Farrell SA, Worton RG. Chromosome loss is responsible for segregation at the *HPRT* locus in Chinese hamster cell hybrids. Somat Cell Genet 1977; 3:539.

91. Albertini RJ, O'Neill JP, Nicklas JA, et al. Alterations of the *hprt* gene in human *in vivo*–derived 6-thioguanine-resistant T-lymphocytes. Nature 1985; 316:369.

92. Turner DR, Morley AA, Haliandros M, et al. *In vivo* somatic mutations in human lymphocytes frequently result from major gene alterations. Nature 1985; 315:343.

93. Bradley WEC, Gareau JLP, Seifert AM, Messing K. Molecular characterization of 15 rearrangements among 90 human *in vivo* somatic mutants shows that deletions predominate. Mol Cell Biol 1987; 7:956.

94. Nicklas J, Hunter TC, O'Neill JP, Albertini RJ. Molecular analysis of the in vivo HPRT mutations

in human lymphocytes. III. Longitudinal study of HPRT gene structural alterations and T-cell clonal origins. Mutat Res 1989; 215:147.

95. Maher VM, Yang J-L, Chen R-H, et al. Use of PCR amplification of cDNA to study mechanisms of human cell mutagenesis and malignant transformation. Environ Mol Mutagen 1991; 18:239.

96. Tindall KR, Whitaker RA. Rapid localization of point mutations in PCR products by chemical (HOT) modification. Environ Mol Mutagen 1991; 18:231.

97. Cariello NF, Swenberg JA, De Bellis A, Skopek TR. Analysis of mutations using PCR and denaturing gradient gel electrophoresis. Environ Mol Mutagen 1991; 18:249.

98. Nicklas JA, Lippert MJ, Hunter TC, et al. Analysis of human *HPRT* deletion mutations with X-linked probes and pulsed field gel electrophoresis. Environ Mol Mutagen 1991; 18:270.

99. Recio L, Cochrane J, Simpson D, et al. DNA sequence analysis of in vivo hprt mutation in human T lymphocytes. Mutagenesis 1990; 5:505.

100. Nicklas JA, O'Neill JP, Hunter TC, et al. In vivo ionizing irradiations produce deletions in the hprt gene of human T-lymphocytes. Mutat Res 1991; 250:383.

101. Nicklas JA, Hunter TC, O'Neill JP, Albertini RJ. Fine structure mapping of the hypoxanthine-guanine phosphoribosyltransferase (HPRT) gene region of the human X chromosome (Xq26), Am J Hum Genet 1991; 49:267.

102. McGinniss MJ, Nicklas JA, Albertini RJ. Molecular analyses of in vivo hprt mutations in human T-lymphocytes: IV. Studies in newborns. Environ Mol Mutagen 1989; 14:299.

103. Fuscoe JC, Zimmerman LJ, Lippert MJ, et al. V(D)J recombinase-like activity mediates hprt gene deletion in human fetal T-lymphocytes. Cancer Res 1991; 51:6001.

104. Albertini RJ, DeMars R. Mosaicism of peripheral blood lymphocyte populations in females heterozygous for the Lesch-Nyhan syndrome. Biochem Genet 1974; 11:397.

105. Jensen RH, Bigbee WL, Langlois RG. Multiple end points for somatic mutations in humans provide complementary views for biodosimetry, genotoxicity and health risks. Prog Clin Biol Res 1990; 340C:81.

106. Stark MH, Tucker JH, Thomson EJ, Perry PE. An automated image analysis system for detection of rare autoradiographically labeled cells in the human lymphocyte HGPRT assay. Cytometry 1984; 5:250.

107. deFazio A, Heneine N, Musgrave EA, Tattersall MH. Enumeration of 6-thioguanine-resistant tumour cells using flow cytometry and comparison with a microtitre cloning assay. Mutat Res 1989; 216:57.

108. DuPont BR, Bigbee WL, Grant SG, et al. Detection of somatic mutations in circulating reticulocytes: Prospects for molecular analysis. Am J Hum Genet 1991; 49(suppl):447.

109. Atwood KC, Scheinberg SL. Somatic variation in human erythrocyte antigens. J Cell Comp Physiol 1958; 52(suppl 1):97.

110. Atwood KC, Pepper FJ. Erythrocyte automosaicism in some persons of known genotype. Science 1961; 134:2100.

111. DuPont BR, Sutton HE. Detection of somatic mutations: Use of the ABO blood group antigen. Am J Hum Genet 1988; 43(suppl):A23.

112. Hakoda M, Hirai Y, Kusunoki Y, Akiyama M. Cloning of in vivo–derived thioguanine-resistant human B cells. Mutat Res 1989; 210:29.

113. Siminovich L. On the nature of hereditable variation in cultured somatic cells. Cell 1976; 7:1.

114. Hall JG. Somatic mosaicism: Observations related to clinical genetics. Am J Hum Genet 1988; 43:355.

115. Penn A. Role of somatic mutation in atherosclerosis. Prog Clin Biol Res 1990; 340C:93.

116. Bishop JM. The molecular genetics of cancer. Science 1987; 235:305.

117. Grant SG. Mutation, segregation, and childhood cancer. Curr Clin Oncol 1992; 2:121.

118. Knudson AG. Hereditary cancer, oncogenes and antioncogenes, Cancer Res 1985; 45:1437.

119. Vogelstein B, Fearon ER, Hamilton SR, et al. Genetic alterations during colorectal-tumor development. N Engl J Med 1988; 319:525.

120. Grant SG, Bigbee WL, Langlois RG, Jensen RH. Allele loss at the human GPA locus: A model for recessive oncogenesis with potential clinical application. Clin Biotech 1991; 3:177.

121. Buetow HK, Murray JC, Israel JL, et al. Loss of heterozygosity suggests tumor suppressor gene responsible for primary hepatocellular carcinoma. Proc Natl Acad Sci USA 1989; 86:8852.

Part III
Red Cell Antibodies

Part III

Red Cell Antibodies

12

Immunological and Physicochemical Nature of Antigen–Antibody Interactions

CAREL J. VAN OSS
State University of New York at Buffalo
Buffalo, New York

I. INTRODUCTION

The binding forces involved in the specific interactions between antigens (Ags) and antibodies (Abs), lectins and carbohydrates, ligands and their receptors, and, in most cases, enzymes and their substrates, are of a noncovalent, purely physicochemical nature. The same (attractive) physicochemical forces that govern Ag-Ab binding also constitute the (repulsive) forces that prevent freely suspended cells, such as red blood cells (RBCs), to approach each other more closely than a given minimum distance (1). Because the distance to which RBCs can approach each other is of crucial importance to a variety of hemagglutination techniques, the rate of decay of the various physicochemical forces, as a function of distance, is especially treated. The difference in the rate of decay as a function of distance of the three major physical forces involved in cell interactions as well as in Ag-Ab bonds is one of the prime reasons for treating the three forces (electrodynamic, electrostatic, and electron-acceptor/electron-donor interactions) separately from each other. The difference in the response of the three types of physical interaction forces to various physical and physicochemical measures taken with an aim, e.g., to dissociate Ag-Ab bonds, is another important reason to maintain a clear distinction between these forces.

Apart from the absence of covalent bonds, Ag-Ab interactions differ in other ways from more conventional chemical reactions. For instance, while the valencies of Abs are known precisely (they are either divalent or decavalent dependent on the antibody class), the valencies of most Ags rarely are well defined. In addition, different valency sites (epitopes) of an Ag often (but not invariably) differ from each other in their chemical composition. Thus, plurivalency of most Ags only has meaning vis-à-vis polyclonal Abs, comprising many Ab populations, where each population has a different antibody-active site (paratope). Even within only one population of Abs that are all directed specifically toward one given epitope, the paratopes, while chemically fairly similar, still vary sufficiently in their amino acid composition to display a wide array of different affinities to that epitope.

Ags can generally combine with their Abs in virtually any proportion, so that the concept of stoichiometry becomes irrelevant to Ag-Ab reactions. Even when the binding energy of an Ag-Ab reaction is determined at the optimal binding, or "stoichiometric" ratio, that binding energy is still strongly proportional to the total dilution of the reagents (2). This phenomenon greatly complicates the experimental conditions under which meaningful Ag-Ab binding energies can be usefully determined and seriously compromises the significance of many of the Ag-Ab binding constants that have been published to date.

The interpretation of Ag-Ab binding affinities is further complicated by hysteresis; i.e., the phenomenon whereby the energy of Ag-Ab *dissociation* is higher than the energy of *association* owing to the gradual formation of additional secondary Ag-Ab bonds of lesser specificity. The role of entropy in Ag-Ab reactions also is somewhat controversial. Although the formation of regular Ag-Ab lattices should reasonably be accompanied by an increase in order, in reality, the formation of Ag-Ab complexes more often than not gives rise to a measurable increase in entropy. Thus, the energetics of Ag-Ab reactions entail difficulties that complicate the discipline of immunochemistry to a greater degree than more conventional fields of chemistry.*

Definitions of abbreviations, symbols, and units used in this chapter are given in Table 1.

II. NATURE OF ANTIGEN-ANTIBODY BINDING FORCES

A. The Ag-Ab Bond

The Ag-Ab bond comprises the following three physicochemical forces: (1) Lifshitz–van der Waals (LW), or electrodynamic, forces; (2) Coulombic, or electrostatic (EL), forces; and (3) electron-acceptor/electron-donor, or polar or (Lewis) acid-base (AB), forces. While in aqueous media LW forces are virtually always attractive, they are practically never quantitatively predominant; they usually represent less than 10% of the total noncovalent interaction.

Ag-Ab bonds thus mainly consist of electrostatic (EL) forces and/or of polar (AB) forces in every conceivable proportion. Some types of Ag-Ab bonds are purely of the EL variety (with a slight background of additional LW forces), whereas others are purely of AB origin (with an equally minor LW background). Also, in a great many cases, Ag-Ab bonds comprise *combinations* of EL and AB forces (with in addition a small LW contribution). It is especially when contemplating dissociation of Ag-Ab bonds that it becomes crucial to take the possibility of a hybrid nature of such bonds into consideration because the conditions favoring the dissociation of EL and AB bonds tend to differ significantly.

B. Lifshitz–van der Waals (LW) Forces

1. Nature of LW Forces

There is a mutual attraction between all atoms and molecules that are brought closely enough together, which is caused by the interaction between the fluctuating dipole occurring in one atom and a second dipole which the first dipole induces in a second atom. The resulting interatomic and intermolecular forces are called van der Waals–London, or dispersion, forces. Of somewhat lesser importance in aqueous media, but by no means necessarily negligible, are two additional van der Waals interactions. These are (1) the interactions between permanent dipoles, called van der Waals–Keesom, or orientation, forces, and (2) the interactions between a permanent dipole and a dipole induced by that permanent dipole, called van der Waals–Debye, or induction, forces. Using the Lifshitz approach, it can be shown that in liquids and solids van der Waals–Keesom and van der Waals–Debye interaction forces obey the same rules as

*The topics on the nature of the Ag-Ab bond, thermodynamics of Ag-Ab interactions, and hemagglutination, treated in this chapter, are closely assimilated to chapters on these subjects written by this author in *Immunochemistry*, edited by C. J. van Oss and M. H. V. Van Regenmortel, Marcel Dekker, New York, in preparation.

Table 1 Abbreviations, Symbols, and Units Used in This Chapter

Antigens and Antibodies

Ab	Antibody
Ag	Antigen
Ag-Ab	Antigen-antibody, or antigen•antibody complex(es)
MAb	Monoclonal antibody
EPI (subscript)	Epitope, or antigenic determinant
PARA (subscript)	Paratope, or antibody-active site
Ig	Immunoglobulin(s): IgA, IgD, IgE, IgG, IgM
Fc	Carboxy terminal Ig moiety
P3	3-azopyridine (hapten)
Blood groups	A, B, D(Rh_0), O, M, N, c

Length

Å	Ångström $= 10^{-8}$ cm $= 0.1$ nm
ℓ	Interparticle or intermolecular distance
ℓ_o	Distance at the minimum equilibrium distance between particles or macromolecules; $\ell_o \approx 1.5$ to 1.6 Å
R	Radius of spheres (also: receptor; gas constant).

Superscripts and Subscripts

LW (superscript)	Lifshitz–van der Waals
AB (superscript)	(Lewis) acid-base, or pertaining to electron acceptor/electron donor interactions; in aqueous systems, also pertaining to Brønsted acid-base interactions
EL (superscript)	Electrostatic (or electrokinetic)
BR (superscript)	Brownian movement
TOT (superscript)	Total
L (subscript)	Liquid
S (subscript)	Solid
i j } (subscript)	Generalization for subscripts, 1, 2, 3

Free Energy, Surface Tension, and Interfacial Tension

ΔG	Free energy of interaction: expressed in energy units (per particle, per mole, per molecule, or per unit surface area)
ΔG_{132}	Free energy change of interaction between materials 1 and 2, immersed in liquid 3 (units: J, erg, kcal, kT [$= 4.04 \times 10^{-21}$ J at 20°C])
ΔG_{131}	Free energy change of interaction between two particles or molecules of material 1, immersed in liquid 3 (units as above)
ΔH	Enthalpy, i.e., heat change component of ΔG (units as above)
ΔS	Entropy, i.e., "disorder" change component of ΔG (units: calories per mole degree)
γ_i	Surface tension of liquids and solids
γ_{ij}	Interfacial tension between two liquids or between a liquid and a solid
$\gamma^{\oplus}$	Surface tension: electron acceptor parameter
$\gamma^{\ominus}$	Surface tension: electron donor parameter
γ^{LW}	Lifshitz–van der Waals component of the surface tension
γ^{AB}	(Lewis) acid-base component of the surface tension:

$$\gamma_i = \gamma_i^{LW} + \gamma_i^{AB}$$

where

$$\gamma_i^{AB} = 2\sqrt{\gamma_i^{+}\,\gamma_i^{-}}$$

(Eq. 6)

(continued)

Table 1 Continued

All surface tensions, their components, and parameters may be expressed in units of tension (e.g., mN/m^2) or, preferably, in units of energy per unit surface area (e.g., mJ/m^2, ergs/cm^2), to bring them on a level comparable to that of ΔG; cf. Eq. 2.

Energy Units and Related Symbols

J	Unit of energy = 10^7 ergs = 0.239 cal
kcal	Kilocalorie = 4.186×10^{10} ergs = 4186 J
mJ/m^2	(= erg/cm^2). The mJ/m^2 is the preferred unit of surface tension (γ_i), interfacial tension (γ_{ij}), and (often) of interfacial free energy (ΔG_{132}, ΔG_{131})
kT	Unit of energy per particle, cell, or molecule (1 kT = 4.04×10^{-21} J at 20°C, or 293° Kelvin)
k	Boltzmann's constant (k = 1.38×10^{-23} J per degree Kelvin, per molecule or particle).
R	Gas constant (R = 1.986×10^{-3} K cal = 8.31×10^{10} ergs = 8.31 J, per degree Kelvin per mole); R = 6.022×10^{23} k, where 6.022×10^{23} equals the number of molecules in 1 mole.
T	Absolute temperature (in degrees Kelvin)

Law of Mass Action

K_a	Association constant (in liters per mole)
K_b	Dissociation constant (in moles per liter)
$k_{1,2}$	Kinetic association constant (in liters per mole/sec.).
$k_{2,1}$	Kinetic dissociation constant (in sec^{-1})
M	Mole, or molar

Other Physical Units, Entities, or Symbols

A	Hamaker, or van der Waals constant, usually in 10^{-21} J, or in 10^{-14} ergs
C	Concentration (usually in moles per liter)
D	Diffusion coefficient
L	Liter
Mw	Molecular weight
R	Receptor
S_c	Contactable surface area, between Ag and Ab, or between any two macromolecules
ΔV	Volume charge
e	Charge of the electron (e = 4.8×10^{10} electrostatic units)
mV	Millivolts
n_i	Number of ion species, i, per cubic centimeter
v_i	Valency of ionic species, i, in solution
ϵ	Dielectric constant (for water at 20°C, ϵ = 80)
θ	Contact angle (in degrees)
ζ	(Electrical) zeta-potential of particles measured at the slipping plane (in millivolts)
κ	Inverse Debye length, or inverse of the thickness of the diffuse ionic double layer
ψ_0	(Electrical) psi-nought potential at the exact interface between particle and liquid.

Waals–London (dispersion) forces, *on a macroscopic scale* (3–5). These forces are collectively alluded to as Lifshitz–van der Waals (LW) forces.

2. *LW Free Energies*

Lifshitz–van der Waals interactions between atoms and/or molecules, when occurring in medium-sized to large molecules or particles, are to a significant degree additive. Their free energy of interaction, ΔG^{LW} (in the configuration of two semi-infinite flat parallel bodies), may thus be expressed as

$$\Delta G^{LW} = \frac{-A}{12\pi \ell^2} \tag{1}$$

where A is the Hamaker coefficient (which is linked to physical properties of the interacting materials, including those of the liquid, when the interaction takes place in a liquid medium) and ℓ is the distance between the two parallel bodies or molecules. For a number of materials, the Hamaker coefficients can be measured and/or calculated (6). Van der Waals–London interactions can be estimated via the Lifshitz approach (6) or via determinations of the Lifshitz–van der Waals surface tension components (4). The free energy, ΔG_{132}^{LW}, of the Lifshitz–van der Waals part of the interaction between two materials 1 and 2 (in a liquid medium 3) can be determined as follows. For $\ell = \ell_o$ (ℓ_o is the minimum equilibrium distance between two parallel bodies or molecules; $\ell_o \approx 1.57\text{Å}$ [4]) $\Delta G_{132}^{LW}G$ is expressed by means of the Dupré equation in condensed media:

$$\Delta G_{132}^{LW} = \gamma_{12}^{LW} - \gamma_{13}^{LW} - \gamma_{23}^{LW} \tag{2}$$

where γ_{ij}^{LW} stands for the interfacial tensions between the materials indicated by the subscripts and where ΔG_{132}^{LW} is the same at ΔG^{LW} given in Eq. 1. Once the LW components of the surface tensions of, e.g., Ag (1), Ab (2), and of the liquid medium (3), γ_1^{LW}, γ_2^{LW}, and γ_3^{LW}, are known, the interfacial tensions of Eq. 2 can be obtained from the LW components of the surface tensions, with an error of less than æ2% (5):

$$\gamma_{ij}^{LW} = (\sqrt{\gamma_i^{LW}} - \sqrt{\gamma_j^{LW}})^2 \tag{3}$$

Based on the Dupré equation (Eq. 2), it can also be shown that the interaction between two similar molecules, or cells, 1, immersed in a liquid, 3, can be expressed as:

$$\Delta G_{131}^{LW} = -2\gamma_{13}^{LW} \tag{4}$$

Eq. 4 is of importance when studying the stability of cells suspended in liquids; e.g., in connection with hemagllutination (see Sect. VI below).

3. *Sign and Relative Unimportance of LW Forces in Ag-Ab Interactions*

ΔG_{132}^{LW} can be negative (attractive) or positive (repulsive) depending on the value of the Hamaker coefficient, A_{33}, of the liquid medium relative to the values of the Hamaker coefficients, A_{11} and A_{22}, of Ag and Ab. Thus, manipulation of some of the properties of the liquid medium may turn an attractive reaction (association) into a repulsive reaction (dissociation) (4). In *aqueous media* however, which have a very low γ^{LW} value ($\gamma? \approx 21.8$ mJ/m^2), the interaction between biological molecules or particles (usually with a $\gamma?$ value of the order of 40 mJ/m^2), ΔG_{131}^{LW} and ΔG_{132}^{LW} always has a negative value; i.e., the LW interactions between biological entities, in aqueous media, virtually always are *attractive* with a maximum value of about –5 mJ/m^2 between two *dry* biological entities (i.e., after expulsion of water of hydration). Between two *hydrated* biological entities, in water, the value of ΔG_{131}^{LW} or ΔG_{132}^{LW} is only about -0.5 mJ/m^2 as the γ^{LW} value of such hydrated entities is of the order of 27 mJ/m^2 versus 21.8 mJ/m^2 for γ^{LW} of water. In *aqueous media*, where essentially all Ag-Ab reactions take place, LW interactions are never the only interaction forces and usually represent less than 10% of the total interaction. The LW interaction energy is just (a usually relatively small) part of the total interaction energy; it is additive to the other components.

4. Minimum Distance Between Ag and Ab Surfaces and Decay with Distance of LW Forces

Owing to the marked increased in the Lifshitz–van der Waals attraction at short distances of interaction (see Eq. 1), LW attractions are stronger, the better the steric fit between an epitope and its complementary paratope.* The overall distance between the epitope and the paratope, as between other macromolecules and/or particles, can be as small as about 2 Å (7,8) and in ideal cases can approach 1.5 Å (4), which is of the order of magnitude of the minimum equilibrium distance, l_o. Up to a distance $\ell \approx 100$ Å, ΔG^{LW} decays with l in proportion to $(\ell/\ell_o)^2$ (see Eq. 2). However, at $\ell \geq 100$ Å, the rate of decay becomes steeper owing to retardation effects in the dispersion component of the LW forces. (For the decay with distance of LW forces in configurations other than the plane-parallel configuration given in Eq. 1, see refs. 1 and 4.)

C. Polar, or Lewis Acid-Base (AB), Forces—Hydrogen-Bonding Interactions

1. Definition and Scope of (AB), or Polar, Interactions

Polar forces may be defined as the forces operating in electron acceptor/electron donor, or Lewis acid-base, interactions. These interactions are designated by the superscript AB for (Lewis) acid-base interactions (4,9,10). (The superscript AB used in this chapter does *not* stand for antibody; antibody is designated as Ab, which is not used as a superscript.) Hydrogen bonds (Brønsted acid-base interactions) are a subclass of polar forces; thus all interactions that take place in a strongly hydrogen-bonding liquid such as water of necessity involve polar interactions.

2. Polar (AB) Free Energies

Polar energies also obey an equation based on the Dupré equation (Eq. 2), but the γ_{ij}^{AB} term is expressed by an equation which is very different from the γ_{12}^{LW} term:

$$\gamma_{ij}^{AB} = 2\left(\sqrt{\gamma_i^+\gamma_i^-} + \sqrt{\gamma_j^+\gamma_j^-} + \sqrt{\gamma_i^+\gamma_j^-} + \sqrt{\gamma_i^-\gamma_i^+}\right) \tag{5}$$

where γ_i^+ and γ_i^- are the electron–acceptor and the electron–donor parameters, of the polar surface tension component γ_i^{AB} (4,10), where:

$$\gamma_i^{AB} = 2\sqrt{\gamma_i^+\gamma_i^-} \tag{6}$$

For homogeneous solids as well as for pure liquids, γ_i^{LW}, γ_i^+ and γ_i^- can be determined; e.g., via contact angle measurements† (liquid/solid) or interfacial tension measurements (liquid/liquid) (4,10). For whole biopolymers, all these parameters can be measured, both in the dry and

---

*The same reasoning holds for the other interaction classes: EL as well as AB forces also both are strongest at the shortest possible distance, $\ell \to \ell_o$.

†This is done by contact angle (θ) determinations on dry (and/or on hydrated layers of cells, proteins, or peptides with three completely characterized liquids, L (two of which liquids must be polar), using the Young equation that can be solved for the three unknown parameters γ_s^{LW}, γ_s^+ and γ_s^- of the solid, S (4,10):

$$(1 + \cos\theta)\,\gamma_L = 2\left(\sqrt{\gamma_s^{LW}\gamma_L^{LW}} + \sqrt{\gamma_s^+\gamma_L^-} + \sqrt{\gamma_s^-\gamma_L^+}\right) \tag{7}$$

This equation should be used three times, with the different values for θ obtained with the three different liquids, L.

in the hydrated state (11). Unfortunately, however, a given epitope on a protein, or on a polysaccharide, is much too small for such measurements.

Based upon the Dupré equation for condensed media (cf. Eq. 2), the polar (AB) free energy of interaction between different biopolymers (and/or cells), 1 and 2, immersed in a liquid, 3, can be expressed as

$$\Delta G_{132}^{AB} = 2[\sqrt{\gamma_3^+}(\sqrt{\gamma_1^-} + \sqrt{\gamma_2^-} - \sqrt{\gamma_3^-})$$

$$+ \sqrt{\gamma_3^-}(\sqrt{\gamma_1^+} + \sqrt{\gamma_2^+} - \sqrt{\gamma_3^+}) - \sqrt{\gamma_1^-\gamma_2^-} - \sqrt{\gamma_2^+}] \qquad (8)$$

3. "Hydrophobic," or Attractive, AB Interactions

The interaction between totally apolar (macro) molecules or particles, when immersed in water, is predominantly (i.e., for $\approx$ 99%) polar and only for about 1% caused by Lifshitz–van der Waals forces (12,13). These interactions are familiar to most under the name of "hydrophobic" interactions, although the designation "interfacial" interactions is more appropriate. There are tables listing the degree of "hydrophobicity" of various amino acids (14,15). These values, however, are only qualitatively linked to the Lifshitz–van der Waals constant and the available electron-acceptor (γ^+) and electron-donor (γ^-) parameters of given amino acids, and do not permit the computation of interaction energies. Thus, it still is difficult to arrive at a quantitative expression of the individual contribution to the attractive "hydrophobic" interaction energy of individual epitopes and especially of their constituent moieties.

However, averaging over the entire biopolymer, or cell surface, when ΔG_{132}^{AB} has a sufficient negative value to make the total value of ΔG_{132}^{TOT} (= $\Delta G_{132}^{LW} + \Delta G_{132}^{AB} + \Delta G_{132}^{EL}$) *negative*, a net attraction occurs. Similarly, when a sufficient number of "hydrophobic" moieties are present in an epitope, *or* in a paratope, ΔG_{132}^{TOT} for such a pair will be negative, and a *specific* attraction will occur.

4. Hydrophilic, or Repulsive, AB Interactions

On the other hand, hydrophilic macromolecules or cells, immersed in water, manifest a net polar AB repulsion averaged over their entire contactable surfaces. In these cases, ΔG_{132}^{TOT} (= $\Delta G_{132}^{LW} + \Delta G_{132}^{AB} + \Delta G_{132}^{EL}$) is *positive*. This repulsion, which is predominantly due to AB forces, is the driving force for the solubility of proteins and for the stability of cells in aqueous media (1,16,17).

5. Specific Ag-Ab Binding and the Interplay Between Attractive and Repulsive Forces

With AB forces in particular and to a lesser degree also in certain cases with EL forces (see below), a marked dichotomy exists between the overall aspecific repulsion among biopolymers and cells, immersed in water, and the attraction occurring, e.g., between epitopes and paratopes, where the specific attraction can prevail over the aspecific repulsion, in such cases where the specificity is sufficiently pronounced and the (specific) binding force sufficiently strong. This dichotomy is the more striking, if one takes into consideration that the forces responsible for the overall aspecific repulsion, and those causing the specific attraction are qualitatively the same noncovalent physicochemical forces; i.e., LW, AB, and EL forces, where the AB forces usually are predominant (18).

Normally, the complete *molecules* of Ag and Ab repel each other ($\Delta G_{\text{Ag-water-Ab}}^{TOT} > 0$), while an attraction exists between epitope (EPI) and paratope (PARA) ($\Delta G_{\text{EPI-water-PARA}}^{TOT} < 0$). For the *specific* Ag-Ab binding (i.e., attraction) to prevail, it is necessary that $\Delta G_{\text{EPI-water-PARA}}^{TOT} > \Delta G_{\text{Ag-water-Ab}}^{TOT}$, *and* that at least one of the specific moieties (usually the epitope) be situated on a prominent site of the (antigen) molecule, *and* that such a site has a small radius of curvature. The latter requirement decreases the overall force of repulsion between an opposing protein (e.g., the antibody) and the site comprising the epitope (on the antigen) when both are still some distance removed from each other. In other words, if the epitope is situated on a prominent and, preferably, on a pointy protuberance of the antigen molecule (or cell), it can optimally pierce the normally existing repulsion field* between Ag and Ab. Contact can then be made, after which the specific attraction of the Ag-Ab (EPI-PARA) bond can prevail. Table 2 illustrates the contrasts and general characteristics of aspecific and specific interaction forces in aqueous media (18). It may be noted that most frequently, in specific Ag-Ab interactions of the "hydrophobic" (AB) variety, the "hydrophobic" moiety in the interacting partnership is usually located on the *paratope* and is then situated in a concavity ("cleft") of the paratope.

In this context, it is useful to remember that while Ags can be proteins or carbohydrates (or even other types of molecules), Abs always are proteins (immunoglobulins). And when comparing surface properties, in contrast to carbohydrates, proteins are the principal biopolymers with "hydrophobic" sites. It thus seems clear that professional biorecognition polymers need to be proteins (and not carbohydrates) in order to enable them to include "hydrophobic" interactions in their repertory of physicochemical binding modes. This is the most likely reason why carbohydrates occur nowhere as *recognition molecules,* such as, e.g., antibodies or lectins (18). Carbohydrates can, however, be easily *recognized* because in attractive "hydrophobic" interactions in aqueous media, only one of the reactants needs to be "hydrophobic"—the other one may be hydrophilic. When "hydrophobic" recognition patches occur on freely circulating proteins (e.g., immunoglobulins), they have to be somewhat hidden in concavities to circumvent the type of accidental aspecific "hydrophobic" binding that would otherwise frequently occur between two proteins with prominent "hydrophobic" sites (18) and thus lead to insolubility in water.

The sites at the surface of proteins that are most exposed to other proteins and/or to other surfaces or cells are more hydrophilic than the sites one finds in the interior of the tertiary structure of native (i.e., undenatured) protein molecules in aqueous solution. The tertiary

Table 2 Comparisons Between Aspecific (Cell-Cell, Cell-Biopolymer, or Biopolymer-Biopolymer) and Specific (Ag-Ab) Interactions

	Aspecific	Specific
Nature of contact sites	Usually rather homogeneous	Often heterogeneous
Surface area of contact	Large (10–100 nm^2)	Small (0.5–5.0 nm^2)
Total size of molecule or particle	May be quite large (up to 10 μm in diameter)	Usually small (1–10 nm Stokes radius, or with processes of a very small radius of curvature)
Influence of Brownian movement	Small	Large
Binding energy	May be repulsive or attractive (+25 mJ/m^2,[a] for erythrocytes)	Attractive (–7 to –25 kT^b per particle, or –10 to –50 mJ/m^2)

[a]Strong repulsive forces of this magnitude can only be overcome by moieties with a very small radius of curvature; hence the smallness or thinness of most molecules comprising a ligand or receptor.
[b]k is Boltzmann's constant (k = 1.38 × 10^{-23}J per degree Kelvin) and T is the absolute temperature in degrees of Kelvin. Thus, at 20°C (= 293° K), 1 kT = 4.04 × 10^{-23}J.
Source: From Ref. 18.

*This repulsion field is principally due to AB interactions (sometimes alluded to as hydration forces), which are in some instances (e.g., in the case of erythrocytes) helped by an additional electrostatic (EL) repulsion. The residual LW attraction in aqueous media is easily overcome by the AB repulsion and in some cases also by EL repulsions if present.

configuration of native protein molecules, when dissolved in water, may be likened to that of micelles, which are spontaneously formed by surfactant molecules: The hydrophilic moieties of the surfactant chains are oriented outward and the "hydrophobic" tails of surfactants are hidden in the interior of micellar structures.

6. Decay of Polar (AB) Forces as a Function of Distance

Polar forces decrease as a function of distance at an exponential rate. The rate of decay with distance of ΔG^{AB} is expressed (in the configuration of semi-infinite flat parallel bodies) as:

$$\Delta G_\ell^{AB} = \Delta G_{\ell_o}^{AB} \exp\left[(\ell_o - \ell)/\lambda\right] \tag{9}$$

where ℓ_o is the minimum equilibrium distance (which may be taken to be of the same order of magnitude as for LW interactions, i.e., $\ell_o \approx 1.5$ Å), and where λ is the correlation length (or decay length) typical for the solvent molecules, which, for liquid water, has an empirical value of the order of 0.6 nm (1) to 1.0 nm (19). Contrary to electrostatic interactions (see below), the decay of AB forces with distance is not influenced by the ionic strength of the liquid medium. (For the decay of AB energies in configurations other than plane-parallel, see refs. 1, 4, and 16.)

7. Direct Hydrogen-Bonding Interactions

Direct hydrogen bonding between Ag and Ab, i.e., between O and C=O, NH and C=O, and NH and OH groups has been identified with certainty in only a few cases; for example, with *o*-substituted benzoate haptens, reacting with anti–*p*-azobenzoate Ab (7). In the case of neutral hydrophilic polysaccharide Ags, such as dextrans, which are strong electron donors (10), ruling out "hydrophobic" as well as electrostatic interactions, they may conceivably specifically interact with Ab-active sites in a direct closely fitting electron donor (Ag) electron acceptor (Ab) mode. However, at least on a macroscopic level, no available electron acceptor activity of immunoglobulins has been demonstrated. Thus, while direct H bonding theoretically could exist in, e.g., dextran-antidextran interactions, it probably does not occur to any significant degree.* Direct hydrogen bonds between Ag and Ab may evolve secondarily in those cases where the primary bond is between a somewhat acidic Ag and a basic Ab, e.g., with DNA–anti-DNA (high-affinity Abs), in which case the primary, electrostatic bond ultimately appears to evolve into a direct hydrogen bond (20,21) (see Sect. III.D).

D. Electrostatic (EL) Forces

1. Nature of EL Forces

Electrostatic (EL), or Coulombic, interactions between Ag and Ab are due to the presence of one or more ionized sites on the epitope and oppositely charged ions on the paratope. These typically are the COO^- and the NH_2^+ groups on polar amino acids of the Ag and Ab molecules (where the Ag is a protein or a peptide or similarly charged moieties on carbohydrate or other nonproteinaceous Ags). In some hapten-AB systems, the number and position of the ionized sites have been determined (7).

---

*While both hydrophobic interactions and direct hydrogen bonds are due to hydrogen bonds, the mechanisms in both cases are quite different. In hydrophobic interactions, the low-energy ("hydrophobic") moieties are "squeezed together" through the hydrogen-bonding energy of cohesion of the surrounding water molecules (12,13). Direct hydrogen bonds, on the other hand, occur through precise C=O-HO binding between the opposing epitope and paratope.

2. EL Free Energies

Short-Range Electrostatic Interactions.   Owing to the shielding effect of the diffuse ionic double layers surrounding the charged sites (which effect varies strongly with the ambient ionic strength and with the distance between charged sites), the calculation of EL interaction energies is a complicated operation. However, as a first approximation, the free energy (ΔG^{EL}) of attraction between a COO^- and a NH_2^+ group, at a distance of about 3 Å, in a medium with an ionic strength $\mu = 0.15$, is of the order of about -7 kcal/mol (22), or about -12 mJ/m^2, for a charge interaction between an opposing epitope-paratope pair with a surface area of ≈ 400 Å^2. This binding energy is of the same order of magnitude as that of a fairly typical interaction between Ag and Ab (Table 3).

This approach to EL binding is analogous to the direct type of AB interaction discussed above (see Sect. C.7). However, with EL bonds, direct binding is the rule because of the fact that, contrary to direct H bonds (which only occur when the most precise optimal alignment between, e.g., H and O can be realized), EL attractions are capable of starting at a distance and grow stronger and also automatically become more precisely aligned upon closer approach.

Long-Range Electrostatic Interactions.   In most in vivo and also in in vitro situations, most biopolymers and cells, being generally negatively charged, undergo at least a certain degree of mutual EL repulsion. The main measurable property of the overall surface charge of a biopolymer or cell is its surface (or ζ) potential. This is most readily measured by electrophoresis, and from the ζ-potential, thus obtained, the fundamental potential (ψ_o-potential) at the exact particle (or molecule)/liquid interface can be obtained. From the ψ_o-potential, ΔG^{EL} as a function of distance, ℓ, can be obtained as follows:

Table 3 Parameters Enhancing ($+$) or Suppressing ($-$) Ag-Ab *Dissociation*[a]

Parameter						
	\multicolumn{6}{Free Energy Component Involved}					
Parameter	ΔH	$T\Delta S$	ΔG^{LW}	ΔG^{AB}	ΔG^{EL}	ΔG^{TOT}
Increase in time			$+$	$+$	$+$	$+$
Increase in temperature	$+$	$-$				0^{b}
Increase or decrease in pH					$+$	$+$
Increase in ionic strength				$(-)$		$++^{c}$
Addition of strong electron donor solvents (DMSO, ethylene glycol, propanol)				$+$		$+$
Addition of strong electron donor polymers (polyethylene glycol)			$-^{d}$	$-^{d}$	$-^{d}$	$-^{d}$
Addition of strong dehydrating agents ($[NH_4]_2 SO_4{}^{e}$: also polyethylene glycol)[f]	$-$			$-^{d}$		$-^{d}$
Addition of epitope-mimicking haptens			$+$	$+$	$+$	$+$
Dilution		$+$	$+$	$+$	$+$	$+$

[a]To obtain the influence on Ag-Ab *association*, use opposite sign.
[b]0 indicates no significant change.
[c]Only leads to real dissociation with exclusively electrostatic Ag-Ab complexes.
[d]Only in the sense of enhancement of *association*.
[e]Caution: May lead to Ag-Ab *dissociation* with exclusively electrostatic Ag-Ab complexes.
[f]Can also cause aspecific protein precipitation.
Source: Data partially derived from Ref. 21.

$$\Delta G^{EL}_{(\ell)} = 1/\kappa \cdot 64 \, nkT\gamma_0^2 \exp(-\kappa\ell) \tag{10}$$

where $1/\kappa$ is the Debye-length, or the electrostatic decay length:

$$1/\kappa = \sqrt{\epsilon kT/(4\pi e^2 \Sigma v_i^2 n_i^2)} \tag{11}$$

and

$$\gamma_0 = \frac{\exp(ve\psi_0/2kT) - 1}{\exp(ve\psi_0/2kT) + 1} \tag{12}$$

(ϵ = dielectric constant of the liquid [for water, $\epsilon = 80$]; k = Boltzmann's constant [k = 1.38 $\times 10^{-23}$J per °K]; T = the absolute temperature in °K; e = charge of the electron [e = 4.8 5 10^{-10} e.s.u.]; v_i = valency of each ionic species in solution in the liquid; n_i = number of ions of each species per cubic centimeter of bulk liquid; v = valency of the counterions dissolved in the liquid) (see, e.g., refs. 23–25). Equation 10 pertains to the interaction between two semi-infinite plane-parallel bodies (for other configurations, see, e.g., refs. 1, 4, and 16); it should be noted that for the EL interaction between spheres with radius, R, ΔG^{EL} is proportional to R, and inversely proportional to ψ_0^2.

3. Decay of EL Forces as a Function of Distance

In general, the rate of decay of EL interactions with distance may be expressed as:

$$\Delta G^{EL}_\ell = \delta G^{EL}_{\ell_0} \exp(-\kappa\ell) \tag{13}$$

It is clear from Eqs. 19 and 11 that the value ΔG^{EL} strongly depends on the ionic strength (see n_i of Eq. 11) of the liquid medium: For a given value of ϕ_0, ΔG^{EL} has the highest absolute value at the lowest salt content. The values for $1/\kappa$ are for 0.1 M NaCl: 10 Å, for 0.01 M NaCL: 100 Å, and for 10^{-5} M NaCl: 1000 Å. At physiological salt concentration (i.e., 0.15 M NaCl), $1/\kappa \approx 8$ Å. Thus, in more dilute salt solutions, EL interactions are measurable at much greater distances than at high ionic strengths (Eq. 9).

From Eqs. 9 and 10, it can be seen that both AB and EL free energies decay exponentially as a function of distance, ℓ, and of a constant (λ, resp. $1/\kappa$). In the case of AB forces, that constant (λ) is relatively invariable and mainly linked to the molecular properties of the liquid (e.g., water). In the case of EL forces, that "constant" ($1/\kappa$) is variable; it changes with the concentration (and kind) of salts dissolved in the (aqueous) liquid. Thus ΔG^{EL} not only is lowest at high salt concentrations, it also decays much more steeply at high ionic strengths.

In the interaction between erythrocytes (which have a fairly respectable ψ_0 potential of about -26 mV [1,16]), the EL repulsion (acting at a distance) between cells (albeit weaker than the AB repulsion) contributes to the total intercellular repulsion (and thus to the stability of RBC suspensions) in a non-negligible manner. The ionic strength of the aqueous medium not only influences erythrocyte stability, it also governs hemagglutination in other ways owing to the variation of the EL interaction energy with distance as a function of ionic strength (see Sect. VI).

4. Calcium Bridging

Purely (or mainly) electrostatic Ag-Ab interactions can occur not only through negatively charged sites on one determinant attracting positive sites on the other but also via the binding of negatively charged epitopes to equally negatively charged paratopes by means of linkage through, for example, Ca^{2+} ions, by analogy with cell-cell interaction and cell-adhesion phenomena. One example of Ca^{2+} bridging, involving synthetic polypeptides (comprising negatively charged polyglutamic acid moieties), has been described by Liberti (26). Ag-Ab complexes of that type can be dissociated with the complexing agent ethylenediaminetetraacetic acid (EDTA). Other Ca^{2+}-dependent reactions have been observed in DNA–anti-DNA interactions (V. Kumar, unpublished observations, 1989) and, in Abs to a marker peptide used in the affinity purification of recombinant proteins (27).

E. Size of Binding Sites

In proteins and peptides, the maximum size of the epitope is close to that of penta- or hexapeptides, yielding a specific surface area varying between 2.5 and 5.0 nm^2 (28–30). However, specific epitope (or hapten) surface areas as small as 0.5–2.5 nm^2 occur quite as frequently. In polysaccharides, the maximum size of epitopes is close to that of penta- or hexasaccharides, corresponding to the same maximum specific surface area as for peptides. Here also much smaller specific epitope surface areas are quite current (30) (see Table 2). It is obvious that the surface areas of epitopes are closely comparable to those of the corresponding paratopes.

F. Occurrence of LW, AB, and/or EL Forces Alone or in Combination

1. Exclusively LW Bonds

The sole occurrence of LW bonds in Ag-Ab reactions is exceedingly rare, particularly if one wishes to limit such LW interactions only to those where any traces of polar (AB) reactivity is to be excluded. Even the epitope polyalanine (28) would only have the appearance of being entirely apolar. The side chains are, of course, apolar (as are those of polyvaline, polyleucine, polyproline), but the backbone of all amino acids consists of polar C=O and NH groups. Even more important is the fact that the interaction between totally apolar molecules, in water, is predominantly due to polar forces* (12,13). However, while no Ag-Ab interaction is likely to be exclusively due to LW forces (at least not when occurring in aqueous media), LW interactions can never be completely disregarded when considering the total Ag-Ab interaction energy, especially in the secondary Ag-Ab interactions (see Sect. III.D).

2. Exclusively AB Bonds

On the other hand, polar (AB) bonds alone occur very frequently in various Ag-Ab reactions. The only requirement for an Ag-Ab reaction to be exclusively polar is that the LW and the EL interaction energies be zero. One clear example is the dextran-antidextran reaction. The electrostatic or ζ-potential of dextran is as close to zero as possible (33), and due to the strong hydration of dextran in aqueous solution, the value of ΔG_{132}^{LW} is also very low, at least as far as the early, primary Ag-Ab encounter is concerned. Interfacial ("hydrophobic") Ag-Ab interactions also can be just about entirely polar, i.e., when the γ^{LW} of the polar moiety is close to the γ^{LW} of water, i.e., in the case of most alkyl groups, and when the ζ-potential of these apolar groups is negligible (which is usually the case). Secondary Ag-Ab interactions (see Sect. III.D) most often also are mainly polar.

3. Exclusively Electrostatic Bonds

Exclusively electrostatic bonds also occur in Ag-Ab reactions. Among the better studied of these is the DNA–anti-DNA system (34). In many protein-antiprotein systems, the bonds are,

---

*Until the early 1980s, we tended to lump attractive polar (hydrophobic) interactions under the general category of "van der Waals bonds" (31). New, more rigorous approaches to the analysis of LW and AB forces yielded the realization that such interactions between apolar moieties, immersed in water, are largely the outcome of (Lewis) acid-base (AB) interactions and are only to a rather minor degree due to Lifshitz–van der Waals (LW) bonds (4,10,12,13) (see also the experimental results of Israelachvili et al. [32]).

at least in the early, *primary* Ag-Ab reaction electrostatic; a common example of this category is the bovine serum albumin (BSA)–anti-BSA system, where at pH 9.5, no precipitate occurs (at equivalence ratios of Ag/Ab) but only small amounts of 10S and 16S complexes can be observed. However, at pH 7.0, pronounced precipitation occurs (35). A more recently reported system is that of the human idiotype–anti-idiotype complex formation which is the cause of the occurrence of immunoglobulin G (IgG) dimers and other IgG oligomers in pooled human plasma gamma globulin fractions. Almost all of these complexes dissociate at pH 4 and about one third of the complexes dissociate in 4 M NaCl, which would indicate that many if not most of the *primary* bonds are exclusively electrostatic in nature, and that even some of the *secondary* bonds are electrostatic (36). (For the differentiation between primary and secondary bonds, see Sect. III.D).

4. Bonds of Combined Origin

The Ag-Ab bonds of many polysaccharide or glycoprotein Ags and of most polypeptide Ags are brought about by a combination of LW, AB, and EL interactions. Thus, in these cases, the "lock and key" mechanism of the Ag-Ab interaction proposed by Emil Fischer in the nineteenth century consists of the best steric fit for optimal LW and AB attraction combined with the most precise juxtaposition of oppositely charged ions for maximum EL attraction. Also, in predominantly EL bonding, as with BSA–anti-BSA (see above), as soon as Ag and Ab are brought closely together by EL attraction (at neutral pH), in most cases, additional LW and AB and polar attractions are subsequently formed secondarily and aspecifically between the epitope and paratope and also between moieties of Ag and Ab immediately adjacent to the epitope and paratope. It is important to realize the multiple origin of the attractive forces in all these cases when attempting to dissociate Ag-Ab complexes of this category (see Sect. III.D).

III. THERMODYNAMICS AND MEASUREMENT OF ANTIGEN-ANTIBODY INTERACTION ENERGIES

A. Nonstoichiometry of Ag-Ab Bonds

As is obvious from the formation of soluble as well as insoluble Ag-Ab complexes, Ags and Abs (37) as well as other complex-forming substances, such as cationic and anionic surfactants (38), can combine in a wide range of proportions. Ag-Ab reactions thus are essentially nonstoichiometric. In view of the nonstoichiometry of Ag-Ab interactions, the determination of the valency of Ags and Abs (see below) has its own peculiar rules.

B. Valency of Ags and Abs

1. Determination of Ag and Ab Valencies

The valency of Ags can be determined with complexes formed in an excess of Ab, while the valency of Abs can only be determined with complexes formed in an excess of Ag. Precipitates obtained at optimal Ag:Ab ratios (37) often have, however, close to stoichiometric Ag-Ab proportions, with possibly a slight excess of Ag.

2. Valency of Abs

Human antibodies of the IgG, IgA, IgD, and IgE classes are divalent; antibodies of the IgM class are decavalent. (Dimeric IgA, humoral or secretory, is, of course, tetravalent.) IgM class Abs are especially prone to steric hindrance, i.e., owing to their sheer size, large Ag molecules, when binding one of the 10 paratopes of IgM, also can prevent one or several more IgM paratopes from binding other Ag molecules of the same specificity. The steric hindrance effect of IgM manifests itself at Ag molecular weights of 2,000 and higher, so that with bigger Ags apparent valencies for IgM were found that were less than 10; the lowest valencies being observed with the highest molecular weight Ags (39).

It is possible to render IgG class Abs monovalent through partial digestion with papain (such monovalent IgG molecules, called Fab fractions, lack the Fc tail).

3. Valencies of Ags

Most protein Ags are plurivalent only vis-à-vis a complete antiserum elicited against them containing antibodies against each of the epitopes. Each different valency site of a protein Ag usually is an epitope with a different configuration from the other valency sites. A given monoclonal Ab can react with only one valency site of such a protein Ag. Some repeating types of biopolymer may be plurivalent, with all the epitopes being identical to each other, e.g., DNA, or tobacco mosaic virus, or they may have only two or three different groups of epitopes that are identical to one another within each group (DNA also can be an example of this type of Ag). On the other hand, other repeating bipolymers may be monovalent, for example, dextran in the ideal, totally unbranched form; its dominant epitope is the terminal nonreducing sugar (28). The immunodominant epitopes of native globular proteins tend to be situated near their carboxyterminal and at *prominent places* on the outer periphery of their tertiary configuration (29). From known valencies of globular proteins and comparable biopolymers (e.g., viruses), it follows that there is roughly one epitope for about every 35–40 amino acids. As a first approximation, one may thus estimate the valency, N, of a given globular protein as $N = (M/5000)^{2/3}$ (40). The valencies (N) thus calculated for a number of Ags with molecular weights (M) varying from 13,000 to 41,000,000 agree well with the reported valencies (41).

C. Thermodynamics

1. Equilibrium Constants and Free Energies of Interaction

Equilibrium Constants. The Ag-Ab interaction may be expressed as:

$$Ag + Ab = Ag–Ab + x \text{ calories} \tag{14}$$

The equilibrium constants of that reaction are

$$K_a = \frac{[Ag - Ab]}{[Ag]. \ [Ab]} \tag{15a}$$

and

$$K_a = \frac{[Ag] \cdot [Ab]}{[Ag - Ab]} \tag{15b}$$

where K_a and K_d signify the association and dissociation constants, respectively, and the terms in brackets indicate concentrations in moles. $K_a = 1/K_d$ only in ideal cases.

In practice, one will almost invariably find that the energy needed to prevent association (corresponding to K_a as far as the primary interaction is concerned; see below) is less than the energy required to dissociate already existing complexes (corresponding to K_d). One of the major reasons of this is the continuing formation of additional secondary bonds after the initial primary Ag-Ab complex formation (21,35,41–43). This phenomenon (also called hysteresis) is discussed in more detail below (see Sect. III.D). Because of the (generally) high molecular weights of Ag and Ab and, therefore, of their very low molar concentrations, molar concentrations can be used here instead of the traditional activities. Depending on the method of measurement used (see below), one obtains either K_a or K_d.

In view of the heterogeneity and multiplicity of epitopes in most Ags, and of the heterogeneity of antibodies in antisera directed against such Ags, Eqs. 14 and 15a and b are oversimplifications. Thus, K_a and K_d should rather be considered to be practical constants, reflecting the average of all the subreactions involved, in all cases except the ideal situation of the reaction of a monovalent hapten with a monoclonal Ab.

Free Energies of Interaction. Once the practical equilibrium association constant, K_a, has been determined, the total free energy change, $\Delta\Gamma^{TOT}$, of the complete reaction can be derived:

$$\Delta G^{TOT} = -RT \ln K_a \tag{16}$$

where R is the gas constant (1.986×10^{-3} kcal, or 8.3144×10^7 erg, or 8.3144 J, per degree Kelvin per mole) and T is the absolute temperature in degrees of Kelvin. It should be emphasized, however that, strictly speaking, Eq. 16 is only valid for standard conditions; i.e., for those cases where unit molar concentrations* of both Ag and Ab were used, and is formally expressed as:

$$\delta\Gamma^\circ = -PT \, \lambda\nu \, K_2^\circ \Delta G^\circ = -RT \ln K_2^\circ \tag{16a}$$

(where the superscripts $^\circ$ indicate that standard conditions prevailed). When the binding energy between single Ag and Ab *molecules* is to be derived, the gas constant, R, must be divided by Avogadro's number, i.e., by 6.022×10^{23}, to obtain Boltzmann's constant, k, so that then:

$$\Delta G = -kT \ln K_a \tag{17}$$

where k is 1.38×10^{-16} erg per degree, or 1.38×10^{-23} J per degree. All association equilibrium constants, K_a (Eqs. 15a and b, 16, 16a, and 17), are expressed in liters per mole; Σ (LM^{-1}); the dissociation constant, K_2° is expressed in moles per liter (ML^{-1}). By measuring K_a at two or more different temperatures, the enthalpy, ΔH, can be calculated:

$$\frac{d \ln K_a}{dt} = \frac{\Delta H}{RT^2} \tag{18}$$

which allows the determination of the entropy, ΔS, by means of van't Hoff's equation:

$$\Delta G^{TOT} = \Delta H - T\Delta S \tag{19}$$

Another way of obtaining just ΔH is via microcalorimetry. If K_a is determined at several temperatures, Eqs. 18 and 19 yield ΔG and ΔS. ΔG, as derived from K_a, usually is expressed in kilocalories per mole, but it can also be expressed in unites of ergs per square centimeter (of mJ/m^2) provided the contactable surface area of the epitope(s) (and of the paratope[s]) is known. ΔG^{TOT} comprises $\Delta G^{LW} + \Delta G^{AB} + \Delta G^{EL}$. If one measures ΔH by equilibrium determinations (yielding K) at different temperatures using Eq. 18, it is advisable to do such determinations at three different temperatures (35).

Contrary to general belief, the binding constant, K_a, as measured by the usual methods, is *not* an invariable parameter uniquely characteristic of a given Ag-Ab reaction. For example, at optimal Ag-Ab ratios, K_a of the BSA–anti-BSA reaction increases from 1.7×10^7 LM^{-1} to 6.5×10^{11} LM^{-1} on 100-fold dilution of both reagents (2). While this increase is undoubtedly due, in part, to the polyclonality of the Ab (where, of course, at greater dilution the higher-affinity Abs are the principal Abs that still bind), this trend will persist even with monoclonal Abs (2). Thus, it must be faced that many, if not most, of the published K_a values for various Ag-Ab (or Ig receptor) interactions reflect the *dilution* at which the measurements were done more stror.,ly than an actual unique binding constant that might be held to be a characteristic property of the system under study. For instance, the high K_a

---

*These are the "standard conditions." Unless otherwise stated, ambient pressure, temperature, and pH are held to be kept constant. It should be realized that owing to the high molecular weight of all Abs and most Ags, unit molar concentrations are not attainable in practice.

values published for the binding of IgE to Fc receptors on basophils and mast cells (44) would be more a function of the very low IgE concentrations which one is normally forced to utilize than of an intrinsically high K_a.

The best solution for obtaining reasonably reliable K_a values, notwithstanding the strong influence of the volume in which the reaction occurs, is to follow the rules given by Van Regenmortel and Hardie (45), which include operating under constant conditions of the percentage of occupied binding sites (e.g., 50% binding sites occupied) and measuring at a wide range of reagent concentrations.

2. Affinity and Avidity

In defining Ab affinity and Ab avidity, it is best to follow Steward (46), who defines affinity as a thermodynamic expression of the binding energy of an antibody-active site for its homologous antigenic determinant. "Experimentally this term has its most precise application in monovalent hapten-anti-hapten systems" (46) and, it should be added, especially when the antibody is monoclonal. Although avidity is based on affinity, it also involves factors such as Ab valency, Ag valency, Ab heterogeneity, and differences in antigenic determinants of a given Ag. ΔG^{TOT} (Eqs. 16 and 19) stands for the affinity of a monoclonal antihapten Ab toward its homologous monovalent hapten, and, in general, for the *affinity* of a monoclonal Ab toward a solitary nonrepeating epitope on a given Ab. However, ΔG^{TOT} can also express the *avidity* of a *family of antibodies* (of one immunoglobulin class; e.g., IgG) toward their (plurivalent) Ag. To distinguish between these two thermodynamic expressions, it may be prudent to label them ΔG_{AFF}^{TOT} and ΔG_{AV}^{TOT}, respectively. Karush (43) calls these two binding energies *intrinsic affinity* and *functional affinity*, respectively (see also ref. 47).

3. Kinetics

The kinetics of the reaction

$$Ag + Ab \underset{k_{21}}{\overset{k_{12}}{\rightleftharpoons}} Ag\ Ab \tag{20}$$

can be determined with temperature-jump relaxation and stopped-flow techniques (48). In hapten-Ab systems the rate constants of *association* are very high (of the order of $k_{12} \approx 10^6$ to 10^8 LM^{-1}/sec). The values of k_{12} do not vary greatly; in most cases, they tend to be of the same order of magnitude. The kinetic constants are related to the binding constant as:

$$K_a = \frac{k_{12}}{k_{21}} \tag{21}$$

Thus, binding constants are mainly determined by the much more variable and much slower *dissociation* rate constants, k_{21} (40–42,49).

4. Measurement Methods*

Theory. The methods for measuring the equilibrium constant (K) of Ag-Ab interactions generally depend on the accurate determination of free and bound forms of the antigen under conditions in which the total antibody concentration is kept constant or is known if varied. The methods for determining these concentrations are described below. Results of the binding experiments are usually analyzed by means of standard Scatchard plots (40,42,47,50) derived from the law of mass action (Eq. 15a). The equations normally used for thermodynamic calculations, using the data from such binding experiments, are not given here; they can be found in Refs. 40 and 41. It should be noted that by the various approaches for plotting the

*Most of the material discussed in this section is based on ref. 40.

data (40,47), K_a can be found, as well as the antibody valency, the antigen valency, and the (Sips) antibody heterogeneity index.

Experimental Approaches. Many techniques are available for determining the binding constants of a particular Ag-Ab interaction. The thermodynamic estimations of Ab affinity require the accurate determination of the concentration of the free and bound Ag or Ab under conditions that do not disturb the equilibrium of the Ag-Ab interaction. In general, quantitation of the required free and bound antigen or antibody concentrations is achieved either physically through the separation of the bound and free components by hemagglutination, dialysis, selective precipitation, centrifugation, gel filtration, or chemically by utilizing changes in the properties of the antigen or antibody (e.g., fluorescence) which occur as a result of binding.

Quantitative Hemagglutination. Quantitative hemagglutination may be done "manually" by hemocytometry or automatically by electronic particle counting. The first work on quantitative hemagglutination was done in the 1940s and 1950s by Wurmser and Filitti-Wurmser (51), who obtained K_a and ΔH values for the ABO blood group system (by measuring concentrations of free blood group antibody as well as concentrations of blood group antibody bound to RBCs of various blood groups, by hemocytometry, at different temperatures). However, the ΔH and ΔS values they obtained for A and B blood group antibodies in homo- and heterozygous systems are open to question because in the 1940s and 1950s an insufficiently precise notion existed about the molecular weights of the various classes of antibodies (so that their assumed antibody concentrations, in moles per liter, were erroneous, and they did not know whether they worked with IgG or IgM class antibodies). Steane (52) reviewed the more recent publications on binding energies of various blood group Abs by quantitative hemagglutination using hemocytometry. Steane (52) also treats the automated approach to quantitative hemagglutination and discusses in particular the results obtained with the ABH and the D and c blood group systems, including the influence of various treatments of the RBCs (e.g., enzymes, polybasic molecules) (see also Sect. IV.A.5.2).

Equilibrium Dialysis and Ultrafiltration. When the antigen is much smaller than the antibody molecule (particularly when hapten-antibody interactions are studied), equilibrium dialysis or ultrafiltration with the aid of a membrane that is permeable to the antigen (or hapten) and impermeable to both the antibody molecules and the antigen-antibody (or hapten-antibody) complexes are the methods most often used. Because of the antibody heterogeneity, such experiments are generally performed using a range of antigen concentrations and a consistent antibody concentration or vice versa.

At equilibrium, the concentration of unbound antigen (or hapten) should be the same on both sides of the partitioning membrane. The amount of hapten on the antibody side of the membrane then represents the total concentration of the free plus bound hapten. By subtraction, the amount of bound antigen (hapten) can be calculated and, from these equilibrium constants, may be obtained (7,28,47).

Precipitation Methods. When the antigen is soluble under conditions where the antibody molecule and hence antigen-antibody complexes are insoluble (e.g., 50% saturated $[NH_4]_2SO_4$ solution, 8% polyethylene glycol), usable data can be obtained. The required concentrations of free and bound components can readily be determined by evaluating the precipitates and supernatants after precipitation. This technique is generally employed when the antigen can be radiolabeled (39). The method is useful for rapid estimations of affinity, has the advantage of not requiring purified antibody, and gives results that compare well with those obtained using equilibrium dialysis. However, for purely electrostatic Ag-Ab complexes, such as DNA–anti-DNA, the use of high salt concentrations is not indicated as the medium- and low-affinity complexes tend to dissociate at high ionic strengths (34).

At equivalent Ag:Ab ratios, equilibrium constants, and thus ΔG, may be obtained by precipitate formation in tubes. It then suffices to have either Ag or Ab radioactively or otherwise labeled to derive [Ag-Ab], as well as [Ag] and [Ab], because at equivalence [Ag] = [Ab] (53).

Analytical Ultracentrifugation.   Analytical ultracentrifugation can be used to yield equilibrium constant values for a variety of antigen-antibody systems (28). The method relies on the fact that antigens, antibodies, and Ag-Ab complexes have different sedimentation velocities so that, upon separation in a gravitation field, they will separate and the amount of each can be quantitated optically (e.g., with schlieren optics) as the surface area under each peak.

Gel Filtration or Sieving.   This technique relies on the molecular weights of the antigen, antibody, and Ag-Ab being different. Consequently, they will elute separately upon gel filtration, thereby permitting an evaluation of the various concentrations. This technique requires that the eluent contain a constant concentration of one of the reagents so as not to disturb the equilibrium; it is generally performed in conditions of antigen excess.

Insoluble Antigen.   When one is dealing with insoluble antigens (e.g., blood group antigens on the surfaces of erythrocytes or antigen covalently coupled to an insoluble matrix [e.g., polystyrene latex]), the amounts of free or bound radio- or fluorescent-labeled antibody can easily be obtained by simple centrifugation, to obtain K values. Hughes-Jones (54–56) used this approach with erythrocytes and radiolabeled Ab to obtain K_a values for the D and c blood group antigens.

Affinity Methods.   Affinity methods, such as affinity electrophoresis (57,58) and affinity diffusion (35,53), depend on the degree to which, for example, Ag, when migrating into an Ab-containing gel, slows down as a function of Ab concentration. The *dissociation* constant, K_d, can be obtained according to

$$\frac{D_0}{D_i} = 1 + \frac{C_i}{K_d} \tag{22}$$

where D_0 is the electrophoretic mobility (or diffusion coefficient) of Ag in the gel without Ab and D_i the electrophoretic mobility (or diffusion coefficient) of Ag in the gel at Ab concentration C_i. When D_0/D_i is plotted on the ordinate versus C_i on the abscissa, one finds $-K_d$ at the intercept of the (straight) line of the function with the abscissa or $1/K_d$ as the slope of the line. The zero Ab concentration diffusion coefficient (D_0) of Ag is found by extrapolation to zero Ab concentration (53). One can obtain K_d (Eq. 15b) only in ideal (totally homogeneous) systems, with Ags with only one specificity of antigenic determinant, and with monoclonal Abs (in which case one would not expect precipitation to occur). With heterogeneous Ag-Ab systems, one finds K_d values (at least with affinity electrophoresis and diffusion methods visualized by an advancing precipitation front) that are several decimal orders of magnitude lower than those found via precipitation in tubes, as one tends mainly to measure the components with the highest K_d value (53). A further reason for the different values found with affinity and equilibrium systems lies in the fact that affinity methods are kinetic systems, where one does not wait for complete equilibrium to set in, so that secondary interactions (see Sect. III.D) may not have had time enough to occur. It is clear that, in the BSA–anti-BSA system, affinity diffusion results also reflect "hydrophobic" interactions; these occur even at pH 9.5, where electrostatic interactions in this system are largely inoperative (35).

Fluorescence.   Fluorescence provides a marker by which the behavior of a fluorescent molecule in a complex mixture can be studied. Fluroescence intensity is strongly influenced by local molecular environment. Changes in fluorescence can provide sensitive and precise information about intermolecular complex formation (e.g., Ag-Ab interactions) (28).

Fluorescence Quenching.   Antibody molecules have a natural fluorescence derived mainly from tryptophan residues in the molecule. When some nonfluorescing haptens bind with the Ab, they cause this fluorescence to decrease. From the relative extents of quenching, the amount of hapten bound by a specifically purified can be calculated and a value for K_a obtained (28). A similar principle can be employed in the case of haptens whose fluorescence is enhanced when they are bound to an Ab. In contrast to the above, however, this method allows impure Ab preparations to be used and values of K_a for weakly bound haptens can also be determined. Kinetic measurements by the temperature-jump method can also be done by spectrofluorometry (59).

Fluorescence Polarization. Fluorescent solutions which are excited with vertically polarized or natural light emit partially polarized fluorescence as viewed at right angles to the incident beam. Polarization of fluorescence is due to the fixed relationship between molecular orientation and absorption and emission of fluorescence. If a small fluorescent hapten is bound by an Ab, there will be marked reduction in the rotational freedom of the hapten and a corresponding increase in polarization. Again, it is possible to obtain relative values of the extent of fluorescence polarization for 100% unbound Ag and to compare these with the extent of polarization for bound haptens and thereby establish equilibrium constants (28,40,41). The common labeling reagents for protein Ags are fluorescein isothiocyanate, rhodamine, and dimethylaminonaphthalenesulfonyl chloride.

Immunoassay Methods. Radioimmunoassay and enzyme immunoassay methods can also be applied to obtain K_a values (see, e.g., ref. 60).

Hapten Inhibition Methods. Several methods exist for obtaining relative values of K_a for both strongly and weakly bound haptens relative to a reference hapten. If the absolute value of K_a for the reference hapten is known from measurements by one of the methods described above, absolute K_a values can be calculated from the relative K_a values. Such methods include hapten inhibition of Ag-Ab precipitation (28,65), hapten inhibition of complement fixation, and several other competitive reactions where the hapten competes with the antigen for binding to the Ab.

Microcalorimetry. Microcalorimetry is the direct way of measuring Ag-Ab binding enthalpies, ΔH; in contrast to the two-temperature method (28,35). By the "batch" microcalorimetric approach one measures, for example, the heat output (in microcalories per second) versus time during the course of an Ag-Ab reaction (61). More versatile and simpler to operate is the flow calorimeter (62), which also records microcalories per second versus time, but which is more suitable for operation with small volumes (≤ 10 ml), with greater ease of mixing and allowing direct determination of ΔH of the reagents, reacting in many different ratios, in a short time (63).

Interfacial Free Energies. Interfacial free energies, obtained by measurement (or estimation) of the surface tensions of the antigenic determinant and the antibody-active site of a purely polar (AB) Ag-Ab system, can give the upper and the lower limits of the free energy of binding; for example, in the dextran-antidextran system (64). Measurement of the surface tensions of double-stranded DNA and of anti-DNA antibodies permits one to determine that the polar (AB) + apolar (LW) components of the reaction energy of the DNA–anti-DNA are so low as to be practically negligible; that system can thus be regarded as a rare example of a purely electrostatic Ag-Ab system (34).

Other Methods. Other methods that utilize disturbances in quantum levels of atoms to indicate energy changes brought about by antigen-antibody binding include nuclear magnetic resonance (NMR) and electron spin resonance (ESR) (28,65).

Via dilatometry, the volume changes (ΔV) occurring during Ag-Ab reactions can be measured. These volume changes go through a maximum when optimal Ag-Ab ratios are reached in nonstoichiometric precipitating systems, whereas hapten-antihapten systems reach a plateau value when saturation is reached. There is a certain proportionality between plateau ΔV values and K_a (66).

5. Order of Magnitude of Ag-Ab Binding Parameters

Order of Magnitude of K_a, k_{12}, k_{21}, *and* ΔG. In general, K_a can vary from 10^3 to 10^{12} LM^{-1} and ΔG from -4 to -13 kcal/mol (40–42). As most Ag-Ab reactions are exothermic, ΔH tends to be negative (usually from 0 to -10 kcal/mol). ΔS can vary from -40 to $+80$ entropy units per degree mole (or calories/degree mole); more often than not, ΔS is positive (for the exceptional case of the $D(Rh_0)$–anti-D system, see below).

As stated in Section III.C.3, the kinetic association constant, k_{12}, is fairly constant, at 10^6 to $10^8 LM^{-1} sec^{-1}$; k_{21} varies much more; from 10^4 to $10^{-4} sec^{-1}$ (40–42). Thus, it is the hypervariable kinetic dissociation rate constant, k_{21}, which causes the variability in K_a (see Eq. 21).

The energies of formation found in Ag-Ab interactions (and in hapten-antihapten interactions) agree well with the order of magnitude of the (relatively weak) physical bonds involved in such reactions. Covalent bonds have higher energies of formation (ΔG of the order of -10 to $-1,000$ kcal/mol).

The wide variability of K_a does *not* correspond to a great variability in ΔG of Ag-Ab interactions. It should be remembered that ΔG is a function of the (natural) logarithm of K_a (see, e.g., Eq. 17; thus, when K_a varies from 10^3 to $10^9 LM^{-1}$, this corresponds only to a variation in ΔG from -6.9 kT to -20.7 kT, or just a threefold increase). Similarly, in terms of kilocalories per mole, ΔG usually varies only between -4 and -12 kcal/mole.

Enthalpic and Entropic Contributions to ΔG. LW, AB, and EL interactions are predominantly enthalpic (13), so that in the attractive Ag-Ab interactions, ΔH generally has a negative value. In the exceptional case where ΔH is *positive*, as in the D–anti-D reaction (67), one must suspect the occurrence of a local phase change (e.g., the "melting" of a lipid moiety), which agrees well with the apparently irreversible denaturation of the D-antigenic site following the D–anti-D reaction (68) (see also Good and Wood [69], who observed that contrary to the A–anti-A and B–anti-B reactions, the D–anti-D interaction appears to be mainly entropy driven).

In most typical Ag-Ab interactions, as the temperature increases, ΔH becomes less negative, while $T.\Delta S$ proportionally increases, leaving ΔG approximately unchanged (see Eq. 19) (35,70). This phenomenon is known as an enthalpy-entropy compensation. It is mainly due to the fact that with an increase in temperature (T)-H bonds (and also EL bonds) become weaker. This gives rise to two phenomena:

1. With an increase in T, there is a *decrease* in the AB ("hydrophobic") and EL binding energies, which are mainly enthalpic* (ΔH).
2. With an increase in T, there is a *decrease in hydration* (which is also due to the decrease in ΔG^{AB}). This gives rise to a decrease in the distance ℓ between epitope and paratope, which thus in its turn causes a largely compensating *increase* in ΔG (cf. Eqs. 1, 8, and 9). This decrease in hydration also is concomitant with a decrease in the number of oriented ("organized") molecules of water of hydration, which manifests itself as an *increase in entropy* ($T\Delta S$).

In many cases, an increase in T, therefore, causes a decrease in ΔH, which is more or less exactly counterbalanced by an increase in $T.\Delta S$ (Eq. 19), leaving ΔG largely unchanged in Ag-Ab interactions.

6. The Law of Mass Action

The law of mass action (Eq. 15a and also pertaining to Eq. 14 or 20) implies that when one changes the Ab (or the Ag) concentration, the amount of Ag-Ab complex also will change. For

---

*Contrary to popular belief, the "hydrophobic" interaction energy is more often than not predominantly *enthalpic*; this is especially the case with the interaction energy between low-energy molecules, which are slightly polar (13).

instance, if (at constant Ag concentration) one decreases the Ab concentration, the amount of Ag-Ab complex formed also will decrease, and if one increases the Ab concentration, the amount of Ag-Ab formed will increase. The same applies to other systems; one pertinent example is the reaction in vivo between the Fc moieties of IgG (Fc) and the Fc receptors (R) of phagocytic leukocytes. The binding constant, K_a, for Fc-R is of the order of 10^6 to 10^8 L/M (71,44). In circulating blood, phagocytic R is bound fairly strongly to IgG, which is normally present in high concentrations, so that it is unlikely that Fc-R–mediated interactions between rather sparse sensitized particles and phagocytes takes place in the *blood stream* to any significant degree. However, in the *spleen*, where Fc-R–mediated interactions play a more important role, the situation is different due to higher cell, and concomitantly lower IgG, concentrations as well as to high local macrophage concentrations (with high densities of R per cell). Thus, Fc-R–mediated interactions between sensitized cells and phagocytes are much more strongly favored in the spleen than in the vascular blood circulation (72). For instance, autoimmune RBC destruction by phagocytes mainly takes place in the spleen and only slightly in the peripheral blood circulation. In the same manner, it is easily understood why depleted blood IgG levels (achieved, e.g., by absorption of peripheral IgG by protein A columns) can have therapeutic antitumor effects in vivo (73), as that treatment causes an increase in free R, which favors their interaction with specific antitumor antibodies of the IgG3 subclass, which are not removed by protein A and have the strongest affinity to R of the four IgG subclasses (72). Conversely, it also becomes easy to understand how massive increases in circulating IgG, brought about by multiple transfusions of gamma globulin solutions, causes a significant (usually temporary) amelioration in the clinical course of autoimmune thrombocytopenic purpura and in autoimmune neutropenia because the sensitized platelets or neutrophils of these patients are less readily destroyed by their phagocytic cells as long as the phagocytes' R are swamped by a large increase in circulating IgG (72). It also becomes clear why the interaction in vitro of Rh_0 (D)–positive human RBCs sensitized with IgG class anti-Rh_0 (D) antibodies, with the Fc-R or monocytes, strongly decreases in the presence of increased concentrations of ambient IgG (72). It is also obvious from Eq. 15a that simple centrifugal washing of phagocytes will more strongly favor detachment of monomeric immunoglobulins the lower the value of K_a. At very high K_a values (of the order of 10^{10}), removal of immunoglobulin (e.g., IgE) by washing becomes virtually impossible (72). Measurement of (Fc) and (Fc-R) done at different dilutions can yield values for K_a as well as for the total number of R per cell, even if R is unknown (72). It should be emphasized that the above considerations are as applicable to antigen-antibody interactions as to other ligand-receptor interactions.

7. *Affinity of Monoclonal and Polyclonal Abs*

Usually, the affinity of monoclonal Abs (MAbs) to a given epitope is lower than that of polyclonal Abs (PAbs) to the same epitope. A lower K_a value of MAbs to multivalent Ags (comprising several different epitopes) is to be expected on account of the lack of cooperative cross-linking that would otherwise prevail with the help of the different paratopes of PAbs. This drawback of MAbs can be overcome by using mixtures of two or more MAbs specific for different epitopes of the same Ag. Single MAbs do not form immune precipitates with Ags, but immunoprecipitation does become possible with mixtures of two or more MAbs (74). Single MAbs, however, can form immune precipitates with large Ags (e.g., plant viruses) with repeating identical epitopes (75). In such cases, however, the distinction between immune precipitation and agglutination becomes hazy and clearly hemagglutination with MAbs is entirely feasible.

The apparent lower affinity (expressed as K_a) of MAbs, in comparison with PAbs, however, is mainly due to the fact that, when measuring K_a of PAbs, one actually mainly measures the K_a of the PAb *components* with the highest affinity even though such high-affinity PAb *components* represent only a small fraction of the total. In other words, high-affinity PAb components are rather rare, as are high-affinity MAbs. Bankert et al. (76) observed that various MAbs directed against 4-azophthalate have a fairly wide array of binding constants (ranging from 4×10^4 to 4×10^7 LM^{-1}), the highest value of which compares well with the higher values obtained, in general, with polyclonal Abs against haptens (77).

8. Influence of Brownian Motion

Regardless of its size, every single detached molecule, cell, or particle (with three degrees of freedom), immersed in a liquid, is endowed with a Brownian energy (ΔG^{BR}) of $+1.5$ kT (78). This repulsive energy helps to keep it in solution or suspension provided the energy of attraction between similar molecules or particles immersed in that liquid is significantly less than -1.5 kT per pair of molecules or particles (see also ref. 79).

For example, a hapten that can react with its specific paratope with an attractive energy ($\Delta G^{LW} + \Delta G^{AB} + \Delta G^{EL}$) of -10 mJ/m^2, and that has a contactable surface area, S_c, of about 0.4 nm^2, undergoes an energy of attraction to the paratope of -1.0 kT, which however then is exactly counterbalanced by a repulsive Brownian energy of $+1.0$ kT (given that in the course of detachment, the hapten may be estimated to have only two degrees of freedom). This then allows the hapten to detach again (on an average) as often as it becomes attached, as the condition is fulfilled here where $\Delta G^{TOT} = \Delta G^{LW} + \Delta G^{AB} + \Delta G^{EL} + \Delta G^{BR} = 0$, so that $K_a = K_d = 1$, and $k_{12} = k_{21}$ (cf. Eqs. 15a, 17, and 21). Thus, small haptens usually need to be attracted to a specific paratope with energies greater than ≈ 10 mJ/m^2. On the other hand, large epitopes, with a contactable surface area $S_c \approx 6.0$ nm^2, which undergo the same attraction to their paratope of -10 mJ/m^2 will, on a molecular scale, be attracted to that paratope with an energy ($\Delta G^{LW} + \Delta G^{AB} + \Delta G^{EL}$) of -15.0 kT. This easily overcomes the Brownian repulsion, $\Delta G^{BR} = +1.0$ kT, so that it will remain rather strongly attached. The condition of $\Delta G^{TOT} = -15.0 + 1.0 = -14.0$ kT gives rise to an equilibrium constant $K_a = 1.2 \times 10^6$ LM^{-1} (see Eq. 17). Thus, while small epitopes need a high-binding energy to overcome the Brownian repulsion and remain attached to their paratope, large epitopes require a much smaller binding energy per unit surface area.

It is clear that it can often be advantageous to express the free energies of Ag-Ab interaction ($\Delta G^{LW} + \Delta G^{AB} + \Delta G^{EL}$) in kT units (Eq. 17); i.e., to express these values on a molecular rather than on a molar level. In so doing, the degree of attractive energy between Ag and Ab can immediately be estimated in relation to the disruptive energy of the Brownian motion, which has a fixed value of about $+1$ kT.

When the total free energy is measured directly (see Sect. III.G.4), the influence of the brownian motion energy is always included; i.e., $\Delta G^{TOT} = \Delta G^{LW} + \Delta G^{AB} + \Delta G^{EL} + \Delta G^{BR}$.

D. Ag-Ab Association and Dissociation

1. Primary and Secondary Bonds: Hysteresis

Primary Bonds. The *specificity* of the bonds between epitope and paratope is principally due to the interactions that occur very early during the Ag-Ab binding process. The early attraction between epitope and paratope while these moieties are still some distance apart results in the primary bond. The distance at which epitope and paratope start attracting each other to a significant degree is somewhat less than 100 Å for electrostatic (EL) and polar (AB or "hydrophobic") interactions (41). However, while the specificity of Ag-Ab interactions is mainly linked to the primary bond, in many cases, the primary bond energy is significantly smaller than the total (primary + secondary) bond energy (21,35,41,42,80).

The primary bond energy can be determined by measuring the energy required to prevent the bond from forming. A few examples of primary bonds can be given. First, to prevent bovine serum albumin (BSA) from reacting with anti-BSA, it suffices to raise the pH from 7.0 to 9.5 (35). However, to *dissociate* BSA–anti-BSA complexes, once formed, it is necessary to raise the pH to 9.5 *and* to add 9.7 M ethylene glycol (80). In a purely polar system, to prevent the interaction between 3-azopyridine (P3), coupled to rabbit serum albumin, with rabbit anti-P3, it suffices to add 1.9 M dimethyl sulfoxide (DMSO), but the energy needed to *dissociate* anti-P3 from P3 requires the admixture of 6.4 M DMSO (80).

In exclusively electrostatic systems, on the other hand (e.g., low- and medium-affinity DNA–anti-DNA systems) (34,81), no difference could be measured between the primary and the total energy of association, as deducted from the equality between the energies of dissociation and of prevention of association.

While primary bonds of the sole Lifshitz–van der Waals variety are virtually nonexistent, instances where the other bond types occur as the sole primary bond are common: (1) primary polar (or "hydrophobic") bonds: P3–anti-P3 (the hapten 3 - azopyridine) and dextran-antidextran; and (2) primary electrostatic bonds: BSA–anti-BSA, and idiotype–anti-idiotype (40–42).

Secondary Bonds; Hysteresis. The much greater energy usually needed for dissociating most Ag-Ab bonds than is required for the prevention of their association (hysteresis) is due to the existence of further secondary bonds that have formed subsequent to the formation of the initial primary Ag-Ab bonds. The difference between the energy of dissociation and the energy required to prevent association of Ag from Ab is equal to the energy of the secondary Ag-Ab bonds. Thus, the energy of the secondary bond (ΔG_{sec}) is obtained as follows (42):

$$\Delta G_{sec} = \Delta G_{dissociation} - \Delta G_{prevention\ of\ association} = \Delta G_{total} - \Delta G_{primary} \qquad (23)$$

Electrostatic bonds rarely occur as secondary bonds. The purely electrostatic DNA–anti-DNA system has been studied from this aspect: The similarities of pH conditions, leading to dissociation or to prevention of association (lack of hysteresis), points to an absence of secondary electrostatic bonds in this system (see above [81]). Secondary electrostatic bonds are likely to be rare occurrences, as the probability of negatively and positively charged amino acids on Ag and Ab (outside of the epitope and paratope) being situated precisely opposite each other is very slight and, in those rare cases where it might occur, such moities would be indistinguishable from the epitope and paratope, and such an Ag-Ab system simply would behave as a system with somewhat larger than usual epitopes and paratopes.

Polar (AB or "hydrophobic") interactions are the most common bonds involved in secondary Ag-Ab bonding. As soon as epitope and paratope have combined in a primary bond, various nonspecific (especially nonpolar) moieties of Ag and/or Ab in the immediate vicinity of epitope and paratope can undergo a "hydrophobic" attraction, approach each other even more closely, and then bind to each other secondarily. Thus, both in cases where the primary bond is mainly polar (e.g., P3–anti-P3) (80) *and* where the primary bond is largely electrostatic (BSA–anti-BSA) (35), secondary bonds of the (AB) "hydrophobic" type almost invariably develop.

With time, a further strengthening of existing (primary as well as secondary) bonds of all categories takes place through the extrusion of interstitial solvent. This results in a shorter distance between epitope and paratope, which considerably enhances the interfacial attraction energy (cf. Eqs. 1, 9, and 13).

2. Conditions Favoring Ag-Ab Association or Dissociation

The conditions favoring association of Ag with Ab usually are, at least qualitatively, the inverse of the conditions favoring their dissociation. For the sake of simplicity it therefore suffices to describe only the various conditions by which dissociation of Ag-Ab complexes can be achieved (see Table 3).

Dissociation usually is most readily achieved by *combining* the admixture of a strong electron-donor organic solvent (e.g., DMSO, ethylene glycol, propanol) to the liquid medium, with an increase (or in some cases with a drastic decrease) in pH (21,42,80). Only relatively weak, purely electrostatic systems dissociate well by just increasing the ionic strength; in systems with mainly "hydrophobic" bonding, however, raising the ionic strength tends to be counterproductive (because high-salt concentrations cause dehydration, which in its turn causes a further increase in surface "hydrophobicity"). Addition of chaotropic salts, on the other hand, favors dissociation of both "hydrophobic" and electrostatic bonds (42) because they have the capacity of increasing the ionic strength as well as of opening up, or of displacing, hydrogen bonds, and thus of dissociating bonds due to "hydrophobic" interactions.

Elution of blood group Abs from RBCs (anti-A, anti-K, anti-D) using the combined DMSO and increased pH approach has been described by van Oss et al. (68), who reviewed some other blood group Ab elution methods. Helmerhorst et al. (82) described the efficiency of various Ab elution approaches (including elution with DMSO *and* pH 9.5; elution at pH 2.8; elution by heating at 56°C; elution with ether), for the elution of granulocyte, platelet, and HLA Abs. Finally, a large number of cases of conditions favoring Ag-Ab dissociation as well as the prevention of Ag-Ab formation were listed by Absolom and van Oss (42), including a number of blood group Ag-Ab systems.

3. Effect of Temperature

It has already been shown that quite often an increase in temperature causes no significant change in ΔG due to the enthalpy-entropy compensatory effect discussed earlier (Sect. C.5.b.).

However, it should be remembered that, other factors remaining equal, a small decrease in $\Delta G^{TOT}/kT$ due to an increase in temperature can result in a more pronounced decrease in K_a (Eq. 17). For instance, an increase in temperature from 20 to 50°C, for an initial value of ΔG^{TOT} of −16 kT (which then becomes reduced to −14.5 kT), results in a 4.4-fold decrease in K_a from 8.9×10^6 LM^{-1} to 2.0×10^6 LM^{-1}. In Ag-Ab reactions, however, other factors do not necessarily remain equal when the temperature increases.

In about 30% of the cases, it proved possible to elute granulocyte or platelet Abs by heating to 56° for 60 minutes (82).

4. Effect of Other Factors

Time. With the lapse of time, the Ag-Ab bond becomes stronger due to secondary interactions. Thus, if one aims at *dissociation* (e.g., with a view to an affinity separation step), it is advantageous to effect the dissociation procedure *as soon as possible* after the Ag-Ab has taken place (see Table 3).

Haptens. The admixture of haptens (Hp), which are identical to the epitope of an Ag in a given Ag-Ab system, will tend to cause a dissociation of Ag-Ab in favor or the association of Hp-Ab. This phenomenon can be used to advantage, especially in dissociating lectin–blood group epitope bonds by means of the addition of the lectin-specific sugar (see Table 3).

Influence of Strong Electron Donor Polymers. Strong electron donor polymers such as polyethylene glycol (PEG) at concentrations of about 3–10% (v/v) will repel most other polymers in aqueous solutions (e.g., serum proteins). This causes an incipient phase separation, which then pushes the proteins into a smaller volume and also partly dehydrates them. This effect favors Ag-Ab association; i.e., the formation of Ag-Ab complexes. However, care must be taken not to overdo the effect because free immunoglobulins will start to precipitate at only slightly higher PEG concentrations than needed for Ag-Ab association (see Table 3).

Influence of Strong Dehydrating Agents. The addition of $(NH_4)_2SO_4$ in molar concentrations will favor the insolubilization of Ag-Ab complexes, through dehydration, especially by enhancing the "hydrophobic" (AB) attraction and by decreasing the distance between epitope and paratope (as also with PEG, see above). However, when the Ag-Ab system is exclusively electrostatic, $(NH_4)_2SO_4$ on the contrary will tend to *dissociate* such complexes (see Sect. II.F.3 and see Table 3).

Dilution. Dilution favors Ag-Ab dissociation, especially of the lower affinity components, although K_a may increase as dilution favors the higher affinity Abs (2). An electric field (electrophoresis) applied to, e.g., Ag-Ab complexes associated with an Ab fixed to an immobilized carrier, will favor dissociation when the Ag can be electrophoretically removed from (and prevented from returning to) the fixed Ab. In such cases, obeying the law of mass action (Eqs. 14 and 15a), continuous removal of one of the reagents (Ag) by electrophoresis (i.e., through artificial dilution of one of the participants) displaces the equilibrium depicted in Eq. 14 to the left, leading to dissociation.

IV. HEMAGGLUTINATION

A. Mechanism of Agglutination

1. Mechanism

Agglutination is the destabilization of a stable suspension* of antigenic particles by cross-linking them with Abs directed to their epitopes. Because destabilization of antigenic particles can be detected with a rather small volume (as little as 0.1 ml of a dilute particle suspension) and because relatively few Ab molecules suffice to achieve destabilization, agglutination is an exceptionally sensitive method for detecting small amounts of antibody (as small as a nanogram). The dimension of antigenic particles used in agglutination may range from a few nanometer to about 10 μm in diameter. Antigenic particles may be cells (e.g., RBCs, bacteria, etc.) carrying their native epitopes or inert particles (e.g., polymer latices) to which antigenic molecules have been adsorbed or covalently attached).

2. Visualization

Sedimentation Velocity. The force resisting sedimentation of a particle or cell in a liquid medium is proportional to its radius, R, while the force inducing sedimentation is proportional to R^3. The net force causing sedimentation is therefore proportional to R^2. Thus, when agglutination causes an increase in linear size by a factor x, the clumps will sediment x^2 times faster than the initial monodispersed cells. For instance, single human erythrocytes, suspended in saline water, sediment at a rate of about 1 cm/hr at ambient gravity, while clumps of agglutinated erythrocytes, comprising an average of 30 cross-linked cells, sediment 1 cm in about 6 min under the same conditions. The visual observation of a 10-fold increase in sedimentation rate of a RBC suspension in a test tube may, therefore, be considered an indication of significant agglutination. The same holds true for accelerated sedimentation in a centrifuge, but as most cells (especially large cells such as erythrocytes) sediment rather quickly, even at relatively low gravitational (g) forces, centrifugation has its usefulness mainly by means of the inspection of the physical properties of sedimented packed agglutinates rather than by observation of the actual sedimentation rate, which is difficult to measure under normal circumstances.

Physical Properties of Agglutinates. When cells (agglutinated or otherwise) have been sedimented by centrifugation, there are a number of ways of recognizing agglutination macroscopically: by the difference in adherence to the rounded bottom of the test tube and by

---

*A suspension of particles or cells is deemed to be "stable" when the particles remain detached from each other through the action of net repulsive forces. Stable particles may *sediment* but they will not agglomerate, agglutinate, or otherwise destabilize or clump without further outside intervention.

the difference in dispersability that may be observed while resuspending the sedimented cells (e.g., by shaking).

Nonagglutinated, monodispersed cells or particles pack very tightly when forced to the bottom of a test tube by centrifugation. Thus, nonagglutinated cells are deposited in a small, round, sharply delineated "button" at the bottom of the tube. Agglutinated cells, on the other hand, form large, open network structures of many cells attached to each other at a few points only; such large agglutinates will not pack tightly, so that they will deposit on and adhere to the entire hemispherical inner surface of the bottom of the test tube. In those cases where too few cells are available for visual inspection of the deposited clumps, resuspension of the cells may be attempted; e.g., by vigorous shaking of the test tubes. Nonagglutinated cells can be completely redispersed in this manner, but agglutinates cannot be dispersed; they remain present as large flocs. With large amounts of cells, this phenomenon is visible with the naked eye, but when relatively few cells are present in each tube, microscopic inspection of the contents of each tube may be necessary.

3. Two-Dimensional Agglutination

Agglutination can be performed on flat plates (e.g., glass, plastic, or cardboard). By this technique, agglutination is recognized visually by the coarse graininess of agglutinated cell or particle clumps in contrast to the smooth aspect of monodisperse cell or particle suspensions. Owing to the exiguity of the third dimension in the conformation of a flat layer of cell or particle suspension, two-dimensional agglutination is much more quickly visible with the naked eye than agglutination in test tubes. Also, much smaller amounts of cells are required and, if desirable, the final test results (e.g., when agglutination is done on a sheet of special paper or cardboard) can be conserved after drying.

4. Agglutination in Gels

Agglutination of very small particles (e.g., sonicated fragments of stromata) can be effected in gels by double diffusion of these very small antigenic particles against specific antisera (83). The main advantage of this approach is that, due to the bidimensional geometry and the peculiar properties of double immunodiffusion (84), it becomes possible to investigate the degree of immunological relationship between, e.g., blood groups C and D, M and N, and blood group A subgroups and their Abs (83,85,86).

5. Quantitative Agglutination

Automated Methods. To quantitate the results of multiple hemagglutination determinations in quick sequence, agglutinated cells should be separated from nonagglutinated cell suspensions. The nonagglutinated RBCs are hemolyzed and the amount of hemoglobin is quantitated in a spectrophotometer; (420 nm wavelength), this will be proportional to the number of nonagglutinated cells. By comparing the difference with the total amount of cells used, a measure of the number of cells that have been agglutinated can be obtained; e.g., as a function of the concentration of antibody (87).

For the quantitation of antibody (or antigen) by latex agglutination, the number of nonagglutinated particles (which all have the same size) may be automatically determined by light scattering, at small forward scattering angles, to assure only the smallest particles are counted (88). (For the use of quantitative hemagglutination to obtain thermodynamic data on blood group Abs affinities and equilibrium constants, see Section III.C.4.c.)

Titration. Titration by hemagglutination is at best, a semiquantitative approach. It is done by serial dilution of the antiserum in saline; constant amounts of RBCs are added and the serum that causes recognizable hemagglutination at the greatest dilution is assumed to have the most Ab (89, p. 4). The Ab titer of the antiserum is the inverse of the dilution of the tube containing the most dilute Ab in which hemagglutination can be observed (for technical details and standardization, see ref. 90). One assumes that for a given number of RBCs, the number of epitopes of a given type is reasonably constant. In certain cases, however, that amount may vary depending, e.g., on the genetic make-up of the RBC donor; this is especially the case with the MN and Rh Ags (89, p. 341) (see below).

Determination of the Number of Epitopes per RBC. Quantitative hemagglutination under conditions of excess of (radioactive) antibodies has been used to determine the number of epitopes of a given blood group specificity per RBC. For instance, homozygous (DD, Rh_0-positive) human RBCs from homozygous (DD) donors have been reported to comprise 10,300 D epitopes, while RBCs from heterozygous (Dd) donors would appear to contain 6400 D epitopes (see ref. 91).

The number of A antigenic determinants on RBCs is much higher: $\approx 1,000,000$ per A_1 RBC. The much greater number of A than of D epitopes per RBC probably is the principal reason for the spiculation of RBCs caused by anti-A, while the interaction of anti-D does not affect their smooth biconcave shape (92,93).

6. Influence of Temperature on Hemagglutination

Hemagglutination usually is stronger at room temperature or at 4°C than at 37°C. Rh antibodies usually hemagglutinate better at 37°C than in the cold (they are called "warm" Abs) (90); the reason for this probably lies in the partially lipidic nature of the Rh epitope (67) (see also ref. 40, p. 345). Thus, to detect all blood groups antibodies, hemagglutination tests should be done in the cold (room temperature) *and* at 37°C.

B. Hemagglutination with IgM and IgG Antibodies

1. "Complete" and "Incomplete" Antibodies

From the early days of the clinical application of blood transfusion, hemagglutination with blood group antibodies has been the principal analytical tool in blood banking and immunohematology. It has long been known that with "complete" IgM antibodies, due to their size as well as to the availability of 10 antibody sites (39) disposed at diametrical distances of about 30 nm, hemagglutination is much more readily achieved than with "incomplete" antibodies of the IgG class, which have only two antibody sites that are maximally about 12–14 nm apart (1,16,37).

However, as "incomplete" IgG antibodies are also of considerable importance among blood group antibodies, much effort has been devoted to modifications of the environment and properties of erythrocytes to facilitate hemagglutination with IgG. With some IgG blood group antibodies (e.g., anti-A and anti-B) on the other hand, hemagglutination is easily achieved; the reasons for this are discussed below.

2. Distance Between Cell Surfaces

Using equations of the type of Eqs. 1, 9, and 13, rather accurate graphs can be made of the values of ΔG_{131}^{LW}, ΔG_{131}^{AB}, and ΔG_{131}^{EL} (cf. Eq. 4), respectively, as a function of the intercellular distance, ℓ (1,16). ΔG_{ℓ}^{LW}, and ΔG_{ℓ}^{AB} values for human erythrocytes can be derived from contact angle determinations with several liquids, on flat layers of stromata, using Eq. 7 (see, e.g., ref. 16). ΔG_{132}^{EL} values are derived from electrokinetic measurements on whole erythrocytes using, interalia, Eqs. 10 and 11. The electrophoretic mobility of erythrocytes yields their potential, from which their ψ_0-potential, and thus ΔG^{EL} can be derived (16) (see Sect. II.D.2.b). Figure 1 shows a ΔG_{131}^{TOT} versus ℓ graph for human erythrocytes in the flat-flat (i.e., rouleau) formation as well as in the edge-edge conformation. The intercellular distances, ℓ, which are depicted in Figure 1, are counted from the distal edges of the cellular glycocalices.

Under physiological conditions of pH and ionic strength, the outer edges of the glycocalyx of erythrocytes cannot approach each other to an intercellular distance, ℓ, smaller than about

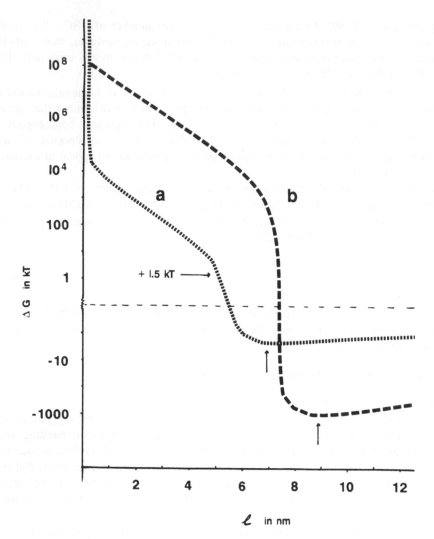

Figure 1 Energy balance of human RBCs, taking ΔG^{EL}, ΔG^{LW}, and ΔG^{AB} into account. The decay length of water is taken to be $\lambda - 0.6$ nm (see Fig. 2 and text). The left-hand curve (a) is computed by assuming a radius of curvature at the approach of two cells of $R = 1.5$ μm. The right-hand curve (b) is based on the interaction between two cells in the flat parallel slab mode, with a surface area of approach $S = 25.9$ μm^2. The vertical arrows indicate the secondary minima of attraction of the two modes a and b. A horizontal arrow indicates the place on curve (a) of $\Delta G = +1.5$ kT, corresponding to $\ell \approx 5.0$ nm, which is the most likely minimum distance between glycocalyx surfaces of two RBCs approaching each other via their convex edges, under the influence of their brownian motion. The relatively slight elastic repulsion engendered by cell–cell encounters at $\Delta G = +1.5$ kT is not taken into account here. (From Ref. 1.)

4–5 nm (1,16), which, however, makes the distance at the secondary minimum of attraction (see Fig. 1) between the actual cell membranes of two opposing erythrocytes about 15–16 nm, which is slightly more than the "reach" of IgG Abs (12–14 nm) but quite sufficient for cross-linking by IgM Abs (27–28 nm) (1) (Fig. 2). The interactions that force erythrocytes to keep a certain distance apart are threefold: an LW attraction ($\Delta G_{\ell_o}^{LW} \approx -0.6$ mJ/m^2); a hydrogen-bonding (AB) repulsion $\Delta G_{\ell_o}^{AB} = +25$ mJ/m^2); and an electrostatic (EL) repulsion ($\Delta G_{\ell_o}^{EL} = +0.5$ mJ/m^2). Each of these interactions follows a different regime in their decay as a function of distance (cf. Eqs. 1, 9, and 13) (16) resulting in a secondary minimum of attraction at a distance between the distal edges of the glycocalices of about 5 nm in the edge-edge conformation (see Fig. 1). As can be seen in Figure 2, IgM Abs can always cross-link RBCs whether the epitopes are situated on the glycocalyx strands (which are at least 5 nm apart) or on the cell membranes (which are at least 15 nm apart). IgG Abs, however, can only cross-link RBCs when the epitopes are situated on the glycocalyx edges (which is the case with ABO blood group Ags) but not when the epitopes are part of the cell membrane (which is the case with Rh blood group Ags). Therefore, to facilitate hemagglutination with anti-Rh Abs (which tend to be of the IgG class), one of two types of measures can be taken: (1) the cells can be pushed closer together, or (2) the "reach" of IgG class Abs may be extended.

3. Methods for Increasing the "Reach" of IgG Abs

Chemical Approach. The maximum distance between the two paratopes on one IgG molecule can be increased by mild reduction followed by alkylation (94), which results in breaking at least some of the inter-heavy chain disulfide bonds ins the hinge region. Not all inter–heavy chain disulfide bonds should be broken because that would result in monovalent Ab pieces, which are incapable of cross-binding. A "reach" of about 15–16 nm must be attained to achieve hemagglutination. It, therefore, seems probable that this method mainly applies to the opening up of IgG3 with its 11 S-S bonds, and to a lesser extent to IgG2 with 4 S-S bonds (95).

Immunochemical Approach. The most important method of increasing the "reach" of IgG class Abs is the *indirect* antiglobulin, or Coombs test (96). By this approach, two or more RBCs monogamously sensitized with IgG Abs are subsequently cross-linked by means of (usually rabbit) antihuman IgG. A schematic illustration of this mode of cross-linking is given in Figure 3. It is a two-step approach, but the end result is that cross-binding occurs through two human IgG molecules (one at each end), each about 12–14 nm long, which are linked together by one (rabbit) antihuman IgG molecule with a "reach" of about 12 nm, resulting in an extended tetravalent Ab, with a total "reach" of $\approx$ 36 nm; i.e., each slightly larger than that of IgM. For all cross-matching tests used for blood transfusions and for other tests for Rh-Abs, the use of the indirect antiglobulin test remains indispensable.

The *direct* antiglobulin test (97), i.e., the testing for in vivo sensitization of RBCs, by means of antihuman IgG is an indispensable test for the detection of sensitization in cases of hemolytic disease of the newborn and autoimmune hemolytic anemia.

4. Methods for Reducing the Intercellular Distance

Decreasing ℓ by Centrifugation. Centrifugation was first used for this purpose by Hirszfeld and Dubiski, who showed that (Rh-positive) RBCs could be brought close enough together for cross-linking with "incomplete" IgG-Abs at 15,000g, but not at 3,750g (98).

Decreasing ℓ by Reduction of the Intercellular Repulsion. Reduction of the intercellular repulsion is mainly effective when especially directed to the polar, hydrogen-bonding (AB) repulsion, as the polar repulsion between RBCs under physiological conditions accounts for at least 90% of the total intercellular repulsive forces (see above). The electrostatic repulsion amounts to only 2–10% of the total repulsive forces and the Lifshitz–van der Waals attraction is only about 2% of the total interaction (all at closest approach).

The polar intercellular repulsion can be decreased by most methods which also cause a decrease in the cells' surface (ζ) potential. It was believed earlier that the stability of cells (and other particles) in aqueous suspension was just due to the balance between the van der Waals (LW) attraction and the electrostatic (EL) repulsion (99). In the case of RBCs, this turns out not to be valid, as the until fairly recently neglected polar (AB) forces have been shown to play the major role (16). Earlier explanations of the destabilization of RBC suspensions through cell

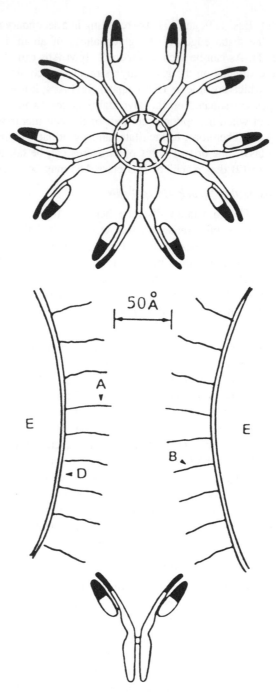

Figure 2 Diagram of the minimum distance of approach of two normal human RBCs, with an IgG and an IgM molecule drawn on the same scale. The curvature of the RBC surfaces has been drawn vastly exaggerated considering the scale: On this scale, the diameter of an RBC would be about 33 ft ($\approx$10 m). E indicates the interior of the RBCs; A, B, and D indicate sites of A, B, and D antigenic determinants. The closest approach between two unsensitized RBCs is $\approx$50 Å between the extremities of the sialoglycoprotein surfaces (drawn here as simple strands), which may be estimated to extend $\approx$50 Å from each cell membrane's lipid bilayer. (From Ref. 37.)

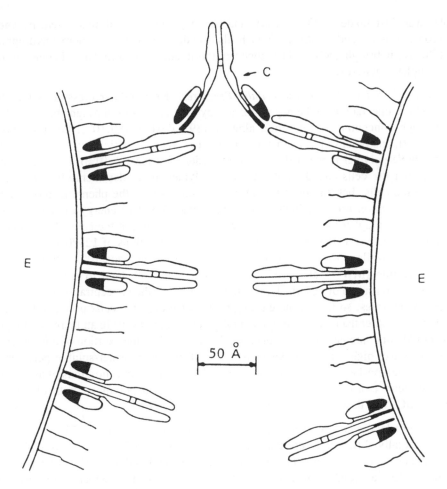

Figure 3 Diagram of the minimum distance of approach of two human RBCs, E, monogamously sensitized with IgG- anti-D. The curvature of the RBC surfaces has been drawn vastly exaggerated considering the scale. The closest approach between sensitized cells is $\approx$40 Å (from Fc tail to Fc tail). The extremities of two opposing IgG Fc tails obviously can easily be cross-linked by another (rabbit-anti-human IgG) IgG molecule, here indicated by C. (From Ref. 37.)

treatment with enzymes or by the addition of plurivalent cations (e.g., La^{3+} ions, see ref. 100; or Al^{3+} ions, see ref. 101), which were based on a decrease in ζ-potential caused by these measures (102,103), must therefore be revised. It is true that treatment of RBCs with neuraminidase, bromelin, or papain, as well as with plurivalent cations, causes a significant decrease in their ζ-potential (103). However, the more important effect of enzymatic or cation treatment of RBCs is that they become *less hydrophilic*, thus decreasing their polar (AB) repulsion, which then results in a decrease in their intercellular distance, ℓ.

Papain is among the most effective enzymes in decreasing the intercellular distance; it is widely used in facilitating hemagglutination with ("incomplete") IgG class Abs. Among salts with multivalent cations, those with the highest valency are the most effective in destabilizing negatively charged particles (23), including RBCs. The connection between a decrease in ζ-potential and increased hydrophobicity has recently become apparent (11,104). The observation that plurivalent cations (which are electron acceptors) cause hydrophilic electron donating materials to become more "hydrophobic" (using phospholipids and Ca^{2+} as an example) was first made by Ohki (105), and was explained as outlined above by van Oss et al. (106). Tannic acid treatment (which also renders erythrocytes more "hydrophobic") also is effective in bringing RBCs closer together; this treatment also enhances hemagglutination with incomplete IgG-Abs.

Decreasing ℓ by Exertion of Extracellular Pressure.   Extracellular pressure is the mechanism by which one facilitates hemagglutination by IgG class Abs through the admixture of relatively high concentrations of serum albumin (89), dextran (89,107,108), polyvinyl pyrrolidone (109), and other water-soluble polymers (110). When a sufficiently high concentration of water-soluble polymer is reached (e.g., of the order of at least 2–10%), a phase separation occurs between the cells and the polymers (the polymer molecules themselves may in part adsorb onto the cells, but that does not alter the mechanism of the phenomenon). When the polymer concentration becomes high enough, the polar (AB) free energy of repulsion of the polymers becomes higher than the polar free energy of repulsion of the cells. This reduces the intercellular distance, ℓ (110). With serum albumin, concentrations of 12–20% (w/v) are used for that purpose, while typically dextran concentrations between 5 and 10% suffice to decrease ℓ. (Higher dextran [MW $\approx$ 500,000] concentrations than 10% tend to restabilize the cells because the concentration of adsorbed dextran then surpasses the concentration of free dextran; this reverses the roles, so that in the ensuing phase-separation the *cells* now exert a stronger pressure on each other than the free polymer molecules, which results in an increase in ℓ [110]).

One should not confound the mechanism for decreasing ℓ by the exertion of outside pressure by means of fairly high concentrations of polar (electron-donor) water-soluble polymers with the hemagglutination-facilitating effect caused by relatively low concentrations of asymmetrical polymers of high molecular weight, or of positively charged polymers, both of which can cross-link RBCs and thus bring them closer together (see below).

Decreasing l by Cross-linking the Cells with Asymmetrical Polymers.   This approach is based on a totally different mechanism from the one discussed above. Cross-linking with polymers occurs at relatively low polymer concentrations and is done with (1) very asymmetrical, high molecular weight neutral or negatively charged polymers which cross-link through adsorption and/or entanglement with two (or more) cells per polymer molecule; or (2) already adsorbed biopolymer molecules which are made insoluble; or (3) positively charged polymers.

Cross-linking with the first types of polymers gives rise to the rouleau-formation type of hemagglutination. Red blood cells *preferentially* attract each other in the parallel disk conformation at an intercellular distance, l, of about 7 nm (1). Figure 1 shows that the energy of attraction of RBCs at the secondary minimum is about three orders of magnitude greater in the parallel disk configuration than in the edge-edge configuration. Red blood cells thus appear to have a natural propensity to form rouleaux. However, in the normal course of events, RBCs will not form stable rouleaux because even minute hydrodynamic disturbances will cause the cells to slide away from each other. It should be remembered that the maximum of attraction occurs when two parallel disks still are about 7 nm apart: when they approach one another only slightly more closely, the attraction turns into an even greater repulsion. Thus, stable rouleau formation only occurs when the energetically favored parallel disk situation can become stabilized in that conformation through the anchoring action of cross-linking stringlike polymer molecules (99). Human RBCs attract each other in the parallel disk conformation, at the "secondary minimum" of attraction, with a given free energy of attraction, whereas slightly different cells (e.g., rabbit erythrocytes) attract each other in the same manner with a somewhat different energy of attraction (99). This can give rise to the phenomenon in which rouleau formation occurring with mixtures of cells of two different species (e.g., human and rabbit RBCs) become totally segregated, each individual rouleau either completely consisting of human or of rabbit RBCs (111). This sort of RBC aggregation can be achieved with a variety of asymmetrical polymers: fibrinogen (112), dextran (112,113), nucleic acids (114), heparin (115), and polymerized albumin (116). The higher the molecular weight of an asymmetrical polymer, the lower the concentration needed to obtain rouleau formation: with dextran MW $\approx$ 100,000, 1% causes rouleau formation, whereas with dextran MW $\approx$ 270,000, a 0.4% concentration of the polymer suffices (112). The cross-linking induced by dextran can be inhibited by glucose (110), which suggests that the strong adsorption of dextran onto the erythrocyte glycocalix may be due to the presence of a lectinlike peptide on the cell surface with glucose specificity. This would then be comparable with the opposite of the lectin-RBC interaction (117).

Cross-linking with a second class of polymers has an entirely different mechanism. It is mediated by the normally occurring aspecific adsorption of euglobulins (mainly of the IgM type from the serum onto the RBCs, which normally occurs under physiological conditions, but which does not, by itself, cause cross-linking. However, when the ionic strength of the suspending medium is lowered, the adsorbed euglobulins precipitate and in so doing interact with each other intercellularly causing cross-linking. When RBCs are washed to remove the adsorbed proteins, this type of cross-binding is no longer possible, but when the eluted euglobulins are added back to the RBC suspension, cross-linking at low ionic strength resumes (118). The aspect of RBCs agglomerated in this manner is different from that of regular rouleaux; some remnants of cell stacks can still be discerned, but all clumps look as though they were painted over (with layers of precipitated euglobulin), as observed by scanning electron microscopy (93). Addition of salt to cells agglomerated in this manner redissolves the euglobulins and allows the cells to redisperse. This method of RBC agglomeration was formerly used as a means for removing the cryoprotectant from previously frozen, newly thawed cells, by sedimenting the agglomerates at ambient gravity, thus avoiding the need for centrifugal washing (119). The elucidation of the mechanism of this class of (low ionic strength) cross-binding of RBCs (118) was at the origin of the development of an automated hemagglutination-enhancing method by Rosenfield et al. (120).

Cross-linking of RBCs with a third class of polymers can occur with positively charged polyelectrolytes (usually of relatively low to medium molecular weight), which cross-link RBCs by direct combination with (and neutralization of) the acid site of the glycocalyx. Complexes of this type are most easily formed at relatively low ionic strengths and redisperse upon the addition of salt. Basic polymers of this type are: Polybrene (poly[hexadimethrine bromide]) (121), protamine, and polylysine (113,122). Polybrene (as well as albumin in high concentrations) induces RBCs to become stomatocytic (i.e., to display only one deep dimple instead of two shallow ones) (110). It should be stressed that neutralization of negatively charged sites on the glycocalyx also makes the cell surfaces more "hydrophobic" (see above) and thus even more prone to agglutination.

Decreasing ℓ by RBC Spiculation. Cell surface processes in the form of spicules or spikes, with a small radius of curvature, undergo a much smaller repulsion than smooth parts of the cell surface. Spicules can therefore approach other cell surfaces much more closely than totally smooth cells. Anti-A as well as anti-B (as well as anti-A lectins) tend to cause spiculation in RBCs, but anti-D does not (92,93,123). Thus, hemagglutination with anti-A or anti-B, even of the IgG class, never is a problem. However, major problems are encountered with anti-D Abs which usually are of the IgG class, and which leave the cells quite smooth. It should be noted that dextran (MW $\approx$ 40,000) also causes spiculation (110), which may be another reason for its usefulness in facilitating hemagglutination with incomplete IgG anti-D. The reason why spiculation occurs with anti-A and anti-B or lectins, and not with anti-D, probably lies in the difference in the numbers of A versus D epitopes per cell—the number of A epitopes being of the order of 10^6, whereas that of D is only of the order of 10^4 per cell (93) (see also Sect. IV.A.5).

Papain treatment also gives rise to surface irregularities in RBCs, but the processes induced by this approach have a larger radius of curvature (i.e., $R \approx 0.5$ µm) than the spicules caused by, e.g., anti-A ($R \approx 0.15$ µm) (93).

REFERENCES

1. van Oss CJ. Surface free energy contribution to cell interactions. In: Glaser R, Gingell D, ed. Biophysics of the Cell Surface. New York: Springer-Verlag, 1990:131.
2. van Oss CJ, Walker J. Concentration dependence of the binding constant of antibodies. Mol Immunol 1987; 24:715.
3. Chaudhury MK. Short-Range and Long-Range Forces in Colloidal and Macroscopic Systems. PhD Thesis, State University of New York at Buffalo.
4. van Oss CJ, Chaudhury MK, Good RJ. Interfacial Lifshitz–van der Waals and polar interactions in macroscopic systems. Chem Rev 1988; 88:927.
5. Good RJ, Chaudhury MK. Theory of adhesive forces across interfaces—1. The Lifshitz–van der Waals component of interaction in adhesion. In Lee LH, ed. Fundamentals of Adhesion. New York: Plenum Press, p. 137.
6. Visser J. On Hamaker constants: A comparison between Hamaker constants and Lifshitz–van der Waals constants. Adv Colloid Interface Sci 1972; 3:331.
7. Pressman D, Grossberg AL. The Structural Basis of Antibody Specificity. Reading, MA: WA Benjamin, 1973.
8. Israelachvili JN. Van der Waals forces in biological systems. Q Rev Biophys 1974; 6:341.
9. Fowkes FM. Role of acid-base interfacial bonding in adhesion. J Adhes Sci Tech 1987; 1:7.
10. van Oss CJ, Chaudhury MK, Good RJ. Monopolar surfaces. Adv Colloid Interface Sci 1987; 28:35.
11. van Oss CJ, Good RJ. Orientation of the water molecules of hydration of human serum albumin. J Protein Chem 1988; 7:179.
12. van Oss CJ, Good RJ. On the mechanism of "hydrophobic" interactions. J Dispersion Sci Tech 1988; 9:355.
13. van Oss CJ, Good RJ. Surface enthalpy and entropy and the physico-chemical nature of "hydrophobic" and hydrophilic interactions. J Dispersion Sci Tech 1991; 12:273.
14. Nemethy G, Scheraga HA. The structure of water and "hydrophobic" bonding in proteins III. The thermodynamic properties of "hydrophobic" bonds in proteins. J Phys Chem 1962; 66:1773.
15. Manavalan P, Ponnuswamy PK. "hydrophobic" character of amino acid residues in globular proteins. Nature 1978; 275:673.
16. van Oss CJ. Energetics of cell-cell and cell-biopolymer interactions. Cell Biophys 1989; 14:1.
17. van Oss CJ. Hydrophilic and "hydrophobic" interactions in proteins. In: Visser J ed. Protein Interactions 1992.
18. van Oss CJ. Aspecific and specific intermolecular interaction in aqueous media. J Mol Recogn 1990; 3:128.
19. Israelachvili JN, Pashley RM. Measurement of the "hydrophobic" interaction between the "hydrophobic" surfaces in aqueous electrolyte solutions. J Colloid Interface Sci 1984; 98:500.
20. van Oss CJ, Smeenk RJT, Aarden LA. Inhibition of association vs. dissociation of high-avidity DNA/anti-DNA complexes: Possible involvement of secondary hydrogen bonds. Immunol Invest 1985; 14:245.
21. van Oss CJ, Good RJ, Chaudhury MK. Nature of the antigen-antibody interaction—Primary and secondary bonds: Optimal conditions for association and dissociation. J Chromatogr 1986; 376:111.
22. Gabler R. Electrical Interactions in Molecular Biophysics. New York: Academic Press, 1978:245.
23. Overbeek JThG. Electrokinetic phenomena. In: Kruyt HR, ed. Colloid Science. Vol 1. Amsterdam: Elsevier, 1952:194.
24. Overbeek JThG, Bijsterbosch BH. The electrical double layer and the theory of electrophoresis. In: Righetti PG, van Oss, CJ, Vanderhoff JW, eds. Electrokinetic Separation Methods. Amsterdam: Elsevier, 1979:1.
25. Hunter RJ. Zeta Potential in Colloid Science. London: Academic Press, 1981.

26. Liberti PA Incremental bonding site filling of anti-polypeptide antibodies. Immunochemistry 1975; 12:303.
27. Prickett KS, Amberg DC, Hopp TP. A calcium-dependent antibody for identification and purification of recombinant proteins. Biotechniques 1989; 7:580.
28. Kabat EA. Structural Concepts in Immunology and Immunochemistry. New York: Holt, Rinehart, Winston, 1968:82.
29. Atassi MZ. Immune recognition of proteins. In: Atassi MZ, van Oss CJ, Absolom DR, eds. Molecular Immunology. New York: Marcel Dekker, 1984:15.
30. Cunningham RK. Immunochemistry of polysaccharide and blood group antigens. In: Atassi MZ, van Oss CJ, Absolom DR, eds. Molecular Immunology. New York: Marcel Dekker, 1984:53.
31. van Oss CJ, Absolom DR, Neumann AW. The "hydrophobic effect": Essentially a van der Waals Interaction. Colloid Polymer Sci 1980; 258:424.
32. Israelachvili JN. Intermolecular and Surface Forces. New York: Academic Press, 1985.
33. van Oss CJ, Fike RM, Good RJ, Reinig JM. Cell microelectrophoresis simplified by the reduction and uniformization of the electroosmotic backflow. Anal Biochem 1974; 60:242.
34. de Groot RR, Lamers MC, Aarden LA et al. Dissociation of DNA/anti-DNA complexes at high pH. Immunol Commun 1980; 9:515.
35. van Oss CJ, Absolom DR, Bronson PM. Affinity diffusion II. Comparison between thermodynamic data obtained by affinity diffusion and precipitation in tubes. Immunol Commun 1982; 11:139.
36. Tankersley DL, Preston MS, Finlayson JS. Immunoglobulin G dimer, an idiotype-antiidiotype complex. Mol Immunol 1988; 25:41.
37. van Oss CJ. Agglutination and precipitation. In: Atassi MZ, van Oss CJ, Absolom DR, eds. Molecular Immunology. New York: Marcel Dekker, 1984:361.
38. van Oss CJ. Specifically impermeable precipitate membranes. Surface Colloid Sci 1984; 13:115.
39. Edberg EG, Bronson PM, van Oss CJ. The valency of IgM and IgG rabbit anti-dextran antibody as a function of the size of the dextran molecule. Immunochemistry 1972; 9:273.
40. van Oss CJ, Absolom DR. Nature and Thermodynamics of antigen-antibody interactions. In: Atassi MZ, van Oss CJ, Absolom DR, eds. Molecular Immunology. New York: Marcel Dekker, 1984:337.
41. van Oss CJ. Antigen-antibody reactions. In: Van Regenmortel MHV, ed. The Structure of Antigens. Boca Raton, FL: CRC Press, 1992:99.
42. Absolom DR, van Oss CJ. Nature of the antigen-antibody bond and the factors affecting its association and dissociation. Crit Rev Immunol 1986; 6:1.
43. Karush R. Multivalent binding and functional affinity. Contemp Top Mol Immunol 1976; 5:217.
44. Froese A. The immunoglobulin-binding receptors of rat mast cells and rat basophilic leukemia cells. In: Froese A, Paraskevas F, eds. Structure and Function of F_c Receptors. New York: Marcel Dekker, 1983:83.
45. Van Regenmortel MHV, Hardie G. Determination of avidity of antiviral antibodies at 50% binding of antibody. J Immunol Methods 1979; 27:43.
46. Steward MW. Immunochemistry. New York: John Wiley & Sons, 1974:42.
47. Steward MW. Affinity of the antibody-antigen reaction and its biological significance. In: Glynn LE, Steward MW, eds. Immunochemistry. New York: John Wiley & Sons, 1977:233.
48. Froese A, Sehon AH. Kinetics of antibody-hapten reactions. Contemp Top Mol Immunol 1975; 4:23.
49. Pecht I. Dynamic aspects of antibody function. In: Sela M, ed. The Antigens. Vol 6. New York: Academic Press, 1982:1.
50. Hardie G, Van Regenmortel MHV. Immunochemical studies of tobacco mosaic virus—I: Refutation of the alleged homogeneous binding of purified antibody fragments. Immunochemistry 1975; 12:903.
51. Wurmser R, Filitti-Wurmser S. Thermodynamic study of the isohaemagglutinins. Prog Biophys Chem 1957; 7:87.
52. Steane EA. Thermodynamic Studies of Erythrocyte Antigen-Antibody Interaction and the Modulation of This Phenomenon by Partial Enzymatic Digestion of the Cell Membrane. PhD Thesis, George Washington University, Washington, DC.
53. van Oss CJ, Bronson PM, Absolom DR. Affinity diffusion. I. Method for measuring dissociation constants of precipitating antibodies. Immunol Commun 1982; 11:129.

54. Hughes-Jones NC. Nature of the reaction between antigen and antibody. Br Med Bull 1965; 19:171.
55. Hughes-Jones NC. The estimation of the concentration and equilibrium constant of anti-D. Immunology 1967; 12:565.
56. Rochna E, Hughes-Jones NC. The use of purified ^{125}I-labelled anti–γ-globulin in the determination of the number of D antigen sites on red cells of different phenotypes. Vox Sang 1965; 10:675.
57. Horejsi V. Affinity electrophoresis. Analyt Biochem 1981; 112:1.
58. Bog-Hansen TC, Takeo K. Affinity electrophoresis. Electrophoresis 1980; 1:67.
59. Haselkorn D, Friedman S, Givol D, Pecht I. Kinetic mapping of the antibody combining site by chemical relaxation spectrometry. Biochemistry 1974; 13:2210.
60. Thorell JI, Larson SM. Radioimmunoassay and Related Techniques. St Louis, MO: CV Mosby, 1978; 14.
61. Steiner RF, Kitzinger C. A calorimetric determination of the heat of an antigen-antibody reaction. J Biol Chem 1956; 222:271.
62. Sturtevant JM. Flow calorimetry. Fractions 1969; 1:1.
63. Johnston MFM, Barisas BG, Sturtevant JM. Thermodynamics of hapten binding to MOPC 315 and MOPC 460 mouse myeloma proteins. Biochemistry 1974; 13:390.
64. van Oss CJ, Neumann AW. Comparison between antigen-antibody binding energies and interfacial free energies. Immunol Commun 1977; 6:341.
65. Kabat EA. Structural Concepts in Immunology and Immunochemistry. 2nd ed. New York: Holt, Rinehart, Winston, 1976.
66. Ohta Y, Gill TJ, Leung CS. Volume changes accompanying the antigen-antibody reaction. Biochemistry 1970; 9:2708.
67. Green FA. Erythrocyte membrane phosphatidylcholine and Rh(D) cryolatency. Immunol Commun 1982; 11:25.
68. van Oss CJ, Beckers D, Engelfriet CP, et al. Illusion of Blood Group Antibodies from Red Cells. Vox Sang 1981; 40:367.
69. Good W, Wood JE. The hydrational effect of alkali metal and halide ions on the Rh–anti-Rh system. Immunology 1971; 20:37.
70. Mukkur TKS. Thermodynamics of hapten-antibody interactions. Crit Rev Biochem 1984; 16:133.
71. Dorrington K, Klein MH. Structure and binding specificity of the $F_c\gamma$ receptors on murine macrophages. In: Froese A, Paraskevas F, eds. Structure and Function of F_c Receptors. New York: Marcel Dekker, 1983:15.
72. van Oss CJ, Absolom DR, Michaeli I. A disquisition on the energetics of immunoglobulin binding to receptors in vivo and in vitro. Immunol Invest 1985; 14:167.
73. Sjögren HO, Wallmark A, Flodgren P, et al. Adsorption of human plasma on protein A-Sepharose: Effects on in vitro parameters of tumor immunity. In: Beyer JH, Borberg H, Fuchs C, Nagel GA, eds. Plasmapheresis in Immunology and Oncology. New York: Karger, 1982:114.
74. Molinaro GA, Eby WC, Molinaro CA, et al. Two monoclonal antibodies to two different epitopes of human growth hormone form a precipitate line when counter diffused as soluble immune complexes. Mol Immunol 1984; 21:771.
75. Halk EL, Hsu HT, Aebig J, Franke J. Production of monoclonal antibodies against three Ilarviruses and Alfalfa mosaic virus and their use in serotyping. Phytopathology 1984; 74:367.
76. Bankert RB, Mazzafero D, Mayers GL. Hybridomas producing hemolytic plaques used to study the relationship between monoclonal antibody affinity and the efficiency of plaque inhibition with increasing concentrations of antigen. Hybridoma 1981; 1:47.
77. Pfeiffer NE, Wylie DE, Schuster SM. Immunoaffinity chromatography utilizing monoclonal antibodies: Factors which influence antigen-binding capacity. J Immunol Methods 1984; 97:1.
78. Einstein A. Theoretical observations on the Brownian motion. Z. Electrochem 1907; 13:41.
79. Van de Ven TGM. Colloidal Hydrodynamics. London: Academic Press, 1989;
80. van Oss CJ, Absolom DR, Grossberg AL, Neumann AW. Repulsive van der Waals forces. I. Complete dissociation of antigen-antibody complexes by means of negative van der Waals forces. Immunol Commun 1979; 8:11.
81. Smeenk RJT, Aarden LA, van Oss CJ. Comparison between dissociation and inhibition of association of DNA/anti-DNA complexes. Immunol Commun 1982; 12:177.

82. Helmerhorst FM, van Oss CJ, Bruynes ECE, et al. Elution of granulocyte and platelet antibodies. Vox Sang 1982; 43:196.

83. Milgrom F, Loza U. Agglutination of particulate antigens in agar gels. J Immunol 1967; 98:102.

84. Ouchterlony Ö. Handbook of Immunodiffusion and Immunoelectrophoresis. Ann Arbor, MI: Ann Arbor Science, 1968.

85. Milgrom F, Loza U. Immunodiffusion tests with Rh antigens and antibodies. Vox Sang 1969; 16:470.

86. Milgrom F, Mohn JF, Loza U. Immunodiffusion studies of blood group A antigen. Vox Sang 1974; 26:147.

87. Greenwalt TJ, Steane EA. Quantitative haemagglutination. II. A method for assaying red cell antigens using the Auto-Analyzer. Br J Haematol 1970; 19:701.

88. Masson PL, Cambiaso CL, Collet-Cassart D, et al. Particle counting immunoassay, Methods Enzymol 1981; 74:106.

89. Race RR, Sanger R. Blood Groups in Man. Oxford, England, Blackwell; 1962.

90. Stratton F, Renton PH. Practical Blood Grouping. Oxford, England: Blackwell, 1958: 30, 167.

91. Masouredis SP. Relationship between Rh_0 (D) genotype and quantity of ^{131}I anti-Rh_0 (D) bound to red cells. J Clin Invest 1960; 39:1450.

92. Salsbury AJ, Clarke JA. Surface changes in red blood cells undergoing agglutination. Rev Franc Etud Clin Biol 1967; 12:981.

93. van Oss CJ, Mohn JF. Scanning electron microscopy of red cell agglutination. Vox Sang 1970; 19:432.

94. Romans DG, Tilley CA, Crookston MC, et al. Conversion of incomplete antibodies to direct agglutinins by mild reduction: Evidence for segmental flexibility within the F_c fragment of immunoglobulin G. Proc Natl Acad Sci USA 1977; 74:2531.

95. Burton DR, Gregory L, Lefferis R. Aspects of the molecular structure of IgG subclasses. In: Shakib F, ed. Basic and Clinical Aspects of IgG Subclasses. Basel: Karger, 1986:7.

96. Coombs RRA, Mourant AE, Race RR. A new test for the detection of weak and "incomplete" Rh agglutinins. Br J Exp Pathol 1945; 26:255.

97. Coombs RRA, Mourant AE, Race RR. In vivo isosensitization of red cells in babies with haemolytic disease. Lancet 1946; 1:264.

98. van Oss CJ. Stability of human red cell suspensions at 300,000xG. J Dispersion Sci Tech 1985; 6:139.

99. van Oss CJ, Absolom DR. Influence of cell configuration and potential energy equilibria in rouleau phenomena. J Dispersion Sci Tech 1985; 6:131.

100. Lerche D, Hessel E, Donath E. Investigation of the La^{3+}-induced aggregation of red blood cells. Stud Biophys 1979; 78:95.

101. Sachtleben P, Ruhenstroth-Bauer G. Agglutination and the electrical surface potential of red blood cells. Nature 1961; 192:982.

102. van Oss CJ, Absolom DR. Zeta potentials, van der Waals forces and hemagglutination. Vox Sang 1983; 44:183.

103. van Oss CJ, Absolom DR. Hemagglutination and the closest distance of approach of normal, neuraminidase- and papain-treated erythrocytes. Vox Sang 1984; 47:250.

104. Holmes-Farley SR, Reamey RH, McCarthy TJ, et al. Acid-base behavior of carboxylic groups covalently attached at the surface of polyethylene: The usefulness of contact angle in following the ionization of surface functionality, Langmuir 1985; 1:725.

105. Ohki S. A mechanism of divalent ion induced phosphatidylserine membrane fission. Biochim Biophys Acta 1982; 689:1.

106. van Oss CJ, Chaudhury MK, Good RJ. Polar interfacial interactions, hydration pressure and membrane fusion. In: Ohki S, Doyle D, Flanagan TD, et al, eds. Molecular Mechanisms of Membrane Fusion. New York: Plenum Press, 1988:113.

107. Grubb R. Dextran as a medium for the demonstration of incomplete anti–Rh-agglutinins. J Clin Pathol 1949; 2:223.

108. van Oss CJ, Arnold K, Coakley WT. Depletion flocculation and depletion stabilization of erythrocytes. Cell Biophys 1990; 17:1.

109. Hummel K. Quantitative Untersuchungen über die Bindung von Polyvinylpyrrolidon an die Erythrozytenoberfläche. Blut 1963; 9:145, 215.

110. van Oss CJ, Mohn JF, Cunningham RK. Influence of various physicochemical factors on hemagglutination. Vox Sang 1978; 34:351.

111. Sewchand LS, Canham PB. Induced rouleau formation in interspecies populations of red cells. Can J Physiol Pharmacol 1976; 54:437.
112. Mollison PL. Blood Transfusion in Clinical Medicine. Oxford, England: Blackwell, 1972:150, 384.
113. van Oss CJ, Coakley WT. Mechanisms of successive modes of erythrocyte stability and instability in the presence of various polymers. Cell Biophys 1988; 13:141.
114. Ishiyama I. Hemagglutination induced by nucleic acids. Nature 1963; 197:912.
115. Jan KM. Red cell interactions in macromolecular suspension. Biorheology 1979; 16:137.
116. Jones JM, Kerwick RA, Goldsmith KLG. Influence of polymers on the efficacy of serum albumin as a potentiator of "incomplete" Rh agglutinins. Nature 1969; 224:510.
117. Perera CB, Frumin AM. Hemagglutination by Fava bean extract inhibited by simple sugars. Science 1966; 151:821.
118. van Oss CJ, Buenting S. Adsorbed euglobulins as the cause of agglomeration of erythrocytes in the Huggins blood-thawing method. Transfusion 1967; 7:77.
119. Huggins CE. Frozen blood-clinical experience. Surgery 1966; 60:77.
120. Rosenfield RE, Spitz C, Bar-Shany S, et al. Low ionic concentration to augment hemagglutination for the detection and measurement of serological incompatibility. Analyt Chem Technicon Symp. Vol 1. Mediad, New York, 1968:173.
121. Lalezari P. A new method for detection of red blood cell antibodies. Transfusion 1968; 8:372.
122. Greenwalt TJ, Steane EA. Quantitative hemagglutination. VI. Relationship of sialic acid content and aggregation by polybrene, protamine and poly-L-lysine. Br J Haematol 1973; 25:227.
123. Rebuck JW. Structural changes in sensitized human erythrocytes observed with the electron microscope. Anat Rec 1953; 115:591.
124. Steane EA, Greenwalt TJ. Erythrocyte agglutination. Sandler SG, Nusbacher J, Schaufield MS, eds. Immunobiology of the Erythrocyte. New York: Alan R Liss, 1980:171.

13

Monoclonal Antibodies to Human Red Blood Cell Blood Group Antigens

MARION L. SCOTT
International Blood Group Reference Laboratory
Bristol, England

DOUGLAS VOAK
East Anglican Blood Transfusion Centre
and University of Cambridge
Cambridge, England

I. INTRODUCTION

The original work of Kohler and Milstein (1), which described the principles of monoclonal antibody (MAb) production, used sheep red blood cells (RBCs) as the antigenic stimulus. The first monoclonal antibodies produced were to RBC determinants. Production of MAbs to human blood group A antigen (2) and the demonstration that such antibodies might be able to replace polyclonal sera as blood grouping reagents (3) were significant breakthroughs in the application of MAb technology to medicine.

Since these early discoveries, MAbs have been produced to a wide variety of structures on the RBC membrane. Their characterization has led to increased understanding of the structures underlying blood group polymorphisms, the interaction of structural components of the RBC membrane in health and disease and the identification of markers on the RBC that are useful tags for molecules in other cell types. Monoclonal antibodies have been developed successfully to replace polyclonal sera as diagnostic blood grouping reagents, and human monoclonal anti-D antibodies are undergoing trials as therapeutic reagents, thereby providing unlimited quantities of high-quality, reproduceable, consistent diagnostic and therapeutic reagents at a fraction of the cost of polyclonal reagents, and avoiding the ethical disadvantages of immunizing humans.

With advances in recombinant DNA technology, we are now poised on the brink of a further new era of using "designer" immunological probes as investigative tools, therapeutic and diagnostic reagents. This chapter reviews the contributions MAb technology has made to our understanding and investigation of human blood groups over the past 17 years and looks forward to the application of genetically engineered antibody fragments in the future.

II. PRODUCTION OF MONOCLONAL ANTIBODIES

A. Rodent Systems

In the original procedure as described by Kohler and Milstein (1), spleen cells from hyperimmunized mice were fused with myeloma cells from other suitable mouse strains and a mouse-mouse hybridoma was established. The sequence of events for the classic method of producing MAbs has been described elsewhere in detail (4,5). In addition to the classic mouse × mouse or rat

× rat hybridomas, fusions have been performed with rat × mouse, rabbit × mouse, and human × mouse. Such cell lines produced by fusion of cells from two different species are called heterohybridomas.

1. Selection of Myeloma Lines

The development of suitable myeloma fusion partners was an important part of the development of monoclonal antibody technology. As the function of the myeloma cell is to confer the property of continuous growth in culture on the hybrid fusion products, it is important that the myeloma cells themselves can be selectively killed in culture, so that they do not outgrow hybrids. To this end, the myeloma cells used are biochemically selected cloned mutants that lack the enzyme hypoxanthine guanine phosphoribosyl transferase (HGPRT). This allows for later selection by the use of aminopterin in culture, which blocks the normal de novo synthesis of bases for nucleic acid production, so that only cells containing enzymes necessary for the production of nucleotides by the salvage pathways, such as HGPRT, can survive and grow. Early myeloma lines, such as P3/X63-Ag8 and P3-NS-1-Ag 4-1, still produced immunoglobulin chains. The first anti-A, W61 (2), gave poor agglutination with A_2B cells because the NS-1 myeloma used produced its own κ light chain that became incorporated in a high proportion of the immunoglobulin M (IgM) anti-A molecules, thus reducing their agglutinating efficiency with RBCs with low antigen site density (3,6). This was called the HLK, or mixed light chain, phenomenon, as HLK hybridomas make a variable mixture of three types of molecules (IgG) or subunits (IgM), HL (totally active), HLK (semiactive), and HK (totally inactive). Subcloning the HLK W61 anti-A cell line produced a useful anti-A–secreting HL cell line. However, the HLK phenomenon was later overcome by using improved myeloma lines, such as NS-0, which did not produce any unwanted heavy or light chains (4). The use of NS-0 in fusions produces only HL types; i.e., all the immunoglobulin is of spleen cell origin.

2. Immunization

Monoclonal antibody technology provides the means for one antibody-secreting cell produced in vivo to be selected and grown in bulk in vitro. Classically, cells producing antibody of required specificity are induced in vivo by immunization procedures.

Red blood cell human blood group–specific MAbs have been induced in mice by immunizing with a variety of immunogens, including whole RBCs, before and after enzyme modifications, fractionated RBC membranes, soluble blood group substances, or synthetic blood group haptens coupled to a suitable carrier molecule. Since the selection and cloning procedures separate MAbs of different specificities, the immunizing antigenic preparation need not necessarily be purified before use. Many blood group–specific MAbs have been made "by mistake" when attempting to make other specificity MAbs to cellular starting material. For example, one of the most avid anti-A MAbs (MHO4) was accidentally made while an attempt was being made to make platelet-specific MAbs—the ABO group of the platelet donors used for the immunizations was not taken into account! A number of different immunization regimens can be used, with variation in the length and timing of the schedule, the use of adjuvants and the route of injection. Generally speaking, as with conventional immunization, shorter schedules tend to lead to the production of lower-affinity IgM antibodies, and longer schedules to higher-affinity IgG isotypes.

As for any immunization procedure to produce antibodies, it is important to understand that an animal may only produce mature antibody-secreting cells if it lacks some of the determinants of the immunogen; i.e., the immunogen is recognised as foreign. In vitro, as opposed to in vivo, immunization can be used where the normal regulation of the immune response might present difficulties in the production of specific antibodies (7), and strains of mice of different H-2 (MHC) haplotypes may give better responses to some antigens. The use of a rat hybridoma system may give rise to different specificity MAbs than can be produced in a mouse system (8).

B. Human Systems

Despite the overall success in the production of rodent MAbs to human blood group antigens, no such MAbs have been produced to the clinically important Rh antigens. This may be because these antigens, which are only expressed on human RBCs, are not recognized by the mouse or rat immune system. Different approaches are obviously required to produce human MAbs from those used in the mouse system. Human myeloma cell lines with comparable attributes to the mouse myeloma lines used for fusion have not been developed. However, certain viruses contain genes that will immortalize cells under specific conditions, allowing their continuous culture in vitro. When used in vitro, the Epstein-Barr virus (EBV) infects and immortalizes peripheral human B lymphocytes, which will thereafter grow continuously in culture as lymphoblastoid cell lines. EBV infection also causes polyclonal activation of peripheral B lymphocytes, with the synthesis and secretion of immunoglobulin. T-cell, accessory cell cooperation, or T-cell–replacing factors are not required to activate the B cells. The immortalization of specific Ig-secreting B lymphocytes was first achieved by Steinitz et al. (9), who reported a stable cloned EBV-containing B-lymphoblastoid cell line producing a human MAb to dinitrophenacetic acid. Since then, human MAbs with a variety of specificities, including anti-Rh(D), have been produced in this way. However, although it is relatively easy to establish lymphoblastoid cell lines producing specific antibody, the antibody production is commonly lost on expansion of the culture. Similarly, specific antibody production is often lost during cloning. Stable EBV-transformed lines producing human monoclonal anti-D have been produced by repeated cloning and selection (10). Improvements in stability of human lines have been achieved by back-crossing human anti-D–secreting EBV lines to a mouse-human heteromyeloma line (11) or to a mouse myeloma line (12). Use of this approach has recently enabled the production of further blood group–specific human MAbs that were not possible to produce in rodent systems, notably MAbs to other Rhesus and Kidd antigens (13,14).

The use of peripheral B lymphocytes from donors known to have been immunized with the antigen in question increases the chances of success from this approach. However, the ethical considerations concerned with deliberate immunization of human subjects make this approach extremely dependent on obtaining fortuitous samples from donors who have been "accidentally" immunized by transfusion or pregnancy. It has recently been shown that SCID (severe combined immunodeficient) mice can be reconstituted with normal human peripheral blood mononuclear cells and produce human antibody in response to antigenic stimulation. Responses to Rh(D) have been achieved in such mice (15). Human B cells from such immunized mice could provide a rich source of antibody-secreting cells for EBV transformation and MAb production in vitro and avoid the ethical limitations involved in immunizing donors.

Although the species of MAbs for use as diagnostic blood grouping reagents or research tools is not significant, the fact that the production of monoclonal anti-D can only be achieved in a human system has been fortuitous when considering potential therapeutic applications (see below). In other fields, genetic engineering techniques have been required to "humanize" MAbs produced in rodent systems for therapeutic use in humans (16).

C. Recombinant Systems

Recent new technologies in molecular biology have shown that parts of antibodies such as single-chain Fv and Fab fragments may be produced in large quantities by bacteria; e.g. *Escherichia coli* (17). The use of phage expression systems and rapid selection of high-affinity antibody fragments mean that this technology could produce large amounts of high-affinity cloned human antibody fragments using source material from unimmunized donors. Manipulation at the DNA level, by site-directed mutagenesis, may lead to the production of "designer" antibody fragment clones, with specificities and affinities that could not be achieved by in vivo immunization procedures. Production of large amounts of "designer" molecules in bacterial systems may further revolutionize blood grouping reagents and procedures.

D. Cloning and Selection of MAb-Producing Cell Lines

Selection is a vital part of any MAb-producing protocol, so that the cells that are selected for further growth are producing antibody with the characteristics required. If a successful fusion has been achieved, the tissue culture laboratory will be faced with an impossible amount of work to keep all the resultant cell lines growing and freeze stocks down. The screening method used must be one that can be completed on a large number of samples in a short time—results should be available on screening within the same day that supernatants are harvested. Delays in screening may result in the loss of cell lines of great potential by overgrowth with other cells. Useful antibodies must be identified rapidly, and the cells producing them cloned away from other cells.

The screening method used should relate to the purpose for which the MAbs are required. If the intention is to produce MAbs that can be used by the "immediate spin" blood grouping technique, there is little point in screening in any other way other than direct agglutination of the appropriate group RBCs after a short incubation time. If, however, one is interested in looking at the distribution and quantity of RBC blood group antigens on different cell types, MAbs that only react by the antiglobulin test (AGT), enzyme tests, or enzyme-linked immunosorbent assay (ELISA) techniques may be worth screening and selecting for.

The specificity of blood group–specific MAbs can generally be rapidly established as part of the screening procedure by conventional serological techniques with appropriate panels of cells. Absolute specificity of antibody produced by stable cell lines should be confirmed after cloning and selection over a range of different, highly sensitive techniques, and dependence for reactivity on conditions of concentration, temperature, pH and ionic strength should be carefully examined (see below).

Screening may also be carried out on a very specific basis for characteristics of the MAbs other than serological specificity. For example, apart from screening fusions for directly agglutinating anti-B, it is possible to make the selection more restrictive for a particular type of anti-B. Many anti-B MAbs tend to precipitate in harvested culture supernatants owing to autoreactivity as structures similar to the B carbohydrate epitope are frequently present on mouse immunoglobulin Fc regions (18). Such precipitation can cause problems in bulk processing and standardization as blood typing reagents. By performing fusions and carefully screening for nonprecipitating anti-B MAbs, better reagent antibodies can be obtained.

Similarly, many MAbs show monolayering effects when used as reagents in plastic tubes or microplates, which again can cause problems if they are to be used as routine blood typing reagents. By careful selection on cloning, it is possible to produce clones producing MAbs that do not tend to monolayer. If a particular class of antibody is required, this can be specifically selected for. A panning technique can be used with magnetic beads coated with anti-IgG or anti-IgM and washing to remove hybridoma cells not producing that class of antibody. Alternatively, cloning supernatants can be screened using class-specific ELISA techniques, with only those cells producing antibody of the correct class being selected for further growth (19).

Such detailed selection can be performed after the first rounds of cloning and selection. Even established monoclonal cell lines produce somatic mutation variants when grown in continuous culture, and advantageous mutations can be selected for by recloning and selecting for the required characteristic. Beckwith et al. (19) have described selection of class-switch variants. Martel et al. (20) have described enrichment of the avidity of anti-A MAbs by panning hybridoma cells on group A RBC-coated plates and selecting those resistant to washing off. Mushens et al. (21) have described selection of sister clone avidity variants of anti-D MAbs.

In our laboratory, we have selected nonmonolayering sister clones of an anti-A cell line that had previously caused severe monolayering problems in plastic microplates.

III. CHARACTERIZATION OF MONOCLONAL ANTIBODIES

Once a stable MAb-producing cell line has been established in culture, the antibody it produces will gradually become better characterized as its performance under different conditions is assessed.

The antibody isotype should first be established. This can be achieved by Ouchterlony, ELISA, or passive haemagglutination methods. When mice are immunized with human RBCs or blood group active substances, MAbs produced are usually of the IgM or IgG type. However, several examples of IgA anti-A and anti-A,B MAbs have been reported (22). Traditional serological methods of distinguishing IgM from IgG antibodies with dithiothreitol are not sufficient to determine the Ig class of MAbs as variable results can be obtained (23,24). It may also be useful to determine the light chain (κ or λ) type of the MAb.

The serological specificity of a blood group MAb can normally be readily determined by the pattern of reactivity in conventional serological techniques against panels of characterised untreated and enzyme-treated RBCs.

Specificity should also be confirmed at high and low concentrations of the MAb by using concentrated culture supernatant, purified concentrated antibody or ascitic fluid, and titration series where neat supernatant gives a negative result. Some aspects of serological specificity that have been described for blood group–specific MAbs are concentration or technique-dependent effects rather than true specificity determinants; e.g., MAD-2 anti-D reacts with category D^V variants at high concentrations, but not at low concentrations, whereas HAM-A anti-D will not react with such variants at any concentration. Specificity against weak variants should be evaluated in titration studies when using IgG antibodies as prozoning may otherwise give rise to a false-negative reaction. The results of the International Society of Blood Transfusion (ISBT) workshops on MAbs antibodies has shown that individual laboratories will evaluate the D variant "specificity" of the same MAb supernatant differently because of differences in techniques.

Reactivity in serological techniques should also be evaluated under a range of conditions with respect to pH and ionic strength. For example, many anti-N MAbs are very dependent on high pH conditions, whereas others will react at neutral pH. For MAbs with specificity to ABO, H, I, Le, or P blood group systems, there are a range of synthetic chemical structures available to determine precise specificities by binding and inhibition assays (25). Some MAbs are dependent on the degree of sialidation of RBC glycosyl sequences for their reactivity—this can be evaluated by reaction patterns pre- and postsialidase treatment of cells.

In situations where a number of MAbs have been generated to one antigenic structure, epitope mapping studies can be undertaken to determine the precise specificity of the MAbs. This is normally achieved by producing Fab fragments of the MAbs by papain digestion and radio- or enzyme labeling them. RBCs are incubated with unlabeled Fab from one MAb, washed, and then incubated with labeled Fab from another MAb. If the binding of the first MAb inhibits the binding of the second MAb, then they are inferred to recognize the same or spatially closely related epitopes on the antigenic structure. By this type of technique, antigens can be "mapped" with different MAbs. For example, complement-reactive MAbs have been mapped to areas of the complement molecule exposed after binding to RBCs (26,27). Different epitopes of the Rh(D) antigen have been proposed (28) as the result of the binding patterns shown by different MAbs. Where an antigen has already been epitope mapped with MAbs, it is useful to characterize any new MAbs in the same way to see if their specificities fit into established epitope groups or if they define a new epitope.

For MAbs with ABO, P, Lewis, and related specificities, the fine specificity of the antibodies can be determined by inhibition with a range of synthetic saccharides. Anti-A and anti-B can be grouped according to their pattern of inhibition with these different substances. Studies with monoclonal antibodies have shown that the A and B epitopes can occur on different chain types on the RBC (25,29). A_1 and A_2 RBCs were shown to differ both quantitatively and qualitatively. Both phenotypes bear A type 2 structure. A_1 RBCs, in addition, also bear A type 3 and type 4 structures, which do not occur on A_2 RBCs (30).

Cultivation of MAb-Secreting Cell Lines

Monoclonal antibodies can be produced by cultivating the selected MAb-secreting cell lines either in a tissue culture system in vitro or by growing intraperitoneally in mice/rats as ascitic tumors in vivo. Although higher concentrations of MAbs can be produced by the in vivo method, the ascitic fluids produced contain contaminating immunoglobulin of host origin and other variable host proteins. For example, mice naturally make anti-A, and their ascitic fluid frequently contains anti-A (31), which is a contaminant of blood group–specific MAbs. Production of ascitic fluid may be difficult from some cell lines that tend to form solid tumors, and yields of fluid are often variable from any one cell line. In addition, production of ascitic fluid in mice should be discouraged for ethical reasons as in vitro alternatives are available.

Before attempting any routine culture of a MAb-producing cell line in vitro, the cells should be screened and shown to be free of microbial infection. Infection that may not be apparent in small-scale culture can cause severe problems when attempts are made to scale up the culture. In particular, mycoplasmal infection may be inapparent in a small-scale culture, but attempts to scale up production result in low cell numbers, high cell death, and low antibody production. In addition, mycoplasmal infections are difficult to cope with in the tissue culture laboratory and are notorious for spreading between different cell cultures even if good aseptic techniques are in use. All cell lines under routine culture in a tissue culture laboratory should be routinely screened regularly for mycoplasmal infection.

Cells should be grown for 2 weeks in antibiotic-free medium, assessed visually for fungal or bacterial infection, and then assayed for mycoplasmal infection. Assays for mycoplasmal infection may be by culture, by fluorescent staining of infected cells, or by the newer DNA probe hybridization techniques. If mycoplasmal infection is detected, the cells should be immediately be disposed of by autoclaving if other stocks that might be mycoplasma free are available. If no mycoplasma-free stocks are available, and it is important to continue growing the cell line, the cells should be treated to attempt to eradicate the mycoplasma. In our laboratory, a successful protocol for treating mycoplasmal infected cells with the antibiotic ciprofloxacin has been developed (R. E. Mushens, unpublished data) based on the work of Schmitt et al. (32). Results of Mowles et al. (33) confirm our observations. Cells are cultured over 2 weeks in the presence of 1, 10, 25, and 50 µg/ml ciprofloxacin. The higher levels of ciprofloxacin will be toxic to the cells, but cytotoxicity varies from cell line to cell line. Cells are recovered from wells containing the highest concentration of ciprofloxacin where there are viable cells. These cells are grown in antibiotic-free medium and retested for mycoplasmal infection. Cells are recloned after ciprofloxacin treatment to ensure that the process has not given rise to nonsecreting cells.

Each cell line producing a MAb has its own characteristics of growth, antibody secretion, and chromosomal stability. The stability and antibody secretion rate of many cell lines can be improved by repeated cloning and selection. Growth rates can be monitored by measuring the change in cell concentration over time and secretion rates measured by estimating the concentration of antibody (by ELISA (34) or radial immunodiffusion) in relation to the cell number. Stability can be assessed by analytical limiting dilution cloning analysis at various stages during cell growth.

Methods used for in vitro culture vary according to the quantity of supernatant required, the degree of postculture purification required, the concentration of antibody required, and the shear stress sensitivity of the cells.

For the generation of small (up to 100–200 ml) quantities of supernatant for evaluation or research, cells are normally grown in static culture in tissue culture flasks. The cells settle onto the base of the flask and secrete antibody into the medium above. This method requires a flat culture vessel such that the cells are not overlaid with a large volume of medium. Sufficient gaseous and nutrient/catabolite diffusion occurs in such a high surface area system. It is, therefore, impractical for generating larger volumes of supernatant. The culture is continued until the cells start to die, and then supernatant is harvested by centrifugation. If the medium used for the cell growth is reliant on bicarbonate/CO_2 for buffering, then HEPES should be added on harvest to avoid the harvested, stored supernatant turning alkaline, which could compromise the activity of the antibody. Addition of 0.1% sodium azide protects the harvested supernatant from microbial infection, although it should be remembered that azide is not stable and will not protect a supernatant indefinitely if stored at 4C! It is good practice to aliquot harvested supernatant according to the average volumes used at one time and prevent microbial challenge as far as possible. Addition of 1 mM EDTA and phenyl methyl sulphonyl fluoride (PMSF) will prevent proteolytic degradation of antibody caused by proteases from senescent cells in the culture, particularly if the cells have been grown in a low concentration of fetal calf serum. Addition of albumin to a final protein concentration of 1.0–2.5% will serve to stabilize the antibody and also prevent protease attack by providing alternative saturating substrate. It may be more practical to store the supernatant in frozen aliquots—preliminary trials should be undertaken first to assess the stability of the antibody to freeze-thaw procedures.

For growth of liter volumes, cells may be grown in spinner flasks, where cells are constantly mixed in a larger volume of medium by a rotating stirrer. Alternatively, roller bottles may be used, where the entire cylindrical culture bottle is constantly rotated. The surface area of the culture vessel is now not important as the cells and medium are being constantly mixed together in equilibrium with the incubator gaseous environment. Mixing is essential to ensure that cells are adequately provided with nutrients and oxygen. Cells that are particularly sensitive to shear stress may not grow well in such a system. Harvesting and storage of supernatant is as above. Concentration of antibody can be achieved by tangential flow ultrafiltration.

For growth of up to 3–5 L of supernatant, a bench-top stirred bioreactor may be used. In such vessels, the pH and dissolved oxygen of the medium are constantly monitored and adjusted, and the level of nutrients, such as glucose and glutamine, can be sampled and adjusted. Again, cells that are particularly susceptible to shear stress may not grow well in such a system.

In larger suspension growth vessels, up to 1,000 L, growth may be maximized by stirred or air-lift systems. Special impellors have now been developed for mammalian cell culture that do not impart as high shear stress on the cells as the original stirrers developed for bulk bacterial cell culture. Alternatively, an air-lift system can be used in which air is injected into the base of the culture vessel to provide oxygen for growth and mixing of the culture.

Various alternative systems have been developed for in vitro bulk culture of static cells. In these systems, the cells are encouraged to grow in a static environment to a high cell density and are fed continously with nutrients while catabolic products are removed. Cells may be retained around hollow fibers in cartridges, where the culture medium is pumped through the lumen of the controlled pore-size fibres. The pore size is sufficient to allow diffusion of essential nutrients, catabolites, and gases but retain cells and, if required, antibody. Alternatively, cells may be retained in microspheres. Such systems do not subject cells to shear stress. Another advantage is that cells may easily be adapted to low-serum or serum-free media when they are growing at high density. This makes the medium costs cheaper and simplifies downstream processing where purified antibody is required; e.g., for therapeutic monoclonal anti-D. Antibody is produced at higher concentrations than is possible in suspension culture systems.

When a new cell line is being considered for bulk culture, it is important to establish first that the cell line will secrete the same MAb stably throughout the projected continuous culture period without giving rise to a large number of variant viable cells that do not secrete antibody and, therefore, have a significant growth advantage over antibody-secreting cells. Bulk culture of an unstable line results in production of a very expensive large volume of supernatant with negligable antibody content! In our laboratory, cells considered for bulk culture are first grown in continuous culture in small static flasks for 3 months, and analytical limiting dilution clonings are performed at the start and finish of the culture period to determine the ratio of MAb secretors to nonsecretors and to check that MAb produced by each cell at the end of the culture period has the same characteristics as MAb produced at the start. Instability detected in this protocol means that the cell line would be recloned and assessed again prior to freezing down master and working cell banks and proceeding to bulk culture.

IV. RANGE OF MONOCLONAL ANTIBODIES PRODUCED TO RED BLOOD CELL BLOOD GROUP ANTIGENS

Monoclonal antibodies have been produced to many of the human RBC blood group antigens and the molecules that bear the polymorphic determinants. Examples are shown in Table 1. This table is not an exclusive list of all MAbs produced to blood group antigens; it merely

Table 1 Examples of MAbs to Human RBC Blood Group Antigens

Antibody Specificity	References
A	2,37,41,42
B	38,40,41
A and B	40,41,43
H	82
I	83
Le[a]	78,84
Le[b]	41
P/P$_1$/P[k]	85–88
LKE	87
M	71,73,88
N	70,71,89
Wr[b]	90
K	91,92
k	93
LW[ab]	94
T	95
T[n]	96
MER-2	97
D	10,12,53,54
C	14,57
c	14,57
E	14,57
e	14,57
Jk[a] / Jk[b]	13
Lu[b]	98
JMH	99
Fy	100

quotes examples of each specificity. Those specificities where monoclonals have been developed and assessed as typing reagents are discussed fully below.

Monoclonal antibodies have also been of great impact in the elucidation of the structures responsible for the different blood group polymorphisms. These aspects are reviewed in Part 1 of this book.

V. USE OF BLOOD GROUP–SPECIFIC MONOCLONAL ANTIBODIES AS DIAGNOSTIC REAGENTS

The use of MAbs for routine major blood grouping reagents was established early in the 1980s. Principles for the selection and evaluation of monoclonal ABO, Rh(D), and antiglobulin reagents evolved during the 1980s. In October 1990, an International Workshop "Reagents for the 1990's" (35) was jointly organized by the U.S. Food and Drug Administration (FDA) and the ICSH (International Committee for Standardization in Haematology)/ISBT (International Society for Blood Transfusion) working party on reagents to review the policies and procedures adopted for the licensing, production, and use of reagents, taking particular account of the use of MAbs. Delegates represented major reagent producers and expert users. Recommendations for the validation of monoclonal-based reagents were agreed, including recommendations for field trials and stability trials. It was generally agreed that once a clone had been well characterized with a wide panel of RBCs and master and working cell banks frozen down, then validation of specificity on each batch of supernatant thereafter produced from those cell banks could be performed with a restricted panel, primarily to check for accidental contamination. Various methods of measuring MAb concentrations were presented, including radial immunodiffusion, ELISA, and passive haemagglutination. These were shown to be helpful in the formulation of standardised reagents. However, it was agreed that the evaluation of each batch of reagent for avidity and potency should be performed by experienced serologists using standard serological techniques, in parallel to agreed standards, and using a defined scoring system to record the various grades of agglutination. In particular, the method for assessing potency of "immediate spin" reagents was debated, and it was agreed that use of a 5-min incubation time prior to centrifugation provided a reasonable time for uniform comparison of reagents. Standardization of centrifugal force and time was also debated, and acceptable combinations agreed as 100–110g for 60 sec, 200–220g for 25–30 sec, 500g for 15–18 sec or 1,000g for 12–15 sec. Accelerated stability studies on monoclonal reagents were shown to give variable results, and it was agreed that there was no substitute for real-time stability data at 4°C. Six months' stability data at 4°C should be acquired before a monoclonal reagent is launched.

Monoclonal reagents should be formulated to exceed, in terms of potency and avidity, current national and international standards. The FDA reference preparations are most widely used by manufacturers. They are only available to licensed manufacturers or international standards organizations. However, FDA-licensed reagents exceed the FDA minimum reference preparations and may be used as guidelines until international reference preparations are available. A working party of the ICSH/ISBT is currently developing, in conjunction with the FDA and the European Commission (EC), international reference preparations that will be available throughout the world. The reference standards to be adopted by the EC for licensing purposes in the mid-1990s should thus be equivalent to those adopted by the ISCH/ISBT and the FDA.

Monoclonal ABO and Rh(D) antibodies have also made possible the development of novel solid-phase cell typing procedures, where the antibody is immobilized on the surface of wells of microplates (23,24,36). These procedures require that the solid phase is coated with a semipurified solution of specific antibody, and this solution must not contain high amounts of other immunoglobulins or proteins that would compete with the specific antibody for binding to the plastic. Monoclonal antibodies provide a ready source of such coating materials.

A. Monoclonal ABO Typing Reagents

In 1980, the first monoclonal blood group antibody used in blood grouping—an anti-A—was described (37). During the next few years, anti-B and anti-A+B monoclonal antibodies were produced (38–43). The antibodies were raised in mice, and human RBCs or natural or synthetic blood group–active substances were used for the immunization. Most of these antibodies are of the IgM type and hence good agglutinators, but strongly agglutinating IgA (22) and IgG antibodies also exist. The first of these MAb reagents were of nearly the same quality as the currently available human polyclonal serum-based reagents or only slightly better. Soon superior MAbs were made and formulated into reagents. Anti-A MAbs were made that readily detected even very weak variants of A, such As A_X, and were superior in performance to human reagents. In 1987, the ISBT arranged an International Workshop on Monoclonal Antibodies. Many of the ABO MAbs then available were tested in laboratories worldwide, and it was concluded that some of these MAbs, either alone or blended with suitable other MAbs, were excellent reagents that were superior to polyclonal reagents. At that time, no satisfactory single anti-A+B MAb was in existence, but such MAbs antibodies have been produced since, and the possibility to use a single MAb for such a reagent was clearly shown in the second ISBT International Workshop on Monoclonal Antibodies (44). It was shown at these workshops that the best reagents were made from MAbs that reacted with all variants of the A structure (for anti-A) or the B structure (for anti-B). Those monoclonals that only reacted with particular types of A or B structure generally performed poorly as reagents.

Some high-affinity anti-A monoclonals (e.g., MH04 and BS63) detect many examples of A_X, and because they are so potent, they also can detect traces of A on the group B cells of people with high levels of galactosyl transferase that show some cross-reactions and make a little A on these group B cells (45). This phenomenon is called the B(A) phenomenon (46–48). The opposite phenomenon, called the $A_1(B)$ phenomenon, has been seen with one high-affinity monoclonal anti-B (BS85) (49). The occurrence of B on group A cells occurs only on adult A_1 and not on A_2 or cord A cells, and the transferase levels of the donors are not elevated (50).

The main characteristics of the B(A) and $A_1(B)$ phenomena are:

1. The B transferases make a little A in (mostly blacks) 0.2–0.8% of Bs. The A transferases make a little B in 1.41% of As.
2. The agglutinates associated with the B(A) and $A_1(B)$ in "spin-tube" and enzyme-enhanced microplate tests are very fragile. The reactions are enhanced by albumin and enzymes.
3. They are specifically inhibited: The B(A) reaction is inhibited by A saliva and the $A_1(B)$ reaction by B saliva.
4. Both phenomena occur at high concentrations of antibody and are prevented by dilution of the antibody.

These powerful monoclonal anti-A and anti-B can be used either diluted and/or blended with other less avid MAbs to make acceptable, highly potent, specific reagents. The dilution of such avid MAbs to avoid the B(A) and $A_1(B)$ phenomena is an extra quality control step in ABO reagent production that was not needed with polyclonal source material.

The other phenomenon noted with these types of very potent monoclonal anti-A and anti-B is that although they are excellent in spin-tube tests, they can cause weaker agglutination reactions than those expected in slide tests with strong phenotype cells (e.g., MH04 anti-A × A_1 cells). This may be because these very avid antibodies produce small agglutinates with low levels of antibody that are insufficient to produce large agglutinates. For these reasons, the best strategy for producing a general-purpose, good-quality monoclonal anti-A or anti-B reagent is to blend supernatant from a high-avidity hybridoma cell line with that from a lower-avidity line. The high-avidity antibody will adequately detect weak phenotypic variants but will be sufficiently diluted to not detect the B(A) or A_1(B) phenomena. The lower-avidity MAb will dilute the higher-avidity antibody and provide a good strength of agglutination with strongly reactive phenotypes using slide tests.

Most monoclonal anti-Bs used for reagents do not detect acquired B (39,51), but MAbs have been described that react well with RBCs of the acquired B phenotype and are inhibited by the deacetylated A structure (25,39).

The use of anti-A,B or anti-(A+B) reagents is now of doubtful utility given the high performance of monoclonal anti-A and anti-B reagents. The use of such a reagent as a "check" is only justifiable if there are doubts about the quality and ability of the anti-A and anti-B to detect all group A variants. However, if it is mandatory to use anti-A,B for blood grouping, selected MAbs—either as blends of anti-A and anti-B, cross-reacting anti-A,B with anti-A capable of detecting A_X or single anti-AB reagents (52)—are more potent and of better reproducible quality than most polyclonal anti-A,B reagents. These potent anti-AB MAbs have been shown to bind to a common part of the A and B antigen, which can be located terminally or at an internal portion of the antigen (25).

Examples of the tube potency titers of some monoclonal anti-A and anti-B supernatants are shown in Tables 2 and 3.

Table 2 Saline Titers of Tissue Culture Supernatant Monoclonal Anti-A Reagents

RBCs	3D3	MH04	BS-63	Polyclonal Commercial Reagent
A_1	1024	1024	512	512
A_2	512	512	512	256
A_1B	512	512	512	512
A_2B	64	256	256	64
A_2B weak	4	256	256	8
A_3B	0	256	128	1
A_3	4	256	128	4
A_x	0	64	32	0

Table 3 Saline Titers of Tissue Culture Supernatant Monoclonal Anti-B Reagents

RBCs	NB1/19	3B4	5A5	BS-85	Polyclonal Commercial Reagent
A_1B	256	64	256	256	64
A_2B	512	128	512	512	64
B	512	128	512	512	128
B cord	256	64	256	256	64
B weak	0	32	64	32	64
A_1	0	0	0	0	0
O	0	0	0	0	0

B. Monoclonal Anti-D Typing Reagents

Human monoclonal IgM and IgG antibodies have been prepared (10,53–55) (for reviews, see refs. 56 and 57).

A major breakthrough has been the large-scale supply of potent, stable, IgM monoclonal anti-Ds as typing reagents. This was first achieved by Thompson et al. (12) using cell lines derived by back-crossing human anti-D–secreting EBV-transformed lymphocytes to mouse myelomas. These cell lines, e.g., MAD-2, FOM-A, FOM-1, HAM-A, and the later lines produced by other groups, e.g., BS 226 (Sonneborn, Biotest) and BAC-9 (CNTS), grow well in tissue culture to give antibody-containing supernatants with saline titers of 128–1024 with R_1r cells in 5-min spin-tube tests. Reagents made from these supernatants enable Rh(D) typing to be performed by simple saline tube or slide tests along with ABO typing, and they work equally well at room temperature or 37C. Selected reagents are excellent for use in microplate or automated systems.

However, unlike the ABO variants where MAbs can be selected that will detect all variants, all MAbs produced to date are directed at limited epitopes of the Rh(D) antigen, and they thus show limited specificity (28,57–59). Table 4 shows the reaction patterns of examples of monoclonal anti-Ds with rare types of RBCs from D categories (D positive with anti-D in their serum), D variants (D positive with missing epitopes but no anti-D), and with weak D (D^u) types. New D variants are being discovered with the increased routine use of monoclonal anti-D reagents, and many of these do not fit with the reaction patterns of known D categories or variants. Evidence suggests that there are at least seven epitopes of the D antigen, and possible overlaps between these epitopes may give rise to many D variants as defined by monoclonal anti-Ds (56,57).

Various strategies have been adopted by reagent manufacturers and users to overcome the pitfalls associated with the specificity limitations of monoclonal anti-Ds.

An early solution to overcome the specificity limitations of IgM monoclonal anti-Ds with category/variant cells and lack of sensitivity with weak D cells was to blend a high-titer monoclonal IgM anti-D supernatant with just sufficient IgG polyclonal anti-D to give reliable second-phase indirect antiglobulin tests with the reagents, as shown by the example in Table 5. This type of blended reagent has been widely available commercially. These reagents are used by simple saline tests for the detection of normal D types and the AGTs performed on negative tests only in manual donor testing and when taking babies' blood samples of D– mothers unless the detection of weak D is mandatory when testing patients' blood samples. The quantity of IgG in the blend must be carefully controlled to ensure that it does not cause

Table 4 Limited Specificity of Monoclonal Anti-D With D Category and D Variant RBCs

	D Category RBCs								D Variant	
	III	IV	IV	V	V	VI	VI	VII	HOW	POL
MAbs (IgM)										
HD-7	3+	0	0	3+	3+	0	0	+	nt	nt
MAD-2	3+	c	c	+	0	0	0	+	0	0
BS-226	c	c	c	0	c	0	0	c	c	c
FOM-1	c	c	c	0	0	0	0	+	c	0
BAC-9	c	c	c	c	c	0	0	3+	0	c
Polyclonal (IgG)	c	c	c	c	c	2+	3+	3+	c	c

Abbreviations: c, complete agglutination; nt, not tested.

Table 5 Examples of a Monoclonal IgM and Polyclonal IgG Anti-D Blend for Saline D Typing and AGT for Weak D (D^u)

	R$_1$R$_1$	R$_1$R$_2$	R$_1$r	Category VI	R$_1^u$r	R$_1^u$r	R$_2^u$r	rr
Saline	c	c	c	0	0	0	0	0
IAT				3+	3+	3+	3+	0

Abbreviation: c, complete agglutination.

prozone (blocking) of the IgM anti-D reaction with the weakest common D type (R$_1$r) cells after extended incubation tests.

Chemical modification of IgG3 monoclonal anti-Ds by reduction and alkylation (60) produces saline-agglutinating monoclonal anti-D that can be used in place of IgM monoclonal anti-D. However, IgG1 MAbs do not form potent agglutinins on reduction and alkylation and cannot be used in this way. A reduced and alkylated monoclonal IgG3 reagent detects D^u very efficiently when the AGT is used as all the antibody is IgG. A further advantage is that the RBCs require limited or no washing prior to the AGT as all the IgG present is anti-D. Detection of further D variants not recognized by the IgG3 antibody can be achieved by blending with IgG1 MAbs with different epitope specificities. Those D variants not detected by the reduced and alkylated antibody will be detected by the AGT.

Further IgM/IgG blends have now been produced where the IgG component also is monoclonal. This gives the advantage, as described for the chemically modified blends, of reducing or obviating the need for washing prior to the addition of antiglobulin serum (AGS). Also in these blends, it is easier during manufacture to exercise tight control of the relative concentrations of IgM and IgG antibodies to avoid problems caused by blocking than it is when using polyclonal material for the IgG component.

All blended reagents suffer from some reduced ability to detect weak D (D^u) in direct tests; this is due to blocking by the IgG component designed to be active in the AGT. These types of reagents are designed to be used by AGT for detection of weak D (D^u) or variants not detectable by the IgM (or chemically modified IgG3) agglutinating component. They do not reliably detect weak D without the AGT.

Some IgM monoclonal anti-Ds can be potentiated to detect weaker D^{u}s in saline tests by the addition of dextran or albumin. However, different potentiated reagents show heterogeneity of reactions with panels of D^u RBCs (Table 6). The level of detection of D^u by any one IgM monoclonal anti-D is affected by the concentration of the antibody (e.g., in the East Anglican Blood Transfusion Center, Cambridge, the use of a BS 226 reagent at 1 in 40 in our 16C Technicon enhanced bromelain methyl cellulose system missed 1/10,000 D^{u}s. The same reagent at 1 in 25 permitted detection of these D^{u}s).

The choice of monoclonal reagents and techniques that have been become available has led to considerable controversy on policies for Rh(D) typing.

In the Netherlands, the discontinuation of the use of the AGT for D^u testing of donors was recommended in 1989 (61) on the grounds that Schmidt et al. (62) had demonstrated that weak D (D^u) was not immunogenic. However, one example of primary and two examples of secondary immunizations were seen in the initial trial over 2 years. Thus, the Dutch developed a quality control protocol by which the combinations of anti-D reagents used for donor blood testing are evaluated against a cell panel of D variants and weak Ds against which the reagents are required to give at least a 1+ grade of reaction by manual spin-tube tests with at least 70% of the panel. The Central Laboratory of the Dutch Red Cross Transfusion Service in Amsterdam (CLB) developed a potentiated IgM monoclonal anti-D and an enzyme test IgG polyclonal anti-D, with a recommendation that this combination of anti-D reagents, and not just monoclonal anti-D reagents, should be used to Rh(D) type donor bloods by simple one-stage direct tests. No further

Table 6 Detection of Weak D (D^u) Types
by Enhanced IgM Monoclonal Anti-D

	Anti-D Reagents		
RBCs	BS-226	BS-226 Dextran	CLB 4319-1 Enhanced
D^u 1	2+	3+	3+
2	2+	2+	2+
3	2+	2+	2+
4	+/2+	+	w
5	+	2+	0
6	0	0	+
7	0	+/2+	0
8	0	+/2+	0
9	0	+	0
10	w	2+	+/2+
R$_1$r	c	c	c
rr	0	0	0

immunizations of Rh(D)-negative patients by weak D donor blood have been reported since the adoption of the reagent quality control procedure.

There is no doubt that sensitive automated donor blood testing by appropriately selected and standardized potentiated anti-D reagents can be achieved without the use of AGT for weak D (D^u) (63). However, the use of manual or microplate D donor typing tests is subject to individual worker skills, especially at the reading stage of the test. The agglutinates associated with weak Ds, at the 1+ or even 2+ level of reaction, are often very fragile and the agglutination is easily destroyed by overagitation of the tests during the reading procedure.

Reactions of monoclonal and polyclonal anti-Ds with the weak D (D^u) RBCs from the donor ("3–41") that caused primary immunization in the Dutch trial are shown in Table 7. Several problems were revealed by direct tests for weak D:

1. The RBCs of the weak D ("3–41") gave very fragile agglutination reactions (1+ to 2+) with the IgM monoclonal anti-Ds that could detect this "immunogenic" weak D (D^u). Thus, staff training to guarantee detection of this weak D would be difficult to assure by manual tests.
2. An IgM + polyclonal IgG blended reagent detected the weak D (D^u) in the short 5-min

Table 7 Detection of an Immunogenic Weak D (3-41) by
"Saline Tube" Tests

	5-min Incubation			15-min Incubation		
	3-41	R1r	rr	3-41	R1r	rr
Reagent						
MAD-2	0	c	0	0	c	0
BS-226	1+/2+	c	0	2+	c	0
4319-1	2+	c	0	1+/2+	c	0
BAC-9	1+/2+	c	0	1+/2+	c	0
Blend	1+/2+	c	0	0	c	0
IgM + IgG				(Blocked)		

test but was negative after a longer 15-min incubation test, as presumably the IgG anti-D had blocked the IgM anti-D reaction. This type of observation has been seen many times (personal communications, J. Case [Gamma Biologicals, Houston, TX] and D. Davies [Ortho Diagnostics, Raritan, NJ]).

3. Conventional polyclonal IgG anti-Ds did not detect saline-suspended or serum-suspended "3–41" RBCs, but if diluted 1:6 with manufacturer's reagent diluent, they would detect the serum-suspended RBCs. These reagents were not standardized to detect weak D by direct tests. They prozone with weak D as they contain a high concentration of IgG anti-D (33–35 Iu/ml) to enable them to work well with normal D by slide as well as tube tests, but they are excellent for detection of weak D by AGT.

The controversies about D typing of donors and patients with regard to weak D and D variants continue. Different centers and countries are developing different policies.

The ISBT/ICSH working party on blood grouping reagents is producing a freeze-dried reference preparation of an IgM monoclonal anti-D to act as a minimum potency reference preparation for direct agglutinating reagents of this type. It is thought that blended reagents should achieve the same minimum direct agglutination potency (titer 64–128 with R_1r cells) as unblended reagents. The working party is also undertaking to prepare a panel of D-variant, D-category, and weak D (D^u) RBCs that are properly evaluated for the assessment of anti-Ds for use in reagents. This will extend the work of van Rhenen et al. (61) and include detailed serology with a panel of monoclonal anti-Ds and determination of the number of D antigen sites with selected IgG monoclonal anti-Ds.

C. Other Rh Monoclonal Reagents

Since the second ISBT workshop, excellent human monoclonal IgM saline agglutinating anti-C, anti-c, anti-E, and anti-e have been produced (14). Recent trials of these antibodies as reagents demonstrated that the anti-C and anti-E (14) are better than conventional reagents for slide, spin-tube, microplate, and automated tests. The anti-c and anti-e were not quite so good, but they were generally better than conventional reagents run in parallel with the 750 tube and 250 slide tests used in a clinical trial by Ortho Diagnostics.

D. Monoclonal Antiglobulin Reagents

Monoclonal antibodies to IgG and complement components are used in the formulation of antiglobulin reagents for the detection of antibody bound to RBCs. Thus, although these monoclonal antibodies are not directed against determinants that are part of the RBC membrane, they are used routinely in blood group serology and merit discussion in this chapter.

In 1983, Downie et al. (64) tried to blend existing monoclonal anti-IgG antibodies to make a satisfactory serological reagent but found that they could not equal the performance of polyclonal reagents, particularly in the detection of weak anti-Fy^a. However, selection of clones specifically for use as antiglobulin reagents has produced single MAbs with equivalent serological performance to the ISBT/ICSH reference preparations R3P and RIIIM (65). Gamma Biologicals now markets an FDA-licensed polyspecific antiglobulin reagent with a single monoclonal anti-IgG component. This MAb detects IgG subclasses 1, 2, and 3 but not subclass 4. Clinical trials have shown that only a very limited number of blood group–specific antibody-containing sera have only an IgG4 component, notably of anti-JMH specificity. Such antibodies are not thought to be clinically significant.

Monoclonal anti-IgGs for serological use should be selected and developed as reagents according to the protocols of the ISBT/ICSH working party on antiglobulin reagents (66,67). Particular attention should be paid to the requirement to avoid prozones with weak anti-D, anti-K, and anti-Fy^a sensitized RBCs while maintaining potency. The monoclonal anti-IgG should be at least as resistant to inhibition by serum (caused by inadequate washing of tests prior to AGS addition) as R3P, the reference AGS. Monoclonal anti-IgG should detect at least the IgG 1, 2, and 3 subclasses, and it should ideally also detect IgG4 (68), although as stated above, a monoclonal that does not detect IgG4 has been used successfully in an FDA-licensed reagent. A monoclonal anti-IgG must also have adequate stability to form the basis of an AGS reagent.

As it is relatively easy to prepare successful antiglobulin reagents from conventional polyclonal rabbit antihuman IgG sera, there is little incentive to move to the monoclonal alternative. However, pressures to move away from the continued use of animals to generate products may cause the production of monoclonal anti-IgG for antiglobulin reagents by more manufacturers.

In comparison, conventional polyclonal anti-C3c/C3d is costly to make and often contains mixtures of antibodies that vary considerably in production from batch to batch. Formulation of the anti-C3d component of a polyspecific antiglobulin reagent is complicated by the delicate balance between achieving adequate potency and the occurrence of "false" positives caused by C3d uptake on to normal RBCs, particularly when the cells are incubated in fresh serum, as in compatibility tests. The use of selected monoclonal anti-C3c blended with monoclonal anti-C3d can produce a reagent with equivalent serological performance to a reagent with polyclonal anti-C3c/d, as shown by the example of RIIIM that is the ISBT/ICSH reference AGS with monoclonal anticomplement components. Alternatively, selected IgM anti-C3d such as BRIC 8 (66,67,69) can provide very potent anticomplement activity without the need to use anti-C3c and are as free of false positives as the reference AGS reagents R3P and RIIIM. Monoclonal anti-C3c and anti-C3d, therefore, offer considerable advantages in the efficient production of reproducible quality polyspecific antiglobulin reagents. Recent claims at the Washington ISBT/ICSH/FDA meeting "Reagents for the 90's" that 3 out of 400 donor bloods showed C3d polymorphism and were negative with some monoclonal anti-C3d deserves further evaluation, but this may reflect quantitative, not qualitative, variation.

E. Other Monoclonal Blood Grouping Reagents

Conventional polyclonal anti-M and anti-N reagents are difficult to make and give poor reproducibility batch to batch. Monoclonal MN typing reagents, therefore, offer considerable advantages. Each monoclonal anti-M or anti-N needs to be carefully assessed for its optimum pH, as M- and N-specific monoclonal antibodies are frequently very pH dependent (70–74). Murine monoclonal anti-N, as with human and rabbit polyclonal anti-N antibodies, reacts with the N-like antigen "N," which is found on glycophorin B and is not a product of the N gene. Fortunately, "N" occurs at a lower site density than the true N product of the N gene on glycophorin A in heterozygotes. Thus, it is relatively easy to make monoclonal anti-N reagents "specific" for N in a particular method by selecting the dilution at which they fail to detect "N" on MM RBCs but have an adequate reaction with MN cells. It is important to use S+ MM RBCs for the negative control in selecting the "specific" anti-N dilution because these cells have approximately 30% more "N" than ss MM RBCs (75–76).

Some murine monoclonal anti-M reagents may be cross-reactive with N, whereas others do not react at all with the N or "N" antigens; e.g., BS-57. However, BS-57 does not detect the variant M^c because presumably glycine is an important of the M structure recognized by BS-57, and it is replaced by glutamic acid in M^c (77). However, this can be a useful discrepancy, as M^c is easily recognized if a second anti-M is selected to ensure that it is reactive with M^c.

Anti-Le^a and anti-Le^b murine monoclonal reagents (78) have been routinely used for several years and should be evaluated as are conventional polyclonal reagents, including an A$_1$ Le^b

cell, to demonstrate if an anti-Le^b requires a high H status for adequate reactions, as is typical of most reagents.

Recently, excellent human IgM monoclonal anti-Jk^a and anti-Jk^b antibodies have been described by Thompson et al. (13). The use of these antibodies as reagents has simplified an IAT typing test to a simple agglutination test.

VI. USE OF BLOOD GROUP–SPECIFIC MONOCLONAL ANTIBODIES AS THERAPEUTIC PRODUCTS

Male volunteers are currently routinely immunized to generate sufficient quantities of high-titer polyclonal anti-D plasma for the production of purified prophylactic IgG anti-D. As for the production of diagnostic reagents, avoidance of immunization of volunteers by the use of MAbs offers considerable ethical advantages. In addition, for therapeutic reagents, the reduction in risk of transmission of human blood-borne viruses achieved by use of a monoclonal product is of high significance.

The mode of action of prophylactic anti-D in suppressing anti-D production in D– mothers of D+ babies is not fully understood (reviewed in ref. 79). However, to be effective, the therapeutic antibody must be capable of not only binding to the antigen on RBcs (via its Fab region) but also interacting with the effector cells of the immune system (via its Fc region). Selection of monoclonal anti-D for therapeutic use, therefore, depends not only on the antigen specificity of the monoclonal antibody (as for diagnostic applications) but also its functional activity in interacting with effector cells.

IgG monoclonal anti-Ds, with serological specificity demonstrated in conventional tests, have been evaluated in various in vitro systems designed to test how effective the MAbs are at interacting with the effector cells of the immune system. These assays involve rosette formation of sensitized cells with monocytes and phagocytes, adherence of sensitized RBCs to monocyte monolayers, antibody-dependent cellular cytotoxicity measurements by radiolabeled chromium release, and chemiluminescent measurements of the oxidative burst caused when monocytes react with sensitized RBCs. Generally, IgG3 antibodies appear to be more important at mediating attachment of sensitized RBCs to effector cells, whereas IgG1 antibodies are more effective at promoting activity. In vitro evidence of synergistic effects between these two subclasses has been obtained (80).

Clinical trials of monoclonal anti-D are currently in progress using selected IgG1 and IgG3 MAbs alone and in combination. Preliminary results in UK trials look promising (81).

VII. CONCLUSIONS

Over the past 10 years, there has been a rapid adoption in the developed countries of MAbs as reproducible, cost-effective, clinically proven replacements for polyclonal human serum–derived material in diagnostic blood transfusion reagents. MAbs are currently being evaluated in clinical trials as replacements for polyclonal human serum–derived IgG in therapeutic reagents. In addition, MAbs have contributed much to the knowledge of the molecular structure and genetics of blood group polymorphisms.

Now that many cell lines have been established, it is to be hoped that monoclonal ABO and anti-D supernatants/reagents may be made readily available in developing countries to provide high-quality reliable blood transfusion diagnostic reagents at low cost.

REFERENCES

1. Kohler G, Milstein C. Continuous culture of fused cells secreting antibody of predefined specificity. Nature 1975; 256:495.

2. Barnstable EJ, Bodmer WF, Brown G, et al. Production of monoclonal antibodies to group A erythrocytes, HLA and other human cell surface antigens: New tools for genetic analysis. Cell 1978; 14:9.

3. Voak D, Lennox E, Sachs S, et al. Monoclonal anti-A and anti-B development as cost effective reagents. Med Lab Sci 1982; 39:109.

4. Galfre G, Milstein C. Preparation of monoclonal antibodies, strategies and procedures. Methods Enzymol 1981; 73:3.

5. Voak D, Lennox E. Principles of monoclonal antibodies in blood Transfusion work. Biotest Bull 1983; 4:281.

6. Voak D, Milstein C, Downie DM, Jarvis J. Monoclonal antibody structure and its importance for the performance of ABO and anti-C3 antibodies. 18th Congress of the International Society of Blood Transfusion, Munich, July 21–28, 1984.

7. Borrebaeck CAK. Human monoclonal antibodies produced by primary in vitro immunization. Immunol Today 1990; 9:355.

8. Smythe J, Gardner B, Anstee DJ. Quantitation of glycophorins C and D on normal red cells using monoclonal antibodies. Transfus Med 1992.

9. Steinitz M, Klein G, Koskimies S, Makel O. EB virus-induced B lymphocyte cell lines producing specific antibody. Nature 1977; 269:420.

10. Kumpel BM, Poole GD, Bradley BA. Human monoclonal anti-D antibodies. Their production, serology, quantitation and potential use as blood grouping reagents. Br J Haematol 1989; 71:125.

11. Bron D, Feinberg MB, Nelson NHT, Kaplan HS. Production of human monoclonal IgG antibodies against Rhesus (D) antigen. Proc Natl Acad Sci USA 1984; 81:3214.

12. Thompson KM, Melamed MD, Eagle K, et al. Production of human monoclonal IgG and IgM antibodies with anti-D rhesus specificity using heterohybridomas.

13. Thompson KM, Barden G, Sutherland J, et al. Human monoclonal antibodies to human blood group antigen Kidd Jk[a] and Jk[b]. Transfus Med 1991; 1:91.

14. Thompson KM, Barden G, Sutherland J, et al. Human monoclonal antibodies to C,c,E and G antigens of the Rh system. Immunology 1991; 71:323.

15. Leader KL, Macht LM, Steers F, et al. Antibody responses to the blood group antigen D in SCID mice reconstituted with human blood mononuclear cells. Immunology 1992; 76:229.

16. Winter G, Milstein C. Man-made antibodies. Nature 1991; 349:293.

17. Marks JD, Hoogenboom HR, Bonnert TP, et al. By-passing immunization. Human antibodies from V-gene libraries displayed on phage. J Mol Biol 1991; 222:581.

18. Judson PA, Smythe JS. Mechanism of cryoprecipitation of anti-blood group B murine monoclonal antibodies. Transfus Med 1991; 1:97.

19. Beckwith M, Moratz CM, Young HA, Mathieson BJ. Analysis of isotype switch variants of a Qa-5 specific hybridoma. J Immunol Methods 1989; 123:249.

20. Martel F, Bazin R, Verrette S, Lemieux R. Characterisation of higher avidity monoclonal antibodies produced by murine B-cell hybridoma variants selected for increased antigen binding of membrane Ig. J Immunol 1988; 141:1624.

21. Mushens RE, Dawes BJ, Scott ML. Comparison of ELISA, AutoAnalyzer and manual serological techniques for the quantitation of monoclonal anti-D. Transfusion Med 1990; 1(suppl 1):61.

22. Guest AR, Scott ML, Smythe J, Judson PA. Analysis of the structure and activity of A and A,B immunoglobulin A monoclonal antibodies. Transfusion 1992; 32:239.

23. Scott ML, Guest AR, King M-J, et al. Characterisation of anti-A monoclonals by liquid-phase and solid-phase serology and radioimmunoassay. Rev Transfus Immunohaematol 1987; 30:443.

24. Scott ML, Guest AR, King M-J, et al. Characterisation of anti-B and anti-A+B monoclonals by liquid-phase and solid-phase serology and radioimmunoassay. Rev Fr Transfus Immunohaematol 1987; 30:515.

25. Oriol R, Samuelsson BE, Messeter L. ABO antibodies serological behaviour and immuno-chemical characterisation. J Immunogenet 1990; 17:279.

26. Dobbie D, Brazier DM, Gardner B, Holburn AM. Epitope specificities and quantitative and serologic aspects of monoclonal complement (C3c and C3d) antibodies. Transfusion 1987; 27:453.

27. Mushens RE, Bakacs T. Inhibition of the classical activation pathway of complement mediated lysis by monoclonal antibodies to complement components C3c and C3d. Transfusion 1992; 32:430.

28. Lomas C, Tippett P, Thompson KM, et al. Demonstration of seven epitopes on the Rh D antigen using human monoclonal antibodies and red cells from D categories. Vox Sang 1989; 57:261.

29. Clausen H, Hakomori SI. ABH and related histo-blood group antigens; immunochemical differences in carrier isotypes and their distribution. Vox Sang 1989; 56:7.

30. Clausen H, Levery SB, Nudelman E, et al. Repetitive A epitope (type 3 chain A) defined by blood group A_1 specific monoclonal antibody TH-1. Chemical basis of qualitative A_1 and A_2 distinction. Proc Natl Acad Sci USA 1985; 82:1199.

31. Shaw MA. Inherent anti-A in mouse ascitic fluids. Med Lab Sci 1986; 43:194.

32. Schmitt K, Daubener W, Bitter-Suermann D, Hadding U. A safe and efficient method for the elimination of cell culture mycoplasmas using ciprofloxacin. J Immunol Methods 1988; 109:17.

33. Mowles J, Moran S, Doyle A. Mycoplasma control. Nature 1989; 340:352.

34. Mushens RE, Scott ML. A fast and efficient method for quantification of monoclonal antibodies in an ELISA using a novel incubation system. J Immunol Methods 1990; 131:83–89.

35. Reagents for the 90's. Convenors P.A. Hoppe and D. Voak. 1st International Meeting of the ISBT/ICSH/FDA and reagent manufacturers. Washington, DC, Nov 7–9, 1990.

36. Scott ML. Principles and applications of solid-phase blood group serology. Transfus Med Rev 1991; 5:60.

37. Voak D, Sachs S, Alderson T, et al. Monoclonal anti-A from a hybrid myeloma: evaluation as a blood grouping reagent. Vox Sang 1980; 39:13.

38. Sachs S, Lennox E. Monoclonal anti-B as a new source of blood typing reagents. Vox Sang 1981; 40:99.

39. Salmon C, Rouger, PH, Doimel C, et al. ABH subgroups and variants. Use of monoclonal antibodies. Biotest Bull 1983; 4:300.

40. Voak D, Lowe AD, Lennox E. Monoclonal antibodies: ABO serology. Biotest Bull 1983; 4:291.

41. Messeter L, Brodin T, Chester MA, et al. Mouse monoclonal antibodies with anti-A, anti-B and anti-A,B specificities; some superior to human polyclonal ABO reagents. Vox Sang 1984; 46:185.

42. Lowe AD, Lennox E, Voak D. A new monoclonal anti-A culture supernatant with the performance of hyperimmune human reagents. Vox Sang 1984; 46:29.

43. Moore S, Chirnside A, Micklem LR, et al. A mouse monoclonal antibody with A(B) specificity which agglutinates A_x cells. Vox Sang 1984; 47:427.

44. Messeter L, Johnson U. (eds). Proceedings of the 2nd ISBT workshop on monoclonal antibodies to human red blood cell and related antigens. Lund, Sweden. J Immunogenet 1990; 17:213.

45. Greenwell P, Yates AD, Watkins WM. Blood group A synthesising activity of the blood group B gene specified 3-galactosyl transferase. In: Schaur R, Boer P, Buddecke E, Kramer MF., eds. Glycoconjugates. Stuttgart: Vliegenthart and Wiegendt, Thieme, 1979:268.

46. Beck ML, Hardman JT, Henry R. Reactivity of a licensed monoclonal anti-A reagent with group B cells. Transfusion 1986; 26:572.

47. Treacy M, Stroup M. (eds). Proceedings of a scientific forum on blood grouping anti-A (murine monoclonal blend) Bioclone. Sept 1986. Raritan, NJ, Ortho Diagnostics DS1-346, 1987.

48. Goldstein J, Lenny L, Davies D, Voak D. Further evidence for the presence of A antigen on group B erythrocytes through the use of specific exoglycosidases. Vox Sang 1989; 57:142.

49. Sonneborn HH, Voak D. Monoclonal antibodies detect overlapping specificities of A and B glycosyl transferases. Poster abstract, Congress Int. Soc. Haemat., Milan, Italy, 1988.

50. Voak D, Sonneborn H, Yates A. The A_1(B) phenomenon: A monoclonal anti-B (BS-85) demonstrates low levels of B determinants on A_1 red cells. Transfus Med 1992; 2:119.

51. Munro AC, Inglis G, Blue A, et al. An evaluation of mouse monoclonal anti-A and anti-B as routine blood grouping reagents. Med Lab Sci 1982; 39:123.

52. Broly H. 2nd International ISBT Workshop on monoclonal antibodies against human red blood cells and related antigens. Lund, Sweden, 1990.

53. Crawford DH, Barlow MJ, Harrison JF, et al. Production of human monoclonal antibody to Rhesus D antigen. Lancet 1983; 1:386.

54. Doyle A, Jones TJ, Bidwell JL, Bradley BA. In vitro development of human monoclonal antibody secreting plasmacytomas. Hum Immunol 1985; 13:199.

55. Goosens D, Champonier F, Rouger PH, Salmon C. Human monoclonal antibodies against blood group antigens. Preparation of a series of stable EBV immortalized clones producing

high levels of antibody of different isotype and specificities. J Immunol Methods 1987; 101:193.

56. Thompson KM, Hughes-Jones NC. Production and characterisation of monoclonal anti-Rh. In: Contreras M, ed. Bailliere's Clinical Haematology. Vol 3, No 2. London: Bailliere Tindall, Harcourt Brace, Jovenovich, 1990: 243–253.

57. Tippett P, Moore S. Monoclonal antibodies against Rh and Rh related antigens. J Immunogenet 1990; 17:309.

58. Voak D, Lennox E. Monoclonal antibodies for laboratory aspects of transfusion practice. In: Cash J, ed. Progress in Transfusion Medicine. Vol 1. Edinburgh: Churchill Livingstone, 1986:1–18.

59. Lowe AD, Green SM, Voak D, et al. A human-human monoclonal anti-D by direct fusion with a lymphoblastoid line. Vox Sang 1986; 51:212.

60. Scott ML, Guest AR, Anstee DJ. Subclass dependence of reduction and alkylation of IgG monoclonal anti-D to complete anti-D. Transfusion 1989; 29:57S.

61. Rhenen DJ van, Overbeeke MAM. Quality control of anti-D sera by a panel of donor red cells with weak reacting D antigens and with partial D antigens by the Federation of the Netherlands Red Cross Blood Banks. Vox Sang 1989; 57:273.

62. Schmidt PJ, Morrison EG, Schol J. The antigenicity of the Rh (D^u) blood factor. Blood 1962; 20:196.

63. Contreras M, Knight RC. The Rh-negative donor. Clin Lab Haematol 1989; 11:317.

64. Downie DM, Voak D, Jarvis J, et al. The use of monoclonal antibodies to human IgG in blood transfusion serology. Biotest Bull 4:348.

65. Voak D, Nilsson U. Report of studies on monoclonal anti-IgG antibodies. J Immunogenet 1990; 17:331.

66. Voak D, Downie DM, Moore BPL, Engelfriet CP. Anti-human globulin reagent specification: The European and ISBT/ICSH view. Biotest Bull 1986; 1:7.

67. Engelfriet CP, Voak D. International reference polyspecific anti-human globulin reagents. Vox Sang 1987; 53:241.

68. Frame T, Bot A, Vlug A, Eijk R. Subclass and epitope specificities of monoclonal anti-IgG antibodies. Second International ISBT Workshop on Monoclonal antibodies to red cell antigens and related determinants, Lund, Sweden, 1990.

69. Holt PDJ, Donaldson C, Judson PA, et al. NBTS BRIC-8. A monoclonal anti-C3d antibody. Transfusion 1986; 25:267.

70. Fraser RH, Munro AC, Williamson AR, et al. Mouse monoclonal anti-N. J Immunol 1982; 9:295.

71. Sonneborn HH, Uthemann H, Munro AC, et al. Reactivity of monoclonal antibodies directed against blood groups M and N. Dev Biol Stand 1984; 67:61.

72. Sonneborn HH, Ernst M. Further characterisation and standardisation of mouse monoclonal antibodies reacting with M/N blood group antigens. Dev Biol Stand 1987; 67:97.

73. Nichols ME, Rosenfield RE, Rubinstein P. Two blood group M epitopes disclosed by monoclonal antibodies. Vox Sang 1985; 49:134.

74. Rubocki R, Milgrom F. Reactions of murine monoclonal antibodies to MN blood group antigens. Vox Sang 1986; 51:217.

75. Voak D, Davies D, Sonneborn H, et al. The application of monoclonal antibodies for the detection of genetic markers of human red cells. Adv Forensic Haemogenet 1988; 2:268.

76. Anstee DJ, Lisowska E. Monoclonal antibodies against glycophorins and other glycoproteins. J Immunogenet 1990; 17:301.

77. Dahr W, Uhlenbruck G, Jansen E, Schmalish R. Different N-terminal amino acids in the MN glycoprotein free MM and NN erythrocytes. Hum Genet 1977; 35:335.

78. Fraser RH, Allan EK, Inglis G, et al. Production and characterisation of mouse monoclonal antibodies to human Le^a blood group structures. Exp Clin Immunogenet 1984; 1:145.

79. Tovey LAD. Towards the conquest of Rh haemolytic disease. Transfus Med 1991; 2:99.

80. Kumpel BM, Wiener E, Urbaniak SJ, Bradley BA. Human monoclonal anti-D antibodies. (ii) The relationship between IgG subclasses, Gm allotype and Fc mediated function. Br J Haematol 1989; 71:415.

81. Thomson A, Contreras M, Gorick B, et al. Clearance of Rh D positive red cells with monoclonal anti-D. Lancet 1990 2(336):1147.

82. Fraser RH, Mackie A, Inglis G, et al. Characterisation of anti-glycoconjugate monoclonal anti-bodies. Rev Fr Transfus Immunohaematol 1987; 30:633.

83. Feizi T. Demonstration by monoclonal antibodies that carbohydrate structures of glycoproteins and glycolipids are oncodevelopmental antigens. Nature 1985; 314:53.

84. Young WW, Johnson HS, Tamura Y. Characterisation of monoclonal antibodies against the human Le[b] blood group antigen. J Biol Chem 1983; 256:13223.

85. Borne AEG von dem, Admiraal LG, Mass CJ, et al. Monoclonal antibodies against antigens of the blood group P system and related structures. In: Rouger P, Salmon C, eds. Monoclonal Antibodies Against Human Red Blood Cell and Related Antigens. Paris: Arnette, 1987:119–145.

86. Kannagi R, Levery SB, Ishigami F, et al. New globoseries glycosphingolipids in human teratocarcinoma reactive with a monoclonal antibody directed to a developmentally regulated antigen, stage specific embryonic antigen 3. J Biol Chem 1983; 258:8934.

87. Tippett P, Andrews PW, Knowles BB, et al. Red cell antigens P (globoside) and Luke: Identification by monoclonal antibodies defining the murine stage specific embryonic antigens -3 and -4 (SSEA-3 and SSEA-4). Vox Sang 1986; 51:53.

88. Fraser RH, Inglis G, Mackie A, et al. Mouse monoclonal antibodies reacting with M blood group-related antigens. Transfusion 1985; 25:261.

89. Fletcher A, Harbour C, Matthews M, et al. Blood grouping with monoclonal anti-N antibodies. Aust J Exp Biol Med Sci 1986; 64:215.

90. Anstee DJ, Edwards PAW. Monoclonal antibodies to human erythrocytes. Eur J Immunol 1982; 12:228.

91. Parsons SF, Judson PA, Anstee DJ. BRIC 18: A monoclonal antibody with a specificity related to the Kell blood group system. J Immunogenet 1982; 9:377.

92. Nichols ME, Rosenfield RE, Rubinstein P. Monoclonal anti-K14 and anti-K2. Vox Sang 1987; 52:231.

93. Sonneborn HH, Uthemann H, Pfeffer A. Monoclonal antibody specific for human blood group k (cellano). Biotest Bull 1983; 4:328.

94. Sonneborn HH, Uthemann H, Tills D, et al. Monoclonal anti-Lw[ab]. Biotest Bull 1984; 2:145.

95. Rahman RAF, Longnecker BM. A monoclonal antibody specific for the Tomsen-Friedenreich cryptic T antigen. J Biol Chem 1982; 129:2021.

96. King M-J, Parsons SF, Wu AM, Jones N. Immunochemical studies on the differential binding properties of two monoclonal antibodies reacting with Tn cells. Transfusion 1991; 31:142.

97. Daniels GL, Tippett P, Palmer DK, et al. MER-2 a red cell polymorphism defined by monoclonal antibodies. Vox Sang 1987; 52:107.

98. Parsons SF, Mallinson G, Judson PA, et al. Evidence that the Lu[b] blood group antigen is located on red cell membrane glycoproteins of 85 and 78 kDa. Transfusion 1987; 27:61.

99. Knowles RW, Yan B, Daniels GL, et al. Monoclonal antibodies recognising high frequency red cell antigens including type 2H and JMH. Transfusion 1981; 21:612.

100. Nichols ME, Rosenfield RE, Rubinstein P. A new human Duffy blood group specificity defined by a murine monoclonal antibody. J Exp Med 1987; 166:776.

14

Structural Analyses of Red Blood Cell Autoantibodies

DON L. SIEGEL and LESLIE E. SILBERSTEIN
University of Pennsylvania School of Medicine
Philadelphia, Pennsylvania

I. INTRODUCTION

Erythrocyte autoantibodies may be benign, present in the plasma of healthy individuals, or pathogenic, causing autoimmune hemolysis (1,2). Autoimmune hemolytic anemia (AIHA) consists of two major clinical disorders: *cold* hemagglutinin disease (cold AIHA) due to an IgM antibody that preferentially agglutinates red blood cells (RBCs) in the cold (4–24°C) and the more common syndrome of *warm* reactive (37°C) immunoglobulin G (IgG)–induced autoimmune hemolytic anemia (warm AIHA).

Previously, the complexity of erythrocyte autoantibodies has been approached by serological examination of the antigen binding properties and by isotype analyses of serum autoantibodies. In this chapter, we discuss these previous investigations as well as the more recent studies using molecular approaches.

II. SPECIFICITY OF RBC AUTOANTIBODIES

The serological specificities of *cold reactive* autoantibodies in cold AIHA are determined by their differential reactivity with normal adult and cord RBCs and the effect of RBC treatment with proteolytic enzymes such as ficin or papain. Using these techniques, specificities termed I, i, Pr, Pr_2, Pr_3, and Gd, and Fl have been defined (3–9). The I/i antigens are branched/unbranched carbohydrate chains attached to either membrane lipids or proteins, whereas the Pr antigens are defined as carbohydrate antigens on sialoglycoproteins. These antibody specificities can also be demonstrated in the plasma of healthy individuals, although the titer is usually much lower in normal subjects (<1:64) than in patients with hemolysis (>1:1000). The serological specificity, however, does not differentiate the harmless cold reactive RBC autoantibodies in healthy subjects from the harmful cold antibodies observed in cold AIHA. The majority of cold agglutinins are immunoglobulins (Ig) of the IgM class and are directed at I/i blood group antigens (2,10). This antigen system comprises oligosaccharide chains composed of repeating N-acetyllactosamine (Gal[β1 → 4]GlcNAc[β1 → 3]) units (13) linked to ceramide or the membrane glycoproteins band 3 and band 4.5 (11,12) (Fig. 1). The best available evidence indicates that the difference between I and i antigens relates to branching of the oligosaccharide chain; anti-i antibodies recognize a linear N-acetyllactosamine oligosaccharide, whereas anti-I antibodies recognize a similar chain that is also branched (13–15). There appears to be a developmentally regulated transition in expression of the I/i antigens; fetal and newborn RBCs express mostly i antigen, whereas adult RBCs demonstrate the opposite pattern (4) (Fig. 1). This transition appears to involve the acquisition of a "branching enzyme" (a [β1 → 6]-N-acetylglucaminyl transferase) (15). It is of interest to note that the conversion of the unbranched i structure to a branched one coincides temporally with the switch from fetal to adult hemoglobin synthesis that has led some researchers to suggest that these processes may be coupled (16).

I and i antigens are also present on human granulocytes, macrophages, platelets, and lymphocytes, and antibodies to these antigens can be lymphocytotoxic (17,18). In addition, they are variably expressed on nonhuman RBCs (19) and cultured cell lines of several animal species (20). On human B lymphocytes, the I/i antigens appear to be carried on a family of high molecular weight glycoproteins (~200 kd) known as the leukocyte common antigen (T200 or CD45) (21), whereas on normal T cells, lower molecular weight (128–140 kd) sialo-glycoproteins express I/i-related structures (21–23). The presence of I/i-related antigens on CD45 is of particular interest because CD45, recently identified as a protein tyrosine phosphatase involved in regulating lymphocyte activation and proliferation (for review, see ref. 24), can exist as isoforms abnormally distributed on cells in autoimmune disease (25,26). The finding that antibodies to CD45 on T or B cells can either inhibit or augment lymphocyte activity in vitro depending on what other membrane receptors are nearby (27) raises interesting questions regarding the effect(s) that autoantibodies to I/i blood group antigens may have on lymphocyte function in vivo.

In contrast, *warm reactive* RBC autoantibodies are characterized by ill-defined serological specificity.

A. Rh-Related Specificities

Many serological studies have suggested that warm-reacting autoantibodies are directed at Rh blood group antigens in a majority of cases by virtue of their "pan-reactivity" with all RBC

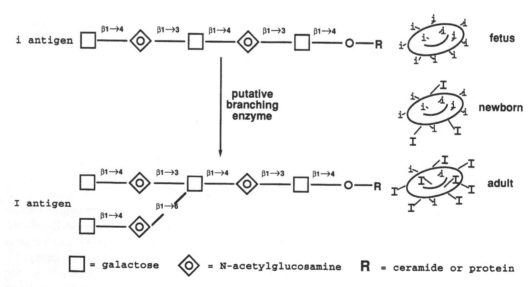

Figure 1 Structure and expression of human I/i blood group antigens.

phenotypes except Rh_{null} cells that lack all Rh components (28–31). This pattern of reactivity has led to the notion of a common "Rh-core" structure to which these antibodies are directed. However, what these serologic observations mean in molecular terms is not at all clear. For example, it is possible that these autoantibodies do not bind to Rh antigens per se but to Rh antigens in combination with some other ubiquitous RBC membrane component(s) (32,33). Alternatively, the autoantigens may not be Rh related at all because Rh_{null} cells, which are misshapen and fragile (34) and display a variety of membrane transport defects (35), have decreased expression of other blood group antigens, including S, s, U, and N (36). In a small number of cases, a "relative Rh specificity" can be observed in which antisera are pan-reactive but display increased reactivity against cells possessing certain Rh antigens such as Rh(e). In still fewer cases, autoantibodies specific for particular Rh antigens have been described (37,38). In these situations, RBCs lacking the corresponding Rh antigen have been found to survive better in vivo than those that express the antigen.

B. Other Specificities

Warm-reacting autoantibodies with specificities apparently unrelated to the Rh system include autoanti-Kell (39), autoanti-Jk_a (40), autoanti-N (41), autoanti-S (42), and a number of others (43). Hemolysis in a patient with warm AIHA presumably mediated by an autoantibody directed against the RBC cytoskeletal protein band 4.1 has been reported (44); however, the patient's serum also contained other RBC autoantibodies including anti-S. In addition, the patient's brother, who had no evidence of hemolytic anemia, had the band 4.1 autoantibody as well, so the significance of these findings remains difficult to interpret.

III. STRUCTURE OF RBC AUTOANTIBODIES

Previous Serological Studies

1. Isotype

In *cold* AIHA, the cold autoantibody is probably a monoclonal antibody (MAb) forming a homogeneous peak on the serum protein electrophoretic pattern (17,45) and contains a single light chain isotype. Cold autoantibodies, present in normal plasma and that are not associated with hemolysis, are also IgM,κ but further characterization as to clonality is lacking. The cold RBC autoantibodies associated with viral infections are usually polyclonal, although in some patients, electrophoretic studies show homogeneous banding patterns suggesting restricted clonality.

The *warm* autoantibodies are primarily IgG, with rare reports of IgM or IgA (43). Antibodies causing immune hemolysis are usually IgG1 and IgG3. Warm autoantibodies are generally considered to be polyclonal, although some evidence suggests that they can be restricted in the Gm allotype (46) and/or light chain type (47).

2. Variable (V) Region

The reason we know more about the specificity and structure of pathogenic cold reactive autoantibodies is that these serum antibodies are present in high amounts as paraproteins and are relatively homogeneous. The presence of high serum concentrations of homogeneous cold reactive RBC autoantibodies has facilitated the study of antibody specificity, idiotypy, and to a limited extent the N terminal amino acid sequences of V regions (48–50). Thus, more extensive structural analyses involving the entire V region were necessary to understand further the contribution of heavy and light chains to antigen binding. More recently, it has been possible to establish in vitro cell lines to study the cellular origin of these antibodies and to examine the diversity of immunoglobulin V region usage at both the molecular and serological (i.e., idiotypic) level. These studies, which are discussed below, have provided important insight into the heterogeneity of pathogenic cold agglutinins, particularly with respect to the role self-antigen may play in their evolution.

In contrast, the nature of the autoimmune response in warm AIHA, a more common and clinically significant disorder, has remained poorly characterized. The major difficulty in studying this disease on a molecular level has been the inability to generate stable Epstein-Barr virus (EBV)–transformed autoreactive B-cell clones from the lymphocytes of affected patients. Although the reason for this technical difficulty is not clear, it may relate to a relative resistance of IgG-producing B cells to EBV-transformation as noted in other systems. Consequently, our understanding of the specificity, structure, and clonality of warm autoantibodies is limited to that provided by serological observations and the analysis of minute quantities of immunoglobulin molecules eluted off the surface of patient RBCs.

IV. IN VITRO PRODUCTION OF MONOCLONAL RBC AUTOANTIBODIES

Both cold and warm AIHA may be idiopathic or secondary to lymphoproliferative disorder, immune deficiency syndromes, collagen vascular disease, infection, or drug therapy. To further understand the biology of these hemolytic syndromes, it became clear that a continuous source of biological material was required. Several approaches have been used to date to establish a sufficient number of autoantibody-producing clones from individual patients that would afford a reasonable assessment of the anti-RBC antibody repertoire in vivo.

The methods involve the hybridoma techniques and the use of the EBV to transform human B cells. Our laboratory has previously used the hybridoma technique, and although cold-reactive RBC autoantibody-producing clones were established from one individual (51), subsequent attempts with the GM4672 cell line were unsuccessful.

The hybridoma technique potentially has two major limitations when applied to the proposed study. These include a low incidence of RBC autoantibody-producing B cells in the spleen and/or peripheral blood and furthermore the unavailability of an optimal *human* fusion partner with a high frequency and growth rate. Additionally, the level of specific antibody production by the fusion partner (plasmacytoma/lymphoblastoid cell line) dilutes the MAb of interest.

In contrast, the method of EBV transformation has been most useful for studying pathogenic cold agglutinins (52,53). The EBV is a herpesvirus capable of infecting human B lymphocytes via membrane receptors related to those for the third component of complement. This infection can then result in transformation allowing the transformed cells to grow virtually indefinitely in vitro. Several laboratories have used this property to establish immunoglobulin-secreting human B-cell lines.

The approaches from different laboratories are quite diverse with respect to the initial seeding density of the lymphocytes, the activation of lymphocytes, the cloning of cells under limiting dilution conditions, and the presence of T lymphocytes. Such variation in method is probably related to the ultimate purposes for which the EBV-transformed B-cell clones will be used. Thus, for example, with regard to the initial seeding density of lymphocytes, it is important to evaluate the probable frequency of the desired (auto)antigen-specific B-cells in the sources of these cells (peripheral blood, lymph node, spleen, bone marrow).

In order to improve the yield of EBV-transformed B cells, several methods have been developed to increase the efficiency of EBV transformation. In particular, polyclonal activators were used to stimulate B cells prior to exposure to EBV. However, there is evidence that polyclonally activated autoantibodies differ from ("unstimulated") autoantibodies present in autoimmune conditions. Since we are interested in antibodies that cause autoimmune disease in vivo, B cells are not stimulated with polyclonal activators in the technique presented here. In contrast, polyclonal activation may be appropriate if the goal is to generate antibodies for use as reagents. The efficiency of transformation is also thought to be increased when performed under limiting dilution conditions. However, this is an extraordinarily labor-intensive approach if clones secreting antibodies with defined specificities are desired. In addition, it is well recognized that EBV-transformed B cells do not grow well when plated as single cells. For this reason, co-culture in the presence of irradiated feeder cells and the use of conditioned media are necessary. Furthermore, under these conditions, the addition of the T-cell mitogen phytohemagglutinin to tissue culture wells containing viable T cells is essential. The latter interventions are thought to induce T-cell–derived growth factors that may promote the growth of EBV-transformed B cells.

The transformation of B cells with or without prior T-cell depletion remains controversial. In the present method, T cells are not depleted to avoid manipulation of the remaining B cells. However, cyclosporin is added to the media during the first week of tissue culture, presumably to counteract unwanted T-cell responses.

The stability of EBV-transformed B-cell lines is very heterogeneous with regard to immunoglobulin production and survival in tissue culture. The factors responsible for this are not known. Nevertheless, cell lines have been generated by several laboratories, including ours, which have stable production for over a year in continuous culture. The subsequent fusion of EBV-transformed clonal cell lines with human lymphoblastoid cell lines or mouse-human hybridomas apparently increases the stability of these cells. The experience with this technique (EBV-hybridoma) has not been uniformly favorable, partly because an ideal nonimmuno-globulin-secreting fusion partner of human origin is not yet available.

Our laboratory is interested in the human immune response to RBC cell antigens, particularly carbohydrate antigens. Over the last several years, we have produced clonal cell lines producing carbohydrate-specific human monoclonal antibodies from a number of patients with cold agglutinin disease. The sera of these patients contain antibodies that preferentially agglutinate RBCs at cold temperatures (i.e., 4C) by recognizing carbohydrate antigens on these cells. By isolating the patient's lymphocytes and transforming them with EBV using the following method, it has been possible to establish stable cell lines that secrete these monoclonal cold agglutinins in vitro.

Methods for EBV Transformation of Human B Lymphocytes (Fig. 2)

1. Conditioned Medium

Human peripheral blood mononuclear cells are isolated by Ficoll-Hypaque density centrifugation and resuspended to a density of 1×10^6/ml in RPMI 1640 containing 2 mM glutamine, 50 μg/ml gentamicin, 2% heat-inactivated human type AB defibrinated plasma, and 1 μg/ml of the T-cell mitogen phytohemagglutinin. Following incubation for 36 hr at 37C, 5% CO_2 the supernatant is collected and stored frozen in aliquots at −70C.

2. Complete Medium

RPMI 1640 containing 20% fetal calf serum 25% conditioned medium, 2 mM glutamine, penicillin (100 U/ml), streptomycin (100 μg/ml), 2% human AB plasma (as above), and Mito+ Serum Extender (Collaborative Research, Bedford, MA).

3. EBV-Containing Medium

The B95-8 marmoset cell line (American Type Culture Collection #ATCC CRL 1612) releases high titers of EBV. The cell line is plated at an initial density of 2×10^4/ml in 25 ml of RPMI 1640 with 10% fetal calf serum, 2 mM glutamine, penicillin (100 U/ml), and streptomycin (100 μg/ml) in a T-75 flask. Following 7 days at 37C, 5% CO_2, the supernatant is collected, filtered through a 0.45-μm cellulose acetate filter, and centrifuged for 30 min at 100,000g using a Beckman Ti60 rotor at 4C. The pellet is resuspended in 100 μl of RPMI 1640 containing 20% fetal calf serum and 0.1–0.2 μg/ml of cyclosporine. The EBV-containing medium is then

1. Ficoll-Hypaque centrifugation of PBL s

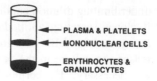

2. 10^7 mononuclear cells + 60 μl EBV-containing supt. of B95-8 cell line

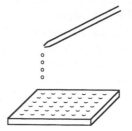

3. Limiting dilution at 10^3 - 10^4 cells/well in 96-well plate

4. Screen after 3 - 4 weeks

5. Subclone

Figure 2   Epstein-Barr virus transformation of human B-lymphocytes.

used immediately for B-lymphocyte transformation. It can also be frozen in aliquots at –70C and used within 6 months; this may not yield optimal results, however.

4. EBV Transformation of Human Lymphocytes

Human peripheral blood mononuclear cells are isolated by density gradient centrifugation, as above (Fig. 2), and either used fresh or are stored frozen in liquid nitrogen in the presence of 5% dimethyl sulfoxide and 95% fetal calf serum. The fresh or rapidly thawed lymphocytes are transferred to a 15-ml round-bottom tissue culture tube. The cells are washed by resuspension in 10 ml of RPMI 1640 followed by centrifugation (200g, 10 min) and aspiration of the supernatant. The pellet is resuspended in 1 ml of complete medium. The cell viability is determined by Trypan blue dye exclusion. Sixty microliters of EBV-containing medium is added per 1.0×10^7 total viable mononuclear cells. Following a 2-hr incubation at 37C, 4 ml of complete medium is added and the cells are incubated undisturbed for an additional 4–5 days.

5. Cloning in 96-Well Plates

Flat- or round-bottom 96-well tissue culture plates are equally effective. The EBV-infected cells are washed four times in complete medium, as above. The cells are resuspended to a density of $2–3 \times 10^5$/ml in complete medium in the presence of irradiated (3,000 rad) normal, random donor human lymphocytes at a density of 1×10^6/ml. The latter are used as feeder cells. This mixed cell suspension is plated into wells of the 96-well plate (100 μl/well). After 5–7 days, 100 μl of fresh complete medium is added to each well. During the subsequent weeks, at appropriate times, 50–100 μl of culture supernatant is removed from each well and replaced with an equal volume of fresh complete medium. The feeding schedule will vary depending on the density, condition, and growth characteristics of the EBV-transformed cells. Discrete colonies are usually visible in 3–6 weeks.

6. Screening for Cold Hemagglutination

Seventy-five to 100 μl of culture supernatant from each well is transferred to round-bottom 96-well plates (sterile, but not tissue culture treated). The plates are incubated on ice for 1 hr and then 50 μl of an ice-cold 1.0–1.5% suspension of RBCs in phosphate-buffered saline (PBS) (pH 7.4) is added. Human blood group A, B, or O RBCs are used that are either untreated or treated with the proteases papain or ficin. The plates are then incubated at 4C for 1 hr. Positive agglutination is defined as large, rigid, or irregular circles; unagglutinated RBCs form a tight "button" at the bottom of the well.

7. Subcloning of EBV-Transformed Cells

Wells containing supernatants that yield strong positive results by cold hemagglutination are chosen for subcloning. The cells from one well are transferred to a 15-ml conical tissue culture tube and washed four times, as above, using RPMI 1640. The cells are resuspended in 0.5–1.0 ml of fresh complete medium and counted. These cells and irradiated donor lymphocytes are mixed and diluted to yield 1×10^5 irradiated donor lymphocytes and 1, 10, or 50 transformed lymphocytes per 100 μl of fresh complete medium. These suspensions are then added to 96-well plates (100 μl/well) and cultured, as above. Typically, two entire 96-well plates are used at 50 cells per well and 4 plates each are used for 10 cells per well and for 1 cell per well. Approximately 2–3 weeks after subcloning, colonies are visible and can be rescreened for cold hemagglutination. Positive wells are gradually expanded into 24 well plates using a minimal amount of media to maintain a high cell density. Feeder cells can also be used at this stage. Wells with growth are then expanded to T-25 flasks, again by maintaining cells at high density but without feeder cells.

V. MOLECULAR AND SEROLOGICAL STUDIES OF V REGION GENES OF RBC AUTOANTIBODIES

A. Autoreactivity to I and i Antigens

The establishment of EBV-transformed B-cell lines secreting either anti-I or anti-i autoantibodies has allowed for nucleotide sequence analyses of the entire expressed variable region genes to further assess the molecular basis for the autoimmune response (54,55). Collectively, the work from two laboratories studying four anti-I and four anti-i cold agglutinins indicates that anti-I as well as anti-i cold agglutinins likely derive from the same $V_H4.21$ (or closely-related) gene segments (54). Furthermore, protein sequencing of another anti-I cold agglutinin has also indicated $V_H4.21$ usage (56).

In contrast, the variable region genes used by the anti-I/i *light* chains do not demonstrate such restriction. Although the anti-I cold agglutinin light chains appear to derive from the VκIII gene family, the anti-i cold agglutinins use light chains from a number of different Vκ families, including VκIII (54). To ask whether the anti-I/i light chains that use VκIII might exhibit similar idiotypic cross-reactivity as observed for the heavy chains, a panel of eight VκIII light chain–dependent monoclonal anti-idiotypic antibodies were raised against an anti-I autoantibody expressing V_H4 and VκIII genes (57). Significant idiotypic heterogeneity was observed among VκIII-expressing cold agglutinin light chains. In addition, the idiotypic heterogeneity could be ascribed to the use of at least three different VκIII gene segments, as well as to somatic diversification of the germline-encoded genes.

The remarkable restriction in the variable region genes used for the anti-I/i heavy chains yet diversification in the associated light chain variable region gene usage suggests a model for the relative contributions of heavy and light chains to antigen binding. The V_H sequence would be required for the global interaction with the I/i antigen complex, whereas the V_L sequence would confer the fine specificity that distinguishes between these distinct yet related carbohydrate structures. This model for cold agglutinin binding to the I/i antigens is currently being tested through the use of bacterial expression systems that permit the mixing and matching of heavy and light chains from different immunoglobulin molecules (see below). From a practical standpoint, the similarities in idiotypic structure among cold agglutinin heavy chain variable regions and the ability to generate anti-idiotypic antibodies specific for these structures suggest exciting potential therapeutic applications for these reagents in downregulating the production of autoantibodies or inhibiting the growth of an underlying malignancy (58).

In this same study by Silberstein et al. described above (54), the expressed variable region genes were also examined for the number and pattern of somatic mutations in order to evaluate the potential role for antigen-mediated selection. It was determined that both the V_H and V_L genes encoding the anti-i antibody were identical to germline sequences, whereas numerous base pair differences were noted in the anti-I response. Compared with its most likely germline precursor, $V_H4.21$, the V_H gene encoding anti-I had only three amino acid differences, two located in framework regions and one in a complementarity-determining region (CDR, or region of antigen contact). In contrast, the V_L sequence of anti-I had a relatively high number of amino acid substitutions (relative to the total number of silent mutations) when compared with its likely precursor germline sequence. These amino acid changes resulted from a *nonrandom* distribution of replacement mutations in the CDRs. Taken together, these results provide evidence that positive selection by antigen led to the accumulation of amino acid substitutions in the light chain of the anti-I antibody studied. If this proves to be a universal feature of anti-I cold agglutinins, it may represent a consequence of differential regulation of the immune responses to the related I/i antigens. Perhaps the high expression of i antigen on fetal RBCs mediates tolerance to i either by clonal anergy or deletion of B cells with anti-i specificity. The expression of I antigen occurs much later in development, so immunologic tolerance for I may differ from that for i. With respect to B-cell function, it was recently demonstrated that IgM autoantibodies found in patients with the Wiskott-Aldrich syndrome, a rare X-linked recessive immunodeficiency disorder, often have anti-i cold agglutinin activity, are encoded by the $V_H4.21$ gene, and recognize a subpopulation of human B cells present early in B-cell ontogeny (59). This same early B-cell population is also recognized by anti-i cold agglutinins isolated from patients with cold agglutinin disease (54). These studies suggest the possibility that the gene product encoded by this highly conserved germline $V_H4.21$ gene may play a physiological role in B-cell development and/or differentiation.

B. Autoreactivity to the Pr₂ Antigen

In contrast to the structural uniformity of anti-I cold agglutinins discussed above, substantial structural differences occur in the two anti-Pr₂ cold agglutinins that have been sequenced (48,53). In the latter case, the heavy chain variable region was 88% homologous to a V_HI germline gene, whereas the light chain variable region was 97% homologous to a VκIII germline gene. Anti-idiotypic antibodies raised against the anti-Pr₂ cold agglutinin from this patient did not show cross-reactivities with RBC autoantibodies from other individuals having anti-Pr or different specificities and were thus unique to this patient's anti-Pr₂ autoantibody (60).

VI. APPROACHES IN DEVELOPMENT

As stated previously, the generation of viable B-cell clones secreting warm reactive RBC autoantibodies has not been successful thus far. Our laboratory as well as others are currently working with a newly described molecular biological approach to express human antibody repertoires in *Escherichia coli*. These systems involve the transfection of bacteria with human heavy chain/light chain constructs that lead to the bacterial secretion of immunoglobulin Fab fragments. Alternatively, heavy chain/light chain protein constructs that bind antigen can be expressed as part of the viral coat proteins of filamentous phage particles (see ref. 61 for recent review). It is anticipated that these approaches will afford the production of antibody molecules with properties resembling those of the serum warm-reactive autoantibodies. This will then make it possible to further elucidate the nature of the corresponding RBC autoantigen(s) and also define the use of V regions required for antibody binding.

An overview of two types of nonmammalian antibody expression systems is presented in Figure 3. Briefly, cDNA is prepared from the mRNA isolated from patient lymphocytes (peripheral blood, splenic, or bone marrow) and the rearranged heavy and light chain DNA segments are amplified using the polymerase chain reaction (PCR) and primers that anneal to conserved regions of the first framework region and constant region. The heavy chain and light chain PCR products are cloned into either a derivative of the λgt11 expression vector (Fig. 2A) (62) or into a novel phagemid expression vector (Fig. 2B) (63). In the former method, the phages are plated on bacterial lawns. Because bacteriophage λ grows lytically, the expressed immunoglobulin molecules (actually Fab fragments) can be screened with nitrocellulose filters by "lifting" the antibody molecules from the resultant phage plaques. The filters can identify the position(s) of phage plaques expressing antibody molecules of interest when incubated with

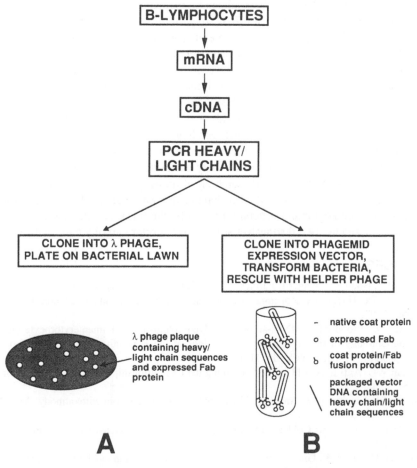

Figure 3   Methods to express human immunoglobulin repertoires in bacteria.

labeled antigen. Since the λ vectors used are modifications of λZapII (64), plasmids can be excised from the plaque-purified phage to permit the high-level expression of MAb molecules in *E. coli* cultures or to provide a source of DNA for nucleotide sequencing. Although this method can provide libraries with as many as 10^8 to 10^9 members, "access" to the library via plaque lifts can be cumbersome. For example, to isolate a particular specificity that is present with a frequency of 1 in 10^6 plaques, over 1,000 Petri dishes would need to be screened. Furthermore, the method of screening the filters with antigen can be problematic when the antigen molecules are not known and/or are not available as soluble proteins as would be the case with membrane-bound RBC autoantigens.

Because of these drawbacks, much of our attention has been directed at adapting the phage display approach (Fig. 3B) to the RBC system (65). In this method, heavy chain and light chain PCR products are cloned into a vector that links them to the DNA sequence for one of the coat proteins of filamentous phage. *E. coli* are transformed with these constructs by electroporation and are then coinfected with filamentous helper phage. Following phage replication, phage assembly takes place during which time heavy chain/light chain–containing vector DNA is packaged into virions coated with copies of native coat protein (provided by the helper phage) and antibody/coat protein fusion product (provided by expression of the initial vector construct). As a result, phagemid libraries of heavy chain/light chain DNA are generated in solution that are coated with antigen binding copies of the expressed immunoglobulin DNA. Screening for RBC binding antibodies can be performed in solution. For example, phagemid libraries with concentrations as high as 10^{13} members/ml can be incubated in solution with RBCs of defined phenotype. Phagemid particles with anti-RBC specificities will bind and sediment with pelleted and washed RBCs. Bound phagemid can be eluted with low pH and used to reinfect fresh *E. coli* for subsequent molecular analysis. This system also allows for the subsequent uncoupling of the antibody molecules from the viral coat protein so that soluble antigen binding protein can be prepared from specific affinity-selected phagemid particles.

As mentioned in the beginning of this section, these new approaches for the in vitro production of human antibodies may provide a means for elucidating both the nature of the RBC autoantibodies, as well as their corresponding autoantigen(s). However, these methods have the potential for providing powerful means of manipulating individual heavy and light chain gene segments to form structures that may not exist normally in nature. One application currently underway is the mixing and matching of anti-I and anti-i heavy and light chains to determine the relative contributions of each chain to antigen binding. The results of these studies may identify the immunoglobulin structures that confer the fine specificity required to distinguish between the I/i antigens, two distinct yet structurally similar carbohydrate molecules.

REFERENCES

1. Tippett P, Noades J, Sanger J. Further studies of the I antigen and antibody. Vox Sang 1960; 5:107.
2. Dacie J. The Haemolytic Anaemias, Congenital and Acquired, 2nd ed. London: Churchill Livingstone, 1967.
3. Anstee DJ. Blood group MNSs-active sialoglycoproteins of the human erythrocyte membrane. In: Immunobiology of the erythrocyte. Proceedings of the Eleventh American Red Cross Scientific Symposium. 67–68. New York: Alan R. Liss.
4. Marsh WL. Anti Ii: A cold antibody defining the I's relationship in human red cells. Br J Hematol 1961; 7:200.
5. Marsh WL, Jenkins WJ. Anti Sp₁: The recognition of a new cold autoantibody. Vox Sang 1968; 15:177.
6. Roelcke D. A review: Cold agglutination. Antibodies and antigens. Clin Immunol Immunopathol 1974; 2:266.
7. Roelcke D, Ebert W, Giesen HP. Anti Pr₃: Serological and immunochemical identification of new anti-Pr subspecificity. Vox Sang 1976; 30:122.

8. Roelcke D. A further cold agglutinin, Fl, recognizing a N-acetyneuraminic acid-determined antigen. Vox Sang 1981; 41:98.

9. Roelcke D, Riesen W, Geisen HP, Ebert W. Serological identification of the new cold agglutinin specificity anti Gd. Vox Sang 1977; 33:304.

10. Weiner AS, Unger LT, Cohen L, et al. Type-specific cold autoantibodies as a cause of acquired hemolytic anemia and hemolytic transfusion reactions. Biologic test with bovine red cells. Ann Intern Med 1956; 44:221.

11. Childs RA, Feizi T, Fukuda M, et al. Blood group I activity associated with band 3, the major intrinsic membrane protein of human erythrocytes. Biochem J 1978; 173:333.

12. Fukuda M, Fukuda MN, Hakomori S. The developmental change and genetic defect in carbohydrate structures of band 3 glycoprotein of human erythrocyte membranes. J Biol Chem 1979; 254:3700.

13. Feizi T, Childs K, Watanabe K, Hakomori S. Three types of blood group specificities among monoclonal anti-autoantibodies revealed by analogues of a branched erythrocyte glycolipid. J Exp Med 1979; 149:975.

14. Niemann H, Watanabe K, Hakomori S, et al. Blood group i and I activities of "lacto-N-nor-hexa-osylceramide" and its analogues; The structural requirements for i-specificities. Biochem Biophys Res Commun 1978; 81:1286.

15. Watanabe K, Hakamori S. Status of blood group carbohydrate chains in autogenesis and oncogenesis. J Exp Med 1976; 144:644.

16. Hakomori S. Blood group ABH and Ii antigens of human erythrocytes: Chemistry, polymorphism, and their developmental change. Semin Hematol 1981; 18:39.

17. Pruzanski W, Shumak KH. Biological activity of cold-reacting antibodies. Parts I and II. N Engl J Med 1977; 297:538, 583.

18. Dunstan RA, Simpson MB, Borowitz MJ. Heterogenous distribution of antigens on human platelets demonstrated by fluorescence flow cytometry. Br J Haematol 1985; 61:603.

19. Wiener AS, Moore-Janowski J, Gordon EB, Davis J. The blood factors I and i in primates including man in lower species. Am J Phys Anthropol 1965; 23:389.

20. Childs RA, Kapadia A, Feizi T. Glycoconjugates. 1979; 518. Stuttgart: Georg Thieme.

21. Omary MB, Trowbridge IS, Battifora HA. Human homologue of mouse T200 glycoprotein. J Exp Med 1980; 152:842.

22. Childs RA, Feizi T. Differences in carbohydrate moieties of high molecular weight glycoproteins of human lymphocytes of T and B origins revealed by monoclonal autoantibodies with anti-I and anti-i specificities. Biochem Biophys Res Commun 1981; 102:1158.

23. Childs RA, Dalchau R, Seudder P, et al. Evidence for the occurrence of O-glycosidically linked oligosaccharides of poly-N-acetyllactosamine type on the human leucocyte common antigen. Biochem Biophys Res Commun 1983; 110:424.

24. Thomas R. The leukocyte common antigen family. Ann Rev Immunol 1989; 7:339.

25. Yamashita Y, Yasuyuki I, Toshiaki O. Poly[N-acetyllactosamine]–type sugar chain in CD45 antigens of adnormal T cells of lpr mice are different from those of normal T cells and B cells. Mol. Immunol 1989; 26:905.

26. Rose LM, Ginsberg AH, Rothstein TL, et al. Selective loss of a subset of T helper cells in active multiple sclerosis. Proc Natl Acad Sci 1985; 82:7389.

27. Sanders ME, Makgoba MW, Shaw S. Immunol Today 1988; 9:195.

28. Weiner W, Vos GH. Serology of acquired hemolytic anemia. Blood 1963; 22:606.

29. Petz LD, Garratty G. Acquired Hemolytic Anemia. New York: Churchill Livingstone, 1980.

30. Eaton RB, Schneider G, Schur PH. Enzyme immunoassay for antibodies to native DNA. Arthritis Rheum 1983; 26:52.

31. Issitt PD, Pavone BG. Critical reexamination of the specificity of auto–anti-Rh antibodies in patients with a positive direct agglutinin test. Br J Haematol 1978; 38:63.

32. Agre P, Cartron JP. Molecular biology of the Rh antigens. Blood 1991; 78:551.

33. Victoria EJ, Pierce SW, Branks MJ, Masouredis SP. IgG red blood cell autoantibodies in autoimmune hemolytic anemia bind to epitopes on red blood cell membrane band 3 glycoprotein. J Lab Clin Med 1990; 115:74.

34. Sturgeon P. Hematologic observations on the anemia associated with blood type Rh_{null}. Blood 1970; 36:310.

35. Lauf PK, Joiner CH. Increased potassium transport and oubain binding in human Rh$_{null}$ red blood cells. Blood 1976; 48:457.

36. Dahr W, Kordowicz M, Moulds J, et al. Characterization of the Ss sialoglycoprotein and its antigens in Rh$_{null}$ erythrocytes. Blut 1987; 54:13.

37. Högman C, Killander J, Sjölin S. A case of idiopathic autoimmune haemolytic anemia due to anti-e. Acta Paediatr Scand 1960; 49:270.

38. Sachs V. Anti-C as a sole autoantibody in autoimmune hemolytic anemia. Transfusion 1985; 25:587.

39. Marsh WL, Øyen E, Alicea E, et al. Autoimmune hemolytic anemia and the kell blood groups. Am J Hematol 1979; 7:155.

40. van Loghem JJ, van der Hart M. Varieties of specific auto-antibodies in acquired hemolytic anemia. Vox Sang 1954; 4:2.

41. Dube VE, House RF, Moulds J, Polesky HF. Hemolytic anemia caused by auto anti-N. Am J Clin Pathol 1975; 63:828.

42. Allessandrino EP, Costamagna L, Pagani A, Coronelli M. Late appearance of autoantibody anti-S in autoimmune hemolytic anemia. Transfusion 1984; 24:369.

43. Mollison PL, Engelfreit CP, Contreras M. Blood Transfusion in Clinical Medicine. 8th ed. Oxford, England: Blackwell, Scientific Publications 1986.

44. Wakui H, Imai H, Kobayashi R. Autoantibodies against erythrocyte protein band 4.1 in a patient with autoimmune hemolytic anemia. Blood 1988; 72:408.

45. Christenson WN, Croucher DJ. Electrophoretic studies on sera containing high-titre cold haemagglutinins: Identification of the antibody as the cause of an abnormal gamma 1 peak. Br J Haematol 1957; 3:262.

46. Litwin SD, Balaban S, Eyster ME. Gm allotype preference in erythrocyte IgG antibodies of patients with autoimmune hemolytic anemia. Blood 1973; 42:241.

47. Leddy JP, Bakemeier RF. Structural aspect of human erythrocytes autoantibodies. J Exp Med 1965; 121:1.

48. Wang AC, Fudenberg HH, Wells JV, Roelcke D. A new subgroup of the kappa chain variable region associated with anti-Pr cold agglutinins. Nature New Biol 1973; 243:126.

49. Gergely J, Wang AC, Fudenberg HH. Chemical analyses of variable regions of heavy and light chains of cold agglutinins. Vox Sang 1973; 24:432.

50. Evans SW, Feizi T, Childs R, Ling NR. Monoclonal antibody against a crossreactive idiotypic determinant found on human autoantibodies with anti-I and -i specificities. Mol Immunol 1983; 20:1127.

51. Schoenfeld YS, Hsu-Lin SC, Gabriels JE, et al. Production of autoantibodies by human-human hybridomas. J Clin Invest 1982; 70:205.

52. Silberstein LE, Goldman J, Kant JA, Spitalnik SL. Comparative biochemical and genetic characterization of clonally related human B-cell lines secreting pathogenic anti-Pr$_2$ cold agglutinins. Arch Biochem Biophys 1988; 264:244.

53. Silberstein LE, Litwin S, Carmack CE. Relationship of variable region genes expressed by a human B-cell lymphoma secreting pathologic anti-Pr$_2$ erythrocyte autoantibodies. J Exp Med 1989; 169:1631.

54. Silberstein LE, Jefferies LC, Goldman J, et al. Variable region gene analysis of pathologic human autoantibodies to the related i and I red blood cell antigens. Blood 1991; 73:2372.

55. Pascual V, Vistor K, Leisz D, et al. Nucleotide sequence analysis of the V regions of two IgM cold agglutinins: Evidence that the V$_H$4-21 gen segment is responsible for the major cross-reactive idiotype. J Immunol 1991; 146:4385.

56. Leoni J, Ghiso J, Goni F, Frangione B. The primary structure of the Fab fragment of protein KAU, a monoclonal immunoglobulin M cold agglutinin. J Biol Chem 1991; 266:2836.

57. Jefferies L, Silverman GJ, Carchidi CM, Silberstein L. Idiotypic heterogeneity of V$_k$III autoantibodies to the related i and I red blood cell antigens. Clin Immunol Immunopathol 1992; 65:119.

58. Stevenson FK, Smith GJ, North J, et al. Identification of normal B-cell counterparts of neoplastic cells which secrete cold agglutinins of anti-I and anti-i specificity. Br J Haematol 1989; 72:9.

59. Grillot-Courvalin C, Brouet JC, Piller F, et al. An anti-B cell autoantibody from Wiskott-Aldrich

syndrome which recognizes i blood group specificity on normal human B cells. Eur J Immunol 1992; 22:1781.

60. Jefferies LC, Stevenson FK, Goldman J, et al. Anti-idiotypic antibodies specific for a pathologic anti-Pr$_2$ cold agglutinin. Transfusion 1990; 30:495.

61. Winter G, Milstein C. Man-made antibodies. Nature 1991; 349:293.

62. Huse WD, Sastry L, Iverson SA, et al. Generation of a large combinatorial library of the immunoglobulin repertoire in phage lambda. Science 1989; 246:1275.

63. Barbas CF, Lerner RA. Combinatorial immunoglobulin libraries on the surface of phage (Phabs): Rapid selection of antigen-specific Fabs. Methods: A Companion to Methods in Enzymol 1991; 2:119.

64. Short JM, Fernandez JA, Sorge JA, Huse WD. Lambda ZAP: A bacteriophage lambda expression vector with in vivo excision properties. Nucleic Acids Res 1988; 16:7583.

65. Siegel DL, Silberstein LE. Production of human red cell antibodies in bacteria by repertoire cloning. Transfusion 1992; 32:455.

IV
Immune Destruction of Cells

15

Complement in Transfusion Medicine

JOHN FREEDMAN and JOHN W. SEMPLE
University of Toronto
Toronto, Ontario, Canada

I. INTRODUCTION

The complement system defines a group of plasma and membrane proteins that interact to produce a number of humoral immune effects, including cell lysis, bacterial opsonization, and signs and symptoms of acute inflammatory response. The complement proteins account for approximately 5% of all plasma proteins. Complement was first identified as a heat-labile bacteriolytic factor in blood in the late nineteenth century. Since the beginning of the twentieth century, complement has been known to play a role in the in vivo destruction of red blood cells (RBCs) by blood group antibodies. In the intervening years, the widespread involvement of complement in immunological processes has been elucidated, including in the fields of immunohematology and blood transfusion. During the 1960s, it was recognized that the anticomplement antiglobulin test (AGT) was useful not only for the diagnosis of autoimmune hemolytic anemia (AIHA) but might also be of value in detecting some RBC alloantibodies. This chapter concentrates on the aspects of complement of particular interest to transfusionists. Since a detailed description of the biochemistry of the complement proteins is beyond the scope of this chapter and can be found elsewhere (1–3), a summary only is given, with attention to the degradation pattern of C3, the component of most interest to immunohematologists.

II. CLASSIC AND ALTERNATIVE PATHWAYS

The number of components involved in the complement system (Table 1) is still increasing. The complement system is an activated enzyme cascade characterized by proteins that circulate as inactive, or zymogen, forms. When a component in the pathway is converted by specific partial proteolysis to its active form, it then cleaves and activates the next zymogen in the pathway. Simply, there are two activation pathways, a single terminal pathway, complement receptors (CR), and a number of amplification and regulatory steps involved in the complement system.

Table 1 Physical and Functional Properties of the Complement Proteins

Pathway	Complement Protein	Cleavage Product	Subunits	MW (kd)	Serum (μg/ml)	Biological Activity
Classic	C1q		18 (6x3 A,B,C)	400	250	Ag-Ab Binding
	C1r		1	85	100	
		Heavy chain		57		
		Light chain		28		Cleavage of C1s
	C1s		1	85	80	
		Heavy chain		57		
		Light chain		28		Cleavage of C4
	C4		3 (α,β,γ)	204	450	Binds C2
		C4a		9		Anaphylatoxin
		C4b		84		Membrane binding
	C2		1	95	20	Active site of $\overline{C4b2a}$
		C2a		65		Binds to C4b
		C2b		30		
Central	C3		2 (α,β)	195	1300	C5 convertase/CR1 binding
Alternative	C3b		2	185		Anaphylatoxin
		C3a		9		
		iC3b		182		CR3/CR4 binding
		C3f		3		
		C3c		145		
		C3dg		40		CR2 binding
		C3d		30		CR2 binding
	B		1	93	150	
		Ba		30		Chemotaxis
		Bb		63		Active site of $\overline{C3bBb}$
	D		1	25	1–2	Cleavage of Factor B
	P		3	145–156	25	Stabilizes C3bBb
Terminal	C5		2 (α,β)	190	80	Chemotaxis/anaphylatoxin
		C5a		11		
		C5b		185		Initiation of MAC
	C6		1	120	50	Subunit of MAC
	C7		1	120	50	Subunit of MAC
	C8		3 (α,β,γ)	150	50	Subunit of MAC
	C9		1	71	50	Subunit of MAC

A. Nomenclature

The proteins of the classic pathway of complement activation are designated by a capital letter C followed by a number; e.g., C1, C4, C2, and so forth. The proteins associated with the alternative pathway of complement activation are designated by capital letters; e.g., factor B, factor D, and so forth. The enzymatically active forms of the components have a bar over the symbol; e.g., $\overline{C1}$.

B. Complement Activation

The activation routes for complement are divided into the classic and alternative pathways. Both pathways are a series of cascade reactions with amplification loops and control proteins and both produce convertases that act on the central component of complement, C3. Basically there are three major steps in complement activation: recognition, activation, and a terminal step known as the membrane attack complex (MAC); these are summarized in Figure 1.

C. The Classic Pathway

1. C1 Activation

The classic pathway of complement activation is initiated by the binding of C1, a complex zymogen protease, to an antigen-antibody (Ag-Ab) complex (4). Only immunoglobulins IgG and IgM isotypes have the ability to bind and activate C1, and studies have shown that although a single IgM molecule is sufficient to carry out this process, at least two molecules of IgG are required (4). It has been estimated that in order for two IgG molecules to be in sufficiently close proximity to activate C1, about 1,000 IgG molecules are required on the cell surface (5). C1 is a three-subunit molecule held together in the presence of ionic calcium. C1q, the subunit that binds the Ag-Ab complex at the antibody CH_2 domains, is composed of 18 chains and has a molecular weight (Mw_r) of 400 kilodaltons (kd). C1q is associated with two additional subunits, C1r and C1s, single chain proenzymes of serine proteases, in a 1:2:2 ratio (6). Subsequent to binding of C1 to the Ag-Ab complex, $\overline{C1q}$ undergoes a conformational change to expose an active serine enzymatic site. This activation is associated with the cleavage of the C1r subunit into a heavy chain of 57 kd and light chain of 28 kd (7). The esterase activity of the $\overline{C1r}$ light chain cleaves C1s in a similar manner, activating the C1s light chain serine protease

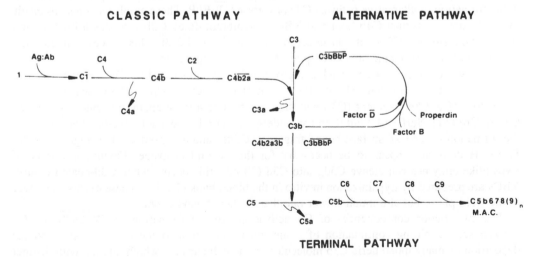

Figure 1   Schematic diagram of complement activation pathways.

(7). C$\overline{1s}$ has broad enzymatic specificity and is responsible for cleavage of C4 and C2, the second series of complement proteins in the classic cascade.

2. Cleavage of C4

C4 is composed of three disulfide-linked chains termed α, β, and γ with Mw$_r$ of 93 kd, 78 kd, and 33 kd, respectively. Activated C$\overline{1s}$ can cleave the α chains of multiple C4 molecules to release C4a (9 kd) molecules. The larger remaining C4b molecules are capable of binding to cell surface membranes via ester or amide bonds in the vicinity of the Ag-Ab-C1 site. These bound C4b molecules have a protective effect on C1 against C1 inactivators (8). This is the first amplification event in the complement cascade and for each antibody molecule bound many molecules of C4b are bound to the cell surface.

3. Cleavage of C2

C2 is a single polypeptide chain of 95 kd that can bind to cell-bound C4b and is subsequently cleaved by C1s in the presence of magnesium. Following cleavage, the larger C2a fragment remains bound to C4b and is the active site of the C4b2a complex, the classic pathway C3 convertase, which catalyses the next stage, cleavage of C3. The C4b2a complex is relatively labile with a half-life of approximately 1 min (3).

4. Cleavage of C3

C3 (195 kd) is a two-chain disulfide-linked glycoprotein (α 120 and β 75 kd) of central importance in the complement system. It is the most abundant complement protein in plasma and is a common link between the classic and alternative pathways. Cleavage of C3 by the C4b2a convertase releases a 9-kd α-chain N terminal C3a fragment that is a potent anaphylatoxin. The larger C3b molecule then undergoes a complex rearrangement of tertiary structure exposing a thiolester site in the C3d region of the α-chain that can bind covalently to hydroxyl groups on a plasma membrane (9); unbound C3b fragments are hydrolyzed and become unreactive. The thioester bond can be broken by water, resulting in a new covalent bond between C3b and the electron pair–donating group. On particles such as RBCs, the formation of ester bonds seems to be favored (10) and many molecules of C3b will incorporate water into the reactive bond for each molecule that is able to bind covalently to the complement-activating surface. Generation of C3b may itself result in further cleavage of native C3 by its participation in the formation of alternative pathway C3 convertase C3bBbP. These amplification steps result in much more C3b than C4b bound to RBCs. Membrane-fixed C3b provides a binding and stabilization site for C5 so it can undergo cleavage by C4b2a3b; this process initiates the formation of the membrane attack complex (MAC) of complement.

C3b is susceptible to further attack that proceeds by several steps (Fig. 2). The first cleavage is made by factor I with factor H and CR1 (see later) as cofactors. This α-chain cleavage results in the loss of a 3-kd fragment (C3f) and the formation of a three-chain molecule, inactivated C3b (iC3b) (11). Surface-bound iC3b can undergo a second cleavage by factor I that results in the formation of a 41-kd surface-bound fragment, C3dg, and a 145-kd soluble fragment, C3c. Factor H does not appear to be necessary for this second cleavage. Finally, a variety of trypsinlike enzymes can cleave C3dg into C3d (30 kd); this occurs when C3d-coated control RBCs are prepared by trypsinization in vitro in the blood bank (12–16). These events can occur in the fluid phase but at a much slower rate than surface-bound events.

The two major consequences of C3 activation are (1) formation of C4b2a3b, or C5 convertase, permitting continuation of complement activation to the C5b-9 MAC; and (2) deposition of many monomeric C3b molecules on the cell surface, which interact with distinct complement receptors on a variety of somatic cells.

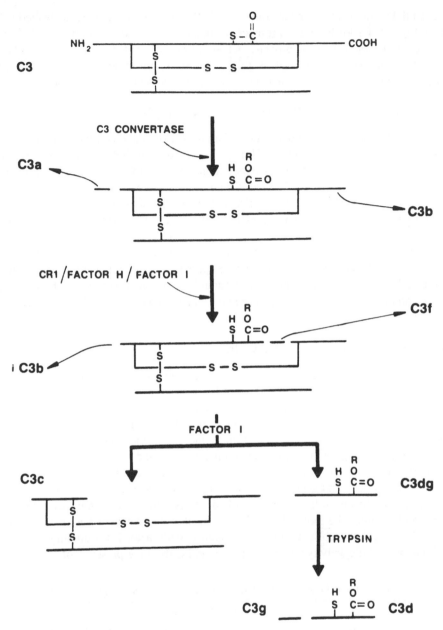

Figure 2 The enzymatic cleavage pathways of C3.

D. The Alternative Pathway

This pathway was originally discovered when it was demonstrated that a yeast cell wall preparation called zymosan could consume C3 at 37°C without affecting the concentrations of C1, C4, or C2 molecules (17). It provides a natural defence system against microorganisms and other pathogens and operates independently of natural antibodies. There are six serum proteins thought to be important in the alternative pathway of complement activation (18), of which three mediate activation and amplification (C3, factor B, and factor D) and the other three (properdin, factor H, and factor I) mediate control functions.

An essential component of the C3 convertase in the alternative pathway is cleaved C3 (C3b) itself (see Fig. 1). Factor B, in the presence of magnesium, forms a complex with C3b and is then cleaved by factor D, a serine protease. Cleavage releases a 30-kd fragment, Ba. The 63-kd Bb fragment, although bound to C3b (C3bBb), has serine protease activity and is capable of cleaving C3 in precisely the same manner as the C4b2a complex of the classic pathway.

E. Cleavage of C5 and the Membrane Attack Complex

Complement activation results in deposition of a number of active complement proteins on the RBC surface. Activation of a single C1 molecule results in deposition of several hundred molecules of activated C3 with consequent augmentation of the numbers of later acting complement components bound. C3b binds C5 and presents the molecule to an adjacent C3bBb or C4b2a3b convertase. Cleavage of C5 releases the anaphylatoxin C5a and exposes membrane and C6 binding sites on the larger fragment, C5b. Cleavage of C5 by either the classic or alternative pathway convertases is the final enzymatic step in the complement cascade. The membrane attack pathway is initiated by formation of C5b and proceeds by sequential assembly of C5b, C6, C7, C8, and C9 into a polymeric complex that, based on its hydrophobic properties can insert itself into the plasma membrane. If enough MACs are driven through the membrane, the cell can no longer maintain ionic balance and ruptures as a result of colloid osmotic lysis—in vivo this results in intravascular hemolysis.

F. Regulation of Complement Activation

Regulation of the classic pathway can occur at several steps (Table 2). C1 inhibitor (C1-Inh) is a single-chain glycoprotein of the serpin family of serine protease inhibitors that can bind to the active site of C1r or C1s to destroy their protease activity. In addition, C4b enzymatic activity is under control of the C4-binding protein (C4bp). On binding to C4b, C4bp exerts two regulatory functions: C4b2a dissociation is increased and C4b becomes susceptible to proteolysis by factor I, generating inactive fragments, C4c and C4d.

C3b on the cell surface is in itself an amplification step. Bound C3bBb can cleave many C3 molecules, thereby generating more C3b and large amounts of anaphylatoxin in the process (1). This pathway thus must be finely controlled. Properdin (P), a gamma globulin, can bind to C3bBb and stabilize the molecule by decreasing its rate of decay. Factor H, on the other hand, can downregulate C3bBb activity by competing with factor B for binding with C3b (19). Factor I has proteolytic activity against both C3b and C4b in the presence of factor H and can

Table 2 Physical and Functional Properties of the Complement Regulatory Proteins

State	Protein	Subunits	MW (kd)	Serum (µg/ml)	Biological Activity
Soluble	C1-INH	1	110	200	
	C4bp	8	500	250	Accelerates decay of C4b2a
	Factor H	1	150	450	Accelerates decay of C4b2a
	Factor I	2 (α,β)	80	35	Cleavage of C3b
	S protein	1	83	500	Binds fluid phase C5b-7
	Sp-40,40	2	70	50	Binds fluid phase C5b-7
Membrane	CR1	1	160–250		Accelerates decay of C3/C5
	DAF	1	70		Accelerates decay of C3/C5
	MCP	1	45–70		Accelerates decay of C3/C5
	HRF/MIP	1	65		Control of MAC formation
	CD59	1	20		Control of MAC formation

thus inactivate both the alternative and classic cascade (20). CR1, which inactivates C3/C5 convertases (see below), membrane cofactor protein (MCP; CD46), which acts on C3b bound to cells, and factor H, whose major substrate is fluid-phase C3b, all have potent cofactor activity for factor I–mediated splitting of C3b to iC3b.

Several phophatidyl-inositol–linked proteins have been reported that influence membrane-bound complement, inhibiting two critical steps; i.e., C3 convertases and MAC formation. These include (1) decay-accelerating factor (DAF; CD55), a glycoprotein that inhibits formation and accelerates decay of the C3 and C5 convertases of the classic and alternative pathways of complement activation (21); (2) MAC-inhibitory protein (MIP), also known as C8-binding protein (C8bp) or as homologous restriction factor (HRF), which inhibits formation of the MAC (22); and (3) protectin (CD59), which also inhibits formation of the MAC on homologous cells (23). Protectin is also known as HRF20, P18, membrane inhibitor of reactive lysis (MIRL), or MAC-inhibitory factor (MACIF) (24,25). The significance of these proteins, anchored to the membrane via glycosylphophatidylinositol, has been elucidated in paroxysmal nocturnal hemoglobinuria (PNH), where a fraction of the blood cells are deficient in these complement inhibitors, resulting in increased susceptibility of the cells to complement. Although protectin has been identified in a number of human tissues, until recently a functional role had been demonstrated only in circulating cells; recent observations suggest that it may also be important in the maintenance of glomerular integrity (26).

III. COMPLEMENT RECEPTORS (Table 3)

Many of the biological functions of complement are mediated by cellular receptors that interact with complement cleavage products (Fig. 3). These interactions culminate in a series of complex biochemical reactions within the cell that trigger various cellular functions. The complement receptors (CRs) are extremely important components of immune function and may be an influence on the state of differentiation on the cells in which they reside. Only a brief description of these receptors is given; more detailed analysis can be found elsewhere (27,28).

A. Receptors for Anaphylatoxins

Receptors for C3a have been identified on mast cells, basophils, lymphocytes, and platelets. Stimulation of C3a receptors leads to degranulation of mast cells, with release of histamine and other mediators of anaphylaxis. C5a, the "classic" complement anaphylatoxin, is 200-fold more potent than C3a in causing anaphylactic reactions and mediates its activities via receptors on

Table 3 Physical and Functional Properties of the Complement Receptors.

Receptor	Subunits	MW (kd)	Cellular Distribution	Biological Activity
CR1 (CD35)	1	190–280	RBC: 1,000 WBC: 5–30,000	C3b receptor
CR2 (CD21)	1	140	B cells Epithelium	C3d/C3dg receptor Epstein-Barr virus receptor
CR3 (CD18)	2 (α,β)	245	Monocytes Lymphocytes Neutrophils Epithelium	iC3b receptor
CR4	2 (α,β)	245	Same as (CR3)	iC3b binding

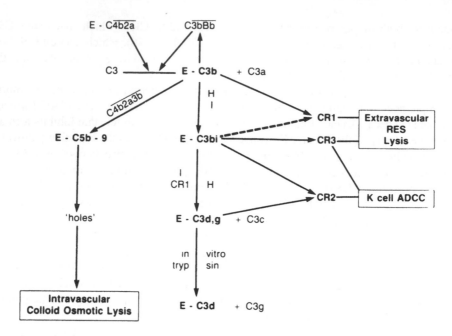

Figure 3 Interrelationship of C3 subcomponents and complement receptors in complement-mediated red cell destruction. (From Freedman, J. The significance of complement on the red cell surface, Transfus Med Rev 1987; 1:58.)

mast cells and basophils. A C5a chemotactic receptor has also been identified on neutrophils and monocytes.

B. Receptors for C3 Fragments

The receptors for several C3 fragments have been shown to be important in stimulating phagocytosis of bacteria, antibody-sensitized RBCs, and other particles (29,30).

1. CR1

All primate RBCs possess immune adherence (C3b) receptors. The isolated C3b receptor (CR1; CD35) is a glycoprotein that exists on the membrane in the form of a hexamer or pentamer (1). There are from 1,000–3,000 CR1 receptors on each RBC and about fivefold higher numbers on various leukocytes. The CR1 receptor has a 1,000-fold higher affinity for C3b than C3, hence allowing C3b to play an important role in mediating phagocytosis. Binding of a C3b-coated target to CR1, however, does not in itself initiate phagocytosis (31). A second signal, usually in the form of IgG interacting with Fc receptors, is required. In addition to phagocytosis, CR1 plays a critical role in the degradation of C3b. C3b binding to CR1 allows the molecule to become accessible to the actions of factor I that cleave receptor-bound C3b to inactivated iC3b (32). CR1 is also important to the processing of circulating immune complexes. C3b readily binds immune complexes that protect C3b from degradation by factors H and I. The C3b-bound immune complexes are effectively removed from the plasma by absorption onto the surface of RBCs and eventually destroyed in the liver (33,34).

2. CR2

CR2 is a 140-kd membrane protein that recognizes C3dg, the breakdown product of C3b after interaction of C3b and factor I. Tryptic enzymes can further break down C3dg to C3d that also interacts with CR2. The receptor is present on all B lymphocytes and may be important in regulating B-cell cycling and differentiation (35). CR2 is also the B-cell acceptor site for the Epstein-Barr virus.

3. CR3

Factor I, in the presence of factor H, cleaves C3b into iC3b. CR3 is the iC3b receptor and is found on epithelial cells, neutrophils, and monocytes, cells that mediate antibody-dependent cell cytotoxicity (ADCC) and natural killer (NK) cell cytotoxicity (28,30). It has two chains of 95 kd (β) and 150 kd (α) and is a member of the integrin family of adhesion proteins (CD18). The receptor is very specific for iC3b and recognizes the characteristic RGD (arg-gly-asp) sequence of the α-chain of C3. Owing to its structure, CR3 is involved in cellular adherence and deficiencies of this receptor result in major cellular adherence defects. With respect to phagocytosis, CR3 acts like CR1 in that it requires a second signal.

4. CR4

CR4 is closely related to CR3 and also recognizes iC3b. Interaction of complement-opsonized RBCs with the surface of phagocytes via these receptors also does not initiate phagocytosis unless a second activation signal is present.

IV. COMPLEMENT AND BLOOD GROUPS

A. Chido/Rodgers

The human immune blood group antibodies, anti-Rodgers (anti-Rg^a) and anti-Chido (anti-Ch^a), define antigenic determinants on the C4d fragment of C4. There are two C4 isotypes, C4A and C4B, which are the products of two homologous closely linked genes on chromosome 6. Individuals who lack either C4A with Rodgers or C4B with Chido may become immunized to these determinants. It appears that all RBCs have some C4d bound, but the mechanism of binding is not understood. The binding of C4d occurs in the absence of an antibody that is usually required to initiate the classic activation pathway. Although in vitro bound C4d is considered to be trypsin insensitive (36), it has been observed that Rg^a and Ch^a determinants on normal RBCs are trypsin sensitive (37,38); Giles has suggested that some of the membrane structures that act as acceptor molecules for C4d (and C3d), such as the MN sialoglycoproteins, are trypsin sensitive (39). The antigenic determinants of C4 are only part of the complex polymorphism demonstrated at the protein level. Anti-Rg^a and anti-Ch^a reagents have been found to be polyspecific in almost every case, and two Rodgers and six Chido high-frequency determinants have been defined; an additional determinant of lower frequency (15–25%) has also been described (37). These determinants are associated with each other in certain combinations and there is a strong association between Rodgers/Chido determinants and the electrophoretic variants of C4 allotypes (40). The C4A and C4B isotypes show more than 99% homology and the main sequence differences reside in the C4d region where the antigenic determinants are located (36). Yu (41) noted that the sequence data of genomic DNA of C4 fitted the antigenic polymorphism rather than the electrophoretic polymorphism and devised a structural model dependent on amino acid sequence variation at four polymorphic sites; the model is composed of sequential and conformational epitopes and has stood the test of time. It remains, however, unclear which sequence variations are responsible for the electrophoretic allotypes of C4 and whether they are located within the C4d fragment.

B. Cromer/Inab

Another complement component that has been of interest to transfusionists is the complement regulatory protein, decay-accelerating factor (DAF). This factor is of interest not only because of its important role in paroxysmal nocturnal hemoglobinuria (PNH), as described later, but also because the Cromer (Cr) complex of blood group antigens has been located on DAF (42). Cells of the Inab phenotype, which lack all Cromer antigens, also lack DAF but are not susceptible, or only minimally more sensitive than normal cells, to complement-mediated hemolysis, a finding that may alter the concept of DAF's functional role (43).

C. Knops/McCoy

The Knops/McCoy (Kn/McC) human RBC blood group system belongs to the category of blood group antigens that generate so-called "high-titer low-avidity" antibodies in immunized transfusion recipients. It has recently been shown that Kn/McC null RBCs have no detectable immunoreactive complement receptor CR1 (C3b/C4b receptor; CD35) in their membranes. Experiments with human antisera to Kn/McC antigens and with monoclonal anti-CR1 antibodies, and studies with isolated human RBC membrane proteins, have indicated that the CR1 protein bears the Kn/McC blood group antigens (44). Similar findings were reported by Moulds et al. (45), who found, in addition, that the Swain-Langley (Sl) and York (Yk) blood group antigens appear to be related to CR1. It is interesting to speculate whether the low numbers or expression of CR1 reported on RBCs from patients with systemic lupus erythematosus (SLE) (46) might correlate with the acquired lack of another high-frequency blood group antigen.

V.   QUANTITATION OF RBC-BOUND C3d

The rate of destruction of RBCs in acquired immune hemolytic anemias is in large measure dependent on the amounts of Ig and complement components on the cell surface. The distinction between strongly and weakly coated RBCs can be made to only a limited extent by the strength or weakness of agglutination in the AGT. The antiglobulin titration score is a more reliable way to assess the degree of RBC sensitization. Because the AGT provides only a semiquantitative index of cell-bound globulins, assays have been developed to quantitate the amount of cell-bound IgG and C3 more definitely. Initial techniques used for quantitation of RBC-bound C3 were C1 fixation and transfer (47) and a modification of the complement-fixation antiglobulin consumption test (48); results were expressed as molecules of C1 fixed per cell because some antisera contained antibodies of at least three C3 specificities and because of uncertainty as to the combining ratio of anti-C3 with cell-bound C3. Although useful in a model system, these tests are indirect and time consuming. In general, studies have depended on the availability of well-characterized antisera specific for the individual antigenic determinants; dependability of results and validity of interpretation have assumed that the antisera were monospecific, potent, and of high-binding affinity. There has been, however, marked variability among anticomplement reagents from different manufacturers, as well as among different lots from the same manufacturer (49,50). The same can be said for reagents produced by individual investigators, although these are generally of better specificity and potency.

Quantitation of C3, or those fragments of C3 that become bound to the RBC surface following complement activation, has been complicated by difficulty in determining the binding ratio between antibody and the specific C3 fragment. Although the C3d/anti-C3d combining ratio was found to be 1 in the fluid phase (50), data were not available on the combining ratio in the fixed phase; i.e., anti-C3d with RBC-bound C3d. Such data are essential to interpretation of results obtained in quantitative experiments of bound C3d. In studies using radiolabeled polyclonal antisera for quantifying the binding ratio, the ratio will likely vary with the extent of fragment degradation, complicating interpretation. In examining the relationship of ^{125}I–anti-antiglobulin C3d-neutralizable cpm to the number of C3d molecules bound per RBC (determined separately by Scatchard analysis using ^{125}I–anti-C3d at antibody excess), Chaplin et al. (51) showed that in the range of 50–500 C3d molecules per cell, the antiglobulin:anti-antiglobulin molar combining ratio was approximately 3. Nonetheless, uncertainty as to the molar combining ratio with polyclonal rabbit reagents makes reference to a calibration curve of questionable value. Recent work using monoclonal anti-C3 antibodies has indicated a binding ratio of 1–2 anti-C3 molecules per C3 fragment when <2,000 anti-C3 molecules are bound; the ratio rises to 3–4:1 when >5,000 molecules are bound (52).

Estimations of the number of bound monoclonal anti-C3 molecules have suggested that agglutination becomes visible microscopically when >100 anti-C3 antibody molecules are bound and is macroscopically complete when >300 molecules are bound (45).

VI. C3d ON NORMAL RBCs

Conventional anti-C3d antiglobulin agglutination tests, which are relatively insensitive, have been reported to be positive on RBCs from 0.01 to 1.0% of normal donors and on RBCs from about 7% of random hospital patients without AIHA or obvious complement-mediated disease (53–56).

Radioactive antiglobulin studies have indicated that small amounts of C3d and C4 are bound to all normal RBCs. The weak false-positive agglutination reactions observed with potent anti-C3d sera may be due to this normal RBC-bound C3d; the reactions may be related to relative potencies of the antisera and may also reflect varying antigen strength on different normal cells. It has been suggested that although such results have been regarded as nonspecific and insignificant, they may be due to abnormal amounts of complement deposited on RBCs and may be useful in predicting the onset of autoimmune hemolysis (57).

Higher levels of RBC-bound C3d have been reported on normal RBCs taken into citrate-phosphate-dextrose (CPD) anticoagulant than on RBCs taken into ethylenediamine-tetraacetic (EDTA) (58); this may reflect the relative inefficiency of CPD as an anticomplementary reagent. Recent studies defining the range of RBC-bound C3d in healthy subjects (51,58–64) showed cord RBCs to have less bound C3d than do RBCs from adults, but no correlation with subject age was found with adults. An increased incidence of positive direct antiglobulin tests (DATs) with anticomplement reagents with increasing age of subjects has been reported (65), but this has not been confirmed in quantitative studies. The reason for lower C3d on cord RBCs remains unexplained, but may be due to lower serum complement levels in newborns or perhaps to less antigenic provocation in the fetus.

The normal range of RBC-bound C3d defined in different studies has ranged from as low as 5–40 to 97–537 C3d molecules/RBC (51,58–64). The lower figures are more likely correct and the differences probably reflect differences in the techniques used, uncertainty as to the combining ratio of RBC-bound C3d and anti-C3d, and differences in specificities of anti-C3d reagents used (66). Although several studies have noted marked differences in C3d/RBC among different healthy individuals, the RBC-bound C3d remained unchanged in individual healthy subjects over prolonged periods of study (51,63).

With newer anticoagulants, blood is being kept for longer periods before transfusion. In contrast to the instability of RBC-bound C3d in vivo, if blood is taken into CPD and maintained at 4°C in autologous plasma, a significant increase in RBC-bound C3d is observed with prolonged storage time (67); the reasons for the difference in vivo and in vitro may relate to differing conditions of enzymic degradation of bound C3d in vitro and in vivo. Older donor blood units, taken into CPD and stored at 4°C as packed RBCs, showed significantly higher levels of RBC-C3d than did units stored for a shorter period of time. In no case, however, did donor unit RBCs give a positive DAT on serological testing with routine anti-C3d. In contrast, RBCs taken into EDTA showed no increase in cell-bound C3d with increased storage time.

Szymanski et al. (68) also suggested that there is a progressive increase in RBC-bound large C3 molecules with increased storage time. The increase in RBC-bound C3d with aging in vitro may be important in the determination of the optimal concentration of anti-C3d in antiglobulin reagents for routine blood bank testing. This may be particularly so for tests using a long serum incubation time because the amount of C3d on RBCs increases after incubation at 37°C even with compatible serum (60). Therefore, anti-C3d should not be used in a concentration high enough to detect normally present RBC-bound C3d.

The mechanism by which C3d molecules are bound in vivo to the RBCs of normal subjects is unknown; the classic complement pathway seems to be involved (51). The physiologic significance of C3d and C4d on normal RBCs remains unclear. The association of the Chido and Rodgers blood group antigens with C4d described earlier complicates the interpretation of the presence of C4d on normal human RBCs. The C4d detected may actually be that which resides in the Chido and Rodgers antigens; on the other hand, the Chido and Rodgers blood group substances may be present because of a low constant level of complement activation. There is, thus far, no parallel explanation for the presence of C3d on normal human RBCs. It may be that continuing low-grade activation of the classic pathway of complement accounts for at least a portion of RBC-bound C3d in normal subjects. Although its clinical significance remains unclear, the presence of RBC-bound C3d in normal subjects is an important consideration in determining the optimal characteristics of the anticomplement component of antiglobulin reagents.

VII. PATHOPHYSIOLOGY OF COMPLEMENT-MEDIATED RBC DESTRUCTION

Proteins of the complement system have a key role in the mediation of immune tissue-damaging reactions in human disease. The intensity of the process and the nature of the inciting stimulus are reflected in the degree of complement activation and the pathway involved. The complement system is one of the principal effectors of the humoral arm of the immune system. Like other components of the immune system, however, complement is a "double-edged sword" and its role in the pathogenesis of disease is of considerable relevance to immunohematologists. Owing to both pathways of activation, complement can mediate various effects that relate to transfusion medicine.

Elucidation of the chemistry of C3 and C4 has been pivotal to understanding the mechanisms of phagocytosis of complement-coated RBCs both in vitro and in vivo. Receptors with different antigen specificities may work synergistically to produce markedly enhanced rosette formation or phagocytosis in vitro when the RBCs are coated with IgG + C3b or IgG + C3d (31,69–71). It would appear that the in vitro observations may, at least in part, be extrapolated directly to the pathogenesis of RBC destruction in vivo in patients with autoimmune and alloimmune hemolysis. When IgG and C3 are bound to the RBCs, the rate and amount of in vivo clearance is often greater than when IgG alone is present. Often, patients with AIHA who have both IgG and C3 on their RBCs require higher dosage of steroids and respond less well to steroids than do patients with only RBC-bound IgG. It would, however, be an oversimplification to conclude that the in vitro studies fully describe the mechanisms of reduced in vivo RBC life span in all circumstances of immune-mediated extravascular hemolysis. Other mechanisms for the damage and destruction of antibody-coated RBCs still need to be explored.

Complement-fixing antibodies affect RBCs in vivo either by (1) producing a membrane lesion resulting in acute osmotic intravascular lysis or (2) by inducing a membrane change resulting in sequestration and extravascular destruction of the altered RBCs by the reticuloendothelial system (RES). The latter mechanism is likely the more important from a clinical viewpoint; i.e., occurs more often.

A. Sequestration of C3b-Coated RBCs in the RES

Early studies in animals indicated the importance of C3b in the sequestration of complement-coated RBCs when complement-fixing antibody is present (48,72). Survival studies in animals as well as in humans, using RBCs coated with antibody and complement, showed that even under conditions such that there was little intravascular lysis, rapid sequestration of the RBCs in the microvasculature occurred with reappearance of the cells in the circulation within several hours. It was postulated that the temporary sequestration involved binding of complement-coated RBCs to C3b receptors on macrophages in the liver; subsequent degradation of the C3b molecule, as described earlier, results in the release of the RBCs into the general circulation again (48,72–75). Mollison (76) showed that although a proportion of RBCs coated by autologous C3 in vitro was rapidly destroyed following transfusion, the remaining RBCs survived normally. In humans, 25–40% of low-ionic strength complement-coated RBCs were removed from the circulation with a T_{50} of 30 sec; the cells began reappearing in the general circulation within 20 min, often entirely reappearing within 3 days. Similar observations have been made in patients with chronic cold hemagglutinin disease (CHAD), but increasing the amount of RBC-bound complement resulted in the permanent elimination of about 30% of the cells, although those reappearing survived normally.

The elegant studies of Jaffe et al. (74) demonstrated the pathophysiological significance of in vivo cleavage of C3b in mediating the release of a proportion of freshly C3-coated RBCs sequestered by C3b receptor–bearing macrophages (primarily Kupffer cells in the liver). Cleavage or degradation of C3b allows the resulting C3d-coated cells to return to the circulation, where they appear to survive normally over a subsequent 20–35 day period of observation. Some of the sequestered RBCs were phagocytosed in the liver, whereas others were released as damaged spherocytic cells. Spherocytes are, however, less commonly seen in complement-mediated immune hemolysis than in hemolysis mediated by IgG. The surviving RBCs, where C3b has been degraded to C3d (C3dg), do not have C3b on their surfaces.

1. C3d-Coated RBCs

It appears that bound C3b is necessary for complement-mediated cell sequestration. Subsequent degradation of C3b to C3d permits the C3d-coated cells to survive normally because there are no C3d receptors on macrophages. There are, however, receptors for C3d on some lymphocyte subpopulations and an effect of RBC-C3d coating on the cytotoxicity of lymphocytes against IgG-coated RBCs has been demonstrated in vitro (71). Although there are several possible explanations for the apparent failure of potentially damaging C3d receptor-bearing cells to affect in vivo survival of C3d-coated RBC, the reasons remain unclear.

Chaplin et al. (77), using quantative assays for RBC-bound C3d, confirmed that the in vivo life span of transfused cells coated with C3d in vitro was normal. RBC-bound C3d was shown to be unstable in vivo, with 90% of the bound C3d antigen disappearing from the normally surviving RBC over a week. It was also shown that subjects who have been kept warm for several days but in whom the RBC are coated with C3d probably have antigen-antibody complexes constantly activating complement, presumably at sublytic levels. Hence, when RBC coating by C3 occurs as an isolated event (e.g., drug-related complement-mediated hemolysis or sensitization by donor plasma alloantibodies), the DAT with anti-C3d would be expected to become much weaker over the course of a few days owing to the disappearance of RBC-bound C3d antigen per se and not necessarily owing to destruction of the complement-coated RBCs. Persistence of a strongly positive anti-C3d antiglobulin reaction, on the other hand, would indicate an ongoing process rather than an isolated-event complement-mediated process. The mechanism by which C3d reactivity is lost from the cell membrane is unclear. RBC-bound C4d antigen disappears more slowly (77).

2. C4-Coated RBC

Phagocytes also have receptors for C4b. C4-coated RBC are, however, in spite of immune adherence, not prematurely destroyed in vivo. Outside of the function of C4 as part of the classic pathway C3 convertase, a role for RBC-bound fragments of C4 (in particular C4d) in immune hemolysis has not been defined.

B. Factors Affecting Complement Uptake and RES Sequestration

1. Immunoglobulin Class

RBC-bound complement usually results from binding of specific antibody to antigens on the RBC membrane. In immunohematologic diseases, IgG and IgM antibody-dependent complement activation is the predominant mechanism, resulting in classic pathway-mediated complement deposition on RBCs. The ability of RBC antibodies to activate complement is thus an important determinant of RBC destruction. Complement-activating capacity is dependent on immunoglobulin class, subclass, affinity for antigen, and number of immunoglobulin molecules bound per cell.

Macrophages carry specific receptors for C1q, C4b, C3b, C3bi, properdin, and factor B; RBCs coated with these complement fragments bind to the phagocytic cell surface. In contrast to IgG Fc receptor macrophage binding, binding to the complement receptor is generally an insufficient signal for ingestion of the complement-coated RBCs and a second signal is required (78). This second signal may be the presence of a few molecules of IgG antibody. Complement thus augments the effect of antibody. When IgG and complement are deposited on the RBCs, these cells are predominantly sequestered in the spleen. If, however, large amounts of antibody and complement are present on the cell surfaces, the cells are sequestered in the liver. Sequestered cells are phagocytosed and do not return to the circulation, presumably because IgG acts as a second signal triggering phagocytosis. With IgG antibodies, it is likely that hundreds to thousands of IgG molecules are required on the RBC surface to be sufficiently close to form an antibody doublet necessary for binding of C1q and consequent initiation of the complement cascade (79).

IgM antibodies almost invariably mediate complement activation. No receptor for the Fc fragment of IgM had been shown on the human phagocytes, and IgM antibody alone does not appear to cause clearance directly. It is the complement deposition on the cell surface that results in shortened in vivo RBC survival. Although IgM antibody-mediated complement deposition on the RBC surface allows for receptor-mediated clearance and phagocytosis, IgM cannot itself provide a second signal for phagocytosis. C3b sensitization alone is a poor stimulus for phagocytosis (78,80). IgM-mediated RBC-bound complement is therefore an inefficient stimulus for phagocytosis. Consequently, spherocytes are not usually seen in large numbers in the peripheral blood of patients with complement-only hemolysis. A single IgM molecule on the RBC surface may allow for C1q binding and initiation of the cascade. However, one complement-activating site is considered to be generally not sufficient to permit sequestration via complement receptor binding and, in experimental systems, 20–40 molecules of IgM antibody per cell are needed before one sees clearance (48,73–75).

IgG3 and IgG1 usually activate complement, IgG2 sometimes does so, and IgG4 rarely if ever activates complement. IgM is more effective than IgG at initiating complement activation, but IgG is more efficient at promoting complement-mediated phagocytosis and extravascular destruction. Although, in theory, IgM antibodies are expected to activate complement more readily than IgG antibodies, in practice, the nature and distribution of antigen sites seems to be more important than immunoglobulin class because the ability of RBC alloantibodies to bind complement is closely related to blood group specificity.

2. Blood Group Antigen Specificity:

Many blood group antibodies activate complement. It has been of interest that, with rare exceptions, antibodies of Rh specificity virtually never bind complement despite usually being of IgG1 or IgG3 subclass. Rosse (81) showed that a system containing multiple anti-Rh antibodies could activate and bind complement to RBCs, supporting the concept that the relatively small number of Rh antigenic sites on the RBCs results in less chance of formation of the IgG doublet necessary for complement activation. This has not, however, been confirmed by others (82) and does not adequately allow for the complement-activating ability of some antibodies to RBC antigens of low surface density; e.g., Kell, Duffy, Kidd. Frank et al. (75) suggested that some IgG anti-D antibodies do cause complement fixation in vitro, although apparently by a mechanism different from IgM mediation, because C3d, but not C3b, was found on the in vitro–sensitized RBCs.

The location of membrane-bound C3b is strongly influenced by the site of activation, and when complement is activated by antibody, this site is in the vicinity of antigens to which the antibody is directed (83). Currie et al. (84), using antibodies to different RBC antigens to fix C3b, determined that the rate of loss of the C3c moiety depends on both the antigen site around which C3b is bound and the number of CR1s per RBC. When C3b was bound by antibodies to antigens on branched-chain glycoproteins, cleavage to C3dg occurred more rapidly than when C3b was bound by antibodies to antigens closer to the red cell lipid bilayer. The rate of cleavage to C3dg correlated with the number of complement receptors (CR1) per RBC, reflecting their role as cofactors in the cleavage of iC3b by factor I. The results suggested that the Jk^a and P blood group antigen sites are physiologically different from the A or I blood group antigen sites. It may be that the Jk^a antigen itself or nearby available C3b binding sites are less exposed, or less mobile, or more sparse than those of the long-chain polysaccharide antigens. These differences in antigen characteristics may thus affect the life span of C3b/iC3b on RBCs; this may be important for determining the rate and mechanism of clearance of C3-coated RBCs.

3. Macrophage Activation

Activation of macrophages may occur in infections allowing phagocytosis of sensitized RBCs via the C3b receptors. It appears that the resting macrophage may bind but not phagocytose C3b-coated RBCs, which are bound to and phagocytosed by activated macrophages (70). It is well known that chronic infection may lead to exacerbation of AIHA; it may be that chronic infection activates macrophages so that C3b receptor triggering leads to phagocytosis in the absence of other triggers of phagocytosis. Monocytes from patients with AIHA have been shown to be more active in vitro than those from normal donors (85,86). Triggering of the fibronectin receptor also enhances phagocytosis of C3b-coated RBCs (87,88); the mechanism for this effect is unknown. Some lymphokines may also act as the second signal.

C. The MAC and Colloid Osmotic Lysis

In immunologically mediated clearance of RBCs, the main role of complement is to allow extravascular sequestration by interaction of complement-coated RBCs with complement (and immunoglobulin) receptor-bearing cells of the RES. When large amounts of complement are activated, however, the full sequence of complement activation may occur with the development of the C5b-9 MAC and its insertion into the RBC membrane resulting in colloid osmotic intravascular hemolysis. Intravascular complement-mediated RBC destruction may be seen in acute hemolytic episodes in CHAD, some warm AIHAs, some drug-induced hemolytic reactions, some alloimmune hemolytic transfusion reactions, and in PNH. The MAC mechanism of the complement system is initiated when C5 becomes activated. Polley et al. (89) observed an ultrastructural lesion in the RBC membrane when C5 is fixed to the surface, and the "doughnut hypothesis" of cytolysis by complement describes an annular structure made up of C5b-9, which is inserted into the lipid bilayer of the cell membrane, thus creating a hole (90). The MAC probably associates with the membrane through hydrophobic nonpolar interactions, but controversy about this process remains. Recent work suggests that C5b-9 complexes, in addition to interacting with the lipid bilayer, may interact with the cytoskeleton of the cell membrane (91). Sung et al. (92) reported that fixation of C3 and C4 subcomponents to the RBC membrane results in increased lipid fluidity of the membrane. Similar pathophysiological mechanisms may occur in immune-mediated neutrophil and platelet diseases.

D. Complement-Fixation and RBC Membrane Deformability

Reactions occurring between RBCs and phagocytic cells depend in part on the size, shape, and deformability of the RBC; alterations in these parameters may affect the fate of the RBCs during such interactions. Complement-coated RBCs adhere to, and are covered by, the exploring metapod of phagocytes. Complement deposition on the RBC surface may affect RBC-phagocyte adherence by altering RBC deformability as well as by affecting membrane receptors. Based on RBC filtration data, Durocher et al. (93) suggested that C3b sensitization results in a decrease in membrane deformability, which returns to normal when C3b is degraded to C3d. Rosse (94), on the other hand, reported no change in membrane deformability with membrane C3b deposition. Sung et al. (92), using newer techniques for assessment of membrane rheology, found that C3 subcomponents bound to the RBC membrane did affect cell deformability. RBCs coated with C3d alone, or C3d plus other complement components, showed significantly increased membrane elasticity and microviscosity; i.e., decreased deformability. Although C3b is probably bound to the exofacial membrane surface, the effects of C3d on the viscoelastic properties of the RBC membrane are probably mediated by its action on the endofacial cytoskeletal protein network.

Since it may result in reduced membrane deformability, C3d deposition may thus render it difficult for the sensitized RBCs to pass through the narrow sinusoids of the RES. It has been observed that older RBCs have more C3d on their surfaces than do young RBCs (67); the decreased deformability may perhaps make it more difficult for senescent cells to traverse the narrow splenic sinusoids and they may be sequestered in the RES by mechanical filtration, thus contributing to other mechanisms of senescent RBC destruction. The impaired deformability of C3d-coated RBCs may possibly play a role in the development of the phlebitis, pulmonary infarction, and gangrene sometimes seen in patients with AIHA. The lung is a rare site of RBC sequestration. In the presence of C5a generation, granulocytes adhere to one another and embolize to the lung. Whether such pulmonary erythrostasis occurs frequently in complement-mediated AIHA remains unknown, but this too may perhaps play a role in the pulmonary infarction occasionally associated with AIHA.

E. C3b and RBC Senescence

Kay et al. suggested that senescent RBCs are cleared from the circulation because a senescent cell antigen (SCA) becomes exposed on the cell membrane that reacts with naturally occurring IgG autoantibodies to the SCA (95); the sensitized cells are then removed by macrophages. The SCA has been characterized and located to band 3 of the RBC membrane (95). IgG autoantibodies to other RBC skeletal proteins have also been found in human sera (96). Dense (old) RBCs have been shown to contain not only increased amounts of IgG but also C3 fragments on their surfaces (67,68,97); both these components may lead to enhanced phagocytosis. Lutz et al. (97) have shown that phagocytosis of senescent RBCs can be enhanced by naturally occurring anti–band 3 antibodies mediating the binding of C3b to the RBC surface, and it was concluded that the opsonization by anti–band 3 antibodies and complement of oxidised RBCs is a relevant mechanism for in vivo clearance of aged RBCs.

VIII. RBC-BOUND COMPLEMENT IN IMMUNOHEMATOLOGICAL DISEASES

Engelfriet et al. (98) showed that RBCs sensitized in vivo with complement in patients with AIHA had the C3d subcomponent of C3 on their surfaces. C4d also is, with rare exceptions, present on such cells, but its significance, and that of fixed C5, is still not completely clear. Although apparently rare, the frequency with which clinically important AIHA results exclusively from alternative pathway activation is as yet undefined. There have been no reports of immune hemolysis due to C4 bound to RBCs in the absence of C3.

A. Amount of RBC-Bound C3

Fischer et al. (62) showed a correlation between the antiglobulin titration score and the number of molecules of C3 per RBC. For a given titration score, however, there were three times as many C3 molecules per RBC on in vitro as on in vivo–sensitized cells. Furthermore, the absolute number of bound C3 molecules was unknown. The presence or absence of hemolysis was not related to the concomitant presence or absence of IgG on the cells but could be roughly related to the amount of complement on the cells. Fischer et al. found that only 14% of patients with <1,100 molecules of C3/RBC had AIHA, whereas 72% of patients with at least 1,100 molecules of C3/RBC had overt hemolysis (62). Thus, the amount of C3 bound to an RBC appears to be an important determinant of in vivo hemolysis.

Quantitative determinations of RBC-bound C3d in randomly selected hospital patients have shown a bimodal distribution curve. Although most hospital patients have normal levels of cell-bound C3d, approximately one third have higher levels not associated with positive DAT (51,63). Chaplin et al. (51), using a radioactive antiglobulin technique, observed that increased RBC-bound C3d is a common reflection of severe illness and that the highest levels of RBC-bound C3d occur in patients with immune-mediated disease. Freedman et al. (57) showed that RBC-bound C3d levels were moderately elevated in patients with a wide variety of diseases in which complement is generally thought to be activated; e.g., lymphoma, infections, tissue injury, collagen vascular disease, malignancy, pregnancy, and renal disease. Generally, patients with only a moderate increase in C3d molecules/RBC had a negative DAT; thus, if one is particularly looking for complement activation and fixation to cells in such situations, a sensitive technique, such as the radioactive antiglobulin method, should be used to detect only slightly increased cell-bound C3d. It was also evident that, similar to reported findings with RBC-bound IgG, some patients may have only slightly elevated levels of RBC-bound C3d and a negative DAT, yet have otherwise unexplained hemolytic anemia.

Patients with AIHA (warm or cold, primary or secondary) usually had high levels of RBC-bound C3d that were associated with a positive DAT with anticomplement reagents. In some patients with severe AIHA, RBC-bound C3b was detectable; this atypical finding may be due to a marked complement activation with saturation of macrophage C3b-receptor sites, thus delaying the destruction of RBC before degradation of C3b to C3dg has been completed. Although differences were small, the C3d/anti-C3d equilibrium constants, or K_0, values in some patients were consistently above or below the normal range; this may be a reflection of slight differences in antigenic specificities of C3d (57). Such differences in specificities have been described for different preparations of soluble and fixed C3d prepared in vitro (66,99). Such small differences in antigen and antibody specificity may have particular relevance with regard to the optimal characteristics of new monoclonal antibodies now being developed.

B. Specific Disease States (Table 4)

RBC-bound complement may be due to autoantibodies, alloantibodies, drug-induced antibodies, complement activation remote from the RBC; e.g., DNA/anti-DNA. Complement activation in immunohematological disease is generally by the classic pathway, but in some diseases, alternative pathway activation may also be operative; e.g., systemic lupus erythematosus (SLE), acquired immunodeficiency syndrome (AIDS), and PNH.

1. Warm AIHA

The incidence of C3 on the RBCs of patients with warm AIHA varies in several large studies. Overall, whereas 40–50% of patients with warm AIHA have IgG and C3 on their RBC surfaces, C3 alone is seen in about 10–20% of cases (55,100). Occasional patients have IgA, IgM, or combinations of these with IgG along with C3 on their RBCs. It appears that most autoantibodies activate complement even when this is not easily demonstrated in vitro tests. Patients with AIHA have been described whose autoagglutinins reacted with aged, but not with fresh, RBCs; the DAT was positive owing to complement sensitization (101,102).

2. Cold AIHA

In CHAD, the causative antibody is usually an IgM agglutinin with specificity in the Ii blood group and typically the DAT with anti-IgG, -IgM, -IgA, and -C3c are negative but DAT with anti-C3d is positive.

3. Paroxysmal Cold Hemoglobinuria (PCH)

Similar to patients with CHAD, patients with PCH have an autoantibody that complexes with the patient's RBCs at low temperatures. The antibody in PCH is, however, IgG. Because the auto–anti-P blood group IgG antibody in PCH binds to the cells typically at low temperatures, the biphasic hemolysin is usually reflected by a complement-only positive DAT, although a modified DAT may reveal the presence of IgG autoantibody on the RBCs.

4. Drug-Induced Immune Hemolysis

In patients on whose RBCs complement-only is detected, drug-induced immune hemolytic anemia of the immune complex mechanism should be considered. In these patients, the DAT will be positive with anticomplement (anti-C3d) reagent but usually negative with anti-IgG. There is a long list of drugs that may cause positive DAT and hemolysis resulting from complement activation associated with immune complex formation. If a patient forms antibody

Table 4 Common Direct Antiglobulin Test Reaction Patterns.

	Reactions with	
	Anti-IgG	Anti-C3
Warm AIHA (1°, 2°)	+	0
	+	+
	0	+
Cold AIHA (1°, 2°)	0	+
Drugs (immune-complex type)	0	+
PNH	0	+
PCH	0	+
Alloantibodies		
P, Le, Jk	0	+
Rh, K, Fy	+	0
K, Fy, Jk	+	+

to these drugs, on subsequent exposure to the drug, an immune complex of drug-antidrug forms. The complex may attach nonspecifically to the cells (e.g., RBCs, platelets, granulocytes) and activate complement leading to intravascular lysis of the cells, often resulting in a profound anemia or thrombocytopenia. The immune complex may be loosely bound to the cell or may detach from it, but activated complement components will bind to "innocent bystander" cells in the microenvironment.

5. *Paroxysmal Nocturnal Hemoglobinuria (PNH)*

This is an acquired clonal stem-cell disorder with defective and deficient hematopoiesis. The characteristic that has been used to define PNH is the unusual hypersensitivity of the blood cells to the hemolytic action of complement. PNH RBCs may have C3b on their surface; on complement activation, they bind more C3b and more C5 than do normal RBCs. The same is true for neutrophils and platelets. Three populations of cells have been defined in PNH relative to their sensitivity to complement lysis (103). The PNH RBCs lack the membrane-associated DAF (CD55) protein, the function of which is to accelerate decay dissociation of both classic and alternative pathways' C3 convertase (C4b2a and C3bBb, respectively) (104,105). Other regulatory protein deficiencies have also been reported in PNH and probably must also be missing to account for the sensitivity of PNH cells to activated complement; i.e., a membrane inhibitor of reactive lysis (MIRL; CD59) and the C8-binding protein or homologous restriction factor, which may be simply a polymeric or altered form of CD59 (106–108). These proteins share the characteristic of having a glycophospholipid anchor. The lack of these regulatory proteins results in inefficient regulation of either the C3/C5–converting enzymes or the MAC, with consequent intravascular hemolysis. The molecular basis of the defect is still unknown.

6. *Hereditary Erythroblastic Multinuclearity with a Positive Acidified Serum Lysis Test (HEMPAS)*

This is a rare disorder encountered by transfusionists. In this syndrome, RBCs are very sensitive to cold agglutinin–induced complement activation and lysis, although the amount of bound antibody is not increased. In contrast to PNH, where fixation of C4 is normal (and fixation of C3 is increased), much more C4 is bound to HEMPAS RBCs than to normal RBCs for a given amount of fixed antibody and fixed C1. The defect in HEMPAS may be due to an inability to synthesize some biantennary lactosaminylglycans of the blood cells (109–112).

7. *Hereditary Deficiencies of Individual Components of Complement*

These have, in general, not been of particular interest to immunohematologists. Hereditary deficiency of the early complement components, e.g., C2, C4, C3, may cause a lupuslike syndrome. C1q-INH deficiency may result in RBC-bound C4, and less commonly bound C3, resulting in a positive DAT, but significant immune hemolysis is not generally seen.

8. *C3 NEF*

Although important in infections and other diseases, activation of the alternative pathway does not play a large role in immunohematological diseases. Positive complement-only DAT has been noted in patients in whom an IgG autoantibody, termed the C3 nephritic factor (C3 NEF), is present. C3 NEF is specific for the alternative pathway C3 convertase creating a stable enzyme complex escaping the regulatory mechanisms of the alternative pathway (113); C3 NEF is found in patients with membranoproliferative glomerulonephritis and in patients with partial lipodystrophy (114).

9. *Hemolytic Transfusion Reactions*

A number of alloantibodies can activate complement; some examples are shown in Table 5. Most clinically important are antibodies within the ABO and Kidd systems; complement binding

Table 5 Examples of Alloantibodies that Activate Complement

Blood Group Antibodies	Complement Coating of RBCs	Complement-Mediated Lysis
ABO	Usually	Usually
Kidd	Often (50–70%)	Sometimes
Vel, PP$_1$P^k	Often	Sometimes
Kell, Duffy	Sometimes (10–30%)	Uncommon
Rh	No	No

by antibodies in the Kidd system is discussed in more detail in Section IX.D. Salama and Mueller-Eckhardt (115) described new findings in patients with delayed hemolytic transfusion reactions (DHTRs) that contradicted traditional concepts. In long-term study of 26 patients with DHTR due to antibodies of the Rh, Kell, and Duffy systems, they found that in only 38% was the DAT positive owing to IgG sensitization. In contrast, the DAT was positive owing to strong complement coating of the RBCs in all cases regardless of the specificity of the antibody. The complement-positive DAT remained positive for weeks and even months after the responsible transfusion. It was suggested that the antibodies attach to autologous as well as allogeneic cells by nonspecific cross-reactivity resulting in classic pathway complement activation. It may be that once antibody-dependent classic pathway generation of C3b has occurred, continued complement activation may occur by amplification of alternative pathway C3 convertase C3bBb. Alternatively, the autologous RBCs may bind C3 as a "bystander" mechanism (116). Cleavage of C3b by plasma C3b inactivators to C3d may protect some of the autologous RBCs from immunologic clearance (115). Such a mechanism may account for the observations of complement fixation by anti-D antibodies described by Frank et al. (75), which are discussed in Section VIII.B.1. A similar hypothesis has been proposed to explain the destruction of the patient's own platelets in posttransfusion purpura. Nonetheless, the findings described by Salama and Mueller-Eckhardt remain at variance with the experience of others (117,118), and Chaplin speculated that since cell-bound C3d is relatively unstable, the presence of C3d on autologous cells long after DHTR suggests a continuously ongoing process, more likely a result of associated autoimmunization at the time of the DHTR (117).

10. Bystander, or Reactive, Hemolysis

Reactive hemolysis refers to RBC lysis differentiated from classic complement lysis in that it occurs in the absence of antibody on the RBCs and can occur in the presence of EDTA (119–121). This was first described, in PNH, by Yachnin and Ruthenberg (122), who suggested that intercurrent infections in patients with PNH might result in complement-activating immune complex formation and lysis of the particularly sensitive RBCs from patients with PNH (see Sect. VIII.B.5); they suggested that this may also occur in some cases of acquired immune hemolytic anemias where immune complexes are present; e.g., in SLE. A complex of C567 is formed as a result of antigen-antibody reaction, and this complex can attach itself to normal RBCs, allowing the RBCs to be lysed by C8 and C9, although the cells have neither antibody nor early complement components bound to their surfaces (119–121). Transfer of the C567 complex can occur from activation on one cell to the binding site on another cell (123). The phenomenon of reactive hemolysis has also been described in autoimmune hemolytic anemia (124) and may occur in drug-induced hemolytic anemia, posttransfusion purpura, hemolytic anemia of malarial and protozoal infections (125), hemolytic transfusion reactions (115,118), and the passenger lymphocyte syndrome, especially in association with ABO-incompatible marrow transplants from unrelated donors (126).

11. Miscellaneous

Hong et al. (127) recently reported that the perfluorocarbon blood substitute Fluosol activates complement resulting in Fluosol-bound Bb, H, and C3d and increased fluid-phase C5a. Paradoxically, lower concentrations of Fluosol caused greater amounts of complement activation, suggesting a complex interaction of activators and inhibitors that changes as the available surface area is decreased. Janatova et al. (128) have shown that biomedical polymers differ in their capacity to activate complement; from a transfusionist's viewpoint, this may be important in relation to plastic storage bags, filters, and apheresis equipment. Heparin-induced extracorporeal low-density lipoprotein precipitation has been shown to activate and deplete complement (129), as has immunoadsorption with staphylococcal Protein A (130,131). Immunoglobulins modified for intravenous use (IVIg) have been recently introduced into clinical immunohematology practice. IVIg appears to have multiple mechanisms of action and it has been reported to interfere with the complement cascade (132,133). IVIg may effectively inhibit deposition of early complement components (activated C3 and C4 fragments) onto antibody-sensitized RBCs (134); it does not appear to interfere with the recognition step of the classic complement pathway (135).

C. Complement and the Platelet "Storage Lesion"

Platelets are able to modulate complement activation by several mechanisms. Platelet α granules contain complement factor H that can inhibit C3bBb (136). The granules also contain C1 inhibitor that can downregulate C1 activation. In addition, platelets carry the receptor for C1q, which can sequester the molecule and inhibit its association with C1r and C1s. Exposure of platelets to the MAC C5b-9 causes α granule and membrane vesicle release but does not appear to activate the platelet (137), and the consequences of this exposure remain as yet unknown. Complement activation in platelet concentrates has also been demonstrated.

With increasing storage time, platelet function declines in platelet concentrates; the time-dependent metabolic and functional "platelet storage lesion" includes abnormal platelet morphology, impaired platelet adhesion, aggregation, and activation, as well as release of platelet α granule proteins into the plasma. Bode et al. (138) have shown that C3a accumulates within stored platelet concentrates; this activation may lead to platelet lesions similar to those described above. The activation event has been attributed to activation of C4 and increase in C3a. C3a levels rise progressively as platelet concentrates are stored, and this has been associated with a concomitant decrease in platelet responsiveness (138). Gyongyossy-Issa et al. (139) have shown that when washed human platelets are exposed to C3a, their ability to respond to arachidonic acid and collagen is completely abrogated. It might, therefore, be possible to inhibit the storage lesion and extend platelet function and/or storage life by developing approaches to inhibit complement activation in platelet units. However, further work needs to be done to identify the activator(s) of complement within this system and to develop methods to specifically downregulate the activation.

IX. ANTICOMPLEMENT ANTIGLOBULIN REAGENTS

In the almost 50 years since the description of the AGT, the test continues to be one of the most widely used tests in blood transfusion practice. Nonetheless, despite recognition of the importance of antiglobulin reagents and their quality control, the provision of standards for anti-IgG, and anti-C3 in particular, has long been the subject of debate (140–144).

The AGT can detect the presence of RBCs coated with complement in vivo; the test thus may be useful for laboratory diagnosis of autoimmune and drug-induced immune hemolytic anemias. There also appear to be some alloantibodies that are detectable only by antiglobulin sera containing anticomplement activity. Although cell-bound C5, C6, and C8 can sometimes be detected on the RBC membrane by AGT, in immunohematology, RBC-bound C3 and C4 have been of most significance. There has, over the years, been considerable controversy over the relative importance of the anticomplement activity in antiglobulin sera designed for routine blood bank use. There has been a concomitant debate about the optimal standards for the anticomplement test and reagents. This has been complicated by the changing complexities of the complement system.

A. Need for Standardization

Discrepancies between the strength of antiglobulin reactions and the rate of RBC destruction are commonly encountered. The relationship of hemolysis in vivo to a positive DAT with anticomplement alone, or with anticomplement plus anti-IgG, is less clear than for RBCs having only IgG detectable on their surfaces. Although some patients with a weakly positive DAT may have significant hemolysis, others with strongly positive DAT due to RBC-bound C3 may have no hemolysis. Although these differences, in part, relate to the mechanism by which complement is fixed to the RBCs, it may also relate to variations in the amount of complement fixed. Discrepancies among results of tests performed with commercially available reagents, and apparent discrepancies among reports using antisera investigators produced themselves, may reflect the lack of accepted criteria for reagent standardization with resultant wide variation in potency and specificity. Although virtually all commercial antiglobulin sera were said to have some reactivity with complement, it became evident in the early 1970s that there was nonuniformity of the reagents related to relative proportions of anti-C3c and anti-C3d in the different reagents (49,141,142). Much experimental work in this area was performed with unstandardized and incompletely characterized reagents, complicating interpretation of individual studies and making it difficult to compare the results from different laboratories.

The data emphasized the need for standardization of antiglobulin sera in order to assure a predictable level of performance. The criteria of potency should recognize the capacity of an antibody to bring about prompt, strong agglutination of RBCs coated with the globulin for which the antiserum is specific. This requires that the amount of specified RBC-bound antigen can be reliably quantified, its binding and antigenic integrity be stable throughout the test, the amount and distribution of the antigen on the RBC surface be standardized, and that the sensitized RBCs not be coated with other immune globulins for which the reagents may contain additional unsuspected antibodies. Methods have been developed for reproducibly preparing RBCs coated with specific subcomponents of C3, along with methods for quantifying the number of specific complement subcomponents on the RBC surfaces. Potent antisera, specific for complement subcomponents, have been developed and methods devised for quantitating these antisera in terms of micrograms of specific anticomplement antibody per milliliter (49,50, 143,145). Hence, standard antiglobulin sera, with known concentrations and equilibrium constants, could be prepared (146).

B. Potential Adverse Effects of Anticomplement in Antiglobulin Sera

It needs to be considered whether the presence of anticomplement activity in an antiglobulin serum may be at all detrimental. It has been suggested that antiglobulin sera containing anticomplement antibodies cause numerous "false-positive" reactions; these have been ascribed to antispecies antibodies or other nonspecific agglutinating components. Issitt et al. (147) found that, with the products of certain manufacturers, the incidence of unwanted positive reactions increased concomitantly with an increase of anticomplement in those reagents, but apparently the reactions were caused by the introduction of antispecies antibodies at the same time as anticomplement levels were increased; recognition of this phenomenon has permitted its correction in commercial products. Although Nasongkla et al. (148) were unable to show any correlation between the false-positive reactions and the amount of C3d on the RBCs, Freedman et al. (149) and Garratty (150) have reported that some antiglobulin sera continue to cause weak agglutination of normal RBCs even after multiple (up to 12) absorptions with washed packed RBCs of mixed A, B, and O groups; such weak agglutination may occur even after considerable dilution of the antisera. The so-called false-positive reaction may, on the other hand, be true but undesirable positive reactions resulting from complement fixation by clinically insignificant cold antibodies or normal incomplete cold antibody.

Probably the most common cause of unwanted reactions with anticomplement antiglobulin sera is due to cold antibodies. Any sample of refrigerated clotted blood may yield a false-positive DAT owing to complement sensitization. This is usually an in vitro phenomenon associated with cold autoantibody-induced complement fixation; occasionally this may occur even at room temperature. Since most anticoagulants are anticomplementary, the phenomenon occurs much less often with anticoagulated blood. Garratty (140) found that the RBCs from about half of refrigerated clots had RBC-bound complement components; 66% reactive with anti-C4 and 23% with anti C3. The RBC-bound complement fragments were predominantly C4d and C3d. However, when segments from units collected into ACD were tested, only 18% reacted with anti-C4 and none reacted with anti-C3 (140). Issitt et al. reported similar findings (142). Hence, samples for DAT should be taken into EDTA. Cold antibodies may cause similar problems in the indirect antiglobulin test (IAT). When clinically insignificant cold autoantibodies or alloantibodies are present, they might sensitize RBCs with complement at room temperature; at 37°C, the antibodies will elute from the RBCs but complement remains, leading to a positive IAT (140). Fortunately, most blood banks no longer consider it necessary to perform a room-temperature phase of the compatibility test, and this should prevent many of the unwanted reactions observed with antiglobulin sera containing anticomplement activity.

In contrast to anti-IgG, which does not usually cause false-positive reactions, anti-C3 levels in antiglobulin sera designed for routine use must be carefully controlled to prevent false-positive reactions occurring as a result of C3d present on normal RBCs. Several studies, using anticomplement sera, have reported positive DAT in approximately 7% of random hospital patients when testing EDTA-treated RBCs. Antibody-mediated complement binding to RBCs always involves C4 as well as C3; because, as described above, anti-C4 in antiglobulin serum results in unwanted false-positive reactions with normal RBCs stored at 4°C, anticomplement in polyspecific antiglobulin serum should contain only anti-C3. In addition, if anti-C4 is present, it can be considered unnecessary because RBC-bound C4d has never been observed in a hemolytic situation without C3d present as well.

C. Potentially Enhanced Detection of IgG Antibodies by Anticomplement

There is evidence that the use of anticomplement in antiglobulin sera may improve the likelihood of antibody detection. Wright and Issitt (151), in a survey of 140 IgG complement-fixing antibodies, found that over 64% were detected with higher titer scores when complement was involved in their detection. Augmented complement activation was described by Müller-Eberhard et al. (2). One bound IgM molecule (or a doublet of IgG molecules) activates many C4 molecules and each C4 then activates many C3 molecules. Thus, although only weak agglutination may be observed using anti-immunoglobulin serum, much stronger agglutination may be seen when using anticomplement serum. The increased sensitivity of the anticomplement antiglobulin test was also shown by Holburn (152), who found that the antibody concentration at the endpoint of the titer for an IgM anti-Le[a] was 1.1 μg/ml with a saline agglutination test, 0.42 μg/ml when an anti-IgM antiglobulin test was used, and 0.04 μg/ml when an anticomplement antiglobulin test was used.

D.　Anti-C3d Versus anti-C3b in Antiglobulin Serum

Anticomplement reagents for routine use have usually been oligospecific; e.g., anti-C3 (C3b + C3d). When monospecific reagents are used, anti-C3d is the most commonly used monospecific anticomplement in the blood bank. One should note that agglutination of RBCs tested with anticomplement sera is enhanced by incubating the tube for 5–10 min at room temperature and then centrifuging; this incubation is particularly important for optimum reactivity when using monoclonal anti-C3d.

Because 10–20% of cases of warm AIHA present with C3d and no IgG on their RBCs, it is generally accepted that anti-C3d is a useful part of the diagnostic workup of patients with warm AIHA. Anti-C3d is essential for detection of CHAD because virtually all cases of CHAD have complement-only on their RBCs. Hence, anti-C3d should be included in all antiglobulin sera used for DAT. The major controversy has involved the necessity for anticomplement in the IAT. A plethora of literature has debated whether clinically significant alloantibodies exist that are detectable in the IAT using anticomplement, which are not detectable by anti-IgG. In brief, it appears that certain blood group alloantibodies do exist that cannot be detected by routine procedures with anti-IgG, yet can be detected by antiglobulin sera containing anti-C3 (possibly as a result of the amplification effect in complement fixation). Many of these antibodies are of specificities considered to be potentially clinically significant; e.g., antibodies of the Kidd blood group system (153–156). These antibodies appear to be relatively uncommon, and one large prospective study of 39,436 random sera from hospital patients found that approximately 1 in 8,000 sera contained an anti-Jk[a] that might not have detected if anti-C3 had not been used (157). Interestingly, Stratton et al. (158) described two cases of hemolytic disease of the newborn, one caused by anti-K and one by anti-Jk[a], where the DAT was positive only with anticomplement reagents. Although any antibody of the Kidd system is generally considered to be potentially serious, the degree of destruction of incompatible RBCs in vivo by Kidd antibodies not detectable by anti-IgG remains unclear. It remains a good principle to avoid a possible delayed hemolytic transfusion reaction by detecting potentially significant antibodies and transfusing blood lacking the appropriate antigens. The low frequency of clinically significant alloantibodies detected by anticomplement alone, however, leaves the decision of whether to include anticomplement in antiglobulin sera designed for the IAT an individual one of balancing potential difficulties, and perhaps cost, with the risk to the patient if one of these antibodies is not detected.

E.　Requirements for Anticomplement Antiglobulin Sera

Minimum requirements for antiglobulin sera were published by the Food and Drug Administration (FDA) in the United States in 1985, and standards were provided for antiglobulin sera, including anti-C3. The Office of Biologic Research and Review of the FDA tests every lot of antihuman globulin with a panel of RBCs minimally coated with a standard preparation of anti-D, anti-Fy[a], C3b, C3d, C4b, C4d, and IgA to confirm acceptable reactivity and specificity. The product label must indicate whether the reagent contains anti-IgG, anti-C3b, anti-C3d, and anti-C4. The reagent must contain adequate anti-C3d to be recommended for use in the DAT. A polyspecific reagent suitable for general-purpose DAT and IAT must contain at least anti-IgG and anti-C3d. Manufacturers are provided with potency standards for anti-IgG and anti-C3d to be used in quality control tests. The International Society of Blood Transfusion and the International Committee for Standardization in Haematology (ISBT/ICSH) Working Party on Standards for Antiglobulin Serum found that levels of anti-C3d necessary for optimal antibody reactivity often cause agglutination of RBCs that have been incubated with normal serum, although collected and stored in ACD or CPD anticoagulants. An ISBT/ICSH reference antiglobulin reagent is available from the central laboratory of the Netherlands Red Cross Blood

Transfusion Service. It provides manufacturers with an optimum reagent for comparison. The FDA reference reagent provides a minimum standard of potency. Additional reagents are being produced and evaluated. In 1982, the ISBT/ICSH approved a polyspecific spin antiglobulin reference reagent called RIII (159), consisting of a blend of polyclonal anti-IgG and monoclonal anticomplement antibodies. The anticomplement component of the reagent was a blend of two murine monoclonal antibodies, anti-C3c and anti-C3d (titer 64 and 2, respectively, with low-ionic C3-coated RBCs). RIII is a comparative standard and its anti-C3 cannot be matched by conventional reagents. The French specification for polyspecific antiglobulin serum requires an anti-C3d level greater than that specified by ISBT/ICSH/FDA criteria but, at these high levels, false-positive reactions may occur.

F. Monoclonal Anticomplement Reagents

Monoclonal anti-C3 antibodies must also be assessed on their individual merits. Because monoclonal reagents tend to show greater prozone effect than do polyclonal reagents, it is important to use the serum to cell ratio recommended by the manufacturer. The exquisite specificity of monoclonal reagents, directed at a single epitope, may explain the observation that monoclonal anti-C3d reactivity is sometimes not as strong as polyclonal anti-C3d when testing RBCs coated with C3b in vitro; the monoclonal C3d specificity may be directed at a receptor hidden on the C3b-coated RBCs. Dobbie et al. (160), using monoclonal antibodies, have described seven different epitopes, four on the C3c and three on the C3d fragment of C3; they noted that the pH is critical for the reactivity of the monoclonal antibodies. It is of interest that in quantitative studies investigators have found markedly fewer C3d molecules/RBC when using monoclonal anti-C3d than on the same RBCs using conventional monospecific anti-C3d (50). The narrow specificity of monoclonal antibodies may permit easier standardization and dissection of complement component specificities but may be too restricted for a reagent for routine clinical use and it may be that a "blend" of monoclonal anti-C3d reagents is required.

X. CONCLUSIONS

In summary, complement sensitization of RBCs may result from allo- and/or autoimmune disease and may cause (1) intravascular RBC destruction, (2) sequestration and phagocytosis in the RES, (3) sequestration with subsequent return to circulation where RBCs may survive normally, or (4) essentially normal survival of RBCs. Much has been learned of the pathophysiological and diagnostic significance of the fragments of C3 bound to RBCs in vivo and in vitro and important strides have been made in the performance characteristics of anticomplement antiglobulin sera designed to detect these fragments. This chapter has concentrated on aspects of particular interest to immunohematologists and transfusionists. For further information on other aspects of complement proteins, and the significance of their activation, the reader is referred to one of the many comprehensive reviews (1–3).

REFERENCES

1. Frank MM, Fries LF. Complement. In: Paul WE, ed. Fundamental Immunology, Second Edition. New York: Raven Press, 1989:679.
2. Müller-Eberhard HJ. Complement. Springer Semin Immunopathol 1983; 6:2.
3. Morgan BP. Complement. Clinical Aspects and Relevance to Disease. London: Academic Press, 1990.
4. Borsos T, Chapuis RM, Langone JJ. Distinction between fixation of C1 and the activation of complement by natural IgM anti-hapten antibody: Effects of cell surface hapten density. Mol Immunol 1981; 18:863.

5. Müller-Eberhard HJ, Nilsson UR, Dalmasso AP, et al. A molecular concept of immune cytolysis. Arch Pathol 1966; 82:205.

6. Colomb MJ, Arloud GJ, Villiers CL. Structure and activation of C1: Current concepts. Complement 1984; 1:69.

7. Schumaker VN, Zavodsky P, Poon PH. Activation of the first component of complement. Annu Rev Immunol 1987; 5:21.

8. Tenner AJ, Frank MM. Activator-bound C1 is less susceptible to inactivation by C1-inhibitor than is fluid phase C1. J Immunol 1986; 137:625.

9. Isenman DE, Cooper NR. The structure and function of the third component of human complement. I. The nature and extent of conformational changes accompanying C3 activation. Mol Immunol 1981; 18:331.

10. Tack BF, Harrison RA, Janatova J. Evidence for presence of internal thioester bond in the third component of human complement. Proc Natl Acad Sci USA 1980; 77:5764.

11. Law SK, Levine RP. Interaction between the third complement protein and cell surface macromolecules. Proc Natl Acad Sci USA 1977; 74:2701.

12. Harrison RA, Lachmann PJ. The physiological breakdown of the third component of complement. Mol Immunol 1980; 17:9.

13. Lachmann PJ, Pangburn MK, Oldroyd RG. Breakdown of C3 after complement activation. Identification of a new fragment, C3g, using monoclonal antibodies. J Exp Med 1982; 156:205.

14. Chaplin H, Monroe MC, Lachmann PJ. Further studies of the C3g component of the a2D fragment of human C3. Clin Exp Immunol 1982; 51:639.

15. Lachmann PJ, Voak D, Oldroyd RG, et al. Use of monoclonal anti-C3 antibodies to characterize the fragments of C3 that are found on erythrocytes. Vox Sang 1983; 45:367.

16. Ross GD, Lambris JD, Cain JA, Newman SL. Generation of three different fragments for factor H vs. CR1 cofactor activity. J Immunol 1982; 129:2051.

17. Pillemer L, Blum L, Lepow IH, et al. The properdin system and immunity. I. Demonstration and isolation of a new serum protein, properdin, and its role in immune phenomena. Science 1954; 120:279.

18. Pangburn MK. Activation of complement via the alternative pathway. Fed Proc 1983; 42:139.

19. Weiler JM, Daha MR, Austen KF, Fearon SL. Control of the amplification convertase of complement by the plasma protein β1H. Proc Natl Acad Sci USA 1982; 73:3268.

20. Pangburn MK, Schreiber RD, Muller-Eberhard HJ. Human complement C3b inactivator: Isolation, characterization, and demonstration of an absolute requirement for the serum protein β1H for cleavage of C3b and C4b in solution. J Exp Med 1977; 146:257.

21. Nicholson-Weller A, Burge J, Fearon DT, et al. Isolation of a human erythrocyte membrane glycoprotein with decay-accelerating activity for C3 convertases of the complement system. J Immunol 1982; 129:184.

22. Schonermark S, Rauterberg EW, Shin ML, et al. Homologous species restriction in lysis of human erythrocytes: A membrane-derived protein with C8 binding capacity functions as an inhibitor. J Immunol 1986; 136:1772.

23. Sugita Y, Nakamo Y, Tomita M. Isolation from human erythrocytes of a new membrane protein which inhibits the formation of complement transmembrane channels. J Biochem (Tokyo) 1988; 104:633.

24. Holguin MH, Fredrick LR, Bernshaw LJ, et al. Isolation and characterization of a membrane protein from normal human erythrocytes that inhibits reactive lysis of erythrocytes of paroxysmal nocturnal hemoglobinuria. J Clin Invest 1989; 84:7.

25. Devine DV. The regulation of complement on cell surfaces. Transfus Med Rev 1991; 5:123.

26. Rooney IA, Davies A, Griffiths D, et al. The complement-inhibiting protein, protectin (CD50 antigen), is present and functionally active on glomerular epithelial cells. Clin Exp Immunol 1991; 83:251.

27. Berger M, Gaither TA, Frank MM. Complement receptors. Clin Immunol Rev 1983; 1:471.

28. Schreiber AD. The chemistry and biology of complement receptors. Springer Semin Immunopathol 1984; 7:221.

29. Ross GD, Medof ME. Membrane complement receptors specific for bound fragments of C3. Adv Immunol 1985; 37:217.

30. Sim RB, Malhotra V, Day AJ, Erdei A. Structure and specificity of complement receptors. Immunol Lett 1986/1987; 14:183.

31. Unkeless JC, Wright SD. Phagocytic cells: Fcγ and complement receptors. Gallin JI, Goldstein IM, Snyderman R, eds. Inflammation: Basic Principles and Clinical Correlates. New York: Raven Press, 1988:343.

32. Ehlenberger AG, Nussenzweig V. The role of membrane receptors for C3b and C3d in phagocytosis. J Exp Med 1977; 145:357.

33. Medof ME, Iida K, Mold C, Nussenzweig V. Unique role of the complement receptor CR1 in the degradation of C3b associated with immune complexes. J Exp Med 1982; 156:1739.

34. Cornacoff JB, Hebert LA, Smead WL, et al. Primate erythrocyte-immune complex-clearing mechanism, J Clin Invest 1983; 71:236.

35. Cooper NR, Moore MD, Nemerow GR. Immunobiology of CR2, the B lymphocyte receptor for Epstein-Barr virus and the C3d complement fragment. Annu Rev Immunol 1988; 6:85.

36. Tilley CA, Romans DG, Crookston MC. Localization of Chido and Rogers determinants to the C4d fragment of human C4. Nature 1978; 276:713.

37. Giles CM. Antigenic determinants of human C4, Rodgers and Chido. Exp Clin Immunogenet 1988; 5:99.

38. Giles CM, Davies KA, Walport MJ. In vivo and in vitro binding of C4 molecules on red cells; a correlation of numbers of molecules and agglutination. Transfusion 1991; 31:223.

39. Giles CM. Three decades of reference serology. Transfus Med 1991; 1:145.

40. Giles CM, Uring-Lambert B, Goetz J, et al. Antigenic determinants expressed by human C4 allotypes; a study of 325 families provides evidence for the structural antigenic model. Immunogenetics 1988; 27:442.

41. Yu CY, Campbell RD, Porter RR. A structural model for the location of the Rodgers and Chido antigenic determinants and their correlation with the human complement component C4A/C4B isotypes. Immunogenetics 1988; 27:399.

42. Telen MJ, Hall SE, Green AM, et al. Identification of human erythrocyte blood group antigen on decay accelerating factor (DAF) and identification of an erythrocyte phenotype negative for DAF. J Exp Med 1988; 167:1993.

43. Merry AH, Rawlinson VI, Uchikawa M, et al. Lack of abnormal sensitivity to complement-mediated lysis in erythrocytes deficient only in decay accelerating factor. Biochem Soc Trans 1989; 17:514.

44. Rao N, Ferguson DJ, Lee S-F, Telen MJ. Identification of human erythrocyte blood group antigens on the C3b/C4b receptor. J Immunol 1991; 146:3502.

45. Moulds JM, Nickells MW, Moulds JJ, et al. The C3b/C4b receptor is recognized by the Knops, McCoy, Swain-Langley, and York blood group antisera. J Exp Med 1991; 173:1159.

46. Ross GD, Yount WJ, Walport MJ, et al. Disease-associated loss of erythrocyte complement receptors (CR[1], C3b receptors) in patients with systemic lupus erythematosus and other diseases involving autoantibodies and/or complement activation. J Immunol 1985; 135:2005.

47. Borsos T, Leonard EJ. Detection of bound C3 by a new immunochemical method. J Immunol 1971; 107:766.

48. Schreiber AD, Frank MM. Role of antibody and complement in the immune clearance and distribution of erythrocytes. I. In vivo effects of IgG and IgM complement-fixing sites. J Clin Invest 1972; 51:575.

49. Chaplin H, Hoffman NL. Radioimmunoassay evaluation of anti-C3d reactivity in broad spectrum commercial antiglobulin reagents. A three year study. Transfusion 1982; 22:6.

50. Chaplin H, Monroe MC. Comparison of pooled polyclonal rabbit anti-human C3d with four monoclonal mouse anti-human C3ds. II. Quantitation of RBC-bound C3d, and characterization of antiglobulin agglutination reactions against RBC from 27 patients with autoimmune anemia. Vox Sang 1986; 50:87.

51. Chaplin H, Nasongkla M, Monroe MC. Quantitation of red blood cell-bound C3d in normal subjects and random hospitalized patients. Br J Haematol 1981; 48:69.

52. Merry AH. Quantitative aspects of the antiglobulin test for red cell-bound IgG, C3d and C3g. Biotest Bull 1986; 1:53.

53. Worlledge SM. The interpretation of a positive direct antiglobulin test. Br J Haematol 1978; 39:157.

54. Freedman J. False-positive antiglobulin tests in healthy subjects and in hospital patients. J Clin Pathol 1979; 32:1014.

55. Petz LD, Garratty G. Acquired Immune Hemolytic Anemias. New York: Churchill Livingstone.

56. Judd WJ, Butch SH, Oberman HA, et al. The evaluation of a positive direct antiglobulin test in pretrans-fusion testing. Transfusion 1980; 20:17.

57. Freedman J, Ho M, Barefoot C. Red blood cell-bound C3d in selected hospital patients. Transfusion 1982; 22:515.

58. Graham H, Davies DM Jr, Tigner JA, et al. Evidence suggesting that trace amounts of C3d are bound to most human red cells. Transfusion 1976; 16:530.

59. Rosenfield RE, Jagathambal. Antigenic determinants of C3 and C4 complement components on washed erythrocytes from normal persons. Transfusion 1978; 18:517.

60. Freedman J, Massey A. Complement components detected on normal red blood cells taken in EDTA and CPD. Vox Sang 1979; 37:1.

61. Freedman J, Massey A. Quantitation of C3 subcomponents on red cells coated with complement in vitro. J Clin Pathol 1980; 37:977.

62. Fischer JT, Petz LD, Garratty G, et al. Correlation between quantitative assay of red cell-bound C3 serologic reactions and hemolytic anemia. Blood 1974; 44:359.

63. Freedman J, Barefoot C. Red blood cell-bound C3d in normal subjects and in random hospital patients. Transfusion 1982; 22:511.

64. Merry AH, Thomas EE, Rawlinson VI, et al. The quantification of C3 fragments on erythrocytes: Estimation of C3 fragments on normal cells, acquired haemolytic anaemia cases and correlation with agglutination of sensitized cells. Clin Lab Haematol 1983; 5:387.

65. Gorst DW, Rawlinson VI, Merry AH, et al. Positive direction antiglobulin test in normal individuals. Vox Sang 1980; 38:99.

66. Freedman J, Massey A. Differences in specificities of anti-C3d sera raised to C3d antigens prepared in different ways. Transfusion 1981; 21:32.

67. Freedman J. Membrane-bound immunoglobulins and complement components on young and old red blood cells. Transfusion 1984; 24:477.

68. Szymanski IO, Odgren PR. Studies on the preservation of red blood cells. Attachment of the third component of human complement to erythrocytes during storage at 4°C. Vox Sang 1979; 36:213.

69. Mantovani B, Rabinovitch M, Nussenzweig V. Phagocytosis of immune complexes by macrophages. Different roles of the macrophage receptor sites for complement (C3) and or immunoglobulin (IgG). J Exp Med 1972; 135:780.

70. Munn LR, Chaplin H, Jr. Rosette formation by sensitized human red cells—Effects of source of peripheral leukocyte monolayers. Vox Sang 1977; 33:129.

71. Kurlander RJ, Rosse WR, Ferreira E. Quantitative evaluation of antibody-dependent lymphocyte-mediated lysis of human red cells. Am J Hemato 1979; 6:295.

72. Schreiber AD, Frank MM. The role of antibody and complement in the immune clearance and destruction of erythrocytes. II. Molecular nature of IgG and IgM complement fixing sites and effects of their interaction with serum. J Clin Invest 1972; 51:583.

73. Atkinson JP, Frank MM. Studies on the in vivo effects of antibody and complement in the immune clearance and distribution of erythrocytes in man. J Clin Invest 1974; 54:339.

74. Jaffe CJ, Atkinson JP, Frank MM. The role of complement in the clearance of cold agglutinin-sensitized erythrocytes in man. J Clin Invest 1976; 58:942.

75. Frank MM, Schreiber AD, Atkinson JP, et al. Pathophysiology of immune hemolytic anemia. Ann Intern Med 1977; 87:210.

76. Mollison PL. The role of complement in the hemolytic process in vivo. In: Wolstenholme GEW, Knight J, eds. Ciba Foundation Symposium: Complement. Boston: Little Brown, 1965:328.

77. Chaplin H, Coleman ME, Monroe MC. In vivo instability of red-blood-cell-bound C3d and C4d. Blood 1983; 62:965.

78. Rosse WJ, De Boisfleury A, Bessis M. The interaction of phagocytic cells and red cells modified by immune reactions. Comparison of antibody and complement coated red cells. Blood 1975; 1:345.

79. Frank MM. Mechanisms of cell destruction in immunohemolytic anemia. In: Bell CA, ed. A

Seminar on Laboratory Management of Hemolysis. Las Vegas. Arlington, VA: American Association of Blood Banks, 1979:29.

80. Brown DL, Lachmann PJ, Dacie JV. The in vivo behavior of complement-coated red cells: studies in C6 deficient, C3-depleted and normal rabbits. Clin Exp Immunol 1970; 7:401.

81. Rosse WJ. Fixation of the first component of complement (C'la) by human antibodies. J Clin Invest 1968; 47:2430.

82. Freedman J, Massey A, Chaplin H, et al. Assessment of complement binding by anti-D and anti-M antibodies employing labelled antiglobulin antibodies. Br J Haematol 1980; 45:309.

83. Opferkuch W, Rapp HJ, Colten HR, Borsos T. Immune hemolysis and the functional properties of the second (C2) and fourth (C4) components of complement. II. Clustering of effective C42 complexes at individual hemolytic sites. J Immunol 1971; 106:407.

84. Currie MS, Pradip K, Wojcieszak R, et al. Effect of antigen site and complement receptor status on the rate of cleavage of C3c antigen from red cell bound C3d. Blood 1988; 71:786.

85. MacKenzie MR. Monocytic sensitization in autoimmune hemolytic anemia. Clin Res 1975; 23:132A (abstr).

86. Kay NE, Douglas SD. Monocyte-erythrocyte interaction in vitro in immune hemolytic anemias. Blood 1977; 50:889.

87. Wright SD, Craigmyle LS, Silverstein SC. Fibronectin and serum amyloid P component stimulate C3b- and C3bi-mediated phagocytosis in cultured human monocytes. J Exp Med 1983; 158:1338.

88. Pommier CG, O'Shea J, Chused T, et al. Studies on the fibronectin receptors of human peripheral blood leukocytes. Morphologic and functional characterization. J Exp Med 1984; 159:137.

89. Polley MJ, Müller-Eberhard HJ, Feldman JD. Production of ultrastructural membrane lesions by the fifth component of complement. J Exp Med 1971; 133:53.

90. Mayer MM. Mechanism of cytolysis by complement. Proc Natl Acad Sci USA 1972; 69:2954.

91. Bauer J, Valet G. Cell volume and osmotic properties of erythrocyte after complement lysis measured by flow cytometry. J Immunol 1983; 130:839.

92. Sung K-LP, Freedman J, Chabanel A, et al. Effect of complement on the viscoelastic properties of human erythrocyte membrane. Br J Haematol 1985; 61:455.

93. Durocher JR, Gockerman JP, Conrad ME. Alteration of human erythrocyte membrane properties by complement fixation. J Clin Invest 1975; 55:675.

94. Rosse WF. Interactions of complement with the red-cell membrane. Semin Hematol 1979; 16:128.

95. Kay MMB. A red cell aging antigen. In: Garratty G, ed. Red Cell Antigens and Antibodies. Arlington, VA: American Association of Blood Banks, 1986:35.

96. Lutz HU, Wipf G. Naturally occurring autoantibodies to skeletal proteins from human red cells. J Immunol 1982; 128:1695.

97. Lutz HU, Fasler S, Stammler P, et al. Naturally occurring anti-band 3 antibodies and complement in phagocytosis of oxidatively-stressed and in clearance of senescent red cells. Blood Cells 1988; 14:175.

98. Engelfriet CP, Pondman KW, Wolders J, et al. Autoimmune hemolytic anemias. III. Preparation and examination of specific antisera against complement components and products, and their use in serological studies. Clin Exp Immunol 1970; 6:721.

99. Freedman J, Chaplin H, Johnson CA. Comparison of low-molecular-weight products following reaction of C3-C3b with C3b inactivator and with trypsin. Vox Sang 1977; 33:212.

100. Petz LD, Swisher SN. Clinical Practice of Blood Transfusion. New York: Churchill Livingstone, 1981:45.

101. Jenkins WJ, Marsh WL. Autoimmune haemolytic anaemia. Lancet 1961; 2:16.

102. Ozer FL, Chaplin H. Agglutination of stored erythrocytes by a human serum. Characterization of the serum factor and erythrocyte changes. J Clin Invest 1963; 42:1735.

103. Rosse WF, Adams JP, Thorpe AM. The population of cells in paroxysmal nocturnal haemoglobinuria of intermediate sensitivity to complement lysis: Significance and mechanism of increased immune lysis. Br J Haematol 1974; 28:181.

104. Parker CJ, Barker PJ, Rosse WF. Increased enzymatic activity in the alternative pathway convertase when bound to the erythro-cytes of paroxysmal nocturnal hemoglobinuria. J Clin Invest 1982; 377:337.

105. Nicholson-Weller A, March JP, Rosenfeld SI, Austen KF. Affected erythrocytes of patients with

paroxysmal nocturnal hemoglobinuria are deficient in the complement regulatory protein, decay accelerating factor. Proc Natl Acad Sci USA 1983; 80:5430.

106. Zalman LS, Wood LM, Frank MM, et al. Deficiency of the homologous restriction factor in paroxysmal nocturnal hemoglobinuria. J Exp Med 1987; 165:572.

107. Holguin MH, Wilcox LA, Bernshaw NJ, et al. Relationship between the membrane inhibitor of reactive lysis and the erythrocyte phenotypes of paroxysmal nocturnal hemoglobinuria. J Clin Invest 1989; 84:1387.

108. Zalman LS, Wood LM, Müller-Eberhard HJ. Isolation of a human erythrocyte membrane protein capable of inhibition expression of homologous complement transmembrane channels. Proc Natl Acad Sci USA 1986; 83:6975.

109. Jarnefelt J, Ruksh J, Li Y-T, Laine RA. Erythroglycan, a high molecular weight glycopeptide with the repeating structure [galactosyl (1-4)-2-deoxy-2 acetaminoglucosyl (1,3)] comparing more than one-third of the protein-bound carbohydrate of the human erythrocyte stroma. J Biol Chem 1978; 253:8006.

110. Fukuda MN, Dell A, Scartezzini P. Primary defect of congenital dyserythropoietic anemia type II. Failure in glycosylation of erythrocyte lactoaminoglycan proteins caused by lowered N-acetyl-aminylglucosetransferase II. J Biol Chem 1987; 266:7195.

111. Fukuda MN, Masri KA, Dell A, et al. Defective glycosylation of erythrocyte membrane glycoconjugates in a variant of congenital dyserythropoietic anemia type II: Association of low level of membrane-bound form of galactyosyltransferase. Blood 1989; 73:1331.

112. Fukuda MN, Masri KA, Dell A, et al. Incomplete synthesis of N-glycans in congenital dyserythropoietic anemia type II caused by a defect in the gene encoding alphamannosidase II. Proc Natl Acad Sci USA 1990; 87:7443.

113. Daha MR, Austen K, Fearon DT. The incorporation of C3 nephritic factor (C3NeF) into a stabilized C3 convertase, C3b, Bb (C3NeF), and its release after decay of convertase function. J Immunol 1977; 119:812.

114. Fine DP. Complement and Infectious Diseases. Boca Raton, FL: CRC Press, 1981:33.

115. Salama A, Mueller-Eckhardt C. Delayed hemolytic transfusion reactions: Evidence for complement activation involving allogeneic and autologous red cells. Transfusion 1984; 24:188.

116. Salama A, Mueller-Eckhardt C. Binding of fluid phase C3b to nonsensitized bystander human red cells: A model for in vivo effects of complement activation on red cells. Transfusion 1985; 25:528.

117. Chaplin H Jr. The complication of red cell-bound complement in delayed hemolytic transfusion reactions (editorial). Transfusion 1984; 24:185.

118. Ness PM, Shirey RS, Thomas SK, Buck SA. The differentiation of delayed serologic and delayed hemolytic transfusion reactions: Incidence, long-term serologic findings, and clinical significance. Transfusion 1990; 30:688.

119. Thompson RA, Rowe DS. Reactive haemolysis—A distinctive form of red cell lysis. Immunology 1968; 14:745.

120. Thompson RA, Lachmann PJ. The complement-mediated lysis of unsensitized cells. I. The characterization of the indicator factor and its identification. J Exp Med 1970; 131:629.

121. Lachmann PJ, Thompson RA. Reactive lysis: The complement-mediated lysis of unsensitized cells. II. The characterization of activated reactor as C56 and the participation of C8 and C9. J Exp Med 1970; 131:643.

122. Yachnin S, Ruthenberg JM. The initiation and enhancement of human red cell lysis by activators of the first component of complement and by first component esterase: Studies using normal red cells and red cells from patients with paroxysmal nocturnal hemoglobinuria. J Clin Invest 1965; 44:518.

123. Gotze O, Müller-Eberhard HJ. Lysis of erythrocytes by complement in the absence of antibody. J Exp Med 1970; 132:898.

124. Salama A, Bahkdi S, Müller-Eberhard C. Evidence suggesting the occurrence of C3-independent intravascular immune hemolysis. Reactive lysis in vivo. Transfusion 1987; 27:49.

125. Woodruff AW, Ansdell VE, Pettitt LE. Cause of anaemia in malaria. Lancet 1979; 1:1055.

126. Petz LD. The expanding boundaries of transfusion medicine. In: Nance SJ, ed. Clinical and Basic Science Aspects of Immunohematology. Arlington, VA: American Association of Blood Banks, 1991:73.

127. Hong F, Shastri KA, Logue GL, Spaulding MB. Complement activation by artificial blood substitutes Fluosol: In vitro and in vivo studies. Transfusion 1991; 31:642.
128. Janatova J, Cheung AK, Parker CJ. Biomedical polymers differ in their capacity to activate complement. Complement Inflamm 1991; 8:61.
129. Wurzner R, Schuff-Werner P, Franzke A, et al. Complement activation and depletion during LDL-apheresis by heparin-induced extracorporeal LDL-precipitation (HELP). Eur J Clin Invest 1991; 21:288.
130. Muroi K, Sasaki R, Miura Y. The effect of immunoadsorption therapy by a protein A column on patients with thrombocytopenia. Semin Hematol 1989; 26:10.
131. Langone JJ, Das C, Bennett D, et al. Generation of human C3a, C4a, and C5a anaphylatoxins by protein A of Staphylococcus aureus and immobilized protein A reagents used in serotherapy of cancer. J Immunol 1984; 133:1057.
132. Basta M, Langlois PF, Marques M, et al. High-dose intravenous immunoglobulin modifies complement-mediated in vivo clearance. Blood 1989; 74:326.
133. Basta M, Kirshbom P, Frank MM, Fries LF. Mechanism of therapeutic effect of high-dose intravenous immunoglobulin. Attenuation of acute, complement-dependent immune damage in a guinea pig model. J Clin Invest 1989; 84:1974.
134. Basta M, Fries LF, Frank MM. High doses of intravenous Ig inhibit in vitro uptake of C4 fragments onto sensitized erythrocytes. Blood 1991; 77:376.
135. Basta M, Fries LF, Frank MM. High doses of intravenous immunoglobulin do not affect the recognition phase of the classical complement pathway. Blood 1991; 78:700.
136. Devine DV, Rosse WF. Regulation of the activity of platelet-bound C3 convertase of the alternative pathway of complement by platelet factor H. Proc Natl Acad Sci USA 1987; 84:5873.
137. Sims PJ, Faioni EM, Wiedmer T, Shattil SJ. Complement proteins C5b-9 cause release of membrane vesicles from the platelet surface that are enriched in the membrane receptor for coagulation factor Va and express prothrombinase activity. J Biol Chem 1988; 263:18205.
138. Bode AP, Miller DT, Newman SL, et al. Plasmin activity and complement activation during storage of citrated platelet concentrates. J Lab. Clin Med 1989; 113:94.
139. Gyongyossy-Issa MIC, Devine DV. Homologous C3a alters human platelet agonist responses. Blood 1990; 76:384a.
140. Garratty G, Petz LD. The significance of red-cell-bound complement components in development of standards and quality assurance for the anti-complement components of antiglobulin sera. Transfusion 1976; 16:297.
141. Garratty G, Petz LD. An evaluation of commercial antiglobulin sera with particular reference to their anti-complement properties. Transfusion 1971; 11:79.
142. Issitt PD, Issitt CH, Wilkinson SL. Evaluation of commercial antiglobulin sera over a two-year period. Part I. Anti-beta 1A, anti-alpha 2D, and anti-beta 1E levels. Transfusion 1974; 14:93.
143. Gardner B, Ghosh S, Brazier DM, et al. Quantitative quality control of antiglobulin reagents. Clin Lab Haematol 1983; 5:215.
144. Petz LD, Garratty G. Antiglobulin sera—Past, present and future. Transfusion 1978; 18:257.
145. Chaplin H, Freedman J, Hughes-Jones NC. Quantitation of antibodies to C3d subcomponent of human C3. Immunology 1977; 32:1007.
146. Giles C, Engelfriet CP. Working party on the standardization of antiglobulin reagents of the expert panel of serology. Vox Sang 1980; 38:178.
147. Issitt PD, Issitt CH, Wilkinson DL. Evaluation of commercial antiglobulin sera over a two year period. II. Anti-IgG and anti-IgM levels and undesirable contaminating antibodies. Transfusion 1974; 14:103.
148. Nasongkla M, Hummert J, Chaplin H. Weak "false positive" direct antiglobulin test reactions with polyspecific antiglobulin reagents. Transfusion 1982; 22:273.
149. Freedman J, Chaplin H, Mollison PL. Further observations on the preparation of antiglobulin reagents reacting with C3d and C4d on red cells. Vox Sang 1977; 33:21.
150. Garratty G. The significance of complement in immunohematology. CRC Crit Rev Clin Lab Sci 1985; 20:25.
151. Wright MS, Issitt PD. Anti-complement and the indirect antiglobulin test. Transfusion 1979; 19:688.
152. Holburn AJ. Quantitative studies with ^{125}I-IgM anti-Le[a]. Immunology 1973; 24:1019.

153. Giblett ER. Blood group alloantibodies: an assessment of some laboratory practices. Transfusion 1977; 17:299.
154. Howell P, Giles CM. A detailed serological study of five anti-Jk^a sera reacting by the antiglobulin technique. Vox Sang 1983; 45:129.
155. Howard JE, Winn LC, Gottlieb CE, et al. Clinical significance of the anti-complement component of antiglobulin antisera. Transfusion 1982; 22:269.
156. Sherwood GK, Haynes BF, Rosse WF. Hemolytic transfusion reactions caused by failure of commercial antiglobulin reagents to detect complement. Transfusion 1976; 16:417.
157. Petz LD, Branch DR, Garratty G, et al. The significance of the anticomplement component of antiglobulin serum (AGS) in compatibility testing. Transfusion 1981; 21:633 (abstr).
158. Stratton F, Rawlinson VI. Complement-fixing antibodies in relation to hemolytic disease of the newborn. Transfusion 1965; 5:216.
159. Voak D, Downie DM, Moore BPL, et al. Antihuman globulin reagent specification. The European and ISBT/ICSH view. Biotest Bull 1986; 1:7.
160. Dobbie D, Brazier M, Gardner B, Holburn AM. Epitopes specificities and quantitative and serologic aspects of monoclonal complement (C3c and C3d) antibodies. Transfusion 1987; 27:453.

16

Macrophage-Mediated Cell Destruction

PETER HORSEWOOD and JOHN G. KELTON
McMaster University Medical Centre
Hamilton, Ontario, Canada

I. INTRODUCTION

The clearance of foreign cells, abnormal host cells (infected cells, malignant cells), and senescent host cells is a pivotal component of the host defense system. The importance of this system is well illustrated by its redundancy and the fact that defects in the ability to destroy foreign or invading cells can be lethal. The potential number of targets that must be cleared is vast, yet the pathways of clearance are limited and surprisingly similar among species. This similarity is probably the best evidence of the overall effectiveness of the host defense system. The ability to recognize many different antigens that are different from the host is the primary responsibility of immunoglobulin and immunoglobulin-bearing cells. The immunoglobulins (especially IgG) bind to antigens on the target cell and this initial antigen-antibody interaction initiates a chain of events that ultimately leads to the clearance of the cell. A series of complex genetic events initiate the formation of the vast array of antibodies capable of binding to virtually every antigen that an individual will ever be exposed to. This chapter focuses on the events that follow the initial interaction of an antibody or other opsonins with the cell or particle that is destined to be cleared.

Because of the ease in obtaining red blood cells (RBCs) for study, the clearance of RBCs by the host defense system has proved to be a highly useful model in studying how this component of the host defense system functions. In this chapter, we focus mainly on RBC clearance, but it is important for the reader to recognize that the clearance of RBCs serves as the model for how any foreign cell is cleared. Indeed, it is an important concept that all cells (normal and abnormal) are cleared in a similar fashion. This explains why the treatment of autoimmune conditions using strong immunosuppressants can result in an increased risk of infection or the development of malignant diseases within the individual.

There are two general routes for the clearance of RBCs. The first is via the binding of antibody (usually IgG) to antigens on the RBC surface. Subsequently, the IgG-sensitized RBCs adhere to and are phagocytized by reticuloendothelial (RE) cells. This is termed extravascular hemolysis because the RBCs are destroyed within phagocytic cells and outside the vasculature. The other pathway of clearance traditionally considered to be important in RBC destruction is through the deposition of complement components on the RBC membrane. Complement activation leads to the insertion of the terminal complement components (the membrane attack complex) directly into the RBC membrane, forming pores in the membrane and lysing the RBCs. This process is termed intravascular hemolysis and although it can occur, for example, as a result of an ABO-incompatible transfusion reaction, it is not a physiological component of cell clearance. Indeed, even by a teleological argument (the intravascular lysis of a cell with the discharging of the cell contents into the vasculature with resulting secondary injury), one can anticipate that this is a highly undesirable event. Far more frequently, complement components steer cells toward extravascular phagocytosis and it is only when there are major disruptions in the host defense system that intravascular lysis results. This occurs when the reticutoendothelial system (RES) is acutely overwhelmed (the transfusion reaction) or there are defects in the complement control system.

The antibody molecules involved in RBC destruction are represented by alloantibodies (hemolytic disease of the newborn, hemolytic transfusion reactions), autoantibodies (IgG- and IgM-mediated autoimmune hemolytic anemia), and drug-induced antibodies (autoantibodies associated with methyldopa and drug-dependent antibodies associated with penicillin and quinine/quinidine). Cell-bound complement and other opsonins also contribute to the cell destruction. Each of these opsonins is recognized by specific receptors present on the cells of the RES. It is to these receptors that the targeted cells bind and ultimately are cleared. The cell destruction occurs either through phagocytosis or, less commonly, antibody-dependent cellular cytotoxicity (ADCC).

In this chapter, we review the components of the RES, summarize some of the techniques used to investigate the RE system, with a major focus being on the recent explosion in information that reflects the molecular study of the receptors and their ligands.

II. THE RETICULOENDOTHELIAL SYSTEM: AN OVERVIEW

The RES is a mononuclear phagocytic system located primarily in the reticular connective tissue framework of the spleen, liver, lungs, bone marrow, and, to a lesser extent, the lymphoid tissue. When the term *reticuloendothelial system* was coined by Aschoff (1), the phagocytic cells were believed to be derived from endothelial cells and to secrete collagenlike substances. We now recognize that both concepts were incorrect: The phagocytic cells are derived from mesenchymal tissue, not endothelium. Furthermore, these cells sit in reticular tissue but do not produce it. However, the term reticuloendothelial system is still used because of general acceptance.

In an attempt to overcome some of the shortcomings of this nomenclature, a new classification was proposed that encompasses the phagocytic, tissue-mononuclear cells and their precursors, and has been termed the mononuclear phagocyte system (MPS (2). The RES and MPS are functionally equivalent; however, for purposes of this chapter, we use the more traditional designation of reticuloendothelial system.

III. THE ORGANS INVOLVED IN RETICULOENDOTHELIAL FUNCTION

A. Spleen

The spleen is involved in clearing aged cells, abnormal cells, antibody- and complement-sensitized cells, microorganisms, and other particles and debris. This is in addition to its roles in hematopoiesis and as a major lymphoid organ. It is the unique vascular structure and anatomy of the spleen that enables it to carry out this clearing function (3) (Fig. 1).

In humans, the spleen consists of an outer capsule that encloses the splenic pulp. A network of trabeculae radiate inward from the capsule and divide the pulp into many interconnected

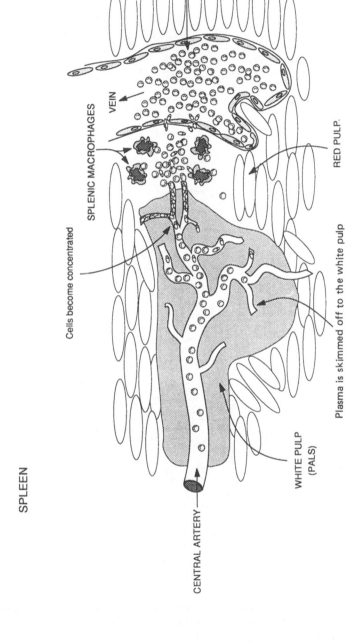

Figure 1 Schematic representation of blood flow through the spleen. The small central arteries are surrounded by periarteriol lymphatic sheaths (PALS) that constitute the white pulp of the spleen. Smaller arteries radiate from the central arteries through the PALS and into the marginal zone. The small arteries "skim off" plasma at the periphery and the central arteries become enriched in cells. The central arteries gradually narrow and terminate in the red pulp close to the sinuses; blood cells percolate through the red pulp and reenter the venous circulation via the sinuses.

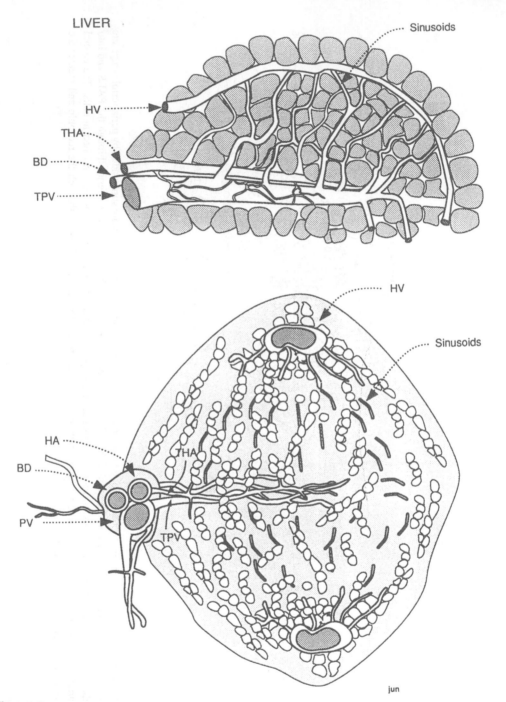

Figure 2 Schematic representation of blood flow through the liver. Blood enters the liver via the portal veins (PV) and hepatic arteries (HA), which, together with the bile ducts (BD), form the portal triads. Small, terminal portal venules (TPV) and hepatic arterioles (THA) radiate from the portal veins and hepatic arteries. These vessels merge with the sinusoids that drain into the efferent hepatic veins (HV). The Kupffer cells reside in the draining sinusoids.

compartments. Arteries enter the spleen where they branch and travel along the trabeculae. Smaller central arteries branch out from the trabecular arteries, and these are surrounded by a reticular meshwork containing lymphoid cells and macrophages. These periarterial lymphatic sheaths (PALS) and the nodules that periodically extend from them constitute the white pulp of the spleen. The central arteries gradually narrow as they pass through a marginal zone into the red pulp, which constitutes the main bulk of the spleen. It is uncertain whether any of these very narrow arteries are in direct continuity with the venous sinuses and form a closed circulatory pathway. The majority appear to terminate in the red pulp where the red cells slowly percolate through the openings between endothelial cells of the venous sinuses (open circulatory pathway) (4).

Small arteries radiate out at right angles from the central arteries, and many of these terminate in the marginal zone between the PALS and the red pulp. Because cellular elements tend to flow in the central axial area of arteries, the smaller radial arteries are able to "skim" plasma off at the periphery (5). Consequently, the blood of the central arteries becomes enriched in cells and depleted of plasma as it passes into the red pulp. This blood has an exceptionally high hematocrit. The separation of the plasma components from the cellular elements plays an important role in the function of the splenic macrophages found in the red pulp. The separation of the IgG from the cellular components means that there is less competition for the IgG-sensitized cells in the binding to macrophage Fc receptors. The biological advantage of these events is described later in this chapter.

The unique architecture and vasculature of the spleen allows direction and trafficking of the fluid and particulate and cellular elements to required areas: Lymphocytes are directed to the white pulp area where they may be retained; soluble plasma antigens are directed to the marginal zones that are rich in antigen-processing macrophages. The concentrated and RBC-rich blood enters the red pulp via the terminal arteries and percolate through "filter beds" rich in macrophages (6). To reenter the circulation, the cells must squeeze through openings, called fenestrations, between the endothelial cells that line the sinus. This environment ensures maximum contact of any antibody-sensitized cells with the splenic macrophages and also prevents cells with defective deformability from squeezing through the sinusoidal spaces and reentering the circulation. RBCs can contain intracellular inclusions that can be physiological (retained nuclear remnants) or pathological (malarial parasites). These inclusions are removed during passage of the RBCs through the endothelial fenestrations.

B. Liver

The liver is surrounded by a thin fibrous capsule that merges with the interior connective tissue and also surrounds the portal triad of biliary duct, hepatic artery, and portal vein. This connective tissue and vascular/biliary system branches extensively within the lobes of the liver subdividing the parenchyma into small segments or lobules. Blood is carried into the liver from both the hepatic artery and the portal vein. The blood of the portal vein is derived from capillaries of the alimentary tract and from the venous drainage of the spleen (7).

The physiology and structure of the liver is viewed in terms of either lobule or acinus units (8). The acinar unit is formed about a vascular axis containing a portal vein, hepatic artery, and bile duct (Fig. 2). Terminal afferent vessels consisting of hepatic arterioles and portal venules radiate at right angles from the hepatic arteries and portal veins. The arterioles and the portal venules merge with the sinusoids to form the acinar microcirculatory unit. The sinusoids are drained by at least two hepatic venules at the periphery of the unit. The capillarylike sinusoids contain the phagocytic cells first described by Kupffer (9,10), which constitute the largest group of fixed macrophages of the body.

Because the liver receives a large blood flow and represents such a large reservoir of phagocytic cells, it is an important clearance organ. This primary function is also due to the anatomical position of the Kupffer cells. They are the first phagocytic cells to encounter blood draining from the gut, a major site for entry of pathogens into the body. As a measure of this phagocytic capacity, it has been shown that after in vivo injection of colloidal carbon, 90% is taken up by the liver. Similarly, after intravenous administration of soluble aggregates of human IgG to human volunteers, Lobatto and coworkers (11) showed the liver to be the predominant clearance organ. This study also showed that RBCs bound many of the aggregates, consistent with their uptake by the CR1 receptors on RBCs. IgG-coated RBCs in the same volunteers were cleared predominantly by the spleen.

Another study by the same group suggested that Fc receptors of the liver Kupffer cells may be less efficient at removing IgG-coated red cells than the phagocytic cells of the spleen (12). However, it is difficult, and probably unnecessary, to proportion the relative contributions of the spleen compared with the liver for overall RE activity. Many other factors contribute to the function of the RES. These include the size of the organs, blood flow, nutritional status, drugs, and the release of activating and depressing modulators. A recent study suggested that calcium is a possible modulator of Kupffer cell phagocytic function (13). Control by calcium and other divalent cations may regulate organ-specific serum opsonins that differentiate between liver and spleen activities. No major change in phagocytosis was seen in a group of patients who had undergone posttraumatic splenectomy, although other macrophage system functions were affected (14). Alterations of the Kupffer cell response to endotoxin following splenectomy has been proposed to result from the loss of the priming effects of splenic lymphokines (15). Kupffer cells are exposed to splenic lymphokines and to other vascular factors through the portal circulation derived from the spleen. Hence, the RES is complex and interconnected on a molecular and macromolecular level.

IV. MACROPHAGES AND MONOCYTES OF THE RES

The role of macrophages in the process of phagocytosis was noted over 100 years ago in the pioneering studies of Metchnikoff (16). He described the large mononuclear phagocytes, which he called macrophages ("large eaters"), and differentiated them from the smaller, phagocytic polymorphonuclear cells, which he termed microphages. Today, we have a greater appreciation of the role of macrophages and other cells of their lineage. They not only function as phagocytes but are intimately involved in many other aspects of the host defense, including (1) defense against microorganisms, (2) antigen processing and interaction with B and T cells, (3) release of regulatory cytokines, (4) release of defensive toxins.

The monocytes (or blood-borne macrophages) and the tissue macrophages trace their origin to the bone marrow pluripotent, hematopoietic stem cell (Fig. 3). Through a series of divisions, the stem cells become increasingly committed, giving rise to a later stem cell that forms cells of both the granulocytic and mononuclear phagocytic series. The bone marrow monoblast is the first identifiable progenitor of the macrophage. It has phagocytic capabilities and displays Fc receptors characteristic of mature cells. The monoblasts divide to produce promonocytes that in turn produce the monocytes. These are released from the bone marrow into the circulation where they have a half-life of about 1–3 days. Migration of the monocytes to tissues throughout the body gives rise to the terminally differentiated tissue macrophages. However, it is possible that a small percentage of tissue macrophages arise by self-proliferation (10,17). Macrophages found in different anatomical sites have different activities, functions, and properties, which are conditioned in part by their environment.

The heterogeneity of macrophages has led to a variety of names and descriptions for the various cells of the lineage. The monocytes of the blood are short-lived, mobile cells, whereas the tissue macrophages derived from the monocytes may be either mobile or fixed.

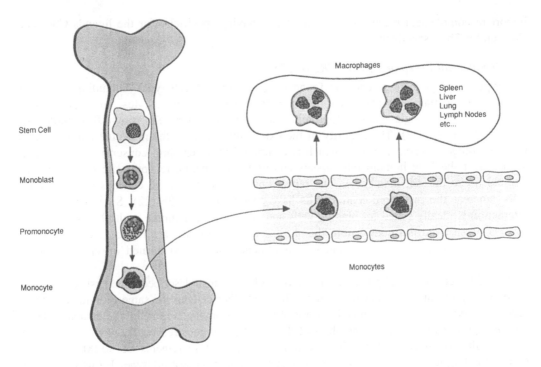

Figure 3 Mononuclear phagocyte cell lineage. Hematopoietic stem cells in the bone marrow give rise to monoblasts that divide and produce promonocytes. The promonocytes differentiate into monocytes that leave the bone marrow and circulate in the blood. The monocytes migrate into tissues where they differentiate into macrophages.

Cells of the monocyte/macrophage lineage have distinctive membrane markers, receptors, and functions, and these allow them to be distinguished from morphologically similar cells. Previously, the cells were identified by their enzymatic activities for nonspecific esterase, lysozyme, and peroxidase. Today, identification focuses on the binding of monocyte/macrophage–specific monoclonal antibodies. The most characteristic functional properties of the macrophages are their ability to recognize foreign or damaged material and to endocytose such material. Endocytosis, whether pinocytosis of soluble matter or phagocytosis of particulate matter, is mediated through binding to specific cell surface receptors. These receptors have both immune and nonimmune functions. It is the complement and Fc receptors that are critically important in the function of macrophage phagocytosis of RBCs. Indeed, the immune-mediated ingestion of cells, bacteria, or immune complexes is the property most identifiable with macrophages. In the next section, we review the properties of several of these phagocytic receptors.

A. Complement and IgG Fc Receptors of Macrophages/Monocytes

1. Complement Receptors

Activation of the complement cascade results in the binding of complement molecules to the cell surface, which promotes their removal either directly through cell lysis or more likely through immune phagocytosis. Cell-bound complement is recognized via specific receptors on phagocytic cells. These receptors recognize cleavage fragments of the C3 and C4 complement molecules and are important in immune clearance and regulation. Macrophages possess two important complement receptors, CR1 and CR3, having specificity for the ligands C3b (and C4b) and iC3b, respectively.

2. Complement Receptor Type 1, CR1 (CD35)

The type 1 complement receptor is found on many human cell types, including RBCs, B lymphocytes, certain T lymphocytes, neutrophils, eosinophils, monocytes, and macrophages (18–20). CR1 is a single-chain glycoprotein whose primary structure is known from molecular cloning studies (21,22). The majority of the extracellular part of the molecule comprise four long homologous repeats, each of which is composed of seven short consensus repeats (Fig. 4). Each of the long homologous repeats constitutes a separate receptor site except for the one closest to the cell membrane. The repeat unit most distal to the cell has specificity for C4b, whereas the two more central units have specificity for C3b (22). Such a multivalent interaction is ideally suited for binding cells and complexes containing multiple C4b and C3b ligands. Conserved positions within the short consensus repeats are found in other C3/C4–binding proteins that together comprise a multigene family (23) located on chromosome 1 (24).

Two different structural polymorphisms for CR1 have been described. The first results from different glycosylation of the CR1 on the RBCs and other cells of the same individual (25). A second allotypic polymorphism is the result of four autosomal codominant alleles that code for CR1 receptors having different numbers of the long homologous repeats (reviewed in ref. 26). This results in allotypes that differ by molecular weight increments of 30,000–50,000 d (corresponding to the long homologous repeats). The commonest allotype, F (also known as A) (gene frequency 0.81) has four long homologous repeats, whereas the S (also known as B) allotype (gene frequency 0.2) has five. Two rare allotypes F' (also known as C) and D are known. Because each of the long homologous repeats encodes a specific binding site for C3b and C4b, it is likely that the different allotypes may have different affinities/capacities for the binding of complement containing immune complexes (26).

CR1 has two major functions that are to a degree opposite to each other. CR1 participates in complement regulation and at the same time helps clear complement-sensitized cells. Regulation of the complement system is achieved through inhibition of C3 and C5 activation. Immune complex clearance in humans and other primates is mediated in large part through the CR1 receptors of RBCs (27). Although RBCs have relatively few CR1 receptors (500–750/cell), the large number of RBCs compared with other cells in the circulation has the net effect of making them the dominant CR1-bearing cell. Soluble immune complexes in the circulation bind to the CR1 receptor on RBCs, which transport them to the liver where many of the complexes will be destroyed. The immune complexes are stripped from the RBCs by the high affinity CR3 receptors on the liver macrophages and the RBCs are returned to the circulation. C3b-containing immune complexes bound to the CR1 receptors on RBCs are susceptible to proteolysis by plasma factor I. The factor I cleaves C3b to produce iC3b. This complement component has a high affinity for the CR3 receptor and explains the transfer of the RBC-bound immune complexes to the phagocytic cells in the liver.

The role of CR1 in immune phagocytosis is multifactorial and requires the cooperation of other mediators. Thus, direct phagocytosis of C3b-coated particles through CR1 on normal resting macrophages does not occur. However, stimulation of the macrophages or target enhancement though the binding of additional opsonins (especially IgG) can trigger CR1-mediated phagocytosis (28–30). The phagocytosis seen after stimulation may be due to increased receptor expression through mobilization of intracellular stores (31). Capping of CR1 receptors has been shown to result in the cocapping of Fc receptors without the latter binding antibody and is dependent on the binding of CR1 to the cytoskeleton (32,33). This synergy is seen in the phagocytosis of oxidatively stressed human RBCs by auto-anti–band 3 antibodies. In the

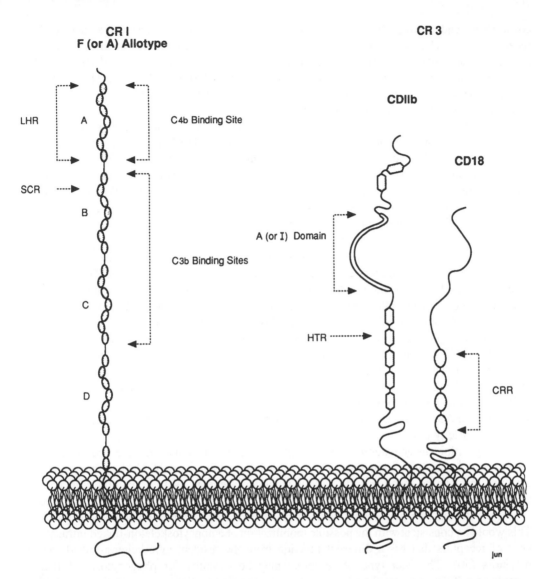

Figure 4 Schematic diagram of the structure of the CR1 and CR3 complement receptors. The CR1 F (also known as A) allotype is shown. It is a single-chain glycoprotein organized into four (A–D) long homologous repeats (LHR) each composed of seven short consensus repeats (SCR). The terminal LHR binds C4b and the two central LHRs bind C3b. CR3 is a noncovalently linked heterodimer composed of an α-chain (CD11b) and a β-chain (CD18). The α-chain (CD11b) contains seven homologous tandem repeats (HTR), the second and third of which are split by an additional A (also called interactive, I) domain that may contain the C3 ligand–binding site. The β-chain (CD18) has a cysteine-rich region (CRR) consisting of four tandem repeats.

absence of bound C3b, the anti–band 3 antibody alone is insufficient to mediate phagocytosis (34). Even though RBCs carry CR1 receptors, they do not participate directly in phagocytosis.

3. Complement Receptor Type 3, CR3 (CD11b/CD18)
Human type 3 complement receptor has specificity for the inactivated third component of complement, iC3b (35). CR3 is widely distributed and found on follicular dendritic cells,

eosinophils, and neutrophils as well as on cells of the monocyte/macrophage lineage. The receptor is a member of the integrin superfamily, and like other members of the superfamily, it exists as a noncovalently linked heterodimer (see Fig. 4). It shares a common β-chain (CD18) with two other heterodimers, LFA-1 (CD11a/CD18) and p150,95 (CD11c/CD18). Together, the three members form the leukocyte adhesion family of receptors (36).

cDNA studies have delineated the primary structure of the α- and β-subunits (37–39). The α-chain of CR3, like other integrin α-chains, contains divalent cation-binding sites that are necessary for receptor conformational stability and ligand binding (40). Calcium binding to the sites may differentiate adhesive and phagocytic functions of the receptor (40). The α-chain contains an approximately 200–amino acid segment on its extracellular region that is termed the I domain. This domain has homology with similar domains in von Willebrand factor, complement components factor B and C2, and collagen proteins (41). Since both factor B and C2 bind C3b, this region may be important in the ligand-recognition site of CR3.

Functional studies have shown that the CR3 receptor can mediate the phagocytosis and lysis of iC3b-coated RBCs (42). It has also been shown that CR3 is active in the natural killer cell–mediated killing of targets carrying surface-attached C3 fragments (43). The effects of monoclonal antibodies on the blocking of receptor function have suggested a multifunctional role for CR3 (44). Thus, although some monoclonal antibodies inhibit binding of iC3b but not spreading or chemotaxis, other monoclonal antibodies show the opposite effect.

The iC3b ligand that binds to CR3 contains an arginine-glycine–aspartic acid (RGD) sequence. RGD has been shown to be involved in the binding of many ligands to integrin receptors (45). The importance of the RGD sequence in mediating ligand-receptor coupling is unknown, although a fibrinogen peptide containing a modified RGD sequence blocked both iC3b and fibrinogen binding to CR3 (46). It is possible that, like other integrin receptors, secondary binding sequences in addition to RGD receptor sites are involved in determining overall specificity (47).

The regulation and activation of CR3 receptors is unknown but may involve a conformational change and intracellular signaling. There is an intracellular pool of CR3 within monocyte granules that can be mobilized via various stimulatory events (48). Activation with phorbol esters shows an increase in both the CR3 number and iC3b binding, but after 1 hour, the binding activity is decreased below resting levels while the receptor number remains increased (49). This would be consistent with the possible mobilization of a noncytoskeleton-linked intracellular pool of receptors that has a different function from the resident cytoskeleton-linked surface receptors (50). The later type of receptors may be essential for phagocytosis of IgG or complement (C4b)–sensitized targets, whereas the former functions in recognition and binding only. Other studies utilizing anti-CD11b monoclonal antibody inhibition of IgG Fc receptor-mediated binding and phagocytosis reached similar conclusions (51). The authors of the study suggested an immobile subset of CR3 existed on monocytes and these were important in binding and ingestion of IgG opsonized targets. That such an immobile subpopulation of CR3 receptors is responsible for phagocytosis of target cells irrespective of their being bound by IgG Fc receptor or CR1 receptor is an intriguing concept. Recent studies have provided further insight into the cytoskeletal requirements in human macrophage-mediated phagocytosis via complement and Fc receptors (52).

4. IgG Fc Receptors

Macrophages carry all of the three classes of IgG Fc receptors. The three classes of receptors have been designated FcγRI, FcγRII, and FcγRIII (reviewed in refs. 53 and 54). Recent studies of the gene structure, transcriptional processing, and resulting proteins indicate that there are large families of molecules composing a more diverse system of receptors than encompassed by the three class systems. This has prompted the proposal of a different classification system based on "groups" of Fcγ receptors to better accommodate the many members (53); however, in this chapter, we will use the more traditional classification.

The diversity of the FcγR is manifested further in terms of ligand specificity, ligand affinity, and cell distribution. How this heterogeneity is reflected in the functional diversity is unclear at the present time. It is to be expected that each of the classes of receptors with their various subtypes would have specific receptor function. In this way, the three receptor types found on macrophages would be employed for specific purposes and not merely serve as back-up systems for one another. However, it also has been proposed that the receptors do not perform specific tasks but rather functionality is determined by the cell type carrying the receptor (55).

Despite the heterogeneity of the various receptors, they share a good deal of homology. All members are membrane-bound glycoproteins of the Ig supergene family whose genes map to the long arm of chromosome 1 (56). The extracellular part of the proteins is composed of immunoglobulin heavy chain second constant region, CH2-like domains (57). The proteins have diverse transmembrane and cytoplasmic structures indicating a role in cell signaling.

5. FcγRI (CD64)

The 70-kd FcγRI is an integral membrane glycoprotein that is expressed predominantly on monocytes and macrophages. It binds human IgG1, IgG3, and IgG4 but has little or no affinity for IgG2 (58). The binding site on human immunoglobulin has been localized to the Cγ2 domain (59). Unlike the other Fc receptors, FcγRI has high affinity for its ligands, binding monomeric IgG with a K_d of 10^{-8} to 10^{-9} M (58,60).

Investigations at the molecular level have described three distinct cDNA clones for FcγRI

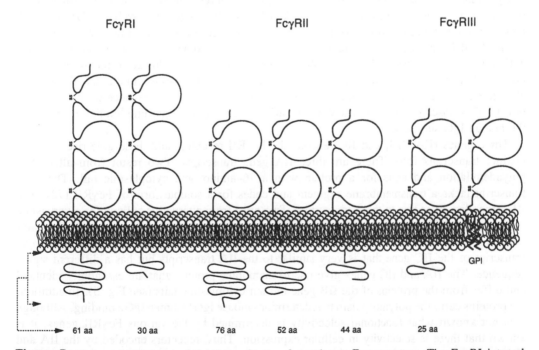

Figure 5 Schematic diagram of the three classes of membrane Fcγ receptors. The FcγRI integral membrane receptors comprise three immunoglobulin Cγ2 domains and a cytoplasmic tail of either 61 or 30 amino acids (aa). The FcγRII integral membrane receptors have two extracellular immunoglobulin domains and a cytoplasmic tail of 76, 52, or 44 amino acids. The integral membrane FcγRIII present on macrophages and NK cells has two immunoglobulin domains and a 25–amino acid cytoplasmic tail. The FcγRIII present on neutrophils is a glycosylphosphatidylinositol (GPI)–linked molecule lacking a cytoplasmic tail, and it has two extracellular immunoglobulin domains.

(61). Two of these code for polymorphic differences and the third produces a molecule having a different intracytoplasmic domain. All code for an extracellular region composed of three Ig-type domains. The first two domains are homologous to the extracellular domains of the FcγRII and FcγRIII receptors but the third shows little homology. The FcRI molecules have a 21–amino acid transmembrane region and a cytoplasmic domain of either 30 or 61 amino acids (Fig. 5).

Interferon gamma (IFN-γ) upregulates the expression of the receptor on monocytes and macrophages (62,63) and the increased expression has been shown to increase antibody-dependent cellular cytotoxicity (64). However, increased expression does not always result in augmented cytotoxicity (55). Furthermore, the receptor has been shown to be effective in mediating phagocytosis of RBC target cells by monocytes and macrophages (65).

6. FcγRII (CD32)

The FcγRII receptor is a 40-kd integral membrane glycoprotein that has low affinity for monomeric IgG. This receptor is very widely distributed, being found on most types of circulating blood cells, including platelets, but it is absent on T cells, RBCs, and natural killer (NK) cells (66). Macrophages have high numbers of FcγRII (30,000–80,000/cell), but unlike FcγRI, there is no increase in receptor number after treatment with cytokines (67). The affinity of binding for IgG, which is too low to measure by direct binding of monomeric IgG, has been estimated to have a K_d of less than 10^{-7} M (68). This property suggests that FcγRII binds only to immune complexes or cells sensitized by many molecules of IgG.

As with FcγRI, there are differences in the specific binding of IgG subclasses to FcγRII. Early studies indicated specificity for IgG1 and IgG3, with IgG2 and IgG4 showing little binding (69). However, another study indicates that FcγRII binds IgG2 equally as well as IgG1, although there was a low binding affinity for IgG4 (70). There is a genetically determined polymorphism of the FcγRII receptor that is manifest by a selective binding of mouse monoclonal IgG1 antibodies by individuals (71). This polymorphism results from a change of the amino acid at position 131 that is critical for the binding of mouse IgG1 (70). More importantly, this change also determines the binding of human IgG2, possibly giving some relevance to the polymorphism. This observation could also explain earlier discrepancies regarding binding affinities of the human IgG subclasses.

Three genes (IIA, IIB, and IIC) encode the FcγRII receptors and these give rise to seven distinct transcripts (56). There are three IIA gene transcripts: Two result from alternative polyadenylation and code for a protein with a 76–amino acid cytoplasmic tail. The third transcript lacks a transmembrane segment and codes for a soluble form of FcγRII (72). The IIB gene also gives rise to three transcripts. Two arise from alternative splicing of cytoplasmic exons and code for proteins with either a 52– or 44–amino acid cytoplasmic tail. The third derives from alternative splicing of the exons encoding the signal sequence. There is a single transcript of the IIC gene that is very similar to the IIA transcripts but has a different signal sequence. The IIA and IIC genes give rise to membrane proteins that are essentially identical and differ from the proteins of the IIB gene in their cytoplasmic tails (see Fig. 5). In addition, the proteins carry the polymorphism that determines mouse IgG1/human IgG2 binding. Although it is not known what functional selectivity is determined by the various FcγRII genes, it is known that there is selectivity in cellular expression. Thus, receptors encoded by the IIA and IIC genes are expressed on monocytes, macrophages, and neutrophils, whereas those of the IIB gene are expressed on monocytes, macrophages, and lymphocytes (72).

The low-affinity FcγRII receptors can mediate many biological functions, including phagocytosis, ADCC, superoxide generation, and lysosomal enzyme release (55,65,73). FcγRII-mediated cytotoxicity is enhanced by IFN-γ, but this does not occur via increased receptor numbers (55). Additionally, the receptor activity has been shown to be enhanced by proteolytic enzymes that cause an increased affinity for ligand binding (74). The in vivo relevance of this phenomena is unclear, but it could result in a controlling mechanism whereby augmentation of ligand binding occurs at inflammatory sites or during macrophage activation when proteases are released.

7. FcγRIII (CD16)

The third type of IgG-binding receptor, FcγRIII, was originally identified as a 50- to 70-kd membrane glycoprotein on neutrophils (75). The diffuse molecular weight is a result of posttranslational glycosylation modifications. On macrophages, where the FcγRIII is an abundant receptor (40,000–100,000/cell), it has a 45- to 65-kd mass (76). In addition, the receptor is present on eosinophils, NK cells, mesangeal cells, trophoblasts, and on a subpopulation of monocytes (77).

FcγRIII, like FcγRII, has low affinity for binding monomeric IgG ($K_d < 10^{-7}$ M) (78). However, recent data (53) suggests that the macrophage FcγRIII receptor may have a higher affinity than originally thought. The binding specificity for human IgG indicates that subclasses IgG1 and IgG3 bind about equally well, whereas IgG2 and IgG4 do not bind (78,79).

Two FcγRIII genes, FcRIIIA and FcRIIIB, have been identified that are selectively expressed in different cells (80). These genes have extensive homology and differ by only 12 nucleotides in the coding regions. The FcRIIIA gene codes for a transmembrane glycoprotein that is expressed on NK cells and macrophages, whereas the FcRIIIB gene codes for a glycosyl-phosphatidylinositol (GPI)–linked molecule that is expressed on neutrophils only (81,82) (see Fig. 5). The FcRIII B gene codes for a transcript with a short 4–amino acid cytoplasmic tail, whereas the FcRIII A gene codes for a longer 25–amino acid cytoplasmic tail. A single, critical amino acid change of phenylalanine to serine between FcRIII A and FcRIII B determines the different membrane anchoring of the two receptors. The serine 203 results in a GPI-linked protein with loss of the short cytoplasmic tail (80,83,84). The expression of the transmembrane form of the receptor, as found on macrophages, is dependent on association with a surface expression regulator (SER). Two regulators that mediate the surface expression have been identified: the γ-chain of the high-affinity IgE receptor and the ζ-chain that is present in the CD3–T-cell receptor complex (83,85,86).

The FcγRIII found on neutrophils, but not on macrophages, carries the NA1/NA2 neutrophil-specific alloantigen system. The molecular basis of the polymorphism has been identified and results in minor amino acid differences between the two allotypes (80,87). One allotype (NA2) has amino acid changes that result in two additional glycosylation sites and enables the two forms to be distinguished by electrophoretic mobilities (88). Macrophages and NK cells express an NA2 form exclusively (88,89).

Conflicting data exist whether the macrophage and the neutrophil FcγRIII receptors can mediate the phagocytosis of IgG-coated RBCs (65,90,91). Although it has been shown that the macrophage FcγRIII receptor can mediate phagocytosis, there is uncertainty about the neutrophil receptor. There are also conflicting reports about the ability of the macrophage receptor to mediate direct cell lysis (76,92). These differences may reflect the different assay systems used to monitor the functions and the actual role played by the FcγRIII in vivo is unknown.

8. Fcγ Receptor Relationships

The presence of three different classes of receptors for IgG on macrophages poses questions about their functional relationships. Data show that these receptors arose via duplication and recombination of an ancestral gene (56). The receptors have considerably homology, but at the same time, they have many differences that enable them to be differentiated both biochemically and biologically. The differences have been delineated under well-defined in vitro conditions that allow dissection of their individual functions. However, for the most part, these conditions are contrived and may not be representative of actual in vivo environments. Under normal physiological conditions, one would expect that the high-affinity Fc receptors (FcγRI) are occupied by monomeric IgG and, therefore, not activated by individual IgG molecules. This suggests that this receptor, like the two low-affinity Fcγ receptors, would be triggered only by clustering through multivalent ligands such as immune complexes or antibody-coated target cells. Although a restricted cellular distribution may result in a defined function for some of the receptors, the presence of all three receptors on the macrophage demands interpretation.

It is possible that the receptors may cooperate with one another and with other surface molecules. Cooperation has been shown for FcγRIII on macrophages and NK cells (83,85,86), and there is evidence that FcγRII can cooperate with FcγRI in binding ligands and activating the FcγRI receptor (93).

It is likely that all classes of receptors become occupied to some extent when targets bearing a high density of bound IgG molecules interact with macrophages. Under these circumstances, the receptors may be performing redundant functions. The description of a family lacking detectable FcγRI on their phagocytic cells, but who showed normal phagocytosis and were healthy, supports this conclusion (94). Other individuals who lacked neutrophil FcγRIII, but were otherwise healthy, also have been identified (95). In contrast to the possible redundant function of the receptors is the finding of a role for a single receptor class in immune clearance. Thus, the infusion of monoclonal anti-FcγRIII antibody inhibited the antibody-dependent destruction of platelets in a patient with immune thrombocytopenic purpura (ITP) (96).

V. OTHER MACROPHAGE RECEPTORS IN PHAGOCYTOSIS

The phagocytosis of opsonin-coated cells occurs primarily through the IgG and complement receptors; however, other molecules capable of mediating phagocytic functions have been described. Adherence of monocytes to collagen activates CR1 and CR3 and enhances Fc receptor–mediated phagocytosis (97). Binding to other extracellular matrix proteins also has been demonstrated to enhance phagocytic activity, and these findings may be relevant to macrophage function at inflammatory sites (98). The receptors responsible for the collagen binding have not been identified, but VLA2 molecules may be involved (97). Other molecules that have homology to collagen have also been shown to enhance FcR and CR1 phagocytic activity. These include C1q, a subunit of the first component of the classic complement pathway, and pulmonary surfactant protein (99). The mannose-binding protein that serves as an opsonin for yeast, bacteria, and fungi also has collagenlike domains (100). The specific receptor or receptors for these collagen homologues have not been identified.

Platelet-activating factor (PAF) has been shown to enhance the monocyte ingestion of diamide-treated human RBCs (101). Using this senescent RBC cell model, PAF was shown to induce protein kinase C translocation, phosphorylation of CR1, and stimulation of CR1-mediated phagocytosis. In this respect, PAF resembles the ability of phorbol esters and extracellular matrix proteins to activate complement receptors. Lymphokines have also been shown to augment macrophage complement receptors (29).

Fibronectin, like other extracellular matrix proteins, increases the clearance of IgG and complement-sensitized cells (28,30,98). However, unlike most of the previously noted opsonins, this large glycoprotein circulates in plasma. As such, it can act as an opsonin by binding to both monocytes/macrophages and to blood-borne targets. Specific receptors on the monocytes/macrophages recognize the arginine, glycine, and aspartic acid sequence (RGD) of the fibronectin molecule (102,103). Although fibronectin binding does not increase the number or affinity of the complement receptors, the enhanced phagocytosis occurs through complement receptor activation (104,105).

Macrophage receptors also recognize and can phagocytize proteins and cells carrying certain advanced glycosylation end products that result from nonenzymatic glycosylation reactions (106). These glycosylated products accumulate on long-lived cells and on cells from diabetic individuals. The receptors may, therefore, play a role in removing senescent cells from the circulation. Removal of senescent thymocytes through cell surface carbohydrates binding to macrophage lectinlike receptors also has been described (107). Phagocytosis by macrophages of senescent human neutrophils having charged molecules on their surface has been reported (108). The phagocytosis was shown not to involve opsonic complement or FcR receptors nor the receptor for the advanced glycosylation products.

A receptor for a lipopolysaccharide-binding protein that binds to lipopolysaccharides inserted into RBC membranes has been described (109). The receptor is present on monocytes and macrophages but not on other leukocytes and is distinct from other opsonic receptors. Binding of coated RBCs by the receptor alone does not cause phagocytosis but it strongly enhances phagocytosis of cells coated with suboptimal amounts of IgG. Low-density lipoprotein has been identified as a regulator of FcRI-mediated phagocytosis (110). The low-density lipoprotein is required for optimal expression of the high-affinity receptors. However, it is not known if the macrophage low-density lipoprotein receptor is involved in this process.

VI. FACTORS IN RES-MEDIATED CELL CLEARANCE

In the normal individual, there is a delicate balance between the various immune mediator molecules and the reticuloendothelial receptors that bind them. Disturbance of this balance can result in either up- or downregulation of the RES. Although many molecules can participate in this process, it is IgG and complement and the respective cellular receptors that are the most important.

Normal cells have small amounts of IgG on their surface, yet circulate without being cleared by the RES. The amount of IgG on normal RBCs is approximately 30 molecules/cell (111,112), which is below the detection limit of the antiglobulin test (113). Similarly, normal circulating platelets have bound IgG, and although there is controversy about the actual amount of IgG on platelets, it is more than on RBCs (114). Levels of 80 to greater than 10,000 IgG molecules per platelet have been reported (115,116).

Complement components also have been detected on the surface of normal RBCs. The amounts, like those of IgG, are low, with values ranging from 5–500 molecules/cell (117–119). It is unlikely that this complement arises from antibody-mediated activation but more likely occurs through other mechanisms. It could, for instance, result from simple adsorbtion of C3 breakdown products. Such products could also bind to the RBC CR1 receptor. The increased level of C3 found on stored RBCs is compatible with either of these mechanisms (120). However, it should be kept in mind that the basal levels for both IgG and complement are the average values. Subpopulations of cells could (and probably do) exist that have levels considerably in excess of the average. These populations could include senescent cells destined for clearance. In addition, patients have been reported whose cells carry large amounts of bound IgG but circulate without apparent interaction with the RES. Conversely, some patients appearing to have immune hemolytic reactions have no detectable antibody on their RBCs.

Considering the basal levels of IgG and complement components on circulating cells, what then are the factors that determine macrophage recognition and destruction in pathological states? Are IgGs of defined specificities, class, and subclass or affinities important? Is the quantity or the antigen distribution a determining factor? Many of these factors have been investigated and have been reviewed recently (121). One factor that has received less attention is the activity of the RES.

A. Antibody Class and Subclass

There are no specific receptors for IgM on phagocytic cells. Consequently, IgM will only mediate cell clearance through activation of complement. This can occur through direct intravascular cell lysis, as can occur in cold agglutinin disease. The IgM binds to RBCs in the cooler, peripheral parts of the circulation and dissociates on reaching the warmer central parts. But before dissociating, the IgM activates the classic complement pathway. The presence of IgM antiplatelet antibodies in immune thrombocytopenia also has been reported (122–124). Whether such antibodies, through complement activation, can result in platelet destruction in the absence of IgG antibodies is unknown.

Specific receptors for IgA have been described on macrophages (125,126). However, they have not been considered to play a major role in immune-mediated cell clearance. The incidence of specific IgA antibodies occurring without IgG antibodies in warm autoimmune hemolytic disease is very low (113,127,128). Nevertheless, several reports have described immune hemolytic anemia associated with IgA antibodies (129–131). Since IgA does not activate complement, the role of specific Fcα receptors in immune clearance may warrant investigation. Alternatively, it may be that low levels of specific IgG accompany the IgA and these might be identified using more sensitive testing methods (132). In support of this possibility is the observation that IgA synergize IgG-mediated cell destruction by antibody-dependent cellular cytotoxicity (133).

There are little data available concerning IgA platelet antibodies in autoimmune thrombocytopenia. In one report IgG, but not IgM or IgA platelet-associated immunoglobulins, were correlated with mean platelet life span (134). This study showed no correlation between splenic or hepatic sequestration patterns and platelet-associated IgM or IgA; although platelets with higher IgG levels were more readily sequestered in the spleen.

The vast majority of antibodies mediating immune cell destruction are IgG, with the IgG1 subclass predominating (132,135). Although there are multiple immunoglobulin classes and subclasses normally present in sera from patients with autoimmune hemolysis, there are cases described where only a single IgG subclass was identified. It is not difficult to understand cell destruction occurring via IgG1 and IgG3 antibodies either in combination with other immunoglobulins or alone. Both activate complement and both readily bind to all types of macrophage Fc receptors. However, autoimmune and alloimmune antibodies of IgG2 subclass that induce hemolytic anemia have been described (121,136,137).

IgG2 activates complement only weakly and does not bind well to Fcγ receptors; therefore, it would not be expected to be a good mediator of cellular clearance. However, one report indicates IgG2 binds well to FcγRII (70). Also, the low-affinity binding of IgG2 may be enhanced in situations in which it can bind in clusters. Thus, IgG2 alone or in conjunction with a low levels of cell-bound complement may be sufficient to cause cell destruction. Alternatively, it may be that low levels of other IgG subclasses accompany the IgG2 but are not detectable by antiglobulin testing.

Examples of IgG4 as the only IgG subclass antibodies (e.g., anti-Ytª) binding to RBCs have been reported (138); these antibodies probably are not clinically significant. It remains unexplained why such antigens should give rise to Ig4 subclass antibodies so frequently. It is generally assumed that the Fcγ receptors bind IgG1 and IgG3 equally well, although there is some uncertainty as to their relative affinities (53,54,66). However, studies with RBCs sensitized with IgG1 and IgG3 suggest that IgG3 is the better opsonin (139–141). The efficiency of the difference is seen particularly well with monoclonal antibody–coated RBCs. One hundred molecules of monoclonal IgG3 anti-D coating initiates macrophage binding, whereas 10,000 molecules of monoclonal IgG1 are required (141). A related study showed that whereas monoclonal IgG1 anti-D antibodies resulted in phagocytosis, IgG3 anti-D antibodies mediated cytotoxic lysis (142). Caution must be used, however, in extrapolating in vitro assays with monoclonal antibodies to actual in vivo conditions. The issues relating to the relative efficiency of IgG1 compared with IgG3, particularly in relation to cases of hemolytic disease of the newborn, have been reviewed by Garratty (135).

B. Quantity of IgG and Complement Required for Cell Clearance

There is a very large literature analyzing the quantity of immunoglobulins on RBCs and how this relates to cell destruction. Recent articles by Garratty have reviewed this literature and have helped to establish some relationships in what previously has been a confusing area (121,135). Under defined conditions, there is generally a direct correlation between the amount of RBC-bound antibody and the destruction of such cells (143,144). However, because of the differences in criteria for assessing hemolysis and the tremendous variability in reagents and methods used to measure bound IgG, there are conflicting data on the validity of immunoglobulin quantitation as a predictor of cell destruction (145). Clearly, some situations arise in which the amount of bound IgG measured by conventional testing is very low, yet there is evidence of hemolysis (146). Conversely, there are examples where cells have significant amounts of bound IgG, yet can circulate without apparent interaction with the RES (147).

It is difficult to reconcile the variability seen with the various levels of RBC-bound IgG and the level of interaction of such cells with the macrophage Fc receptors. Incomplete correlation in many cases may be explained through a lack of knowledge of the particular classes and subclasses of IgG bound. The state of activation of the RES also is a factor that is rarely considered, particularly because most correlations have involved noncellular in vitro testing methods. To overcome these limitations, assays have been devised in an attempt to simulate better in vivo conditions (148–150). One study compared several methods to correlate serological, quantitative IgG levels and cell-mediated functions of alloantibodies with the severity of hemolysis in newborns (151). The results suggested that monocyte-based functional assays were the best predictors of hemolysis. The amount of IgG binding to RBCs may also affect whether phagocytosis or cytotoxic lysis by macrophages occurs. In one study, low levels of IgG anti-D were found to induce phagocytosis, whereas high levels induced cytolysis (152).

Assays that measure platelet-bound IgG have shown increases in platelet IgG in most cases of immune thrombocytopenia (153–155). Studies of alloimmune posttransfusion purpura also have demonstrated increased levels of IgG on the surface of the patients' platelets (156–157). Caution must be used in correlating these results with immune mechanisms of platelet removal because increased levels of platelet-associated IgG have been found in cases of nonimmune thrombocytopenias. Additionally, there is a large range in the level of platelet-associated IgG reported by different investigators (114). However, in general, there is an inverse relationship between the amount of platelet-bound IgG and the platelet count implying more efficient removal of the more heavily sensitized platelets (153,158).

Assays have been developed that might better represent in vivo removal of opsonized platelets. Salch and associates have described assays to investigate platelet surface–bound IgG and the ability of monocytes to bind to these platelets (159). They found that normal donors had less than 400 molecules of IgG per platelet, whereas 90% of patients with new-onset immune thrombocytopenia had greater than 800 molecules per platelet. The pathophysiological relevance of this amount of platelet-bound IgG was shown by the fact that in vitro sensitization of platelets with PlA[1] alloantibodies required greater than 800 molecules of IgG per platelet to bind to human monocytes. However, they did not observe a correlation between the amount of platelet surface–bound IgG and the severity of thrombocytopenia.

The role of bound complement in addition to bound IgG is frequently neglected. However, studies by Ehlenberger and Kurlander have underscored the role of complement in cell clearance

(160,161). These investigators showed that small amounts of IgG on RBCs could not induce phagocytosis. But, if the target cells also had bound complement, then phagocytosis occurred. Other studies also have shown a synergistic effect of complement with IgG for Fc receptor–mediated phagocytosis (34).

There is a general correlation between the amount of complement on the RBCs cells and the severity of immune-mediated hemolytic anemia (162,163). Complement alone does not normally result in immune clearance. However, only a few IgG molecules are necessary in addition to complement to bring about immune clearance. This effect can be explained by a targeting role of the bound complement. In the presence of plasma containing large amounts of competing IgG, the Fc receptors of macrophages are either occupied (FcγRI) or inhibited from binding (FcγRII and RcγRIII). The macrophage complement receptors, which are specific for breakdown products of C3, are not inhibited by plasma C3. The complement receptors bind the cells bearing complement components and ensure that the Fc receptors can interact with the cell-bound IgG. This mechanism can be bypassed in cases where cell-bound antibodies occur at high local density. Then Fc receptors can directly interact with the clustered IgG with little competition from plasma IgG. A study showing the priming of monocytes for FcR-mediated phagocytosis by CR1 cross-linking supports this concept (164). In this study, no priming was seen when the CR3 receptor was cross-linked.

The ability of auto- and alloantiplatelet antibodies to activate complement and mediate the immune destruction of platelets is controversial. Some, but not all, studies have demonstrated elevated levels of platelet-associated C3 in autoimmune thrombocytopenia (165,166). Sometimes the complement level was correlated with surface IgG levels (167–169). However, it is possible that nonspecifically bound plasma C3 could account for the elevated complement levels. Some investigators have shown that platelets from patients with autoimmune thrombocytopenia have high levels of albumin (170). This raised the possibility that binding of small amounts of platelet-specific antibodies could "activate" the platelets such that they became "sticky" and bound plasma proteins. This results in increased levels of surface-bound albumin and immunoglobulins (nonspecific) and presumably also of bound C3, which is an abundant plasma protein.

Some cases of elevated platelet surface–bound complement presumably arise from antibody-mediated activation. Here the complement components found on the surface are not normal plasma constituents and are detected by antisera specific for complement activation. Thus, markedly increased levels of C3d and the terminal membrane complex, C5,6–9, were seen on platelets sensitized with drug-dependent platelet antibodies and moderate levels with platelet autoantibodies (169).

C. Affinity and Specificity of the Antibodies

There is little information available regarding the effects of antibody affinities on cell destruction. The most obvious cases involve low-affinity IgM cold agglutinins. These antibodies bind their targets in the cooler, peripheral regions of the circulation but dissociate at warmer body temperature. At some intermediate temperature, complement activation occurs and the cells are lysed intravascularly or bind to the CR1 and CR3 receptors of macrophages, particularly in the liver. There is some evidence that antibodies with increased affinity lead to increased RBC destruction (171). However, there is no convincing data relating antibody-binding equilibrium constants to the efficiency of cell removal. Perhaps more important than affinity is avidity, whereby multivalent antigens are better able to bind antibody. Avidity is related to the target antigen, its geometry, and the antibody specificity. Surface glycoproteins containing repeat epitope sequences could result in antibody clustering and efficient binding to macrophage Fc receptors. Similarly, high-density antigens such as the blood group ABO molecules will give rise to high numbers of closely bound antibodies. Low-density antigens such as Rh result in widely spaced antibody binding. Not only will the antibody density affect the interaction with the Fc receptors but it will also determine the extent of complement deposition. Although a single IgM molecule can initiate complement activation, several IgG molecules must be sufficiently close for complement activation.

Several of the requirements necessary for IgG-mediated Fc receptor interactions have been studied by Walker and coworkers (172). They found that rosette formation between FcRII-bearing Daudi cells and RBCs sensitized with antiglycophorin monoclonal antibodies did not correlate with the level of sensitization. However, the extent of rosette formation did correlate with the proximity of the epitopes to the RBC membrane. Those monoclonal antibodies recognizing epitopes close to the membrane surface were poor at rosette formation, whereas those recognizing epitopes further away were better. Binding of monoclonal antiplatelet antibodies to platelet FcRII receptors have similarly been shown to be independent of the level of binding but critically dependent upon the target molecule (173). There is no known correlation between the specificity of antiplatelet autoantibodies and severity of thrombocytopenia. Neonatal thrombocytopenia occurs most frequently with alloantibodies against the PLA^1 antigen located on glycoprotein IIIa (GPIIIa). GPIIIa is the most abundant platelet glycoprotein. However, $Br^{a/b}$, another frequently found alloantigen system causing neonatal thrombocytopenia, is found on the low-abundance GPIa glycoprotein (174). Thus, it appears that factors other than antigen abundance play a role in platelet destruction.

D. Activity of the RES

In the past, efforts to understand the destruction of cells by the RES have centered on factors such as amount and type of antibody, its subclass, specificity, and so forth. In recent years, it has become apparent that the state of activity of the RES is equally important. Clearance studies of sensitized RBCs have shown that there is a considerable interindividual variation in monocyte and macrophage activities. The variation is considerable among normal, healthy individuals and there is even larger variation among patients. In these individuals, there is often an imbalance of the cytokines and inflammatory mediators that control the level and activity of the receptors important in cell destruction. Alterations in the RES can either enhance or impair cell destruction.

E. Enhanced RES Function

Cytokines and several other biological mediators are important in the upregulation and modulation of RES receptors. Interferon gamma enhances macrophage phagocytic activity and antibody-dependent cell cytotoxicity (63,64,175). This cytokine increases the expression of macrophage FcγRI both in vitro and in vivo (62,63,176). In addition, INF-γ results in increased activation of FcγII without increasing the number of receptors (92). Similarly, interleukin-6 has been shown to enhance FcγRI-mediated ADCC without increasing receptor number (177). The biological activity of FcγRII can be enhanced by proteolytic enzymes through a mechanism that increases the receptor affinity without increasing its expression (74). Increased biological activity of the CR1 receptor occurs through the action of T-cell cytokines and through chemotactic agents (29). Chemotactic agents have also been shown to upregulate the expression of CR3 receptors (48).

The effect of cytokines and other biological mediators suggests that the activity of the RES could be dramatically increased in certain pathological states or under certain stimulatory condition. Release of interferons and other cytokines occurring with viral or bacterial infections could trigger some episodes of autoimmune cell destruction. For instance, acute autoimmune thrombocytopenia in children is thought to involve a viral initiation event (178). The disorder can also be induced by immunization with live vaccine (178,179). Autoimmune hemolytic anemia also has been observed following vaccination (113,180).

Studies of RE function using in vitro assays to monitor monocyte-RBC interactions have shown that there is increased reactivity in patients with autoimmune hemolytic anemia (181,182). Whether these increases are a result or a cause of the condition is unknown; it could be that a preexisting activation results in an autocatalytic effect whereby the RES is further activated.

F. Impaired RES Function

In general, defective IgG-mediated clearance is seen in disease states associated with circulating immune complexes. Perhaps the best studied of these diseases is systemic lupus erythematosus (SLE) in which a profound defect in Fc receptor–specific clearance occurs (182,184). Frank and colleagues found that patients with SLE have an impaired clearance of IgG-sensitized autologous RBCs and clearance rates were correlated with the level of disease activity (183). Aggregated human serum albumin clearance in these patients was normal and indicated that the macrophage defect was Fc receptor specific. The defective Fc receptor function impairs the clearance of immune complexes that may contribute to the disease pathogenesis. Similar findings have been found in other autoimmune diseases, including mixed connective tissue disease (185) and Sjögren's syndrome (186). In these patient groups, there were less dramatic correlations between RES function and immune complex levels. Therefore, RE blockade by immune complexes does not appear to be absolute and other factors such as the nature of the complex may be important in determining the extent of the blockage.

Studies of Fc receptor function in patients with rheumatoid arthritis have shown only minimal clearance defects (12,187). However, the liver-spleen uptake ratio of IgG-sensitized cells in patients with rheumatoid arthritis was increased (12,188). These results suggest that Fc receptors on Kupffer cells are less efficient at removing IgG-coated RBCs than splenic macrophages. These results are in keeping with the general understanding of the spleen being the major organ for sequestration and removal of IgG-sensitized cells. On the other hand, the liver is the major organ for sequestration of IgM-sensitized cells. The IgM-sensitized cells activate complement and the cells bind to the Kupffer cell complement receptors with subsequent further enzymatic cleavage to C3d and release of the cells back into the circulation (189).

One group of investigators studied the relationships among platelet-associated IgG, platelet life span, and RE cell function (100). These studies indicated that some patients with elevated levels of platelet-bound IgG had a normal platelet survival. This finding was explained on the basis of an impairment of the RES. Therefore, unless normal RE function is evaluated, it is not appropriate to conclude that elevated platelet-associated IgG is a nonspecific finding in a nonthrombocytopenic patient or a patient whose platelet life span is normal.

In addition to the blockading effect of immune complexes, plasma IgG levels would be expected to influence RES function (191). Results of several studies confirm this expectation. Patients with hypergammaglobulinemia have been shown to have delayed Fc-specific immune clearance, whereas patients with hypogammaglobulinemia have enhanced clearance (192). In one study, the rapid clearance seen in a patient with hypogammaglobulinemia returned to normal after treatment with gamma globulin. Similarly, other investigators have shown a delayed clearance of anti-Rh–sensitized autologous RBCs in immune thrombocytopenic patients treated with intravenous gamma globulin (IV IgG) (193,194). The delayed clearances were accompanied by concomitant rises in the platelet count that was mediated by a blockade of the RES. However, further studies showed that monocytes from patients receiving IV IgG had decreased affinity for IgG without decreased receptor numbers, which persisted after removal of the IV IgG (195). Thus, the effect of IV immunoglobulin may modify macrophage function through alternate or additional mechanisms to Fc receptor blockade.

IgG anti-D has been used to treat immune thrombocytopenia, and the effect is believed to result from a reversible blockade of macrophage Fc receptors (196,197). It has also been hypothesized that the effect of IV IgG and anti-D may be mediated by the presence of anti-HLA antibodies in the preparations (198). These antibodies have been shown to specifically inhibit immune phagocytosis by an Fc-dependent mechanism (198,199).

The role played by Fc receptor–mediated functions in the abnormalities associated with diabetes mellitus have been reviewed (200). Impaired mononuclear phagocytic function in diabetics appears to be multifactorial. Modulation of FcR expression by insulin results in decreased antibody-dependent cytotoxicity (201). In addition, there are effects on Fc receptor number and on increased catecholamine levels that in turn are associated with depressed phagocytosis (200,202).

Depressed RES function has been observed in patients receiving methyldopa (203). Many patients receiving this drug develop a positive direct antiglobulin test, yet few of these develop hemolytic anemia. In the nonhemolyzing population, a delayed clearance of anti-Rh–sensitized autologous RBCs has been reported and this was postulated to result from drug-induced impairment of the RES. Also, corticosteroids have been shown to modify the clearance of IgG-coated cells and change the expression of Fc receptors (204). The exact mode of action of the drugs in modulating macrophage function is unknown and likely is multifactorial. Corticosteroids, for instance, have been shown to inhibit antibody-dependent cellular cytotoxicity and phagocytosis and to inhibit monocyte chemotaxis and migration (205,206).

Danazol is an attenuated androgen that has been used successfully in the treatment of both immune thrombocytopenia and autoimmune hemolytic anemia (207,208). Monocytes from thrombocytopenic patients receiving danazol have significantly decreased numbers of IgG-binding sites. Hence, the effect of danazol resembles corticosteroids in this regard (209).

The use of anti–Fc receptor–specific monoclonal antibodies would be expected to be an efficient way of blocking or downregulating macrophage Fc receptor function. Recently, Clarkson and associates have used this strategy in the treatment of refractory immune thrombocytopenia purpura (96). They found that infusion of an anti-FcγRIII monoclonal antibody caused a dramatic, but transient, rise in the platelet count in one patient. Further studies are necessary to determine the exact mechanism of this treatment to exclude effects by contaminating aggregates or formation of opsonized neutrophils that might block Fc receptors. Studies with Fab or F(ab')$_2$ fragments are warranted.

Certain autoimmune diseases in which there is impaired mononuclear phagocytic clearance are associated with a HLA-B8/DRw3 haplotype. Delayed Fc-mediated clearance has also been shown in normal volunteers with HLA-B8/DRw3 haplotype (210). However, no defect in Fcγ receptor expression was found in such individuals based either on receptor numbers or affinity (211). Impaired RES clearance has also been shown with normal individuals who have HLA-DR2 and MT-1 haplotypes (212).

REFERENCES

1. Aschoff L. Das reticulo-endotheliale system. Ergeb inn Med Kinderheilk 1924; 26:1–119.
2. van Furth R, Cohn ZA, Hirsh JG, et al. The mononuclear phagocyte system: A new classification of macrophages, monocytes, and their precursor cells. Bull WHO 1972; 46:845–852.
3. Groom AC, Schmidt EE. Microcirculatory blood flow through the spleen. In: Bowder AJ, ed. The Spleen: Structure, Function and Clinical Significance. London: Chapman and Hall, 1990:45–102.
4. McCusky RS, McCusky PA. In vivo and electron microscopic studies of the spleen microvasculature in mice. Experientia 1985; 41:179–187.
5. Weiss L. The structure of the intermediate vascular pathways in the spleen of rabbits. Am J Anat 1963; 113:51–91.

6. Weiss L, Geduldig U, Weidanz WP. Mechanisms of splenic control of malaria: Reticular cell activation and the development of a blood-spleen barrier. Am J Anat 1986; 176:251–285.

7. Millward-Sadler GH, Jezequel AM. Normal histology and ultrastructure. In: Wright R, Millward-Sadler GH, Alberti KGMM and Martan S, eds. Liver and Biliary Disease. London: Bailliere Tindall, 1985: 13–44.

8. Rappaport AM. The structure and functional unit in the human liver (liver acinus). Anat Rec 1958; 130:673–686.

9. Wake N. Perisinusoidal stellate cells (fat-storing cells, interstitial cells, lipocytes), their related structure in and around the liver sinusoids, and vitamin A–storing cells in extrahepatic organs. Int Rev Cytol 1980; 66:303–353.

10. Wake K, Decker M, Kirn A, et al. Cell biology and kinetics of Kupffer cells in the liver. Int Rev Cytol 1989; 118:173–229.

11. Lobatto S, Daha MR, Voetman AA, et al. Clearance of soluble aggregates of human immunoglobulin G in healthy volunteers and chimpanzees. Clin Exp Immunol 1987; 69:133–141.

12. Lobatto S, Breedveld, Camps JAJ, et al. Mononuclear phagocyte system Fc-receptor function in patients with seropositive rheumatoid arthritis. Clin Exp Immunol 1987; 67:461–466.

13. Moghimi SM, Patel HM. Calcium as a possible modulator of Kupffer cell phagocytic function by regulating liver-specific opsonic activity. Biochim Biophys Acta 1990; 1028:304–308.

14. Simon M, Djawari D, Hohenberger W. Impairment of polymorphonuclear leukocyte and macrophage function in splenectomized patients. N Engl J Med 1985; 313:1092.

15. Billiar TR, West MA, Hyland BJ, Simmons RL. Splenectomy alters Kupffer cell response to endotoxin. Arch Surg 1988; 123:327–332.

16. Metchnikoff ME. Sur la lutte des cellules de l'organisme contre l'invasion des microbes. Ann Inst Pasteur 1887; 1:321–336.

17. Bouwens L, Baekeland M, Wisse E. Importance of local proliferation in the expanding Kupffer cell population of rat liver after zymosan stimulation and partial hepatectomy. Hepatology 1984; 4:213–219.

18. Fearon DT. Identification of the membrane glycoprotein that is the C3b receptor of the human erythrocyte, polymorphonuclear leukocyte, B lymphocyte and monocyte. J Exp Med 1980; 152:20–30.

19. Fischer E, Capron M, Prin L, et al. Human eosinophils express CR1 and CR3 complement receptors for cleavage fragments of C3. Cell Immunol 1986; 97:297–306.

20. Wilson JG, Tedder TF, Fearon DT. Characterization of human T lymphocytes that express the C3b receptor. J Immunol 1983; 131:684–689.

21. Klickstein LB, Wong WW, Smith JA, et al. Human C3b/C4b receptor (CR1): Demonstration of long homologous repeating domains that are composed of the short consensus repeats characteristic of C3/C4 binding proteins. J Exp Med 1987; 165:1095–1112.

22. Klickstein LB, Bartow TJ, Miletic V, et al. Identification of distinct C3b and C4b recognition sites in the human C3b/C4b receptor (CR1,CD35) by deletion mutagenesis. J Exp Med 1988; 168:1699–1717.

23. Holers VM, Cole JL, Lublin DM, et al. Human C3b and C4b regulatory proteins: A new multigene family. Immunol Today 1985; 6:188–192.

24. Weis JH, Morton CC, Bruns GA, et al. A complement receptor locus: Genes encoding C3b/C4b receptor and C3d/Epstein-Barr virus receptor map to 1q32. J Immunol 1987; 138:312–315.

25. Lublin DM, Griffith RC, Atkinson JP. Influence of glycosolation on allelic and cell specific Mr variation, receptor processing and ligand binding in the human complement C3b/C4b receptor. J Biol Chem 1986; 261:5736–5744.

26. Wong WW. Structural and functional correlation of the human complement receptor type 1. J Invest Dermatol 1990; 6:64S–67S.

27. Cornacoff JB, Herbert LA, Smead WL, et al. Primate erythrocyte-immune complex-clearing mechanism. J Clin Invest 1983; 71:236–247.

28. Pommier CG, Inada S, Fries LF, et al. Plasma fibronectin enhances phagocytosis of opsonized particles by human peripheral blood monocytes. J Exp Med 1983; 157:1844–1854.

29. Griffin JA, Griffin FM. Augmentation of macrophage complement receptor function in vitro. I.

Characterization of the cellular interactions required for the generation of a T lymphocyte product that enhances macrophage complement receptor function. J Exp Med 1979; 150:653–675.

30. Wright SD, Craigmyle LS, Silverstein SC. Fibronectin and serum amyloid P component stimulate C3b- and C3bi-mediated phagocytosis in cultured human monocytes. J Exp Med 1983; 158:1338–1343.

31. Changelian PS, Jack RM, Collins LA, Fearon DT. PMA induces the ligand-independent interalization of CR1 on human neutrophils. J Immunol 1985; 134:1851–1858.

32. Jack RM, Fearon DT. Altered surface distribution of both C3b receptors and Fc receptors on neutrophils induced by anti-C3b receptor or aggregated IgG. J Immunol 1984; 132:3028–3033.

33. Jack RM, Ezzel RM, Hartwiz J, Fearon DT. Differential interaction of the C3b/C4b receptor and MHC class 1 with the cytoskeleton of human neutrophils. J Immunol 1986; 137:3996–4003.

34. Lutz H, Bussolino F, Flepp R, et al. Naturally occurring anti-band 3 antibodies and complement together mediate phagocytosis of oxidatively-stressed human red blood cells. Proc Natl Acad Sci USA 1987; 84:7368–7372.

35. Wright SD, Rao PE, van Voorhis WC, et al. Identification of the C3bi receptor of human monocytes and macrophages by using monoclonal antibodies. Proc Natl Acad Sci USA 1983; 80:5699–5703.

36. Hynes RO. Integrins: A family of cell surface receptors. Cell 1987; 48:681–690.

37. Corbi AL, Kishimoto TK, Miller LJ, Springer TA. The human leukocyte adhesion glycoprotein Mac-1 (complement receptor type 3 CDIIb) alpha subunit: Cloning, primary structure and relation to the integrins, von Willebrand factor and factor B. J Biol Chem 1988; 263:12403–12411.

38. Pytela R. Amino acid sequence of the murine Mac-1 α chain reveals homology with the integrin family and an additional domain related to von Willebrand factor. EMBO J 1988; 7:1371–1378.

39. Law SKA, Gagnon J, Hildreth JEK, et al. The primary structure of the β-subunit of the cell surface adhesion glycoproteins LFA-1, CR3 and p150,95 and its relationship to the fibronectin receptor. EMBO J 1987; 6:915–919.

40. Graham IL, Brown EJ. Extracellular calcium results in a conformational change in Mac-1 (CD11b/CD18) on neutrophils. J Immunol 1991; 146:685–691.

41. Larson RS, Corki AL, Berman L, Springer TA. Primary structure of the LFA-1 alpha subunit: An integrin with an embedded domain defining a protein superfamily. J Cell Biol 1989; 108:703–712.

42. Rothlein R, Springer TA. Complement receptor type three-dependent degradation of opsonized erythrocytes by mouse macrophages. J Immunol 1985; 135:2668–2672.

43. Ramos OF, Kai C, Yefenof E, Klein E. The elevated natural killer sensitivity of targets carrying surface-attached C3 fragments require the availability of the iC3b receptor (CR3) on the effectors. J Immunol 1988; 140:1239–1243.

44. Anderson DC, Miller LJ, Schmalstieg FC, et al. Contributions of the Mac-1 glycoprotein family to adherence-dependent granulocyte functions: Structure-function assessments employing subunit-specific monoclonal antibodies. J Immunol 1986; 137:15–27.

45. Ruoslahti E, Pierschbacher MD. New perspectives in cell adhesion. RGD and integrins. Science 1987; 238:491–497.

46. Wright SD, Witz JI, Huang AJ, et al. Complement receptor type three (CD11b/CD18) of human polymorphonuclear leukocytes recognizes fibrinogen. Proc Natl Acad Sci USA 1988; 85:7734–7738.

47. Kloczewiak M, Timmons S, Lukas TJ, Hawiger J. Platelet receptors recognition site on human fibrinogen: Synthesis and structure-function relationship of peptides corresponding to the carboxy-terminal segment of the gamma chain. Biochemistry 1984; 23:1767–1774.

48. Miller LJ, Bainton DF, Borregaard N, Springer TA. Stimulated mobilization of monocyte Mac-1 and p150,95 adhesion proteins from an intracellular vesicular compartment to the cell surface. J Clin Invest 1987; 80:535–544.

49. Wright SD, Meyer BC. Phorbol esters cause sequential activation and deactivation of complement receptors on polymorphonuclear leukocytes. J Immunol 1986; 136:1759–1764.

50. Graham IL, Gresham HD, Brown EJ. An immobile subset of plasma membrane CD11a/CD18 (Mac-1) is involved in phagocytosis of targets recognized by multiple receptors. J Immunol 1989; 142:2352–2358.

51. Brown EJ, Bohnsack JF, Gresham HD. Mechanism of inhibition of immunoglobulin G-mediated phagocytosis by monoclonal antibodies that recognize the Mac-1 antigen. J Clin Invest 1988; 81:365–375.

52. Newman SL, Mikus LK, Tucci MA. Differential requirements for cellular cytoskeleton in human macrophage complement receptor- and Fc receptor-mediated phagocytosis. J Immunol 1991; 146:967–974.

53. van de Winkel JGJ, Anderson CL. Biology of human immunoglobulin G Fc receptors. J Leukocyte Biol 1991; 49:511–524.

54. Unkless JC. Function and heterogeneity of human Fc receptors for IgG. J Clin Invest 1989; 83:355–361.

55. Fanger MW, Shen L, Graziano RF, Guyre PM. Cytotoxicity mediated by human Fc receptors for IgG. Immunol Today 1989; 10:92–99.

56. Qiu WQ, de Bruin D, Brownstein BH, Pearse R, Ravetch JV. Organization of the human and mouse low-affinity FcγR genes: Duplication and recombination. Science 1990; 248:732–735.

57. Williams AF, Barclay AN. The immunoglobulin superfamily—Domains for cell surface recognition. Ann Rev Immunol 1988; 6:381–405.

58. Anderson CL, Abraham N. Characterization of the Fc receptor for IgG on a human macrophage cell line, U937. J Immunol 1980; 125:2735–2741.

59. Duncan AR, Woof JM, Partridge LJ, et al. Localization of the binding site for the human high-affinity Fc receptor on IgG. Nature 1988; 332:563–564.

60. Kurlander RJ, Batker J. The binding of human immunoglobulin G1 monomer and small, covalently cross-linked polymers of immunoglobulin G1 to human peripheral blood monocytes and polymorphonuclear leukocytes. J Clin Invest 1982; 69:1–8.

61. Allen JM, Seed B. Isolation and expression of functional high-affinity Fc receptor cDNAs. Science 1989; 243:378–380.

62. Perussia B, Dayton ET, Lazarus R, et al. Immune interferon induces the receptor for monomeric IgG1 on human monocytic and myeloid cells. J Exp Med 1983; 158:1092–1113.

63. Guyre PM, Morganelli, Miller R. Recombinant immune interferon increases immunoglobulin G Fc receptors on cultured human mononuclear phagocytes. J Clin Invest 1983; 72:393–397.

64. Shen L, Guyre PM, Fanger MW. Polymorphonuclear leukocyte function triggered through the high affinity Fc receptor for monomeric IgG. J Immunol 1987; 139:534–538.

65. Anderson CL, Shen L, Eicher DM, et al. Phagocytosis mediated by three distinct Fcγ receptor classes on human leukocytes. J Exp Med 1990; 171:1333–1345.

66. Ravetch JV, Anderson CL. In: Metzger H, ed. Fc Receptors and the Action of Antibodies. American Society of Microbiology, Washington, DC: 1990:211–235.

67. Liesveld JL, Abboud CN, Looney RJ, et al. Expression of IgG Fc receptors in myeloid leukemic cell lines. J Immunol 1988; 140:1527–1533.

68. Karas SP, Rosse WF, Kurlander RJ. Characterization of the IgG-Fc receptor on human platelets. Blood 1982; 60:1277–1282.

69. Rosenfeld SI, Anderson CL. Fc receptors of human platelets. In: George JN, ed. Platelet Immunology, Philadelphia; JB Lippincott, 1989:337–353.

70. Warmerdam PAM, van der Winkel JGJ, Vlug A, et al. A single amino acid in the second Ig-like domain of the human Fcγ receptor II plays a critical role in human IgG2 binding. J Immunol 1991; 147:1338–1343.

71. Tax WJ, Williams HW, Reekers PP, et al. Polymorphism in mitogenic effect of IgG1 monoclonal antibodies against T3 antigen on human T cells. Nature 1983; 304:445–447.

72. Brooks DG, Qiu WQ, Luster A-D, Ravetch JV. Structure and expression of human IgG FcRII (CD32): Functional heterogeneity is encoded by the alternatively spliced products of multiple genes. J Exp Med 1989; 170:1369–1386.

73. Willis HE, Browder B, Feister AJ, et al. Monoclonal antibody to human IgG Fc receptors. Cross-linking of receptors induces lysosomal enzyme release and superoxide generation by neutrophils. J Immunol 1988; 140:234–239.

74. van der Winkel JGJ, van Ommen R, Huizinga TWJ, et al. Proteolysis induces increased binding affinity of the monocyte type II FcR for human IgG. J Immunol 1989; 143:571–578.

75. Fleit HB, Wright SD, Unkeless JC. Human neutrophil Fc-γ receptor distribution and structure. Proc Natl Acad Sci USA 1982; 79:3275–3279.

76. Klaassen RJL, Ouwehand WH, Huizinga TWJ, et al. The Fc-receptor III of cultured human monocytes. J Immunol 1990; 144:599–606.

77. Passlick B, Flieger D, Ziegler-Heitbrock HWL. Identification of and characterization of a novel monocyte subpopulation in human peripheral blood. Blood 1989; 74:2527–2534.
78. Simmons D, Seed B. The Fcγ receptor of natural killer cells is a phospholipid-linked membrane protein. Nature 1988; 323:568.
79. Hunzinga TWJ, Kent M, Nuijens JH, et al. Binding characteristics of dimeric IgG subclass complexes to human neutrophils. J Immunol 1989; 142:2359–2364.
80. Ravetch JV, Perussia B. Alternative membrane forms of FcγRIII (CD16) on human NK cells and neutrophils: Cell-type specific expression of two genes which differ in single nucleotide substitutions. J Exp Med 1989; 170:481–497.
81. Selvaraj P, Rosse WF, Silker R, and Springer TA. The major Fc receptor in blood has a phosphatidylinositol anchor and is deficient in paroxysmal nocturnal haemoglobinuria. Nature 1988; 333:565–567.
82. Hunzinga TWJ, van der Schoot CE, Jost C, et al. The P1-linked receptor FcRIII is released on stimulation of neutrophils. Nature 1988; 333:667–669.
83. Lanier LL, Cwirla S, Yu G, et al. Membrane anchoring of a human IgG Fc receptor (CD16) determined by a single amino acid. Science 1989; 246:1611–1613.
84. Scallon BJ, Scigliano E, Freedman VH, et al. A human immunoglobulin G receptor exists in both polypeptide-anchored and phosphatidylinositol-glycan-anchored forms. Proc Natl Acad Sci USA 1989; 86:5079–5083.
85. Hibbs ML, Selvaraj P, Carper O, et al. Mechanisms for regulating expression of membrane isoforms of FcγRIII (CD16). Science 1989; 246:1608–1611.
86. Lanier LL, Yu G, Phillips JH. Co-association of CD3ζ with a receptor (CD16) for IgG Fc on human natural killer cells. Nature 1989; 342:803–805.
87. Ory PA, Clark MR, Kwoh EE, et al. Sequences of complementary DNAs that encode the NA1 and NA2 forms of Fc receptor III on human neutrophils. J Clin Invest 1989; 84:1688–1691.
88. Huizinga TWJ, Kleijer M, Roos D, von dem Borne AEGKr. Differences between FcRIII of human neutrophils and human K/NK lymphocytes in relation to the NA antigen system. In: Knapp W et al, eds. Leukocyte Typing IV. New York: Oxford University Press, 1989, p582.
89. Tetteroo PAT, van der Schoot CE, Visser FJ, et al. Three different types of Fcγ receptors on human leukocytes defined by workshop antibodies: FcγR low of neutrophils, FcγR low of K/NK lymphocytes and FcγRII. In: McMichael AJ et al, eds. Leukocyte Typing III. New York: Oxford University Press, 1987:702–706.
90. Clarkson SB, Ory PA, CD16 developmentally regulated IgG Fc receptors on cultured human monocytes. J Exp Med 1988; 167:408–417.
91. Salmon JE, Kapur S, Kimberly. Opsonin-independent ligation of Fc gamma receptors. The 3G8-bearing receptors on neutrophils mediate the phagocytosis of conconavalin A-treated erythrocytes and nonopsonized Escherichia coli. J Exp Med 1987; 166:1798–1813.
92. Fanger MW, Shen L, Graziano RF, Guyre PM, cytotoxicity mediated by human Fc receptors for IgG. Immunol Today 1989; 10:92–99.
93. Koolwijk P, van der Winkel JGJ, Pfefferkorn LC, et al. Induction of intracellular Ca^{2+} mobilization and cytotoxicity by hybrid mouse monoclonal antibodies. J Immunol 1991; 147:595–602.
94. Ceuppens JL, Baroja ML, van Vaeck F, Anderson CL. A defect in the membrane expression of high affinity 72 kD Fc receptors on phagocytic cells in four healthy subjects. J Clin Invest 1988; 82:571–578.
95. Huizinga TWJ, Kuijpers RWAM, Kleijer M, et al. Maternal genomic neutrophil FcRIII deficiency leading to neonatal isoimmune neutropenia. Blood 1990; 76:1927–1932.
96. Clarkson SB, Bussel JB, Kimberly RP, et al. Treatment of refractory immune thrombocytopenic purpura with an anti-Fcγ receptor antibody. N Engl J Med 1986; 314:1236–1239.
97. Newman SL, Tucci MA. Regulation of human monocyte/macrophage function by extracellular matrix. J Clin Invest 1990; 86:703–714.
98. Brown EJ. The role of extracellular matrix proteins in the control of phagocytosis. J Leuk Biol 1986; 39:579–591.
99. Tenner AJ, Robinson SL, Borchelt J, Wright JR. Human pulmonary surfactant protein (SP-A), a protein structurally homologous to C1q, can enhance FcR- and CR1-mediated phagocytosis. J Biol Chem 1989; 264:13923–13928.

100. Kuhlman M, Joiner M, Ezekowitz RAB. The human mannose-binding protein functions as an opsonin. J Exp Med 1989; 169:1733–1745.
101. Bussulino F, Fischer E, Furrini F, et al. Platelet-activating factor enhances complement-dependent phagocytosis of diamide-treated erythrocytes by human monocytes through activation of protein kinase C and phsophorylation of complement receptor type one (CR1). J Biol Chem 1989; 264:21711–21719.
102. Brown EJ, Goodwin JL. Fibronectin receptors of phagocytes. Characterization of the Arg-Gly-Asp binding proteins of human monocytes and polymorphonuclear leukocytes. J Exp Med 1988; 167:777–793.
103. Wright SD, Meyer BC. Fibronectin receptor of human macrophages recognizes the sequence Arg-Gly-Asp-Ser. J Exp Med 1985; 162:762–767.
104. Bohnsack JF, O'Shea JJ, Takahashi T, Brown EJ. Fibronectin-enhanced phagocytosis of an alternative pathway activator by human culture-derived macrophages is mediated by the C4b/C3b complement receptor (CR1). J Immunol 1985; 135:2680–2686.
105. Wright SD, Licht MR, Craigmyle LS, Silverstein SC. Communication between receptors for different ligands on a single cell: Ligation of fibronectin receptors induces a reversible alteration in the function of complement receptors on cultured human monocytes. J Cell Biol 1984; 99:336–339.
106. Vlassara H, Valinsky J, Brownlee M, et al. Advanced glycosylation endproducts on erythrocyte cell surface induce receptor-mediated phagocytosis by macrophages. J Exp Med 1987; 166:539–549.
107. Duvall E, Wyllie AH, Morris RG. Macrophage recognition of cells undergoing programmed cell death (apoptosis). Immunology 1985; 56:351–358.
108. Savill JS, Henson PM, Haslett C. Phagocytosis of aged human neutrophils by macrophages is mediated by a novel "charge-sensitive" recognition mechanism. J Clin Invest 1989; 84:1518–1527.
109. Wright SD, Tobias PS, Ulevitch RJ, Ramos RA. Lipopolysaccharide (LPS) binding protein opsonizes LPS-bearing particles for recognition by a novel receptor on macrophages. J Exp Med 1989; 170:1231–1241.
110. Bigler RD, Khoo J, Lund-Katz S, et al. Identification of low density lipoprotein as a regulator of Fc receptor-mediated phagocytosis. Proc Natl Acad Sci USA 1990; 87:4981–4985.
111. Jeje MO, Blajchman MA, Steeves K, et al. Quantitation of red cell-associated IgG using an immunoradiometric assay. Transfusion 1984; 24:473–476.
112. Merry AH, Thomsen EE, Rawlinson VI, Stratton F. A quantitative antiglobulin test for IgG for use in blood transfusion serology. Clin Lab Haematol 1982; 4:393–402.
113. Petz LD, Garratty G. Acquired Immune Hemolytic Anemias. Churchill New York: Livingstone, 1980.
114. Sinha RK, Kelton JG. Current controversies concerning the measurement of platelet-associated IgG. Trans Med Rev 1990; IV121–135.
115. Gottschall JL, Collins J, Kunicki TJ, et al. Effect of hemolysis or apparent values of platelet-associated IgG. Am J Clin Pathol 1987; 87:218–222.
116. Lynch DM, Lynch JM, Howe SE. A quantitative ELISA procedure for the measurement of membrane-bound platelet-associated IgG (PAIgG). Am J Clin Pathol 1985; 83:331–336.
117. Rosenfield RE, Jagathambal K. Antigenic determinants of C3 and C4 complement components on washed erythrocytes from normal persons. Transfusion 1978; 18:517–523.
118. Chaplin H, Nasongkla M, Monroe MC. Quantitation of red blood cell-bound C3d in normal subjects and hospitalized patients. Br J Haematol 1981; 48:69–78.
119. Merry AH, Thomben EE, Rawlinson VI, Stratton F. The quantification of C3 fragments on erythrocytes: Estimation of C3 fragments on normal cells, acquired hemolytic anemia cases and correlation with agglutination of sensitized cells. Clin Lab Haematol 1983; 5:387–397.
120. Szymanski IO, Odgren PR, Valeri CR. Relationship between the third component of human complement (C3) bound to stored preserved erythrocytes and their viability in vivo. Vox Sang 1985; 49:34–41.
121. Garratty G. Effect of cell-bound proteins on the in vivo survival of circulating blood cells. Gerentology 1991; 37:68–94.
122. Cines DB, Wilson SB, Tomaski A, Schreiber AD. Platelet antibodies of the IgM class in immune thrombocytopenic purpura. J Clin Invest 1985; 75:1183–1190.

123. Winiarski J, Holm G. Platelet-associated immunoglobulins and complement in idiopathic thrombocytopenic purpura. Clin Exp Immunol 1983; 53:201–207.
124. Nel JO, Stevens K, Mouton A, Pretorius FJ. Platelet-bound IgM in autoimmune thrombocytopenia. Blood 1983; 61:119–124.
125. Fanger MW, Pugh J, Bernier G. The specificity of receptors for IgA on human peripheral polymorphonuclear cells and monocytes. Immunology 1981; 60:324–334.
126. Gauldie J, Richards C, Lamontagne L. Fc receptors for IgA and other immunoglobulins on resident and activated alveolar macrophages. Mol Immunol 1983; 20:1029–1037.
127. Worlledge SM, Blajchman MA. The autoimmune haemolytic anemias. Br J Haematol 1972; 23:61–69.
128. Issitt PD, Pavone BG, Goldfinger D. Anti-Wr[b], and other autoantibodies responsible for positive direct antiglobulin tests in 150 individuals. Br J Haematol 1976; 34:5–18.
129. Sturgeon P, Smith LE, Chun HMT, et al. Autoimmune hemolytic anemia associated exclusively with IgA of Rh specificity. Transfusion 1979; 19:324–328.
130. Clark DA, Dessypris EN, Jenkins DE, Krantz SB. Acquired immune hemolytic anemia associated with IgA erythrocyte coating: Investigation of hemolytic mechanisms. Blood 1984; 64:1000–1005.
131. Reusser P, Osterwalder B, Burri H, Speck B. Autoimmune hemolytic anemia associated with IgA-diagnostic and therapeutic aspects in a case with long-term follow-up. Acta Haematol 1987; 77:53–56.
132. Sokol RJ, Hewitt S, Booker DJ, Bailey A. Red cell autoantibodies, multiple immunoglobulin classes and autoimmune hemolysis. Transfusion 1990; 30:714–717.
133. Shen L, Fanger. Secretory IgA antibodies synergize with IgG in promoting ADCC by human polymorphonuclear cells, monocytes, and lymphocytes. Cell Immunol 1981; 59:75–81.
134. Panzer S, Niessner H, Lechner K, et al. Platelet-associated immunoglobulins IgG, IgM, IgA and complement C3c in chronic idiopathic autoimmune thrombocytopenia: Relation to the sequestration pattern of [111]Indium labelled platelets. Scand J Haematol 1986; 37:97–102.
135. Garratty G. Factors affecting the pathogenicity of red cell auto- and alloantibodies. In: Nance JJ, ed. Immune Destruction of Red Cells. Arlington, VA: American Association of Blood Banks, 1989: 109–169.
136. Dacie JV. Autoimmune hemolytic anemia. Arch Intern Med 1975; 135:1293–1300.
137. Nance S, Bourdo S, Garratty G. IgG2 red cell sensitization associated with autoimmune hemolytic anemia (abst). Transfusion 1983; 23:413.
138. Vengelen-Tyler V, Morel PA. Serologic and IgG subclass characterization of Cartwright (Yt) and Gerbich (Ge) antibodies. Transfusion 1983; 23:114–116.
139. Engelriet CP, Beckers ThAP, van't Veer MB, et al. Recent advances in immune haemolytic anemia. International Congress ISH-ISBT, Budapest (1982). In: Holland SR, ed. Recent Advances in Haematology, Immunology and Blood Transfusion. 1983:235–252.
140. Zupanska B, Thompson E, Brojer E, Merry AH. Phagocytosis of erythrocytes sensitized with known amounts of IgG1 and IgG 3 anti-Rh antibodies. Vox Sang 1987; 53:96–101.
141. Wiener E, Atwal A, Thompson KM, et al. Differences between the activities of human monoclonal IgG1 and IgG3 subclasses of anti-D(Rh) antibody in their ability to mediate red cell-binding to macrophages. Immunology 1987; 62:401–404.
142. Wiener E, Jolliffe VW, Scott HCF, et al. Differences between the activity of human monoclonal IgG1 and IgG3 anti-D antibodies of the Rh blood group system in their abilities to mediate effector functions of monocytes. Immunology 1988; 65:159–163.
143. Mollison PL, Crome P, Hugh-Jones NC, Rochna E. Rate of removal from the circulation of red cells sensitized with different amounts of antibody. Br J Haematol 1965; 11:461–470.
144. Rosse WF. Quantitative immunology of immune hemolytic anemia. II. The relationship of cell-bound antibody to hemolysis and the effect of treatment. J Clin Invest 1971; 50:734–743.
145. Chaplin H. Red cell-bound immunoglobulin as a predictor of severity of hemolysis in patients with autoimmune hemolytic anemia. Transfusion 1990; 30:576–578.
146. Issitt PD, Gutgsell NS. Clinically significant antibodies not detected by routine methods. In: Nance SJ, ed. Immune Destruction of Red Blood Cells. Arlington, VA: American Association of Blood Banks, 1989:77–108.

147. Garratty G, Nance SJ. Correlation between in vivo hemolysis and the amount of red cell-bound IgG measured by flow cytometry. Transfusion 1990; 30:617–621.

148. Engelfriet CP, Ouwehand WH. ADCC and other cellular bioassays for predicting the clinical significance of red cell alloantibodies. Bailliere Clin Haematol 1990; 3:321–337.

149. Shanfield MS, Stevens JO, Bauman D. The detection of clinicaly significant erythrocyte alloantibodies using a human mononuclear phagocyte assay. Transfusion 1981; 21:571–576.

150. Nance SJ, Arndt P, Garratty G. Predicting the clinical significance of red cell alloantibodies using a monocyte monolayer assay. Transfusion 1987; 27:449–452.

151. Hadley AG, Kumpel BM, Leader KA, et al. Correlation of serological, quantitative and cell-mediated functional assays of maternal alloantibodies with the severity of haemolytic disease of the newborn. Br J Haematol 1991; 77:221–228.

152. Engelfriet CP, von dem Borne AEG Kr, Becker D, et al. Immune destruction of red cells. Proceedings of the 34th Annual Meeting of the American Association of Blood Banks, Chicago, 1981.

153. Dixon R, Rosse W, Ebbert L. Quantitative determination of antibody in idiopathic thrombocytopenic purpura. N Engl J Med 1975; 292:230–236.

154. Karpatkin S. Autoimmune thrombocytopenic purpura. Blood 1980; 56:329–343.

155. Kelton JG, Powers PJ, Carter CJ. A prospective study of the usefulness of the measurement of platelet-associated IgG for the diagnosis of idiopathic thrombocytopenic purpura. Blood 1982; 60:1050–1053.

156. Cines DB, Schreiber AD. Immune thrombocytopenia—Use of a Coombs antiglobulin test to detect IgG and C3 on platelets. N Engl J Med 1979; 300:106–111.

157. Pegels JG, Bruynes ECE, Engelfriet CP, von dem Borne AEG. PTP: A serological and immunochemical study. Br J Haematol 1981; 49:521–530.

158. Mueller-Eckhardt C, Kayser W, Mersch-Baumert K, et al. The clinical significance of platelet associated IgG: A study on 298 patients with various disorders. Br J Haematol 1980; 46:123–131.

159. Saleh MN, Moore DL, Lee JY, LoBuglio AF. Monocyte-platelet interaction in immune and nonimmune thrombocytopenia. Blood 1989; 74:1328–1331.

160. Ehlenberger AG, Nussenzweig V. The role of membrane receptors for C3b and C3d in phagocytosis. J Exp Med 1977; 145:357–371.

161. Kurlander RJ, Rosse WF. Monocyte-mediated destruction in the presence of serum of red cells coated with antibody. Blood 1979; 54:1131–1139.

162. Fischer JT, Petz LD, Garratty G, Cooper NR. Correlations between quantitative assay of red cell-bound C3, serologic reactions and hemolytic anemia. Blood 1974; 44:359–373.

163. Freedman J, Ho M, Barefoot C. Red blood cell-bound C3d in selected hospital patients. Transfusion 1982; 22:515–520.

164. Waytes AT, Malbran A, Bobak DA, Fries LF. Pre-ligation of CR1 enhances IgG-dependent phagocytosis by cultured human monocytes. J Immunol 1991; 146:2694–2700.

165. Nel JD, Stevens K. A new method for the simultaneous quantitation of platelet-bound immunoglobulin (IgG) and complement (C3) employing an enzyme linked immunoabsorbent assay (ELISA) procedure. Br J Haematol 1980; 44:281–290.

166. von dem Borne AEGKr, Helmhorst EF, van Leewen EF, et al. Autoimmune thrombocytopenia: Detection of platelet autoantibodies with the suspension immunofluorescence test. Br J Haematol 1980; 45:319–327.

167. Hauch TW, Rosse WF. Platelet-bound complement (C3) in immune thrombocytopenia. Blood 1977; 50:1129–1136.

168. McMillan R, Martin M. Fixation of C3 to platelets in vitro by antiplatelet antibody from patients with immune thrombocytopenic purpura. Br J Haematol 1981; 47:251–256.

169. Kiefel V, Salama A, Mueller-Eckhardt C. In vitro fixation of C3d and C5b-9 on platelets by human platelet reactive antibodies. Blut 1989; 58:33–37.

170. Kelton JG, Steeves K. The amount of platelet-bound albumin parallels the amount of IgG of washed platelets from patients with immune thrombocytopenia. Blood 1983; 62:924–927.

171. Schwartz RS, Costea N. Autoimmune hemolytic anemia: Clinical correlations and biological implications. Semin Hematol 1966; 3:2–26.

172. Walker MR, Woof JM, Brüggemann M, et al. Interaction of human IgG chimeric antibodies with

the human FcRI and FcRII receptors: Requirements for antibody-mediated host cell-target cell interaction. Mol Immunol 1989; 26:403–411.

173. Horsewood P, Hayward CPM, Warkentin TE, Kelton JG. Investigation of the mechanisms of monoclonal antibody-induced platelet activation. Blood 1991; 78:1019–1026.

174. Smith JW, Kelton JG, Horsewood P, et al. Platelet specific alloantigens on the platelet glycoprotein Ia/IIa complex. Br J Haematol 1989; 72:534–553.

175. Mannel DN, Falk W. Interferon γ is required in activation of macrophages for tumor cytotoxicity. Cell Immunol 1983; 79:396–402.

176. Guyre PM, Campbell AS, Kniffin W, Fanger MW. Monocytes and polymorphonuclear neutrophils of patients with streptococcal pharyngitis express increased numbers of type I IgG Fc receptors. J Clin Invest 1990; 86:1892–1896.

177. Erbe DV, Collins JE, Shen L, et al. The effect of cytokines on the expression and function of Fc receptors for IgG on human myeloid cells. Mol Immunol 1990; 27:57–67.

178. McClure PD. Idiopathic thrombocytopenic purpura in children: Diagnosis and management. Pediatrics 1975; 55:68–74.

179. Carpentieri U, Haggard ME. Thrombocytopenia and viral diseases. Tex Med 1975; 71:81–83.

180. Rosse WF. Correlation of in vivo and in vitro measurements of hemolysis in hemolytic anemia due to immune reactions. Prog Hematol 1973; 8:51–75.

181. Kay NE, Douglas SD. Monocyte-erythrocyte interaction in vitro in immune hemolytic anemias. Blood 1977; 70:889–897.

182. Gallagher MT, Branch Dr, Mison A, Petz LD. Evaluation of reticuloendothelial function in autoimmune hemolytic anemia using an in vitro assay of monocyte-macrophage interaction with erythrocytes. Exp Hematol 1983; 11:82–89.

183. Frank MM, Hamburger MI, Lawley TJ, et al. Defective reticuloendothelial system Fc-receptor function in systemic lupus erythematosus. N Engl J Med 1979; 300:518–523.

184. Hamburger MI, Lawley TJ, Kimberly RP, et al. A serial study of splenic reticuloendothelial system Fc-receptor functional activity in systemic lupus erythematosus. Arthritis Rheum 1982; 25:48–54.

185. Hamburger MI, Moutsopoulos HM, Lawley TJ, et al. Reticuloendothelial system Fc receptor function in mixed connective tissue disease. Arthritis Rheum 1979; 22:618.

186. Hamburger MI, Moutsopoulos HM, Lawley TJ, Frank MM. Sjögren's syndrome: A defect in reticuloendothelial system Fc-receptor-specific clearance. Ann Intern Med 1979; 91:534–538.

187. Fields TR, Gerardi EN, Ghebreihiwet B, et al. Reticuloendothelial system Fc receptor function in rheumatoid arthritis. J Rheumatol 1983; 10:550–557.

188. Malaise MG, Foidart JB, Hauwaert C, et al. In vivo studies on the mononuclear phagocyte system Fc receptor function in rheumatoid arthritis. Correlations with clinical and immunological variables. J Rheumatol 1985; 12:33–42.

189. Frank MM, Schreiber AD, Atkinson JP, Jaffe CJ. Pathophysiology of immune hemolytic anemia. Ann Intern Med 1977; 87:210–222.

190. Kelton JG, Carter CJ, Rodger C, et al. The relationship among platelet-associated IgG, platelet lifespan and reticuloendothelial cell function. Blood 1984; 63:1434–1438.

191. Segal DM, Dower SK, Titus JA. The role of non-immune IgG in controlling IgG-mediated effector functions. Mol Immunol 1983; 11:1177–1189.

192. Kelton JG, Singer J, Rodger C, et al. The concentration of IgG in the serum is a major determinant of Fc-dependent reticuloendothelial function. Blood 1985; 66:490–495.

193. Fehr J, Hofmann V, Kappelar V. Transient reversal of thrombocytopenia in idiopathic thrombo-cytopenic purpura by high dose intravenous gammaglobulin. N Engl J Med 1982; 306:1254–1258.

194. Bussel JB, Kimberly RP, Inman RD. Intravenous gammaglobulin treatment of chronic idiopathic thrombocytopenic purpura. Blood 1983; 62:480–486.

195. Kimberley RP, Salmon JE, Bussel JB, et al. Modulation of mononuclear phagocyte function by intravenous gammaglobulin. J Immunol 1984; 132:745–750.

196. Salama A, Kiefel V, Amberg R, Mueller-Eckhardt C. Treatment of autoimmune thrombocytopenic purpura with Rhesus antibodies [Anti-Rh$_0$(D)]. Blut 1984; 49:29–35.

197. Salama A, Kiefel V, Mueller-Eckhardt C. Effect of IgG anti-Rh$_0$(D) in adult patients with chronic autoimmune thrombocytopenia. Am J Hematol 1986; 22:241–250.

198. Neppert J, Clemens M, Mueller-Eckhardt C. Immune phagocytosis inhibition by commercial immunoglobulins. Blut 1986; 52:67–72.

199. Neppert J, Marquard R, Mueller-Eckhardt C. Murine monoclonal antibodies and human alloantisera specific for HLA inhibit monocyte phagocytosis of anti-D-sensitized human red blood cells. Eur J Immunol 1985; 15:559–563.

200. Abrass CK. Fc receptor-mediated phagocytosis: Abnormalities associated with diabeis mellitus. Clin Immunol Immunopathol 1991; 58:1–17.

201. Bar RS, Kohn CR, Koren HS. Insulin inhibition of antibody-dependent cytotoxicity and insulin receptors in macrophages. Nature 1977; 265:632–635.

202. Rhodes J. Modulation of macrophage Fc receptor expression in vitro by insulin and cyclic nucleotides. Nature 1975; 257:597–599.

203. Kelton JG. Impaired reticuloendothelial function in patients treated with methyldopa. N Engl J Med 1985; 313:596–600.

204. Friedman D, Nettl F, Schreiber AD. Effect of estodiol and steroid analogues on the clearance of immunoglobulin G-coated erythrocytes. J Clin Invest 1985; 75:162–167.

205. Petroni KG, Shen L, Guyre PM. Modulation of human polymorphonuclear leukocyte IgG Fc receptors and Fc receptor-mediated functions by IFN-γ and glucocorticoids. J Immunol 1988; 140:3467–3472.

206. Rinehart JJ, Balcerzak SP, Sargone AL, LoBuglio AF. Effect of corticosteroids on human monocyte function. J Clin Invest 1974; 54:1337–1343.

207. Aahn YS, Harrington WJ, Simon SR, et al. Danazol for the treatment of idiopathic thrombo-cytopenic purpura. N Engl J Med 1983; 308:1396–1399.

208. Ahn YS, Harrington WJ, Mylvaganum R, et al. Danazol therapy for autoimmune hemolytic anemia. Ann Intern Med 1985; 102:298–301.

209. Schreiber AD, Chien P, Tomaski A, Cines DB. Effects of danazol in immune thrombocytopenic purpura. N Engl J Med 1987; 316:503–508.

210. Lawley TJ, Hall RP, Fauci AS, et al. Defective Fc-receptor functions associated with the HLA-B8/Drw3 haplotype. N Engl J Med 1981; 304:185–192.

211. Fries LF, Hall RP, Lawley TJ, et al. Monocyte receptors for the Fc portion of IgG studied with monomeric human IgG1: Normal in vitro expression of Fcγ receptors in HLA-B8/DRw3 subjects with defective Fcγ-mediated in vivo clearance. J Immunol 1982; 129:1041–1049.

212. Kimberley RP, Gibofsky A, Salmon JE, Fotino M. Impaired Fc mediated mononuclear phagocyte system clearance in HLA-DR2 and MT-1 positive healthy young adults. J Exp Med 1983; 157:1698–1703.

17

Cellular Immunoassays and Their Use for Predicting the Clinical Significance of Antibodies

BARBARA ŻUPAŃSKA
Institute of Hematology and Blood Transfusion
Warsaw, Poland

I. INTRODUCTION

Red blood cells (RBCs) antibodies are detected and characterized in different serological tests. Such tests, however, may not always distinguish between clinically significant and clinically benign antibodies (1,2). The reason lies in the immunological mechanism of extracellular RBC destruction by noncomplement-binding immunoglobulin G (IgG) antibodies. Such antibodies do not cause the damage to the RBCs themselves, but sensitized RBCs are phagocytosed and/or lysed in the spleen by cells of the mononuclear phagocytic system (MPS) (3–6). The in vitro cellular immunoassays aim to reflect this interaction (Fig. 1). Unfortunately, it is not possible to simulate the environment in which RBCs are destroyed in vivo. Thus, the cellular immunoassays are performed in a relatively simple way by mixing sensitized cells with peripheral blood Fc receptor (FcR)–bearing cells, usually monocytes, incubating them and assessing different stages of the interaction. The interactions are adherence as measured by the rosette assay (RA), phagocytosis (and usually also adherence) by the monocyte monolayer assay (MMA), the metabolic response of monocytes during erythrophagocytosis in the chemiluminescence test (CLT), and extracellular lysis by the antibody-dependent cellular cytotoxicity (ADCC) assay (Fig. 1).

The cellular immunoassays were developed for better evaluation of the clinical significance of antibodies. The distinction between clinically significant and clinically benign antibodies is important in patients with alloantibodies of questionable clinical significance who require blood transfusion when a compatible donor is not available and in alloimmunized women to predict the severity of hemolytic disease of the newborn (HDN). Such distinction might also be helpful in patients with suspected autoimmune hemolytic anemia (AIHA). The cellular immunoassays can also be used for investigating the in vitro mechanisms of RBC interactions with FcR-bearing cells.

This chapter presents the general characteristics and immunological basis of cellular immunoassays and the main factors that can influence their results. We show how the use of the cellular immunoassays expanded our knowledge of the in vitro interaction between RBCs sensitized with polyclonal or monoclonal antibodies and FcR-bearing cells. The practical

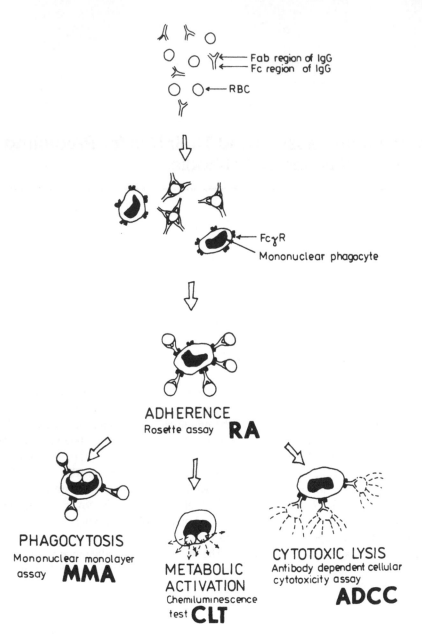

Figure 1   Interaction of sensitized RBCs with Fc receptor–bearing cells and how it is reflected in the cellular immunoassays.

application of cellular immunoassays in AIHA, in HDN, and in alloimmunized patients to be transfused will be discussed.

II.   HISTORICAL BACKGROUND

A review of the literature indicates that interest in the demonstration of cell involvement of RBC destruction is very old. Observations on the phagocytosis of RBCs by monocytes can be traced back to the end of the nineteenth and the beginning of the twentieth centuries. Ehrlich

(7) and Rowey (8) reported that peripheral blood smears of patients with hemolytic anemia contained mononuclear cells with ingested RBCs. This was followed by the report of Buchan and Conrie (9) describing the same phenomenon in HDN. The old observations were, however, forgotten for almost 60 years and not rediscovered until the 1960s.

The first application of a cellular immunoassay to study RBCs coated with alloantibodies was described by Archer in 1964 (10) and 1965 (11). He demonstrated phagocytosis of anti-A–, anti-B–, and anti-Rh–sensitized RBCs in vitro. These findings were explored in more detail by LoBuglio et al. (12) in 1967. They observed that the binding of sensitized RBCs to the monocytes was not always a prelude to erythrophagocytosis, but it nevertheless caused morphological injury to RBCs, as manifested by sphering, increased osmotic fragility, deformation, and fragmentation. They also found that this binding was inhibited by fluid-phase IgG in serum, and since then monocyte-erythrocyte interactions have usually been studied in the absence of fluid-phase IgG. Investigations of FcR-bearing cells and RBCs were facilitated during the 1970s by the introduction of density gradient centrifugation procedures for the preparation of homogeneous populations of mononuclear cells from peripheral blood (13).

Interest in the ability of different cellular immunoassays to correlate with the clinical significance of RBC antibodies began by the end of 1970s. The first clinical study on autoantibodies was carried out almost in parallel by Kay and Douglas (14) and Engelfriet's group (15) and on alloantibodies by Schanfield (16,17) using the RA and monocyte monolayer assay (MMA). Since then, several groups of investigators applied the MMA to AIHA (18–24), to HDN (25–28) and to alloimmunized patients for whom no compatible blood was readily available (29–34).

The clinical application of ADCC with lymphocytes (K cells) and monocytes was introduced by Urbaniak et al. (35,36) and Ouwehand et al. (37), respectively, at the beginning of the 1980s and followed by others (38–40). These tests were used on sera from alloimmunized pregnant women to predict the severity of HDN.

The newest cellular immunoassay, introduced by Hadley et al. (41) in 1988, is the chemiluminescence test, which has also been used to predict the severity of HDN (39).

Cellular immunoassays are useful tools for investigating the function of Fc receptors on different cells. The investigations performed at the end of 1970s and beginning of 1980s used RBCs sensitized with polyclonal anti-D antibodies as a model [42–44] and in recent years monoclonal anti-D antibodies were used (45,46). The latter have also been used in studies to evaluate their efficacy as a replacement for plasma-derived anti-D in Rh prophylaxis.

III. CHARACTERISTICS OF CELLULAR IMMUNOASSAYS

A. Rosette Assay

The RA reflects the attachment of sensitized RBCs to FcR-bearing cells. It is usually performed with peripheral blood monocytes (15,44) but other FcR-bearing cells can also be used, such as monocyte-like U937 cells (39), peripheral lymphocytes (43,44), and granulocytes (45). Apart from peripheral blood monocytes, other cells are not usually used for clinical assessment of antibodies. They are, however, use for the investigations of FcRs on effector cells.

The RA is simple in that a suspension of sensitized RBCs is mixed with a suspension of effector cells, centrifuged slowly, incubated for a short time at room temperature, and resuspended gently. The sensitized RBCs adhere to the effector cell and thereby form rosettes that can be counted using a microscope (Fig. 2). The results are expressed as the percentage of effector cells that form rosettes (usually with at least three adherent RBCs). In negative controls, no rosettes should be found.

Although the RA is easy to perform and rapid, it has some technical disadvantages—the

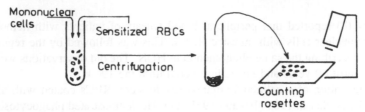

Figure 2   Schematic representation of the rosette assay.

reading is laborious and subjective and sometimes many RBCs adhere to a single monocyte and form clumps in which the number of rosettes is difficult to count (Table 1).

The RA has only rarely been used for assessing the clinical significance of antibodies, usually in patients with AIHA. This was probably due to the technical disadvantages mentioned above and to the fact that the test only reflects the adherence of RBCs to monocytes, whereas for RBC destruction, in vivo phagocytosis presumably plays the more important role.

B.   Monocyte Monolayer Assay

The MMA reflects adherence and/or phagocytosis of sensitized RBCs by peripheral blood monocytes (24,25). Cultured monocytes (46) or peritoneal macrophages (17) may also be used as effector cells.

The test is also known as the phagocytosis assay (47,48), macrophage binding assay (46), or phagocytic monolayer assay (49). However, the most often used name is the MMA (19) because the test involves making a monolayer of monocytes (by adhering mononuclear cells to plastic or glass surface) before the suspension of sensitized RBCs is added. Phagocytosis proceeds for approximately 2 hr at 37°C, and then RBCs that are not bound to monocytes are removed by washing. After fixing and staining, most workers assess the percentage of monocytes with internalized or adherent RBCs (Fig. 3). Some authors assess only phagocytosed RBCs after lysis (50) of adherent cells or without such lysis (21).

Most investigators express results as percentage of monocytes with internalized RBCs plus those with adhering cells (percentage of active monocytes, percentage of reactivity) (19,47,48). Others count the number of RBCs interacting with 100 monocytes (the total association index, the associated RBC values) (17,23) or the number of phagocytosed RBCs (the phagocytosis index) (21,29). Schanfield (22) took another approach—he counted all interacting RBCs but expressed the results as the percentage of a positive control; i.e. RBCs sensitized with anti-D serum. This approach was said to reduce the interassay coefficient of varation (CV). In negative

Table 1   Technical Advantages and Disadvantages of Cellular Immunoassays

Assay	Advantages	Disadvantages
RA	Simple, rapid	Evaluation of results: subjective, laborious, sometimes difficult
MMA	Simple, does not require isotopes nor special equipment, slides can be preserved and later evaluated	Evaluation of results: subjective, laborious, high interassay coefficient of variations
CLT	Simple, rapid semiquantitative, objective, does not require laborious counting of results	Less sensitive than MMA, requires lumino-meter
ADCC	Objective, quantitative, does not require laborious counting of results	Requires isotopes

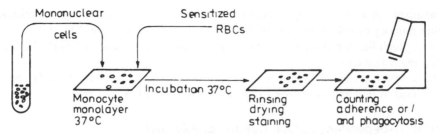

Figure 3 Schematic representation of the monocyte monolayer assay.

controls, i.e., with nonsensitized RBCs, phagocytosis and adherence should not be observed, a result above 3% reactivity is usually regarded as positive.

The MMA is performed by many laboratories because it is a simple test that does not require radioisotopes (like the ADCC) nor special equipment (like the CLT). Another advantage of the test is that the results can be preserved for later evaluation or comparison. On the other hand, the MMA is more labor intensive, and the interassay CV is high, with subjectivity involved in recording adherence and phagocytosis of RBCs (see Table 1).

The MMA has been the most commonly applied in vitro test for the assessment of clinical significance of antibodies. It has been used in patients with alloantibodies for whom compatible blood was difficult to obtain (17,31–33), for prediction of the severity of HDN in babies of alloimmunized women (16,25–28,40), and in patients with AIHA (19–24).

C. Chemiluminescence Test

The monocyte response to antibody-coated RBCs can be assessed by luminol-enhanced chemiluminescence (41,51). This approach also is used to measure monocyte responses to sensitized granulocytes and platelets (52). During erythrophagocytosis and following activation of the respiratory burst, monocytes produce oxygen radicals, which react with a substance called luminol. The product of this chemical reaction is a generation of light that is measured every 5 min for a total of 1 h at 37C in a luminometer (Fig. 4). The results are compared with the chemiluminescence generated by monocytes incubated with nonsensitized RBCs. Thus, the opsonic activity of test sera may be expressed as a ratio or opsonic index. The opsonic index of normal sera should be 1.0 ± 0.1 (mean ± 1 SD). To reduce interassay variation, opsonic indices may be expressed as a percentage of a positive control (RBCs sensitized with human monoclonal IgG1 anti-D or appropriate dilution of polyclonal anti-D antibodies).

The CLT provides a simple, rapid and semiquantitative means of assessing monocyte response to sensitized RBCs. The advantage of this method compared with the MMA is that it is faster, objective, and does not require laborious counting of cells under the microscope. The disadvantage is that it is not as sensitive as the MMA and requires a luminometer that might

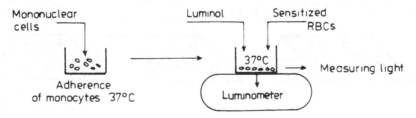

Figure 4 Schematic representation of the chemiluminescence test.

not be available in every routine laboratory (see Table 1). Test sensitivity is optimized by incubating monocytes before addition of RBCs in IgG-free medium for 2 hr at 37°C to allow release of cytophilic, serum-derived IgG to give maximum vacancy of FcR (Hadley AG, personal communication).

The CLT was introduced for the clinical evaluation of antibodies only recently, and it has only been used in immunized women to predict the severity of HDN (39).

D. Antibody-Dependent Cellular Cytotoxicity Assays

The ADCC assay measures the lysis of sensitized RBCs by monocytes (37) or lymphocytes (53–55) (monocyte-driven ADCC—ADCC(M) and K cell–dependent ADCC—ADCC(L)).

The principle of the assay is to label RBCs with ^{51}Cr, sensitize them with antisera, and then to measure the radioactivity released into the supernatant from a mixture of RBCs and effector cells incubated together at 37°C (Fig. 5). The ^{51}Cr released from sensitized RBCs is determined after subtracting spontaneous chromium release and expressed as a percentage of the total released from RBCs by triton. Variability of the test can be minimized by the use of a calibration curve obtained using dilutions of a standard anti-D serum. The number of units of anti-D in the undiluted standard serum is arbitrarily defined as 100 U/ml. Specific lysis greater than 3% is considered positive.

There are some technical differences between the ADCC(M) and the ADCC(L). Although the former is always done with presensitized RBCs (37), the latter is usually performed with serum directly added to the culture (53). Moreover, for the ADCC(L), enzyme-treated RBCs (with papain or bromelin) are used (53).

The ADCC is an objective and quantitative method. The main disadvantage is that it requires radioisotopes (see Table 1).

In clinical practice, the ADCC assay has been used to predict the severity of HDN (35–40).

IV. IN VITRO FACTORS AFFECTING CELLULAR IMMUNOASSAYS

Cellular immunoassays are more difficult to standarize than serological tests. The results are influenced by several factors. This section only emphasizes the most important variables that generally apply to all tests (Table 2). A more detailed discussion can be found elsewhere (56).

A. Effector Cells

The results of cellular immunoassays are influenced by the source of effector cells and the variation among cells from different individuals or the same person but on different occasions.

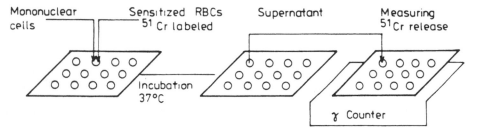

Figure 5   Schematic representation of the antibody-dependent cellular cytotoxicity assay.

Table 2   Variables Affecting the Results of Cellular Immunoassays

Effector cells:
    source of cells
    variation among different donors
    freshness of cells
    enhancement of activity by culturing with INF-γ or release of cytophilic
       IgG to culture medium
Target cells:
    number of antigenic determinants (zygosity)
    RBC to serum ratio
    incubation time and temperature
    enzyme treatment
Target to effector cell ratio
Other variables:
    effect of complement
    incubation atmosphere
    reproducibility in counting results
    expression of results

The freshness of cells and whether their activity is stimulated in vitro may also affect their activity.

Effector cells are generally isolated from peripheral blood, although macrophages obtained from peritoneal fluid of patients on dialysis (17) or monocytes cultured in vitro (14,57) have been used for the MMA and RA. Such cells are regarded as more active, although are not easily available. The monocyte-like cell line U937 (58) has been used for the RA, MMA, and CLT, but it has mainly been used for investigating the immunological basis of cellular immunoassays. The activity of effector cells can be enhanced by culturing them with interferon gamma for several days (57) or by release of cytophilic IgG to IgG-free cultured medium (Hadley AG, personal communication).

Since in practice peripheral blood monocytes are the main source of effector cells for cellular immunoassays, the results of the tests are influenced by the variation in activity of monocytes from different donors (59,60). A considerable variation was also observed if cells from a single donor were tested over a 3-year period (59). Some investigators have tried to circumvent this problem by using frozen monocytes prepared from the pooled buffy coats of 50–100 U for the ADCC (37), or a mixture of monocytes from two to six donors (39,48,61), or the patient's own monocytes (20,21,23,56) for other tests.

If the tests are performed with fresh peripheral monocytes, the cells should be used as soon as possible after blood is drawn. If the storage of monocytes cannot be avoided, the blood should be stored at room temperature. However, after storage for 24 hr, monocytes have a reduced activity, especially toward weakly sensitized RBCs (56,59). If the patient's monocytes have to be mailed, control monocytes should always be sent in addition.

B. Target Cells

It has been shown that the number of IgG molecules on the RBC can influence the results of cellular immunoassays (37,45,48,61,62). The strength of RBC sensitization depends on the number of antigenic determinants on the RBC (e.g., homozygous versus heterozygous donors) (18,22), the RBC to serum ratio used for the sensitization (22), and the incubtion time and temperature. In general, the conditions used for sensitization of RBCs for cellular immunoassays are no different from those used for routine serology.

RBCs can be treated with enzymes (e.g., papain or bromelin) before they are used in cellular assays. In practice, it is restricted to the ADCC(L). The reason why such cells work better in this assay is not clear, but is unlikely to be due to increase binding of the number of antibodies to the RBC.

C. Target to Effector Cells Ratio

The ratio of RBCs to monocytes may greatly influence the results of cellular immunoassays results. In the MMA and CLT using RBCs sensitized with IgG1 or IgG3 anti-D, results were dependent on the IgG subclass of sensitizing antibodies (see Sect. V.B). However, although all investigators agree that the adherence (42,60,61) and lysis (37) of RBCs is greater for IgG3 antibodies, published data concerning the relative abilities of IgG1 and IgG3 anti-D in mediating phagocytosis are contradictory, and both IgG1 (64) and IgG3 (48,60,62,63) have been reported to be the most active. Hadley and Kumpel (50) have shown that the reason for these discrepancies may lie in the ratio of RBCs to monocytes used in the assays. They observed that at high RBC to monocyte ratios, IgG1 anti-D was the more active subclass, and at low ratios, IgG3 anti-D was more active at mediating phagocytosis. These investigators have also shown that the results of the CLT were optimal at high ratios of IgG1-sensitized RBCs and low ratios of IgG3-sensitized RBCs to monocytes. It seems very probable that the depressed phagocytosis at high concentrations of IgG3-sensitized RBCs may be due to the large number of cells that bind to the exterior of each monocyte—the involvement of large areas of the membrane in RBC binding may stabilize it rendering the cell incapable of phagocytosis.

D. Other Factors that May Influence the Results of Cellular Immunoassays

It has been shown that the predictive value of the MMA for antibodies of some specificities (e.g., anti-Lan, anti-Jk[a], anti-Fy[a]) depends on the presence of fresh human serum in the RBC sensitization phase (29,33,34,56,65,67). It is most likely that the enchanced reactivity of such antibodies is due to complement (56), although Issitt et al. (66) do not agree with this hypothesis.

Among other factors considered to influence the results of the MMA is the incubation atmosphere. Although most investigators use CO_2-enriched environment, Garratty (56,59) produced evidence that the MMA may be performed without the use of a CO_2 incubator, which is very important from practical point of view because many laboratories do not have such incubators.

It has also been found that the results of the MMA are influenced by the reproducibility in counting monocytes with adhering and phagocytosed RBCs. The CV was considerably reduced when many monocytes were evaluated (at least 200 monocytes should be evaluated if the results are above 20%, and 600 monocytes if the results are lower than 20% (56,59).

It is possible to interpret the results of a cellular immunoassay in several ways. A result may be considered positive if reactivity is greater than that seen with nonsensitized RBCs. However, such positivity may not relate to in vivo significance. For predicting clinical significance, it is more reasonable to assign threshold values above which RBC destruction is predicted (see Sect. VI).

This section emphasizes how many variables can affect the cellular immunoassays. Before using assays in clinical practice, laboratories must carefully standarize assays, preferably with reference antibodies of known clinical significance.

V. IMMUNOLOGICAL BASIS OF CELLULAR IMMUNOASSAYS

Although rapid progress has been made in elucidating the mechanism of the interaction between sensitized RBCs and monocytes and lymphocytes in vitro, many questions remain unanswered.

Nevertheless a great deal of information has been accumulated that allows us to understand at least some factors that play an important role in the interaction of sensitized RBCs with effector cells in vitro.

Since sensitized RBCs interact with effector cells via the Fc portions of antibody molecules on the RBC (68) and FcR on effector cells (4–6), the mechanism of this interaction is mainly dependent upon the nature of FcγR (distribution, affinity, geometry) (69,70) and the quantity and quality of antibody on the RBC (5). Other factors also can play an important role in this interaction, such as the repulsive forces between target and effector cells and the topography of antigens on the RBC (1,5,71).

A. Fc γ Receptors

The characteristics of three distinct but closely related classes of FcγR (69,70,72–74), all belonging to the Ig supergene family, are presented in Table 3.

In early experiments, RAs performed simultaneously with different FcγR-bearing cells (monocytes, granulocytes, and lymphocytes) showed that monocytes required much lower numbers of IgG molecules per RBC than other cells for adherence (45,61). Subsequent elucidation of the nature of FcγRs on different cells suggested that this is due to the presence on monocytes, but not on granulocytes or lymphocytes, of FcγRI that has a high affinity for monomeric IgG.

The FcγRI seems to be predominantly, or perhaps solely, responsible for the attachment of sensitized RBCs to monocytes, although they also express FcγRII and, as recent investigations have shown, 10% of these cells also express FcγRIII (75). The evidence was gained from the experiments in which the expression of different FcγRs was upregulated, downregulated, or blocked (58). It appears that (1) the treatment of monocyte-like U937 cells with interferon gamma, which increases FcγRI expression, also increases rosette formation; (2) treatment of U937 cells with dibutyryl cyclic adenosine monophosphate (AMP), which upregulates FcγRII expression and downregulates FcγRI expression, decreases rosette formation; (3) rosette formation by U937 cells is inhibited to a greater extent by murine mIgG2a myeloma protein, which binds preferentially to FcγRI than by IgG1 myeloma protein, which has a higher binding affinity for FcγRII; and, finally, (4) rosette formation is not observed with the FcγRII-bearing Daudi cell line.

FcγRI plays a crucial role not only in rosette formation but also in all other monocyte-based functional assays (76,77). The blocking of both FcγRII and FcγRIII on macrophages by monoclonal antibodies has no effect on the lysis of anti-D–sensitized RBCs, whereas blocking

Table 3   General Characteristics of IgG Fc γ Receptors (FcγR)

Fc class	Mol Wt (kDa)	CD	Affinity for IgG	Ligands	Distribution
FcγRI	72	CD64	High	3>1>4>>>2	Monocytes, macrophages, neutrophils (IFN-induced), U937 cell line
FcγRII	40	CD32	Low	3>1=2>>>4	Monocytes, macrophages, neutrophils, B cell, platelets, U937 cell line, Daudi cell line
FcγRIII A B	50–80	CD16	Medium Low	1=3>>>2,4	Monocytes (subpopulation), macrophages, neutrophils, NK cells, T cell (subpopulation)

of FcγRI by mouse IgG2a completely inhibits such lysis (76). If RBCs are sensitized with murine monoclonal antibody against glycophorin A, the blocking of FcγRII, but not of FcγRIII, results in partial inhibition. However, the number of anti-glycophorin antibodies bound is far greater than the number of anti-D molecules. Hence, the FcγRI is probably the only receptor that can induce lysis of RBCs sensitized with human IgG antibodies except perhaps for those sensitized with IgG anti-A and anti-B that can give very high sensitization levels (76).

FcγRI on monocytes appears to recognize and bind IgG antibody via the CH_2 domain of immunoglobulin just below the hinge region (Fig. 6). Woof et al. (78) found that amino acid residues 233–237 are crucial for FcγRI recognition.

It has also been shown that the carbohydrate on the IgG molecule is important for the interaction with FcγRI on the monocyte (80). RBCs sensitized with aglycolysated IgG monoclonal anti-D do not form rosettes with U937 cells and are also inactive in the CLT (79,81). Although the carbohydrate is not accessible for direct interaction (see Fig. 6), its role may be to stabilize the CH_2 domain structure and to maintain the tertiary conformation that is essential for functional activities (79).

Lymphocytes do not possess FcγRI, but natural killer (NK) cells form rosettes with anti-D–sensitized RBCs, probably via FcγRIIIA (70,82). This receptor has medium affinity for IgG.

K-cell dependent ADCC is presumably mediated by FcγRIIIA; lysis can be abolished by monoclonal anti-FcγRIII antibody (79). However, it has been reported that not all anti-D antibodies that are capable of forming rosettes are capable of mediating K-cell lysis (83). The reason for this difference lies in the nature of the interaction of IgG with FcγRIII. It has been found that different IgG domains are responsible for the attachment and for the induction on lytic signal (Fig. 7). The first event involves CH_3 domain (408–416 residues), whereas the killing is triggered through CH_2 domain (274–301 residues) (84,85). In other words, an additional signal is required to activate lymphocytes for lysis (83). These data are consistent with observations on rosette formation and ADCC activity with lymphocytes using aglycosylated anti-D monoclonal antibodies for RBC sensitization. Such antibodies lack CH_2 domain carbohydrate. The rosette formation was not affected by removing the carbohydrate, whereas the lytic activity was abolished (81).

The differences between FcRs with respect to their affinity for monomeric IgG are important in relation to the inhibition of the interaction with sensitized RBCs with FcR-bearing cells by

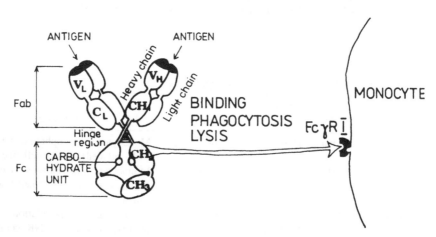

Figure 6   Interaction between FcγRI on the monocyte and CH_2 domain of IgG.

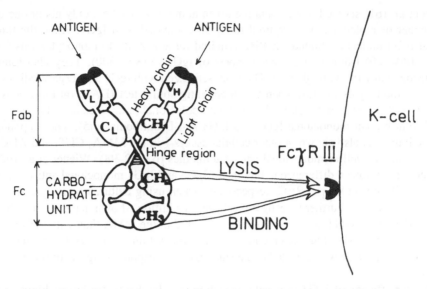

Figure 7   Interaction between FcγRIII on lymphocyte and CH2 and CH3 domain of IgG.

fluid-phase serum IgG. Thus, the use of monocytes necessitates the use of sensitized washed RBCs (37), whereas K-cell assays may be performed in the presence of serum (53,54,86).

Contrary to the well-established role of FcγRs in cellular immunoassays, the role of complement receptors (CRs) is much less known (Table 4). It is very likely that RBCs coated with C3b or iC3b adhere to CR1 and CR3 on monocytes and marcophages and act synergistically with coated IgG. It is also possible that C3d (C3d,g) in addition to IgG on RBCs may play a synergistic role in the macrophage-RBC interaction (? with CR3) (87–91).

B. Antibodies

The IgG subclass of sensitizing antibodies affect immunoassay results. Only IgG1 or IgG3-coated RBCs interact wih FcR-bearing cells. RBCs sensitized with IgG2 and IgG4 antibodies were not shown to interact, which is in agreement with clinical observations (3,4).

In all assays performed with mononuclear phagocytes, IgG3 anti-D antibodies appeared to be more efficient than IgG1 antibodies. Douglas et al. (60) found that 500 IgG1 molecules but only 100 IgG3 molecules per RBC were required to obtain monocyte-mediated phagocytosis.

Table 4   General Characteristics of Complement Receptors (CR)

CR	Mol Wt (kDa)	CD	Reactive with	Distribution
CR1	160–260	CD35	C3b>C4b>iC3b	Monocytes, macrophages, neutrophils, RBCs, B cells, some T cells
CR2	145	CD21	C3d part of iC3b= =C3dg>C3d>C3b	B cells, lymph node follicular dendric cells
CR3				
chain	165	CD116	iC3b, possibly	Monocytes
chain	95		C3dg	Neutrophils, large granular lymphocytes
CR4	?	?	iC3b(?), C3dg(?)	Neutrophils

Zupanska et al. (61) showed that to obtain a given number of rosettes, only about one-quarter of the number of molecules was required for IgG3 compared with IgG1. Also, the threshold number of IgG3 molecules bound per RBC required for adherence to monocytes was found to be lower (180–460) from the required numbers of IgG1 (1180–4300). They also found that RBCs sensitized in vitro with IgG3 anti-D but not sensitized with IgG1 anti-D antibodies showed adherence to monocytes in vitro when the direct antiglobulin test (DAT) on those RBCs was negative (61). The foregoing results obtained with polyclonal antibodies have been confirmed using different human monoclonal IgG1 and IgG3 anti-D antibodies (45). The preponderance of IgG3 activity was also shown in other cellular assays—in the MMA, CLT, and ADCC (M) using polyclonal as well as monoclonal anti-D antibodies (62, 92–98). Wiener et al. (92) have found a more pronounced difference in binding of IgG3 and IgG1 monoclonal anti-D antibodies (100 and 10000 molecules per RBC, respectively) when using cultured monocytes stimulated with interferon gamma. Further investigations have, in addition, shown that the interaction with RBCs sensitized with IgG3 anti-D was much more rapid in the MMA than with cells sensitized with IgG1 antibodies. Maximum interaction was achieved within 30 mins and 2 hrs, respectively (99). This difference also was reflected in the kinetics of CL response to IgG1- or IgG3-sensitized RBCs (41).

The greater efficacy of IgG3 in rosette formation may be due to the longer hinge region of IgG3 (100–150Å) enabling it to bridge the gap between two negatively charged cells more effectively than IgG1 (hinge region—20Å) (58,100) (Fig. 8). This hypothesis is consistent with the greatly enhanced rosette formation observed when monocytes or U937 cells were treated with neuraminidase or bromelain, procedures shown to reduce the ζ potential of these cells (58).

IgG3 is similarly more effective than IgG1 in promoting RBC binding to enzyme-treated monocytes; but when steric disadvantages of the shorter hinge region of IgG1 are circumvented, IgG1 is more efficient at activating lytic and metabolic responses (58). These observations are consistent with a synergistically increased monocyte's chemiluminescence to RBCs sensitized

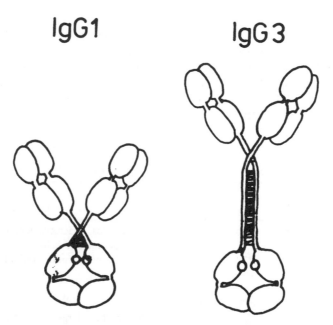

Figure 8 Difference in the hinge region of IgG1 and IgG3.

with a blend of IgG1 and IgG3 monoclonal anti-D antibodies; such effect was not noticed if RBCs sensitized with only IgG1 and only IgG3 were mixed (94).

Taking all these observations into account, it seems very likely that a function dichotomy exists between IgG3 and IgG1; the former being efficient at bridging between two cells and the latter in activating monocytes for further processes (metabolic activity, phagocytosis, lysis). The first event requires that the immunoglobulin should have a long hinge region, whereas other events require the repeated triggering of FcγRs by target-bound IgG molecules. Such triggering might be more efficient because of the relative proximity between the antigen- and FcγR-binding sites of IgG1 molecules, as a result of which the lateral mobility of membrane receptors is limited.

Although the role of IgG subclass composition of antibodies in cellular immunoassays with monocytes has been characterized, their role in the interaction with lymphocytes is less clear. Most authors found IgG3 anti-D polyclonal and monoclonal antibodies to be more active in adherence than IgG1 antibodies (43–45,61). IgG3 antibodies were, however, not found to be active in the ADCC (with one exception of monoclonal anti-c), whereas IgG1 anti-D were efficient in activation of the lysis, although not all IgG1 antibodies were able to do so (93,95,96). These observations are not surprising in light of the involvement of different IgG domains in adherence and lysis by lymphocytes discussed above.

C. Antigens

There are little data about how the results of cellular assays depend on antigens. The number of antigenic determinants influences the number of IgG molecules of an antibody bound to the RBC (zygosity of RBC donors was already mentioned in Sect. IV.B). The quantitative evaluation of RBC sensitization with polyclonal and monoclonal anti-D antibodies has revealed that there is a correlation between the number of IgG-bound antibody molecules and the results of the RA, MMA, CLT, and ADCC(M) (37,45,48,61–63).

It is not clear whether the specificity of an antigen can influence cellular assays results. It was reported that the CL response was higher using anti-K compared with anti-D containing sera at comparable sensitization levels (39). It was suggested that the topography of the K antigen on the RBC membrane may orientate antibody for more efficient cross-linking to monocyte FcγR (39). Although there is not direct evidence for this, such a possibility seems to be likely in the light of experiments with RBCs coated with monoclonal antibody recognizing the hapten 5-iodo-4-hydroxy-3-nitrophenacetyl (anti-NIP) (79). Although rosetting could not be achieved with anti-D antibody–coated RBCs even when the effector cells (Daudi cells) were treated with bromelin, rosetting occurred with RBCs coated with anti-NIP. It is possible that NIP coating will yield antigen at varying distances from the RBC membrane,

Table 5 Immunological Basis of Cellular Immunoassays

Assay	Effector cells	FcγR	Interacting IgG domain with FcR	Activity of IgG1 vs IgG3
RA	Monocyte	FcγRI	CH$_2$	IgG3>IgG1
	Lymphocyte	FcγRIII	CH$_3$	IgG3>IgG1
MMA	Monocyte	FcγRI	CH$_2$	IgG3,IgG1 depending on RBCs:monocyte
CLT	Monocyte	FcγRI	CH$_2$	IgG3>IgG1, synergistic effect
ADCC	Monocyte	FcγRI	CH$_2$	IgG3>IgG1
	Lymphocyte (K cell)	FcγRIII	CH$_3$,CH$_2$	Some IgG1 are active, IgG3(?)

which allows antibody binding to FcγRII easier, whereas the D antigen is attached to the cycloskeleton and hence is not easily accessible.

VI. CLINICAL APPLICATION OF CELLULAR IMMUNOASSAYS FOR PREDICTING THE SIGNIFICANCE OF RBC ANTIBODIES IN VIVO

A. Autoimmune Hemolytic Anemia

Among persons with a positive DAT, there are some who are hemolyzing and some who do not show obvious signs of RBC destruction. Standard clinical criteria and routine laboratory tests are usually sufficient to assess whether or not the patient is hemolyzing. In certain cases, however, the rate of RBC destruction is difficult to evaluate and RBC survival studies with the use of ^{51}Cr-labeled RBCs that provide the most objective results cannot always be performed.

The question arises whether cellular assays could assess the likelihood of RBC destruction in vivo in such patients. The answer would be especially helpful if the decision has to be undertaken whether the treatment should be applied or discontinued.

We may also ask whether a cellular assay may be useful in patients suspected of immune destruction of RBCs when serological tests do not detect autoantibodies i.e. in patients with the so-called Coombs-negative AIHA.

Patients with AIHA were examined using the RA and the MMA in which their RBCs were used as target cells and either monocytes from healthy individuals or autologous monocytes were used as effector cells.

Tables 6 and 7 give the results of the RA and the MMA in DAT-positive persons with and without increased hemolysis in vivo. Although the observations made by different investigators are not easy to compare (different ways of expressing results, different estimates of hemolysis), in most patients with increased hemolysis, the results are higher than those obtained in individuals showing no obvious signs of increased RBC destruction (15,18–24). However, exceptions, such as patients with hemolysis and a negative result of the cellular assay (false negative) and patients without hemolysis but with a positive result of cellular assay (false positive), have been reported by almost all the investigators (15,18–24). The reasons for these discrepancies are not obvious, but we can suggest certain factors such as the treatment, the autoantibodies that can be less strongly bound to reticulocyte-rich young RBC subpopulation (101) (which may be responsible for false-negative MMA results), and the enhanced or diminished activity of the reticuliendothelial system (102–107).

The role played by the last of these was examined by replacing monocytes from healthy

Table 6 Comparison Between RA Results and Hemolysis in Vivo in Patients with Positive Direct Antiglobulin Test

Rosette assay	Hemolysis in vivo		Treatment	Ref.
	increased	not increased		
Positive	22	0	Nontreated	15
Negative	0	20		
Positive	6	4	Prednisone—treated	
Negative	3	6		
Positive	8	2	Nontreated or	18
Negative	0	5	Prednisone <30 mg	
Positive	1	1	Treated with	
Negative	7	1	Prednisone >30 mg	

Table 7 Comparison Between MMA Results and
Hemolysis in Vivo in Patients with Positive Direct
Antiglobulin Test

| No. of cases | Hemolysis in vivo | | Ref. |
	increased MMA pos/neg	not increased MMA pos/neg	
7[a]	1/1	1/4	20
44[b]	18/1	0/25	19
28[c]	18/0	0/10	21
38[d]	22/2	4/10	23
66[e]	33/4	4/25	24

[a]Percent reactive monocytes: positive >3%.
[b]Percent reactive monocytes: positive >3%; mean total
reactivity: hemolysis: 11.4%; no hemolysis: 3.8%.
[c]Number of phagocytosed RBCs by 100 monocytes: positive
>2.
[d]Number of adherent and phagocytosed RBCs by 100 monocytes: positive >2; hemolysis: 1–212, mean 42; no hemolysis: 1–47, mean 7.
[e]Percent reactive monocytes: positive >5%.

donors by patient's monocytes in the MMA. In certain cases, hemolysis in vivo was better
reflected by the MMA with patient's own monocytes (Table 8). Although Zupanska et al. (24)
have shown that in most patients the differences between the MMA results with autologous and
allogenic monocytes were similar to the differences observed if monocytes from different healthy
individuals were used.

MacKenzie (102) suggested that an unknown factor(s) might play an important role in
monocyte activation in patients with AIHA. Fries et al. (103) demonstrated that the number of
FcγR on monocytes was increased in patients with AIHA and that glucocorticoid administration
was associated with a decrease of the monocytes FcγR number. Sunada et al. (104) proposed
that the activation of monocytes in AIHA patients might be caused by their sensitization by
anti-RBC antibodies ("armed" monocytes). These investigators observed that the IgG antibodies
eluted from patients' RBCs conferred on normal monocytes the ability to bind and phagocytoze
nonsensitized RBCs and enhanced the phagocytosis of sensitized erythrocytes. These investigators also observed that the phagocytosis index was lowered significantly to the level of that
observed with normal monocytes after corticosteroid treatment.

Although in patients with AIHA, the use of autologous monocytes is supposed to decrease
false-negative results, in certain cases it appears that the use of autologous monocytes diminishes

Table 8 Results of the MMA Performed with
Normal Allogenic and Autologous Patient's
Monocytes

No. of cases	No. of cases with better results with autologous monocytes	Ref.
7	1	20
7	3	21
2	2	104
12	3	23
33	2	24

the MMA result. This may happen in patients receiving methyldopa (107) or in patients with systemic lupus erythematosus (106). In the latter group of patients, anti-D–sensitized RBCs survived relatively better, probably due to the blockade of the reticuloendothelial system with immune complexes.

Although there are already many arguments for using autologous monocytes in the cellular immunoassays, the real importance of using autologous monocytes needs further confirmation. It should also be remembered that these monocytes are not often easily available.

The introduction of the MMA for the assessment of autoantibodies in AIHA aroused much hope that this test might be helpful in the diagnosis of the so-called Coombs-negative AIHA. However, when we consider the results obtained until now, this hope does not seem realistic. The only investigators who have reported elevated results in 7 out of 11 DAT-negative patients are Gallagher et al. (21), but 6 of these patients had a weakly positive DAT when anti-C3d was used. Other investigators who examined DAT-negative patients did not find a positive MMA (19,23). Garratty (56) summarizes his laboratory experience based on published and unpublished observations and states that although occasionally positive results in DAT-negative patients are obtained (sometimes only with autologous monocytes), in most cases the MMA is noninformative. His laboratory thus abandoned using the MMA routinely in Coombs-negative patients.

It can be concluded that the data available are still not sufficient to say that the cellular assays have a real practical value in patients with AIHA. More observations are needed, especially in patients who should be monitored for a longer period of time during the acute phase and the remission. This would permit us to see whether the results of the MMA can be helpful in controlling the treatment. Our findings (24) in nine patients examined on separate occasions, although only preliminary, showed that in all of these patients the results of the MMA were always high during active hemolysis and became very low or negative during remission.

B. Hemolytic Disease of the Newborn

Despite immune prophylaxis with anti-D immunoglobulin, new cases of HDN due to immunization with the D antigen still occur and mortality in such newborns has not been eliminated. The prediction of the outcome of potential HDN is based on the history of previous pregnancies, the measurements of maternal antibodies (usually in indirect antiglobulin test [IAGT] or AutoAnalyzer [AA]) and, in many cases, on amniocentesis or fetal blood sampling by cordocentesis. The last two procedures are invasive and they can even stimulate further immunization. There is thus a need for noninvasive methods that would reliably predict the severity of HDN. Moreover, there are HDN cases due to antibodies other than anti-D in which such methods also would be very useful because the outcome of HDN is sometimes not known yet.

All known cellular immunoassays have been used for predicting the severity of HDN. Donor RBCs sensitized with maternal antibodies were used as the target cells and mononuclear phagocytes or lymphocytes were used as the effector cells.

The following questions may be asked: (1) whether cellular assays can be helpful in predicting the outcome of HDN; and if so, (2) whether they can predict the outcome of HDN better than a serological evaluation of antibodies in the maternal serum; (3) whether the tests can replace the invasive methods; (4) which cellular assay correlates best with the severity of HDN; and (5) when the cellular assays should be performed.

Tables 9, 10, and 11 present data from publications that analyze more than 10 cases of HDN examined using cellular assays. These data are difficult to compare because the results of the assays are often expressed in different ways and because the severity of HDN is assessed using

Table 9 Results of the MMA in HDN

No. of cases	Summary of results	Comparison with other tests	Ref.
50[a] (31)	PV of neg MMA—94% PV of pos MMA—76%	PV of neg MMA better than PV of IAGT	25
70[b]	Unaffected—always neg; severe—always pos, 95% cases-MMA even >50%; moderate –neg and pos results	PV of MMA better than that of IAGT, similar to that of radiometric antiglobulin test	27
16[b]	PV of neg MMA—100% PV of pos MMA—92%	PV of MMA better than that of amniocentesis	26
75[a] (42)	97% PV in unaffected and mild HDN 60% PV in infants requiring transfusion	Poor correlation of MMA and IAGT and AA	28

Abbreviations: PV, predictive value; IAGT, indirect antiglobulin test; AA, AutoAnalyzer.
[a]These groups contain HDN due to antibodies of different specificities; number of HDN Rh(D) in parentheses.
[b]HDN Rh(D) only.

Table 10 Results of the ADCC in HDN

No. of cases	Summary of results	Comparison with other tests	Ref.
11[a,c]	Good prediction for mild and severe HDN	Better prediction than with AA and amniocentesis	36
80[a]	Good prediction in 53% of moderate and 95% in severe HDN	Better prediction than with IAGT and cytofluoremetric lysis of anti-D	37
167[a]	<30% lysis-unaffected and mild HDN; 30–50% lysis—various cases; >50% lysis—severe and very severe HDN (but exceptions)	Better prediction than with IAGT	49
80[b]	<10% lysis—unaffected; 10–45% lysis—various cases; >45% lysis—severe HDN (only three cases)		38

[a]HDN Rh(D)
[b]HDN(ABO)
[c]ADCC(L), other ADCC(M)

different criteria. Some investigators consider all the cases that require transfusion(s) to be severe (25,26,28); others distinguish different grades of HDN severity (based on the exchange transfusion[s] [27,37,39], intrauterine transfusion[s] [27,37,39], stillbirths [27,37,39], and level of cord hemoglobin [27]). Moreover, some investigators include, in the same group, not only Rh(D) HDN but also HDN caused by other antibodies and not indicate the predictive value of tests in relation to the antibody specificity (25,28).

In spite of all these problems, the cellular immunoassays with mononuclear phagocytes (the MMA, ADCC, CLT) seem to be helpful in predicting the outcome of the HDN, although they are not fully reliable. It should be stressed that positive results can be obtained if the fetus is Rh negative (26,37,39). This is the main reason why the predictive value of negative results is better than that of positive results (see below).

Table 11 Comparison of the Predictive Value of Various Cellular Immunoassays in HDN Rh(D)

No. of cases	Assays	Comparison of results	Ref.
29	CLT, ADCC(M), ADCC(L), RA	ADCC(M) and CLT differentiate infants who require exchange transfusion from mildly affected or unaffected better than ADCC(L) and RA	39
11	CLT, MMA, ADCC(M)	ADCC(M), ADCC(L), and CLT correlate with HDN severity better than MMA	108
40[a]	ADCC(M), MMA	ADCC(M) correlate with fetal anemia (packed cell volume deficit) better than MMA	40

[a]Only severe cases.

All authors agree that the MMA, ADCC(M), and CLT can predict the severity of HDN better than assessment of anti-D strength by the IAGT (25,27,37,49) or with an AA (36). However, it seems that when anti-D are assessed by quantitative methods (the radiometric antiglobulin test [27], enzyme-linked immunosorbent assay [ELISA] [39], cytofluoremetric analysis [37]), the superiority of the predictive value of cellular assays is less obvious.

At this time, it would be too optimistic to recommend replacing amniocentesis with the cellular immunoassays. Although Nance et al. (26) obtained a better predictive value with the MMA than with amniotic fluid analysis, especially where negative results of the MMA were concerned (56), their observations were not confirmed in a larger series. Our previous observations suggested that amniocentesis could have been avoided in seven cases in which the results of the MMA were below 20% in spite of an antibody titer greater than 32 (27). However, when we performed the MMA in 29 women in parallel with 46 amniocenteses (unpublished observations), the predictive value of positive and negative MMA results was about 80% and the predictive value was only better than that of amniotic fluid analysis if negative MMA results were obtained.

One of the reasons why the cellular immunoassays could not replace amniocentesis is that the activity of antibodies may rise rapidly at the end of pregnancy and the results obtained before the thirty-second week of gestation might not be reliable (37,39,49). Further observations are necessary to see whether the use of the cellular assays may at least reduce the number of amniocenteses needed, especially when the cellular immunoassay result is negative.

As has already been mentioned, in general, the predictive value of negative results (<20% reactivity in the MMA [25,27], <30% lysis in the ADCC [49], <10% of positive control in the CLT [39]) of the cellular immunoassays is better than that of positive results. In other words, it is easier to predict that a baby will be unaffected than how severe the HDN will be. But from practical point of view, the former prediction is more important because the main question to answer is whether the fetus or the infant will require transfusion(s). In very severe cases, however, the results of cellular immunoassays were usually very high (>50% reactivity in the MMA [27], >50% lysis in the ADCC [49]). Recently, Garner et al. (40) have investigated a group of severe cases and even though in most of them the results of the MMA and ADCC were very high, they were not very helpful in assessing the packed RBC volume deficit obtained by ultrasound-guided needling from the umbilical vein.

Occasionally, mothers with a high level of anti-D, active in cellular immunoassays, deliver unaffected Rh-positive children in whom the DAT gives strongly positive results (49,108). This was shown to be due to the presence of IgG alloantibodies in the maternal serum, which were capable of blocking the FcγR function of the infant's monocytes thereby making them incapable of destroying the sensitized RBCs (49,109). These antibodies are still being investigated.

Although all cellular assays—the MMA, ADCC, CLT—have been found helpful in predicting the severity of HDN, it seems that the ADCC yields a better predictive value than the MMA (40,108). It also seems that the predictive value of the CLT is similar to that of the ADCC (39,108). However, the CLT has been used only recently and there have been fewer observations gathered than in other tests (39).

The severity of HDN has also been predicted using the lymphocyte-driven ADCC (35,36,39,108). It is difficult to draw a final conclusion about the predictive value of this assay because not many cases were examined. According to Urbaniak et al. (35,36), the severity of HDN may be predicted by the ADCC(L) results better than by the assessment of anti-D antibodies in the AutoAnalyzer and by amniotic fluid analysis. The Report from Nine Collaborative Laboratories (108) (but only two of them tested sera in the ADCC[L] and few cases were investigated) also states that this test predicted the severity of HDN correctly, and the prediction is similar to that obtained from the ADCC(M) (57 and 60, respectively). The prediction was better in cases that did not require transfusions. Hadley et al. (39), on the other hand, reported that the ADCC(L) failed to correlate with disease severity. Like other cellular immunoassays, the ADCC(L) cannot predict correctly the delivery of an unaffected Rh-negative baby.

As had already been mentioned, the results of the cellular immunoassays may depend on the week of gestation. Therefore, they may fail to predict reliably the HDN outcome unless testing is performed regularly and frequently up to the delivery time (49).

The predictive value of the cellular immunoassays in HDN caused by antibodies other than anti-D has been much less investigated. The usefulness of the ADCC(M) was evaluated in 80 cases of ABO incompatibility, but only a few infants were severely affected (38). Just as in HDN due to anti-D, negative (<10% lysis) and very high results (>45% lysis) were more reliable in predicting unaffected and severely affected babies, respectively, than the results that were in between. Since the number of A and B antigens on infants RBCs also appeared to be a very important factor in hemolysis in vivo, the degree of hemolysis was determined by the combination of both the ADCC activity of maternal antibodies and the number of antigens expressed on fetal RBCs.

Whether the cellular immunoassays are useful in HDN caused by antibodies of other specificities is difficult to answer because the number of cases for each specificity is too small for generalization. In most cases, however, the positive test correlated with the need for transfusion (34,110–116).

In conclusion, the cellular immunoassays can be helpful in predicting the severity of HDN; however, there is no evidence that they can replace the invasive methods.

C. Predicting the Clinical Significance of Alloantibodies in Transfused Patients

In the majority of patients with RBC alloantibodies, their serological reactivity is quite sufficient for predicting the survival of transfused cells. Usually the specificity and/or thermal amplitude of an alloantibody is all that is needed to forecast its clinical significance. There are, however, antibodies of questionable clinical significance, which are often against antigens of very high frequency (e.g., anti-Ge, anti-Lan, anti-Yt^a). We may ask the question whether in such patients a cellular immunoassay can predict if the antibody will destroy transfused, incompatible RBCs because very often a compatible donor is not available.

Until now, only the MMA has been used for predicting the clinical significance of alloantibodies in patients who require transfusions. The assay is performed with RBCs with an appropriate antigen sensitized with the patient's antibodies. Results higher than 3% are usually regarded as positive.

Such studies are very hard to perform. First of all, alloantibodies of questionable clinical significance are rare, so it is difficult to collect a sufficient number of cases within a short period of time. Second, although by doing the assay, it is easy to assess whether a given antibody is potentially a danger, it is difficult to find out whether this antibody is actually clinically significant. This can only be done when the patient receives incompatible blood either as small aliqouts labeled with ^{51}Cr and a RBC survival is measured or as a unit of blood and the patient is followed up.

Table 12 presents the results of the MMA in patients with alloantibodies of different specificities in relation to their clinical significance.

Practically in all the cases, the MMA results correlated very well with the clinical significance of the antibodies (17,30–34,117–122). Negative results were observed in patients who had

Table 12 Comparison Between MMA Results and Clinical Significance of Alloantibodies

MMA	No.of cases	Specificity[a]	Clinical significance	Ref.
–	12	Kn^a,Yt^a(2),Yk^a,Ch^a(2)	Normal ^{51}Cr	17
		Yt^a,Jr^a,Yk^a(2),Kn^a,Sd^a	No HTR	
+	2	Yt^a	Reduced ^{51}Cr	
		Hy^a	HTR	
–	5	McC^a(2),JMH,Kn^a,Hy^a	Normal ^{51}Cr reduced t$_{1/2}$	117
–	4	Yt^b	Normal ^{51}Cr	30
		Ge,Vel,Jk^b	No HTR	
+	4	Ge,M	Reduced ^{51}Cr + HTR	
		Jk^a(2)	DHTR	
–	5	Sd^a,Sl^a,P1,HTLA	Expected Ht rise	32
		Lu^b	Reduced ^{51}Cr	
+	11^b	c(2),c+E,K,Kp^b,Jk^a,Jk^b,Gy^a	HTR/DHTR	
		Kp^b,Gy^a,Vel	Reduced ^{51}Cr	
–	5	E,K,Jk^b,M,Sd^a+I	Normal ^{51}Cr	31
+	7	G,E,K(2),Jk^a,D(2)	Reduced ^{51}Cr	
–	6	Ge,Yt^a	Normal ^{51}Cr	33
		Lan,Ge,Yt^a(2)	No Htr, expected Hb/Ht rise	
+	6	Ge,Yt^a(2),Lan(2),Yt^b	Reduced ^{51}Cr	
–	11^c	Yk^a,Cs^a,MnC^a,Yt^a(4)	No HTR, expected Hb rise	118
+	1	Yt^a	Reduced ^{51}Cr	119
+	1	Cr^a	Normal ^{51}Cr,reduced t$_{1/2}$	120
–	1	Ge	No HTR, expected Hb rise	34
+	2	c	DHTR	
		LW^{ab}	Reduced ^{99m}Tc	
–	1	Yt^a	No HTR	121
–	1	Tc^a	Normal ^{51}Cr	122

Abbreviations: HTR, hemolytic posttransfusion reaction; DHTR, delayed hemolytic posttransfusion reaction; ^{51}Cr, short-term (1 h/24 h) chromium-labeled RBC survival studies; t$_{1/2}$, long-term (half-life) chromium-labeled RBC survival studies; ^{99m}Tc, 1 h labeled RBC survival studies; Hb, hemoglobin; Ht, hematocrit.

[a]Number of cases in parentheses.

[b]In three cases, MMA positive only with post transfusion sera and negative with pretransfusion sera.

[c]Author did not mention the number of cases of each specificity.

normal 1-hr or 24-hr ^{51}Cr RBC survival or in patients who showed no clinical signs of rapid RBC destruction (e.g., no immediate posttransfusion reaction or expected hemoglobin and/or hematocrit rise). On the other hand, positive results were obtained in patients with a reduced RBC survival or in patients in whom immediate or delayed posttransfusion reaction was observed. In some cases (i.e., anti-Lan), the MMA results only predicted its clinical significance if the test was performed with fresh human serum (33,65). In other cases (i.e., anti-M) the prediction was only correct when monocytes from healthy individuals were replaced by autologous monocytes (30). However, it is worth noting that in spite of negative or slightly elevated (5%) MMA results and a normal short-term RBC survival in some patients, the long-term t_{1_2} survival was reduced (33,117,120,123).

In general, it may be concluded that negative MMA results allow us to transfuse incompatible blood without much risk in patients with antibodies against high-frequency antigens and of questionable clinical significance (such as anti-Ge, -Lan, -Yt^a) if a compatible donor is not available. However, it is not certain whether the RBCs transfused in patients with negative or slightly elevated results will survive as long as compatible RBCs. It should be noted that since an antibody of given specificity can behave as clinically significant in one patient and as benign in another, we cannot exclude that such an antibody may change its activity in a given patient (e.g., anti-Tc^a IgG1, IgG2, IgG4 active in the MMA became negative when the antibody lost its IgG1 component [122]). Hence, it is important to revaluate the reactivity of an antibody in the MMA before each transfusion.

Application of the MMA should be limited to the cases when compatible blood is difficult to obtain. In all other cases, even though the MMA results are negative, compatible blood should be given otherwise the risk of anamnestic response with subsequent delayed hemolytic reaction is high. This is consistent with observations of Wren et al. (32) that in spite of a negative MMA result obtained with pretransfused serum from patient with anti-c antibody, the test became positive when the serum was taken after the transfusion of incompatible blood and the patient developed a delayed posttransfusion hemolytic reaction.

VII. COMMENTS

The experience with cellular immunoassays allows us to say that these tests are useful for predicting whether patients with alloantibodies of questionable clinical significance may be transfused with incompatible blood if compatible donors are not available and for predicting the severity of HDN. In the latter, however, there is no evidence that the assays can replace the invasive methods. The cellular immunoassays have also been used in patients with AIHA, but here their practical value is less documented than in the two other situations.

There are still many questions that remain unanswered and further investigations are needed. For instance, it is difficult to say which of the tests is more informative in clinical practice. The observations in HDN suggest that the correlation between in vivo and in vitro RBC destruction is better in the monocyte-driven ADCC and CLT than in the MMA. However, such comparisons have not been done in alloimmunized patients to be transfused and in AIHA patients; hence, it would be too early to say that the MMA should be replaced by other cellular assays. It is likely that a test which best reflects the severity of HDN may not be best in other cases. Moreover, there are not enough data on the K cell-driven ADCC assay. Contrary to mononuclear phagocytes, the role of lymphocytes in immune RBC destruction is still controversial but is not excluded and should be further elucidated.

The cellular immunoassays have expanded our knowledge of the role played by FcγRs on mononuclear cells and that played by antibody IgG subclasses in their in vitro interaction with sensitized RBCs.

Moreover, the application of polyclonal as well as monoclonal anti-D antibodies in cellular immunoassays allowed us to compare their efficacy. Their functional activity seems to be similar, and this observation opens the possibility of a clinical trial to see whether the monoclonal anti-Ds can replace plasma-derived anti-D in Rh prophylaxis.

There is no doubt that the cellular immunoassays reflect to some extent the destruction of sensitized RBCs in vivo. However, we are still far from having a test that is fully reliable in predicting the clinical significance of noncomplement-binding antibodies. This is not surprising when we bear in mind that all cellular assays do not take into account the many factors that may influence extracellular hemolysis in vivo (5). Cellular immunoassays are performed with peripheral cells, whereas RBC destruction occurs mainly in the spleen, whose unique anatomy favors the interaction between sensitized RBCs and macrophages. Moreover, the characteristics of FcγRs on macrophages is not quite the same as that on peripheral monocytes; not to mention that their activity in patients may differ from the activity of monocytes from healthy individuals that are usually used in vitro. Among other in vivo factors, we also can consider the blocking effect of FcγR by alloantibodies or by immune complexes. Finally, although it is known that FcγRI on mononuclear phagocytes is the main receptor interacting with sensitized RBCs in vitro, it is not certain whether in vivo all interactions proceed in the same way because of the blocking effect of FcγRI by fluid-phase IgG.

We still hope that further development of immunology and future improvements in investigation methods will allow us to work out tests that will better reflect the RBC destruction.

ACKNOWLEDGMENTS

I would like to express my thanks to Prof. H. Seyfried (Warsaw, Poland) and Dr. A.G. Hadley (Bristol, England) for valuable discussion.

REFERENCES

1. Mollison PL, Engelfriet CP, Contreras M. Blood Transfusion in Clinical Medicine. 8th ed. Blackwell Scientific, 1987.
2. Garratty G. Predicting the clinical significance of alloantibodies and determining the in vivo survival of transfused red cells. In: Judd WE, Barnes A, eds. Clinical and Serological Aspects of Transfusion Reactions. A Technical Workshop, 1982:91.
3. van Loghem JJ, van der Muelen FW, Fleer A, et al. The importance of the Fc receptor for red cell destruction under the influence of non-complement-binding antibodies. In: Mohn F, ed. Human Blood Groups. 5th International Convocation in Immunology Buffalo, Basel: Karger, 1977:75.
4. Engelfriet CP, van dem Borne AEG Kr., Fleer A, et al. In vivo destruction of erythrocytes by complement-binding and non-binding antibodies. Prog Clin Biol Res 1980; 43:213.
5. Garratty G. Factors affecting the pathogenicity of red cell auto- and alloantibodies. In: Nance SJ, ed. Immune Destruction of Red Blood Cells. Arlington, VA: American Association of Blood Banks, 1989:109.
6. Anderson DR, Kelton G. Mechanisms of intravascular and extravascular cell destruction. In: Nance SJ, ed. Immune Destruction of Blood Cells. Arlington, VA: American Association of Blood Banks, 1989:1.
7. Ehrlich P. Farben analitische Untersuchungen Zur Histologie und Klinik des Blutes. Berlin: Hirschwald, 1891.
8. Rowley MW. A fatal anaemia with enormous number of circulating phagocytes. J Exp Med 1908; 10:78.
9. Buchan AH, Conrie JB. Congenital anemia: Four cases with jaundice and enlargement of the spleen. J Pathol 1908; 13:389.
10. Archer GT. Erythrophagocytosis. Mod Med Aust 1964; 10:55.

11. Archer GT. Phagocytosis by human monocytes of red cells coated with Rh antibodies. Vox Sang 1965; 10:590.
12. LoBuglio AF, Contran RS, Jandl JH, et al. Red cells coated with immunoglobulin G: Binding and sphering by mononuclear cells in man. Science 1967; 158:1582.
13. Boyum A. Separation of leucocytes from blood and bone marrow. Scand J Clin Lab Invest 1968; 21(suppl 97):77.
14. Kay NE, Douglas SD. Monocyte-erythrtocyte interaction in vitro in immune hemolytic anemias. Blood 1977; 50:889.
15. van der Meulen FW, van der Hart M, Fleer A. The role of adherence to human mononuclear phagocytes in the destruction of red cells sensitized with non-complement binding IgG antibodies. Br J Haematol 1978; 38:541.
16. Schanfield MS, Schoeppner SL, Stevens JO. New approaches to detecting clinically significant antibodies in the laboratory. In: Sandler SG, Nusbacher J, Schanfield M, ed. Immunobiology of Erythrocyte. New York: AR Liss 1980:305.
17. Schanfield MS, Stevens JO, Bauman D. The detection of clinically significant erythrocyte alloantibodies using a human mononuclear phagocyte assay. Transfusion 1981; 21:571.
18. Brojer E, Zupanska B, Michalewska B. Adherence to human monocytes of red cells from autoimmune haemolytic anaemia and red cells sensitized with alloantibodies. Haematologia 1982; 15:135.
19. Nance S, Garratty G. Correlation between an in vitro monocyte monolayer assay and autoimmune hemolytic anemia (AIHA) (abstr). Transfusion 1982; 22:410.
20. Hunt JS, Beck ML, Tegtmeir G, Bayer WL. Factors influencing monocyte recognition of human erythrocyte autoantibodies in vitro. Transfusion 1982; 22:35.
21. Gallagher MT, Branch DR, Mison A, Petz LD. Evaluation of reticuloendothelial function in autoimmune hemolytic anemia using an in vitro assay of monocyte-macrophage interaction with erythrocytes. Exp Hematol 1983; 11:82.
22. Schanfield MS. The role of mononuclear phagocytes in RBC destruction: In vitro test systems. In: Chaplin H Jr, ed. Immune Hemolytic Anemias. New York: Churchill Livingstone, 1985:135.
23. Herron R, Clark M, Young D, Smith DS. Correlation of mononuclear phagocyte assay results and in vivo haemolytic rate in subjects with a positive direct antiglobulin test. Clin Lab Haematol 1986; 8:199.
24. Zupanska B, Brojer E, Thomson EE, et al. Monocyte-erythrocyte interaction in autoimmune haemolytic anaemia in relation to the number of erythrocyte-bound IgG molecules and subclass specificity of autoantibodies. Vox Sang 1987; 52:212.
25. Nance S, Nelson J, O'Neill P, Garratty G. Correlation of monocyte monolayer assays, maternal antibody titers, and clinical course in hemolytic disease of the newborn (HDN) (abstr). Transfusion 1984; 24:415.
26. Nance SJ, Nelson JM, Horenstein J, Garratty G. Monocyte monolayer assay: An efficient noninvasive technique for predicting the severity of hemolytic disease of the newborn. Am J Clin Pathol 1989; 92:89.
27. Zupanska B, Brojer E, Richards Y, et al. Serological and immunological characteristics of maternal anti-Rh(D) antibodies in predicting the severity of haemolytic disease of the newborn. Vox Sang 1989; 56:247.
28. Bromilow IM, Duguid JKM. Monocyte monolayer assas, autoanalyser values, and haemolytic disease of the newborn. Br J Haematol 1991; 78:588.
29. Branch DR, Gallagher MT, Mison AP, et al. In vitro determination of red cell alloantibody significance using an assay of monocyte-macrophage interaction with sensitized erythrocytes. Br J Haematol 1984; 56:19.
30. Branch DR, Gallagher MT. Correlation of in vivo alloantibody significance or insignificance with an in vitro monocyte-macrophage phagocytosis assay. Br J Haematol 1986; 62:783.
31. Schoeppner-Esty S, Chin J, Mallory D. A comparison of the monocyte monolayer assay (MMA) to the ^{51}chromium (^{51}Cr) red cell survival for determining the clinical significance of red cell alloantibodies (abstr). Blood 68:(suppl 1):302a.
32. Wren MR, Issitt PD. The monocyte monolayer assay and in vivo antibody activity (abstr). Transfusion 1986; 26:548.

33. Nance SJ, Arndt P, Garratty G. Predicting the clinical significance of red cell alloantibodies using a monocyte monolayer assay. Transfusion 1987; 27:449.

34. Zupanska B, Brojer E, McIntosh Y, et al. Correlation of monocyte-monolayer assay results, number of erythrocyte-bound IgG molecules, and IgG subclass composition in the study of red cell alloantibodies other than D. Vox Sang 1990; 58:276.

35. Urbaniak SJ, Greiss MA, Crawford RJ, Ferguson MCJ. Prediction of the severity of Rhesus haemolytic disease of the newborn by an ADCC assay (letter). Lancet 1981; 2:142.

36. Urbaniak SJ, Greiss MA, Crawford RJ, Ferguson MCJ. Prediction of the outcome of rhesus haemolytic disease of the newborn: Additional information using an ADCC assay. Vox Sang 1984; 45:323.

37. Ouwehand WH, Mallens TEJM, Huiskes E, et al. Predictive value of a monocyte-driven cytotoxicity assay for the severity of rhesus (D) haemolytic disease of the newborn; a comparison with two other techniques. In: Ouewhand WH, ed. The Activity of IgG1 and IgG3 Antibodies in Immune-Mediated Destruction of Red Cells. Doctoral thesis, Amsterdam: Rodopi University, 1984:87.

38. Brouwers HAA, Overbeeke MAM, van Ertbruggenm I, et al. What is the best predictor of the severity of ABO-haemolytic disease of the newborn? Lancet 1988; 2:641.

39. Hadley AG, Kumpel BM, Leader KA, et al. Correlation of serological, quantitative and cell-mediated functional assays of maternal alloantibodies with the severity of haemolytic disease of the newborn. Br J Haematol 1991; 77:221.

40. Garner SF, Weiner E, Contreras M, et al. Mononuclear phagocyte assays, AutoAnalyzer quantitation and IgG subclasses of maternal anti-RhD in the prediction of the severity of haemolytic disease in the fetus before 32 weeks gestation. Br J Haematol 1992; 80:97.

41. Hadley AG, Kumpel BM, Merry AH. The chemiluminescence response of human monocytes to red cells sensitized with monoclonal anti-Rh(D) antibodies. Clin Lab Haematol 1988; 10:377.

42. Maslanka K, Zupanska B. Ripley-like serum and other anti-Rh sera in detection of Fc receptor-bearing lymphocytes. Vox Sang 1981; 40:273.

43. Zupanska B, Maslaka K, van Loghem E. Importance of IgG subclasses of anti-Rh antibodies for the detection of Fc receptor-bearing human lymphocytes. Vox Sang 1982; 43:243.

44. Zupanska B, Brojer E, Maslanka K, Hallberg K. A comparison between the receptors for IgG1 and IgG3 on human monocytes and lymphocytes using anti-Rh antibodies. Vox Sang 1985; 49:67.

45. Merry AH, Brojer E, Zupanska B, et al. Ability of monoclonal anti-D antibodies to promote the binding of red cells to lymphocytes, granulocytes and monocytes. Vox Sang 1989; 56:48.

46. Armstrong SS, Weiner E, Garner SF, et al. Heterogeneity of IgG1 monoclonal anti-Rh(D): An investigation using ADCC and macrophage binding assays. Br J Haematol 1987; 66:257.

47. Hunt JS, Beck ML, Wood GW. Monocyte-mediated erythrocyte destruction. A comparative study of current methods. Transfusion 1981; 21:735.

48. Zupanska B, Thompson E, Brojer E, Merry AH. Phagocytosis of erythrocytes sensitized with known amount of IgG1 and IgG3 anti-Rh antibodies. Vox Sang 1987; 53:96.

49. Engelfriet CP, Ouwehand WH. ADCC and other cellular bioassays for predicting the clinical significance of red cell alloantibodies. Baillieres Clin Haematol 1990; 3:321.

50. Hadley AG, Kumpel BM. Phagocytosis by human monocytes of red cells sensitized with monoclonal IgG1 and IgG3 anti-D. Vox Sang 1989; 27:150.

51. Downing I, Templeton JG, Mitchell R, Fraser RH. A chemiluminescence asssay for erythrophagocytosis. J Biolumin Chemilumin 1990; 5:243.

52. Hadley AG, Holburn AM. The detection of anti-granulocyte antibodies by chemiluminescence. Clin Lab Haematol 1984; 6:351.

53. Urbaniak SJ. ADCC (K-cell) lysis of human erythrocytes with rhesus alloantibodies: II. Investigation into the mechanism of lysis. Br J Haematol 1979; 42:315.

54. Show GM, Levy PC, LoBuglio AF. Human lymphocyte antibody-dependent cell-mediated cytotoxicity (ADCC) towards human red blood cells. Blood 1978; 52:696.

55. Randazzo B, Hirschberg T, Hirschber H. Cytotoxic effects of activated human monocytes and lymphocytes to anti-D–treated human erythrocytes in vitro. Scand J Immunol 1979; 9:351.

56. Garratty G. Predicting the clinical significance of red cell antibodies with in vitro cellular assays. Transfus Med Rev 1990; 4:297.

57. Wiener E, Garner SF. The use of macrophages stimulated by immune interferon as indicator cells in the mononuclear phagocyte assay. Clin Lab Haematol 1987; 9:399.

58. Kumpel BM, Hadley AG. Functional interactions of red cell sensitized by IgG1 and IgG3 human monoclonal anti-D with enzyme-modified human monocytes and Fc-R bearing cell lines. Mol Immunol 1990; 27:247.

59. Garratty G, Nance S, O'Neill P. Factors that affect interpretation of monocyte monolayer assays (abstr). Transfusion 1986; 26:570.

60. Douglas R, Rowthorne NV, Schneider JV. Some quantitative aspects of the human monocyte erythrophagocytosis and rosette assays. Transfusion 1985; 25:535.

61. Zupanska B, Thomson E, Merry AH. Fc receptors for IgG1 and IgG3 on human mononuclear cells; an evaluation with known levels of erythrocyte-bound IgG. Vox Sang 1986; 50:97.

62. Hadley AG, Kumpel BM, Leader K, et al. An in vitro assessment of the functional activity of monoclonal anti-D. Clin Lab Haematol 1989; 10:377.

63. Zupanska B. Rosetting, phagocytosis and immune red cell damage. Clin Lab Haematol 1990; 12:309.

64. Wiener E, Jolliffe VM, Scott HCF, et al. Differences between the activities of human monoclonal IgG1 and IgG3 anti-D antibodies of the Rh blood group system in the abilities to mediate effector function of monocytes. Immunology 1988; 65:159.

65. Judd WJ, Oberman HA, Silenicks A, Steiner EA. Clinical significance of anti-Lan. Transfusion 1984; 24:181.

66. Issitt PD, Gutgsell NS, Hervis L. Some stored antibodies give inreliable results in the monocyte monolayer assay (letter). Transfusion 1988; 28:399.

67. Nance SJ, Arndt PA, Garratty G. The effect of fresh normal serum on monocyte monolayer assay reactivity (letter). Transfusion 1988; 28:398.

68. von dem Borne AEG. Kr., Beckers D, Engelfriet CP. Mechanisms of red cell destruction by non-complement–binding IgG antibodies: Essential role in vivo of the Fc-part of IgG. Br J Haematol 1977; 36:485.

69. Anderson CL, Looney RL. Human leucocyte IgG Fc receptors. Immunol Today 1986; 7:264.

70. van de Winkel JGJ, Anderson CL. Biology of human immunoglobulin G Fc receptors. J Leuk Biol 1991; 49:511.

71. Oss CJ, van Mohn JF, Cunningham RK. Influence of various physicochemical factors on hemaglutination. Vox Sang 1978; 34:351.

72. Hogg N. The structure and function of Fc receptors. Immunol Today 1988; 9:185.

73. Kinet JP. Antibody-cell interactions: Fc receptors. Cell 1989; 57:351.

74. Schreiber AD, Gomes F, Levinson AI, Rossman MD. The Fc receptors on human macrophages. Transfus Med Rev 1989; 3:282.

75. Passlick B, Flieger D, Siegler-Heitbrock HWL. Identification and characterization of a novel monocyte subpopulation in human peripheral blood. Blood 1989; 74:2527.

76. Klaasen RJL, Ouwehand WH, Huizinga TWJ, et al. The Fcγ receptor III of cultured human monocytes. J Immunol 1990; 144:599.

77. Van de Winkel JGJ, Boonen GJJC, Janssen PLW, et al. Activity of two types of Fc receptors, Fcγ RI and FcγRII in human monocyte cytotoxicity to sensitized erythrocytes. Scand J Immunol 1989; 29:23.

78. Woof JM, Partridge LJ, Jefferis R, Burton DR. Localisation of the monocyte binding region on immunoglobulin G. Mol Immunol 1986; 23:319.

79. Jefferis R, Lund J, Pound J. Molecular definition of interaction sites on human IgG for Fc receptors (huFcγR). Mol Immunol 1990; 27:1237.

80. Walker MR, Lund J, Thompson KM, Jefferis R. Aglycosylation of human IgG1 and IgG3 monoclonal antibodies can eliminate recognition by human cells expressing FcγRI and/or FcγRII receptors. Biochem J 1989; 259:347.

81. Leader KA, Kumpel BM, Hadley AG, Bradley BA. Functional interactions of aglycosylated monoclonal anti-D with FcgammaRI+ and FcgammaRIII+ cells. Immunology 1991; 72:481.

82. Hadley AG, Zupanska B, Kumpel B, Leader KA. The functional activity of FcγRII and FcγRIII on human lymphocyte subsets. Immunology 1992; 76:446.

83. Rozsnyay X, Sarmay G, Walker M, et al. Distinctive role of IgG1 and IgG3 isotypes in Fcγ R-mediated function. Immunology 1989; 66:491.

84. Sarmay G, Jefferis R, Klein E, et al. Mapping the functional topography of Fc with monoclonal antibodies: localization of epitopes interacting with the binding sites of Fc receptor on human K cells. Eur J Immunol 1985; 15:1037.

85. Sarmay G, Benczur M, Petranyi G, et al. Ligand inhibition studies on the role of Fc receptors in antibody-dependent cell-mediated cytotoxicity. Mol Immunol 1984; 21:43.

86. Kurlander RJ, Rosse WF. Monocyte-mediated destruction in the presence of serum of red cells coated with antibody. Blood 1979; 54:1131.

87. Ehlenberger AG, Nussenzweig V. The role of membrane receptors for C3b and C3d in phagocytosis. J Exp Med 1977; 145:357.

88. Wright SD, Rao WC, van Voormis LS, et al. Identification of the C3bi receptor on human leukocytes and macrophages by using monoclonal antibodies. Proc Natl Acad Sci USA 1983; 80:5699.

89. Inada G, Brown EJ, Gaither TA, et al. C3d receptors are expressed on human monocytes after in vitro cultivation. Proc Natl Acad Sci USA 1983; 81:2351.

90. Hogg N, Ross GD, Jones DB, et al. Identification of an anti-monocyte antibody that is specific for membrane complement receptor type one (CR1). Eur J Immunol 1984; 14:236.

91. Gattegno L, Saffar L, Vaysse J. Inhibition by monoclonal anticomplement receptor type 1 in interactions between senescent human red blood cell and monocytic-macrophagic cells. J Leuk Biol 1989; 45:422.

92. Wiener E, Atwal A, Thomson KM, et al. Differences between the activity of human monoclonal IgG1 and IgG3 subclasses of anti-D(Rh) antibody in their ability to mediate red cell-binding to macrophages. Immunology 1987; 62:401.

93. Kumpel BM, Wiener E, Urbaniak SJ, Bradley BA. Human monoclonal anti-D antibodies: II. The relationship between IgG subclass, Gm allotype, and Fc mediated function. Br J Haematol 1989; 71:415.

94. Hadley AG, Kumpel BM. Synergistic effect of blending IgG1 and IgG3 monoclonal anti-D in promoting the metabolic response of monocytes to sensitized red cells. Immunology 1989; 67:550.

95. Kumpel BM, Leader KA, Merry AH, et al. Heterogeneity in the ability of IgG1 monoclonal anti-D to promote lymphocyte-mediated red cell lysis. Eur J Immunol 1989; 19:2288.

96. Kumpel BM. Functional activity of human Rh monoclonal antibodies (MABS). Workshop 3B. J Immunogenet 1990; 17:321.

97. Urbaniak SJ, Stewart GM. ADCC activity of monoclonal anti-D antibodies. Rev Fr Trans Immunohematol 1988; 31:237.

98. Walker MR, Kumpel BM, Thompson K, et al. Immunogenic and antigenic epitopes of im-munoglobulins. Binding of human monoclonal anti-D antibodies to FcRI on the monocyte-like U937 cell line. Vox Sang 1988; 55:222.

99. Brojer E, Merry AH, Zupanska B. Rate of interaction of IgG1 and IgG3 sensitized red cells with monocytes in the phagocytosis assay. Vox Sang 1989; 56:101.

100. Michaelsen TE, Frangione B, Franklin EC. Primary structure of the "hinge" region of human IgG3. J Biol Chem 1977; 252:883.

101. Branch DR, Shulman IA, Hian ALSS, Petz LD. Two distinct categories of warm autoantibody reactivity with age fractionated red cells. Blood 1984; 63:177.

102. MacKenzie MR. Monocyte sensitization in autoimmune hemolytic anemia (abstr). Clin Res 1975; 23:132a.

103. Fries LF, Brickman CM, Frank MM. Monocyte receptors for the Fc portion of IgG increase in number in autoimmune hemolytic anemia and other hemolytic states and are decreased by glucocorticoid therapy. J Immunol 1983; 131:1240.

104. Sunada M, Suzuki S, Ota Z. Reticuloendothelial cell function in autoimmune hemolytic anemia (AIHA): Studies on the mechanism of peripheral monocyte activation. Acta Med Okayama 1985; 39:375.

105. Kelton JG, Siger J, Rodger C, et al. The concentration of IgG in the serum is a major determinant of Fc-dependent reticuloendothelial function. Blood 1985; 66:490.

106. Frank MM, Hamberger MI, Lawley TJ, et al. Defective reticuloendothelial system Fc-receptor function in systemic lupus erythematosus. N Engl J Med 1979; 300:518.

107. Kelton JG. Impaired reticuloendothelial function in patients treated with methyldopa. N Engl J Med 1985; 313:596.

108. Mollison PI. Results of tests with different cellular bioassays in relation to severity of RhD haemolytic disease. Report from Nine Collaborating Laboratories. Vox Sang 1991; 60:225.

109. Dooren ME, Kuijpers RWAM, Joekes EC. Protection against immune haemolytic disease of newborn infants by maternal monocyte-reactive IgG alloantibodies (anti-HLA-DR). Lancet 1992; 339:1067.

110. Garner SF, Devenish A, Barber H. Severe haemolytic disease of the newborn (HDN) due to anti-E in a good responder during pregnancy (abstr). Transfus Med 1990; 1(suppl 1):57.

111. Kaye EM, Williams EM, Garner SF, et al. Anti-Sc1 in pregnancy. Transfusion 1990; 30:439.

112. Powell V, Habash J, Pizzarro I, et al. Anti-Wr^b and/or En^{a}FR detected in the serum of a Mi^V/M^k antenatal patients (abstr). Transfus Med 1990; 1(suppl 1):26.

113. Leak M, Poole J, Kaye T, et al. The rare M^{k}M^k phenotype in a Turkish antenatal patient and evidence for clinical significance of anti-En^a (abstr). Transfus Med 1990; 1(suppl 1):26.

114. Portugal CL, Pinho MO, Barbosa M, et al. The first example of severe haemolytic disease in an infant born to an Rh null proposita (abstr). In: Book of Abstracts from the ISBT & AABB Joint Congress. Los Angeles, 1990:81.

115. Habash J, Lubenko A, Pizzaro I, et al. Studies on a chilean Mi^V/M^k proposita and her family (abstr). In: Book of Abstracts from the ISBT/AABB Joint Congress. Los Angeles. 1990:155.

116. Shirey RS, Ness PM, Feng T, et al. Fatal erythroblastosis fetalis (EBF) due to anti-c (abstr). In: Book of Abstracts from the ISBT/AABB Joint Congress. Los Angeles. 1990:160.

117. Baldwin ML, Ness PM, Barrasso C, et al. In vivo studies of the long-term ^{51}Cr red cell survival of serologically incompatible red cell units. Transfusion 1985; 25:39.

118. Gutgsell NS, Issitt LA, Issitt PD. Transfusion of antigen-positive, serologically-incompatible blood in immunized patients, based solely on the results of a monocyte monolayer assay (abstr). Transfusion 1988; 28:32S.

119. AuBuchon JP, Brightman A, Anderson HJ, Kim B. An example of anti-Yt^a demonstrating a change in its clinical significance. Vox Sang 1988; 55:171.

120. Leatherbarrow MB, Ellisor SS, Collins PA, et al. Assessing the clinical significance of anti-Cr^a and anti-M in a chronically transfused sickle cell patients. Immunohematology 1988; 4:71.

121. Montanaro-Kitzke H, Julius H, Rajagopalan C, et al. Case report of anti-Yt^a of IgG subclass 2 showing no increased destruction of (Yt^{a+}) RBCs by monocyte monolayer assay (abstr). In: Book of Abstracts from the ISBT & AABB Joint Congress, 1990:152.

122. Anderson G, Gray LS, Mintz PD. Red cell survival studies in a patient with anti-Tc^a. Am J Clin Pathol 1991; 95:87.

123. Levy GJ, Selset G, McQuiston D, et al. Clinical significance of anti-Yt^b. Report of a case using a ^{51}Chromium red cell survival study. Transfusion 1988; 28:265.

18

Autoimmune Hemolytic Anemia

GEORGE GARRATTY

*American Red Cross Blood Services
and University of California, Los Angeles
Los Angeles, California*

I. INTRODUCTION

Autoimmune hemolytic anemia (AIHA) was the first autoimmune disease to be described in which the autoantibody was clearly proven to cause the disease. It would seem to be the easiest model of autoimmune disease for investigators to study, yet it is often ignored by immunologists, even those specializing in autoimmune disease. AIHA is said to occur in 1 per 40,000–80,000 of the population (1,2). It can be associated with autoantibodies reacting optimally at 37°C, causing the so-called warm AIHA (WAIHA), or autoantibodies that react optimally at 0–5°C but capable of reacting up to temperatures (e.g., 30°C) achieved in the peripheral circulation. The latter group are composed of the more common cold agglutinin syndrome (CAS) and the rarer paroxysmal cold hemoglobinuria (PCH). A small percentage of patients present with features of both warm and cold AIHA. Both warm and cold AIHA can occur as primary idiopathic conditions or secondary to other diseases (Tables 1 and 2). Although most drug-induced immune hemolytic anemias are associated with drug-induced autoantibodies, reacting optimally at 37°C, and thus can be classified as WAIHA, we prefer to classify them separately (3). Table 1 shows one way of classifying the immune hemolytic anemias. Table 2 lists some of the diseases most commonly associated with AIHA.

In a series of 347 patients with immune hemolytic anemia (IHA) due to autoantibodies or drug-dependent antibodies, we found 70% to have WAIHA; 16% had CAS; 1.7% had PCH, and 12% had drug-induced IHA (3). Seventy percent of the drug-induced IHA were associated with warm autoantibodies. Dacie and Worlledge reported similar findings (4). In a study of 865 patients, Sokol et al. (5) found only 41% had WAIHA; 32% had CAS; 18% had drug-induced IHA; 2% had PCH, and 7% were classified as mixed AIHA. AIHA showing features of both warm and cold AIHA (combined or mixed AIHA) have been reported as representing 6–8% of all AIHAs (5–8).

The serological techniques most useful for the differential diagnoses of the immune hemolytic anemias have been described in detail in various publications (3,9,10) and are not discussed here. The results obtained after applying these serological tests are given below.

493

Table 1 Classification of Immune Hemolytic Anemias

Autoimmune hemolytic anemia (AIHA)
  warm AIHA
    primary/idiopathic
    secondary
  cold AIHA
    cold agglutinin syndrome
      primary/idiopathic
      secondary
    paroxysmal cold hemoglobinuria
      primary/idiopathic
      secondary
  Combined warm + cold AIHA
    primary/idiopathic
    secondary
Drug-induced immune hemolytic anemia
Alloimmune hemolytic anemia
  hemolytic transfusion reactions
  hemolytic disease of the fetus/newborn

Table 2 Diseases Commonly Associated with Autoimmune Hemolytic Anemia

Warm AIHA
  reticuloendothelial neoplasms (especially chronic lymphatic leukemia and lymphoma)
  myelodysplastic syndromes
  systemic lupus erythematosus (SLE)
  infection (especially viral syndromes in children)
  immunological diseases (especially autoimmune and immune deficiency states)
Cold agglutinin syndrome
  Mycoplasma pneumoniae infection
  lymphoma
  infectious mononucleosis
  Waldenström's macroglobulinemia
Paroxysmal cold hemoglobinuria
  Viral infection
  syphilis[a]

[a]Commonly mentioned in older literature but not noted in series reported during last 20 years.

II. SEROLOGICAL/IMMUNOLOGICAL CHARACTERISTICS OF WARM AIHA

A. Red Blood Cell–Bound Proteins

Patients with WAIHA usually have immunoglobulins and/or complement detectable on their red blood cells (RBCs) by the direct antiglobulin test (DAT). Up to 10% may have a weakly positive or a negative DAT, and more sensitive methods may be needed to detect the cell-bound immunoglobulins (see below). Table 3 shows the results of testing RBCs from 104 patients with anti-immunoglobulins (Ig) anti-IgG, anti-IgM, anti-IgA, and anti-C3 (containing anti-C3dg). Most laboratories use only anti-IgG and anti-C3. Using these antiglobulin sera (AGS) to test the RBCs of 244 patients with WAIHA, we found 67% had RBC-bound IgG and C3; 20% had RBC-bound IgG but no C3; and 13% had RBC-bound C3 but no IgG (3). Sokol et al. (5) found reversed findings to us in the IgG + C3 (24%) and IgG alone (61%) groups. This might reflect on the amount of anti-C3dg in the anti-C3 used for the DAT.

Table 3 Direct Antiglobulin Test Results in 104 Patients with Warm AIHA Using Anti-IgA, Anti-IgM, Anti-IgG, Anti-C3 (3)

	%
IgG only	18.3
C3 only	10.6
IgA only	1.9
IgM only[a]	0
IgG and C3	46.2
IgG and C3 & IgA	12.5
IgG and C3 & IgA & IgM	1.9
IgG and IgA	2.9
IgG and IgM	0
IgG and IgM & C3	3.9
IgG and IgA & IgM	0
C3 and IgA	1.9
C3 and IgM	1.9
IgG present alone or together with other proteins	85.6
C3 present alone or together with other proteins	78.9
IgA present alone or together with other proteins	21.2
IgM present alone or together with other proteins	7.7

[a]Since this study (3) was completed, we have encountered rare patients with only IgM on their RBCs.

Hsu et al. (11) studied 34 patients with positive DATs using an AutoAnalyzer (Technician Corporation, Terrytown, NY), which was more sensitive than the routine DAT. None of the 16 patients without hemolytic anemia had RBC-bound C3 or IgM; 88% had RBC-bound IgG; 25% had RBC-bound IgA (2 patients had only IgA detected on the RBCs). RBC-bound IgG was detected on the RBCs of 11 of 13 patients (85%) with AIHA; 61% had RBC-bound C3; 69% had RBC-bound IgA; 61% had RBC-bound IgM. These investigators (11) emphasized that hemolytic anemia appeared to be associated commonly with RBC-bound C3, IgA, and IgM in addition to IgG in contrast to the patients without hemolytic anemia. They noted that RBC-bound IgM was not detected when the hemolytic anemia was in partial or complete remission. It should be emphasized that the AutoAnalyzer may detect RBC-bound proteins not detectable by the routine DAT even when anti-IgM is used. It is interesting to note that Lalezari et al. (12) found that the RBCs from patients with hemolytic anemia due to methyldopa therapy had RBC-bound IgM (and C1q) in addition to IgG. When the hemolysis stopped, no RBC-bound IgM was detectable. Patients with positive DATs but no hemolytic anemia did not have RBC-bound IgM. The RBC-bound IgM was only detectable using an AutoAnalyzer. It was suggested that the RBC-bound IgM was monomeric.

Ben-Izhak et al. (13) suggested that the presence of more than one class of immunoglobulin on RBCs, detectable by the standard DAT, was associated with severe hemolytic anemia. They found that 36% of 25 patients with AIHA had IgM or IgA in addition to IgG on their RBCs. These patients appeared to respond less well to steroid therapy. Using an enzyme-linked antiglobulin test (ELAT), Sokol et al. (14) showed that multiple immunoglobulins could be detected on 37% of 218 samples from patients with AIHA. Only 15% showed the same results when the standard DAT was used. Using ELAT, the following immunoglobulins were detected: 23% of the RBCs were sensitized with IgG and IgM; 5.8% were sensitized with IgG + IgA; 8% were sensitized with IgG, IgM, and IgA. RBC-bound IgG was present in larger amounts than IgM or IgA in 63% of the samples. Compared with IgG sensitization alone, multiple immunoglobulins were significantly associated with larger quantities (>800 molecules/RBC) of IgG, multiple IgG subclasses, IgG + C3d bound to RBCs, and with serum haptoglobin levels of <0.1 g/L. The latter association was still significant when higher levels of RBC-bound IgG and IgG subclass pattern were taken into account. In RBC samples with multiple immunoglobulin sensitization, there was no significant relationship ($P > 0.05$) between haptoglobins of <0.1 g/L and RBC-bound C3d or multiple IgG subclasses. These investigators (14) concluded that RBC sensitization with multiple immunoglobulin classes, even when undetected by the DAT, may be an important factor in the severity of hemolytic anemia associated with AIHA.

1. IgG Subclass of RBC-Bound IgG

We studied the IgG subclass of the autoantibody on RBCs of 167 individuals with positive DATs (46 patients with AIHA and 32 patients and 89 blood donors with a positive DAT but no hemolytic anemia [15]). Table 4 shows the results. In all three groups, the RBCs were sensitized with predominantly IgG1 autoantibodies (89, 85, and 87%, respectively); usually IgG1 was the only subclass present. IgG2 was present alone, or together with other subclasses, on the RBCs of 5.8% of donors and 15.6 and 26.2%, respectively, of the RBCs from patients without and with AIHA. IgG2 was not found often as the only subclass on the RBCs, but it is interesting to note that one patient with hemolytic anemia had only IgG2 detected on the RBCs (see below). IgG3 was detected on the RBCs of 7% of donors and 15% and 29%, respectively, of the RBCs of patients without and with AIHA; similar to IgG2, it was unusual to find IgG3 alone on the RBCs. IgG4 was detected on the RBCs of 12% of donors and 13% and 24%, respectively, of the RBCs from patients without and with AIHA; it was detected as the sole sensitizing subclass in only five cases, and all were blood donors. Dacie (16) found a similar distribution of IgG subclasses on the RBCs of 57 patients with AIHA. Most of our results were similar to those reported by Engelfriet et al. (17) except for our one unusual case of IgG2-associated AIHA and the cases with IgG3 sensitization associated with no obvious hemolytic anemia. Engelfriet et al. (17) found that IgG3 sensitization was always associated with overt hemolysis. As can be seen in Table 4, although IgG3 sensitization was far more common (29%) in patients with hemolytic anemia than in donors or patients without AIHA, we found six (7%) DAT-positive blood donors and four (13%) patients with IgG3 RBC sensitization but no obvious signs of hemolytic anemia. Engelfriet et al. (18) recently reported on the subclass of RBC-bound IgG of 746 patients with a positive DAT. The patients were not categorized into those with and those without hemolytic anemia. Ninety-four percent had IgG1

Table 4 IgG Subclass of Autoantibodies on RBCs of Blood Donors and Patients With and Without AIHA

IgG subclass (n = 46)	Blood donors (%) (n = 89)	Patients (%) No AIHA (n = 32)	AIHA
IgG1 alone	81.0	72.0	50.0
IgG2 alone	1.3	6.3	2.2
IgG3 alone	2.6	6.3	6.6
IgG4 alone	6.5	0.0	0.0
IgG1 with other subclasses	7.9	12.5	37.0
IgG2 with other subclasses	4.5	9.4	24.0
IgG3 with other subclasses	4.5	6.3	22.0
IgG4 with other subclasses	5.6	12.5	24.0

Source: From Ref. 15.

on their RBCs; 12% had IgG2, 13% had IgG3, and 3% had IgG4 on their RBCs. Although 74% had only IgG1 on their RBCs, IgG2, IgG3, and IgG4 were usually present with other subclasses (0.7% had only IgG2, 2% had only IgG3, and 0.9% had only IgG4 on their RBCs).

B. RBC Autoantibodies Detectable in the Patient's Sera

Most sera contain detectable autoantibody if sensitive enough procedures are used. Because the patient's RBCs are continually adsorbing autoantibody in vivo, the serum antibodies are often of relatively low titer. Table 5 shows the results if untreated sera and sera adjusted to a pH of 6.5–6.8 with added complement are tested. The immunoglobulin classes of antibodies detected in the serum are similar to those detected on the RBCs (see Table 3). IgG autoantibodies are the most commonly detected but some sera contain IgM and/or less commonly IgA autoantibodies. IgM and IgA autoantibodies are usually found together with IgG but on rare occasions they are the only class of autoantibody present. Although 35% of sera contain IgM cold auto-agglutinins in addition to the warm autoantibodies, these cold agglutinins most often are of normal titer and do not react at 30C or above; thus they are probably not pathogenic (3). On some occasions they can be of high titer and/or thermal range and may be potentially pathogenic, adding to the in vivo hemolysis caused by the IgG autoantibody (3,5–8) (see below).

C. Specificity of Autoantibodies

RBC-bound autoantibodies have been shown to react with a variety of antigens. The most common are RBC-blood group antigens, but sometimes membrane components unrelated to blood group antigens, or epitopes on the IgG autoantibody molecule, have been shown to be the targets for the RBC-bound IgG (19). This subject has been comprehensively reviewed elsewhere (19).

1. Blood Group Antigens as Targets

The first target described for autoantibodies was Rh. In the early 1950s, a series of reports described warm autoantibodies with seemingly Rh specificity because they did not react with -D- or certain primate RBCs or routine serology appeared to show definite Rh specificity, such

Table 5 Results of Serum Screening in 244 Patients with Warm AIHA

	% Reacting	
	Serum (% positive reactions)	Acidified serum + acidified complement (% positive reactions)
20°C Untreated RBCs		
lysis	0.4	0.8
agglutination	34.8	34.8
20°C enzyme-treated RBCs		
lysis	1.6	2.5
agglutination	78.6	78.6
37°C untreated RBCs		
lysis	0.4	.04
agglutination	4.9	4.9
IAT	57.4	57.4
37°C enzyme-treated RBCs		
lysis	8.6	12.7
agglutination	88.9	88.9

Source: From Ref. 3.

as anti-e or anti-c (19). Later, Weiner and Vos showed that over 70% of antibodies appeared to react weaker or not at all with Rh_{null} cells (20). This led to the assumption that most warm autoantibodies had Rh specificity. Since then, the story has become a great deal more complex. In 1967, Celano and Levine (21) showed that all eluates tested that were nonreactive with Rh_{null} RBCs contained anti-LW; and in 1972, Marsh et al. (22) showed that some of the antibodies that were nonreactive with Rh_{null} cells were anti-U, not Rh. In 1973, Vos et al. (23) reported that if one tested eluates using adsorption and elution and RBCs of very rare phenotype, for instance, the one example of Rh_{null} that was U negative, then anti-U could be shown to be present in three of eight eluates. They also confirmed Celano and Levine's finding that auto-anti-LW was very common; six of eight eluates were found to contain anti-LW. These specificities were only discernable by using adsorption-elution studies with exotic cells. Other findings have suggested that we should be careful in putting too much faith in specificities based on serological findings. For instance, Victoria et al. (24) labeled warm autoantibodies eluted from RBCs of patients with AIHA and studied their binding characteristics. Epitope-bearing membrane polypeptides were identified after immunoprecipitation of labeled proteins followed by immunoblotting. They showed that all the 12 autoantibodies studied bound to band 3 glycoprotein and that there was no evidence of Rh specificity based on the finding that there was a failure to immunoprecipitate 30-kd Rh-bearing polypeptides. Two of the eluates showed serological evidence for "Rh" specificity in that they did not react with Rh_{null} cells. It was suggested that the apparent serological Rh specificity may be due to a defect in band 3 of Rh_{null} RBCs.

Many specificities other than Rh, LW, and U have now been ascribed to warm autoantibodies. Table 6 lists the specificities and reference 19 reviews the data concerning these specificities.

Autoantibodies are sometimes encountered that appear to have a simple specificity such as anti-E, but the patient appears to lack the E antigen even though anti-E has been eluted from the RBCs. Such antibodies have been termed *mimicking* antibodies. Issitt et al. (25) suggested that such antibodies are not really reacting with a simple target such as E but a more complex target such as Hr or Hr_0, that happens to occur in greater amounts on E+ RBCs, leading us to misinterpret our initial serological results, where only E+ RBCs reacted. Such antibodies can be adsorbed by E+ and E− RBCs, and thus are only mimicking anti-E in our routine serology.

In addition to mimicking another specificity, autoantibodies may mimic alloantibodies in

Table 6 Blood Group Antigens Shown to Be Targets for Warm Autoantibodies

"Rh" (antibody nonreactive with Rh_{null} RBCs)
D, C, E, c, e, f
LW
M*, N, S, U, En^a, Pr, Wr^b, Ge
K, Kp^b, Js^b*, K13, K_x*
Jk^a, Jk^b, Jk3
Fy^b
Xg^a*
Vel
Sc1, Sc3
Co*
An/Wj
R_x
I^t
A, B, Le^a*
Senescent cell antigen

*Not yet proven to cause hemolytic anemia.

that an antibody, such as anti-Kp^b, may be found in a patient's serum and the patient's RBCs found to lack or to have a weakened expression of the putative antigen; for instance, the Kp^b antigen. This can occur when the patient has a negative or weakly positive DAT; thus all results seem to indicate an alloantibody. Later in the course when the patient's hemolytic anemia is in remission, and the antibody is no longer in the serum, the patient can now be shown to possess the antigen in normal strength, and the original stored serum now reacts with the patient's RBCs, suggesting that the antibody is really an autoantibody. Many specificities have been associated with this phenomenon (Rh, LW, Kell, Ge, An/Wj, Duffy, Kidd, En^a, Co, Sc1). One has to believe that it is much more common than the number of reports reflects as it is not common to recheck antigen status and retest the original serum months after the initial tests. There are some data in the literature that suggest this phenomenon right not be restricted to AIHA. In 1984, Salama and Mueller-Eckhardt (26) published a provocative paper concerning delayed transfusion reactions, in which they presented findings that differed considerably to what we had been teaching our students for years. One of the most interesting findings was that the DAT remained positive for over 97 days in six or seven cases followed for 312 days. Anti-K could be eluted from the RBCs of one patient for 299 days following transfusion. The antibody eluted off the RBCs of all these cases had a specificity similar to the original serum alloantibody, yet no antigen-positive transfused cells could possibly have been present at this time. In 1990, Ness described very similar findings in the United States (27). Thus, antibodies such as allo–anti-E, allo–anti-K, and allo–anti-Jk^a can be eluted, over 100 days following transfusion, from DAT-positive red cells, which are presumably the patient's own antigen negative RBCs. These antibodies are showing the same characteristics as the mimicking antibodies that we find associated with AIHA. Neither Salama and Mueller-Eckhardt (26) nor Ness et al. (27) tried adsorbing these antibodies with antigen-negative and antigen-positive RBCs. If these antibodies are not adsorbed by antigen-negative cells, thus fitting the definition of alloantibodies, then one has to question why they are present on the patient's own RBCs.

After reviewing the literature up to 1980, Petz and Garratty (3) concluded that there was ample clinical and experimental evidence to suggest that transfusion may lead to the development of autoantibodies. It now appears from the work of Salama and Mueller-Eckhardt (26) and Ness et al. (27) that the presence of RBC-bound IgG and complement are commonly found for months following delayed transfusion reactions without obvious hemolytic anemia. Most of the antibodies eluted from the antigen-negative RBCs had not broadened their specificity and were well-defined E, K, and Jk^a antibodies eluted from antigen-negative RBCs, but Ness et al. (27) found that a few developed into the typical pan reactions of autoantibodies. At this time, all of this is a great puzzle and is a rich area for investigation.

2. *Targets on Membrane Components that Are Not Blood Group Antigens*

Some target antigens for autoantibodies seem to be associated with the age of the RBCs. For instance, antigens appearing in vivo on senescent cells, antigens appearing in vitro on stored RBCs, and antigens present on younger RBCs. Many investigators have demonstrated the presence of IgG on the RBCs of healthy and sick individuals without any signs of hemolytic anemia (15,28). At least some of this IgG appears to be naturally occurring IgG autoantibody to a senescent cell antigen (SCA) that develops as cells age (see Chapter 7). Some workers, such as Kay, believe that SCA is on band 3 of the cell membrane (29), whereas others believe that anti-SCA are galactosyl antibodies (30). This RBC-bound IgG is usually not detectable by the routine DAT. In 1984, Branch et al. (31) performed studies on age-fractionated RBCs from 24 DAT-positive patients. Seventy-nine percent of the autoantibodies appeared to have reacted preferentially in vivo with the older RBCs, and it was suggested that these antibodies might represent augmented production of the physiological autoantibody responsible for clearing senescent cells. Since 1952, there have been reports of some antibodies, often associated with

AIHA, that would react in vitro much stronger, or sometimes only, with stored RBCs. In 1989, we reported on a case of AIHA associated with a "stored cell" autoantibody (32). The antibody showed the following characteristics: (1) it reacted much stronger with stored, heated, or enzyme-treated RBCs; (2) it showed "mixed field" reactions with antiglobulin sera (AGS); (3) it reacted stronger with older RBCs than younger RBCs separated from fresh blood; (4) we were able to show that the antibody was inhibited by synthetic SCA (kindly supplied by Dr. Marguerite Kay). A retrospective study of some other warm autoantibodies, reactive with enzyme-treated RBCs, showed similar characteristics to anti-SCA. We believe that the ubiquitous anti-SCA can be pathogenic, just as the ubiquitous anti-I, and that anti-SCA specificity may be more common than previously expected.

Although Branch et al. (31) did not find any of the 24 autoantibodies that they studied reacted better with the younger RBC population in the DAT-positive age-fractionated cells, other workers have documented such antibodies. Hauke et al. (33) and Mangan et al. (34) described patients with severe AIHA who had autoantibodies directed against antigens that were present on early erythroid progenitors but not on mature RBCs; autoantibodies against mature RBCs also were present. Thus, it seems that aplastic crises in some patients with AIHA may be due to autoantibodies against targets present on erythroid progenitors, which would not be detected by routine serology. In 1990, we presented an interesting case of cold agglutinin syndrome in which the cold agglutinin appeared to prefer younger RBCs (35); this was first noticed because of preferential clumping of polychromatic RBCs on the stained peripheral blood smear.

Other than reports of autoantibodies to band 3 and galactosyl residues associated with cell aging, autoantibodies to other membrane components have been reported. Lutz et al. (36) detected autoantibodies to spectrin, actin, and band 6 in the sera from all 10 healthy donors that were tested. As these proteins are not present on the surface of the RBC membrane, one would think that RBC-bound IgG autoantibodies to such proteins would not be detected on RBCs, but Wiener et al. (37) eluted IgG antispectrin from the RBCs of patients with β-thalassemia but not from the RBCs of patients with sickle cell anemia or normal donors. They suggested that this IgG may play a role in the increased rate of destruction of RBC in thalassemic patients. Wakui et al. (38) recently described an autoantibody to RBC protein 4.1 in a patient with AIHA. This antibody was detected, together with anti-"En^a-like" and anti-S, in the patient's serum. Unfortunately, an eluate from the patient's RBCs was not tested for antiprotein 4.1 activity.

One of the most interesting areas that impacts on the source of RBC-bound IgG is that concerning the reaction of autoantibodies with RBC membrane phospholipid. In 1940, the antibody responsible for positive syphilis serology was found to react with a lipid extract of bovine heart muscle termed cardiolipin. In the next 30 years, the immunochemistry of cardiolipin, and its immune reactions, were elaborated on; cardiolipin antibodies were found to cross-react with negatively charged phospholipids. In the early 1980s, an association between anticardiolipin and systemic lupus erythematosus (SLE) was established. The so-called "lupus anticoagulant" was found to be anticardiolipin. More recently, a clinical syndrome of recurring thrombosis and fetal loss has been termed antiphospholipid syndrome. RBC- and platelet-bound autoantibodies to phospholipid have been reported to lead to thrombocytopenia, positive DATs, and even AIHA (39–43). For many years, the etiology of the RBC-bound IgG and/or complement found in patients with SLE has been controversial. It now seems probable that antibody against phospholipid may sometimes be binding to phospholipid moieties on the RBC membrane and may also activate complement in the process.

Sometimes RBC-bound IgG autoantibody is not directed against the RBC membrane but against the IgG autoantibody itself. Using adsorption studies and radiolabeled eluted RBC autoantibodies, we found that eluates from DAT-positive blood donors contained more IgG than could be accounted for by autoantibody bound to RBC antigens (44). It was postulated that the extra IgG was due to an IgG antibody directed at the IgG autoantibody bound to RBC antigens. Masouredis and his coworkers went on to prove that this antibody was directed against the idiotype of the RBC-bound autoantibody and that this could be demonstrated by its cross-reactivity with IgG Rh alloantibodies (45). Eluates from the RBCs were shown to contain two populations of antibodies (Fig. 1). As expected, one population, the RBC autoantibody, reacted by indirect antiglobulin test (IAT) with untreated RBCs but did not directly agglutinate them or IgG(Rh)-coated RBCs. The other population that was said to be anti-idiotype did not react with uncoated RBCs, but would directly agglutinate IgG(Rh)-coated red cells (Fig. 1). Perhaps the most provocative finding was that the few DAT-positive patients with AIHA that were tested, in contrast to the DAT-positive donors, did not appear to have anti-idiotype present on their RBCs, and it was suggested that anti-idiotype may provide some protective function and explain why donors with strongly positive DATs do not have hemolytic anemia. It could be argued that Masouredis et al. (45) did not prove that the antibody directed against the autoantibody was anti-idiotype and that it would be more correctly termed an anti-Fab autoantibody.

D. WAIHA Associated with a Negative DAT

Some patients present with all the clinical and hematological signs of WAIHA, yet have a negative DAT and no serum antibodies when tested with routine procedures. Chaplin reported that 2–4% of patients with AIHA show this phenomenon (46). During a 10-year period when we studied 347 patients with obvious AIHA (244 were WAIHA), we encountered 27 other patients who appeared to have WAIHA but had a negative DAT (3). This represents about 10% of the WAIHA and 7% of all the immune hemolytic anemias we encountered (3). Sometimes, this phenomenon appears to be associated with the presence of low-affinity IgG autoantibodies that elute from the RBCs during the in vitro washing of the RBCs. Sometimes, small amounts of RBC-bound IgG can be detected by methods more sensitive than the antiglobulin test.

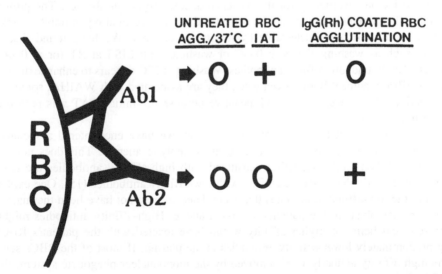

Figure 1 Eluates from RBCs of DAT-positive blood donors contained two antibody populations: Ab1 and Ab2. Ab1 was the RBC autoantibody that reacted with untreated RBCs by IAT but did not agglutinate them or IgG(Rh)-coated RBCs. Ab2 was an IgG autoantibody to an epitope on the IgG RBC autoantibody (said to be anti-idiotype). Ab2 did not react with untreated RBCs but directly agglutinated Ig(Rh)-coated RBCs (45).

Sometimes, RBC-bound IgA and IgM can be shown to be present on the RBCs when appropriate reagents are used.

1. Low-Affinity IgG Autoantibodies

When the routine DAT is performed, the patient's RBCs are washed in large volumes of saline three or four times at room temperature (RT). Sometimes, because cold autoagglutinins are noted, the RBCs are washed with 37C saline. We have encountered rare patients in whom a DAT that is negative or weakly positive by the routine procedure becomes strongly positive when processed under different conditions. We studied 24 patients with AIHA associated with low-affinity autoantibodies; 19 of these patients were sent to us as "DAT-negative" AIHA (47). Thirteen of the 19 patients had a negative DAT if the RBCs were washed with saline at RT but the DATs were positive if the RBCs were washed with ice-cold (0–4C) saline and/or low ionic strength saline (LISS). When the RBCs were washed with cold saline, they were always tested with 10% albumin (as a negative control), in addition to antiglobulin sera, to control that cold autoagglutinins were not causing the positive test result.

The 11 patients (6 of these were sent to us as DAT-negative AIHA) who were DAT positive when their RBCs were washed at RT had stronger positive DATs when the RBCs were washed at 4C but were much weaker or negative when the RBCs were washed at 37C. When RBCs from some of these patients were washed and allowed to stand at RT for 20–160 min before performing the DAT, all DATs were much weaker or negative. When 22 random DAT-positive RBC samples were subjected to the same conditions, DAT titration scores appeared similar to those of the RBCs that were tested immediately following washing; none of the positive DATs became negative (47).

Although low-affinity autoantibodies appear to be uncommon, we believe they may sometimes cause technical problems in obtaining an accurate DAT result and possibly may cause a false-negative IAT in addition to a false-negative DAT. Low-affinity autoantibodies (and possibly alloantibodies) may be dissociated from the RBCs by the process of washing for the DAT (and possibly the IAT). We would suggest that part of the "workup" of a DAT-negative AIHA should include evaluating for the presence of low-affinity antibodies. The presence of low-affinity alloantibodies should also be considered when investigating hemolytic transfusion reactions with no antibodies detectable by routine procedures. We have found that simple approaches such as washing RBCs at 0–4C or washing with LISS at RT (or at 0–4C) will help detect RBC-bound low-affinity antibodies. Washing at 37C appears to enhance dissociation of IgG low-affinity autoantibodies even when they are associated with WAIHA; some cases of "DAT-negative" AIHA were only DAT negative because the initial DAT was performed on RBCs washed at 37C.

It is of interest to add that some of the cases that we have encountered associated with low-affinity autoantibodies have had quite severe hemolytic anemia. This does not seem to agree with published work that RBCs sensitized with high-affinity antibodies are destroyed much more efficiently than those sensitized with low-affinity antibodies (15). One explanation may be that the low-affinity antibodies that were detected may not have been the major cause of the severe hemolysis in the patients discussed above. High-affinity antibodies might have been present and being of higher affinity would have reacted with the patient's RBCs first leaving predominately lower-affinity antibodies in the plasma. If most of the RBCs sensitized with the high-affinity antibody were removed by the mononuclear phagocyte system, then the only RBCs left circulating might be those sensitized with low-affinity autoantibodies. This is a good example of where the results of our in vitro tests may not correlate with the clinical course observed in the patient.

Although low-affinity antibodies appear to be uncommon, the above results emphasize that when we wash RBCs, we are creating conditions very different than those in vivo. The antiglobulin test must be performed immediately following washing of the RBCs. If RBCs are washed at 37C, one should remember that some DATs may be weaker or even negative when low-affinity antibodies are present; on rare occasions, even RBCs washed at RT may yield false weak positive or negative DATs.

2. *RBCs Sensitized with a Small Amount of IgG that Is Below the Threshold of the Routine Antiglobulin Test*

We and others have demonstrated that an obviously positive DAT (e.g., 1+) is only noted when there are about 200 IgG molecules/RBC (3). Using good technique and potent anti-IgG, as little as 100 IgG molecules/RBC can, on occasion, be detected (3). Gilliland et al. (48,49) suggested that sometimes the routine DAT does not detect the quantity of RBC-bound IgG that will interact with macrophages in vivo. Using an assay (a complement-fixation antiglobulin consumption assay [47]) that was more sensitive than the DAT, Gilliland et al. (49) detected IgG on the RBCs of patients with DAT-negative AIHA. Petz and Garratty (3) confirmed that some of the DAT-negative AIHAs had RBC-bound IgG detectable by the assay described by Gilliland et al. (48,49). This RBC-bound IgG usually became undetectable when the patient's hemolytic anemia was in remission and thus seemed to be responsible for the AIHA. In more recent years, other approaches have been used to detect and/or quantitate the small amounts of RBC-bound IgG. Tests that have been used include enzyme-linked antiglobulin tests (15,50–54), radiolabeled anti-IgG (54–56), flow cytometry (51), and various serological approaches (50,51,57).

In 10 years we studied 259 cases of hemolytic anemia of unknown origin in which an immune basis was suspected by the hematologist but the DAT was reported as negative (51). Twenty-five of 259 (10%) referred DAT-negative patients had positive DATs (IgG) when tested by the routine DAT method in our laboratory. Five modifications of the DAT (flow cytometry [FC] with fluorescein-conjugated anti-IgG; direct enzyme-linked antiglobulin test [ELAT] with alkaline phosphatase–conjugated anti-IgG; direct Polybrene [hexadimethrine bromide] test; direct polyethylene glycol [PEG] test; and DAT with cold washes); a concentrated eluate from the RBCs; and a monocyte monolayer assay (MMA) were used to detect RBC-bound IgG. Table 7 shows the results. Eighty of 234 (34%) patients were positive by at least one method. It is of interest that the simple direct Polybrene test was as efficient as complex assays such as FC and ELAT. However, in some patients RBC-bound IgG was detectable by FC and/or ELAT but not Polybrene (the opposite was also true). No one test was optimal; a battery of tests seems to be the most efficient approach to aid in the diagnosis of DAT-negative AIHA.

Table 7 Comparison of Tests Used for Detecting RBC-Bound IgG When DAT Is Negative

Test	No. of Patients	No./% Positive
Flow cytometry	70	15/21
Direct Polybrene	205	38/19
Direct ELAT	201	32/16
Direct PEG	160	16/10
Concentrated eluate	162	15/9
DAT using cold saline washes	209	7/3
MMA	105	4/4

Source: Ref. 51.

3. RBC-Bound IgA and IgM

Routine polyspecific AGS are not standardized to react with IgA- or IgM-sensitized RBCs; they are only required to detect IgG and C3 (C3d). We have found that most of the polyspecific AGS used routinely for DATs do contain anti-IgA, but they sometimes only react following the 5- to 10-min incubation period recommended by the manufacturers to enhance anti-C3 reactivity (58). Anti-IgA and anti-IgM that are standardized for the DAT are not readily available. One can standardize immunological reagents, but as agglutination is far more sensitive than many immunological procedures, great care has to be taken to avoid specificity problems with heterophilic antibodies and anti-light chain cross-reactivity (3). Anti-IgM does not work well by the DAT even when a reagent that is potent by other criteria is used (3). Recently, we have been quite successful detecting RBC-bound IgA and IgM using flow cytometry (unpublished observations).

On rare occasions, WAIHA can be associated with IgA and IgM autoantibodies without the presence of IgG. For the reasons discussed above, they can sometimes present as DAT-negative AIHA.

4. WAIHA Associated with IgA Autoantibodies

The clinical, hematological, and serological features of patients with AIHA associated with IgA autoantibodies are very similar to the AIHA associated with warm IgG autoantibodies (58–67). The patients also respond to the same therapy (i.e., steroids and/or splenectomy). The greatest puzzle is how the IgA-sensitized RBCs are destroyed in vivo (15). Macrophages were originally said not to have, or to have very inefficient, receptors for IgA, but there has been increasing data suggesting that sometimes IgA participates in phagocytosis (68–70) and antibody-dependent cellular cytotoxicity (ADCC) (71). Recently, a human Fc receptor (FcαR) for IgA was cloned (72). The monoclonal antibody used to isolate the clone was capable of inhibiting any binding of IgA and phagocytosis of IgA-coated targets (72). Clark et al. (73) studied the mechanism of hemolysis in a patient with WAIHA associated with an IgA autoantibody. The patient pursued a clinical course (spherocytosis, splenic sequestration of RBCs, response to corticosteroids, and splenectomy) very similar to that of individuals with pure IgG WAIHA, which suggests that the mechanism of hemolysis may be similar to that occurring in WAIHA associated with IgG autoantibodies. Second, the patient's eluate produced antibody-dependent cell-mediated cytotoxicity (ADCC) toward sensitized RBCs that appeared to be IgA dependent; i.e., the ADCC-promoting effect of the eluate was blocked by a solid-phase anti-IgA immunosorbent and by fluid-phase normal IgA. Third, the effect was dependent on the dose of IgA eluate used to sensitize RBCs. Fourth, the patient's eluate promoted phagocytosis of sensitized RBCs by normal mononuclear phagocytes. Fifth, both ADCC and phagocytosis promoted by the patient's eluate were complement independent. Sixth, the patient's eluate failed to produce complement-mediated hemolysis, and complement components could not be detected on sensitized RBCs in vitro or in vivo. Taken together, these observations suggested a possible mechanism for what appeared, clinically, in this patient to be a warm AIHA mediated by IgA; i.e., a complement-independent interaction of IgA-coated RBCs with the patient's mononuclear phagocytes.

Salama et al. (74) studied a 6-year-old patient with AIHA, who had a strongly positive DAT due predominately to IgA, although small amounts of RBC-bound IgG were also detected; no RBC-bound C3 was detected. This patient had severe hemolysis associated with an upper respiratory tract infection. Evidence was presented that C3-independent intravascular immune hemolysis had occurred through "reactive hemolysis." Reactive hemolysis involves C3-independent binding of C5b-9 complexes in addition to IgA (and IgG) but no C3. Salama et al. (74) pointed out that several reports of AIHA associated with IgA autoantibodies appeared to have signs of intravascular lysis (57,59,62) and perhaps reactive lysis could play a role in the hemolytic process.

5. Warm AIHA Associated with IgM Autoantibodies

The in vivo role of IgM autoantibodies that react in vitro at 37° is controversial. IgM warm autoantibodies may agglutinate untreated and/or enzyme-treated RBCs, hemolyze untreated and/or enzyme-treated RBCs, and sensitize RBCs so that IgM and/or complement is detectable by the antiglobulin test. Patients seem to fall into four groups.

Patients with Easily Detectable IgG Autoantibodies and IgM Autoantibodies that Are Not Defined by Routine Tests. If routine procedures are used to test the RBCs and serum of this group, the results would be those most commonly found in idiopathic WAIHA (e.g., IgG or IgG + C3 detected on the RBCs; agglutination and perhaps lysis of enzyme-treated RBCs; a positive IAT with untreated and enzyme-treated RBCs). These results are obtained because anti-IgM is not used routinely for the DAT and IAT, and the immunoglobulin class of the serum antibody(ies) is not usually determined. When anti-IgM was used, Petz and Garratty (3) found that RBC-bound IgM was detected on 8% of the RBCs of patients with warm AIHA. None of the 104 patients had only IgM on the RBCs; 2% had IgG + IgA + C3 + IgM; 4% had IgG + IgM + C3; 2% had IgM + C3 (see Table 3). If more sensitive tests are applied, then RBC-bound IgM is detected more often. Vos et al. (75) showed that 42% of eluates prepared from the RBCs of 55 patients with WAIHA contained IgM and/or IgA in addition to the IgG detected by the DAT. Using the AutoAnalyzer, Hsu et al. (11) found that 8 of 11 (73%) patients with WAIHA associated with IgG positive DATs had RBC-bound IgM present in addition. None of 16 DAT-positive patients without AIHA had RBC-bound IgM. Using ELAT, Sokol et al. (52) detected IgM on the RBCs of 39 of 102 (38%) patients with WAIHA associated with IgG-positive DATs.

Petz and Garratty (3) found that 5% of sera from patients with warm AIHA would agglutinate and 0.4% would hemolyze untreated RBCs at 37°C. Ninety percent of the sera would agglutinate enzyme-treated RBCs and 9–13% would hemolyze enzyme-treated RBCs at 37°C. von dem Borne et al. (76) showed that autoantibodies that hemolyze enzyme-treated RBCs at 37°C are IgM, and that such antibodies by themselves cause only slight to moderate in vivo RBC destruction (77). Wolf and Roelcke (78) recently studied eight sera containing warm hemolysins against enzyme-treated RBCs; none of these agglutinated or hemolyzed untreated RBCs at 37°C. Seven of the eight antibodies were shown to be IgM (one had an IgG component and one an IgA component in addition); one appeared to be IgG without IgM or IgA. In three sera, the IgM antibodies were shown to be monoclonal proteins (κ light chains only). Only one of these eight patients had RBC-bound IgG detectable by the DAT; five had a positive DAT due to RBC-bound complement and two had negative DATs. Wolf and Roelcke (79) also presented evidence to suggest that the targets for IgM warm hemolysins belong to a newer group of phospholipase susceptible RBC antigens, and that this specificity emphasizes that they are a separate category of warm autoantibodies.

Patients with Warm IgM Autoantibodies Associated with RBC-Bound Complement. Routinely, RBCs are only tested with anti-IgG and anti-C3 (C3d). Six to 13% of RBCs from patients with WAIHA have been reported to react with anti-C3 (C3d) but not anti-IgG (3,5). In most cases, it is not known how the C3 came to be on the RBCs. If anti-IgM is used for the DAT, sometimes RBC-bound IgM can be detected, and it is assumed that the IgM autoantibody may have activated complement causing RBC-bound C3 (C3d). Petz and Garratty (3) found that 2% of patients with WAIHA-associated RBC-bound C3 also had RBC-bound IgM. Sokol et al. (5) only found 1 of 355 patients with warm AIHA to have IgM + C3 on their RBCs. Several cases of WAIHA due to IgM warm autoantibodies associated with a positive DAT due to RBC-bound C3 (C3d) have been reported (78,80–89). Sometimes the IgM was only detectable by tests more sensitive than the DAT (83). IgM autoantibodies were detectable in the serum of most patients and sometimes in eluates made from the patients' RBCs. Some investigators commented on the difficulty of obtaining reactive eluates. Dorner et al. (87) could only demonstrate the RBC-bound IgM autoantibody if it was eluted into albumin or serum. Ellis et al. (90) studied the most suitable elution method for IgM in 42 patients with AIHA associated with RBC-bound IgM; heat (56C) elution was found superior to acid stromal, organic solvent, or freeze-thaw methods. Although all of the patients' sera contained pentameric forms of IgM and 64% contained oligomeric forms of IgM, only pentameric IgM was eluted from the RBCs. Thus, it was concluded that low molecular weight IgM was not the cause of in vivo hemolysis in these 42 patients.

Patients with Warm IgM Autoantibodies and a Negative DAT. As mentioned previously, some investigators have demonstrated IgM on the RBCs of patients who have AIHA but have a negative routine DAT (11,51,52). This IgM was sometimes detectable by the DAT using anti-IgM and sometimes only detectable by more sensitive procedures. Sokol et al. (52) studied 219 patients suspected of having AIHA with DAT and ELAT. DAT and ELAT results were the same in 61 patients; in 43 cases, the ELAT detected additional immunoglobulin classes; in 33 cases, the DAT only showed RBC-bound C3 (C3d) but ELAT showed RBC-bound IgM in 16 (50%) of these. In five of 16 cases, the DAT was negative and the ELAT detected RBC-bound IgM. Kay et al. (91) and Szymanski et al. (92) detected low molecular weight (monomeric) IgM on patients' RBCs. Salama and Mueller-Eckhardt (83) reported on 12 children (8 of whom were infants) with relatively severe AIHA associated with noncomplement-binding IgM autoantibodies. The routine DATs were negative in 11 cases and positive owing to RBC-bound C3d in one case. All patients were shown to have RBC-bound IgM when a radioimmune assay was used; two cases also had IgA and/or IgG detected by this assay. An unusual finding with these patients was that no antibodies were detected in the patients' sera by conventional serology or the radioimmune assay. Eluates from RBCs of all 11 patients were nonreactive by conventional serology, but two reacted with anti-IgM by the radioimmune assay.

Severe (Sometimes Fatal) Hemolytic Anemia Associated with Warm IgM Autoantibodies Directed Against Sialidase-Sensitive Determinants. We know of five cases of warm AIHA associated with IgM antibodies directed against sialidase-sensitive determinants (En[a] [85–87], Pr [87], and Wr[b] [93]). These were all associated with severe hemolysis, and all but one showed signs of intravascular lysis; in three cases, the hemolysis was fatal. Table 8 summarizes the data. It should be noted that the patients' RBCs spontaneously agglutinated when centrifuged in two of the cases that led to difficulties in performing DATs and RBC typing. Treatment of the RBCs with dithiothreitol (DTT) overcame the spontaneous agglutination but because of the effect of DTT on RBC-bound IgM, the DAT using anti-IgM were unreliable. Further work using anti-IgM by flow cytometry, which does not involve centrifugation of the RBCs, showed that RBC-bound IgM could be detected by this approach (86).

Several points are worth emphasizing concerning the serology. Although these antibodies were very effective in vivo, they had unusual in vitro characteristics. Two of the DATs were only weakly positive and one was negative. Although the serum antibodies agglutinated RBCs strongly, they sometimes did not react by the IAT; thus they appear to be low-affinity antibodies susceptible to the washing process. We have also encountered this phenomenon with an IgM allo–anti-En[a] that caused a fatal hemolytic transfusion reaction (94). Two of the auto–anti-En[a] that caused fatal hemolysis reacted only at low pH (e.g., 6.5) or in the presence of 30% albumin (86,87). Although the auto–anti-Wr[b] caused fatal hemolysis, it was detected poorly in systems using normal ionic strength saline (93).

III. SEROLOGICAL/IMMUNOLOGICAL CHARACTERISTICS OF COLD AGGLUTININ SYNDROME

Cold agglutinin syndrome (CAS) is a very different disease than WAIHA. The pathogenic autoantibody is IgM. It is an efficient agglutinating and complement-activating antibody that

Table 8 Results of Testing RBCs and Sera from Patients with Warm IgM Autoantibodies Directed Against Sialidase Sensitive Determinants

Case No. (Ref.)	RBCs		Spontaneous Agglutination	Serum	Clinical Course
	DAT	Eluate			
1 (86)	Negative		No	4+ IgM agglutinin at 37°C; (IAT at 37°C was negative); anti-En^a	? Pure red cell aplasia. Remission of AIHA.
2 (86)	2+ (C3), no IgG	IgM 37°C reactive (3+) agglutinin	Yes	3+ IgM agglutinin at 37°C; anti-En^{a}FS. Only reactive at low pH (e.g., pH 6.5) or in the presence of albumin.	Intravascular lysis → Hematocrit <2%; died.
3 (87)	3+ (C3), no IgG, IgM or IgA	Nonreactive	No	2+ IgM agglutinin at 37°C; 37°C lysin; anti-En^{a}FR. Better reactions at low pH or in the presence of albumin.	Lymphoma. Died following transfusion of 5 U.
4 (87)	½+ C3. No IgG, IgM or IgA by DAT but IgM by flow cytometry.	IgM 37°C reactive (4+) agglutinin	Yes	3+ IgM agglutinin at 37°C; no lysin; anti-Pr.	Intravascular lysis. Plasma exchange. IVIG. Remission.
4 (93)	1+ (IgG + C3)	Anti-Wr^b reacting by IAT	Not recorded	4+ IgM agglutinin and 4+ IAT at 37°C (LISS); 37°C lysin (LISS only); anti-Wr^b	Hemoglobin dropped from 7 g to 4 g% in 24 hr. Patient died.

sensitizes RBCs optimally at 0–4°C. The antibody usually reacts up to 30°C, and on rare occasions, it can react at 35–37°C. In most cases, the antibody causes a clinical problem only when the patient's peripheral temperature cools to below 35°F. When this occurs, the antibody can react with the patient's RBCs. The RBCs may be agglutinated in the peripheral circulation causing acrocyanosis of the ears, fingers, nose tip, and toes. Thus, the patient may present with Raynaud's phenomenon. In rare cases, an associated gangrene has been reported (3). Complement activation usually occurs, and the RBCs in the peripheral circulation may be coated with IgM and complement. Conditions are not usually optimal for complement activation to lead to direct lysis of the RBCs; thus hemoglobinemia and hemoglobinuria are uncommon findings in patients with CAS. The RBCs sensitized in the peripheral cooler circulation rapidly move to a 37°C environment and the IgM cold autoantibody elutes from the RBCs into the patient's plasma. The C3b remains bound to the RBCs, but it soon becomes cleaved by factors I and H to become iC3b and finally C3dg. Macrophages have receptors (CR1 and CR3) for C3b and iC3b, thus C3b- and iC3b-coated RBCs may be destroyed in the mononuclear phagocytic system (particularly within the liver); this is probably the major mechanism for the hemolytic anemia in CAS (i.e., extravascular rather than intravascular destruction) (15). As there are no receptors for C3dg on the macrophage, once RBCs are coated with C3dg, they may survive relatively normally. The C3dg-sensitized RBCs may survive better than RBCs not coated with complement as the complement components cluster around the I antigen sites hindering further uptake of anti-I (3,15).

A. RBC-Bound Proteins

If RBCs are taken from patients with CAS and washed at 37°C so that the RBCs represent circulating RBCs, they will be found to have a positive DAT owing to C3 (C3dg) sensitization; no IgG, IgA, or IgM is usually detected. Some investigators using more sensitive procedures have demonstrated the presence of RBC-bound IgG, IgA, and IgM (95–97).

B. RBC Autoantibodies Detected in the Patient's Serum

In contrast to WAIHA, in which the patient's RBCs are continually adsorbing autoantibody at 37°C, leaving limited antibody in the serum, sera from patients with CAS invariably contain large amounts of autoantibody. The antibodies are almost always IgM, but there may be IgG and/or IgA components. The antibodies will agglutinate RBCs to high titer at 4°C and will have a high thermal amplitude, usually up to 30°C (3). Most of the antibodies are capable of hemolyzing RBCs in vitro under optimal conditions. For instance, only 2% of CAS sera will hemolyze untreated RBCs at 20°C, but if fresh inert human serum is added as a source of complement and the pH is adjusted to 6.5–6.8, then 14% of sera causes hemolysis of untreated RBCs (3). If enzyme-treated RBCs are used, then 25% of untreated sera and 94% of sera with added complement will cause hemolysis at 20°C (3). Hemolysis rarely occurs at 37°C. Petz and Garratty (3) found that under optimal conditions, none of 57 CAS sera caused hemolysis of untreated RBCs at 37°C but 10% hemolyzed enzyme-treated RBCs. The IAT is usually negative if the tests are carried out strictly at 37°C; only 5% of sera yield a positive IAT at 37°C (3).

Garratty et al. (98) found that an essential serological finding to distinguish pathogenic from nonpathogenic cold autoagglutinins was their ability to react in vitro at 30°C in the presence of 30% bovine albumin. They found that detection of cold hemolysins, reacting at 20°C, and the cold agglutinin titer at 4°C (using saline or albumin-suspended RBCs), did not always correlate with in vivo hemolysis, but the thermal range correlated well. Sera from all 28 patients with CAS caused lysis of enzyme-treated RBCs at 20°C, but sera from 3 of 4 patients with high-titer cold agglutinins but no hemolytic anemia also contained cold hemolysins. Four patients with complement on their RBCs had abnormal cold agglutinin titers (320, 320, 320, and 1280, respectively) but no hemolytic anemia. Sera from all 28 patients with hemolytic anemia (CAS) reacted with RBCs at 30C in the presence of albumin; only 15 of 28 (54%) sera reacted at 30C without albumin. None of the sera from the four patients with high-titer antibodies and no hemolytic anemia reacted at 30C even in the presence of albumin. Sniecinski et al. (99) described one unusual patient with an IgM monoclonal κ cold antibody, with a titer of 4096 at 4C and reacting up to 37C, who had no hemolytic anemia over 3 years of observation.

The specificities reported to have been associated with CAS are listed in Table 9. (Further discussion of these specificities can be found in refs. 17 and 100 and in Chapter 3 of this book.)

1. Immunochemistry of Pathogenic Cold Autoagglutinins

With rare exceptions, pathogenic cold autoagglutinins are IgM. They exhibit a reversible, thermal-dependent equilibrium reaction with RBCs, with association being favored at lower temperatures. The thermal amplitude depends on the concentration and equilibrium constant of the antibody. The cold agglutinins associated with the chronic idiopathic CAS found in older individuals are almost always monoclonal IgM proteins. Antibodies of the most common specificity (anti-I) almost always have only κ light chains; rare examples of anti-i often have only λ light chains (101–106). The demonstration of the exclusive, or virtually exclusive, occurrence of κ-chains in anti-I cold agglutinins was the first example of a relationship between antibody specificity and light chain type. Amino acid sequence studies, and studies of the N terminal amino acid, of light chains isolated from cold agglutinin light chains, identified glutamic acid as the N terminal amino acid, indicating that they belong to the subgroup VκII (107–108). A restriction within the heavy μ-chains has also been demonstrated by peptide mapping heavy chains of 14 isolated cold agglutinins (109). Thirteen of the 14 belonged to one μ subgroup, as shown by the lack of a particular peptide in 40% of monoclonal M-globulins without known antibody activity (109).

Further immunochemical studies of the heavy chains of IgM cold agglutinins indicated that the μ-chains of different cold agglutinins share antigenic determinants not found on IgM molecules lacking cold agglutinin activity. These specific antigenic determinants appeared to be present on the heavy chains of monoclonal proteins of both anti-I and anti-i specificities (110), and there is one report of similar structural characteristics of a restricted polyclonal protein from a patient with *Mycoplasma pneumoniae* infection (111). Furthermore, antisera specific for the heavy chains of IgM cold agglutinins cross-react with heavy chains of IgA cold agglutinins, which suggests that there is a common idiotypic specificity (110).

Gergely et al. (112) studied the variable regions of four anti-I and two anti-Pr cold

Table 9 Blood Group Antigens Shown to Be Targets for Cold Autoantibodies

I, i, I^T
A*, B, IA, IB, IH*, iH*
Lewis
P
Sialidase-sensitive/protease resistant targets (Gd, Fl, Vo*, Li*)
Sialidase-sensitive/partially protease inactivated targets (Lud, Sa)
Sialidase and protease sensitive targets (Pr)
Miscellaneous (e.g., M, N, R_x, Me, Ju, Om, LW^a*, D)

*Not yet proven to cause hemolytic anemia.

autoagglutinins. Results showed that the heavy chains of four IgM anti-I cold agglutinins were exclusively V_HI subgroups and their light chains were exclusively VκII subgroups. In contrast, the light chains of two cold agglutinins with anti-Pr specificity were not VκII, whereas their heavy chains were not restricted to a single subgroup. The amino acid sequences at the first hypervariable region of light chains (positions 25–35) were similar in two of the four anti-I cold agglutinins. These sequences were different from that of the light chain of another cold agglutinin with anti-Pr specificity. These results supported the concept that only antibodies with the same specificity can share similar primary structure at their antigen-combining sites.

IgG V_H genes are classified into families according to sequence homology. At first it was thought that most of them could be assigned to three major groups: V_HI, V_HII, and V_HIII. Recently, DNA analysis has revealed the presence of three additional V_H families: V_HIV, V_HV, and V_HVI. The V_HIV family was described by Lee et al. (113) as a separate entity from the previously reported V_HII subgroup. Pascual et al. (116) and Silberstein et al. (117) confirmed that pathologenic anti-I cold autoagglutinins are encoded by the $V_H4.21$ heavy chain gene. Pascual et al. (116) showed that a nucleotide change in H chain CDR1 results in the substitution of an asparic acid residue for glycine at position 31, suggesting that this amino acid might be critical to the recognition of I antigen on the RBC. Silberstein et al. (117) studied anti-I and anti-i cold agglutinins from B-cell clones and from the peripheral circulation of patients with lymphoprolifera-tive syndromes. Sequence analyses of expressed variable region genes indicated that both anti-i and anti-I specificities from B-cell clones from two patients were encoded by the $V_H4.21$ or a very closely related V_H4 heavy chain gene, whereas the expressed light chain genes differed. The anti-i–secreting B cells expressed unmutated germline-encoded $V_H4.21$ and VκI gene sequences. The V_H region gene encoding anti-I has the closest homology (97%) to the $V_H4.21$ germline gene and differs at the protein level by only three amino acids. In contrast, although V_L region gene encoding anti-I is most homologous (96%) to the VκIII, kv328 germline gene, there are seven amino acid differences due to nonrandom replacement mutations, which suggests a role for antigen-mediated selection in the anti-I response of this individual. These studies were extended by a structural survey of 20 additional cold agglutinins using antipeptide antibodies specific for determinants V_H and V_L regions. All anti-I and anti-i cold agglutinins were shown to express V_H4 heavy chains, and 14 of 17 cold agglutinins expressed a previously described V_H4 second hypervariable region determinant, termed VH-4-HV2a. It was also found that 13 of 14 anti-I cold agglutinins used VκIII light chains, whereas the anti-i cold agglutinins used light chains from at least three V_L families. Taken together, the data show that anti-i and anti-I cold agglutinins probably both derive from the $V_H4.21$ gene (or a closely related gene). Furthermore, the restricted V_H and different V_L gene use in anti-i and anti-I may reflect the close structural relationship of the i and I antigens. Silverman et al. (114) demonstrated that many anti-I have κIII L chains that express primary sequence-dependent Id determinants linked to the germline gene Humkv325 or a nearly identical gene. By employing antibodies that identified structural determinants within the first framework regions, they found that 10 of 10 κIII anti-I used H chains of protein subgroup II. In another report, the same workers showed that the κIII anti-I cold agglutinins exclusively used heavy chains derived from the V_H4 family (115). Furthermore, these autoantibody heavy chains all expressed the same primary sequence-defined idiotype, corresponding to the second hypervariable region. The structural and genetic correlates of this Id were revealed by the use of a new set of antipeptides corresponding to the sequences of recently reported germline configuration V_H genes. Silberstein discusses more of his work in this area in Chapter 14.

Although most cold agglutinins are IgM, some are IgA (95,118–121) and IgG (95–97,122–128). Cold agglutinins in some patients with infectious mononucleosis and angioimmunoblastic lymphadenopathy have been mixed IgG-IgM. Only occasionally are cold agglutinins cryo-precipitable. Cryoprecipitable anti-I has been observed, but at least one third of anti-i cold agglutinins are cryoprecipitable (129). In 50 patients with CAS, the total concentration of IgM varied from 0.7 to 24.5 mg/ml (130). In most of the patients, the cold agglutinin accounts for the entire elevation of serum IgM above normal levels. In two patients studied by Harboe (130), a homogeneous protein remained in the serum after adsorption with RBC stroma in the cold. This finding was shown to be due to the presence of an additional monoclonal protein without cold agglutinin activity, thus indicating that these were instances of biclonal gammopathy.

Many investigators have noted similarities of laboratory findings in patients with CAS and patients who have monoclonal IgM proteins without cold agglutinin activity. In both instances, bone marrow findings may consist of increased numbers of abnormal lymphoid and plasma cells (131), although Dacie (132) and Firkin et al. (133) reported no excess of plasma cells in patients with CAS. Schubothe (134) analyzed 14 patients with CAS and found 9 had bone marrow lymphocyte counts exceeding 25%; it exceeded 40% in six patients. In one patient, there was an impressive progression of lymphocytic infiltration of the marrow 4 years after the onset of the disease. On the basis of these similarities, some investigators think that a typical case of CAS is probably a variant of Waldenström's macroglobulinemia in which the IgM M-component has cold agglutinin activity (129). However, there are many differences between CAS and patients with macroglobulinemia without cold agglutinin activity (3).

In 1982, Crisp and Pruzanski (135) reported on patients with cold autoagglutinins. Among 78 patients with persistent cold agglutinins, 31 had lymphoma, 13 had Waldenström's macroglobulinemia, 6 had chronic lymphocytic leukemia, and 28 had chronic CAS. The average age was over 60 years. Patients with chronic CAS had more hemolytic crises, bleeding, and Raynaud's phenomena and less frequently lymphadenopathy or hepatosplenomegaly. The frequency of anemia, positive DAT test results, cryoglobulinemia, and Bence Jones proteinuria was similar in the various groups. Survival time from diagnosis was on average 2 years in lymphoma, 2.5 years in Waldenström's macroglobulinemia, more than 6 years in chronic lymphocytic leukemia, and more than 5 years in chronic CAS. Anti-I was common in chronic CAS (74%) and rare in other groups (32–33%). Anti-i and other cold agglutinins were rare in chronic CAS and common in lymphoma and Waldenström's macroglobulinemia. In chronic cold agglutinin disease and in Waldenström's macroglobulinemia, cold agglutinins usually had κ light chains—92 and 71%, respectively, whereas in lymphoma, 71% of cold agglutinins had λ light chains. The type of light chains related to the specificity of cold agglutinins: 58% of IgM/κ were anti-I and 75% of IgM/λ had other specificities. Cold agglutinins were cytotoxic to autologous and allogeneic lymphocytes. Occasionally, more autologous than allogeneic cells were killed, implying that the former may be precoated in vivo with the antibodies. Crisp and Pruzanski (135) concluded that conditions with persistent cold agglutinins are a spectrum that varies from "benign" autoimmunelike chronic cold agglutinin disease to malignant lymphoma. Marked differences in the light chain type of cold agglutinins, specificity toward membranous antigens, and severity of clinical manifestations were noted in benign and malignant varieties.

IV.   SEROLOGICAL/IMMUNOLOGICAL CHARACTERISTICS OF PAROXYSMAL COLD HEMOGLOBINURIA

Paroxysmal cold hemoglobinuria (PCH) is the rarest of the AIHAs. Most commonly encountered is the transient PCH in young children that occurs secondary to infection (3,136,137). The idiopathic chronic form of PCH is rarely seen; we have only encountered four cases in 30 years of studying AIHA.

Because PCH can present so dramatically, it was the first hemolytic anemia to be described, and the diagnostic test (the Donath-Landsteiner test) was the first immunohematological test to be performed (3). Although a cold autoantibody, unlike the antibody causing CAS, the antibody causing PCH is usually IgG, does not agglutinate RBCs efficiently, but activates complement efficiently, and acts as a biphasic hemolysin. This biphasic hemolysin sensitizes RBCs only at a low temperature (it rarely sensitizes RBCs in vitro above 20°C) and causes lysis of the RBCs when they are warmed to 37°C.

Because the IgG antibody is a cold antibody, one would expect it to react in vivo similarly to the IgM antibody associated with CAS. That is to say, one would expect it to sensitize the patient's RBCs when the patient's peripheral circulation falls to a temperature that allows the IgG autoantibody to sensitize the patient's RBCs, but this is not always the case. Patients with PCH often present with hemolysis when their peripheral temperature could not have fallen to the in vitro thermal amplitude (e.g., 15°C) of the biphasic hemolysin. As the IgG autoantibody is an efficient activator of complement and appears to resist elution from the RBCs better than the IgM antibody in CAS, patients often present with signs of intravascular hemolysis (e.g., hemoglobinemia, hemoglobinuria). When the RBCs recirculate to 37°C, the IgG cold auto-antibody elutes from the patient's RBCs into the plasma.

The above theoretical concepts fit fairly well with the clinical/hematological/serological results usually observed with the rare cases of idiopathic chronic PCH in older persons. These patients usually present with a history of intravascular hemolysis following cold exposure. Like most cases of chronic idiopathic CAS, their hemolysis can usually be controlled by keeping them warm. The degree of hemolysis usually parallels the thermal amplitude of the autoantibody. The clinical/hematological/serological findings of the more commonly observed acute transient PCH associated with childhood viremia do not fit well with the theoretical concepts above. These children hemolyze dramatically without necessarily any cold exposure and often keep hemolyzing even when kept warm. Their in vitro serological findings appear similar to the findings of the sera from idiopathic PCH. It is hard to understand why an IgG antibody that will only sensitize RBCs in vitro up to 15°C causes such marked intravascular hemolysis in a patient who is kept at a temperature above 37°C. It would seem that the viral infection plays a role here. Perhaps the RBC membrane is affected to become more susceptible to small amounts of complement activation or the macrophages become hyperactive, although the latter would not explain the dramatic complement-mediated intravascular hemolysis.

A. RBC-Bound Proteins

The DAT result is similar to that of CAS in that only RBC-bound complement (C3dg) is detected. If RBCs are washed at 37°C, no RBC-bound IgG is detected.

B. RBC Autoantibodies Detected in Patients' Sera

The autoantibody associated with PCH is termed a biphasic hemolysin; that is, it sensitizes RBCs in the cold but only hemolyzes them when the RBCs reach 37°C. The diagnostic test is the Donath-Landsteiner (DL) test in which RBCs are incubated with the patient's serum at 0°C (e.g., melting ice) and then moved to 37°C for a further incubation. No lysis occurs following the incubation at 0°C, and no lysis occurs if the incubation is carried out only at 37°C. The thermal amplitude of this antibody is usually less than 20°C; that is, the antibody will still give a positive DL test when the initial incubation is less than 20°C; stronger results will occur as the temperature of the initial incubation is lowered. Rare patients have been described when their DL antibody would sensitize RBCs up to 37°C (139–140).

The autoantibody may sometimes agglutinate RBCs in addition to giving a positive DL test. The agglutination is usually of low titer (<64) at 4°C and of low thermal amplitude (<20°C). The antibody is IgG but is usually only detectable by the IAT if the RBCs are washed with ice-cold saline and ice-cold antiglobulin serum is used following incubation of the patient's serum and RBCs at 0°C. Rare patients have been described whose IgG DL antibody could be detected by the IAT even when the RBCs were washed with saline at RT (139,140).

The DL test is said to be diagnostic for PCH, but on occasions it can be positive when using serum from patients with CAS. These are false-positive results due to the presence of strong monophasic lysins rather than demonstrating the presence of cold biphasic hemolysins. We believe that only about 2% of CAS sera will give a false-positive DL test if untreated RBCs are used, but if enzyme-treated RBCs are used, as suggested by some investigators (136), the false-positive rate will be higher (141).

We found an interesting correlation with positive DL tests and the in vitro reaction of RBCs from patients having positive tests with monocytes (141). Macrophages and monocytes have Fc receptors for IgG1 and IgG3 and the complement receptors CR1 and CR3. The CR1 receptor will interact with C3b, iC3b, and C4b. The CR3 receptor will only react with iC3b. It is said that C3dg and C3d do not interact with mononuclear phagocytes. Thus, we would not expect RBCs from patients with CAS or PCH to react with monocytes or macrophages. Indeed, there is good in vivo evidence that when RBCs reach this state in patients with CAS, they survive relatively normally in vivo. Over the last 10 years, we have tested RBCs from several patients with CAS by a direct MMA and were not surprised to find them nonreactive. More recently, we were surprised to find that RBCs from a patient with PCH that were coated with complement but not IgG reacted quite strongly in the MMA. We studied four more patients with PCH and nine patients with CAS (142). The four cases of PCH all had moderate to strongly C3-coated RBCs; one case had microscopically detectable IgG. All had positive DL tests. All of the selected patients with CAS had moderate to strongly positive DATs due to C3 sensitization; no IgG was detectable. Six of the patients had what appeared to be false-positive DL tests. One case of CAS was studied during a time when the patient was actively hemolyzing and also in remission.

When one speaks of a false-positive DL test, one is usually referring to the finding of lysis in the control tube that has been kept strictly at 37°C and controls for the presence of a warm hemolysin, which may be an alloantibody such as anti-Le^a. The DL test is a test for biphasic hemolysins; that is, ones that sensitize RBCs in the cold and hemolyzes them at 37°C. About 15% of sera from patients with CAS contain monophasic cold hemolysins that will hemolyze untreated RBCs directly at around 20°C (3). Up to 95% of such sera will cause direct lysis of enzyme-treated RBCs at 20°C (3). Thus, theoretically the monophasic cold hemolysin could give a false-positive DL test, and it should be emphasized that no control is usually set up for this when performing the DL test. In practice, we have found only a small percentage of sera from patients with CAS do yield a false-positive DL test, but we should caution that if enzyme-treated RBCs are used for the DL test, then many more false positives may occur, and a control for monophasic lysis set up in parallel should be mandatory.

We retrospectively tested 20 sera from patients with CAS who had monophasic cold hemolysins against untreated RBCs and found only three of them to give false-positive DL tests (141). We have since found that one patient had a trace positive DL test and had monophasic hemolysins only detected with enzyme-treated RBCs. It is difficult to classify this as a false-positive DL test because untreated RBCs were used for the DL test, but perhaps the very weak nature of the positive DL test accounts for this one anomaly. In all other aspects, these six patients had symptoms and serology that was typical of CAS rather than PCH. It should be emphasized that many other patients with CAS did not have positive DL tests even when powerful monophasic cold lysins were present in their sera. Our data suggest that only 2% of all patients with CAS might be expected to give a false-positive DL test if untreated RBCs are used. RBCs from three of the four patients with PCH reacted strongly in the direct MMA (DMMA). That is to say, when their washed RBCs were added to a monocyte monolayer, phagocytosis and/or RBC adherence to the monocytes were seen. The normal range is 0–3%, and the results with the reactive PCH RBCs were 76, 28, and 41%. The RBCs of one patient with PCH did not react with the monocytes, but it should be pointed out that this was a case of virus-induced PCH and the tests were carried out on RBCs taken 10 days following the acute hemolysis and the DL test at that time was very weakly positive. Of great interest was the fact that all six of the RBC samples from the patients with CAS with a positive DL test reacted in the DMMA; results ranged from 7 to 65% reactivity. RBCs from four patients with CAS with negative DL tests all gave less than 3% reactivity in the DMMA. It is of some interest to mention that the first of these four patients is a patient with CAS secondary to *Mycoplasma pneumoniae* infection whose RBCs initially reacted in the DMMA. At the first time of testing, the cold agglutinin titer was 2000 at 4°C and the DL test and the DMMA were positive; 6 weeks later when the hemolytic anemia was in remission and the cold agglutinin titer had dropped to 64 at 4°C and the DL test was negative, the DMMA also was negative. Of interest is the fact that the DAT appeared to be of the same strength (2+ with anti-C3) at both times of testing, but further quantitative analysis was not performed. To confirm what the literature suggests and what we found in our early days of setting up the MMA, we retrospectively examined all our DMMA results from the last few years, with particular reference to any patients whose RBCs were sensitized with C3. We performed DMMAs on 51 patients with only C3 sensitizing their RBCs. Only three gave greater than 3% direct DMMA activity. Two of the three direct MMA results were borderline, being 3.3 and 3.5%, and one was only 4.2%. The DL tests were negative on all three cases (141).

We are left with several questions. Why do patients with PCH have acute intravascular lysis when their biphasic lysins only have an in vivo thermal amplitude of 10–20°C? We and others have found that the MMA correlates quite well with in vivo RBC cell destruction (141). Thus, it is of interest that in vivo complement-sensitized RBCs rarely reacted in the direct MMA unless the associated serum gave a positive DL test. We do not know what makes the RBCs in these cases more palatable to mononuclear phagocytes because the DAT does not differentiate them from the cells that are not reacting. Could the reactive RBCs have C3b or iC3b on the membrane in addition to C3dg? From what we know about the kinetics of C3 breakdown, this is hard to accept. In addition, we did test RBCs from one of the patients with anti-C3c and found the cells to be nonreactive, indicating that the RBCs from this case, which reacted with monocytes, did not have C3b on them. It is also hard to accept that the reactions are due to small amounts of RBC-bound IgG below the threshold of the DAT; we have not found the direct MMA to be an efficient method to detect small amounts of RBC-bound IgG. In addition, one of the reactive RBC samples was tested by ELAT and IgG was not detected by this sensitive procedure. In conclusion, we found that RBCs from patients who have a positive DL test that appear to be coated with C3dg and not IgG react in vitro with monocytes by the MMA regardless of whether the patient has PCH. At present, we do not know why these RBCs are reacting so efficiently with monocytes or why there is a correlation with an in vitro test for biphasic hemolysins in the serum. It will be of great interest to find out whether there is any relationship between these findings and the clinical course in the patients.

The majority of antibodies associated with PCH have P specificity. In 1963, Levine et al. reported that sera from six cases of PCH failed to hemolyze Tj(a-) RBCs by the Donath-Landsteiner test (143). This suggested that the specificity was PP_1P^K. Worlledge and Rousso (144) later showed that RBCs of the rare P^K phenotype were also nonreactive with 11 PCH sera, suggesting that the cold biphasic autohemolysins detectable by the Donath-Landsteiner test were anti-P. Other workers have confirmed these findings (3,145). There are only rare reported cases of any other specificity associated with PCH; these include one example each of anti-I (146), anti-p (147) (which may be anti-Gd) (146), and anti-"Pr-like" (149); Weiner described one example that was originally thought to be anti-HI but was later thought to be another undefined specificity (150). Recently, a case of AIHA associated with IgM monoclonal cold autoagglutinins and monophasic hemolysins with anti-P specificity was described (151). The structure of P system antigens has been well-documented and the P antigen is known to be the glycosphingolipid globoside (GalNAc β[1→3] Gal α[1→4] Gal β[1→4] Glc-Cer). Antibodies causing PCH are inhibited by globoside and Forssman glycolipids (152). Forssman-like antigens are commonly found on bacterial membranes. Judd et al. have described an example of a pH-dependent anti-P (153) and two examples of anti-P that were reactive only at low ionic strength (154).

V. AUTOIMMUNE HEMOLYTIC ANEMIA ASSOCIATED WITH BOTH WARM AND COLD AUTOANTIBODIES

Unusual patients have been described who appear to have serology typical of both WAIHA and CAS (3). These patients usually have IgG and C3 on their RBCs; their serum usually contains an IgG warm autoantibody and a high-titer, high thermal amplitude (e.g., reacting up to 30C) cold agglutinin.

More commonly patients are encountered with IgG warm autoantibodies and IgM cold autoagglutinins that have a normal titer at 4C (<64) but have a high thermal amplitude (i.e., react at 30 or 37C). Some investigators have classified these separately as combined, or "mixed-type" AIHA; these seem to represent 6–8% of all AIHAs (5–8).

VI. AUTOIMMUNE HEMOLYTIC ANEMIA ASSOCIATED WITH CHILDHOOD

Most of the data discussed in previous sections mainly related to adult populations. AIHA presents rather differently in childhood, both clinically and serologically. There are several excellent reviews on childhood AIHA (3,155–159). The results from these and other publications are summarized in Table 10. Differences worth emphasizing between childhood and adult AIHA are the marked increase in transient acute AIHA, the associations with infection, and the much higher incidence of positive Donath-Landsteiner tests in childhood AIHA.

Table 10 Typical Findings Associated with Childhood AIHA that Differ from Adult AIHA[a]

	%	(mean)
Acute AIHA	36–77	(54)
Hemoglobinemia/hemoglobinuria	20	(71% of cases with sudden onset)[b]
Warm AIHA	70–100	(86)
Associated with infection	33–68	(51)
Mortality	6–32	(13)[c]
Positive DL test	5[b]	

[a] Based on 200 children reported in Ref. 156–159.
[b] Reported by Habibi et al. (156).
[c] Some investigators showed that many of these deaths were due to causes other than the hemolytic anemia.

REFERENCES

1. Pirofsky B. Autoimmunization and the Autoimmune Hemolytic Anemias, Baltimore: Williams & Wilkins, 1969.
2. Bottiger LE, Westerholm B. Acquired haemolytic anaemia. Acta Med Scand 1973; 193:223.
3. Petz LD, Garratty G. Acquired Immune Hemolytic Anemias. New York: Churchill Livingstone, 1980.
4. Dacie JV, Worlledge SM. Auto-immune hemolytic anemias. Prog Hematol 1969; 6:82.

5. Sokol RJ, Hewitt S, Stamps BK. Autoimmune haemolysis: An 18-year study of 865 cases referred to a regional transfusion centre. Br Med J 1981; 282:2023.

6. Sokol RJ, Hewitt S, Stamps BK. Autoimmune haemolysis: Mixed warm and cold antibody type. Acta Haematol 1983; 69:266.

7. Shulman IA, Branch DR, Nelson JM, et al. Autoimmune hemolytic anemia with both cold and warm autoantibodies. JAMA 1985; 253:1746.

8. Kajii E, Miura Y, Ikemoto S. Characterization of autoantibodies in mixed-typed autoimmune hemolytic anemia. Vox Sang 1991; 60:45.

9. Garratty G. Laboratory investigation of drug-induced immune hemolytic anemia. In: A Seminar on Laboratory Management of Hemolysis. Washington, DC: American Association of Blood Banks, 1979:1 (suppl).

10. Petz LD, Branch DR. Serological tests for the diagnosis of immune hemolytic anemias. In: McMillan, ed. Immune Cytopenias. New York: Churchill Livingstone, 1983:9.

11. Hsu TCS, Rosenfield RE, Burkart P, et al. Instrumented PVP-augmented antiglobulin tests. Vox Sang 1974; 26:305.

12. Lalezari P, Louie JE, Fadlallah N. Serologic profile of alphamethyldopa-induced hemolytic anemia: Correlation between cell-bound IgM and hemolysis. Blood 1982; 59:61.

13. Ben-Izhak C, Shechter Y, Tatarsky I. Significance of multiple types of antibodies on red blood cells of patients with positive direct antiglobulin test: A study of monospecific antiglobulin reactions in 85 patients. Scand J Haematol 1985; 35:102.

14. Sokol RJ, Hewitt S, Booker DJ, Bailey A. Red cell autoantibodies, multiple immunoglobulin classes, and autoimmune hemolysis. Transfusion 1990; 30:714.

15. Garratty G. Factors affecting the pathogenicity of red cell auto- and alloantibodies. In: Nance SJ, ed. Immune Destruction of Red Blood Cells. Arlington, VA: American Association of Blood Banks, 1989:109.

16. Dacie JV. Autoimmune hemolytic anemia. Arch Intern Med 1975; 135:1293.

17. Engelfriet CP, von dem Borne AEGKr, Beckers D, et al. Immune destruction of red cells. In: Bell CA, ed. A Seminar on Immune-Mediated Cell Destruction. Washington, DC: American Association of Blood Banks, 1981:93.

18. Engelfriet CP, Overbeeke MAM, von dem Borne AEGKr. Autoimmune hemolytic anemia. Semin Hematol 1992; 29:3.

19. Garratty G. Target antigens for red-cell-bound autoantibodies. In: Nance ST, ed. Clinical and Basic Science Aspects of Immunohematology. Arlington, VA: American Association of Blood Banks, 1991:33.

20. Weiner W, Vos GH. Serology of acquired hemolytic anemias. Blood 1963; 22:606.

21. Celano MJ, Levine P. Anti-LW specificity in autoimmune acquired hemolytic anemia. Transfusion 1967; 7:265.

22. Marsh WL, Reid ME, Scott EP. Autoantibodies of U blood group specificity in autoimmune haemolytic anaemia. Br J Haematol 1972; 22:625.

23. Vos GH, Petz LD, Garratty G, Fudenberg HH. Autoantibodies in acquired hemolytic anemia with special reference to the LW system. Blood 1973; 42:445.

24. Victoria EJ, Pierce SW, Branks MJ, Masouredis SP. IgG red blood cell autoantibodies in autoimmune hemolytic anemia bind to epitopes on red blood cell membrane band 3 glycoprotein. J Lab Clin Med 1990; 115:74.

25. Issitt PD, Zellner DC, Rolih SD, Duckett JB. Autoantibodies mimicking alloantibodies. Transfusion 1977; 17:531.

26. Salama A, Mueller-Eckhardt C. Delayed hemolytic transfusion reactions. Transfusion 1984; 24:188.

27. Ness PM, Shirey RS, Thomas SK, Buck SA. The differentiation of delayed serologic and delayed hemolytic transfusion reactions: Incidence, long-term serologic findings, and clinical significance. Transfusion 1990; 30:688.

28. Garratty G. The effect of cell-bound proteins on the in vivo survival of circulating blood cells. Gerontology 1991; 37:68.

29. Kay MMB. Senescent cell antigen: A red cell aging antigen. In: Garratty G, ed. Red Cell Antigens and Antibodies. Arlington, VA: American Association of Blood Banks, 1986:35.

30. Galili U, Flechner I, Knyszynski A, et al. The natural anti-galactosyl IgG on human normal senescent red blood cells. Br J Haematol 1986; 62:317.

31. Branch DR, Shulman IA, Sy Siok Hian AL, Petz LD. Two distinct categories of warm autoantibody reactivity with age-fractionated red cells. Blood 1984; 63:177.

32. Arndt P, O'Hoski P, McBride J, Garratty G. Autoimmune hemolytic anemia associated with an antibody reacting preferentially with "old" red cells. Transfusion 1989; 29:48S (asbtr).

33. Hauke G, Fauser AA, Weber S, Maas D. Reticulocytopenia in severe autoimmune hemolytic anemia (AIHA) of the warm antibody type. Blut 1983; 46:321.

34. Mangan KF, Besa EC, Shadduck RK, et al. Demonstration of two distinct antibodies in autoimmune hemolytic anemia with reticulocytopenia and red cell aplasia. Exp Hematol 1984; 12:788.

35. Kosmin M, Tarantolo S, Arndt P, Garratty G. Cold agglutinin syndrome associated with an autoagglutinin reacting preferentially with young red cells (abstr). In: Book of Abstracts from the ISBT/AABB Joint Congress. Arlington, VA: American Association of Blood Banks, 1990:86.

36. Lutz HU, Wipf G. Naturally occurring autoantibodies to skeletal proteins from human red blood cells. J Immunol 1982; 128:1695.

37. Wiener E, Hughes-Jones NC, Irish WT, Wickramasinghe SN. Elution of antispectrin antibodies from red cells in homozygous β-thalassaemia. Clin Exp Immunol 1986; 63:680.

38. Wakui H, Imai H, Kobayashi R, et al. Autoantibody against erythrocyte protein 4.1 in a patient with autoimmune hemolytic anemia. Blood 1988; 72:402.

39. Out HJ, de Groot PG, van Vliet M, de Gast GC, et al. Antibodies to platelets in patients with anti-phospholipid antibodies. Blood 1991; 77:2655.

40. Hazeltine M, Rauch Y, Danoff D, et al. Antiphospholipid antibodies in systemic lupus erythematosus: Evidence of an association with positive Coombs' and hypocomplementemia. J Rheumatol 1988; 15:80.

41. Sthoeger Z, Sthoeger D, Green L, Geltner D. The role of anti-cardiolipin autoantibodies in the pathogenesis of autoimmune hemolytic anemia (abstr). Blood 76 (suppl):392a.

42. Cabral AR, Cabiedes J, Alarcon-Segovia D. Hemolytic anemia related to an IgM autoantibody to phosphatidylcholine that binds in vitro to stored and to bromelain-treated human erythrocytes. J Autoimmun 1990; 3:773.

43. Arvieux J, Schweizer B, Roussel B, Colomb MG. Autoimmune haemolytic anaemia due to anti-phospholipid antibodies. Vox Sang 1991; 61:190.

44. Masouredis SP, Branks MJ, Garratty G, Victoria EJ. Immunospecific red cell binding of iodine-125-labeled immunoglobulin G erythrocyte autoantibodies. J Lab Clin Med 1987; 110:308.

45. Masouredis SP, Branks MJ, Victoria EJ. Antiidiotypic IgG crossreactive with Rh alloantibodies in red cell autoimmunity, Blood 1987; 70:710.

46. Chaplin H, Jr. Clinical usefulness of specific antiglobulin reagents in autoimmune hemolytic anemias. Prog Hematol 1973; 7:25.

47. Garratty G, Arndt P, Nance S, Postoway N. Low affinity autoantibodies—a cause of false negative direct antiglobulin tests. In: Book of Abstracts from the ISBT/AABB Joint Congress (abstr). Arlington, VA: American Association of Blood Banks, 1990:87.

48. Gilliland BC, Leddy JP, Vaughan JH. The detection of cell-bound antibody on complement-coated human red cells. J Clin Invest 1970; 49:898.

49. Gilliland BC, Baxter E, Evans RS. Red-cell antibodies in acquired hemolytic anemia with negative antiglobulin serum tests. N Engl J Med 1971; 285:252.

50. Garratty G, Postoway N, Nance S, Brunt D. The detection of IgG on the red cells of "Coombs negative" autoimmune hemolytic anemias (abstr). Transfusion 1982; 22:430.

51. Garratty G, Postoway N, Nance S, Arndt P. Detection of IgG on red cells of patients with suspected direct antiglobulin test negative autoimmune hemolytic anemia (AIHA) (abstr). Book of Abstracts from the ISBT/AABB Joint Congress. Arlington, VA: American Association of Blood Banks, 1990:87.

52. Sokol RJ, Hewitt S, Booker DJ, Stamps R. Enzyme linked direct antiglobulin tests in patients with autoimmune haemolysis. J Clin Pathol 1985; 38:912.

53. Gutgsell NS, Issitt PD, Tomasulo PA, Hervis L. Use of the direct enzyme-linked antiglobulin test (ELAT) in patients with unexplained anemia (abstr). Transfusion 1988; 28:36S.

54. Sokol RJ, Hewitt S, Booker DJ, Stamps R. Small quantities of erythrocyte bound immunoglobulins and autoimmune haemolysis. J Clin Pathol 1987; 40:254.

55. Schmitz N, Djibey I, Kretschmer V, Mahn I, Mueller-Eckhardt C. Assessment of red cell autoantibodies in autoimmune hemolytic anemia of warm type by a radioactive anti-IgG test. Vox Sang 1981; 41:224.

56. Yam P, Petz LD, Spath P. Detection of IgG sensitization of red cells with ^{125}I staphylococcal protein A. Am J Hematol 1982; 12:337.

57. Owen I, Hows J. Evaluation of the manual hexadimethrine bromide (Polybrene) technique in the investigation of autoimmune hemolytic anemia. Transfusion 1990; 30:814.

58. Sturgeon P, Smith LE, Chun HMT, et al. Autoimmune hemolytic anemia associated exclusively with IgA of Rh specificity. Transfusion 1979; 19:324.

59. Wager O, Haltia K, Räsänen JA, Vuopio P. Five cases of positive antiglobulin test involving IgA warm type autoantibody. Ann Clin Res 1971; 3:76.

60. Stratton F, Rawlinson VI, Chapman SA, et al. Acquired hemolytic anemia associated with IgA anti-e. Transfusion 1972; 12:157.

61. Suzuki S, Amano T, Mitsunaga M, et al. Autoimmune hemolytic anemia associated with IgA autoantibody. Clin Immunol Immunopathol 1981; 21:247.

62. Wolf CFW, Wolf DJ, Peterson P, et al. Autoimmune hemolytic anemia with predominance of IgA autoantibody, Transfusion 1982; 22:238.

63. Clark DA, Dessypris EN, Jenkins DE Jr, Krantz SB. Acquired immune hemolytic anemia associated with IgA erythrocyte coating: investigation of hemolytic mechanisms. Blood 1984; 64:1000.

64. Kowal-Vern A, Jacobson P, Okuno T, Blank J. Negative direct antiglobulin test in autoimmune hemolytic anemia. Am J Pediatr Hematol Oncol 1986; 8:349.

65. Reusser P, Osterwalder B, Burri H, Speck B. Autoimmune hemolytic anemia associated with IgA—Diagnostic and therapeutic aspects in a case with long-term follow-up. Acta Haematol 1987; 77:53.

66. Göttsche B, Salama A, Mueller-Eckhardt C. Autoimmune hemolytic anemia associated with an IgA autoanti-Gerbich. Vox Sang 1990; 58:211.

67. Girelli G, Perrone MP, Adorno G, et al. A second example of hemolysis due to IgA autoimmunity with anti-e specificity. Haematologica 1990; 75:182.

68. Fanger MW, Goldstine SN, Shen L. Cytofluorographic analysis of receptors for IgA in human polymorphonuclear cells and monocytes and the correlation of receptor expression with phagocytosis. Mol Immunol 1983; 20:1019.

69. Shen L, Maliszewski CR, Rigby WFC, Fanger MW. IgA-mediated effector function of HL-60 cells following treatment with calcitriol. Mol Immunol 1986; 23:611.

70. Yeaman GR, Kerr MA. Opsonization of yeast by human serum IgA anti-mannan antibodies and phagocytosis by human polymorphonuclear leucocytes. Clin Exp Immunol 1987; 68:200.

71. Shen L, Fanger MW. Secretory IgA antibodies synergize with IgG in promoting ADCC by human polymorphonuclear cells, monocytes, and lymphocytes. Cell Immunol 1981; 59:75.

72. Maliszewski CR, March CJ, Schoenborn MA, et al. Expression cloning of a human Fc receptor for IgA. J Exp Med 1990; 172:1665.

73. Clark DA, Dessypris EN, Jenkins DE, Jr, Kurtz SB. Acquired immune hemolytic anemia associated with IgA erythrocyte coating: investigation of hemolytic mechanisms. Blood 1984; 64:1000.

74. Salama A, Bhakdi S, Mueller-Eckhardt C. Evidence suggesting the occurrence of C3-independent intravascular immune hemolysis. Transfusion 1987; 27:49.

75. Vos GH, Petz LD, Fudenberg HH. Specificity and immunoglobulin characteristics of auto-antibodies in acquired hemolytic anemia. J Immunol 1971; 106:1172.

76. von dem Borne AEGKr, Engelfriet CP, van der Kort-Henkes G, et al. Autoimmune haemolytic anaemias: II. Warm haemolysins: Serological and immunochemical investigations and ^{51}Cr studies. Clin Exp Immunol 1969; 4:333.

77. von dem Borne AEGKr, Engelfriet CP, Reynierse E, et al. Autoimmune haemolytic anaemias. VI. 51-Chromium survival studies in patients with different kinds of warm autoantibodies. Clin Exp Immunol 1973; 13:561.

78. Wolf MW, Roelcke D. Incomplete warm hemolysins. I. Case reports, serology, and immunoglobulin classes. Clin Immunol Immunopathol 1989; 51:55.

79. Wolf MW, Roelcke D. Incomplete warm hemolysins. II. Corresponding antigens and pathogenetic mechanisms in autoimmune hemolytic anemias induced by incomplete warm hemolysins. Clin Immunol Immunopathol 1989; 51:68.

80. Freedman J, Newlands M, Johnson CA. Warm IgM anti-I^T causing autoimmune haemolytic anaemia. Vox Sang 1977; 32:135.

81. Schanfield MS, Pisciotta A, Libnock J. Seven cases of hemolytic anemia associated with warm IgM autoantibodies (abstr). Transfusion 1978; 18:623.

82. Freedman J, Wright J, Lim FC, Garvey MB. Hemolytic warm IgM autoagglutinins in autoimmune hemolytic anemia. Transfusion 1987; 27:464.

83. Salama A, Mueller-Eckhardt M. Autoimmune haemolytic anaemia in childhood associated with non-complement binding IgM autoantibodies. Br J Haematol 1987; 65:67.

84. Shirey RS, Kickler TS, Bell W, et al. Fatal immune hemolytic anemia and hepatic failure associated with a warm-reacting IgM autoantibody. Vox Sang 1987; 52:219.

85. Garratty G, Brunt D, Greenfield T, et al. An auto anti-En^a mimicking an allo anti-En^a associated with pure red cell aplasia, Transfusion, 23:408 (abstract).

86. Garratty G, Arndt P, Clarke A, and Domen, R. Fatal hemolysis associated with an IgM anti-En^a warm autoagglutinin. In: Book of Abstracts from the ISBT/AABB Joint Congress (abstr). Arlington, VA: American Association of Blood Banks, 1990:154.

87. Arndt P, Clarke A, Domen R, et al. Two cases of severe warm type autoimmune hemolytic anemia associated with IgM anti-En^a and anti-Pr (abstr). Transfusion 31:28S.

88. Dorner IM, Parker CW, Chaplin H Jr. Autoagglutination developing in a patient with acute renal failure. Br J Haematol 1968; 14:383.

89. Kuipers EJ, van Imhoff GW, Hazenberg CAM, Smit J. Anti-H IgM (kappa) autoantibody mediated severe intravascular haemolysis associated with malignant lymphoma. Br J Haematol 1991; 78:283.

90. Ellis JP, Sokol RJ. Detection of IgM autoantibodies in eluates from red blood cells. Clin Lab Haemat 1990; 12:9.

91. Kay NE, Douglas SD, Mond JJ, et al. Hemolytic anemia with serum and erythrocyte-bound low-molecular-weight IgM. Clin Immunol Immunopathol 1975; 4:216.

92. Szymanski IO, Huff SR, Selbovitz LG, Sherwood GK. Erythrocyte sensitization with monomeric IgM in a patient with hemolytic anemia. Am J Hematol 1984; 17:71.

93. Dankbar DT, Pierce SR, Issitt PD, et al. Fatal intravascular hemolysis associated with auto anti-Wr^b (abstr). Transfusion 1987; 27:534.

94. Postoway N, Anstee DJ, Wortman M, Garratty G. A severe transfusion reaction associated with anti-En^{a}TS in a patient with an abnormal alpha-like red cell sialoglycoprotein. Transfusion 1988; 28:77.

95. Ratkin GA, Osterland CK, Chaplin H. Jr. IgG, IgA, and IgM cold-reactive immunoglobulins in 19 patients with elevated cold agglutinins. J Lab Clin Med 1973; 82:67.

96. Dellagi K, Brouet JC, Schenmetzler C, Praloran V. Chronic hemolytic anemia due to a monoclonal IgG cold agglutinin with anti-Pr specificity. Blood 1981; 57:189.

97. Silberstein LE, Berkman EM, Schreiber AD. Cold hemagglutinin disease associated with IgG cold-reactive antibody. Ann Intern Med 1987; 106:238.

98. Garratty G, Petz LD, Hoops JK. The correlation of cold agglutinin titrations in saline and albumin with haemolytic anaemia. Br J Haematol 1977; 35:587.

99. Sniecinski I, Margolin K, Shulman I, et al. High-titer, high-thermal-amplitude cold autoagglutinin not associated with hemolytic anemia. Vox Sang 1988; 55:26.

100. Roelcke D. Cold agglutination. Transfus Med Rev 1989; 3:140.

101. Harboe M, Lind K. Light chain type of transiently occurring cold haemagglutinins. Scand J Haematol 1966; 3:269.

102. Harboe M, Furth R, van Schubothe H, et al. Exclusive occurrence of ξ-chains in isolated cold agglutinins. Scand J Haematol 1965; 2:259.

103. Cooper AG, Worlledge SM. Light chains in chronic cold hemagglutinin disease. Nature 1967; 214:799.

104. Feizi T. Lambda chains in cold agglutinins. Science 1967; 156:1111.

105. Capra JP, Kehoe JM, Williams RC Jr, et al. Light chain sequences of human IgM cold agglutinins. Proc Natl Acad Sci Wash 1972; 69:40.

106. Cooper AG, Chavin SI, Franklin FC. Predominance of a single mu chain subclass in cold agglutinin heavy chains. Immunochemistry 1970; 7:479.
107. Edman P, Cooper AG. Amino acid sequence at the N-terminal end of a cold agglutinin kappa chain. Fed Eur Biochem Soc Lett 1968; 2:33.
108. Cohen S, Cooper AG. Chemical differences between individual cold agglutinins, Immunology 1968; 15:93.
109. Cooper AG, Chavin SI, Franklin EC. Predominance of a single mu chain subclass in cold agglutinin heavy chains. Immunochemistry 1970; 7:479.
110. Williams RC, Jr. Cold agglutinins: Studies of primary structure, serologic activity, and antigenic uniqueness. NY Acad Sci Ann 1971; 190:330.
111. Jacobson LB, Longstreth GF. Clinical and immunologic features of transient cold agglutinin hemolytic anemia. Am J Med 1973; 54:514.
112. Gergely J, Wang AC, Fudenberg HH. Chemical analyses of variable regions of heavy and light chains of cold agglutinins. Vox Sang 1973; 24:432.
113. Lee KH, Matsuda F, Kinashi T, et al. A novel family of variable region genes of the human immunoglobulin heavy chain. J Mol Biol 1987; 195:761.
114. Silverman GJ, Goni F, Chen PP, et al. Distinct patterns of heavy chain variable region subgroup use by human monoclonal autoantibodies of different specificity. J Exp Med 1986; 168:2361.
115. Silverman GJ, Carson DA. Structural characterization of human monoclonal cold agglutinins: Evidence for a distinct primary sequence-defined V_H4 idiotype. Eur J Immunol 1990; 20:351.
116. Pascual V, Victor K, Lesz D, et al. Nucleotide sequence analysis of the V regions of two IgM cold agglutinins. J Immunol 1991; 146:4386.
117. Silberstein LE, Jefferies LC, Goldman J, et al. Variable region gene analysis of pathologic human autoantibodies to the related i and I red blood cell antigens. Blood 1991; 78:2372.
118. Garratty G, Petz LD, Brodsky I, et al. An IgA high-titer cold agglutinin with an unusual blood group specificity within the Pr complex. Vox Sang 1973; 25:32.
119. Roelcke D. Specificity of IgA cold agglutinins: Anti-Pr$_1$, Eur J Immunol 1973; 3:206.
120. Roelcke D, Dorow W. Besonderheiten der Reaktionswerte eines mit Plasmocytom-y A-Paraprotein identischen Kalteagglutinins. Klin Wachenschr 1968; 46:126.
121. Angevine CD, Bajtai G. A cold agglutinin of the IgA class. J Immunol 1966; 96:578.
122. Tonthat H, Rochant H, Henry A, et al. A new case of monoclonal IgA kappa cold agglutinin with anti-Pr$_1$d specificity in a patient with persistent HB antigen cirrhosis. Vox Sang 1976; 30:464.
123. Mullinax F, Mullinax GL, Himrod B, Brandt CW. Cold agglutination syndrome associated with IgA monoclonal gammopathy (abstr). Arthritis Rheum 1968; 11:500.
124. Tschirhart DL, Kunekl L, Shulman IA. Immune hemolytic anemia associated with biclonal cold autoagglutinins, Vox Sang 1990; 59:222.
125. Ambrus M, Bajtai G. A case of an IgG-type cold agglutinin disease. Haematologia 1969; 3:225.
126. Goldberg LS, Barnett EV. Mixed IgG IgM cold agglutinin, J Immunol 1967; 99:803.
127. Silberstein LE, Shoenfeld Y, Schwartz RS, Berkman EM. A combination of IgG and IgM autoantibodies in chronic cold agglutinin disease: Immunologic studies and response to splenectomy. Vox Sang 1985; 48:105.
128. Szymanski IO, Teno R, Rybak ME. Hemolytic anemia due to a mixture of low-titer IgG lambda and IgM lambda agglutinins reacting optimally at 22C. Vox Sang 1986; 51:112.
129. Pruzanski W, Shumak KH. Biologic activity of cold-reacting autoantibodies. N Engl J Med 1977; 297:538 and 583.
130. Harboe M. Cold auto-agglutinins. Vox Sang 1971; 20:289.
131. Ritzmann SE, Levin WC. Cold agglutinin disease: A type of primary macroglobulinemia: A new concept. Tex Rep Biol Med 1962; 20:236.
132. Dacie JV. The Haemolytic Anaemias, 2nd ed. London: Churchill, 1962.
133. Firkin BG, Blackwell JB, Johnston GA. Essential cryoglobulinaemia and acquired haemolytic anaemia due to cold agglutinins. Aust Ann Med 1959; 8:151.
134. Schubothe H. The cold hemagglutinin disease. Semin Hematol 1966; 3:27.
135. Crisp D, Pruzanski W. B-cell neoplasms with homogeneous cold-reacting antibodies (cold agglutinins). Am J Med 1982; 72:915.

136. Wolach B, Heddle N, Barr RD, et al. Transient Donath-Landsteiner haemolytic anaemia. Br J Haematol 1981; 48:425.

137. Göttsche B, Salama A, Mueller-Eckhardt C. Donath-Landsteiner autoimmune hemolytic anemia in children. Vox Sang 1990; 58:281.

138. Ries CA, Garratty G, Petz LD, Fudenberg HH. Paroxysmal cold hemoglobinuria: Report of a case with an exceptionally high thermal range Donath-Landsteiner antibody. Blood 1971; 38:491.

139. Lindgren S, Zimmerman S, Gibbs F, Garratty G. An unusual Donath-Landsteiner antibody detectable at 37C by the antiglobulin test. Transfusion 1985; 25:142.

140. Nordhagen R. Two cases of paroxysmal cold hemoglobinuria with a Donath-Landsteiner antibody reactive by the indirect antiglobulin test using anti-IgG. Transfusion 1991; 31:190.

141. Garratty G, Nance S, Arndt P, Postoway N. Positive direct monocyte monolayer assays associated with positive Donath Landsteiner tests (abstr). Transfusion 1989; 29:49S.

142. Garratty G. Predicting the clinical significance of red cell antibodies with in vitro cellular assays. Transfus Med Rev 1990; 4:297.

143. Levine P, Celano MJ, Falkowski F. The specificity of the antibody in paroxysmal cold hemoglobinuria (PCH). Transfusion 1963; 3:278.

144. Worlledge SM, Rousso C. Studies on the serology of paroxysmal cold haemoglobinuria (PCH), with special reference to its relationship with the P blood group system. Vox Sang 1965; 10:293.

145. Heddle NM. Acute paroxysmal cold hemoglobinuria. Transfus Med Rev 1989; 3:219.

146. Bell CA, Zwicker H, Rosenbaum DL. Paroxysmal cold hemoglobinuria (PCH) following mycoplasma infection: Anti-I specificity of the biphasic hemolysin. Transfusion 1973; 13:138.

147. Engelfriet CP, Beckers D, von dem Borne AEGKr, et al. Haemolysins probably recognizing the antigen P. Vox Sang 1971; 23:176.

148. Roelcke D. Cold agglutination. Transfus Med Rev 1989; 3:140.

149. Judd WJ, Wilkinson SL, Issitt PD, et al. Donath-Landsteiner hemolytic anemia due to anti-Pr-like biphasic hemolysin. Transfusion 1986; 26:423.

150. Weiner W. The specificity of the antibodies in acquired haemolytic anaemias. In: Proceedings of the Joint Meeting of the 10th Congress of the International Society of Haematology/10th Congress of the International Society of Blood Transfusion, Stockholm 1964:24.

151. von dem Borne AEGKr, Mol JJ, Joustra-Maas N, et al. Autoimmune haemolytic anaemia with monoclonal IgM (K) anti-P cold autohaemolysins. Br J Haematol 1982; 50:345.

152. Schwarting GA, Kundu SK, Marcus DM. Reaction of antibodies that cause paroxysmal cold hemoglobinuria (PCH) with globoside and Forssman glycosphingolipids. Blood 1979; 53:186.

153. Judd WJ. A pH-dependent auto-agglutinin with anti-P specificity. Transfusion 1975; 15:373.

154. Judd WJ, Steiner EA, Capps RD. Autoagglutinins with apparent anti-P specificity reactive only by low-ionic-strength salt techniques. Transfusion 1982; 22:185.

155. Zuelzer WW, Mastrangelo R, Stulberg CS, et al. Autoimmune hemolytic anemia. Natural history and viral-immunologic interactions in childhood. Am J Med 1970; 49:80.

156. Habibi B, Homberg J-C, Schaison G, Salmon C. Autoimmune hemolytic anemia in children. Am J Med 1974; 56:61.

157. Zupanska B, Lawkowicz W, Gorska B, et al. Autoimmune haemolytic anaemia in children. Br J Haematol 1976; 34:511.

158. Buchanan GR, Boxer LA, Nathan DG. The acute and transient nature of idiopathic immune hemolytic anemia in childhood. J Pediatr 1976; 88:780.

159. Carapella de Luca E, Casadei AM, di Piero G, et al. Auto-immune haemolytic anaemia in childhood. Vox Sang 1979; 36:13.

19

Drug-Induced Immune Hemolytic Anemia

GEORGE GARRATTY

American Red Cross Blood Services
and University of California, Los Angeles
Los Angeles, California

I. INTRODUCTION

Drugs were first suspected as a cause of immune hemolytic anemia (IHA) in 1953 (1) when Snapper described a patient who developed pancytopenia with hemolytic anemia, associated with a positive direct antiglobulin test (DAT), following infestion of mephenytoin (Mesantoin). Harris (2) was the first to document carefully the history and serology of a case of immune hemolytic anemia (IHA) due to a drug. The drug, stibophen, was used to treat schistosomiasis. The patient had received a course of stibophen injection 10 years previously with no problems. During the second course of infections, the patient developed acute intravascular hemolysis. The DAT was positive, and the patient's serum was shown to react with allogeneic RBCs only when the drug was present. The stibophen was stopped and the patient's hemoglobin returned to normal in 20 days; the serology became negative after about 60 days.

In 1967, Dausset and Contu (3) reviewed the literature on drug-induced IHA and found only 34 published cases due to 15 drugs. In 1969, Worlledge (4) added six more cases but no other drugs to the list. By 1980, we had found reports of approximately 33 drugs as causes of IHA (5). In 1989, the list had grown to over 50 drugs that were reasonably well-documented as causes of IHA (6); many more less well-documented examples also have appeared in the literature. Table 1 shows the latest list of 71 drugs with reasonable published evidence that they have caused IHA and/or positive DATs.

Although 30% of fatal blood dyscrasias are said to be due to drugs (7), drug-induced IHA is quite rare; drug-induced immune thrombocytopenia is much more common. If 1 in 80,000 of the population has autoimmune hemolytic anemia (AIHA) and about 10% of these are due to drugs (5), then drug-induced IHA probably occurs in about 1 case per million of the population. It is not clear whether the rare patients that have drug-induced IHA are different because only rare patients make drug antibodies or whether these antibodies are more pathogenic in some special individuals.

II. THE IMMUNE RESPONSE TO DRUGS

Drugs are small molecular weight substances (e.g., penicillin has a molecular weight of 300 kd). Because of their size, it is usually assumed that drugs act as haptens to evoke an immune

Table 1 Drugs that Have Caused Immune Hemolytic Anemia
and/or Positive Direct Antiglobulin Tests (DATs)[a]

Acetaminophen	Cianidanol	Methysergide
Amphotericin B	Cisplatin	Nafcillin
Ampicillin	Cyclofenil	Nomifensine
Antazoline	Diglycoaldehyde	p-aminosalicylic acid
Apronal	Dipyrone	Penicillin G
Butizide	Erythromycin	Phenacetin
Carbenicillin	Fenoprofen	Podophyllotoxin
Carbimazole	Fluorouracil (5-FU)	Probenecid
Carbromal	Fluorsemide	Procainamide
Cefamandole	Glafenine	Pyramidon
Cefazolin	Hydralazine	Quinidine
Cefotaxime	Hydrochlorothiazide	Quinine
Cefotetan	9-Hydroxy-methyl-	Ranitidine
Cefoxitin	ellipticinium	Rifampicin
Ceftazidime	Ibuprofen	Sodium pentothal
Ceftriaxone	Insulin	Streptomycin
Cephalexin	Isoniazid	Sulphoamides
Cephaloridine	Latamoxef	Teniposide
Cephalothin	Levodopa	Tetracycline
Chlorinated	Mefenamic acid	Thiopental
hydrocarbons	Melphalan	Tolbutamide
(insecticides)	Methadone	Tolmetin
Chlorpropamide	Methicillin	Triamterene
Chlorpromazine	Methotrexate	Trimellitic anhydride
	Methyldopa	Zomepirac

[a]Drugs were included only when reasonable evidence was presented in the
literature to support that they caused the immune reaction. There are many
more reported, but the evidence that they caused a positive DAT or drug-
induced HA is often minimal or totally lacking.

response. If a hapten forms stable bonds with macromolecules (e.g., protein), the resulting drug-protein conjugate may be immunogenic (8–10). Haptens that form stable bonds with proteins do so with nucleophilic groups on proteins. Nucleophilic groups on proteins include lysyl and cysteinyl residues and the imidazole and phenol groups present in histidine and tyrosine, respectively (10). De Weck (11) points out that since Landsteiner's original observations (8), many immunologists have come to consider haptens as substances of low molecular weight and the word *conjugate* as implying covalent binding between the haptenic group and the carrier molecule. However, in its original meaning as used by Landsteiner, the term *hapten* (from the Greek ηαπεν to fasten) did not imply a notion of size for the haptenic molecule. It did not imply covalent binding between the haptenic group and the carrier. Although the classic concepts of an immune response to low molecular weight substances involves covalent bonding, exceptions have been described. The Forssman hapten, for example, becomes immunogenic upon binding to an immunogenic carrier (or Schlepper) through noncovalent bonds. Nucleic acids and oligonucleotides, which are acidic polymers, can be immunogenic if complexed to basic protein carriers (e.g., methylated bovine albumin) (11–13); thus, it would appear that multiple salt linkages may be sufficient to allow a haptenic response.

The immune response to drugs is affected by the nature of the carrier molecule, the degree of conjugation (epitope density), and the nature of the chemical bond. Administration of benzylpenicillin (BP) to rats at doses up to 2.7 mmol/kg (1g/1kg) does not evoke antibodies to the benzylpenicilloyl (BPO) determinant, but a 1 million-fold lower dose of BP conjugated to a foreign protein is readily immunogenic (14). Kristoffersen et al. (15) reported that a conjugate that contained 11 penicillyl residues per each bovine serum albumin molecule induced a significant antibody response in mice after a single injection. When the ratio is less than 1, as may be anticipated during therapeutic administration, there is no detectable response even after three injections.

The haptenic group formed by small reactive substances generally represents only a portion of the antigen determinant, which may also encompass part of the macromolecular carrier (8,16). A good example of this is represented in Figure 1, which shows the heterogeneity of the combining sites of antibodies to p-azobenzoate coupled to protein (16). Drugs that are hydrolysed rapidly will not function as effective haptens (10). The chemical structure of the antigenic determinant comprising the drug, or its metabolite, and carrier component may be quite different from that of the parent drug, and the antibodies formed may not react with the parent drug in vitro (see below).

Most of the drugs listed in Table 1 probably do not form stable (e.g., covalent) bonds with proteins. This is simply illustrated by the fact that RBCs cannot be coated in vitro with most of the drugs (i.e., they are removed by simply washing the RBCs after incubation in the drug), presumably because the drugs do not combine well with membrane proteins. A few of the drugs (e.g., quinidine) have been studied by more sophisticated methods and have been proven to have a low affinity for protein (see below). Penicillin, and probably closely related drugs such as some of the cephalosporins, do form stable covalent bonds with protein (e.g., on RBC membranes). Penicillins contain a structure that reacts with nucleophilic amino, hydroxy, mercapto, and histidine groups. A number of sites on the penicillin molecule are open to nucleophilic attack and, therefore, a number of antigenic determinants may be formed. The major haptenic determinant is the BPO group (17–25). Cephalosporins are related to penicillins in that both contain a β-lactam ring; cephalosporins have a dihydrothiazine ring, whereas penicillins have a thiazolidine ring. Cephalosporins probably form a cephalosporyl group equivalent to the penicilloyl group, but there is no conclusive evidence for this. The chemistry of hapten formation by cephalosporins has been hindered by the fact that a number of unstable intermediates are formed during aminolysis of cephaloporins (10).

A few other drugs have been shown to combine with RBC membranes efficiently enough

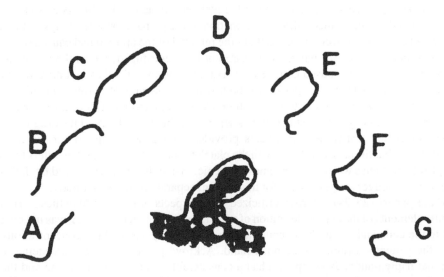

Figure 1 Portions of the van der Waal's outline of the p-azobenzoate group coupled to protein that are reactive with various antibodies (16), A–G = antibody combining sites of different antibody molecules.

Table 2 Drugs that Have Been Shown to
Combine with the RBC Membrane in Vitro
Efficiently Enough to Withstand Multiple
Washes

Penicillins (most)
Cephalosporins (some)
Cisplatin
Carbimazole
Carbromal
Cianidanol
Erythromycin
Streptomycin
Tolbutamide

to withstand multiple washes, but the exact mechanism of cell binding is unknown. Table 2 lists these drugs.

A major question is how do drugs that are not listed in Table 2 act as immunogens? In 1949, Ackroyd described a case of thrombocytopenia due to apronal (Sedormid) (26). Ackroyd suggested an immune basis for apronal-induced thrombocytopenia. In a series of papers, he suggested that the apronal, acting as a hapten, bound loosely to the platelet membrane modifying it sufficiently to render it autoantigenic (26–29). It was noticed that if the platelets were washed in saline after being allowed to react with the patient's serum and the drug in the absence of complement, both the antibody and the drug (apronal) were removed from the platelets. This observation suggested a simple method by which it might be possible to discover the role of apronal in the reaction causing platelet agglutination and lysis and complement fixation. It was assumed that as apronal was so loosely attached to platelets, it might be possible to remove it from combination with platelets and antibody by dialysis. This was found to be so. It was also found that if platelets that had been suspended in the serum of a sensitive patient in the presence of apronal, but in the absence of complement, were washed not in saline but in a saturated solution of apronal in saline, then the antibody remained in contact with the platelets. Platelets that had been treated in this way were then dialysed against saline. Examination of the preparation after dialysis showed that not only had dialysis removed the apronal but the removal of the apronal had caused dissociation of platelets and antibody; for when the preparation was centrifuged, the antibody was found in the supernatant fluid and caused complement fixation if further platelets and drug were added. These experiments, which were performed both with the platelets of apronal-sensitive patients and of normal individuals, seem to demonstrate clearly that apronal acts as a link between the platelet and the antibody because the platelets separate from the antibody, if the drug is removed. Ackroyd suggested that these experiments provided considerable support for the hypothesis outlined above that the drug combines with the platelets and, acting as a hapten, alters the surface of the platelet in such a way that it becomes antigenic. When the drug is removed by dialysis, the platelets are no longer antigenic and, for this reason, separate from the antibody.

In these papers (26–29) Ackroyd criticized some aspects of his own hypothesis. He agreed that some elements of the classic definition of a hapten were not met. The drug was not covalently bound to the cells and the antibody could not be inhibited by adding high concentrations of the drug to the patient's serum. On the other hand, Ackroyd pointed out that Landsteiner (8) had shown that hapten-antibody complexes had a considerable tendency to dissociate and thus very high concentrations of drug were sometimes necessary to inhibit the antibody. Kabat had also pointed out that it may need 1000 molecules in solution to inhibit the action of a single artificially conjugated hapten molecule (28). Ackroyd (28) suggested that perhaps the simplest explanation of the high concentrations of the drug that may be required for in vitro and in vivo reactions is that these high concentrations are needed to force the drug into combination with the platelets to form the antigen. In order to explain why these concentrations do not inhibit the reaction, it would seem necessary further to postulate that the antibody is incapable of reacting with the drug alone and can react only with the drug-platelet conjugate. With reference to the binding of the drug to protein (e.g., membrane protein) as mentioned earlier, it is well-established now that covalent bonding to protein is not necessary for immunogenicity of low molecular weight chemicals. In addition, Park et al. (10) have pointed out that the ability of drug to conjugate to proteins in vitro does not necessarily reflect the potential of the compound to form haptens in vivo because numerous alternative biotransformations may be available that will either preclude reactive metabolite formation or deactivate an electrophilic species once formed. A number of drugs that are associated with hypersensitivity reactions of one form or another have the potential to form haptens as a consequence of enzyme-catalyzed biotransformations in vivo (10). Park et al. (10) suggest that interindividual variations in the ability and capacity to perform a variety of biotransformations are important determinants of drug-protein conjugation in vivo. They also emphasize that much of the information concerning the immunogenicity of various substances has been obtained in animal models designed to be especially sensitive to small doses of putative immunogen and adjuvants are often used (10). Therefore, caution should be exercised when extrapolating to humans.

During the 1970s and the 1980s, Ackroyd's theory that drugs formed a labile combination with cellular proteins, and that the drug and the altered cell membrane acted as an immunogen, fell out of favor. Shulman (30–33) criticized the haptenic hypothesis suggested by Ackroyd (27–29). Shulman proved that drugs such as quinine and quinidine did not bind firmly to platelet membranes; quinidine could be removed by a single washing of the platelets (30). He reported that concentrations of drug in the order of 1 million times the concentration of membrane sites for antibody fixation did not interfere with antibody reactions (32). Using equilibrium dialysis, Shulman showed that the association between cells and drug was much too weak to account for the large amount of antibody that the same cells adsorbed (3). On the other hand, drug antibodies were shown to combine efficiently with drug in the absence of cells; the association constants of the drug antidrug complexes for quinidine, quinine, and apronal were in the range of 10^7 to 10^8 L/mol (31). Thus, Shulman suggested that the patient makes an antibody against a stable complex of the drug with some soluble noncellular macromolecule and when the drug is received again, drug-antidrug immune complexes form and these attach to platelets non- specifically, activating complement and leading to thrombocytopenia. This theory was extended to explain drug-induced IHA (4,5,34). It is interesting to note that Miescher and coworkers proposed an immune complex mechanism to explain apronal-induced thrombocytopenia in 1952 (35). Miescher et al. also showed that rabbits immunized with foreign proteins had immune complexes attached to their platelets and that this led to their destruction by macrophages; they suggested that a similar mechanism might be operating in drug-induced thrombocytopenia (36–38).

In 1975, Ackroyd (29) objected to the immune complex concept because the clinical effects observed in animals with immune complexes on their platelets bears no resemblance to the drug hypersensitivity syndrome observed in humans. Ackroyd (29) referred to work by Cronin (39), who immunized rabbits with apronal conjugated to protein. He achieved this by substituting one of the amino groups of the apronal molecule with an amino-phenyl group. He then coupled the amino-phenyl–substituted compound to protein by diazotization. Rabbits immunized with this protein conjugate developed precipitating antibodies to it. Precipitate formation was inhibited by unmodified apronal showing that the immunological reactivity of the apronal molecule had not been altered by the chemical manipulations employed. However, the rabbit antibody had no effect on rabbit or human platelets in vitro even in the presence of apronal. Moreover, when the aminophenylated apronal compound was diazotized to human albumin, no reaction could be demonstrated between this antigen and the antibody in the serum of a apronal-sensitive patient These experiments, therefore, provided no support for the hypothesis that the antibody in this type of drug hypersensitivity was stimulated by a stable union of the drug with a soluble macromolecule and that absorption of drug immune complexes to platelets caused their lysis. More recently, Salama et al. (40) described a patient who developed acute intravascular hemolysis while receiving carbimazole (1-carbethoxy-3-methyl-2-thiomidazole), a drug that is used for treating hyperthyroidism. The drug is rapidly hydrolyzed to methimazole either in plasma or at an alkaline pH and only the biologically active metabolite methimazole is detectable in plasma. The patient had immunoglobulin G (IgG) and C3 on her RBCs, and IgG autoantibody was elutable from her RBCs. The serum contained carbimazole-dependent antibodies reacting with untreated reagent RBCs when carbimazole was added and also reacting with carbimazole-treated RBCs. The antibody did not react with the metabolite methimazole. This was notable because carbimazole cannot be detected in plasma following oral administration owing to its rapid hydrolysis to methimazole. Thus, it poses the question of how did the patient form antibodies to carbimazole but not the circulating metabolite methimazole? Although the patient's serum reacted with RBCs in the presence of carbimazole, no reactions occurred if the patient's serum was allowed to incubate with the drug before RBCs were added. One would not expect this if drug-antidrug immune complexes were formed. In addition, although the patient's serum did not contain carbimazole, the drug could be detected on circulating RBCs from the patient.

Salama et al. (40) interpreted these and other findings to indicate that a significant amount of carbimazole was rapidly bound to RBCs in such a fashion that the molecular sites at which hydrolysis takes place in the plasma were protected on the RBC membrane. This binding then might maintain the antigenic sites needed for immunogenicity and reactivity. In this case study, the authors seem to have ruled out the possibility that the drug or its metabolite combined with soluble macromolecules (carriers) in the plasma to induce an immune response. They suggested that the drug combined with the RBC membrane; antibodies were induced to the drug-RBC complex, and these antibodies reacted with the drug-RBC membrane complex, activating complement, and inducing in vivo hemolysis. It is also of interest that RBC autoantibodies, reacting against all reagent RBCs without the presence of drug, were also eluted from the patient's RBCs, which suggests that some of the antibody activity was directed solely against the RBCs. These findings and hypotheses correlate closely with Ackroyd's work on platelets.

Shulman and Miescher's "immune complex" theory reigned supreme for about 20 years. Recently, the theory has come under constant attack. Some "new" hypotheses have been suggested (6,41–46). Unfortunately, most of the "new" hypotheses are very similar to Ackroyd's original suggestions, and none of the hypotheses (new or old) fit all of the clinical, immunological, and serological findings. The newer findings that add to the controversy are (1) some drug-dependent antibodies, such as quinidine antibodies, have been shown to bind to platelets by their Fab domain; (2) many drug-induced antibodies appear to show specificity for certain cell lines or specific epitopes on platelets or RBCs; and (3) many patients have now been described who seem to have antibodies with in vitro characteristics of more than one of the previously accepted mechanisms.

A.   Quinine/Quinidine–Dependent Antibodies Appear to Bind to Platelets by Their Fab Domains

In 1985, Christie et al. (47) showed that platelets coated with quinine- or quinidine-induced antibodies form rosettes around protein A–Sepharose beads and normal platelets form rosettes about protein A–Sepharose beads coated with these antibodies. These reactions occurred only in the presence of the sensitizing drug. Platelets also formed rosettes about protein A–Sepharose beads coated with an anti-Pl^{A1} antibody but drug was not required. Formation of rosettes between antibody-coated platelets and protein A–Sepharose was inhibited by F(ab′)$_2$ fragments directed against the F(ab′)$_2$ portion of the IgG molecule. Since binding of IgG to protein A is known to occur via the Fc region, these findings suggest that binding of drug-induced antibodies to platelets occurs at the Fab domains of the IgG molecule

Using a different approach, Smith et al. (48) came to similar conclusions. The antibody domain controlling reactions between platelet membranes and drug-dependent antibodies from patients with thrombocytopenia induced by cinchona alkaloids was studied using F(ab′)$_2$, Fab, and Fc fragments made from purified drug-dependent antibody. By direct binding radioimmunoassay (RIA) measurements, 20,000–50,000 antibody molecules bound per platelet equivalent of purified platelet membranes at apparent saturation with three different antibodies. F(ab′)$_2$ and Fab fragments bound to platelet membranes drug dependently but Fc fragments did not. The ability of drug-dependent IgG fragments to compete with intact IgG was quantitatively measured by RIA and by complement fixation. F(ab′)$_2$ and Fab competed with intact IgG at an 8:1 and > 50:1 molar ratio, respectively, in RIA, and at a 1.6-3:1 and 44-75:1 ratio, respectively, by complement fixation assays. Fc did not compete with IgG in either assay. Smith et al. (48) concluded that the Fab domain supported attachment of drug-dependent antibody to the platelet membrane.

Jordan et al. (49) presented evidence that a tolmetin-dependent antibody associated with severe intravascular hemolysis bound to RBCs by its Fab domain. Serum from a patient with acute intravascular hemolysis was found to contain a drug-dependent IgM antibody that caused complement fixation and agglutination and a drug-dependent IgG antibody that could be detected only by indirect antiglobulin testing. Jordan et al. (49) found that the receptor for the drug-dependent reaction was on all RBCs of a standard commercial panel, as well as on O$_h$, Rh$_{null}$, K$_o$, Jk(a-b-), and i adult cells. Reactions of cells from cord blood were quantitatively the same as adult RBCs. Thus, none of these blood group antigens was the receptor for the tolmetin antibody. Solubilized RBC membranes were transferred by Western blot and incubated with drug-dependent antibody followed by a second incubation with either ^{125}I–protein A or ^{125}I–anti-IgG, all in the presence of drug. The drug-dependent antibody receptor could not be identified this way. However, when ^{125}I-labeled RBC membranes reacted with drug-dependent antibody, were solubilized, precipitated by staphylococcal protein A, eluted, reduced, and electrophoresed in sodium dodecylsulfate–polyacrylamide gel electrophoresis (SDS-PAGE), they produced an autoradiographic line primarily at the level of band 3. An antibody specific for band 3 produced the same pattern as drug-dependent antibody by this technique. ^{125}I-F(ab)$_2$ fragments, prepared by pepsin digestion of diethylaminoethyl (DEAE) chromatographed IgG and chloramine T labeling, bound to RBCs in drug-dependent fashion the same as drug-dependent IgG. Proof that the bound material was drug-dependent F(ab)$_2$ and not a possible contaminant was obtained by eluting bound drug-dependent ^{125}I-labeled protein from RBCs and performing SDS-PAGE followed by autoradiography. More than 90% of the eluted protein had a molecular weight of 100,000. The apparent association constant of the drug-dependent ^{125}I-F(ab)$_2$ binding was approximately $2 \times 10^{8-1}$ M and equal to that of intact IgG from which it was made. These results (49) suggested a similar Fab-dependent mechanism for RBCs as for platelets (47,48).

B. Specificity for Certain Cell Lines or Specific Epitopes on Platelets and RBCs

Drug-dependent antibodies appear to be highly specific for certain cell lines. For instance, many drugs (e.g., quinidine, phenacetin) have been documented to cause thrombocytopenia and hemolytic anemia, but usually in a single patient only one cell line is affected. When two cell lines are affected in one patient, the antibodies, reacting with each cell type, can usually be separated, and prove to be different antibody populations (33,50).

Quinidine- and quinine-dependent antibodies, reactive with platelets, appear to react with specific epitopes on platelet membrane glycoproteins GP Ib/IX and/or GPIIb/IIIa. In 1978, Kunicki et al. (51) showed that quinine/quinidine–dependent antibodies failed to react with platelets from patients with the Bernard-Soulier syndrome. This was confirmed by others (50,52). Platelets from patients with the Bernard-Soulier syndrome are known to be deficient in the GP1b/IX complex, GPV, and at least one other protein. Several investigators produced evidence that quinine/quinidine–dependent antibodies react with epitopes on the GP1b/IX complex (50,53–55). Christie et al. (56) showed that some antibodies react with GPIIb/IIIa. More recently, Visentin et al. (57) studied sera from 13 patients with quinidine- or quinine-induced thrombocytopenia. They found 10 of 13 sera contained IgG antibodies specific for both GPIb/IX and GPIIb/IIIa, 2 reacted with GPIb/IX alone, and 1 reacted with GPIIb/IIIa alone. In all cases, the drug was required for binding of IgG to target GPs. Quinidine and quinine consist of linked quinoline and quinuclidine ring structures and are lipophilic molecules. Visintin et al. (57) suggested that as such molecules are known to accumulate at amphophilic surfaces, they might concentrate preferentially in hydrophobic pockets within the chymotryptic-resistant protein of the GPIIIa molecule (Fig. 2), where they might induce structural changes

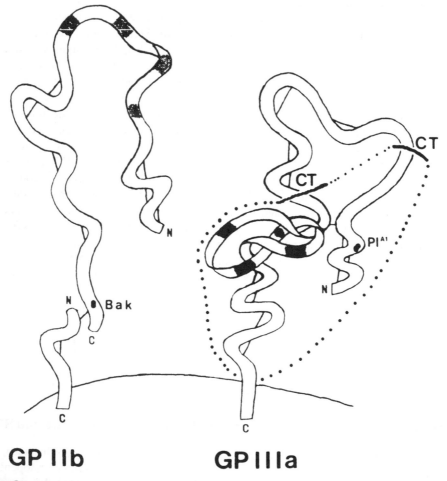

GP IIb   GP IIIa

Figure 2   Schematic representation of the GPIIb complex in the membrane of intact platelets. Dark bands designate cysteine-rich regions of GPIIIa responsible for intrachain disulfide bonding. The encircled part of the GPIIIa molecule is thought to approximate the 61-kd fragment resistant to chymotrypsin digestion (57).

(neoantigens) that are immunogenic in certain individuals. They suggested that antibody bound to such determinants might stabilize the drug-GP complex so that the drug is not readily dissociated from the molecule by washing. The findings of Christie et al. (58) that tritiated quinidine is stabilized in the platelet membrane by the binding of quinidine-dependent antibody is consistent with this possibility.

Increasing numbers of drug-dependent antibodies, reacting with RBCs, with blood group specificity, are being reported. In 1977, Martinez et al. (59) reported a case of immune hemolytic anemia (IHA) induced by streptomycin. The patient's serum reacted with streptomycin-treated RBCs and reacted with untreated RBCs when streptomycin was added to the serum. The streptomycin-treated RBCs only reacted with the patient's serum when D–M+ RBCs were used to treat with streptomycin. It was said that streptomycin-treated D–M– RBCs did not react, but no details were given on how many different samples of various phenotypes were tested. In 1981, Duran-Suarez et al. (60) described five examples of drug-dependent antibodies that would react with RBCs in the presence of drug but only when the RBCs were rich in I antigen (i_{cord}, i_{adult} RBCs were nonreactive). The drugs involved were rifampicin, nitrofurantoin, and an antihistamine (dexchlorphenyramine maleate). Habibi et al. (61) and Salama and Mueller-Eckhardt (62) have also found drug-dependent antibodies that reacted with adult RBCs in the presence of drug (thiopental anesthetic and nomifensine, respectively) and did not react with cord RBCs. Sandvei et al. (63) described a drug-dependent antibody that did not react with cord RBCs but reacted with i_{adult} RBCs as strongly as I_{adult} RBCs. In 1991, Pereira et al. (64) described a single case of IHA and renal failure due to rifampicin-dependent antibodies with anti-I specificity. The antibodies reacted equally well with I+ RBCs of common phenotype or rare phenotypes (Rh_{null}, pp, U–, K_0); cord RBCs did not react. Habibi (65) extended these findings by testing 19 antibodies induced by 11 different drugs against RBCs lacking high-incidence antigens. Five antibodies did not react with –D– RBCs. Two antibodies did not react with P– RBCs; five antibodies did not react with Lu(a-b-) RBCs. One antibody did not react with K_0 RBCs. Only six (32%) antibodies reacted equally well with all phenotypes. Salama and Mueller-Eckhardt (62) tested 30 nomifensine-induced antibodies against RBCs of common and rare phenotypes in the presence of nomifensine. They found that 14 of the 30 (47%) antibodies reacted with all RBCs tested. Nine (30%) were similar to drug-independent autoantibodies, being nonreactive or reacting weaker with Rh_{null} RBCs. Three (10%) did not react with cord RBCs and could be inhibited by soluble I substance. The specificities of the remaining four antibodies, although nonreactive with some RBCs, could not be identified. In 1984, we described a case of chlorpropamide-induced IHA associated with Jk^a specificity (66). The patient's serum contained drug-dependent anti-Jk^a that showed enhanced reactivity in the presence of chlorpropamide. Eventually, the anti-Jk^a was only detectable in the presence of chlorpropamide (Fig. 3).

It is interesting to note that Claas et al. (67) found that none of 10 drug-dependent antibodies associated with thrombocytopenia reacted with all platelets in a panel from donors of different HLA types. No HLA specificity could be determined but Claas et al. believed genetic factors played a role (67).

In addition to some drug-induced antibodies associated with IHA showing blood group specificity, there are several examples of antibodies to chemicals that have shown blood group specificity. Beck et al. (68) and Dube et al. (69) described caprylate-dependent autoagglutinins of anti-c and anti-e specificity. Reviron et al. (70) described an anti-I autoagglutinin that was enhanced in the presence of sodium azide. In 1982, we described an anti-Jk^a that at first appeared to be a low ionic strength saline (LISS) solution–dependent antibody (71). It was later determined that the reactivity was independent of ionic strength but dependent on a preservative (paraben) added to the commercial LISS. Paraben is a methyl ester of hydroxybenzoic acid. The anti-Jk^a

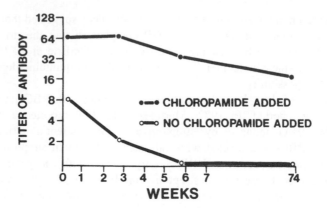

Figure 3 The AGT scores of reactivity with Jk(a+) RBCs when chlorpropamide is added as compared with AGT scores without chlorpropamide (66).

would only react with Jk(a+) RBCs when methyl esters of hydroxybenzoic acid were added to the patient's serum. The Jk(a+) patient had no signs of hemolytic anemia and was transfused with Jk(a+) RBCs with no ill effects (71). Judd et al. (72) reported three more examples of similar autoantibodies.

C. Serological Characteristics of Different Mechanisms Occuring in the Same Patient

Until relatively recently, most reports of individual patients with drug-induced IHA described antibodies showing characteristics associated with either autoantibodies (e.g., methyldopa), the drug adsorption mechanism (e.g., penicillins), or the so-called immune complex mechanism (e.g., quinidine). A few reports suggested antibodies showing characteristics of more than one mechanism. For instance, Muirhead et al. (73), who described a case of acute hemolytic anemia associated with exposure to an insecticide containing chlorinated hydrocarbons. The patient's serum contained a RBC drug-independent autoagglutinin and an antibody that caused in vitro hemolysis of RBCs sensitized with the insecticide. In 1969, Hart and Mesara (74) described a case of hemolytic anemia associated with phenacetin that appeared to be due to an antibody that they thought was a phenacetin-dependent antibody, but a drug-induced autoantibody was also thought to be present. It is not clear whether the antibodies reacting with the patient's own RBCs in these two reports represented a true autoantibody. We have found that sera from patients with drug antibodies working through the "immune complex" mechanism can sometimes react with RBCs in vitro without the presence of added drug (75–77). This can mimic autoantibody by causing agglutination of all RBCs. We believe this is due sometimes to the presence of preformed drug-immune complexes in the patient's serum. This phenomenon can be easily differentiated from true autoantibody. Once the drug is stopped, the immune complexes are cleared rapidly from the plasma by the reticuloendothelial system (RES); thus, the in vitro reactions caused by the drug complexes are usually not seen when serum is tested 24 hr following drug cessation. In contrast, true autoantibodies would still be present. The first of two well-documented cases describing two possible mechanisms in one patient was a report of a streptomycin-induced hemolytic anemia (78). Florendo et al. (78) described a patient whose serum contained an RBC autoantibody that was clearly separable from an antibody that reacted only with streptomycin-treated RBCs. Habibi et al. (79) described a patient with acute intravascular hemolysis and renal failure due to teniposide, a semisynthetic derivative of podophyllotoxin used for cancer chemotherapy. This patient's serum reacted in vitro with RBCs in the presence of teniposide to a titer of 2024 but contained a weaker (titer of 8) RBC autoantibody that reacted without the presence of the drug. The autoantibody in this case was found to persist for 5 months, thus was not caused by the mimicking effect of immune complexes discussed above. Bird et al. (80) described two patients who developed positive DATs while on azapropazone. Both patients' sera contained two distinct antibodies. One was an IgG autoantibody and the other an IgM drug-dependent antibody.

More recently, Habibi (42) and Salama and Mueller-Eckhardt (81,82) presented convincing data that more than one mechanism can operate in a patient. Habibi (42) described four patients with drug-induced acute hemolytic anemia and renal failure. The patients were shown to have drug-dependent antibodies to galfenine, latamoxef, and teniposide together with drug-dependent RBC autoantibodies. Salama and Mueller-Eckhardt (81) studied 31 patients who developed IHA due to nomifensine. The majority of these patients' (23 cases) sera contained IgG and/or IgA antibodies reacting to a highly variable extent with RBCs only in the presence of the drug and/or its metabolites. Sera of six patients contained only IgG RBC autoantibodies, which reacted in the absence of the drug. Three patients had drug-specific and RBC autoantibodies in their sera. The patients with only autoantibodies had a less severe clinical course than those with drug-dependent antibodies, reacting by the immune complex mechanism. Salama and Mueller-Eckhardt (82) also described six patients who had severe hemolytic anemia due to cianidanol, a flavoid used for treating hepatitis. Four patients developed drug-dependent IgM and/or IgG antibodies. One patient developed only IgG RBC autoantibodies, and another patient developed a combination of IgG drug-dependent antibodies and IgG autoantibodies. All drug-dependent antibodies reacted in vitro with RBCs in the presence of the drug (i.e., typical of immune complex mechanism) but unexpectedly also reacted with drug-coated RBCs (i.e., typical of drug-adsorption mechanism). When drug was added to the patient's serum in vitro (i.e., hapten inhibition test), it did not prevent the reactions with drug-coated RBCs.

In 1990, Salama et al. (83) described two patients with acute IHA caused by diclofenac. Both patients had developed IgG drug-independent antibodies and drug-dependent antibodies. The serum of one patient reacted with RBCs only in the presence of urine (ex vivo antigen/metabolite) from patients receiving diclofenac. The serum did not react with RBCs in the presence of diclofenac or its known metabolites. Serum from the other patient reacted with RBCs in the presence of ex vivo antigen as well as in the presence of the drug itself and its main metabolite. The sera of two patients with tolmetin-induced IHA were shown to contain drug-dependent and drug-independent antibodies (84,85). Another closely related drug (zome-pirac) also led to production of drug-dependent and drug-independent antibodies in a patient described by Schulenburg et al. (86).

Recently, the second- and third-generation cephalosporins have been associated with severe IHA (87). Several of these cases have been associated with drug-induced antibodies that have characteristics of several mechanisms (75,77,87–92). Table 3 lists the drugs that have been reported to be associated with antibodies showing characteristics of more than one mechanism.

D. Drug-Induced Autoantibodies

Methyldopa was the first drug to be proven to cause in vivo production of RBC autoantibodies. Such autoantibodies show similar characteristics (e.g., class, subclass, specificity) to those associated with idiopathic warm autoimmune hemolytic anemia (WAIHA) (93). Several theories have been suggested to explain production of RBC autoantibodies. Worlledge (94) and Green et al. (95–97) suggested that methyldopa alters components of the RBC membrane creating new epitopes that are recognized as foreign. There are little data to support this theory. Methyldopa-induced autoantibodies will react with RBCs that have not been treated with the

Table 3 Drugs Associated with Antibodies Showing Characteristics
of More than One Mechanism[a]

Drug	Mechanism[a]	Ref.
Chlorinated hydrocarbons	AA + DA + IC	73
Phenacetin	AA + IC	74
Streptomycin	AA + DA	59,78
Azapropazone	AA + DA	80
Teniposide	AA + IC	42,79
Galfenine	AA + IC	42
Latamoxef	AA + IC	42
Nomifensine	AA + IC	81
Cianidanol	AA + DA + IC	82
Diclofenac	AA + IC	83
Carbimazole	AA + IC	40
Tolmetin	AA + IC	84,85
Zomepirac	AA + IC	86
Cefotaxime	DA + IC	75
Ceftazidime	DA + IC	91
Cefotetan	AA + DA and DA + IC	77,89,90,92

[a]Mechanisms are those described in the literature as (1) autoantibody (AA), (2)
drug-adsorption (DA), (3) "immune complex" (IC).

drug and appear to be directed against antigens present on normal RBCs such as Rh antigens
(e.g., e antigen). Wurtzel's group (98,99) suggested that methyldopa causes aggregation of IgG
with subsequent adsorption of IgG on RBC membranes. Other workers were not able to repeat
these experiments (5,94), and the blood group specificity of many methyldopa-induced
autoantibodies would seem to refute this theory. Finally, Kirtland et al. (100) suggested that
methyldopa alters the immune system by causing a persistent increase in lymphocyte cyclic
adenosine monophosphate (AMP) which inhibits suppressor T-cell functions leading to
unregulated autoantibody production by B cells in some patients.

Kirtland et al. (100) measured cyclic AMP produced in vitro by lymphocytes from healthy
donors after adding methyldopa and by lymphocytes from patients who were receiving
methyldopa. Significantly higher lymphocyte cyclic AMP concentrations were generated by
both sets of lymphocytes compared with lymphocytes from healthy donors without methyldopa
present. To measure the effect of methyldopa on suppressor cells, Kirtland et al. (100) used an
assay of suppressor activity described by Lipsky et al. (101). The assay is based on the finding
that preincubation of lymphocytes before mitogen stimulation in culture leads to less IgG being
generated by B cells. This is purported to be due to enhancement of suppressor T-cell activity
after the in vitro preincubation phase. Kirtland et al. (100) confirmed the results of Lipsky et
al. (101) that less IgG was produced following preincubation of lymphocytes. They showed
that if methyldopa was added during the preincubation phase, then the inhibition of IgG
generation during mitogen-stimulated culture was negated. The amount of IgG generated in
vitro, following addition of methyldopa to the preincubation phase, was significantly greater
than the IgG generated without a preincubation phase. Similar differences were observed when
lymphocytes from patients receiving methyldopa were compared with lymphocytes from healthy
donors. These results were interpreted to show that methyldopa interfered with the normal
function of suppressor T cells to moderate IgG autoantibody production by B cells. Using
similar techniques to those used by Kirtland et al. (100), we also confirmed the effect of
preincubation on in vitro generation by B cells reported by Lipsky et al. (101). We could not
confirm the findings of Kirtland et al. (100) that methyldopa had any effect on suppressor

functions, as defined by the in vitro production of IgG following a preincubation phase (102,103). We agreed with the findings of Kirtland et al. (100) that methyldopa depressed the proliferative response of mononuclear cells to mitogen stimulation.

Procainamide also induces autoantibodies, including RBC autoantibodies (104,105). The following hypotheses have been proposed for the induction of autoantibody production by procainamide: (1) it interacts with nucleoprotein to form a neoantigen (106,107); (2) it acts as an adjuvant for polyclonal activation of autoantibody producing clones (108); (3) it inhibits T-cell DNA methylation inducing T-cell autoreactivity (109); and (4) it interferes with immunoregulation (110–114). The reported effects on cellular immune function are conflicting and the described effects were small and required relatively high concentrations of procainamide. Ochi et al. (115) showed that procainamide impaired generation of suppressor T-cell activity but exerted no enhancing effect on helper T-cell, B-cell, or macrophage activities. Some members of this same group (115) later published findings that conflicted somewhat with their previous conclusions (114). They found that patients on long-term procainamide therapy have normal numbers and ratios of helper and suppressor T cells and normal mitogen-induced suppressor cell activity. A significant reduction in mitogen-induced IgG-secreting cells was attributed to a decrease in both helper T- and B-cell activity in 50% of the patients and only a B-cell activity decrease in 25% of the patients. Ochi et al. suggested that the defects in B- and T-cell function may result from the ability of procainamide to inhibit membrane depolarization by a mechanism similar to that observed in the cardiac conduction system (116). Procainamide may nonspecifically suppress lymphocyte function through the action of the hydrophobic parts of the molecule analogues to the anesthetic effect of its analogue procaine (116).

Miller and Salem (112) found normal suppressor cell function in 14 patients receiving procainamide. However, total in vitro IgG generation from their mitogen-stimulated lympho-cytes was significantly increased compared with healthy controls and patients with systemic lupus erythematosus (SLE). Separated T cells from patients taking procainamide did not affect in vitro suppressor function of T cells from healthy individuals. They postulated that procainamide induced autoantibodies by enhancing helper T-cell function rather than impairing suppression. DeBoccardo et al. (113) found that procainamide inhibited in vitro IgG secretion and generation of IgG plaque-forming cells. The drug inhibited differentiation of B cells to plasma cells rather than production and secretion of IgG. They postulated that procainamide inhibits pokeweed mitogen (PWM)–induced B-cell maturation to plasma cells by inhibiting production of cytokines by helper cells. These results contrasted with those reported by Ochi et al. (115), but it should be pointed out that DeBoccardo et al. (113) used much higher concentrations of procainamide than those used by Ochi et al. (115), which were within the usual therapeutic plasma range. Bluestein et al. (110) found a biphasic response when they studied the effect of different concentrations of procainamide on mitogen-induced lymphocyte proliferation. Marked suppression was observed at a high concentration of the drug but at lower doses of the drug enhanced proliferation was observed. The lower concentrations of procainam-ide were nearer those found in plasma following therapy. We found that therapeutic levels (30 μg/ml) of procainamide did not significantly affect phytohemagglutinin (PHA)–induced lymphocyte proliferation. This result did not agree with the results of Bluestein et al. (111) but agreed with Ochi et al. (115), who reported that procainamide concentrations ranging from 10 to 40 μg/ml did not have any significant effect on PWM-induced proliferation, as measured by tritiated thymidine incorporation. Using the assay described by Lipsky et al. (101) and Kirtland et al. (100), we found that procainamide did not affect suppressor cell activity. These results agree with Miller and Salem (112), DeBoccardo et al. (113), and Yu and Ziff (114) but do not agree with Ochi et al. (115).

We conclude from the above data that there is little evidence to suggest that therapeutic doses of methyldopa or procainamide affect suppressor cell function. Although there is good evidence that both of these drugs (especially procainamide) may affect the immune system, much more work is necessary to clarify the mechanisms involved in the production of drug-induced RBC autoantibodies.

E.   Current Thoughts on the Immune Response to Drugs Associated with Cytopenia

Everyone agrees that a patient may make drug-dependent or drug-independent antibodies following administration of a wide range of drugs. These two types of antibodies may appear alone or together. Drug-independent antibodies appear to be autoantibodies, often indistinguishable from those associated with idiopathic autoimmune cytopenias. It is not obvious whether drug-independent antibodies that always appear alone (e.g., those associated with methyldopa or procainamide) are different from those that appear together with drug-dependent antibodies (e.g., those shown in Table 3). It is my opinion that they may have a different etiology and I will keep them separate when discussing their serological characteristics later.

Drug-dependent antibodies can be divided into two types depending on their serological and clinical characteristics. The first type is only represented by antibodies to the penicillins and closely related drugs, such as some of the cephalosporins. Penicillin and cephalosporins will bond firmly to RBC membranes, and their antibodies will react with drug-coated RBCs but will usually not react when the serum is mixed with drug and RBCs (the so-called "drug adsorption" mechanism [5]). The second type is associated with the majority of drugs. Most of these drugs do not bond well to cell membranes, and thus the antibodies cannot be detected using drug-coated cells; the antibodies are detected by mixing the patient's serum with drug and RBCs (the so-called "immune complex" mechanism). It is interesting to note that some drugs, other than penicillins and cephalosporins, bond firmly to RBC membranes (see Table 2) and can be detected in vitro by their reactions with drug-coated RBCs but cause clinical reactions similar to the so-called immune complex type. As penicillin-induced IHA is associated with such consistent serological and clinical characteristics, I prefer to classify it separately from the other drugs in Table 2.

For the reasons discussed on pp. 528–533, the immune complex hypothesis, suggested by Miescher et al. and Shulman (30–33), has lost favor recently. Many workers are returning to variations of the original hypothesis suggested by Ackroyd (26–29).

In 1985, Habibi (42) suggested that following ingestion of a particular drug, the formation of both autoantibodies and drug-dependent antibodies could be explained by the well-known hapten and carrier specificities commonly developed in animals immunized with hapten-carrier conjugates (8,9). He believed that formation of drug-cell conjugates must be the initial step of most drug-induced cytopenias. He suggested that the rare incidence of this disorder is probably due to the fact that only few individuals are capable either of coupling drugs to their cells in vivo to form efficient immunogens or of mounting an unusually strong immune response to such conjugates. These suggestions were almost identical to those suggested by Ackroyd more than 30 years previously (26–29). Mueller-Eckhardt and Salama (44,46) have also suggested a unifying concept that is basically similar to those of Ackroyd and Habibi regarding the proposed immune response to drugs. They suggested that the immune process is always initiated by a primary interaction of the drug and/or its metabolites with constituents of blood cell membranes. This interaction provides the composite antigenic structure, which provokes the production of two types of antibodies: drug-dependent and/or drug-independent antibodies. The specificity of drug-dependent antibodies is determined by elements of both drug and cell membrane (drug-dependent neoantigen). These antibodies cannot bind sufficiently tight to either one alone. If one part is removed (by dialysis in vitro, by discontinuance of drug administration, and by subsequent excretion in vivo) the immune reaction subsides. Drug-independent antibodies are elicited by a subtle alteration of the membrane by the drug, but their binding sites are sufficiently similar to, or comprise enough unaltered structures of, normal blood cell membranes to support drug-independent binding to the patient's as well as to normal cells (drug-independent neoantigen). Such antibodies behave like autoantibodies and cannot be distinguished from "true" autoantibodies; i.e., of warm AIHA. Mueller-Eckhardt and Salama (44) believe that only one hypothesis is necessary to explain all the phenomenon we observe. They not only criticized the immune complex hypothesis but also criticized the drug-adsorption mechanism (5) and the theory that some drugs (e.g., methyldopa and procainamide) cause autoantibody production by directly affecting the immune system.

I agree that most drugs probably are capable of binding loosely, or sometimes firmly, to circulating cells and that sometimes this leads to an immune response. The factors influencing the strength of the immune response are numerous and complex; they probably include the affinity of the drug for the particular cell and genetic components. The antibodies formed may react with the drug and/or the drug plus a membrane component. Figure 4 illustrates these variations. The concept is based on Landsteiner's original work (8) and the data gathered by Kitagawa et al. (16); it is similar to that suggested by Habibi (42). Antibodies against the drug would react with drug-coated RBCs and be inhibited by the drug. This antibody would be similar to that previously classified as reacting by the "drug adsorption" mechanism (e.g., penicillin antibodies). Antibodies against the drug plus membrane component(s) may be a response mainly to the drug or mainly to membrane components. These may present differently in vitro. The former might react like those classified as reacting by the "immune complex" mechanism as they would require antibody, drug, and cells (i.e., membrane component) to be present; they would not be inhibited by the drug alone. The antibodies reacting mainly with membrane components might present as drug independent antibodies, or autoantibodies, because they react predominately with membrane components and may not need any drug present to react. They may also show blood group specificity if the putative antigens are present on the membrane component combining with the drug to form the immunogen.

In contrast to Mueller-Eckhardt and Salama (44,46), I do not believe that we can explain all the findings with a single hypothesis. I believe that the drug-independent antibodies, which

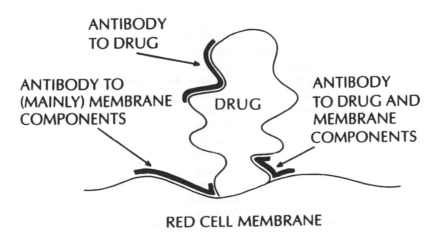

Figure 4   The thicker, darker lines represent antigen-binding sites on the F(ab) region of the drug-induced antibody. Drugs (haptens) bind loosely or firmly to cell membranes and antibodies may be made to (1) the drug (producing in vitro reactions typical of a drug adsorption [penicillin-type] reaction); (2) membrane components or mainly membrane components (producing in vitro reactions typical of autoantibody); or (3) part-drug, part-membrane components (producing an in vitro reaction typical of the so-called immune complex mechanism) (45).

react like autoantibodies, formed by the mechanism illustrated in Figure 3 are different than those induced by drugs such as methyldopa, mefenamic acid, and procainamide. The antibodies induced by these drugs always act as autoantibodies and are never accompanied by drug-independent antibodies. In contrast, the other drug-independent antibodies (e.g., nomifensine and the newer cephalosporins) reported recently (Table 4) always occur together with drug-dependent antibodies. This would fit well with the concept illustrated if Figure 3 that several populations of antibodies are likely to be formed. Although it is possible for only one antibody population to be formed in an individual patient, I would find it hard to accept that methyldopa and procainamide always only induce the single population mainly reacting with membrane components. Although our findings (102,103) suggested that methyldopa and procainamide did not affect suppressor cell function, as measured by Kirtland et al. (100), I believe these drugs do affect immune function in some way to allow proliferation of autoantibody. I also believe that the immune complex hypothesis should not be completely discarded.

III. SEROLOGICAL AND CLINICAL CHARACTERISTICS OF DRUG-INDUCED IHA

Hemolytic anemia caused by drugs by an immune mechanism is due to RBCs being destroyed intravascularly by a complement-mediated process or extravascularly by a complement or IgG-mediated interaction between macrophages and RBCs sensitized with complement and/or IgG-sensitized RBCs. This process of immune RBC destruction is identical to that associated with autoimmune hemolytic anemia (5,117,118). The mechanism causing the RBC sensitization (positive DAT) and the possible subsequent destruction of those RBCs are controversial, and the same arguments that were discussed in the previous section on the immune response to drugs can be applied to the arguments regarding the mechanisms. Regardless of the theoretical concepts the serological and clinical characteristics appear to fall into four distinct categories:

Table 4 Drugs that Have Been Reported to Induce RBC Drug-Independent Antibodies (i.e., Autoantibodies)

Group I[a]	Group II[c]
Methyldopa	Azapropazone
Levodopa	Carbimazole
Mefenamic acid	Cefoxitin
Procainamide	Cefotetan
Catergen[b]	Chlorinated hydrocarbons
Chaparral[b]	Cianidanol
Cyclofenil[b]	Diclofenac
Ibuprofen[b]	Galfenine
	Latamoxef
	Nomifensine
	Phenacetin
	Streptomycin
	Teniposide
	Tolmetin

[a]These drugs induce drug-independent antibodies only.
[b]More evidence is needed to prove that these drugs really can induce RBC autoantibodies.
[c]These drugs induce drug-independent antibodies together with antibodies reacting by different mechanisms (see Table 3).

(1) the penicillin-type drug-dependent antibodies; (2) "nonpenicillin"-type drug-dependent antibodies; (3) drug-independent (auto)antibodies; and (4) nonimmunological adsorption of proteins onto cells.

A. Drug-Dependent Antibodies

Drug-dependent antibodies appear to fall into two groups serologically: those that react with drug-coated RBCs (see Table 2), and those that are only detected when drug, RBCs, and antibody are mixed. Of the drugs listed on Table 2, only the penicillins and sometimes the cephalosporins (e.g., cephalothin) present with consistent characteristics that are different from most other drugs. Three to 5% of patients receiving large doses of the drug intravascularly develop a positive DAT and a small percentage of these develop IHA associated with IgG-mediated extravascular hemolysis. In contrast, the other drug-dependent drugs listed on Table 2 are usually associated with clinical symptoms more typical of the so-called immune-complex mechanism (i.e., acute complement-mediated intravascular hemolysis sometimes associated with renal failure).

1. Penicillin Antibodies

Penicillin antibodies were first detected by Ley et al. (119), who found that a patient's serum reacted with RBCs from a pilot tube of a bottle of donor blood but not with RBCs from the unit itself. This was found to be due to penicillin that had been added to the pilot tube to prevent in vitro infection. Penicillin was found to bind firmly to RBCs, resisting multiple washes. Penicillin antibodies could be detected easily by reacting the patient's serum with the penicillin-coated RBCs and looking for hemolysis, agglutination, and reactions with antiglobulin sera.

Using rabbit antipenicillin, Levine and Redmond (120) showed penicillin was present on the RBCs of 30% of patients receiving 1.2–2.5 million U/day and on the RBCs of all patients taking 10 million or more units per day. When sensitive techniques are used, penicillin antibodies can be detected in over 90% of patients' sera (121). Most sera contain IgM antibodies alone (approximately 80%); approximately 13% contain IgG antibodies as well. These antibodies are usually neutralized by BPO hapten. The antibodies associated with immune hemolytic anemia due to penicillin are IgG and are not easily neutralized by BPO hapten, but inhibition is invariably observed if dilutions of the high-titer pathogenic penicillin antibody are used for the inhibition tests. The high percentage of penicillin antibodies in the normal population is probably due to the continual exposure to penicillin in our modern environment.

In approximately 3% of the patients who receive massive doses of intravenous penicillin, positive DATs will develop (122,123); and in a small percentage of these, hemolytic anemia will develop. The mechanism of the positive DAT and hemolytic anemia seems clear (124,125). The drug is adsorbed to the RBCs and the antipenicillin present in the patient's plasma will react with the penicillin on the RBCs. The quantity of penicillin (BPO) antibody sensitizing the RBC is limited by the number of BPO haptenic groups on the cell, the plasma concentration of BPO-specific antibodies, and the avidity of the antibodies (125). Intravascular hemolysis rarely occurs (126–128); IgG-sensitized RBCs are removed extravascularly by the reticuloendothelial system in the same way as Rh(IgG)-sensitized cells (115,117,118). It is interesting to note that although intravascular lysis rarely occurs, penicillin antibodies often hemolyze penicillin-coated RBCs in vitro (the hemolytic antibodies are always of low titer), and complement is detectable on 40% of the RBCs from patients with a positive DAT due to penicillin antibodies (5).

There is no direct correlation between the presence of IgG and IgM penicillin hemagglutinating antibodies and allergic reactions. Most workers have found no correlation at all, but a few have found that high-titer IgG antibodies occur more often in the allergic group (129,130).

The clinical and laboratory features of penicillin-induced immune hemolytic anemia are quite constant and are listed in Table 5.

Some cephalosporins can also cause drug-induced positive DATs and IHA by a mechanism that appears the same as that for penicillin: Cephalothin (131–138), cephaloridine (139,140), cephalexin (141,142), and cefamandole (143). All of the patients with hemolytic anemia (135–138,142,143) had RBCs sensitized with IgG antibodies to the appropriate cephalosporin, and their sera reacted with cephalosporin-coated RBCs; no intravascular hemolysis was observed. These results were in contrast to the more dramatic complement-mediated intravascular hemolysis associated with some of the newer second- and third-generation cephalosporins (see below).

2. Drug-Dependent Antibodies Other than "Penicillin Type"

This group that often is classified as of the "immune mechanism" type contains the largest number of drugs, but many of them are represented by a single case report in the literature. Table 6 shows the clinical and serological characteristics of this group.

The group is characterized by acute intravascular hemolysis, and in 30–50% of the patients renal failure also occurs. The patients' RBCs are often sensitized with only complement components (e.g., C3dg), but IgG is sometimes also present; on rare occasions, only IgG is detected. The patient's serum will react with RBCs in the presence of the drug and/or a metabolite of the drug. It is usually not possible to prepare drug-coated RBCs using drugs from this group without using chemical coupling techniques (e.g., cross-linking reagents) (144–146); thus, RBCs pretreated with drug do not react with the patient's serum. The drug-dependent antibodies may be IgG and/or IgM; they almost always activate complement. They may cause lysis and/or agglutination and/or sensitization of RBCs detectable by the antiglobulin test in the presence of the drug. Enzyme-treated RBCs almost always react much stronger than untreated RBCs.

B. Drug-Independent Antibodies

Drug-independent antibodies appear as autoantibodies by serological testing; that is, the antibodies are proven to be induced by a drug but react in vitro without drug being present. Table 4 lists drugs that have been reported to cause autoantibody production. It is difficult to prove that a particular drug is responsible for appearance of autoantibodies. As the antibodies react in vitro with RBCs in an identical way to non–drug-induced autoantibodies, they cannot

Table 5 Characteristics Associated with Penicillin-Induced Hemolytic Anemia

1. Hemolysis typically develops only in patients who are receiving very large doses of penicillin (at least 10 million units daily or a week or more).
2. Three percent of patients receiving intravenous penicillin develop a positive DAT but only a small percentage develop hemolytic anemia.
3. Hemolytic anemia is usually less acute in onset than that caused by other drug-dependent antibodies but may be life-threatening if the etiology is unrecognized and penicillin administration is continued.
4. A high titer (>1000) IgG penicillin antibody is present in the serum.
5. The DAT is strongly positive owing to sensitization with IgG. Complement is detected on the RBCs, in addition to IgG, in 40% of the DAT positive patients (5). On rare occasions, complement activation may contribute to the immune hemolysis (126–128).
6. Antibody eluted from the patient's RBCs will react only against penicillin-treated RBCs.
7. Cessation of penicillin therapy is followed by complete recovery, but hemolysis of decreasing severity may persist for several weeks.
8. Other manifestations of penicillin allergy are not necessarily present.

be differentiated serologically. It is not acceptable to blame a drug just because a patient forms RBC autoantibodies following drug administration; this could be coincidental, and it often is. If a patient forms autoantibodies following drug administration and hemolysis resolves following discontinuation of the drug, the evidence is better, but it still does not prove the drug caused the hemolysis. Once again, the two events could be a coincidence. Often the patient is also treated with steroids and remission may not be due to discontinuation of the drug.

A good example of this is the cimetidine story. Two cases of IHA due to cimetidine have been described but the drug was blamed only because of a temporal relationship between drug therapy and hemolytic anemia. Petz et al. (147) published an important paper describing two patients who developed IHA following administration of cimetidine and resolution of their hemolytic anemia and serology following cessation of drug therapy. Both patients were started on the drug again and followed (for up to 24 months in one patient), with no recurrance of hemolytic anemia or autoantibodies. This almost certainly proved that the drug had nothing to do with the symptoms, and that the start and finish of hemolysis paralleling the beginning and end of drug therapy was coincidence. Unfortunately, it is very hard to perform such important confirmatory in vivo experiments and, indeed, could be dangerous in a patient whose initial symptoms included acute intravascular hemolysis rather than only a positive DAT or milder extravascular RBC destruction.

Table 4 divides the drugs into two groups. Those that induce drug-independent antibodies alone and those that induce drug-independent antibodies together with drug-dependent antibodies. I believe that the two groups have a different etiology and the respective antibodies may sensitize the RBCs through a slightly different mechanism. The most thoroughly investigated drugs known to induce RBC autoantibodies are methyldopa and procainamide. In a 10-year period (1970–1980) studying immune hemolytic anemias, Petz and Garratty (5) reported that almost 70% of the drug-induced hemolytic anemias they encountered were due to methyldopa (23% were due to penicillin). Methyldopa is not used as much in the 1990s, and there are no reports on a large series similar to Petz and Garratty's (5) that would reflect on the incidence of methyldopa-induced hemolytic anemia in the 1990s. Table 7 lists the characteristics associated with methyldopa-induced RBC autoantibodies.

There are two unanswered questions regarding methyldopa-induced autoantibodies: (1) Why do up to 15% of patients receiving methyldopa make autoantibodies to their own RBCs? (2) Why do only 0.5% of patients with a positive DAT due to methyldopa have hemolytic anemia?

van der Meulen et al. (148) suggested that there was an in vivo hemolytic quantitative threshold. They used flow cytofluorometry to study 29 patients with positive DATs due to IgG1 autoantibodies; 17 of the patients had signs of overt hemolysis and 12 had no obvious hemolysis. Twelve of the patients were receiving methyldopa; seven of these had overt hemolysis, whereas the other five had no hemolytic anemia. They were able to show a distinct difference in the

Table 6 Characteristics Associated with Drug-Dependent Antibodies Other than the "Penicillin Type"

1. Patient need only take a small amount of the drug.
2. Acute complement-mediated hemolysis often occurs; 30–50% of patients have associated renal failure.
3. The patient's RBCs are often sensitized with only complement but RBC-bound IgG and/or IgM can be present.
4. Patient's serum will react with RBCs in the presence of the drug and/or its metabolite. Antibodies are often IgM, but IgG antibodies can be present alone or together with IgM. Antibodies may cause hemolysis, agglutination, and/or sensitization of RBCs in the presence of drug.
5. After the drug is stopped, hematological remission is rapid.

Table 7   Characteristics Associated with Methyldopa-Induced RBC Autoantibodies

1. Ten to 30% of patients taking methyldopa develop RBC autoantibodies (i.e., positive DAT) within 3–6 months of therapy.
2. Incidence of positive DAT is dose-dependent.
3. Only about 0.5% of patients develop hemolytic anemia.
4. Serological findings are similar to those associated with idiopathic AIHA, particularly those with only IgG on their RBCs:
    IgG autoantibody on RBCs (17% have weak C3 sensitization in addition to IgG)
    IgG autoantibody often present in serum
    Usually "Rh" specificity
5. Following cessation of drug therapy, the hemolytic anemia resolves quickly (usually within 2 weeks) but DAT may keep positive for up to 2 years.

number of IgG molecules on the RBCs of patients with and without AIHA. There appeared to be a "threshold"; i.e., a critical degree of sensitization above which increased RBC destruction in vivo became apparent. Only two discrepant results were found, one in each group of patients; neither of these were patients taking methyldopa. van der Meulen et al. (148) concluded that the quantity of IgG1 autoantibody on the RBCs of DAT-positive patients taking methyldopa was the determining factor for in vivo hemolysis to occur. We (149) also used flow cytometry to study 104 individuals with positive DATs, with and without AIHA, and were unable to confirm this conclusion. We confirmed that flow cytometry was much better than the antiglobulin test (AGT) (i.e., titration scores) in differentiating RBCs with different amounts of IgG on them, particularly when they were strongly (3–4 +) sensitized. Although our results confirmed that the mean amount of RBC-bound IgG was always higher in patients with hemolytic anemia due to autoantibodies (idiopathic and methyldopa-induced) or alloantibodies (hemolytic disease of the newborn), compared with those without hemolytic anemia, we were unable to select a distinct "hemolytic threshold" to differentiate these groups. The range of RBC-bound IgG showed considerable overlap in each group of patients studied.

The method van der Meulen et al. (148) used was similar to the one we (149) used but was not identical; for instance, they used a different flow cytometer. We do not believe the difference in technique explains our different results. The differences between our conclusions and those of van der Meulen et al. (148) could not be explained by the subjects with the RBC-bound IgG. We have no explanation for the different conclusions reached by van der Meulen et al. (148) but would emphasize that our series (149) was larger (104 cases versus 29 cases) and contained a more diverse population of hemolytic anemias (i.e., 12 of the 17 cases of hemolytic anemia studied by van der Meulen et al. [148] were due to methyldopa; our series of 28 patients with hemolytic anemia was composed of 7 idiopathic, 8 methyldopa-induced, and 13 with hemolytic disease of the newborn). Our conclusions were the same when the methyldopa-induced group was analyzed separately to the total group of hemolytic anemias. In conclusion, although we believe there is good evidence to suggest that the amount of RBC-bound IgG is a major factor in determining the degree of in vivo RBC destruction, we do not believe it fully explains the discrepancies between the amount of RBC-bound IgG and the degree of in vivo hemolysis seen in many cases.

C.   Positive DATs Due to Nonimmunological Adsorption of Protein onto RBCs

Some drugs appear to affect the RBC membrane so that proteins are adsorbed nonspecifically leading to a positive DAT. The first drug to be described as causing this effect was cephalothin (131,132). Other cephalosporins may be capable of the same effect but very little has been published on other cephalosporins. Molthan et al. (131) reported that 75% of 31 patients; Gralnick et al. (132) reported 40% of 20 patients; and Perkins et al. (133) reported 38% of 143 patients receiving cephalothin had positive DATs. In an extensive study in 1971, Spath et al. (134) found only 4% of 320 DATs performed on 97 patients receiving cephalothin had positive DATs. They suggested that there may be several explanations for the difference between their results and others. First, the nature of the antiglobulin sera may be of significance. In order that these results might be readily duplicated by others, the initial AGTs were performed with a readily available commercial antiglobulin serum that had previously been evaluated and shown to be potent with respect to anti-IgG and angi-C3 antibodies. This antiglobulin serum did not contain antialbumin, whereas some commercial antisera were shown to have potent antialbumin antibodies. In vitro results indicated that albumin was readily absorbed onto cephalothin-sensitized erythrocytes and could be the cause of false-positive AGTs if an antiserum rich in antialbumin antibodies was used. Second, patient selection may greatly influence the results. The dosage and duration of therapy are likely to influence the incidence of positive reactions. The studies of Spath et al. (134) were carried out in consecutive unselected patients in a community hospital and neither the mean daily cephalothin dosage (6.3 g), the mean duration of therapy (5.5 days), nor the incidence of renal insufficiency were high. The distribution of BUN levels in their patients was as follows: 80% normal levels, 12% in the range of 20–30 mg%, 4% between 30 and 50 mg%, and 4% higher than 50 mg%. Three of the four patients with positive direct Coombs' tests in their series had elevated BUN levels. A greater incidence of positive AGTs may logically be anticipated in referral centers or infectious disease units caring for more selected patients. This may be especially true if a large percentage of patients studied have renal disease, as in the reports of Molthan et al. (131), Gralnick et al. (132), and Perkins et al. (133). Such patients may have a positive DAT unrelated to cephalothin therapy (150). Gralnick et al. (132) and Perkins et al. (133) did not report results of pretreatment DATs and did not present specific immunological data indicating that the positive DATs were caused by cephalosporin administration. Thus, in any series of patients, and particularly in patients with renal disease, control series indicating the incidence of positive DAT in a similar group, pretreatment AGTs, or specific immunological data in each patient (such as the elution of specific antibody from the patients' RBCs) are necessary before the positive DATs may be attributed to the cephalosporin therapy. The method of performing the AGT also is of importance. Spath et al. (134) read their tests microscopically. By doing so, a high incidence of clinically insignificant weakly positive tests might be recorded.

Although Spath et al. (134) confirmed that cephalothin can cause nonimmunological adsorption of protein, three of four patients with a positive DAT (but no hemolytic anemia) had demonstrable IgG anticephalothin antibodies on their RBCs. Thus, most of the positive DATs appeared to be due to an immune mechanism, although additional nonimmunological uptake of protein was not excluded. In a companion paper, Spath et al. (151) studied optimal conditions for detecting cephalothin and penicillin antibodies. The studies confirmed earlier work that penicillin bound to RBCs optimally at around pH 10. A penicillin antibody reacted to a titer of 200, 400, and 3200 with penicillin-coated RBCs prepared at a pH of 7.3, 8.2, and 10, respectively. A cephalothin antibody with a titer of 3200 showed no significant difference when RBCs were coated with cephalothin at pH 7.3, 8.2, or 10.0 (151).

Although it was suggested that cephalothin changed the RBC membrane (132,135), there are very little data to support this. Sirchia et al. (152) and Ferrone et al. (153) showed that cephalothin-treated RBCs act in some ways like RBCs from patients with paroxysmal nocturnal hemoglobinuria (PNH). The treated RBCs had similar enzymatic and metabolic activities to PNH RBCs and were similarly sensitive to the action of complement. PNH RBCs are known to have several membrane abnormalities (154). For instance, phosphatidylinositolglycan (GPI)–anchored proteins are absent or markedly deficient in PNH RBCs (see Chapter 4). Petz and Branch (146) reported that some cephalosporins (cephalexin, cefazolin, cefamandole) did not cause nonimmunological binding of protein to RBCs, but they did not give any data regarding concentration of drugs used to demonstrate this. They suggested that the nonimmunological adsorption of protein may not occur because the RBC membrane is changed by the cephalosporin. They suggested that proteins bind to the exposed β-lactam group of the cephalosporin group and then the cephalosporin-protein conjugate binds to the RBC membrane. Petz and Branch showed that there is much less nonspecific binding of proteins at a lower pH (146). Ninety-seven percent of 133 normal sera reacted by indirect AGT, with RBCs coated with cephalothin at pH 8.5 but only 4 of 87 (4.6%) reacted weakly with RBCs coated with cephalothin at pH 6.0. It was suggested that a low pH cephalothin may still bind to RBCs (unlike penicillin) but the β-lactam ring will be much less likely to undergo nucleophilic attack that would permit binding of proteins when the RBCs are incubated with serum or plasma.

More recently, it has been suggested that some other drugs may affect the RBC membrane in such a way as to allow nonimmunological binding of plasma proteins. Jamin et al. (155) showed that diglycoaldehyde (INOX), an intravenous chemotherapeutic agent used to treat children with malignancies, caused positive DATs in all eight patients receiving the drug. IgG and albumin were found to bind to human RBCs when they were incubated in vitro with normal plasma and INOX or glutaraldehyde. INOX is the periodate oxidation product of the purine nucleoside inosine in which carbons 21 and 31 have been oxidized to formyl groups. Glutaraldehyde is similar in structure to INOX in that it contains two free formyl groups. In vitro studies have shown that proteins can bind to formyl groups by a Schiff's-type reaction. Glutaraldehyde has previously been shown to form Schiff's type reactions with proteins. Jamin et al. (155) postulated that when INOX or glutaraldehyde is incubated with RBCs in an alkaline medium, one aldehyde group could form a Schiff's base with an amino group of the RBC membrane. The other aldehyde group would be free to form a Schiff's base with an amino base of a plasma protein. They further suggested that there may not be associated in vivo hemolysis because the IgG may be covalently attached to the RBCs via the formation of Schiff's bases; as the IgG was not attached by the Fab portion, the Fc portion may not be properly accessible to macrophages.

In theory, any drug containing two or more aldehyde or acid groups capable of reacting with proteins can produce a positive DAT (155). These may include the following: actinorhodine, aztreonam, citric acid, diglycoaldehyde, Evans blue, folic acid, glutamic acid, glutaraldehyde, glutaric acid, glyceryl trinitrate (nitroglycerin), glyoxal, iodipamide (Cholografin), maleic acid, menadiol sodium diphosphate (Synkayvite), pamoic acid, penillic acid, phthalic acid, picric acid, stibophen, sodium iodomethamate (Iodoxyl), terephthaldicarboxaldehyde, and terephthalic acid. Indeed, a later report (156) by the same group reported that suramin caused in vitro adsorption of IgG onto RBCs associated with positive AGTs. Suramin contains six reactive sulfonic acid carbonyl groups and is a reverse transcriptase inhibitor that has been used in treating acquired immunodeficiency syndrome (AIDS). Jamin et al. (156) postulated that suramin causes the nonimmunological adsorption of protein onto RBCs by the formation of amide linkages, whereby the sulfonic acid groups of suramin react with the amino groups of plasma and RBC proteins. It should be emphasized that larger concentrations of suramin had to be used in vitro to cause a positive AGT than would be circulating in vivo. Jamin et al. (156) did not describe any in vivo induction of positive DATs due to suramin administration.

Zeger et al. (157) showed IgG could be adsorbed nonimmunologically onto RBCs treated in vitro with cisplatin, an anticancer chemotherapeutic agent. They also suggested that a positive DAT due to IgG and complement sensitization, which developed in a patient taking cisplatin, was due to nonimmunological protein adsorption in vivo. There was no evidence that this nonimmunological adsorption caused hemolytic anemia even when the patient was rechallenged with the drug. Others (158–161) have described cisplatin-induced hemolytic anemia in six

Table 8 Characteristics Associated with Drug-Induced Nonimmunological Adsorption of Proteins onto RBCs

1. Patients have positive DAT but usually do not have hemolytic anemia.
2. Positive DAT may be due to a multitude of proteins on RBC surface (e.g., IgG, IgM, IgA, C3, albumin).
3. Eluate is usually nonreactive with untreated or drug-treated RBCs.
4. Serum may not react with drug-coated RBCs or with untreated RBCs in the presence of drug.

patients, but only one of these patients had demonstrable cisplatin antibodies. The report by Zeger et al. (157) suggests that positive DATs associated with cisplatin may be due to a nonimmunological mechanism and may be coincidental to the findings of hemolytic anemia; it is possible that the cisplatin-induced hemolysis in the patients described in references 158–161 was nonimmune and not associated with RBC antibody sensitization; it is a pity their sera were not investigated more thoroughly. Table 8 lists the characteristics associated with drug-induced nonimmunological adsorption of proteins onto the RBCs.

REFERENCES

1. Snapper I, Marks D, Schwartz L, Hollander L. Hemolytic anemia secondary to Mesantoin. Ann Intern Med 1953; 39:619.
2. Harris JW. Studies on the mechanism of a drug-induced hemolytic anemia. J Lab Clin Med 1956; 47:760.
3. Dausset J, Contu L. Drug-induced haemolysis. Ann Rev Med 1967; 18:55.
4. Worlledge SM. Immune drug-induced haemolytic anaemias. Semin Hematol 1969; 6:181.
5. Petz LD, Garratty G. Acquired Immune Hemolytic Anemias. New York: Churchill Livingstone.
6. Garratty G. Current viewpoints on mechanisms causing drug-induced immune hemolytic anemia and/or positive direct antiglobulin tests. Immunohematology 1989; 5:97.
7. Hine LK, Gertsman BB, Wise RP, Tsong Y. Mortality resulting from blood dyscrasias in the United States. 1984, 1990; Am J Med 1990; 88:151.
8. Landsteiner K. The Specificity of Serological Reactions. Rev ed. Cambridge, MA: Harvard University Press, 1947:185.
9. Eisen HN, Carsten ME, Belman S. Studies of hypersensitivity to low molecular weight substances. III. The 2,4-dinitrophenyl group as a determinant in the precipitin reaction. J Immunol 1954; 73:296.
10. Park BK, Coleman JW, Kitteringham NR. Drug disposition and drug hypersensitivity. Biochem Pharmacol 1987; 36:581.
11. De Weck AL. Low molecular weight antigens. In Sela M, ed., The Antigens. Vol II. New York: Academic Press, 1974:142.
12. Plescia OJ, Palczuk NC, Braun W, Cora-Figueroa E. Antibodies to DNA and a synthetic polydeoxyribonucleotide produced by oligodexyribonucleotides. Science 1965; 148:1102.
13. Plescia OJ, Palczuk NC, Cora-Figueroa E. Production of antibodies to soluble RNA (sRNA). Proc Natl Acad Sci USA 1965; 54:1281.
14. Kitteringham NR, Christie G, Coleman JW, et al. Drug-protein conjugates—XII. A study of the disposition, irreversible binding and immunogenicity of penicillin in the rat. Biochem Pharmacol 1987; 36:601
15. Kristofferson A, Ahlstedt S, Svard PO. Antigens in penicillin allergy. II. The influence of the number of penicilloyl residues on the antigenicity of macromolecules as determined by radioimmunoassay (RIA), passive cutaneous anaphylaxis (PCA) and antibody induction. Int Arch Allergy Appl Immunol 1977; 55:23.
16. Kitagawa M, Yagi Y, Pressman D. The heterogeneity of combining sites of antibodies as determined by specific immunoadsorbents. II. Comparison of elution patterns obtained with anti-P-azobenzoate antibodies by different kinds of immunoadsorbent and eluting hapten. J Immunol 1965; 95:455.

17. De Weck AL. Studies on penicillin hypersensitivity. I. The specificity of rabbit "anti-penicillin" antibodies. Int Arch Allergy Appl Immunol 1965; 21:20.

18. De Weck AL. Newer developments in penicillin immuno-chemistry. Int Arch Allergy Appl Immunol 1963; 22:245.

19. Levine BB, Ovary Z. Studies on the mechanism of the formation of the penicillin antigen. III. The N-(D-alpha-benzylpenicilloyl) group as an antigenic determinant responsible for hypersensitivity to penicillin G. J Exp Med 1961; 114:875.

20. Levine BB, Price VH. Studies on the immunological mechanisms of penicillin allergy. II. Antigenic specificities of allergic wheal-and-flare skin responses in patients with histories of penicillin allergy. Immunology 1964; 7:542.

21. Levine BB, Redmond AP. Minor haptenic determinant-specific reagents of penicillin hypersensitivity in man. Int Arch Allergy Appl Immunol 1969; 35:445.

22. Parker CW, Shapiro J, Kern M. et al. Hypersensitivity to penicillenic acid derivatives in human beings with penicillin allergy. J Exp Med 1962; 115:821.

23. Parker CW, De Weck AL, Kern M. et al. The preparation and some properties of penicillenic acid derivatives relevant to penicillin hypersensitivity. J Exp Med 1962; 115:803.

24. Siegel BB, Levine BB. Antigenic specificities of skin-sensitizing antibodies in sera from patients with immediate systemic allergic reactions to penicillin. J Allergy 1964; 35:488.

25. Thiel JA, Mitchell S, Parker CW. Specificity of hemagglutination reactions in human and experimental penicillin hypersensitivity. J Allergy 1964; 35:399.

26. Ackroyd JF. The pathogenesis of thrombocytopenic purpura due to hypersensitivity to sedormid. Clin Sci 1949; 7:249.

27. Ackroyd JF. The immunological basis of purpura due to drug hypersensitivity. Proc R Soc Med 1962; 55:30.

28. Ackroyd JF, Rook AJ. Allergic drug reactions. In: Gell PGH, Coombs RRA, eds. Clinical Aspects of Immunology. 2nd ed. Oxford, England: Blackwell Scientific, 1968:693.

29. Ackroyd JF. Immunological mechanisms in drug hypersensitivity. In: Gell PGH, Coombs RRA, Lachmann PJ, eds. Clinical Aspects of Immunology. 3rd ed. Oxford, England: Blackwell Scientific, 1975:913.

30. Shulman NR. Immunoreactions involving platelets. I. A steric and kinetic model for formation of complex from a human antibody, quinidine as a hapten, and platelets; and for fixation of complement by the complex. J Exp Med 1958; 107:665.

31. Shulman NR, Rall JE. Mechanism of blood cell destruction in individuals sensitized to foreign antigens. Trans Assoc Am Physicians 1963; 76:72.

32. Shulman NR. Mechanism of blood cell damage by adsorption of antigen-antibody complexes. In: Grabar P, Miescher PA, eds. Immunopathology, 3rd International Symposium, La Jolla, CA. Basel: Schwabe, 1963:338.

33. Shulman NR. A mechanism of cell destruction in individuals sensitized to foreign antigens and its implications in auto-immunity. Ann Intern Med 1964; 60:506.

34. Garratty G, Petz LD. Drug-induced immune hemolytic anemia: Am J Med 1975; 58:398.

35. Miescher PA, Meischer A. Die sedormid-anaphylaxie. Schweiz Med Wochenschr 1952; 82:1279.

36. Miescher PA, Gorstein F. Mechanisms of immunogenic platelet damage. Johnson SA, Monto RW, Rebuck JW, Horn RC, eds. Blood Platelets. London: Churchill, 1961; 671.

37. Miescher PA, Pepper JJ. Drug-induced immunologic blood dyscrasias. In: Miescher PA, Müller-Eberhard HJ, eds. Textbook of Immunopathology. 2nd ed. Philadelphia: WB Saunders, 1976:421.

38. Miescher PA, Pola W. Haematological effects of non-narcotic analgesics. Drugs 1986; 32(suppl 4):90.

39. Cronin AE. The Immunology of Allergic Drug Reactions. Doctoral thesis, Cambridge, MA: University of Cambridge, 1965.

40. Salama A, Northoff H, Burkhardt H, Mueller-Eckhardt C. Carbimazole-induced immune haemolytic anaemia: role of drug-red blood cell complexes for immunization. Br J Haematol 1988; 68:479.

41. Garratty G. Drug-induced immune hemolytic anemia and/or positive direct antiglobulin tests. Immunohematology 1985; 2:1.

42. Habibi B. Drug induced red blood cell autoantibodies co-developed with drug specific antibodies causing haemolytic anaemias. Br J Haematol 1985; 61:139.

43. Petz LD. Drug-induced immune hemolytic anemia. In: Nance SJ, ed. Immune Destruction of Red Cells. Arlington, VA: American Association of Blood Banks, 1989:53.

44. Mueller-Eckhardt C. Drug-induced immune cytopenias: A unifying pathogenic concept with special emphasis on the role of drug metabolites. Transfus Med Rev 1990; 4:69.

45. Garratty G. Target antigens for red-cell-bound autoantibodies. In: Nance SJ, ed. Clinical and Basic Science Aspects of Immunohematology. Arlington, VA: American Association of Blood Banks, 1991:33.

46. Salama A, Mueller-Eckhardt C. Immune-mediated blood cell dyscrasias related to drugs. Semin Hematol 1992; 29:54.

47. Christie DJ. Mullen PC, Aster RH. Fab-mediated binding of drug-dependent antibodies to platelets in quinidine- and quinine-induced thrombocytopenia. J Clin Invest 1985; 75:310.

48. Smith ME, Reid DM, Jones CE, et al. Binding of quinine- and quinidine-dependent drug antibodies to platelets is mediated by the Fab domain of the immunoglobulin G and is not Fc dependent. J Clin Invest 1987; 79:912.

49. Jordan JV, Smith ME, Reid DM, et al. A tolmetin-dependent antibody causing severe intravascular hemolysis binds to erythrocyte band 3 and requires only the $F(ab)_2$ domain to react (abstr). Blood 1985; 66 (suppl):104a.

50. Chong BH, Berndt MC, Koutts J, Castaldi PA. Quinidine-induced thrombocytopenia and leukopenia: Demonstration and characterization of distinct antiplatelet and anti-leukocyte antibodies. Blood 1983; 62:1218.

51. Kunicki TJ, Johnson MM, Aster RH. Absence of the platelet-receptor for drug-dependent antibodies in the Bernard-Soulier syndrome. J Clin Invest 1978; 62:712.

52. van Leeuwen EF, Engelfriet CP, and von dem Borne AEGKr. Studies on quinine- and quinidine-dependent antibodies against platelets and their reaction with platelets in the Bernard-Soulier syndrome. Br J Haematol 1982; 51:551.

53. Kunicki TJ, Russell N, Nurden AT. Further studies of the human platelet receptor for quinine- and quinidine-dependent antibodies. J Immunol 1981; 126:398.

54. Berndt MC, Chong BH, Bull HA, et al. Molecular characterization of quinine/quinidine drug-dependent antibody platelet interaction using monoclonal antibodies. Blood 1985; 66:1292.

55. Devine DV, Rosse WF. Identification of platelet proteins that bind alloantibodies and autoantibodies. Blood 1984; 64:1240.

56. Christie DJ, Mullen PC, Aster RH. Quinine- and quinidine platelet antibodies can react with GPIIb/IIIa. Br J Haematol 1976; 67:213.

57. Visentin GP, Newman PJ, Aster RH. Characteristics of quinine- and quinidine-induced antibodies specific for platelet glycoproteins IIb and IIIa. Blood 1991; 77:2668.

58. Christie DJ, Aster RH. Drug-antibody-platelet interaction in quinine- and quinidine-induced thrombocytopenia. J Clin Invest 1982; 70:989.

59. Martinez J, Letona J, Barbolla L, et al. Immune haemolytic anaemia and renal failure induced by streptomycin. Br J Haematol 1977; 35:561.

60. Duran-Suarez JR, Martin-Vega C, Argelagues E, et al. Red cell I antigen as immune complex receptor in drug-induced hemolytic anemias. Vox Sang 1981; 41:313.

61. Habibi B, Basty R, Chodez S, Prunat A. Thiopental-related immune hemolytic anemia and renal failure. N Engl J Med 1985; 312:353.

62. Salama A, Mueller-Eckhardt C. On the mechanisms of sensitization and attachment of antibodies to RBC in drug-induced immune hemolytic anemia. Blood 1987; 69:1006.

63. Sandvei P, Nordhagen R, Michaelsen TE, Wolthius K. Fluorouracil (5-FU) induced acute immune haemolytic anaemia. Br J Haematol 1987; 65:357.

64. Pereira A, Sanz C, Cervantes F, Castillo R. Immune hemolytic anemia and renal failure associated with rifampicin-dependent antibodies with anti-I specificity. Ann Hematol 1991; 63:56.

65. Habibi B, Bretagne Y. Blood group antigens may be the receptors for specific drug-antibody complexes reacting with red blood cells. C R Acad Sci (D) (Paris), 296:693.

66. Sosler SD, Behzad O, Garratty G, et al. Acute hemolytic anemia associated with a chlorpropamide-induced apparent auto anti-Jk[a]. Transfusion 1984; 24:206.

67. Claas FHJ, Langerak J, van Rood JJ. Drug-induced antibodies with restricted specificity. Immunol Lett 1981; 2:323.

68. Beck ML. A fatty-acid dependent antibody with Rh specificity. In: Book of Abstracts from the ISBT/AABB Joint Congress. Arlington, VA: American Association of Blood Banks, 1972:6.

69. Dube VE, Zoes C, Adesman P. Caprylate-dependent auto-anti-e. Vox Sang 1977; 33:359.

70. Reviron M, Janvier D, Reviron J, Lagabrielle JF. An anti-I cold autoagglutinin enhanced in the presence of sodium azide. Vox Sang 1984; 46:211.

71. Halima D, Garratty G, Bueno R. An apparent anti-Jk^a reacting only in the presence of methyl esters of hydroxybenzoic acid. Transfusion 1982; 22:521.

72. Judd WJ, Steiner EA, Cochran RK. Paraben-associated autoanti-Jk^8 antibodies. Transfusion 1982; 22:31.

73. Muirhead EE, Groves M, Guy R, et al. Acquired hemolytic anemia, exposure to insecticides and positive Coombs test dependent on insecticide preparations. Vox Sang 1959; 4:277.

74. Hart MN, Mesara BW. Phenacetin antibody cross-reactive with autoimmune erythrocyte antibody. Am J Clin Pathol 1969; 52:695.

75. Shulman IA, Arndt PA, McGehee W, Garratty G. Cefotaxime-induced immune helolytic anemia due to antibodies reacting in vitro by more than one mechanism. Transfusion 1990; 30:263.

76. Garratty G., Houston M., Petz LD, Webb M. Acute immune intravascular hemolysis due to hydrochlorothiazide. Am J Clin Pathol 1981; 76:73.

77. Garratty G, Nance S, Lloyd M, Domen R. Fatal immune hemolytic anemia due to cefotetan. Transfusion 1992; 32:269.

78. Florendo NT, MacFarland D, Painter M, Muirhead EE. Streptomycin-specific antibody coincident with a developing warm autoantibody. Transfusion 1980; 20:662.

79. Habibi B, Lopez M, Serdaru M. et al. Immune hemolytic anemia and renal failure due to teniposide. N Engl J Med 1982; 306:1091.

80. Bird GWG, Wingham J, Babb RG, et al. Azapropazone-associated antibodies. Vox Sang 1984; 46:336.

81. Salama A, Mueller-Eckhardt C. Two types of nomifensine-induced immune haemolytic anaemias: Drug-dependent sensitization and/or autoimmunization. Br J Haematol 1986; 64:613.

82. Salama A, Mueller-Eckhardt C. Cianidanol and its metabolites bind tightly to red cells and are responsible for the production of auto- and/or drug-dependent antibodies against these cells. Br J Haematol 1987; 66:263.

83. Salama A, Göttsche B, Mueller-Eckhardt C. Autoantibodies with drug- or metabolite-dependent antibodies in patients with diclofenac-induced immune haemolysis. Br J Haematol 1990; 77:546.

84. Squires JE, Mintz PD, Clark S. Tolmetin-induced hemolysis, Transfusion 1985; 25:410.

85. van Dijk BA, Rico PB, Hoitsma A, Kunst VAJM. Immune hemolytic anemia associated with tolmetin and suprofen. Transfusion 1989; 29:638.

86. Schulenburg BJ, Beck ML, Pierce SR, et al. Immune hemolysis associated with Zomax™ (abstr). Transfusion 1983; 23:409.

87. Garratty G. Severe immune haemolytic anaemia associated with newer cephalosporins. Lancet 1991; 338:119.

88. Toy E, Nesbitt R, Savastano G, et al. Warm autoantibody following plasma apheresis, complicated by acute intravascular hemolysis associated with cefoxitin-dependent antibody resulting in fatality (abstr). Transfusion 1989; 29:51S.

89. Weitekamp LA, Johnson ST, Fueger JT, et al. Cefotetan-dependent immune hemolytic anemia due to a single antibody reacting with both drug coated and untreated red cells in the presence of drug. In: Book of Abstracts from the ISBT/AABB Joint Congress. Arlington, VA: American Association of Blood Banks, 1990:33.

90. Wojcicki RE, Larson CJ, Pope ME, Sullivan CM. Acute hemolytic anemia during cefotetan therapy. In: Book of Abstracts from the ISBT/AABB Joint Congress. Arlington, VA: American Association of Blood Banks, 1990:33.

91. Chambers LA, Donovan LM, Kruskall MS. Ceftazidime-induced hemolysis in a patient with drug-dependent antibodies reactive by immune complex and drug adsorption mechanisms. Am J Clin Pathol 1991; 95:393.

92. Gallagher MT, Schergen AK, Sokol-Anderson ML, et al. Severe immune mediated hemolytic anemia secondary to treatment with cefotetan. Transfusion 1992; 32:266.

93. Carstairs KC, Breckenridge A, Dollery CT, Worlledge SM. Incidence of a positive direct Coombs test in patients on α-methyldopa. Lancet 1966; 2:133.

94. Worlledge SM. Autoantibody formation associated with methyldopa (Aldomet) therapy. Br J Haematol 1969; 16:5.

95. Green FA, Jung CY, Rampal A, Lorusso DJ. Alpha-methyldopa and the erythrocyte membrane. Clin Exp Immunol 1980; 40:554.

96. Green FA, Jung CY, Hui H. Modulation of alpha-methyldopa binding to the erythrocyte membrane by superoxide dismutase. Biochem Biophys Res Commun 1980; 95:1037.

97. Owens NA, Hui HL, Green FA. Induction of direct Coombs' positivity with alpha-methyldopa in chimpanzees. J Med 1982; 13:473.

98. Wurzel HA, Silverman JL. The effects of alpha-methyl-3, 4-dihydroxyl-L-phenylalanine (methyldopa, Aldomet) on erythrocytes. Transfusion 1968; 8:84.

99. Gottleib AJ, Wurzel HA. Proetin—quinone interaction: In vitro induction of indirect antiglobulin reactions with methyldopa. Blood 1974; 43:85.

100. Kirtland HH, Mohler DN, Horwitz DA. Methyldopa inhibition of suppressor-lymphocyte function. N Engl J Med 1980; 302:825.

101. Lipsky PE, Ginsburg WW, Finkelman FD, Ziff M. Control of human B lymphocyte responsiveness: Enhanced suppressor T cell activity after in vitro incubation. J Immunol 1978; 120:902.

102. Garratty G, Arndt P, Prince H, Shulman I. In vitro IgG production following preincubation of lymphocytes with methyldopa and procainamide (abstr). Blood 68: 108a.

103. Garratty G, Arndt P, Prince HP, Shulman IA. The effect of methyldopa and procainamide on suppressor cell activity. Br J Haematol 1992 (In Press).

104. Kleinman S, Nelson R, Smith L, Goldfinger D. Positive direct antiglobulin tests and immune hemolytic anemia in patients receiving procainamide. N Engl J Med 1984; 311:809.

105. Rubin RL. Autoimmune reactions induced by procainamide and hydralazine. In: Kammuller ME, Bloksma N, Seinen W, eds. Autoimmunity and Toxicology. New York: Elsevier Science, 1989; 119.

106. Blomgren SE, Condemi JJ, Vaughan JH. Procainamide-induced lupus erythematosus: Clinical and laboratory observations. Am J Med 1972; 52:338.

107. Gold EF, Ben-Efraim S, Faivisewitz A, et al. Experimental studies on the mechanism of induction of anti-nuclear antibodies by procainamide. Clin Immunol Immunopathol 1977; 7:176.

108. Schoen RT, Trentham DE. Drug-induced lupus: An adjuvant disease? Am J Med 1981; 71:5.

109. Cornacchia E, Golbus J, Maybaum J, et al. Hydralazine and procainamide inhibit T cell DNA methylation and induce autoreactivity. J Immunol 1986; 140:2197.

110. Bluestein HG, Weisman MH, Zvaifler N, Shapiro RF. Lymphocyte alteration by procainamide: Relation to drug-induced lupus erythematosus syndrome. Lancet 1979; 2:816.

111. Bluestein HG, Redelman D, Zvaifler NJ. Procainamide-lymphocyte reactions. Arthritis Rheum 1981; 24:1019–1023.

112. Miller KB, Salem D. Immune regulatory abnormalities produced by procainamide. Am J Med 1982; 73:487.

113. De Boccardo G, Drayer D, Rubin AL, et al. Inhibition of pokeweed mitogen-induced B cell differentiation by compounds containing primary amine or hydrazine groups. Clin Exp Immunol 1985; 59:69.

114. Yu C-L, Ziff M. Effects of long-term procainamide therapy on immunoglobulin synthesis. Arthritis Rheumat 1985; 28:276.

115. Ochi T, Goldings EA, Lipsky PE, Ziff M. Immunomodulatory effect of procainamide in man. J Clin Invest 1983; 71:36.

116. Seeman P. The membrane actions of anesthetics and tranquilizers. Pharmacol Rev 1972; 24:583.

117. Garratty G. Mechanisms of immune red cell destruction, and red cell compatibility testing. Hum Pathol 1983; 14:204.

118. Garratty G. Factors affecting the pathogenicity of red cell auto- and alloantibodies. In: Nanee SJ, ed. Immune Destruction of Red Blood Cells. Arlington, VA: American Association of Blood Banks, 1989:109.

119. Ley AB, Harris JP, Brinkley M, et al. Circulating antibodies directed against penicillin. Science 1958; 127:1118.

120. Levine BB, Redmond A. Immunochemical mechanisms of penicillin induced Coombs positivity and hemolytic anemia in man. Int Arch Allergy Appl Immunol 1967; 31:594.

121. Levine BB, Fellner MJ, Levytska V. Benzylpenicilloyl specific serum antibodies to penicillin in man. J Immunol 1966; 96:707.

122. Abraham GN, Petz LD, Fudenberg HH. Immunohaematological cross-allergenicity between penicillin and cephalothin in humans. Clin Exp Immunol 1968; 3:343.

123. Petz LD. Immunologic reactions of humans to cephalosporins. Postgrad Med J 1971; 47(suppl):64.

124. Petz LD, Fudenberg HH. Coombs-positive hemolytic anemia caused by penicillin administration. N Engl J Med 1966; 274:171.

125. Levine B. Immunochemical mechanisms of penicillin induced Coombs' positive and hemolytic anemia in man. Int Arch Allergy Appl Immunol 1967; 31:594.

126. Kerr RO, Cardamone J, Dalmasso AP, Kaplan ME. Two mechanisms of erythrocyte destruction in penicillin-induced hemolytic anemia. N Engl J Med 1972; 287:1322.

127. Reis CA, Garratty G, Petz LD, Fudenberg HH. Massive intravascular hemolysis in penicillin-induced immune hemolytic anemia. JAMA 1975; 233:432.

128. Funicella T, Weinger RS, Moake JL, et al. Penicillin-induced immunohemolytic anemia associated with circulating immune complexes. Am J Hematol 1977; 3:219.

129. Levine BB, Redmond AP, Fellner MJ, et al. Penicillin allergy and the heterogeneous immune responses of man to benzylpenicillin. J Clin Inevt 1966; 45:1895.

130. De Weck AL, Blum G. Recent clinical and immunological aspects of penicillin allergy. Int Arch Allergy Appl Immunol 1965; 27:221.

131. Molthan L, Reidenberg MM, Eichman MF. Positive direct Coombs tests due to cephalothin. N Engl J Med 1967; 277:123.

132. Gralnick HR, Wright LD Jr, McGinniss MH. Coombs' positive reactions associated with sodium cephalothin therapy. JAMA 1967; 199:135.

133. Perkins RL, Mengel CE, Saslaw S. Direct Coombs' test reactivity after cephalothin or cephaloridine in man and monkey. Proc Soc Exp Biol Med 1968; 129:397.

134. Spath P, Garratty G, Petz LD. Studies on the immune response to penicillin and cephalothin in humans. II. Immunohematologic reactions to cephalothin administration, J Immunol 1971; 107:860.

135. Gralnick HR, McGinnis M, Elton W, McCurdy P. Hemolytic anemia associated with cephalothin. 217:1193.

136. Jeannet M, Bloch A, Dayer JM, et al. Cephalothin-induced immune hemolytic anemia. Acta Haematol 1976; 55:109.

137. Rubin RN, Burka ER. Anti-cephalothin antibody and Coombs' positive hemolytic anemia. Ann Intern Med 1977; 86:64.

138. Moake JL, Butler CFR, Hewell GM, et al. Hemolysis induced by cefazolin and cephalothin in a patient with penicillin sensitivity. Transfusion 1978; 18:369.

139. York PS, Landes RR, Seay LS. Coombs' positive reactions associated with cephaloridine therapy. JAMA 1968; 206:1086.

140. Fass RJ, Perkins RL, Saslow S. Positive direct Coombs' tests associated with cephaloridine therapy. JAMA 1970; 213:121.

141. Schwartz S, Gabl F, Huber H, Spath P. Positive direct antiglobulin (Coombs') test caused by cephalexin administration in humans. Vox Sang 1975; 29:59.

142. Manoharan A, Kot T. Cephalexin-induced haemolytic anaemia. Med J Aust 1987; 147:202.

143. Branch DR, Berkowitz LR, Becker RL et al. Extravascular hemolysis following the administration of cefamandole. Am J Hematol 1985; 18:213.

144. Orenstein AA, Yakulis V, Eipe J, Costea N. Immune hemolysis due to hydralazine. Ann Intern Med 1977; 86:450.

145. Petersen BH, Graham J. Immunologic cross-reactivity of cephalexin and penicillin. J Lab Clin Med 1974; 83:860.

146. Petz LD, Branch DR. Drug-induced immune hemolytic anemia. In: Chaplin H Jr, eds. Immune Hemolytic Anemias. New York: Churchill Livingstone, 1985:47.

147. Petz LD, Gitlin N, Grant K, Rodvien R, Brotman M. Cimetidine-induced hemolytic anemia: The fallacy of clinical associations. J Clin Gastroenterol 1983; 5:405.

148. van der Meulen FW, de Bruin HG, Goosen PCM, et al. Quantitative aspects of the destruction of

red cells sensitized with IgG1 autoantibodies: An application of flow cytofluorometry. Br J Haematol 1980; 46:47.

149. Garratty G, Nance S. Correlation between in vivo hemolysis and the amount of red cell-bound IgG measured by flow cytometry. Transfusion 1990; 30:617.

150. Garratty G. The clinical significance (and insignificance) of red cell-bound IgG and complement. Wallace ME, Levitt J, eds. Current Applications and Interpretations of the Direct Antiglobulin Test. Arlington, VA: American Association of Blood Banks, 1988:1.

151. Spath P, Garratty G, Petz L. Studies on the immune response to penicillin and cephalothin in humans. I. Optimal conditions for titration of hemagglutinating penicillin and cephalotin antibodies. J Immunol 1971; 107:854.

152. Sirchia G, Murcuriali F, Ferrone S. Cephalothin-treated normal red cells: A new type of PNH-like cells. Experientia 1968; 24:495.

153. Ferrone S, Zanella A, Mercuriali F, Pizzi C. Some enzymatic and metabolic activities of normal human erythrocytes treated in vitro with cephalothin. Eur J Pharmacol 1968; 4:211.

154. Rosse WF. Phosphatidylinositol-linked proteins and paroxysmal nocturnal hemoglobinuria. Blood 1990; 75:1595.

155. Jamin D, Demers J, Shulman I, et al. An explanation for nonimmunologic adsorption of proteins onto red blood cells. Blood 1986; 67:993.

156. Jamin D, Shulman I, Lam HT, et al. Production of a positive direct antiglobulin test due to Suramin. Arch Pathol Lab Med 1988; 112:898.

157. Zeger G, Smith L, McQuiston D, Goldfinger D. Cisplatin-induced nonimmunologic adsorption of immunoglobulin by red cells. Transfusion 1988; 28:493.

158. Getaz EP, Beckley S, Fitzpatrick J, Dozier A. Cisplatin-induced hemolysis. N Engl J Med 1980; 302:334.

159. Levi JA, Aroney RS, Dalley DN. Haemolytic anaemia after cisplatin treatment. Br Med J 1981; 282:2003.

160. Cinollo G, Dini G, Franchini E, et al. Positive direct antiglobulin tests in a pediatric patient following high-dose cisplatin, Cancer Chemother Pharmacol 1988; 21:85.

161. Nguyen BV, Lichtiger B. Cisplatin-induced anemia. Cancer Treat Rep 1981; 65:1121.

20

Hemolytic Disease of the Newborn

JOHN M. BOWMAN
University of Manitoba Health Sciences Centre
Winnipeg, Manitoba, Canada

I. INTRODUCTION

Hemolytic disease of the fetus and newborn (HDN) was first described in 1609 by a French midwife, Louyse Bourgeois. She reported the birth of twins. The first infant was bloated with fluid (hydropic) and died shortly after birth; the second infant appeared well at birth but rapidly became deeply jaundiced (icterus gravis), lay in a position of opisthotonos, became apneic, and died at a few days of age (kernicterus). These two conditions, hydrops fetalis (watery fetus; Fig. 1) and kernicterus (yellow staining of the brain; Fig. 2) were described in detail by the pathologists in the 1890s and early 1900s but were not thought to be the same disease entity. In 1921, Von Gierke (1) hypothesized that kernicterus and hydrops might be related. However, it was Diamond et al. in 1932 who showed that hydrops fetalis, icterus gravis, and kernicterus were different spectra of the same disease (2) characterized by hemolytic anemia, extramedullary erythropoiesis, hepatosplenomegaly (Fig. 3) and the outpouring of immature nucleated red blood cells (RBCs) (erythroblasts; Fig. 4), from which they coined the name erythroblastosis fetalis. They had no idea what caused the hemolysis.

In 1938, Dr. Ruth Darrow, who had lost a baby owing to kernicterus, introduced her fetal hemoglobin hypothesis (3). She theorized that fetal RBCs, containing fetal hemoglobin, traversed the placenta into the maternal circulation. The mother's immune system recognized the fetal hemoglobin as foreign and produced a fetal hemoglobin antibody. The antifetal hemoglobin in turn passed across the placenta into the fetal circulation causing destruction of the fetal RBCs. Her hypothesis was correct except for her specific antigen-antibody. Since we all have very small amounts of fetal hemoglobin in our RBCs, fetal hemoglobin is not a foreign antigen and antifetal hemoglobin is not produced.

In 1939, Levine and Stetson reported a severe transfusion reaction in a woman who had a postpartum hemorrhage following delivery of an hydropic stillborn infant (4). The woman, who had not been transfused previously, was transfused with her husband's blood. Levine and Stetson hypothesized that she had been sensitized to a RBC antigen that the fetus had inherited from its father.

In 1940, the experiment of Landsteiner and Wiener disclosed the true offending antigen (5).

553

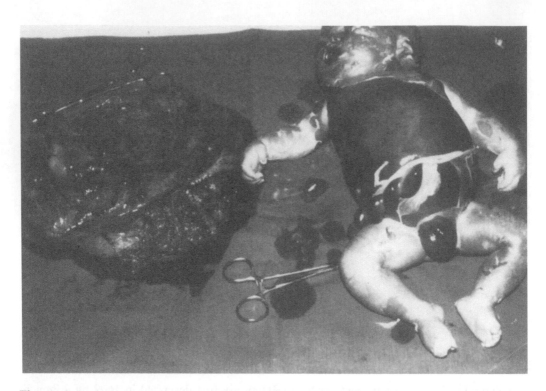

Figure 1   Stillborn fetus with hydrops fetalis; note the edema and markedly enlarged placenta. (From Bowman JM. Rh-Isoimmunization 1977. Mod Med Can 1977; 32:17.)

They injected guinea pigs and rabbits with rhesus monkey RBCs. The guinea pigs and rabbits produced rhesus monkey RBC antibodies. When they took blood samples from a group of white individuals and mixed them with their antirhesus RBC sera, they found that 85% of the white individuals had RBCs that were agglutinated by the sera (i.e., were rhesus positive); the remaining 15% had RBCs that were not agglutinated by the sera (i.e., were rhesus negative). This experiment was a major milestone in medicine. It became the cornerstone of modern immunohematology and also allowed the unraveling of the cause of hemolytic disease. It formed the basis for the science of human anthropology and produced the framework upon which safe blood transfusion is based.

Levine promptly obtained some of Landsteiner and Wiener's antirhesus serum. He determined that his and Stetson's patient was rhesus (Rh) negative (6) her husband was rhesus positive (Rh+). The patient had a powerful antibody that not only agglutinated her husband's RBCs but also agglutinated the RBCs of Landsteiner and Wiener's Rh+ individuals and did not agglutinate those of their Rh– individuals. Although, as we all know now, the monkey antigen called LW and its antibody, anti-LW, are not the same as the human Rh(D) antigen and Rh(D) antibody, this difference does not detract from the importance of Landsteiner and Wiener's discovery.

The etiology of hemolytic disease of the fetus and newborn was established. An Rh(D)– woman, after exposure to Rh(D)+ RBCs produces anti-D. The anti-D, if immunoglobulin G-(IgG), traverses the placenta, coats the fetal D+ RBCs, and hemolyses them, setting in train the chain of events leading to icterus gravis and kernicterus or, in its most severe form, hydrops fetalis.

II.   RH BLOOD GROUP SYSTEM

A.   Nomenclature and Inheritance

The Rh blood group system is still the most common cause of hemolytic disease of the newborn. The system is made up of a family of inherited antigens. Although Wiener and Wexler's theory

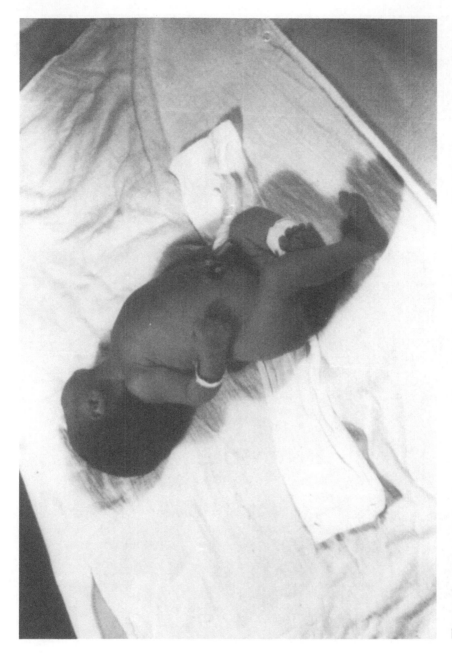

Figure 2 Infant with kernicterus; note spasticity and opisthotonos. (From Bowman JM. Rh-Isoimmunization 1977. Mod Med Can 1977; 32:17.)

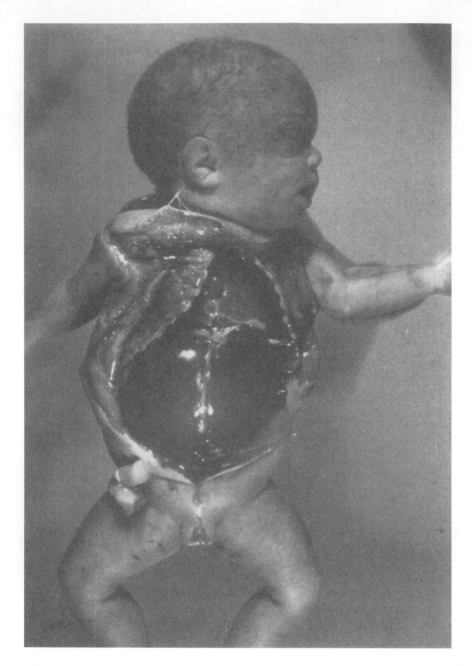

Figure 3 Hydropic neonate who died a few minutes after birth. Note extreme enlargement of the liver and moderate enlargement of the spleen. (From Bowman JM. Blood-group incompatibilities. In: Iffy L, Kaminetzky HA, eds. Principles and Practice of Obstetrics and Perinatology, New York, John Wiley & Sons, 1981; 70:1193.)

of a single gene locus occupied by a pair of complex agglutinogens is probably the most accurate (7), and the numbering nomenclature of Rosenfield et al. is the most straightforward (8), the nomenclature and theories of inheritance of Fisher and Race are simpler and more practical for clinical use (9). They theorize that there are three pairs of Rh antigens; commonly Dd, Cc, Ee. The presence of D indicates a D+ person. The absence of D, not the presence of d, which has

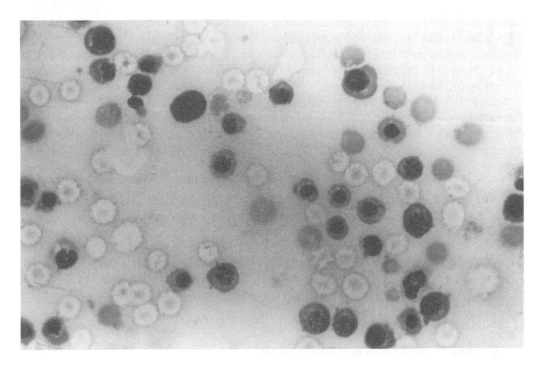

Figure 4 Cord blood of baby with severe Rh erythroblastosis fetalis who required multiple fetal transfusions and exchange transfusions. Smear treated by Kleihauer technique and Wright's stain. Note adult donor ghost RBCs, dark fetal RBCs, and early fetal erythroid series from erythroblasts through to normoblasts. (From Bowman JM. The management of Rh-Isoimmunization. Obstet Gynecol 1978; 52:1–16.)

never been shown to exist, denotes a D– person. The production of anti-D in D– women causes hemolytic disease in D+ fetuses. The antigens are inherited in two sets of three; one set from each parent. CDe(R^1), c(d)e(r), and cDE(R^2) are the most common sets (Table 1). CDE(R^z) is uncommon in whites but not rare in North American Indians. C(d)E(r^y) is exceedingly rare.

Slightly less than half of D+ people are homozygous for the D antigen (i.e., they have inherited a set of antigens containing D from both sets of parents). The remainder are

Table 1 Rh Gene Frequencies in a White Canadian Population of 2000 Unrelated Adults

Gene Complex	Frequency (%)
CDe(R^1)	41
c(d)e(r)	39
cDE(R^2)	16
cDe(R^0)	2.2
C(d)e(r′)	1.1
c(d)E(r″)	0.6
CDE(R^z)	0.08
C(d)E(r^y)	0.00

Source: From Lewis M, Kaita H, Chown B. The inheritance of the Rh blood groups: Frequencies in 1000 unrelated caucasian families consisting of 2000 parents and 2806 children. *Vox Sang* 1971; 20:502.

heterozygous for D (i.e., they have inherited a D-containing set from only one parent). The zygosity for D of the D+ man who impregnates a D– woman is important. If he is homozygous, all of their children will be D+; if he is heterozygous, there is an equal chance that the fetus will be D– or D+. Only D+ fetuses can cause Rh immunization and only Rh+ fetuses are affected by the Rh antibody produced.

Because anti-d has never been detected, the zygosity of the man for D can only be determined if he fathers two infants who have received different sets of antigens from him. Because some sets of antigens are more common than others (see Table 1), the determination of the presence or absence of the other Rh antigens C, E, c, and e, will indicate the likely, but not certain, zygosity of the father for D (Table 2).

There are at least 43 more antigens in the Rh system than the five described. C^w, an allele of C, and D^u, an allele of D, are not uncommon. There are two kinds of D^u individuals, one who is genetically D+ but because of the presence of C on the opposite chromosome has reduction in strength of the D antigen; and the other, who is missing some part of the D antigen mosaic, a so-called D variant. Very uncommonly, a D-variant mother carrying a D+ fetus may produce anti-D, which on at least one occasion has been reported to cause hydrops fetalis (10). Even more rarely, an Rh– mother carrying a D^u fetus may become Rh immunized. D variants are more common in blacks. Tippett and Sanger have described six degrees of D variants in these partially Rh+ people (11).

B. Rh Antigen Structures and Distribution

The Rh antigen D has recently been isolated and characterized (12,13). It is a polypeptide proteolipid with a molecular weight of 28,000–33,000. The Rh antigens are believed to be present only in the RBC membrane, although there is a recent report that placental trophoblast

Table 2 Zygosity for Rh(D) of D+ Father (D– Mother)

Antigens Present in Father	A (Most Likely Rh Genotype)	B (Less likely (Rh Genotype)	C (Least likely Rh Genotype)
1. CDe	$CDe/CDe(R^1R^1)^a$ Homozygous	$CDe/Cde(R^1r')$ Heterozygous	
2. CDce	$CDe/cde(R^1r)$ Heterozygous	$CDe/cDe(R^1R^0)$ Homozygous	$cDe/Cde(R^0r')$ Heterozygous
3. CDEce	$CDe/cDE(R^1R^2)$ Homozygous	$cDE/Cde(R^2r')$ $CDe/cdE(R^1r'')$ $CDE/cde(R^zr)$ Heterozygous	$CDE/cDe(R^zR^0)$ Homozygous
4. DEc	$cDE/cDE(R^2R^2)^a$ Homozygous	$cDE/cdE(R^2r'')$ Heterozygous	
5. DEce	$cDE/cde(R^2r)$ Heterozygous	$cDE/cDe(R^2R^0)$ Homozygous	$cDe/cdE(R^0r'')$ Heterozygous
6. Dce	$cDe/cde(R^0r)$ Heterozygous	$cDe/cDe(R^0R^0$ Homozygous	

[a]Genotypes 1A and 4A cannot be proved because the infant will be of only one paternal genotype (CDe in 1A and cDE in 4A). The remainder of the father's possible genotypes can be proved only if he produces children of two different genotypes.
Source: Bowman JM, Friesen RF. Rh-isoimmunization. In: Goodwin JW, Godden JO, Chance G, eds. Perinatal Medicine. Baltimore, 1976. Williams & Wilkins.

may contain Rh antigenic determinants (14). Rh antigens are an essential component of the RBC membrane. Rare people without any Rh antigens (Rh$_{null}$) have defective RBC membranes and some degree of hemolytic anemia.

Rh negativity is a trait of white individuals. In most whites, the incidence is 15–16%. In Finland, it is only 11–12%. In Basques, its prevalence is about 35%. Millennia ago, races other than white, were probably all Rh(D) positive. They owe their present incidence of Rh negativity to intermingling of white genes, (North American Indians and Eskimos, about 1%; American blacks 7–8%; IndoEurasians, about 2%; Asiatic Chinese and Japanese, almost zero).

III. PATHOGENESIS OF RH IMMUNIZATION

With the rapid institution of universal Rh-compatible blood transfusion, there was surprisingly very little reduction in the incidence of Rh immunization. What was noted, however, was that Rh immunization almost exclusively appeared in parous D– women who had usually had at least one previous unaffected pregnancy. This observation led Wiener, in 1948, to resurrect Darrow's fetal transplacental hemorrhage (TPH) theory (15); i.e., D+ fetal RBCs cross the placenta into the D– mother during pregnancy and at the time of delivery, and it is this mode of exposure that produces Rh immunization (Fig. 5). Darrow's and Wiener's TPH theory was proven by Chown in 1954 (16). A D– primigravida with no anti-D at the time of delivery gave birth to a very anemic infant with many circulating erythroblasts and with hepatosplenomegaly. However, THE RBCs of the infant were direct antiglobulin test (DAT) negative and the woman after delivery appeared to be weakly D+. Differential agglutination methods and quantitative fetal hemoglobin measurements, by alkaline denaturation techniques, showed that 8% of her circulating RBCs were D+ and of fetal origin, proving that a very large fetal TPH had occurred. Within 20 days after delivery, the woman produced a strong anti-D and subsequently had very severely affected erythroblastotic infants.

Although Chown's observation proved that Rh immunization occurred as a result of fetal TPH, knowledge concerning the frequency and size of fetal TPH had to await the development

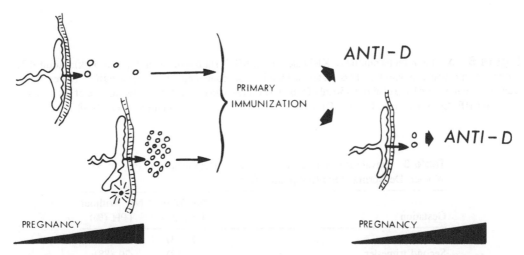

Figure 5 Diagrammatic representation of the hypothesis (Darrow 1938, Ref. 3; Wiener 1948, Ref. 15) (proved by Chown 1954, Ref. 16) that Rh(D)- fetal RBCs traverse the placenta (small amounts during pregnancy, larger amounts at delivery) and into the maternal circulation. If Rh(D)-, the mother responds by producing anti-D. The anti-D, if IgG, traverses the placenta into the fetal circulation, coats the fetal D-RCCs and hemolyzes them.

of the acid elution test of Kleihauer et al. in 1957 (17). This test, which depends upon the resistance of fetal hemoglobin to acid elution (Fig. 6), can detect one fetal RBC in 200,000, adult RBCs. Using this technique, the frequency and size of fetal TPH have been determined (Table 3) (18): 3% in the first trimester, 12% in the second trimester, 45% in the third trimester, and 64% immediately after birth. In 25% of pregnancies, no fetal RBCs can be detected at any time [18]. Unfortunately, the Kleihauer acid elution test is not a test that lends itself to routine blood bank use. The size of fetal TPH increases as pregnancy progresses. Less than 1% of women will have >5 ml and <0.25% will have >30 ml of fetal blood in their circulations.

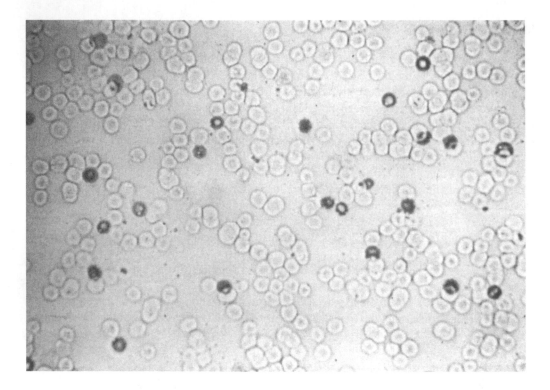

Figure 6   Acid elution technique of Kleihauer. Fetal RBCs stain with eosin (appear dark). Adult RBCs do not stain (appear as ghosts). This maternal blood smear contained 11.2% fetal RBCs, representing a transplacental hemorrhage of about 450 ml of blood. (From Bowman JM. Hemolytic disease of the newborn. In: Conn HF, Conn RB, eds. Current Diagnosis 5. Philadelphia, WB Saunders, 1977:1098.)

Table 3   Prevalence of Fetal Transplacental Hemorrhage (TPH) in 33 Women Delivering ABO-Compatible Babies

Gestation	No. With TPH (%)	No. Without TPH (%)
First trimester	1 (3)	32 (97)
Second trimester	4 (12)	29 (88)
Third trimester	15 (45)	18 (55)
Postdelivery	21 (64)	12 (36)
At any time during pregnancy and delivery	25 (76)	8 (24)

Source: From Ref. 18.

Certain obstetrical situations increase the risk of TPH: antepartum hemorrhage, toxemia of pregnancy, external version, cesarean section, and manual removal of the placenta. Amniocentesis, particularly if not carried out under ultrasound guidance, is a hazard (11.2% before ultrasound in one series) (19). Even with the use of ultrasound, TPH occur in about 2.5% of cases after amniocentesis (20).

A significant number of abortions, both spontaneous and therapeutic, are associated with fetal TPH. The Rh antigen is well developed by 30 to 45 days of gestation. After therapeutic abortion, about 4% of women may have TPH in excess of 0.2 ml of fetal blood.

A. Rh Immune Response

1. Primary Immune Response

The primary immune response develops slowly. In experimental Rh immunization of male volunteers, an antibody may be noted as early as 4 weeks after injection but usually 8 to 9 weeks will elapse before the response is apparent. Indeed, it may not be detectable for 6 months.

The primary response is frequently weak and often IgM in nature. IgM anti-D does not cross the placenta and does not cause fetal RBC hemolysis. The majority of D– women quickly convert to IgG anti-D production. IgG anti-D traverses the placenta and produces fetal RBC hemolysis.

2. Secondary Immune Response

Once the primary response has occurred, a second exposure to Rh+ RBCs produces a very rapid increase in anti-D, which is for the most part IgG. Subsequent exposure may produce even higher levels. If the intervals between antigen exposure are long, the subsequent exposure is often associated with a marked increase in Rh antibody titer and increased avidity (binding constant) of the antibody for the Rh antigen. The greater the avidity of the Rh antibody for the Rh antigen (its binding constant), the greater will be the severity of Rh erythroblastosis.

B. Dose of Rh Antigen Necessary to Produce Rh Immunization

1. Rh Immunizing Experiments

Amounts of D+ blood required to produce Rh immunization may be small. In one study, 50% of volunteers were immunized by 10 ml of blood. In other experiments, two thirds were immunized by five injections of 3.5 ml; 80% by one injection of 0.5 ml of D+ RBCs (21) and 30% by repeated injections of 0.1 ml of RBCs (22). The prevalence of Rh immunization depends on the dose of D+ RBCs; 15% after 1 ml and 65–70% after 250 ml. Secondary immune responses may occur after exposure to much smaller amounts (as little as 0.03 ml of D+ RBCs).

C. Rh Immunization Clinical Studies

Serial fetal cell studies using the Kleihauer technique during pregnancy and immediately after delivery allow the determination of the risk of Rh immunization in relation to the presence and size of fetal TPH. If the TPH is always <0.1 ml of RBCs, the prevalence of Rh immunization detectable up to 6 months after delivery is 3% (22); when volumes exceed 0.4 ml, the prevalence is 22% (21). Because in 75–80% of pregnancies TPH (if any) are always <0.1 ml, the majority of women are Rh immunized as a result of small or undetectable transplacental hemorrhages.

D. Frequency of Rh Immunization

The prevalence of Rh immunization demonstrable within 6 months after delivery of the first Rh+ ABO compatible infant is 8–9%. Nevanlinna noted that about the same number of those who had no detectable Rh antibodies 6 months after delivery demonstrated that they also were Rh immunized by the previous D+ pregnancy by mounting a secondary immune response in the next D+ pregnancy; a phenomenon he called "sensibilization" (23). The true incidence of Rh immunization as a result of the first Rh+, ABO-compatible pregnancy is of the order of 16%.

A woman not immunized by the first such pregnancy is at approximately the same risk in a second D+, ABO-compatible pregnancy. However, as parity increases and the number of women capable of an Rh immune response diminishes because they have become immunized, the number who mount a primary immune response will decrease because of a greater residual number of "nonresponders." By the time an Rh− woman has completed her fifth ABO-compatible, Rh+ pregnancy, there is about a 50% probability that she will be Rh immunized. Before the Rh prevention era, 0.8–1.0% of pregnant women in Manitoba were Rh immunized. About 25–30% of D− women are nonresponders. They do not become Rh immunized despite many D+ pregnancies, although some may become Rh immunized following exposure to a large (massive) amount of D+ blood.

ABO incompatibility confers partial protection against Rh immunization. The prevalence of Rh immunization 6 months after delivery of an ABO incompatible, D+ infant is 1.5–2% (21). Partial protection is probably due to rapid intravascular hemolysis of the ABO-incompatible, D+ RBCs, with sequestration of D+ stroma in the liver, an organ with poor antibody-forming potential; in contrast to the spleen, which is the site of RBC stroma sequestration when extravascular RBC destruction occurs. Although ABO incompatibility confers substantial protection against the primary Rh immune response, it confers no protection against the secondary Rh immune response (24).

Rh immunization during pregnancy, once considered to be a rare phenomenon, is not uncommon. In Winnipeg, 1.8% (62 of 3533) of Rh− women without evidence of Rh immunization in early pregnancy were Rh immunized during pregnancy or within 3 days after delivery (Table 4) (25). Rh immunization during pregnancy accounts for one-seventh of Rh− women who will be Rh immunized by an Rh+ pregnancy. Therefore, Rh immunization during pregnancy is an important factor as far as Rh immunization prevention is concerned.

The risk of Rh immunization occurring after a spontaneous abortion is about 1.5–2.0%, increasing the later in gestation abortion occurs. It is considerably higher after therapeutic abortion, being 4–5%, Women who are Rh immunized following the small TPH that occur at the time of abortion are good responders. They often have very severely affected infants in subsequent pregnancies. Although the risk of immunization after abortion at 6–8 weeks of gestation is small, it becomes significant by the tenth to the twelfth week.

Table 4 Rh Immunization During Pregnancy or Within 3 Days After Delivery (Manitoba, March 1, 1967, to December 15, 1974)

Blood Group of Infant	No. of Rh− Pregnant Women	No. Rh Immunized (%)
Rh+, ABO compatible	2859	58 (2.0)
Rh+, ABO incompatible	674	4 (0.6)
Total of all women*	3533	62 (1.8)

[a]Primigravidas and multigravidas given RhIG after every preceding Rh+ pregnancy and abortion.
Source: From Ref. 25.

IV. PATHOGENESIS OF RH HEMOLYTIC DISEASE

Erythropoiesis is present in the yolk sac of the human embryo by the third week of gestation. Rh antigen has been found in the RBC membrane by the sixth week. By 8–10 weeks of gestation, RBC production has begun in the liver and spleen. Under normal conditions, erythropoiesis has shifted to and is confined to the bone marrow by the sixth month. In the presence of fetal anemia, either due to hemolysis or blood loss, erythropoiesis may persist in the liver and spleen and may be extreme.

The fundamental cause of erythroblastosis fetalis is maternal Rh(D) IgG antibody coating of D+ fetal RBCs and their destruction. Hemolysis causes fetal anemia, which stimulates the production of erythropoietin. Erythropoiesis increases. Fetal marrow RBC production cannot keep up with RBC destruction and extramedullary erythropoiesis (spleen, liver, kidneys, adrenals) recurs. Hepatosplenomegaly (see Fig. 3) is a hallmark of erythroblastosis fetalis.

In the presence of extramedullary erythropoiesis, RBC maturation is poorly controlled. Immature nucleated RBCs from normoblasts to early erythroblasts (see Fig. 4) are poured into the circulation.

A. Mechanism of RBC Hemolysis

1. Complement Mediated Hemolysis

When antibody fixes complement, such as anti-A and anti-B, severe RBC damage occurs. Large defects are produced in the RBC membrane. Intravascular hemolysis with hemoglobinemia and hemoglobinuria occurs. RBC debris is picked up for the most part in the liver, where it is phagocytosed by the reticuloendothelial cells in the microcirculation.

2. Non-Complement Mediated Hemolysis

When antibodies do not fix complement, such as anti-D, either IgG or IgM, the mechanism of hemolysis is quite different. It is more subtle but in the end is as destructive as that of anti-A or anti-B. When anti-D attaches itself to the D antigen in the RBC membrane, the attraction of macrophages to the coated RBCs, (chemotaxis) is increased. The coated RBCs adhere to the macrophages forming rosettes. RBC adherence and formation of rosettes occur particularly in the spleen, where the circulation slows and the hematocrit increases bringing RBCs and macrophages into close apposition. Electron microscopy reveals macrophage pseudopods attaching to the RBC membrane, puckering, and invaginating it (26). A portion of the membrane breaks off, and the defect seals. However, loss of membrane substance causes sphering of the RBCs with greater rigidity and loss of deformability. Even if the RBC escapes the macrophage, it is damaged with greater osmotic fragility and likelihood of lysis. Rh antibody–mediated RBC destruction follows the chain of events outlined: rosette formation around macrophages in the spleen, loss of RBC membrane with sphering and rigidity, and osmotic fragility with lysis and phagocytosis of RBC fragments.

A correlation has been established between lysis by K lymphocytes of RBCs sensitized in utero and the severity of hemolytic disease of the newborn (27). When RBCs sensitized with IgG antibodies adhere to receptors for the Fc portion of IgG on K cells, monocytes, or macrophages, phagocytosis and particularly cytotoxic RBC destruction occurs. Engelfriet et al. (28) have shown that phagocytosis and cytotoxic RBC lysis are independent mechanisms and that cytotoxicity is due to the release of lysosomal enzymes by monocytes/macrophages at their point of contact with sensitized red cells causing the RBCs to lyse. When the fetal RBC population is suddenly coated by a potent antibody, a back-up occurs in the spleen, which causes RBCs converted to spherocytes to be released into the peripheral blood (29). Having escaped once, these abnormal RBCs are now in double jeopardy; as well as being coated with antibody, they have become rigid, less deformable, and are easily trapped in the spleen (30).

3. IgG Subclasses and Severity of Hemolytic Disease

As already noted, the first stage in RBC destruction caused by non–complement binding antibodies such as anti-D, is adherence of the IgG-coated RBCs to the Fc receptors of monocytes. The capacity of RBC-bound IgG3 antibodies to bind to these Fc receptors is greater than that of IgG1 antibodies. One might presume, therefore, that IgG3 anti-D is a more potent and lethal RBC antibody than IgG1 anti-D and this is probably true because clearance of Rh+ RBCs is caused by fewer molecules of IgG3 anti-D than IgG1 anti-D (31). The increased potency of IgG3 versus IgG1 is borne out by studies, which show that IgG1 and IgG3 anti-D in combination caused more severe hemolytic disease than IgG1 anti-D alone (32,33).

IgG3 anti-D alone without accompanying IgG1 anti-D is observed much less often and is often of low titer. In one series (32), IgG3 alone was invariabily of low titer and produced mild disease only. In another series (33), IgG3 along produced Rh disease as severe as that caused by IgG1 alone but less severe than that caused by IgG1 and IgG3 in combination of equal titer.

In contradiction to the two observations of greater severity of hemolytic disease when IgG1 and IgG3 anti-D are both present (32,33), there is a report of greater severity of hemolytic disease when IgG1 alone was present with the Gm allotype G1m (4): 44% severity compared with 31% severity when IgG1 and IgG3 were both present and 8% severity when only IgG3 was present (34). Taken on balance, it appears that IgG3 anti-D is a more dangerous antibody in respect to fetal D+ RBC hemolysis than IgG1 anti-D, but it is usually found in significant concentration only when accompanied by IgG1 anti-D.

V. MATERNAL ALLOANTIBODIES CAUSING FETAL HEMOLYTIC DISEASE

A. Alloantibodies Other Than Anti-A and B

Anti-D in the Rh blood group system is still the most common antibody causing severe hemolytic disease. However, Rh preventive measures have produced a striking reduction in D alloimmunization (84% reduction in Manitoba by 1988).

In Manitoba (population 1 million), the mean annual occurrence of D alloimmunization in pregnant women dropped from 194 in the 5-year period ending October 31, 1967, to 28 in the 6-year period ending October 31, 1988. In the same two periods, the mean annual occurrence of detected non-D alloimmunization in pregnant women, excluding ABO alloimmunization, increased from 14 to 88 (35). This increase is partially due to the increased screening of pregnant D+ women. It is also due to a real increase in the occurrence of non-D alloimmunization because of the increased frequency of blood transfusion (transfused blood being only ABO and D compatible). For this reason, non-D alloantibodies have assumed greater importance in the causation of hemolytic disease. Mollison et al. (36) list the following alloantibodies as having been reported to cause hemolytic disease: (1) within the Rh system, anti-D, -c, -C, -C^w, -C^x, -e, -E, -E^w, -ce, -Ce^s, -Rh32, -Go^a, -Be^a, -Evans, -LW; (2) outside the Rh system, anti-K, -k, -K^u, Kp^a, -Kp^b, -Js^a, -Js^b, -Fy^a, -Fy^3, -Jk^a, -Jk^b, -M, -N, -S, -s, -U, -Vw, -Far, -M^v, -Mit, -Mt^a, -Mur, -Hil, -Hut, -En^a, -PP$_1$P^k, -Lu^a, -Lu^b, -Lu^9, -Di^a, -Di^b, -Yt^a, -Yt^b, -Do^a, -Co^a, -Wr^a; (3) antibodies due to low incidence antigens, anti-Bi, -By, -Fr^a, -Good, -Rd, -Re^a, -Zd; and (4) antibodies to high incidence antigens, anti-At^a, -Jr^a, -Lan, -Ge. They state that of all the multitude of antibodies implicated in producing HDN, those reported to produce moderate to severe hemolytic disease are all of those in the Rh blood group system plus anti-K, -Jk^a, -Js^a, -Js^b, -Ku, -Fy^a, -M, -N, -s, -U, -PP$_1$P^k, -Di^b, -Lan, -LW, -Far, -Good, -Wr^a, and -Zd.

This list appears intimidating but must be considered in conjunction with the frequency with which such antibodies occur and the frequency with which they cause significant hemolytic disease of the newborn.

The increase in occurrence of non-D alloimmunization is reflected in the changing ratio of D to non-D alloimmunization in pregnant patients from outside Manitoba referred to the Rh Laboratory for fetal treatment (Table 5). Although those with anti-D still predominate, the numbers referred with non-D alloimmunization have increased from 2 in the 10-year period ending December 31, 1973, to 19 in the 10-year period ending December 31, 1988. The non-D alloantibodies observed in pregnant Manitoban women during the 26-year period ending October 31, 1988, are listed in Tables 6 and 7. Although anti-E and anti-K were the most common (350 and 337, respectively), only 13 of the 108 affected infants (cord RBCs direct antiglobulin positive) due to anti-E and only 2 of the 8 affected infants due to anti-K required exchange transfusion and/or phototherapy. None of them was severely affected. Anti-c, when present, was more likely to cause hemolytic disease (65% versus 31 and 2.4% for anti-E and anti-K), and in those affected it was more likely to cause disease requiring exchange transfusion and/or phototherapy (29% versus 12 and 25% for anti-E and K). Anti-c was the only non-D alloantibody in the 26-year period that caused disease so severe that it ended in hydropic stillbirth, fetuses

Table 5 Non-Manitoba Patients Referred to the Winnipeg Rh Laboratory with Severe Fetal Hemolytic Disease (January 1, 1964, to December 31, 1988: Antibody Specificity)

5-Year Period	No. of Anti-D Patients	No. of Non–anti-D Patients (%)	Non–anti-D Specificity
1964–1968	57	0	
1969–1973	59	2 (3.3)	1K, 1E
1974–1978	24	1 (4.0)	1K
1979–1983	23	6 (20.7)	1K, 4c, 1Fy[a]
1984–1988	60	13 (17.8)	6K, 3c, 1k, 1cE, 1Jk[a], 1CC[w]

Source: From Ref. 35.

Table 6 Severity of Hemolytic Disease: Manitoba—26 Years (November 1, 1962, to October 31, 1988) Except for Anti-D (November 1, 1975, to October 31, 1988)

Alloantibody Specificity	No. of Patients	Affected (%)	% No Treatment Required	% Phototherapy and/or Exchange Transfusion Required	% Stillborn Hydropic or Hgb <60 g/L
D (13 yr)	420	201 (48)	49	32	19
E	350	108 (31)	88	12	–
c, cE	183	119 (65)	62	29	9*
C, Ce, C[w]	108	34 (32)	79	21	–
Kell	337	8 (2.4)	75	25	–
Kp[a]	6	2 (33)	50	50	–
k	1	1 (100)		100	–
Fy[a]	23	5 (22)	80	20	–
S	14	8 (57)	75	25	–

*Anti-c, other than D, was the only cause of hydrops in Manitoba patients in the 26-year period.
Source: From Ref. 35.

Table 7 Antibodies Associated with No
Treatment Required or No Clinical
Disease—Manitoba

Not affected	
Lu^a	15
Lu^b	1
P	25
Le^a (Le^b)	88
Wr^a	18
Multiple/rare	11
Nonspecific or high incidence	11
Affected but no treatment required	
Fy^b	1 of 3
Jk^a	4 of 7
Jk^b	1 of 2
s	1 of 2
M	2 of 82
LW	1 of 2
Autoantibody	3 of 27

Source: From Ref. 35.

requiring intrauterine transfusions, or infants born with cord hemoglobin levels <60 g/L (6 g/dl).

In a more recent study of K alloimmunization in Manitoban women encompassing the years 1944–1990 (37), 20 infants born of K-alloimmunized mothers were K+ and affected with hemolytic disease. Twelve of the 20 were so mildly affected that they required no treatment. Four were moderately affected and required either exchange transfusion or phototherapy. Four were severely affected (all born before 1955); three were hydropic and died; one, left untreated in a rural hospital, developed kernicterus and died (37).

Anti-C, -Ce, -C^w, -Kp^a, -k, -Fy^a, and -S (see Table 6) on rare occasions caused hemolytic disease severe enough to require treatment after birth, but in no instance was disease so severe that hydrops developed or that fetal transfusions were required. Other blood group antibodies in these pregnant Manitoban patients (see Table 7) produced either no clinical disease or mild clinical disease that did not require treatment.

The experience of the Rh Laboratory over the past 25 years with 22 pregnant non-D alloimmunized women referred from outside Manitoba, a highly selected group with very severely affected fetuses, drawn from a much greater population base, is somewhat different (Table 8). In these referred women, there were examples of the following antibodies: K (nine), c (seven), k (one) (38), Jk^a, Fy^a, CC^w, and E (one each), which produced hemolytic disease so severe intrauterine treatment was required. There are rare instances of other alloantibodies, usually benign, causing severe hemolytic disease (e.g., anti-Kp^b (39), anti-M (40)).

B. ABO Hemolytic Disease

ABO hemolytic disease of the newborn is very different from hemolytic disease either due to anti-D or other blood group antibodies. Anti-A and anti-B, which bind complement in adults, produce violent, life-threatening intravascular hemolysis after transfusion of ABO-incompatible blood. Fetal ABO hemolytic disease is nearly always much milder than Rh, c, K, and some other forms of "atypical" hemolytic disease. Although kernicterus may develop if the baby with ABO hemolytic disease is left untreated, hydrops rarely if ever occurs, and anemia at birth is

Table 8 Twenty-two Non–anti-D Out of Province Referrals to Rh Laboratory

Alloantibody Specificity	No. of Patients	Antigen Negative	Present Pregnancy Hydrops in Pregnancy	Hydropic Deaths	IUT Traumatic Deaths
K	9	1	8	4[a]	0
c	7	0	1	0	2[a]
cE	1	0	0	0	0
Fy[a]	1	0	0	0	0
Jk[a]	1	0	1	0	0
CC[w]	1	0	0[b]	0	0
k	1	0	0[c]	0	0
E	1	0	0[b]	0	1

[a]Three K and 1 c death not treated in Winnipeg.
[b]Prior hydropic death.
[c]Hgb 60 g/L.
Source: From Ref. 35.

never more than moderate. There are extremely rare reports of hydrops fetalis due to ABO erythroblastosis (41,42), but in every reported instance, the possibility of nonimmune hydrops superimposed upon ABO erythroblastosis could not be excluded.

Several reasons can be listed for the paradoxical mildness of ABO hemolytic disease. First, there are a smaller number of A and B antigenic sites on the fetal RBC membrane. Also, anti-A and anti-B do not bind complement on the fetal RBC membrane (43). Second, anti-A and anti-B are mostly IgM, which does not traverse the placenta. Third, the small amounts of IgG anti-A and anti-B that do cross the placenta have a myriad of antigenic sites over than on RBCs, other tissues and secretions, to which they may bind. Only a very small proportion of the minor amount of anti-A or anti-B that crosses the placenta adheres to antigen on the RBC membrane. Because there is very little antibody on the RBC, the cord blood direct antiglobulin test (DAT) in ABO hemolytic disease is only weakly positive and may be negative unless a sensitive test is used. Not infrequently, capillary blood taken when the infant is 2 or 3 days old yields a negative result no matter how sensitive the test used.

In about 25–30% of ABO-incompatible babies, cord blood RBCs are weakly DAT+ at delivery. Only a very small fraction of these infants develop clinical evidence of hemolytic disease (early and severe jaundice). In one hospital of 9000 ABO-incompatible babies delivered from 1954 to 1965, 2500 had weakly DAT+ RBCs and only 41 (<2%) required exchange transfusion (44).

VI. SEVERITY OF FETAL HEMOLYTIC DISEASE

As one might expect, there is a wide spectrum of severity of hemolytic disease (Table 9). About 50% of affected fetuses are so mildly affected that they survive without treatment, as they did in the early 1940s before any treatment was available. Of the remainder, about one-half (25% of the total) will be born alive at or near term in good condition. However, unless they are treated promptly after birth, they will develop kernicterus. Ninety percent will die; the remaining 10% will be left with severe neurological damage, neurosensory deafness, spastic choreoathetosis, and some degree of mental retardation. The remaining 25% will become hydropic and die in utero; about one-half between 18 weeks and 34 weeks' gestation and the other half after 34 weeks' gestation. Although hydrops was once considered to be due to anemic hypervolemic

Table 9 Classification of Severity of Rh Hemolytic Disease

Degree of Severity	Description	Incidence (%)
Mild	Indirect bilirubin does not exceed 300–340 μmol/L (17.5–20.0 mg/100 ml); no anemia; no treatment needed	45–50
Moderate	Fetal hydrops does not develop; moderate anemia; severe jaundice with risk of kernicterus unless treated after birth	25–30
Severe	Fetal hydrops develops in utero	20–25
	Before 34 weeks' gestation	10–12
	After 34 weeks' gestation	10–12

Source: From Ref. 46.

fetal heart failure, in most instances, heart failure is a secondary factor that develops after delivery and treatment. The primary cause is almost certainly hepatic: extreme hepatosplenomegaly, portal hypertension with the development of ascites; hepatocellular damage producing hypoalbuminemia; and generalized anasarca (45).

VII. PREDICTIVE PARAMETERS DETERMINING SEVERITY OF FETAL HEMOLYTIC DISEASE

The problem of investigative and treatment measures in alloimmunized pregnant women is that they carry some risk to the fetus. Therefore, it is important that the severity of fetal disease be determined as precisely as possible and that investigative measures be confined to pregnancies in which the fetus is at risk and treatment measures be restricted to fetuses who require them in order to survive.

Several investigative parameters can be useful in predicting severity of fetal hemolytic disease. These measures include:

1. History of severity of hemolytic disease in previous infants
2. Maternal antibody titers
3. Cell-mediated maternal antibody functional assays
4. Amniotic fluid spectrophotometry
5. Fetal ultrasonography
6. Percutaneous fetal blood sampling

A. Past Pregnancy History

Up to 1961, the only measures available to assess severity of hemolytic disease were the degree of severity of hemolytic disease in previous pregnancies and maternal antibody titers. Although it is usually correct that the severity of hemolytic disease remains the same or increases in severity during subsequent affected pregnancies, occasionally disease may be less severe. With a past history of hydrops, a subsequent affected fetus has a better than 90% but not a 100% chance of becoming hydropic. If hydrops is going to develop, it will do so usually at the same gestational age or earlier, but occasionally later. With a prior history of hydrops and a father heterozygous for the offending antigen, the physician is in a dilemma. The fetus may be antigen negative and unaffected or antigen positive and very severely affected. In a first D-sensitized pregnancy, in which there is no prior history of hemolytic disease, there is an 8–10% likelihood of hydrops developing.

B. Maternal Alloantibody Titers

Although antibody titrations carried out in the same laboratory by the same experienced personnel and using the same methods and test cells are reproducible and do give the physician some indication of risk, they are not of such accuracy by themselves to allow potentially hazardous fetal treatment measures to be undertaken. In an 8-year period, 1954–1961, in which 426 Rh-immunized women came to delivery at the Winnipeg General Hospital, 54 fetuses survived only because they were induced and delivered early. Sixty-seven perinatal deaths occurred. Of the 67 deaths, 34 were potentially salvageable using management measures available at that time (26 with earlier delivery, 8 with later delivery) if the degree of severity of disease had only been better known. When we assessed these 121 most severely affected pregnancies, it was apparent that our accuracy of prediction of severity of hemolytic disease was only 62% (46).

C. Cell-Mediated Maternal Antibody Functional Assays

Because of the relatively poor correlation between blood group antibody titrations and severity of hemolytic disease, various functional assays have been developed that reflect the binding constant or avidity of the antibody for the antigen on the RBC cell membrane and, therefore, its ability to produce severe hemolytic disease. These assays include the monocyte monolayer assay (MMA) (33,47) and the antibody-dependent cellular cytotoxicity (ADCC) using lymphocytes (48), monocytes (49), and monocyte chemiluminescence (50).

Each one of these assays has its proponents. Three recent papers have compared the functional assays. Hadley et al. (51) compared monocyte chemiluminescence, K cell lymphocyte ADCC, monocyte-macrophage ADCC, and a rosette assay using U937 cells. They found that monocyte-based (i.e., monocyte chemiluminescence and monocyte ADCC) functional assays predicted severity of disease better than lymphocyte-based assays (U937 cells and K-lymphocyte ADCC). Similarly, Zupanska et al. (33) found that a monocyte-based assay (MMA) correlated better with clinical severity of hemolytic disease than did rosette assays using either lymphocytes or monocytes. A survey of nine European laboratories carrying out functional assays reported by Mollison (52) testing sera from mothers deliverying babies with varying degrees of hemolytic disease revealed correct results as follows: ADCC (monocytes) 60%, ADCC (lymphocytes) 57%, chemiluminescence 51%; rosetting and phagocytosis[a] with peripheral monocytes 41%, [b] with U937 cells or cultured macrophages 32%. The assays appeared to be more helpful in predicting mild or minimal disease rather than predicting very severe disease. Obviously, since all of these assays measure the potential lethality of the maternal antibody, they are quite incapable of differentiating the unaffected antigen-negative fetus from the affected antigen-positive fetus.

Recently, there has been a report that casts doubt on the ability of the monocyte-macrophage (MMA) assay to predict severity of hemolytic disease of the newborn (53). In sera from 41 pregnant women with potentially dangerous blood group antibodies who delivered affected babies, there was no correlation between the hematocrit of a fetal blood sample obtained at cordocentesis and the MMA (53).

Thus, in summary, although the functional tests listed may be helpful in more accurately determining the fetus at risk and, therefore, in some pregnancies, precluding the need for invasive measures such as amniocentesis and fetal blood sampling, they in no way replace such invaluable perinatal management aids in ultimately differentiating the fetus who requires treatment in utero from the fetus who does not.

D. Amniotic Fluid Spectrophotometry

In 1969, Liley reported the use of amniotic fluid spectrophotometry as a means of determining severity of hemolytic disease (54). Although Bevis, in 1956, was the first to use amniotic fluid spectrophotometry (55), Liley was the first to develop a method of measurement, the deviation from linearity at 450 nm, the absorption spectrum of bilirubin, i.e., the ΔOD 450 reading, which allowed communication from one center to another of an easily interpreted reading, readily giving an accurate determination of severity of hemolytic disease. Readings falling into very high zone 2 or zone 3 (Fig. 7) indicate severe disease, with hydrops present or developing within 7–10 days; readings falling into zone 1 indicate either no disease or no anemia but a 10% chance of requiring exchange transfusion; readings in zone 2 indicate moderate disease, becoming more severe as the zone 3 boundary is approached. The overall amniotic fluid accuracy of prediction of hemolytic disease severity is 95%; this accuracy can only be achieved with serial ΔOD 450 measurements. Amniotic fluid ΔOD 450 readings reflect severity of disease more accurately in the third trimester than they do in the second trimester. In the second trimester, the zone boundaries have not been as accurately determined (56,57); again pointing out the need for serial measurements (often weekly for several weeks). Final readings falling in zone 1 and zone 3 have an accuracy of prediction rate of 98%, but final readings falling in zone 2 have an accuracy of prediction rate of only 90%.

Recently, we have modified the Liley zone boundaries before 24 weeks' gestation by inclining the boundaries downward at the same angle of declination as the angle of inclination after 24 weeks' gestation (58), reflecting the observation that ΔOD 450 readings (i.e., bilirubin levels) in pregnancies unaffected by hemolytic disease peak at 23–24 weeks' gestation (56) (Fig. 8). Because fetal blood sampling, followed if necessary by intravascular fetal transfusions, is, respectively, the most accurate means of determining the presence and severity of Rh hemolytic disease and the preferred method of transfusion in utero if necessary, amniotic fluid ΔOD 450 measurements are used to determine the need for fetal blood sampling. Specifically, fetal blood

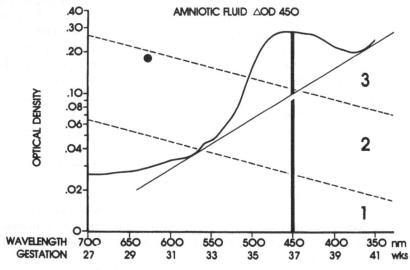

Figure 7   Amniotic fluid spectrophotometric reading: Liley method. ΔOD 450 0.200 (in this example) falls high in zone 2 at 29 1/2 weeks' gestation, indicating severe Rh erythroblastosis. Curved line indicates analysis of OD on patient's liquor; full straight line indicated OD baseline. (From Bowman JM.) Haemolytic disease of the newborn (erythroblastosis fetalis). In: Roberton NRC, ed. Textbook of Neonatology. Edinburgh, Churchill Livingstone, 1986:469.

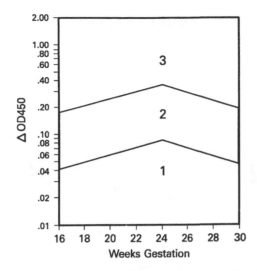

Figure 8 Modification of Liley ΔOD 450 reading zone boundaries before 24 weeks' gestation; zone boundary angle of declination before 24 weeks' gestation is the same as the zone boundary angle of inclination after 24 weeks' gestation. (From Bowman JM. Rhesus haemolytic disease. In: Wald NR, ed. Antenatal and Neonatal Screening. 2nd ed. Oxford, England, Oxford University Press, 1993 [in press].)

sampling should be carried out when a single or final ΔOD 450 reading is at the 65–75% level of zone 2, modified before 24 weeks' gestation.

Amniocentesis is not without hazard. In the preultrasound era, there was a 10% risk of placental trauma (19) placing blood in the amniotic fluid, producing 580-, 540-, and 415-nm oxyhemoglobin peaks (Fig. 9), obscuring the 450-nm peak, making the fluid valueless from the standpoint of predicting severity of hemolytic disease. Even more serious, placental trauma carries a high probability of producing a fetomaternal transplacental hemorrhage exposing the mother to more fetal RBC antigen, increasing her antibody level, and increasing the severity of fetal hemolytic disease. With the advent of ultrasound placental localization, the risk of placental trauma at amniocentesis has been sharply reduced but not removed altogether (residual incidence 2.5% [20]).

E. Perinatal Ultrasonography

The development of ultrasound imaging techniques in the late 1970s was a major advance in the management of maternal blood group alloimmunization (59). Ultrasound allows an estimate of placental and hepatic size and the presence or absence of edema, ascites, and other effusions (i.e., hydrops fetalis) (Fig. 10). It is of great benefit in assessing fetal well-being. It has increased the accuracy of placental localization and has reduced the incidence of placental trauma at amniocentesis. It is essential in directing the transfusion needle with the least possible risk at both intraperitoneal and intravascular fetal transfusions. Following intraperitoneal fetal transfusion, ultrasound confirms the presence of blood in the fetal peritoneal cavity and serial examinations monitor its absorption. At the time of a direct fetal intravascular transfusion, ultrasound observation of turbulence within the fetal umbilical vessel as the blood is injected confirms that it is being transfused into the fetal circulation. Unfortunately, although ultrasound makes the diagnosis of hydrops with great accuracy, it may not make the diagnosis of impending hydrops until hydrops has developed. However, after fetal transfusions, ultrasound biophysical

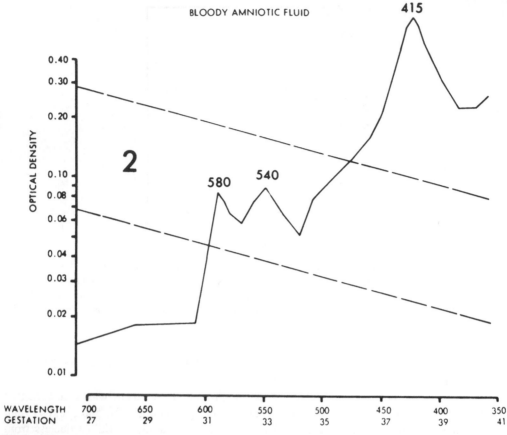

Figure 9 Spectrophotometric curve (Liley method) of amniotic fluid grossly contaminated with blood. Note sharp peaks at 580, 540, and 415 nm, which obscure the 450-nm rise. (From Bowman JM. Hemolytic disease of the newborn. In: Conn HF, Conn RB, eds. Current Diagnosis 5. Philadelphia, WB Saunders, 1977:1098.)

scoring provides an accurate assessment of fetal well-being and whether improvement or deterioration is occurring.

F. Percutaneous Umbilical Blood Sampling (PUBS)

With the development of sophisticated ultrasound equipment and the availability of peri-natologists skilled in its use, percutaneous fetal umbilical blood sampling became feasible in the mid 1980s (60) (Fig. 11). This procedure allows measurements of all blood parameters that can be measured after birth (hemoglobin, hematocrit, blood groups, DAT, serum bilirubin levels, platelet and leukocyte counts, serum protein levels, erythropoietin levels, and fetal blood gases). Fetal blood sampling is the most accurate means of determining the degree of severity of fetal hemolytic disease in the absence of hydrops. The procedure is relatively benign, carrying with it a traumatic fetal mortality rate of a fraction of 1% (60). Since it does carry with it a great likelihood of fetomaternal hemorrhage, it should only be undertaken when serial amniotic fluid ΔOD 450 readings rise into the upper 65–75% of modified zone 2 or when an anterior placenta cannot be avoided at amniocentesis and maternal pregnancy history and/or maternal

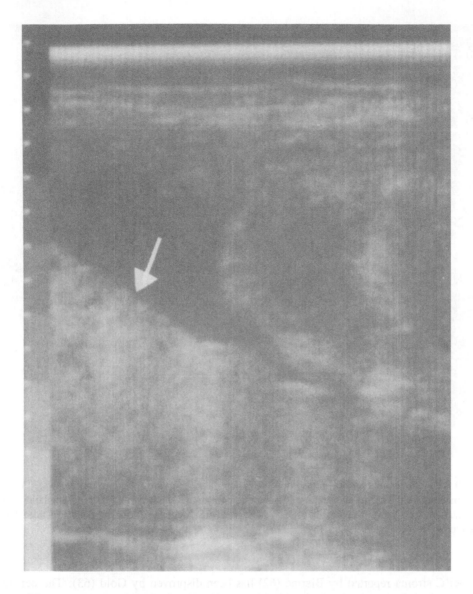

Figure 10　Sonogram of fetus with hydrops fetalis. Placenta is enormously thickened and edematous (white arrow). The fetal abdomen, which is grossly distended with ascitic fluid, is lateral to the arrow. (From Ref. 44.)

antibody titers place the fetus at risk. Fetal blood sampling may be possible as early as 18 weeks' gestation; it usually is feasible by 20–21 weeks' gestation. The preferred sampling site is from the umbilical vessel (preferably the vein) at its insertion into the placenta. For this reason, the procedure is technically easier if the placenta is implanted on the anterior uterine wall.

VIII.　MANAGEMENT OF MATERNAL ALLOIMMUNIZATION

Since the mid 1940s, efforts have been made to suppress the strength of already developed maternal RBC immunization. Rh hapten has been shown to be worthless (61). The value of

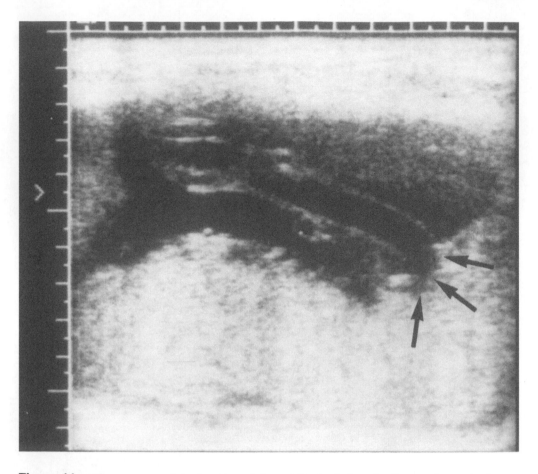

Figure 11   Ultrasonogram of the insertion of the umbilical vein into the placenta (arrows), the target area of insertion of the needle at direct intravascular transfusion. (From Bowman JM. Maternal blood group immunization. In: Creasy RK, Resnik R, eds. Maternal-Fetal Medicine: Principles and Practice. 2nd ed. Philadelphia, WB Saunders 1989:613.

Rh+ RBC stroma reported by Bierme (62) has been disproven by Gold (63). The benefit of administration of promethazine hydrochloride touted by Gusdon (64) has been refuted by others. Administration of Rh immune globulin (RhIG), of great value in Rh prevention, has been shown to be quite ineffective in suppressing Rh immunization, no matter how weak, once Rh immunization has begun (65,66).

The two measures probably of benefit in reducing maternal antibody levels and ameliorating hemolytic disease are (1) intensive plasma exchange (67,68) and (2) the administration of intravenous immune serum globulin (IGIV) (69,70). With intensive plasma exchange, alloantibody levels can be lowered by as much as 75%. In the author's experience, after 6–8 weeks, even with continued plasma exchange, antibody levels tend to rebound. Venous access becomes difficult with the need for placement of arterial venous shunts. The plasma must be replaced, partially with blood fractions (albumin and IGIV), in order to reduce antibody feedback rebound and to keep maternal serum albumin and IgG at adequate levels. Plasma exchange is tedious, costly, and uncomfortable. It is not without minor risk to the mother. The only expectation with the use of intensive plasma exchange is that fetal treatment measures may be delayed until the fetus is at >22 to 24 weeks' gestation. The institution of plasma exchange does not obviate the need for investigative measures such as amniocentesis and/or fetal blood sampling. Plasma exchange should be reserved for the mother with a father homozygous for the antigen to which she is immunized and with a prior history of hydrops at or before 24–26 weeks' gestation. Intensive plasma exchange should be started at 10–12 weeks' gestation when transfer of maternal IgG is beginning, with initial amniocentesis at 18 weeks' gestation, and/or fetal blood sampling at 19–22 weeks' gestation.

There have been reports of the value of high-dose IGIV administration in the severely alloimmunized pregnant woman (69,70). Circulating maternal alloantibody levels can be halved because of the negative feedback produced by total circulating maternal IgG levels of 25–30 g/L, readily achieved by a dose of 2 g/kg body weight. Further benefits of IGIV therapy may be a result of interference with transfer of maternal antibody across the placenta by trophoblastic Fc receptor saturation and reduction of IgG-coated RBC hemolysis by fetal reticuloendothelial Fc receptor saturation with the injected IGIV. If IGIV therapy is considered, it should be used in the same situation as intensive plasma exchange beginning at 10–12 weeks' gestation. The recommended dose is 400 mg/kg maternal body weight for 5 days and repeated at 3-week intervals. Again, amniotic fluid and/or fetal blood sampling assessment of fetal disease at 18–20 weeks' gestation is essential.

A. Neonatal Management

Initial treatment measures in the 1940s were directed toward the close to term, live-born infant who was not hydropic but was doomed to develop kernicterus. Simple transfusion of antigen-negative RBCs was ineffective because hyperbilirubinemia, the cause of kernicterus, was not prevented. With the introduction of exchange transfusion in 1945 by Wallerstein at Jewish Memorial Hospital in New York City (71) in which the infant's antibody-coated antigen-positive hemolyzing RBC were replaced with antigen-negative RBCs, which maintained hemoglobin levels and removed the source of bilirubin, kernicterus became preventable and perinatal mortality from hemolytic disease was reduced from 50 to 25%. Wallerstein removed D+ blood from the sagital sinus of the infant and transfused D– blood into a saphenous vein. The intermittent removal of aliquots of D+ blood and transfusion of aliquots of D– blood via a catheter in the umbilical vein (introduced by Diamond) (72) rapidly became the exchange transfusion method of choice.

Other postdelivery therapeutic measures developed since 1945, such as phototherapy, phenobarbital, and albumin infusion, have reduced the need for exchange transfusion. More sophisticated laboratory methods (albumin saturation indices, reserve albumin binding capacity measurements, free bilirubin measurements) have been developed to define more precisely the risk of kernicterus and thereby restrict the use of exchange transfusions to infants more accurately determined to be at risk. Nevertheless, exchange transfusion has been the keystone in the treatment of the live-born infant with hemolytic disease, and it is exchange transfusion, first carried out 47 years ago, that halved the mortality from hemolytic disease in the late 1940s and early 1950s.

B. Fetal Treatment

1. Induced Early Delivery

The primary problem since 1945 has been the management of the fetus destined to become hydropic in utero. In 1952, Chown hypothesized that induced early delivery might be the solution for the fetus destined to become hydrophic after 32–34 weeks' gestation (50% of all hydrops); that is, accept the considerable risk from prematurity instead of the much greater risk from hemolytic disease. He was proven correct (73). By 1961, the perinatal mortality from hemolytic disease in Manitoba was 16%. Until 1961, the major problem with early delivery was the inability to predict severity of hemolytic disease accurately. With the introduction of amniotic fluid ΔOD 450 measurements, by Liley in 1961 (54), this problem was partially solved. By 1964, the perinatal mortality from Rh hemolytic disease in Manitoba had been reduced to 13%.

2. Intrauterine Transfusions for Fetal Hemolytic Disease

Intraperitoneal Fetal Transfusions   In 1961, induced early delivery could not be undertaken before 31–32 weeks' gestation without encountering prohibitive mortality from prematurity and severe Rh disease. Eight percent of fetuses become hydropic before 32 weeks' gestation. In 1963, the introduction of intraperitoneal fetal transfusions (IPT) by Liley (74) completely altered the prognosis for these most severely affected fetuses.

It has been known since the turn of the century that RBCs placed in the peritoneal cavity are absorbed and function normally. At one time, IPT was a favorite method of transfusing children with thalassemia. IPT was abandoned in favor of vascular transfusions because of the severe discomfort that it caused. Absorption is via the subdiaphragmatic lymphatic lacunae up the right lymphatic duct into the venous circulation. Fetal breathing movements are necessary for absorption to occur (75). In the absence of hydrops, 10–12% of infused RBCs are absorbed daily. The presence of ascites per se does not prevent absorption, although the rate of absorption is more variable (76). If the fetus is not breathing, absorption of RBCs will not occur (75).

A 16-gauge, 18-cm Tuohy needle is directed under ultrasound guidance into the fetal abdomen (Fig. 12). An epidural catheter is then threaded down the needle and the needle is withdrawn on to the maternal abdomen. The proper placement of the catheter tip is confirmed radiographically by the injection of 1.0–1.5 ml of radiopaque contrast medium, with the demonstration of contrast under the diaphragm and around loops of small bowel (Fig. 13). Prior to the ultrasound era (before 1978), visualization of the contrast diffusing into a large volume of ascitic fluid (Fig. 14) was often the way the initial diagnosis of hydrops fetalis was made.

Although IPT was a major advance in the management of severe erythroblastosis fetalis, there were serious problems. The procedure is of no value for the nonbreathing moribund hydropic fetus (75). The RBCs are not absorbed and the fetus dies. If the placenta is implanted on the anterior uterine wall and must be transfixed by the Tuohy needle, the traumatic death rate per procedure is 7% in Winnipeg. Following IPT, there is a 30% spontaneous labor rate per patient. Fortunately, most of such deliveries occur after 30 weeks' gestation. Finally, although serial amniotic fluid ΔOD 450 measurements increase the accuracy of prediction of severity of hemolytic disease, inaccuracies do occur, the occasional only moderately affected fetus despite a zone 3 reading and, less commonly, a hydropic fetus despite a moderate zone 2 reading.

Direct Intravascular Fetal Transfusion   Attempts at direct intravascular transfusions (IVT) either into a fetal or placental blood vessel approached via a hysterotomy incision, were attempted in the mid 1960s (77–79). The results were poor because the women almost invariably went into labor. In 1981, Rodeck reported direct fetal transfusions through a fetoscope (80). Few others have achieved his skill with the fetoscope. Blood or meconium or other turbidity in the amniotic fluid makes fetoscopic visualization of the fetal blood vessels impossible.

With the introduction of fetal blood sampling by the early to mid 1980s, it became feasible to follow the sampling procedure with direct IVT (81–86). Under ultrasound guidance, the tip of a 22- or 20-gauge spinal needle is introduced into an umbilical blood vessel, preferably the

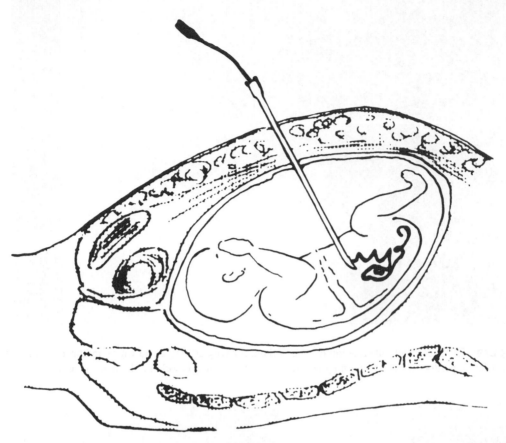

Figure 12 IPT diagram. The Tuohy needle has been inserted across the maternal abdominal wall and uterine wall into the fetal peritoneal cavity, and the epidural catheter has been threaded into the peritoneal cavity of the fetus. The safest position for the fetus at IPT is not with the abdomen anterior (as shown in this diagram) because the umbilical fetal vessels then lie in the center of the target area. (From Bowman JM. In: Iffy L, Kaminetzky HA, eds. Blood-group incompatibilities. Principles and Practice of Obstetrics and Perinatology. New York, John Wiley & Sons, 1981; 70:1143.)

vein but occasionally the artery, at its insertion into the placenta or rarely at its insertion into the fetal abdomen.

In the absence of hydrops, direct measurement of fetal blood parameters is the most accurate method of determining severity of hemolytic disease, being more accurate than amniotic fluid ΔOD 450 measurements and ultrasonographic assessments. The latter two procedures, however, plus past history and maternal antibody titers, indicate the fetus at risk who requires a fetal blood-sampling procedure.

Direct intravascular fetal transfusion does not depend upon diaphragmatic movement to increase hemoglobin levels. Therefore, it is capable of salvaging the moribund, nonbreathing fetus provided the fetus still has umbilical blood flow. Direct IVT increases circulating hemoglobin levels in the fetus immediately rather than in the 8–10 days required for IPT.

In Winnipeg, the venipuncturist, under the direction of the ultrasonographer, places the tip of a 22- or 20-gauge spinal needle in an umbilical blood vessel. Once the needle tip appears to be in the vessel, blood is aspirated and determined to be fetal by a rapid alkaline denaturation test. The correct position of the needle tip is confirmed by the observation of turbulence coursing down the vessel following the injection of sterile isotonic saline. If fetal movements are likely

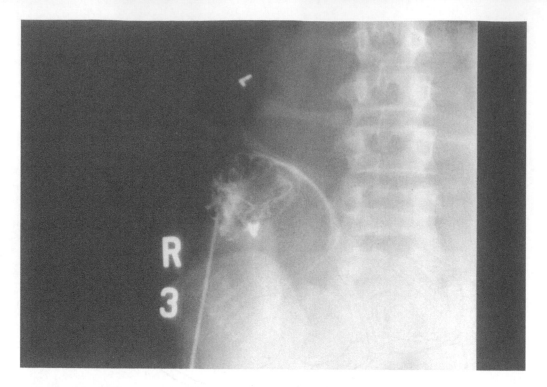

Figure 13 Successful catherization of fetal peritoneal cavity at IPT, as shown by radiopaque contrast agent in the peritoneal cavity, outlining negative shadows of small bowel and the liver. (From Ref. 35.)

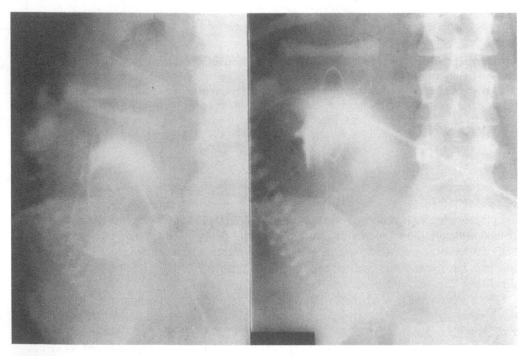

Figure 14 Hydrops fetalis at intrauterine transfusions. Note radiopaque contrast medium infusing into a large volume of fluid in the fetal abdomen at both transfusions. The fetus, hydropic at birth with a cord hemoglobin of 9 g/100 ml and all donor RBCs, survived. (From Ref. 35.)

to disturb the needle insertion, the fetus is paralyzed by the intravenous injection of pancuronium.

While the venipuncturist holds the needle hub and the blood transfusion tubing connector very firmly and the ultrasonographer watches the blood flow turbulence in the fetal blood vessel, the transfusionist (the third member of the team) transfuses compatible packed RBCs in 10-ml aliquots over 1–2 min until the desired transfusion volume is attained (mean 50 ml/kg estimated nonhydropic fetal weight). If there is evidence of significant bradycardia or marked ventricular dilation (a rare event), the transfusion is discontinued before the full volume is administered.

IVT survival rates in Winnipeg (Table 10) are superior to IPT survival rates in every category: 88 versus 76% overall, 94 versus 87% in nonhydropic fetuses, and 76 versus 60% in hydropic fetuses.

There can be no doubt that if IVT is feasible, it is the procedure of choice. Only through IVT can the moribund nonbreathing hydropic fetus be salvaged; 8 of 12 (67%) survived in Winnipeg. What is gratifying is the much lower overall risk with IVT versus IPT (0.8 versus 3.5% per procedure).

Despite the great advantages of IVT, there are two situations in which IPT may be necessary and, therefore, the need for skill in carrying out IPT must be maintained. One is the rare situation early in pregnancy (before 20–21 weeks' gestation) in which the cord vessels may be too small for a successful venipuncture. The second more common situation is the one in which later in pregnancy, after 30 weeks' gestation and after several successful IVTs, increasing fetal size obscures a posterior cord vessel insertion making venipuncture impossible.

IX. PREVENTION OF RH IMMUNIZATION

A. Historical Background

The ability to prevent Rh immunization is a major medical milestone. In 1900, the year that Landsteiner discovered the ABO blood group system and 40 years before his and Wiener's discovery of the Rh blood group system, Von Dungern performed an experiment that pointed the way to the prevention of Rh immunization (87). He injected rabbits with ox RBCs. They produced ox RBC antibodies. He then injected a second group of rabbits with RBCs (antigen) from the same ox and followed this with an injection of sera (antibody) from the first group of rabbits. The second group did not develop ox RBC antibodies. Von Dungern proved the axiom that the presence of passive antibody to an antigen prevented active immunization to the antigen.

One would have thought that Wiener or Levine, remembering these observations, would have realized that prevention of Rh immunization was possible almost immediately after the discovery of the Rh blood group system and the etiology of Rh immunization. It is a commentary

Table 10 Intrauterine Fetal Transfusions Winnipeg—ULTRASOUND ERA

	IPT 204 July 1980–October 1986		IVT 389 May 1986–October 1991	
	Total	Alive (%)	Total	Alive (%)
Fetuses	75	57 (76)	98	86 (88)
Nonhydrops	45	39 (87)	65	61 (94)
Hydrops	30	18 (60)	33	25 (76)
Nonmoribund	22	18 (82)	21	17 (81)
Moribund	8	0 (0)	12	8 (67)

on the slowness with which basic scientific knowledge is applied clinically that more than 20 years elapsed before this information was put to practical use.

B. Rh Prevention Experiments

In 1961, Stern et al. (88) carried out the first experiment using anti-D. They injected 16 Rh– men with ABO-compatible, D+ RBCs, coated in vitro with anti-D sufficient to produce a strongly positive direct antiglobulin (Coombs') reaction. Fourteen men were injected five times; two were injected four times. None of the 16 developed anti-D. When 10 of the 16 were subsequently injected with D+ RBCs not coated with anti-D, 5 (50%) became D immunized.

Promptly after the experiments of Stern et al., studies on the use of anti-D in Rh prevention were begun in Liverpool, England (89), and New York (90) and shortly after in Winnipeg, Canada (91). Zipursky and Israels (91) injected 2 ml of D+, ABO-compatible cord blood RBCs into 18 male, D– volunteers. Six were given nothing further; six were given 1 ml of an immune serum globulin prepared from the plasma of D-immunized women with high anti-D titers; and the remaining six were given 5 ml of the same immune serum globulin (ISG). The RhIG had an anti-D concentration of about 50 μg/ml. Three of the six volunteers (50%) who were given the D+ cord RBCs became immunized; none of the 12 who received the RBCs plus RhIG (either 50 or 250 μg) showed any evidence of D immunization.

The Liverpool group used plasma with high titers of incomplete anti-D (titers of 128–2048); only 3 of 21 volunteers (14%) treated after exposure to D+ RBCs became immunized compared with 11 of 21 volunteers (52%) not given the plasma after exposure to the same volume of D+ RBCs (89).

Experimental studies carried out by the New York group (90), using D antibody in the form of RhIG, produced similar results. Five volunteers given 2 ml of D+ blood followed by 5 ml of RhIG (about 1500 μg of anti-D) showed no evidence of D immunization, whereas four of five volunteers receiving the same volume of D+ blood only were D immunized. In a further study of 14 volunteers given 10 and 5 ml of D+ blood on two occasions, each time followed by 5 ml of RhIG, none showed evidence of Rh immunization compared with 8 immunized of 13 volunteers (62%) given two injections of blood but no RhIG.

These experiments demonstrated that, under experimental conditions, D antibody in the form of RhIG was safe and effective in preventing D immunization.

C. Clinical Trials of Rh Prophylaxis

A trial was begun in Liverpool in 1964 (92) administering about 1000 μg of anti-D after delivery to D–, unimmunized women with >0.2 ml of fetal blood in their circulation and about 200 μg to D– women with <0.2 ml of fetal blood in their circulation. The trial was controlled and was carried on, where possible, through two D+, ABO-compatible pregnancies. Of the treated mothers going through two such pregnancies, 2.3% in the >0.2 ml fetal transplacental hemorrhage (TPH) group and 2.8% in the <0.2 ml fetal TPH group were D immunized compared with 31.4 and 12.3%, respectively, in the untreated control groups. These figures indicated that Rh prophylaxis after delivery was effective in preventing Rh immunization from occurring as a result of two Rh+, ABO-compatible pregnancies.

Clinical trials were carried out in the United States by Columbia University and other centers using an RhIG prepared by Ortho Diagnostic (Raritan, NJ) and administered 72 hrs after delivery (93). Initially 4000–6000 μg of anti-D were given, but very early in the trial, the dose was reduced to 300 μg. The trial was confined to D–, unimmunized mothers delivering ABO-compatible, D+ infants. By the time the treated mothers had undergone two D+ pregnancies, 1.2% were D immunized compared with 11.1% immunized in similar but untreated women.

In the Western Canada Trial (94), 1216 women delivering D+, ABO-compatible infants, who had no evidence of D immunization by a sensitive screening technique (a two-stage papainized RBC method), given RhIG in doses varying from 145 to 435 μg, had no evidence of D immunization when screened by the same technique 6 months after delivery. Of 500 similar women not treated with RhIG, 36 (7.2%) had evidence of D immunization 6 months after delivery.

It was on the basis of these clinical trials, and similar trials carried out in Australia and various European countries, that RhIG was licensed for Rh prophylaxis in 1968. Administration of RhIG will always prevent Rh immunization with two provisos: (1) it must be given before Rh immunization has begun and (2) it must be given in adequate dose.

D. Mechanism Whereby RhIG Prevents Rh Immunization

1. Antigen Deviation and Clearance

The belief that antigen deviation away from the immunological system is the reason RhIG produces suppression of D immunization is elegant in its simplicity. The marked reduction in the prevalence of D immunization that occurs when the D+ fetus is ABO incompatible with the Rh– mother is explained on this basis. Intravascular hemolysis of ABO-incompatible RBCs occurs with uptake of RBC debris primarily in the liver, an organ poorly endowed with potential immunocytes. However, antigen clearance with immune deviation is not the means by which Rh antibody prevents D immunization. D antibody–medicated RBC destruction is extravascular and occurs primarily in the spleen, the most important antibody-forming organ in the body. Indeed, D immunization can only occur after the antigen has left the circulation and is present in the spleen and lymph nodes.

2. Antigen Blocking-Competitive Inhibition

The early theory that D antibody prevents active immunization by covering or blocking all D antigen sites on the RBC membrane is also untenable. Fab fragments that bind to antigen are not effective in preventing active immunization except when used in very large doses (95).

Also, it has been shown that a dose of D antibody sufficient to prevent D immunization does not cover all of the antigen sites (96). Therefore, the concept of antibody binding the antigen and blocking its exposure to receptor sites on the immunocyte is not, by itself, the mechanism whereby D antibody prevents primary D immunization.

3. Antigen Blocking—Central Inhibition

Pollack and Gorman have evolved a central control, or "immunostat," hypothesis that they believe is the mechanism of Rh prevention (97). In this hypothesis, antigen is trapped within the anatomical sites where immune responses occur; i.e., the spleen primarily and lymph nodes secondarily. The immunostat theory depends upon the understanding that antigen recognition and the humoral immune response to antigen require cooperation between T helper lymphocytes and specific B lymphocytes. This interaction occurs on structural surfaces such as macrophages membranes and dendritic cell processes within the splenic white pulp and lymph node follicles.

According to Pollack and Gorman, control of the immune response is determined by positive or negative feedback producing on/off signals transmitted by hormonelike molecules produced by T helper or T suppressor cells and/or macrophages. This feedback system cannot switch off already established antibody synthesis. However, it prevents clones of antibody-producing plasma cells from forming and, therefore, prevents the primary immune response.

When RhIG is injected intramuscularly, the anti-D enters the circulation via the lymphatics.

The anti-D is distributed between plasma and the extravascular fluid compartment, which has twice the volume of the plasma compartment. Depending upon the dose of antibody and the volume of Rh+ RBCs, a certain amount of antibody is bound, binding only a fraction of the antigen sites.

If the bound anti-D has intact Fc fragments, the D+ fetal RBCs are removed predominantly by the spleen and to a lesser extent by the lymph nodes. This removal is caused by the weblike filter of dendritic cell membranes and the T and B lymphocytes that are interdigitated by the dendritic cell membranes. As antibody-coated RBCs are filtered into the spleen and lymph nodes, they increase in concentration within a relatively small volume of plasma. This produces, in effect, an affinity column in which more Rh antibody is removed as the plasma passes through the highly concentrated mass of D+ RBCs, increasing the percentage of bound D antigen sites (96).

Prevention of D immunization is not simply the lack of an immune response but is a dynamic suppression of the immune response by a feedback mechanism requiring antigen and antibody. The lymph node follicles in the spleen are richly endowed with B cells, T cells, macrophages, and dendritic cells with and without Fc receptors (97). Those cells without Fc receptors act as immunological augmentors, whereas those with Fc receptors, when the Fc receptor is bound by antigen-antibody complexes, appear to stimulate suppressor T-cell responses and prevent antigen-induced B-cell proliferation and conversion to antibody-producing plasma cells. The immune complexes (antibody plus RBC membrane antigen) trapped by the dendritic cells are in close contact with T and B cells and macrophages. The antibody Fc piece in the antibody-antigen complex is involved in negative information transfer, probably through the production and release of a lymphokine, soluble immune response suppressor (SIRS) (97). In summary, according to Pollack and Gorman, Rh prevention is due to the formation of anti-D D-antigen immune complexes that set into action negative mediation of the primary immune response.

Pollack and Gorman's central inhibition theory does not explain the observation of Woodrow et al. (98). In order to test the belief that suppression of active immunization was antibody specific, they injected 62 D−K− male volunteers, each with 1 ml of D+K+ RBCs, on two occasions. Thirty-one of the volunteers were each given 14 μg of anti-K IgG at the time of each RBC injection; the remaining 31 received only the RBCs. Whereas 11 of 31 controls (35.5%) became D immunized, only one of 31 given anti-K IgG (3.3%) became D immunized.

The protection against D immunization produced by anti-K could not be explained on the basis of deviation of the D+K+ RBCs away from the spleen because the injected RBCs were radiolabeled and were taken up by the spleen. Because anti-K–coated, D+K+ RBCs are still readily agglutinated by anti-D, K and D antigenic sites in the RBC membrane are not so closely situated that the protective effect of anti-K could be explained on the basis of the K antibody rendering the D antigen sites unavailable to the antigen receptors on the immunocytes. At present, there is no explanation for Woodrow et al.'s observation, which makes the immunostat theory suspect.

4. Original Rh Prevention Recommendations

The clinical trials upon which Rh prevention programs were based were carried out on the assumption that although a current pregnancy was likely to be the immunizing one, primary Rh immunization developed sometime after delivery. It is for this reason that both clinical trial protocols and after licensure recommendations were that one prophylactic dose of RhIG, 300 μg in the United States, should be given to a D−, unimmunized mother within 72 hr after delivery of a D+ infant. Although ABO incompatibility reduces the incidence of D immunization by about 90%, since protection is not absolute, it was recommended that RhIG should be given to all D–, unimmunized women irrespective of the ABO status of their D+ infants.

E. Residual Problems in Rh Prophylaxis

With the licensure of RhIG and comprehensive programs of universal administration in many developed countries, one would have expected that by 1992, 24 years after licensure, Rh prophylaxis would have wiped out D immunization altogether. There has been a gratifying reduction in numbers of D–immunized pregnancies, in Manitoba by 83.7%, from 442 in 1968 through 1970 to 72 in 1985 through 1987. However, some problems still remain, including the following:

1. Compliance after delivery
2. Failure to give RhIG after abortion
3. Failure to give RhIG after amniocentesis
4. Massive TPH
5. Rh immunization during pregnancy–antenatal prophylaxis
6. Augmentation of Rh immunization
7. Rh immunization in infancy, the grandmother theory
8. Weak Rh immunization, attempts at reversal

Compliance after delivery and abortion will not be discussed further.

1. Failure to Give RhIG After Amniocentesis

Before ultrasound placental localization, fetal TPH occurred in 10–11% of patients following amniocentesis (19). Ultrasound placental localization and restriction of the performance of amniocentesis to skilled obstetricians has markedly reduced the incidence of fetal TPH after amniocentesis. Nevertheless, fetal TPH due to amniocentesis still occurs; in 2.6% of 974 women after genetic amniocentesis, in 2.3% of 1215 women having amniocentesis to determine pulmonary maturity, and in 1.9% of 257 women having amniocentesis carried out to determine severity of Rh disease (20).

Every D–, unimmunized woman undergoing amniocentesis at any gestation, for any reason, must be given a full prophylactic dose of RhIG (300 µg) at the time of amniocentesis. This dose should be repeated at 12-week intervals until delivery. There is abundant evidence that RhIG given during pregnancy does not harm the fetus (25).

2. Massive Transplacental Fetal Hemorrhage

The protective effect of RhIG is dose dependent. It has been shown that one prophylactic dose of 300 µg will prevent D immunization up to an exposure of about 30 ml of Rh+ blood (99). If the exposure is greater, protection is partial. The incidence of D immunization following injection of 30–450 ml of D+ blood into D– male volunteers followed by administration of one dose of 300 µg of RhIG is about 30% (100). Of 15,795 pregnancies studied at delivery in Winnipeg, only 0.24% of women had fetal TPH in excess of 30 ml of blood.

Therefore, the D immunization rate due to failure to diagnose massive TPH and administration of only one 300-µg dose of IgG anti-D will be very low: 0.24% of 30%, or 0.07% of all D– women treated. Although routine fetal TPH screening at delivery is recommended, it is apparent that failure to diagnose and treat massive fetal TPH is a rare cause of failure of D prophylaxis.

Massive TPH usually occurs at the time of delivery. If diagnosed after delivery of a D+ infant, multiple doses of RhIG (300 µg) should be given intramuscularly (IM) as follows: two vials if the TPH is between 25 and 50 ml of blood, three vials if between 50 and 75 ml, and so on. It is recommended that the contents of four vials (1200 μg) be given IM every 12 hrs until the total dose has been administered. Following administration of the total dose of RhIG, the result of the Kleihauer test should be negative and passive anti-D should be present in the maternal circulation.

3. Rh Immunization During Pregnancy

In the Manitoban part of the Western Canada Clinical Trial of Rh prophylaxis, 5 of 210 D– primigravidas who initially presented with no evidence of D immunization and had delivered ABO-compatible, D+ infants were immunized at the time of delivery. Postpartum administration of RhIG to these five women was too late to be protective. Two of the five have subsequently had D+ infants. Both infants suffered from hemolytic disease; one required fetal transfusions. Because of these findings, we explored the problem further (25).

During the period March 1, 1967, to December 15, 1974, 3533 D– pregnant women, either primigravidas with no history of abortion or multigravidas given RhIG after every abortion or D+ delivery were followed. Sixty-two, or 1.8% (see Table 4), showed evidence of D immunization during pregnancy or within 3 days after delivery. Five of the 62 (8%) were found to be D immunized before 28 weeks' gestation; one, a primigravida, as early as 11 weeks. She may represent a rare instance of maternofetal transplacental hemorrhage at the time of her own delivery because her mother is D+ (the "grandmother" theory). Rh antibody was first found in the other four (two primigravidas and two multigravidas) between 23 and 28 weeks' gestation. None of these five women would have been protected if RhIG had been administered at 28 weeks' gestation. In 10 (16%), the antibody was discovered between 28 and 34 weeks' gestation and in the remaining 47 (76%) between 34 weeks' gestation and 3 days postdelivery. Therefore, the incidence of D immunization detected between 28 weeks' gestation and 3 days after delivery was 1.6% (57 of 3528).

Our observations that 1.8% of D– women delivering D+ infants are D immunized during pregnancy or within 3 days after delivery are supported by other investigators (see Table 11). The Hamilton and Swedish groups report a 1.9 and 1.6% incidence, respectively (101). In Finland, the incidence is only 0.71% (101). However, the prevalence of Rh negativity and D immunization is lower in the Finns than it is in other white populations.

Rh immunization has been reported from the United States. Twenty-two D– primigravidas became sensitizied before delivery in one report (102). Because the D– primigravida population base from which these 22 arose is unknown, we do not know the incidence of D immunization developing during pregnancy in this series.

D immunization during pregnancy carries with it a serious prognosis for future D+ infants.

Table 11 Rh Immunization During Pregnancy

Study	No.	%
Manitoba	62/3533	1.8
Hamilton	12/621	1.9
Sweden	21/1277	1.6
Total	95/5431	1.75
Finland	156/21966	0.71

Source: From Ref. 101.

In 24 subsequent D+ pregnancies, 11 infants (46%) required phototherapy and/or exchange transfusion. Five of the 11 (21% of the total) were very severely affected; three underwent fetal transfusions and all five required early delivery and exchange transfusions.

Antenatal Rh Prophylaxis Clinical Trial.   Because of accumulating evidence that D immunization during pregnancy was an important cause of residual immunization, the Rh Laboratory, in December 1968, began a clinical trial of antenatal anti-D prophylaxis (25). D– primigravidas slated to deliver at one tertiary and one urban community hospital were offered antenatal prophylaxis. Those scheduled to deliver at the other tertiary hospital, the other three community hospitals, and all rural hospitals in Manitoba were not offered antenatal prophylaxis. From this latter untreated group came the bulk of the 62 women who were Rh immunized during pregnancy. Initially, after informed consent, those in the treatment group were given 300 μg of RhIG IM at 34 weeks' gestation. In May 1969, because of evidence that some women were becoming immunized between 28 and 34 weeks' gestation, the trial was altered to an injection at 28 weeks' gestation and one at 34 weeks' gestation. In January 1972, all Rh– urban women were offered antenatal prophylaxis, with rural women continuing to act as controls. The trial was completed June 30, 1975. Further postdelivery testing was carried out until August 1976. All D– women (treated and untreated antenatally) were given 300 μg of RhIG after delivery if they believed Rh+ infants. Those delivering Rh– infants were removed from the trial. Women treated antenatally reentered the trial in subsequent pregnancies.

Although we knew that RhIG is IgG and will cross the placenta, we were sure that the small amount of anti-D that crossed would not damage the large numbers of Rh+ RBCs in the fetal circulation. In 45 years of experience, the Rh Laboratory has never observed affected D+ infants born to D-immunized mothers with circulating anti-D levels the same as those found following an injection of 300 μg of RhIG. The safety of antenatal Rh prophylaxis was confirmed in the clinical trial. Although 28% of ABO-compatible infants in the trial had RBCs that were weakly DAT+, none showed any anemia or more than the usual degree of physiological jaundice.

The clinical trial was successful (25). Of the 1357 women given antenatal prophylaxis who delivered Rh+ infants, none showed evidence of active Rh immunization at delivery. Of the 1004 women examined 4–12 months after delivery, none showed evidence of active Rh immunization.

Rh Antenatal Prophylaxis Service Program.   Because of the successful clinical trial, a service program of antenatal Rh prophylaxis was begun in Winnipeg on July 1, 1975, and was extended to rural Manitoba on February 1, 1976 (103). Based on a half-life of IgG1 of about 21 days, the calculation was made that about 20 μg of anti-D would still be present in the mother 12 weeks after injection of 300 μg of RhIG. For this reason, the service program consisted of a single injection of 300 μg of RhIG at 28 weeks' gestation.

Because the 28 weeks' gestation service program covers every D– pregnant woman in the province of Manitoba, some women will be treated who were not given RhIG antenatally or, rarely, postpartum or postabortion in previous pregnancies. Therefore, one would expect that the occasional woman given RhIG at 28 weeks' gestation in a current pregnancy but already sensitized ("sensibilized") owing to inadequate prophylaxis during or after a prior pregnancy will show evidence of Rh immunization after 28-week prophylaxis in her current pregnancy.

The results of the service program bear this out (104). Administration of RhIG antenatally and postnatally to 9295 negative unimmunized women who delivered D+ infants reduced the prevalence of D immunization developing between 28 and 40 weeks' gestation from the expected

149 (1.6% of 9295) to 17. Thus, there was a protection rate against the development of D immunization in this period of 88.6%. Combined antenatal and postnatal RhIG prophylaxis in these 9295 women reduced the overall incidence of D immunization after 28 weeks' gestation from the expected 601 to 17, a protection rate of 97.2%. Antenatal Rh prophylaxis has now become a standard treatment measure in North America.

Although arguments against antenatal prophylaxis have been based on the risk to donors from hyperimmunization with D+ RBCs and plasmapheresis (105) and on the even more speculative risk to the fetus from its exposure to IgG anti-D passively administered to the mother (106), these arguments are without foundation. In 21 years of hyperimmunizing D-immunized sterile women by the Rh Laboratory (over 150 in all), none has shown harmful effects. Some plasma donors have been plasmapheresed at weekly intervals more than 40 times yearly for 23 years. None has shown any untoward side effects.

The argument put forward that exposure of the fetus to passive RhIG containing all kinds of IgG might adversely affect subsequent immunological status later in life (106) is specious. All fetuses are exposed to much larger amounts of foreign passive IgG produced by their mothers. This IgG has a protective effect and does not have a damaging effect. There is no reason to believe that the small amount of IgG that crosses the placenta after the mother is given RhIG will have a harmful effet on the fetal and neonatal immune system. Although we have not studied the immunological status of the 24,000 infants delivered in Manitoba after their mothers received antenatal RhIG, we have had no untoward effects reported to us.

4. Augmentation of D Immunization

Whether the risk of D immunization increases when the level of circulating passive antibody drops below a critical level has been debated. An increased incidence of Rh immunization when male volunteers received 10 µg of RhIG with 2.2 ml of R^2R^2 RBCs (5 ml of blood) observed by Columbia Presbyterian investigators (107) could not be confirmed by English investigators (108). However, the latter group found evidence of an increased incidence of D immunization (i.e., augmentation) when male volunteers were injected with 1 µg of Rh antibody and 1 ml of R^2R^2 RBCs (109).

It is, therefore, possible that in some D− pregnant women, the level of persisting passive anti-D may be in the augmenting range rather than the protecting range if their pregnancies extend for more than 12 weeks after their 28 weeks' gestation injection, particularly if they have had a significant TPH. In some of our antenatal prophylaxis failures, the interval between antenatal prophylaxis and delivery was as much as 13.5–15.0 weeks. Because we believe that augmentation can occur, we recommend that the woman given antenatal Rh prophylaxis also receive a second antenatal injection 12 weeks later if she has not delivered. A postpartum dose is not given if delivery occurs within 3 weeks of the second dose provided that there is no evidence of a significant fetal TPH (>0.1 ml of fetal RBCs).

5. Immunization in Infancy—Grandmother Theory

The "grandmother" theory, i.e., the reverse passage of maternal D+ RBCs into the circulation of the pregnant D− woman when she was a fetus and newborn, with subsequent D immunization during infancy, has been hypothesized as a cause of D immunization appearing in such a woman during her first pregnancy. Sixty percent of mothers of D− infants are D+. Initial reports of a high incidence of maternofetal TPH were based on cord blood studies that were inaccurate. Studies of capillary blood samples taken at 1–2 days of age showed that the incidence of maternofetal TPH was about 2% (3 out of 160 infants studied) (110,111). The TPHs were very small, being the equivalent of 0.005 ml of a fetomaternal hemorrhage, which is about one-twentieth of the amount that produces a 3% incidence of maternal primary D immunization.

However, there has been one report of hydrops fetalis produced by massive maternofetal hemorrhage that caused polycythemia, hypervolemia, hyperviscosity, and heart failure in the fetus (112). Fortunately, in that case, both mother and fetus were D+. Reports of a very high incidence of D immunization in D− infants born of D+ mothers (5% (113), 11% (114), and 22% (115)) have been refuted (102,111). We found no examples in 94 infants studied. Based upon the success of antenatal prophylaxis, D immunization due to maternofetal TPH must be exceedingly rare. We do not recommend that RhIG be given to D− infants delivered of D+ mothers.

6. Suppression of Weak D Immunization

If D immunization is demonstrable by an indirect antiglobulin test (IAT), attempts at reversal by administration of RhIG are ineffective (65). The ability of RhIG to suppress or reverse very much weaker D immunization is controversial. One group of investigators reported disappearance of D antibody in 11 of 12 very weakly D-immunized women 6 months after administration of RhIG (116). None of the 11 was followed through another D+ pregnancy. Another group of investigators reported one woman who had a D antibody weakly demonstrable by IAT and by two manual enzyme methods immediately after delivery of her first D+ infant, just before administration of 100 μg of RhIG. Three years later, on nine occasions during and at the end of her second D+ pregnancy, this woman had no demonstrable anti-D when tested by enzyme, indirect antiglobulin, albumin, and saline methods. These investigators believe that administration of RhIG to this woman had reversed her D-immune state (117). We have had a very different experience with a similar patient (65). One of the five patients immunized during pregnancy, described in the Manitoba part of the Western Canada Rh Prevention Trial (25), had a D antibody detected weakly by enzyme and a capillary saline technique, but not by IAT, for the first time 3 days after delivery, just before injection of 270 μg of RhIG. The antibody was not demonstrable immediately after delivery and was no longer detectable at 13 and 17 weeks' gestation in her next pregnancy. At 37 weeks' gestation, she had a secondary immune response antibody to a titer of 4 in albumin, 8 in saline, which indicated that RhIG administration 3 days after delivery of her first infant had not reversed her Rh-immune state. Her antibody titer at the end of her second pregnancy was 16 in albumin, 4 in saline. Although her second infant did not require treatment, her third required intrauterine transfusions (65).

Clinical Trial of Anti-D Suppression. Because of conflicting evidence in respect to anti-D immune suppression by RhIG, we carried out a clinical trial of D immunization suppression between 1969 and 1977. From Rh Laboratory statistics encompassing 39 years, the natural history of weak D immunization was determined in women not treated with RhIG in the preprevention era and in women given RhIG, some at 28 weeks' gestation and after delivery, others only after delivery (65). Thirty-six women were given RhIG (300 μg) when very weak D immunization was first detected (i.e., the antibody could be detected only by enzyme and/or by a timed indirect antiglobulin screen after more than 5 min). The dose was repeated at 6-week intervals until delivery or until D immunization was shown to be progressing (65). Twenty-one (66%) went on to full-blown D immunization despite 300 μg of RhIG administered every 6 weeks, an incidence of progression no different from the 86 of 131 (66%) in the intreated historical control group who went on to fully developed D immunization.

In another study, 14 sterile D− women with weak D immunization were given 0.28 ml of D+ RBCs (66). Seven of the 14 were given 500 μg of anti-D. The other seven were not given anti-D. The secondary D-immune response was just as great in those given the RhIG as it was in those given only D+ RBCs (66).

From the above data, it is almost certain that many of the reported failures of postpartum D prophylaxis are due to the fact that the women were already D immunized but at too low a level for antibody detection ("sensibilization") when they were given RhIG. It is most likely that the one-third of women who do not have progression of their weak D alloimmunization, whether they are given RhIG or not, fail to progress because they have not had any further exposure to a significant number of D+ RBCs (18).

F. Ion Exchange–Prepared RhIG for Intravenous Use

RhIG is usually prepared by the Cohn cold ethanol method. RhIG made by this process is effective and has a low incidence of untoward reactions. It does contain small amounts of IgA and IgM and traces of other plasma proteins. After a second or third injection, some women will develop transient rashes and pain and swelling at the injection site. There is one report of severe anaphylaxis after the use of Cohn-prepared RhIG in an IgA-deficient woman who had developed anti-IgA (118). Cohn-prepared RhIG is anticomplementary and must not be given intravenously (IV). The yield of anti-D in the RhIG prepared by the Cohn method may be as low as 35% of that in the starting plasma. Hoppe et al. have produced RhIG by an ion exchange column method using DEAE (diethylaminoethyl [cellulose]) Sephadex A50 (Pharmacia, Uppsala, Sweden (119) (Fig. 15) This method has been adapted for use in North America. An RhIG prepared by ion exchange is licensed in Canada (120). Anti-D prepared by ion exchange is very pure; it has a very low total protein content, and there is no demonstrable IgA or IgM. Its anticomplementary activity is very low and it may be given IV. Also, it may be given safely to IgA-deficient women. It has been shown to be safe from transmitting viral infection. The efficiency of yield of anti-D in the ion exchange preparation is 85–90%.

Clinical trials and service programs, in which thousands of doses of ion exchange, anti-D have been given IV, show that it is at least as successful in preventing Rh immunization as Cohn cold ethanol–produced RhIG. The advantages of ion exchange RhIG are as follows: (1) greater purity and, therefore, less likelihood of production of a reaction; (2) less cost because the efficiency of yield is greater; and (3) less dose and less discomfort because it is given IV.

G. Production of Monoclonal Anti-D

At present, all RhIG is produced from the plasma of hyperimmunized D– volunteers; either from sterile women initially Rh immunized by pregnancy or from deliberately immunized male volunteers. With time, D–, naturally immunized women, the best source of high-titer anti-D plasma, will disappear and only male volunteers who will require deliberate D immunization will remain. Rh immunization of such male volunteers has been criticized owing to the minor hazards involved. Also, the majority exposed to such hazards do not achieve acceptable anti-D levels.

In the not too distant future, RhIG will undoubtedly be produced in tissue culture. Success has been reported with the production of anti-D by the Epstein-Barr virus transformation of lymphoblastoid cell lines taken from D-immunized donors (121,122) and by fusion of similar transformed cell lines with mouse-human heteromyelomas (hybridomas) (123,124). Once multiple stable monoclonal anti-Ds are produced in quantity, tissue culture RhIG undoubtedly will be prepared from them. This will be the RhIG of the future.

X. TOTAL PREVENTION OF RH IMMUNIZATION, POSSIBLE OR IMPOSSIBLE?

Since the clinical trials of D prophylaxis, great strides have been made in reducing the incidence of D immunization. With total compliance and universal antenatal, postnatal, postabortion, and

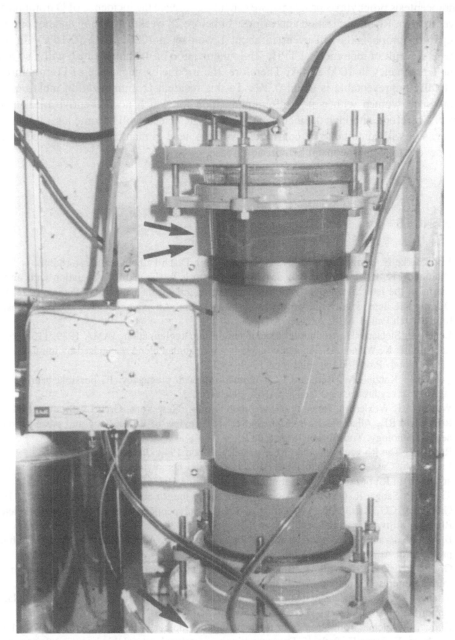

Figure 15 DEAE A-50 Sephadex column. High-titer Rh immune plasma (double arrow) runs through the column. All plasma proteins except IgG stick to the Sephadex. Very pure IgG, with a high anti-D content, runs out of the bottom of the column (single arrow).

postamniocentesis prophylaxis programs, we can further reduce the incidence of D immunization but never to zero. Rh immunization appearing at or before 28 weeks' gestation and not prevented by antepartum prophylaxis will occur in about 1 woman in 1000 at risk (0.10%). In a rare instance as a result of maternofetal TPH, Rh immunization of unknown cause will also appear in about 1 pregnancy in 1000 at risk. Therefore, the irreducible incidence of D immunization that is totally unpreventable is about 0.2%. To this residual D immunization must be added those pregnant women with non-D alloimmunization for which no preventive measures are available. Therefore, although the incidence of hemolytic disease will become less, it will never disappear. We will continue to be confronted with the need to maintain the skills necessary to manage severe fetal and neonatal hemolytic disease.

REFERENCES

1. Von Gierke E. Kernicterus und erythroblastose. Verh Dtsch Pathol Ges 1921; 18:232.
2. Diamond LK, Blackfan KD, Baty JM. Erythroblastosis fetalis and its association with universal edema of the fetus, icterus gravis neonatorum and anemia of the newborn. J Pediatr 1932; 1:269.
3. Darrow RR. Icterus gravis (erythroblastosis neonatorum. An examination of etiologic considerations). Arch Pathol 1938; 25:378.
4. Levine P, Stetson RE. An unusual case of intra-group agglutination. JAMA 1939; 113:126.
5. Landsteiner K, Weiner AS. An agglutinable factor in human blood recognized by immune sera for rhesus blood. Proc Soc Exp Biol Med 1940; 43:223.
6. Levine P, Katzin EM, Burnham L. Isoimmunization in pregnancy: Its possible bearing on the etiology of erythroblastosis fetalis. JAMA 194; 116:825.
7. Wiener AS, Wexler IB. Heredity of the Blood Groups. New York, Grune & Stratton 1958.
8. Rosenfield RE, Allan FH Jr, Swisher SN, et al. A review of Rh serology and presentation of a new terminology. Transfusion 1962; 2:287.
9. Race RR. The Rh genotype and Fisher's theory. Blood 1948; 3:(special issue):27.
10. Lacey PA, Caskey CR, Werner DJ, Moulds JJ. Fatal hemolytic disease of the newborn due to anti-D in an Rh positive D^u variant mother. Transfusion 1983; 23:91.
11. Tippett P, Sanger R. Observations on subdivisions of the Rh antigen D. Vox Sang 1962; 7:9.
12. Gahmberg CG, Karhi KK. Association of $Rh_0(D)$ polypeptides with the membrane skeleton in $Rh_0(D)$-positive human red cells. J Immunol 1984; 133:334.
13. Brown PJ, Evans JP, Sinor LT, et al. The Rhesus D antigen. A dicyclohexylcarbodiimide-binding proteolipid. Am J Pathol 1983; 110:127.
14. Goto S, Nishi H, Tomoda A. Blood group Rh-D factor in human trophoblast determined by immunofluorescent method. Am J Obstet Gynecol 1980; 137:707.
15. Wiener AS. Diagnosis and treatment of anemia of the newborn caused by occult placental hemorrhage. Am J Obstet Gynecol 1948; 56:717.
16. Chown B. Anemia from bleeding of the fetus into the mother's circulation. Lancet 1954; 1:1213.
17. Kleihauer E, Braun H, Betke K. Demonstration von fetalem haemoglobin in den erythrozyten eines blutausstriches. Klin Wochenschr 1957; 35:637.
18. Bowman JM, Pollock JM, Penston LE. Fetomaternal transplacental hemorrhage during pregnancy and after delivery. Vox Sang 1986; 51:117.
19. Peddle LJ. Increase of antibody titer following amniocentesis. Am J Obstet Gynecol 1968; 100:567.
20. Bowman JM, Pollock JM. Transplacental fetal hemorrhage after amniocentesis. Obstet Gynecol 1985; 66:749.
21. Woodrow JC. Rh immunization and its prevention. The immune response in the mother. In: Jensen KG, Killmann SA, eds. Series Hematologica III. Copenhagen, Munksgaard, 1970:3–33.
22. Zipursky A, Israels LJ. The pathogenesis and prevention of Rh immunization. Can Med Assoc J 1967; 97:1245.

23. Nevanlinna HR. Factors affecting maternal Rh immunization. Ann Med Exp Biol 1953; 31 (Fenn suppl 2):1.

24. Bowman JM. Fetomaternal ABO incompatibility and erythroblastosis fetalis. Vox Sang 1986; 50:104.

25. Bowman JM, Chown B, Lewis M, et al. Rh-isoimmunization during pregnancy: Antenatal prophylaxis. Can Med Assoc J 1978; 118:623.

26. Lobuglio AF, Cotran RS, Jandl JH. Red cells coated with immunoglobulin G: Binding and sphering by mononuclear cells in man. Science 1967; 158:1582.

27. Urbaniak SJ. Lymphoid cell dependent (K-cell) lysis of human erythrocytes sensitized with Rhesus alloantibody. Br J Haematol 1976; 33:409.

28. Engelfriet CP, Borne AEG, Beckers DO, et al. Immune destruction of red cells. In A Seminar on Immune-Mediated Cell Destruction. Washington, DC, American Association of Blood Banks, 1981:113.

29. Cooper RA. Loss of membrane components in the pathogenesis of antibody-induced spherocytosis. J Clin Invest 1972; 51:16.

30. Pollock JM, Bowman JM, Manning FA, Harman CR. Fetal blood sampling in Rh Hemolytic Disease. Vox Sang 1987; 53:139.

31. Thomson A, Contreras M, Gorick B, et al. Clearance of Rh D-positive red cells with monoclonal anti-D. Lancet 1990; 336:1147.

32. Pollock JM, Bowman JM. Anti-Rh(D) IgG Subclasses and severity of Rh hemolytic disease of the newborn. Vox Sang 1990; 59:176.

33. Zupanska B, Brojer E, Richards Y, et al. Serological and immunological characteristics of maternal anti-Rh(D) antibodies in predicting the severity of haemolytic disease of the newborn. Vox Sang, 1989; 56:247.

34. Parinaud J, Blanc M, Grandjean H, et al. IgG subclasses and Gm allotypes of anti-D antibodies during pregnancy: Correlation with the gravity of the fetal disease. Am J Obstet Gynecol 1985; 151:1111.

35. Bowman J. Treatment Options for the fetus with alloimmune hemolytic disease. Transfus Med Rev 1990; IV:191.

36. Mollison PL, Engelfriet CP, Contreras M. Chapt. 14, Hemolytic disease of the newborn. In: Mollison PL, ed. Blood Transfusion in Clinical Medicine. 8th ed. Oxford, England, Blackwell Scientific, 1987:639.

37. Bowman JM, Pollock JM, Manning FA, et al. Maternal Kell blood group alloimmunization. Obstet Gynecol 1992, 79:239.

38. Bowman JM, Harman CR, Manning FA, et al. Erythroblastosis fetalis produced by anti-k. Vox Sang 1989; 56:187.

39. Dacus JV, Spinnato JA. Severe erythroblastosis fetalis secondary to anti-Kp^b sensitization. Am J Obstet Gynecol 1984; 150:888.

40. MacPherson CR, Christiansen MJ, Newton WA, et al. Anti-M antibody as a cause of intrauterine death. Am J Clin Pathol 1961; 35:31.

41. Cox MT, Sheils L, Masel D, Blumberg N. Fetal hydrops due to anti-B. Transfusion 1991; 31 (suppl) S98:29S.

42. Miller DF, Petrie SJ. Fatal erythroblastosis fetalis secondary to ABO incompatibility: Report of a case. Obstet Gynecol 1963; 22:773.

43. Brouwers HAA, Overbeeke MAM, Huiskes E, et al. Complement is not activated in ABO-haemolytic disease of the newborn. Br J Haematol 1988; 68:363.

44. Bowman JM. ABO hemolytic disease. In Creasy RK, Resnick R, eds. Maternal-Fetal Medicine: Principles and Practice. Philadelphia, WB Saunders 1989:652.

45. James LS. Shock in the newborn in relation to hydrops, The Rh problem. Robertson JG, Dambrosio F, eds. Proceedings of the International Symposium on the Management of the Rh Problem. Milan, Instituti Clinici di Perfezionamento 1970:193.

46. Bowman JM, Pollock JM. Amniotic fluid spectrophotometry and early delivery in the management of erythroblastosis fetalis. Pediatrics 1965; 35:815.

47. Nance SJ, Nelson JM, Horenstein J, et al. Monocyte monolayer assay: An efficient noninvasive

technique for predicting the severity of hemolytic disease of the newborn. Am J Clin Pathol 1989; 92:89.

48. Urbaniak SJ, Greiss MA, Crawford RJ, et al. Prediction of the outcome of Rhesus haemolytic disease of the newborn: Additional information using an ADCC assay. Vox Sang 1984; 46: 323.

49. Engelfriet CP, Brouwers HAA, Huiskes E, et al. Prognostic value of the ADCC with monocytes and maternal antibodies for haemolytic disease of the newborn (abstr). Book of Abstracts. XXIst Congr ISH and XIXth Congr ISBT, Sydney 1986:162.

50. Hadley AG, Kumpel BM, Merry AH. The chemiluminescent response of human monocytes to red cells sensitized with monoclonal anti-Rh(D) antibodies. Clin Lab Haematol 1988; 10:377.

51. Hadley AG, Kumpel BM, Leader KA, et al. Correlation of serological, quantitative and cell-mediated functional assays of maternal alloantibodies with the severity of haemolytic disease of the newborn. Br J Haematol 1991; 77:221.

52. Mollison P. Results of tests with different cellular bioassays in relation to severity of RhD haemolytic disease. Report from Nine Collaborating Laboratories. Vox Sang 1991; 60:225.

53. Brown SJ, Perkins JT, Sosler SD, et al. The monocyte-monolayer assay does not predict severity of hemolytic disease of the newborn. Transfusion 1991; 31(suppl):S193, p. 53S.

54. Liley AW. Liquor amnii analysis in management of pregnancy complicated by rhesus immunization. Am J Obstet Gynecol 1961; 82:1359.

55. Bevis DCA. Blood pigments in haemolytic disease of the newborn. J Obstet Gynaecol Br Emp 1956; 63:68.

56. Nicolaides KH, Rodeck CH, Mibashan MD, et al. Have Liley charts outlived their usefulness? Am J Obstet Gynecol 1986; 155:90.

57. Ananth U, Queenan JT. Does midtrimester ΔOD 450 of amniotic fluid reflect severity of Rh disease? Am J Obstet Gynecol 1989; 161:47.

58. Bowman JM. Rhesus haemolytic disease. In: Wald NJ, ed. Antenatal and Neonatal Screening. 2nd ed. Oxford, England, Oxford University Press, 1992.

59. Chitkara U, Wilkins I, Lynch L, et al. The role of sonography in assessing severity of fetal anemia in Rh- and Kell-isoimmunized pregnancies. Obstet Gynecol 1988; 71:393.

60. Daffos F, Capella-Pavlovsky M, Forestier F. Fetal blood sampling during pregnancy with use of a needle guided by ultrasound: A study of 606 consecutive cases. Am J Obstet Gynecol 1985; 153:655.

61. Carter BB. Preliminary report on a substance which inhibits anti-Rh serum. Am J Clin Pathol 1947; 17:646.

62. Biermé SJ, Blanc M, Abbal M, et al. Oral Rh treatment for severely immunized mothers. Lancet 1979; 1:604.

63. Gold WR Jr, Queenan JT, Woody J, et al. Oral desensitization in Rh disease. Am J Obstet Gynecol 1983; 146:980.

64. Gusdon JP Jr, Caudle MR, Herbst GA, et al. Phagocytosis and erythroblastosis: 1. Modification of the neonatal response by promethazine hydrochloride. Am J Obstet Gynecol 1976; 125: 224.

65. Bowman JM, Pollock JM. Reversal of Rh alloimmunization. Fact or Fancy? Vox Sang 1984; 47:209.

66. De Silva M, Contreras M, Mollison PL. Failure of passively administered anti-Rh to prevent secondary Rh immune responses. Vox Sang 1985; 48:178.

67. Graham-Pole J, Barr W, Willoughby MLN. Continuous flow plasmapheresis in management of severe Rhesus disease. Br Med J 1977; 1:1185.

68. Robinson EAE, Tovey LAD. Intensive plasma exchange in the management of severe Rh disease. Br J Haematol 1980; 45:621.

69. Berlin G, Selbing A, Ryden G. Rhesus haemolytic disease treated with high-dose intravenous immunoglobulin (letter). Lancet 1985; 1:1153.

70. Margulies M, Voto LS, Mathet E, et al. High-dose intravenous IgG for the treatment of severe Rhesus alloimmunization. Vox Sang 1991; 61:181.

71. Wallerstein H. Treatment of severe erythroblastosis by simultaneous removal and replacement of blood of the newborn. Science 1946; 103:583.
72. Diamond LK. Replacement transfusion as a treatment for erythroblastosis fetalis. Pediatrics 1948; 2:520.
73. Chown B, Bowman WD. The place of early delivery in the prevention of foetal death from erythroblastosis. Pediatr Clin North Am 1958; May:279.
74. Liley AW. Intrauterine transfusion of fetus in hemolytic disease. Br Med J 1963; 2:1107.
75. Menticoglou SM, Harman CR, Manning FA, et al. Intraperitoneal fetal transfusion: Paralysis inhibits red cell absorption. Fetal Ther 1987; 2:154.
76. Lewis M, Bowman JM, Pollock JM, et al. Absorption of red cells from the peritoneal cavity of a hydropic twin. Transfusion 1973; 13:37.
77. Adamsons K Jr, Freda VJ, James LS, et al. Prenatal treatment of erythroblastosis fetalis following hysterotomy. Pediatrics 1965; 35:848.
78. Asensio SH, Figueroa-Longo JG, Pelegrina A. Intrauterine exchange transfusion. Am J Obstet Gynecol 1966; 95:1129.
79. Seelen J, Van Kessel H, Eskes T, et al. A new method of exchange transfusion in utero:Cannulation of vessels on the fetal side of the human placenta. Am J Obstet Gynecol 1966; 95:872.
80. Rodeck CH, Holman CA, Karnicki J, et al. Direct intravascular fetal blood transfusion by fetoscopy in severe rhesus isoimmunization. Lancet 1981; 1:625.
81. De Crespigny LC, Robinson HP, Quinn M, et al. Ultrasound- guided blood transfusion for severe rhesus isoimmunization. Obstet Gynecol 1985; 66:529.
82. Berkowitz RL, Chikara U, Goldberg JD, et al. Intrauterine intravascular transfusions for severe red blood cell isoimmunization: Ultrasound guided percutaneous approach. Am J Obstet Gynecol 1986; 155:574.
83. Nicholaides KH, Soothill PW, Clewell W, et al. Rh disease: Intravascular fetal blood transfusion by cordocentesis. Fetal Ther 1986; 1:185.
84. Seeds JW, Bowes WA. Ultrasound-guided intravascular transfusion in severe rhesus immunization. Am J Obstet Gynecol 1986; 154:1105.
85. Grannum PAT, Copel JA, Moya FR, et al. The reversal of hydrops fetalis by intravascular intrauterine transfusions in severe isoimmune fetal anemia. Am J Obstet Gynecol 1988; 158: 914.
86. Harman CR, Bowman JM, Manning FA, et al. Intrauterine transfusion—Intraperitoneal versus intravascular approach: A case-control comparison. Am J Obstet Gynecol 1990; 162:1053.
87. Von Dungern F. Beitrage zur immunitatslehr. Munch Med Wochenschr 1900; 47:677.
88. Stern K, Goodman HS, Berger M. Experimental iso-immunization to hemo-antigens in man. J Immunol 1961; 87:189.
89. Clarke CA, Donohoe WTA, McConnell RB, et al. Further experimental studies in the prevention of Rh-haemolytic disease. Br Med J 1963; 1:979.
90. Freda VJ, Gorman JG, Pollack W. Successful prevention of experimental Rh sensitization in man with an anti-Rh gamma 2-globulin antibody preparation: A preliminary report. Transfusion 1964; 4:26.
91. Zipursky A, Israels LG. The pathogenesis and prevention of Rh immunization. Can Med Assoc J 1967; 97:1245.
92. Combined study (1966). Prevention of Rh-haemolytic disease: Results of the clinical trial. A combined study from centres in England and Baltimore. Br Med J 1966; 2:901.
93. Pollack W, Gorman JG, Freda VJ, et al. Results of clinical trials with Rhogamin women. Transfusion 1968; 8:151.
94. Chown B, Duff AM, James J, et al. Prevention of primary Rh immunization: First report of the Western Canadian Trial. Can Med Assoc J 1969; 100:1021.
95. St Sinclair NR. Regulation of the immune response. I. Reduction in ability of specific antibody to inhibit long-lasting IgG immunological priming after removal of the Fc-fragment. J Exp Med 1969; 129:1183.
96. Pollack W. Mechanisms of Rh immune suppression by Rh immune globulin. In: Garratty G, ed.

Hemolytic Disease of the Newborn. Arlington, VA, American Association of Blood Banks, 1984:53.

97.   Pollack W, Gorman JG. Rh immune suppression: An immunostat hypothesis. In: Scientific Symposium: Rh Antibody Mediated Immunosuppression. Raritan, NJ, Ortho Research Institute of Medicine and Science, 1976:115.

98.   Woodrow JC, Clarke CA, Donohoe WTA, et al. Mechanisms of Rh prophylaxis: An experimental study on specificity of immunosuppression. Br Med J 1975; 2:57.

99.   Pollack W. Ascari WQ, Crispin JF, et al. Studies on Rh prophylaxis: II. Rh immune prophylaxis after transfusions with Rh-positive blood. Transfusion 1971; 11:340.

100. Pollack W, Ascari WQ, Kochesky RJ, et al. Studies on Rh prophylaxis: I. Relationship between doses of anti-Rh and size of antigenic stimulus. Transfusion 1971; 11:333.

101. Blajchman M, Zipursky A, Bartsch RR, et al. Rh immunization during pregnancy, McMaster conference on prevention of Rh immunization, September 28–30. Vox Sang 1977; 36:50.

102. Scott JR, Beer AE, Guy LR, et al. Pathogenesis of Rh immunization in primigravidas: Fetomaternal versus maternofetal bleeding. Obstet Gynecol 1977; 49:9.

103. Bowman JM, Pollock JM. Antenatal-Rh prophylaxis 28 weeks' gestation service program. Can Med Assoc J 1978; 118:627

104. Bowman JM, Pollock JM. Failures of intravenous Rh immune globulin prophylaxis: An analysis of the reasons for such failures. Transfus Med Rev 1987; 1:101.

105. Nusbacher J, Bove JR. Sounding board. Rh immuno-prophylaxis: Is antepartum therapy desirable? N Engl J Med 1980; 303:935.

106. Hensleigh PA. Preventing rhesus isoimmunization. Antepartum Rh immune globulin prophylaxis versus a sensitive test for risk identification. Am J Obstet Gynecol 1983; 146:749.

107. Pollack W, Gorman JG, Hager HJ, et al. Antibody-mediated immune suppression to the Rh factor: Animal models suggesting mechanism of action. Transfusion 1968; 8:134.

108. Contreras M, Mollison PL. Failure to augment primary Rh immunization using a small dose of "passive" IgG anti-Rh. Br J Haematol 1981; 49:371.

109. Mollison PL. Can primary Rh immunization be augmented by passively administered antibody? In: Frigoletto FD Jr, Jewett JF, Konugres AA, eds. Rh Hemolytic Disease–New Strategy for Eradication. Boston, Hall, 1982:161.

110. Cohen R, Zuelzer WW. The transplacental passage of maternal erythrocytes into the fetus. Am J Obstet Gynecol 1965; 93:566.

111. Bernard B, Presley M, Caudillo G, et al. Maternal fetal hemorrhage: Incidence and sensitization (abstr). Pediatr Res 1977; 11:467.

112. Bowman JM, Lewis M, de Sa DJ. Hydrops fetalis caused by massive maternofetal transplacental hemorrhage. J Pediatr 1984; 104:769.

113. Hindemann P. Maternofetal transfusion during delivery and Rh sensitization of the newborn (letter). Lancet 1973; 1:46.

114. Bowen FW, Renfield M. The detection of anti-D in Rho (D)-negative infants born of Rho (D)-positive mothers. Pediatr Res 1976; 10:213.

115. Carapella-de Luca E, Casadei AM, Pascone R, et al. Maternofetal transfusion during delivery and sensitization of the newborn against rhesus D-antigen. Vox Sang 1978; 34:241.

116. Godel JC, Buchanan DI, Jarosch JM, et al. Significance of Rh-sensitization during pregnancy: Its relation to a preventive programme. Br Med J 1968; 4:479.

117. Tovey LAD, Scott JS. Suppression of early rhesus sensitization by passive anti-D immunoglobulin. Vox Sang 1980; 39:149.

118. Rivat L, Parent M, Rivat C. Accident survenu apres injection de gamma-globulines anti-Rh du a la presence d'anti-corps anti-yA (letter). Presse Med 1970; 78:2072.

119. Hoppe HH, Mester T, Hennig W, et al. Prevention of Rh-immunization: Modified production of IgG anti-Rh for intravenous application by ion exchange chromatography (IEC). Vox Sang 1973; 25:308.

120. Bowman JM, Friesen AD, Pollock JM, et al. WinRho: Rh immune globulin prepared by ion exchange for intravenous use. Can Med Assoc J 1980; 123:1121.

121. Crawford DH, Barlow MJ, Harrison JF, et al. Production of human monoclonal antibody to rhesus D antigen. Lancet 1983; 1:386.

122. Crawford DH, McDougall DCJ, Mulholland N, et al. Further characterisation of a human monoclonal antibody to the rhesus D antigen produced in vitro. Behring Inst Mitt 1984; 74:55.

123. Bron D, Feinberg MB, Teng NNH, et al. Production of human monoclonal IgG antibodies against rhesus (D) antigen. Proc Natl Acad Sci USA 1984; 81:3214.

124. MacDonald G, Primrose S, Biggins K, et al. Production and characterization of human-human and human-mouse hybridomas secreting Rh(D)-specific monoclonal antibodies. Scand J Immunol 1987; 25:477.

21

Alloimmune Refractoriness to Transfused Platelets

SHERRILL J. SLICHTER
Puget Sound Blood Center
and University of Washington School of Medicine
Seattle, Washington

I. EXPECTED RESPONSE TO TRANSFUSED PLATELETS

Before discussing the criteria for diagnosing alloimmune platelet refractoriness, it is important to identify the expected response to homologous platelet transfusions in thrombocytopenic patients. There are two parameters that characterize the platelet response—the initial platelet recovery or corrected count increment and the subsequent survival of the transfused platelets.

A. Initial Posttransfusion Platelet Recovery or Corrected Count Increment

1. Posttransfusion Platelet Recovery

The posttransfusion platelet recovery (PPR) can be calculated as follows:

$$\frac{\text{Platelet Increment} \times \text{Patient's Weight (kg)} \times \text{Blood Volume Estimated at 75 ml/kg} \times 100}{\text{Platelet Count of Infused Platelets} \times \text{Volume of Platelets (ml)}}$$

Platelet increment is calculated by subtracting the pretransfusion platelet count from the posttransfusion platelet count drawn within 10–60 min after transfusion (1). Sixty ± 15% of transfused homologous platelets are recovered in the circulation of thrombocytopenic patients, and this is equivalent to that seen for autologous platelets in normal volunteers, i.e., 66 ± 8% (2).

The 40% of platelets that do not circulate are pooled in the spleen (3). Thus, in asplenic individuals, the posttransfusion platelet recovery approaches 100%, whereas in hypersplenism, the recovery is reduced in proportion to the size of the spleen.

2. Corrected Count Increment

As an alternative measure of initial platelet response, a corrected count increment (CCI) can be calculated.

$$\text{CCI} = \frac{(\text{Platelet Increment}) \times (\text{Body Surface Area in m}^2)}{\text{Number of Platelets Transfused} \times 10^{11}}$$

A CCI of 30×10^9/L represents 100% recovery (4), and a CCI corresponding to a 60% recovery would be 18×10^9/L.

B. Posttransfusion Platelet Survival

At platelet counts of $<100 \times 10^9$/L, there is a direct relationship between platelet count and platelet survival (2). Platelets are lost from circulation by two mechanisms: (1) an estimated 7.1×10^9/L, or 17% of the $41.2 \pm 4.9 \times 10^9$/L, platelets lost daily are randomly removed; and (2) the remaining platelets (approximately 83%) are removed by senescent mechanisms. Presumably, the random platelet removal is a consequence of platelets that are used in an endothelial supportive function.

In normal subjects with an average platelet count of $258 \pm 44 \times 10^9$/L, this random platelet utilization of 7.1×10^9 platelets/day accounts for <3% of the circulating platelet pool. However, as the platelet count falls to levels of 100×10^9/L and below, this random platelet loss represents a significant and ever-increasing fraction of the circulating platelets that directly reduces platelet survivals. For example, in six clinically stable, nonalloimmunized thrombocytopenic patients with average baseline platelet counts of $19 \pm 6 \times 10^9$/L, platelet survivals were only 3.4 ± 1.1 days with a range of 2.3–5.0 days, compared with normal autologous platelet survivals of 9.6 ± 0.06 days with a range of 8.5–10.4 days measured in nonthrombocytopenic volunteers (2).

II. DEFINITION OF ALLOIMMUNE PLATELET REFRACTORINESS

Alloimmune platelet refractoriness is present when there is a significant reduction in platelet recovery and/or survival in association with alloantibodies. Although this definition appears straight forward, it is often difficult to determine mechanisms of platelet refractoriness in any given patient. There are two reasons for this: (1) there are many additional factors that may be associated with poor platelet recoveries and survivals besides alloimmunization—such as fever, infection, drugs, and splenomegaly, (5,6); and (2) just the presence of antibodies does not necessarily mean that these antibodies are causing the patient's poor response to transfused platelets. In order to conclusively demonstrate that alloimmunization is the cause of platelet refractoriness, antigen-compatible platelets must be given and show a better response than unselected platelets. If a compatible platelet transfusion does not improve a patient's response to platelets, then the patient may still be alloimmune refractory but there must be additional factors that are impairing the response to any transfused platelets.

A. Abnormal Platelet Responses

Guidelines of <30% recovery at 1hr or a survival of <2 days can be used as indicators of an abnormal response. These values correspond to less than half the expected recovery measurement, and the survival is shorter than that seen in thrombocytopenic patients (2).

By the CCI criterion, an unsuccessful transfusion is a CCI of <7.5, or $<10.0 \times 10^9$/L (depending on the investigator), within 1 hr of a transfusion, and <4.5, or $<7.5 \times 10^9$L, at 18–24 hr (4,7–10). A CCI of $7.5–10.0 \times 10^9$/L is equivalent to a 25–30% recovery, and a CCI of $4.5–7.5 \times 10^9$/L equals 15–25% recovery. Thus, the two reported criteria for determining abnormal platelet responses, based on either platelet recovery or CCI measurements, are roughly equivalent.

On a practical level, the number of platelets transfused is often not counted, and, therefore, it is not possible to calculate either platelet recovery or CCI. In these circumstances, an increment of $<5 \times 10^9$ platelets/L after two sequential transfusions of 6 U of platelet concentrates is sufficiently reduced to identify clearly patients who are in need of further evaluation to identify causes and management of their platelet refractoriness.

B. Detection of Platelet Alloantibodies

As HLA antigens are the major immunogens present on the surface of platelets, lymphocytotoxic antibodies to HLA antigens expressed on lymphocytes are often used as a marker of platelet alloimmunization. However, there have been major improvements in direct platelet antibody testing using a variety of techniques (11,12), and there are several advantages to this approach. Some HLA antigens may not be as well expressed on platelets as lymphocytes (13–16). Thus, detecting a strong lymphocytotoxic antibody against HLA antigens on lymphocytes may not necessarily correlate with platelet transfusion outcomes. In addition, there is increasing interest in the role of platelet-specific, non-HLA antigens in alloimmune platelet refractoriness (17–22). These types of antibodies can only be detected by direct platelet antibody assays.

As another guide to the significance of any alloantibodies detected, there are several studies demonstrating that the higher the frequency of antibody reactivity with panel lymphocytes or platelets, the more likely is the patient to demonstrate poor responses to pooled random-donor platelet transfusions (1,7,23). Thus, the more panreactive the antibody, the more likely is any platelet unresponsiveness due to alloimmunization.

III. PREVENTION OF PLATELET ALLOIMMUNIZATION

Before proceeding to a discussion of how to manage the alloimmunized platelet refractory patient, it is important to recognize that there may be effective methods of preventing platelet alloimmunization so as to avoid this complication of platelet therapy. Although these prevention of platelet alloimmunization techniques have associated expenses that are greater than providing pooled random-donor platelet transfusions, they may be less expensive than the costs of providing antigen-compatible platelet donors if the patient becomes alloimmunized.

A. Immunosuppress the Platelet Transfusion Recipient

Patients with malignant disorders have a much lower rate of immunization to platelet transfusions than do patients with aplastic anemia. In one study, only 20 of 65 (31%) of the transfused patients with acute myelogenous leukemia (AML) developed alloantibodies compared with 7 of 8 (88%) of the patients with aplastic anemia (24). The difference is likely due to the potentially immunosuppressive chemotherapy given to patients with leukemia while they are being transfused. In addition, the high-dose steroids received by patients with acute lymphocytic leukemia (ALL) compared with patients with AML may produce a lower incidence of alloimmunization; i.e., 18% for patients with ALL versus 44% for AML; $p < 0.0002$ (25). However, in another study, immunization frequency was the same—38% in AML and 35% in ALL (26). In neither study were the doses of the chemotherapeutic agents used detailed, and there may be clear differences in immunization rates depending on the patients' chemotherapy (24,26). Overall, in a series of studies (24,25,27–31), 380 of 944 (40%) patients with malignant disorders receiving chemotherapy developed alloantibodies.

In a dog platelet transfusion model, none of the nine recipients given cyclosporine A therapy became refractory to platelets from a single random-donor dog—even after 8 weekly transfusions. Furthermore, six of nine recipients (67%) remained responsive to an additional 8 weekly transfusions after the cyclosporine was stopped (32). In six of seven baboons (86%) given either prednisone, antithymocyte globulin, or a combination of these two agents, platelet refractoriness did not occur after repeated weekly platelet transfusions from a single random-donor baboon (33).

In summary, it is unlikely that specific immunosuppressive therapy given to prevent platelet alloimmunization—as was done in the animal transfusion experiments—would ever be accepted for patients because of the increased infectious disease and tumor recurrence risks that might result from such therapy. However, it is quite likely that patients with malignancy who are receiving chemotherapy have a reduced rate of immunization because of the immunosuppressive effect of some of their treatments. Furthermore, it is also possible that some of the other methods that have been used to prevent platelet alloimmunization such as modifying the transfused blood products (outlined below) are, in part, successful because the transfused patients are at least partially immunoincompetent because of their disease or its treatment.

B. Limit the Number of Transfusions Provided

Unfortunately, to limit the number of transfusions provided to patients is not a very practical approach as the patients for whom the development of platelet alloantibodies represents a significant detriment to their care are also those who are likely to have prolonged periods of thrombocytopenia, and they will usually require multiple transfusions. In addition, all chronically thrombocytopenic patients also receive red blood cell (RBC) transfusions either because of failure to produce RBCs—usually for the same condition that has produced their thrombocytopenia or because the thrombocytopenia results in blood loss.

It takes at least 10–14 days for a naive transfusion recipient to form an antibody (24,25,27–31), and the patient may require many or few platelet transfusions during that time period—depending on their clinical condition. The time required for antibody development may explain why some investigators have demonstrated a relationship between the number of platelet transfusions and the development of alloantibodies if the patients being studied had periodic transfusions over time (23,24,29,34,35), whereas others have found that even a few transfusions may result in alloimmunization (25,28,36).

C. Limit the Number of Donors

There have been three prospective randomized trials to determine the relative benefits of providing single random-donor apheresis platelets compared with pooled random-donor platelet transfusions to prevent platelet alloimmunization (37–39) (Table 1). Only one of these studies showed a significant decrease in rates of platelet refractoriness and lymphocytotoxic antibody formation (39) in spite of the fact that the number of donor exposures for the patients who received pooled random-donor platelets was up to 10 times that of the patients receiving single random apheresis platelets.

In a dog platelet transfusion model, recipient dogs were given either repeated transfusions of a pool of platelets obtained from the same six random-donor dogs, or they received transfusions from a single random donor until they became platelet refractory, and then a new donor was used (40). There was no difference in the frequency of platelet refractoriness for either transfusion program; 17 of 22 (77%) of the recipients of pooled random-donor platelets became refractory to all 6 donors compared with 6 of 10 (60%) of the dogs who received platelets individually from 6 random donors; $p > 0.05$. However, it required significantly fewer pooled random-donor transfusions (5.5 ± 1.0) compared with single random-donor transfusions (14.0 ± 5.0) to develop refractoriness; $p < 0.01$. Thus, single random-donor platelet transfusions in the dog delay, but do not prevent, platelet refractoriness.

As only about 40% of chronically transfused patients with malignant disorders become alloimmunized (41), the question becomes whether it is worthwhile to provide all chronically thrombocytopenic patients with the more expensive single-donor apheresis transfusions when

Table 1 Transfusions of Single Random-Donor Apheresis Platelets versus Pooled Random-Donor Platelet Concentrates

Reference	Pooled random-donor platelet concentrates						Single random-donor apheresis platelets						
	patients (No.)	transfusion[a] events (No.)		platelet refractory		alloantibodies	patients (No.)	transfusion[a] events (No.)		platelet refractory		alloantibodies	
		Platelets	RBCs	No.	(%)	No. (%)		Platelets	RBCs	No.	(%)	No.	(%)
Sintnicolass et al. (37)	17	2.4 (1–75) (NS)	8 (3–20) (NS)	NI		2　12 (NS)	17	1.7 (1–75)	5 (2–19)	NI		1	6
Kakaiya et al. (38)	7	8 ±6 (NS)	NI	NI		2　29 (NS)	9	10 ±9	NI	NI		5	56
Gmur et al. (39)	27	5.5 ±3.0 (NS)	10.7 ±5.5 (NS)	14	52 (<0.005)	15　56 (p < 0.002)	27	6.0 ±3.0	12.8 ±6.0	4	15	4	15

Abbreviations: NI, no information; NS, not significant.
Significance values compare the results of transfusions with pooled random donor platelet concentrates to single random-donor apheresis platelets.
[a]Average transfusions per patient (range) ±1 SD. In the studies by Sintnicolaas or Kakaiya, each pooled random donor transfusion consisted of 10 platelet concentrates, and for Gmur's study, 5–10 platelet concentrates/transfusion were given. In Sintnicolaas' study, all RBCs were buffy coat poor, and in Gmur's study, the RBCs were made leukocyte poor by filtration.

only a fraction of the patients need protection and, at best, alloimmunization is likely to be only delayed rather than prevented. However, it is clear that there are more single-donor platelet transfusions being provided in the United States. Based on the latest statistics available, 11% of the platelets transfused in 1980 were from single donors, and this percentage increased to 25% in 1987 (42). How much of this increase was due to a requirement to collect more platelets to meet blood center inventory needs, as an attempt to reduce donor exposures to reduce the risk of virus transmission, or as a result of planned single-donor transfusion programs to prevent platelet alloimmunization is unknown. It is likely that all of these factors may have contributed to the observed changes in platelet products transfused.

D. Select Compatible Donors

1. ABO Compatibility

A and B antigens are expressed on the surface of platelets (43). To determine the effect of ABO mismatching on platelet alloimmunization, 40 leukemic patients undergoing induction chemotherapy were randomly assigned to receive two sets of paired transfusions of ABO-compatible or ABO-incompatible pooled random-donor platelet transfusions (44). Although there was no difference in platelet recoveries with the first set of transfusions, the CCI for the second ABO-compatible transfusion averaged 14.9×10^9/L compared with 9.5×10^9/L for the ABO-incompatible transfusion ($p < 0.0007$), whereas survivals were similar. Eleven patients had serial isohemagglutination titers for anti-A and anti-B antibodies performed, and in the six patients with consistently poor results to ABO-incompatible platelets, the relevant anti-A or anti-B titers were either elevated at baseline or became elevated after the incompatible transfusions (isohemagglutination titers were 256–1024). In contrast, only one of the five patients with consistently good responses to ABO-incompatible platelets had elevated titers.

In another study of 26 patients undergoing treatment for acute leukemia or autografting for relapsed Hodgkin's disease who were randomly assigned to receive either ABO-compatible or ABO-incompatible platelets, platelet refractoriness was significantly lower in the group receiving ABO-compatible platelets—not only because patients did not increase their anti-A or anti-B isohemagglutinin titers but also the ABO-compatible recipients had a much lower incidence of lymphocytotoxic and platelet-specific alloantibodies (45). Nine of the 13 patients (69%) who were given ABO-mismatched platelet transfusions became platelet refractory compared with only 1 of 13 patients (8%) who received ABO-compatible platelets; $p < 0.0014$

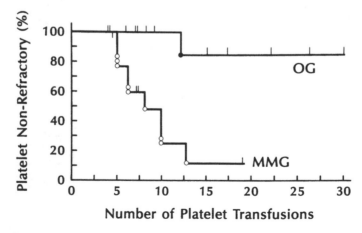

Figure 1   Estimated survival curves of refractoriness by number of platelet transfusions. Ordinate: Probability (%) of not becoming refractory. Log rank statistic = 10.3 ($p = 0.0014$). MMG = mismatched ABO group platelets; OG = own ABO group platelets. (From Ref. 45.)

(Fig. 1). The repeated administration of ABO-mismatched platelets produced a significant rise in anti-A/B titers in 7 of 13 patients (54%) that were generally correlated with poor platelet increments. In addition, 5 of 13 recipients (38%) of the ABO-mismatched platelets developed lymphocytotoxic antibodies, and 4 of 13 (31%) developed platelet-specific alloantibodies compared with only 1 of 13 (8%) and 1 of 13 (8%), respectively, of the recipients of ABO-compatible platelets. The close temporal association between the development of HLA and platelet-specific alloantibodies and rises in anti-A/B titers suggests that, in the process of responding to the ABO-incompatible antigens, recognition of other antigen incompatibilities also occurred. Data from these two studies suggests that provision of ABO-compatible platelets may be a simple method of reducing the incidence of alloimmune platelet refractoriness.

2. HLA Compatibility

As HLA antigens are the predominant immunogens expressed on the surface of platelets and the major cause of refractoriness to ABO-compatible platelets, in two transfusion trials the benefits of HLA compared with random single-donor apheresis platelet transfusions were evaluated (46,47). In one trial (46), 18 patients with cancer receiving chemotherapy for a variety of malignant disorders received only HLA-matched platelets and another 15 patients received single-donor platelets mismatched for one or more HLA-antigens. There was no significant difference between total number of platelet transfusions per patient (median 3 versus 5, respectively; $p = 0.076$), number of platelet transfusions per thrombocytopenic episode (median of 3.0 versus 3.5, respectively; $p = 0.28$), or in days between transfusions (median of 2 versus 2, respectively; $p > 0.4$). Only one study patient developed antiplatelet antibodies.

In the other study, 30 patients with newly diagnosed acute leukemia were given RBC and platelet apheresis transfusions that were both made leukocyte poor prior to transfusion (47). Nineteen patients received single random-donor apheresis transfusions, and 11 patients received apheresis transfusions compatible for at least three out of the 4 HLA-A and B locus antigens. The single random-donor apheresis group received a mean of 33 units of RBCs and 19 random apheresis transfusions compared with 23 units of RBCs and 9 HLA-matched apheresis transfusions. Three of the 19 recipients (16%) who were given random single-donor apheresis platelets developed lymphocytotoxic antibodies, and 1 of 19 (5%) became platelet refractory compared with 0 of 11 and 0 of 11, respectively, for the recipients of the HLA-selected transfusions. There were no significant differences in platelet refractoriness or antibody development between the groups. Thus, in neither of these two studies was there evidence that provision of HLA-matched apheresis platelets provided an additional benefit over that achieved with single random-donor apheresis transfusions.

E. Modification of the Transfused Platelets and RBCs to Reduce Their Immunogenicity

For some of the investigations to be discussed, only the transfused platelets were modified and evaluated. However, it should be remembered that chronically thrombocytopenic patients require both RBC and platelet transfusions, and transfusion studies modifying both products will be needed to determine the efficacy of any of these methods in preventing platelet alloimmunization.

1. Leukocyte Reduction

It has been well-documented that alloantigen recognition requires the expression of both class I and class II HLA antigens on the surface of the transfused cells (48,49). As platelets, in contrast to white blood cells (WBCs), express only class I but not class II HLA antigens and RBCs do not express HLA antigens, the question of whether leukocyte-poor blood components will prevent platelet alloimmunization has been investigated. Early animal studies in both rats (48) and mice (50) demonstrated that leukocyte-depleted platelets were not associated with alloantibody development.

In humans, administration of $<5 \times 10^6$ leukocytes did not result in lymphocytotoxic antibody formation following a limited number of injections (51,52) (Table 2). Although centrifugation techniques have been used to produce leukocyte-poor blood products, in the last several years, a number of very efficient leukocyte-reduction filters have been developed. A review of the literature between 1980 and 1990 provides data on the residual leukocyte levels in RBC and platelet products using these filters (53). In fact, the efficacy of some of these leukocyte-reduction filters is so good that newer techniques are required to count accurately the very low number of WBCs remaining in the filtered products (54).

To date, there have been six prospective randomized clinical trials in 299 patients evaluating the efficacy of leukocyte-poor RBCs and platelets in preventing platelet alloimmunization (Tables 3 and 4) (47,55–59). There was substantial variability in patient selection, methods of leukocyte reduction, and endpoint criteria used in these trials (Table 3). Not unexpectedly, there were also differences in the leukocyte concentration of the control blood products and the leukocyte-poor blood products, as well as in the results of these transfusion trials (Table 4). Four of the six studies showed a reduction in the development of lymphocytotoxic antibodies in patients given leukocyte-poor products; however, in the three studies that tested for platelet-specific alloantibodies, there was no difference between the control and leukocyte-poor arms. The incidence of clinical refractoriness to transfused platelets was reduced by leukocyte-poor blood products in only 3 of 6 of the trials.

Two recent editorials have suggested caution in interpreting the data from these leukocyte-poor transfusion trials because of the small numbers of patients in these studies and conflicting data on the levels of leukocytes that either produce or prevent platelet alloimmunization and/or platelet refractoriness (60,61). Furthermore, in another recent study, although the 27% incidence of antibody formation in 71 previously-pregnant females was the same as the 19% found in 264 nonpresensitized patients (all patients were receiving leukocyte-poor RBC and platelet products), the rate of platelet refractoriness was significantly higher in the previously pregnant women—15 of 71 (21%) compared with 16 of 264 (6%) in the nonpresensitized patients; $p < 0.001$ (62). This suggests that the subgroup of patients with prior antigenic exposure through pregnancy or probably as well by transfusions—although the latter patients were excluded from the trial—may not clinically benefit from filtration procedures.

One technical issue that has been raised in the performance of these trials is the timing of the leukocyte reduction. One investigator suggested that an intact WBC is required for induction of an immune response (48), whereas another found WBC fragments were immunogenic (63). As WBCs break down during storage and there is no information on whether the leukocyte-reduction filters will remove these fragments, it may be important to filter the blood products shortly after collection to prevent the transfusion of potentially immunogenic fragments. The question of the immunogenicity of WBC fragments has been evaluated in rabbit transfusion

Table 2 Leukocyte Threshold for Alloimmunization

Reference	No. WBC/Injection	No. Injections	No. Immunized/ No. Transfused (%)	
Fisher et al. (51)	1.5×10^7	3[a]	5/12	(42)
	$<5.0 \times 10^6$	3[a]	0/12	(0)
Petranyi et al. (52)	$<1.0 \times 10^5$	2[b]	0/5	(0)

[a]Injections given every 2 weeks to patients in renal failure.
[b]Injections given every 6 weeks to normal volunteers.

Table 3 Leukocyte-poor Transfusion Trials—Methods

Reference	Patient's diagnosis	Leukocyte-Poor product preparation		Endpoint criteria		
		RBCs	Platelets	lymphocytotoxic antibody positive	platelet antibody positive	clinically platelet refractory
Schiffer et. al. (55)	AML	Frozen, washed[a]	Centrifugation	Positive with ≥20% of a panel of 80–100 lymphocytes	NT	Required HLA-matched donors
Murphy et. al. (47)	Acute leukemia	Immugard IG 500	Centrifugation	Positive with at least 1 of a panel of 20 HLA-selected lymphocytes	Positive using PIFT with at least 1 of 2 donors	Platelet recovery 0% at 20 hr posttransfusion in the absence of clinical factors
Sniecinski et. al. (56)	Hematologic malignancy or AA	Immugard IG 500	Immugard IG 500	Positive with ≥10% of a lymphocyte panel	Positive using ^{125}I staphylococcal protein A test with at least 1 of a panel of 20 platelets	Two consecutive platelet transfusion recoveries of <20% of predicted value at 1 hr posttransfusion in the absence of clinical factors
Andreu et. al. (57)	Hematologic malignancy or refractory anemia	Immugard IG 500	Immugard IG 500	Positive with >10% of a panel of 30 lymphocytes	NT	Two consecutive platelet transfusions with recoveries of <20% at 18 hr posttransfusion
Oksanen et. al. (58)	AML, ALL	Cell Select	Immugard IG 500	Positive with at least 1 of a panel of 24 HLA-selected lymphocytes	Positive using PIFT test with at least 1 of a random panel of 8 platelets	CI of <2.5 × 10⁹/U transfused at 1 hr post transfusion
van Marwijk Kooy et al. (59)	AML, ALL	Cell Select[a]	Cell Select	Positive with >10% of a panel of 30 HLA-selected lymphocytes	NT	Two consecutive platelet transfusions with recoveries of <20% at 1 hr posttransfusion in the absence of clinical factors

Abbreviations: NT, not tested; PIFT, platelet immunifluorescence test; AA, aplastic anemia.
[a]RBC's for both treated and control arms were prepared in the same fashion.

Table 4 Leukocyte-Poor Transfusion Trials—Results

Reference	Patients (No.)	Control platelets (WBCs × 10^6)	Control RBC (WBCs × 10^6)	Leukocyte-Poor Platelets (WBCs × 10^6)	Leukocyte-Poor RBC (WBCs × 10^6)	Antibody positive Lymphocytotoxic control (%)	Lymphocytotoxic Leukocyte Poor (%)	Platelet control (%)	Platelet Leukocyte Poor (%)	Clinically platelet refractory control (%)	Clinically platelet refractory Leukocyte poor (%)
Schiffer et al. (35)	56	65	Frozen[b] Washed	12	Frozen,[b] Washed	42	20		NT	19	16
							$p = 0.07$				NS
Murphy et al. (47)	50	5830[c]	NI	90–220[c]	≤8	48	16	10	11	23	5
							$p < 0.02$		NS		NS
Sniecinski et al. (54)	40	530	3900	6	50	50	15	35	15	50	15
							$p < 0.01$		NS		$p < 0.01$
Andreu et al. (57)	69	477–678	2300	47–151	61	31	12		NT	47	21
							$p < 0.05$				$p < 0.05$
Oksanen et al. (58)	31	800	1000	0.2	0.1	26	13	33	31	26	13
							NS		NS		NS
van Marwijk Kooy et al. (59)	53	35[d]	<5[d]	<5	<5	42	7		NT	46	11
							$p < 0.004$				$p < 0.005$

Abbreviations: NI, no Information; NT, not tested; NS, no significant difference between control and leukocyte-poor data.

[a] Leukocyte data are reported as average number or range of residual WBCs per transfusion event for platelets or per unit of RBCs transfused.

[b] Frozen washed RBCs have no identifiable intact WBCs.

[c] Single random-donor apheresis transfusions were given rather than the pooled random-donor transfusions used in all other studies except for Andreu et al., where one of four trial sites used single random-donor apheresis transfusions.

[d] Control platelets leukocyte reduced by centrifugation and RBCs made leukocyte poor by filtration.

models (63,64). In one study (64), 24 control rabbits received 8 weekly fresh whole blood transfusions prepared from a single donor of a different strain. At the end of 8 weeks, platelets from the donor rabbit were radiolabeled and given to the recipient of the whole blood transfusions. Donor platelet survivals averaged 18.5 hr compared with autologous platelet survivals of 41.9–75.1 hr. The platelet refractory rate (defined as a donor platelet survival of <42 hr) was 96% in these recipients. In contrast, immediate leukocyte depletion and storage of the whole blood for 1 week prior to transfusion resulted in mean donor platelet survivals of 54.7 hr and a refractory rate of 33%. However, if the blood was stored for 1 week and then leukocyte depleted and transfused, after 8 weekly transfusions of the poststorage leukocyte-depleted whole blood, donor platelet survivals were only 31.0 hr, and 67% of the recipients were platelet refractory (p <0.05 for both endpoints) compared with prestorage leukocyte-depleted transfusions. During the week of storage, the WBC count in the unfiltered blood decreased by approximately 20%. In the other study (63), rabbits received RBCs made leukocyte poor immediately after collection or after 3 days of storage, or they received frozen/thawed deglycolized RBCs. None of the recipients of the immediately filtered blood developed lymphocytotoxic antibodies, whereas all the recipients of the other blood products became immunized.

One other note of caution concerning the use of leukocyte-poor blood products in the management of leukemic patients is the observation that although the patients admitted to one of these transfusion trials (47) had the same survival rate regardless of their blood product assignment, leukemia remission duration was significantly better in the group receiving standard blood components (65). Projected actuarial relapse-free survival rates for the recipients of the standard blood components was 50% and for the leukocyte-free blood component recipients 9% (p <0.001). A possible explanation for these findings is the development of transient engraftment and unrecognized graft-versus-host disease (GVHD) from the contaminating leukocytes in the standard blood components; GVHD has an antileukemic effect (66). However, these results have not been confirmed in other studies that also involved small numbers of patients (59,67,68) (58, 52, and 70 patients, respectively). Resolution of the effects of the type of blood products transfused on leukemia status will require much larger clinical trials (69).

2. Ultraviolet Irradiation (UVR)

Instead of removing WBCs from the transfused blood products—with the inherent problems of complete and effective removal, another approach would be to alter the transfusions to eliminate their immunogenicity. In that regard, a very important observation demonstrated that UVR renders lymphocytes unable either to stimulate or respond in mixed lymphocyte culture (MLC) even though HLA antigens are still expressed on the surface of the UV irradiated lymphocytes (70). It has been known for some time that γ- irradiation prevents lymphocytes from responding in MLC, but γ-irradiated cells are still able to act as stimulating cells in MLC. Several explanations were postulated for the failure of UVR-treated lymphocytes to stimulate in MLC: (1) other unrecognized antigens on the cell surface important for MLC reactivity are altered by UVR; (2) lymphocytes release mediators for the MLC reaction that are inhibited by UVR; or (3) the motility of UV-irradiated cells is impaired preventing appropriate cell-to-cell interaction—a function known to be required for MLC reactivity. It is of interest that since this initial publication, all of these potential mechanisms for failure of UV-irradiated cells to stimulate in MLC have been evaluated, and more than one of these mechanisms may be involved in producing the UVR effect (71).

In a dog transfusion model, 11 of 12 recipients (92%) of UV-irradiated donor platelets did not become platelet refractory after 8 weekly single random-donor transfusions (p <0.01) compared with unmodified controls in which only 3 of 21 (14%) were not refractory (32). In addition, when unmodified platelet transfusions were continued from the same random donor, tolerance to the unmodified platelets was observed in 8 of 11 (73%) of the nonrefractory recipient dogs. To determine if the tolerance induced was specific to the platelets of only the treated donor, the eight nonrefractory recipients were also given unmodified transfusions from at least two other random-donor dogs (called secondary donors). A high degree of nonspecific tolerance to platelets from other donors had been induced in these transfused animals—10 of 23 (43%) of the secondary donors were tolerated by the dogs who had previously received UV-irradiated platelets.

These encouraging results in the dog model have led to several recent studies to evaluate the effects of UVR on human platelets. The in vivo viability and function of human platelets remains intact after the platelets have been UV irradiated in special plastic bags that permit adequate UV penetrance (Table 5) (72–74). Furthermore, platelets were able to be UV-B irradiated and then stored with no adverse effects on poststorage platelet viability.

In a pilot study (75), four patients undergoing bone marrow transplantation for advanced hematologic malignancies were given UV-B–treated platelet concentrates. None of these patients showed any adverse effects after the transfusion of UV-B–exposed platelets. In the patients whose platelet counts increased after a transfusion, bleeding was effectively controlled. One of these four patients was a previously transfused patient who was refractory to platelet transfusions when the UV-B–treated platelet concentrates were first initiated. The remaining three patients received only UV-B–irradiated platelet concentrates. One of the latter patients became refractory after 14 platelet transfusions, and the other two patients each became refractory after 10 transfusions. However, all three of these patients were clinically ill with transplant-related complications such as septicemia and hepatic failure, suggesting that their refractoriness may well have been due to platelet consumption rather than alloimmunization. This hypothesis was supported by the fact that none of the patients developed lymphocytotoxic or antiplatelet antibodies in spite of the fact that they were concurrently receiving standard unmodified RBC transfusions. However, it is important to note that these patients were also receiving immunosuppressive therapy to allow engraftment and prevent GVHD. This therapy would have contributed to any immune unresponsiveness that was induced by the UV-irradiated platelet transfusions.

A large multi-institutional trial sponsored by the National Heart, Lung, and Blood Institute has recently been initiated in the United States to explore the relative merits of leukocyte reduction and UV-B irradiation in the prevention of platelet alloimmunization (76). Certainly either of these two approaches—which require only a manipulation of the product prior to transfusion to prevent platelet alloimmunization—is to be preferred over the other approaches discussed previously that would involve either some type of immunosuppression of the recipient or donor selection.

3. Storage of Blood Products

To determine whether stored blood products are less immunogenic than fresh, rhesus monkeys were given either fresh whole blood, whole blood stored for 1–4 weeks, or platelets stored for 1 week (77). Three injections were given during a 1-week period, and samples were drawn 1 week later for lymphocytotoxic antibody testing against the donor's lymphocytes. All but 1 of the 15 animals who received blood stored for <2 weeks developed antibodies (93%) compared with 50% of the 10 animals who received blood stored for 3 weeks or longer; $p < 0.05$. After injections of 1-week-old platelets, only two of the eight recipients (25%) formed antibodies compared with recipients of blood stored ≤2 weeks ($p < 0.01$). Possible explanations for these findings may be a loss of lymphocyte viability (78), loss of class II antigen expression on lymphocytes associated with decreased ability to stimulate in MLC (79), or an accumulation

Table 5 UV-B Irradiation: In Vivo Evaulation of Platelet Concentrates

Reference	Irradition/ storage bag	Platelet product	UV-B irradiation (mJ/cm²)	No. of observations	Storage time (Days)	Normal volunteer autologous radiolabeled platelet studies				Patient studies			
						recovery (%)		survival (days)		platelet increment (× 10⁹/L)		bleeding time correction (min)	
						Control	UV-B	Control	UV-B	Control	UV-B	Control	UV-B
Pamphilon et al. (72)	Stericell (Dupont)	Standard PC	300	8	5[a]	35 ± 12	40 ± 7	7.8 ± 0.6	7.6 ± 0.5				
Andreu et al. (73)	Stericell (Dupont)	Standard PC	1500	4	1[b]	75 ± 3	74 ± 1	7.8 ± 0.4	7.0 ± 0.5				
Buchholz et al. (74)	PC 269[c] (Fenwal)	Standard PC	2600	10	1[b]	44 ± 8	42 ± 12	7.9 ± 1.6	6.9 ± 1.3				
	PC 269[c] (Fenwal)	Standard PC	2600	10	5[b]	45 ± 8	48 ± 10	6.4 ± 1.0	5.7 ± 1.0				
	PC 269[c] (Fenwal)	CS 3000 Apheresis	2600	4	1[b]	44 ± 2	57 ± 17	5.0 ± 1.0	5.9 ± 1.0				
	NI	NI	2600	7	NI					19 ± 5	20 ± 8	<6 (3/4)[d]	<6 (5/5)[d]

Abbreviations: NI, no information; PC, platelet concentrate.
The first five studies were paired autologous experiments using radiolabeled platelets in normal volunteers. In the last study, non–UV-irradiated or UV-irradiated platelets from the same donor were given to thrombocytopenic patients.
[a]UV-B irradiated prestorage.
[b]UV-B irradiated poststorage.
[c]UV-B irradiation bag; storage bag not identified. Other studies storage and UV-B irradiation all done in same bag.
[d]Number of bleeding times corrected to <6 minutes/ # tested.

of plasma factors during storage that impairs the lymphocyte-proliferative response in MLC (80).

4. Pretreatment of Platelet Recipients with Antibody-Coated Cells

Prior administration of either antibody-coated RBCs or lymphocytes to rats prevented the subsequent development of lymphocytotoxic or antiplatelet antibodies following platelet transfusions (81). Failure to develop an immune response to the transfused platelets was directly related to the amount of antibody used to coat the donors' RBCs or lymphocytes. The immunosuppressive effect was transferable by giving a serum immunoglobulin G (IgG) fraction from pretreated animals to naive recipients prior to transfusing platelets, suggesting that the mechanism of suppression was related to the induction of a broadly reactive regulatory IgG.

Cyclosporine Loading of Donor Platelets. In a dog transfusion model, donor platelets were incubated with cyclosporine prior to injection. Five of nine recipients (56%) given cyclospor-ine-loaded donor platelets from a single unrelated donor dog were not immunized by 8 weekly platelet transfusions compared with only 3 of 21 control recipients (14%) who were not immunized; $p <0.05$ (32). Furthermore, four of the five nonimmunized recipients remained responsive to their primary donors' platelets even when the transfusions were continued without cyclosporine loading. These four persistently nonrefractory recipients also were nonresponsive to platelets from all six other random donors tested, whereas recipients refractory to platelets from their primary donor also became refractory to platelets from all other random-donor dogs tested. Cyclosporine loading did not impair platelet viability in the dog (32), and platelet function is unaffected by cyclosporine loading in humans (82).

IV. MANAGEMENT OF PLATELET ALLOIMMUNIZATION

There are two basic approaches to the management of alloimmunized patients if the prevention of platelet alloimmunization strategies outlined in the previous section have not been suc-cessful—either select compatible donors or attempt to reverse alloimmunization.

A. Select Compatible Donors

ABO, HLA, and platelet-specific antigens are all expressed on platelets and identification of compatible platelets may require matching for one or more of these systems. Such matching can be accomplished either by typing the patient's platelets and selecting antigen-compatible donors or by using cross-match testing to identify compatible donors.

1. Antigen Matching

ABO Matching. Before proceeding to the more complex situations of selecting either HLA or platelet-specific antigen-compatible donors, it is important to document that the patient is still refractory after receiving platelets from ABO-compatible donors. ABH antigens on platelets consist of type 2 heavy chains that are intrinsic to the membrane as well as soluble type 1 heavy chains that are adsorbed from the plasma (43,83,84). There are approximately equal amounts of the two types of heavy chains on the platelet surface.

The relevance of ABH antigens to platelet transfusion compatibility was first reported in 1965 (85). Radiolabeled A_1 platelets, when given to group O normal recipients, resulted in average recoveries of 19% compared with 63% recoveries for ABO-compatible platelets. However, when group B platelets were given to O recipients, the average recovery was maintained at 57%. When group A_1B platelets were given to group O recipients the average recovery was only 8%. Furthermore, ABO-incompatible platelet recovery was inversely related to the isohemagglutination titers of the transfused recipient. A later study confirmed these results (86), and another study demonstrated that the amount of incompatible A or B antigen on donor platelets also influenced the transfusion results (87). In two group O patients with high-titer anti-A antibodies, group A_2 platelets—which expressed 38-fold less A antigen than A_1 platelets—were compatible both in vitro by platelet cross-match testing and in vivo by transfusion responses.

Several large platelet transfusion studies have established the transfusion relevance of donor-recipient ABO antigen-compatibility. Ninety-one patients who were refractory to random-donor platelets received 389 HLA-matched or selectively mismatched single-donor apheresis platelet transfusions (88). For the HLA-matched donor-recipient combinations, ABO-compatible platelets resulted in average recoveries of 73 ± 4% at 1 hr compared with 55 ± 5% for ABO-mismatched transfusions (p <0.01), and data at 24 hr posttransfusion were 37 ± 3% versus 29 ± 4%, respectively (p <0.05). In a second, similar study of 51 patients refractory to pooled random-donor platelets who received 316 HLA-selected donor apheresis transfusions, ABO-compatible platelet transfusions gave average CCIs of 10 × 10^9/L for ABO-compatible transfusions and 5.9 × 10^9/L for platelets incompatible with the recipient's plasma antibodies (p < 0.01) (89). When the donor's plasma contained ABO antibodies incompatible with the recipient's platelets, there was an intermediate increment of 8.2 × 10^9/L. The authors suggested that the donor's antibody bound to the recipient's plasma-incompatible antigens and the resulting immune complexes compromised donor platelet increments. However, the incompatible plasma results were not significantly different from either the ABO-compatible or ABO-incompatible platelet transfusin results.

Although all of the above studies showed no effect of ABO incompatibility on platelet survival but only on recovery, a recent report has demonstrated markedly reduced platelet survivals when ABO-incompatible platelets were given to two group O recipients with high titers of immune (IgG) anti-A or anti-B antibodies (90). Thus, there may be certain situations in which survival, as well as recovery, is compromised with the transfusion of ABO-incompatible platelets.

Other studies (6,91–93) have not demonstrated an effect of ABO-incompatibility on transfusion responses. However, failure to observe an effect in these studies may be related to other immune and nonimmune factors that influenced platelet responses in these patients, the amount of ABO-incompatible antigen expressed on donor platelets or the titer of the ABO-incompatible isohemagglutinin in the recipient.

Although blood group antigens Le^a, I, i, and P have been demonstrated on platelets (94–96), platelet refractoriness related to donor-recipient incompatibility for these antigens has not been reported. The Rh, Duffy, Kell, Kidd, and Lutheran antigens are not present on platelets (97).

HLA Matching

Avoid Incompatibile Donor HLA Matching. Although many patients develop broadly reactive HLA antibodies, some patients demonstrate limited antibody specificity. Screening patients' serum against a panel of HLA-typed lymphocytes will identify those patients who can easily be supported by avoiding the specific HLA antigens to which they have developed alloantibodies. However, most patients will require the more difficult task of selecting HLA-matched donors because they have multispecific anti-HLA antibodies.

Select HLA Antigen–Compatible Donors. The HLA-A and HLA-B antigens are the major immunogens expressed on the surface of the platelet (98). In contrast, the HLA-C, HLA-D, and HLA-DR antigens are either not present or only weakly expressed on the platelet surface. Incompatibility for these latter antigens has not been documented to cause refractoriness to platelet transfusions (99,100). Yankee (4,101) was the first to demonstrate the value of using HLA-matched donors either from within the family or an unrelated population to achieve compatible transfusion responses for patients who had become alloimmune refractory to pooled random-donor platelets. However, the complexity of the HLA system makes it very unlikely that HLA-matched donors will be available for most refractory patients without the availability of large HLA-typed donor pools (see below). Therefore, Duquesnoy (102) evaluated the effectiveness of donor platelets that were selectively mismatched for cross-reactive HLA antigens. Of 421 single-donor apheresis transfusions administered to 59 alloimmunized platelet-refractory patients, either grade B1 donors (where three donor and recipient antigens were matched but the fourth donor antigen was either unknown [BIU] or cross-reactive [B1X]), or B2-matched donors (where the donor and recipient shared two HLA antigens but the third and fourth donor antigens were either unknown or cross-reactive) were as successful as A-matched donor-recipient combinations where donor and recipient shared all four HLA antigens.

In addition to demonstrating the ability to expand the compatible donor base by means of cross-reactive antigens, there were two other important observations from this study. The first observation was that approximately 30% of even the best-matched donors (A, B1, or B2 matches) produced unsuccessful posttransfusion platelet increments. Although it is possible that there were clinical factors that compromised the transfusion results, the patients were specifically selected to be without fever, sepsis, splenomegaly, or coagulopathy at the time of the transfusion. Possible immunological explanations for these incompatible transfusion results are the presence of (1) platelet-specific antibodies (to be discussed later) or (2) antibodies against cross-reactive HLA antigens. The other observation was that failure of cross-reactive antigens to produce compatible platelet responses may be due to the development of intragroup antibodies. Cross-reactivity, as defined in HLA serology, is based upon the in vitro observation that one serum may react with a single antigen, whereas another serum may react consistently with the same antigen and with additional antigens of the same locus. The original and the additional antigens became known as a cross-reactive group. Such cross-reactive groups are now known to define HLA public determinants that are on the heavy chain of the HLA molecule, and they are distinct from the allelic determinants (103,104). In fact, there is increasing evidence that the highly reactive antisera produced by many patients, often with few transfusions, may show definite relationships to public epitopes. There is now substantial interest in trying to determine whether public antigen–matching between donor and recipient is possibly a simpler and more useful method of identifying compatibility within the HLA system.

Establish HLA-Typed Community Donor Platelet Apheresis Panels. In order to provide for HLA-matched donors, an adequate-sized panel of HLA-typed donors must be available. Although family members represent a good source of HLA-compatible donors, they frequently cannot meet a patient's total transfusion needs as only one or two suitable donors are often identified. In addition, if a marrow transplant is a consideration, family platelet donations should be avoided pretransplant to reduce the incidence of graft rejection due to the development of alloantibodies to minor histocompatibility antigens (105). Thus, most blood centers have established HLA-typed platelet apheresis panels by recruiting members from among whole blood donors. The major questions concerning HLA-typed platelet apheresis panels are how large should they be and are they cost effective.

Duquesnoy first estimated HLA-typed donor pool sizes required to provide compatible donors and the benefits of using cross-reactive antigens to increase donor availability (106). Based on a study of transfusion results in 48 patients and varying the donor pool size between 500 and 5000, it was found that the available donors increased by 150-fold if cross-reactive antigens were considered compatible compared with the donors available if only HLA-A–, HLA-B1U–, or HLA-B2U–matched donors were used. With a pool size of approximately 1000 reliable donors, the majority of alloimmunized thrombocytopenic patients could be supported. In a subsequent study by Schiffer (107), although most patients had an average of 9 donors available with no mismatched antigens within a pool of 2470 donors, donor availability was significantly related to the phenotype frequency of the patient's antigens. For the 39 patients with relatively common phenotypes (HLA phenotypes A1, B8; A3, B7; A2, B7; A2, B12 [or B44, B45]), there would have been 74 A-, B1-, or B2-matched donors available. However, for the 61 patients who did not have a common phenotype, only 10 would have had 10 or more potential donors. For the latter patients, family member platelet support may well be needed. In another study, data from 4338 platelet apheresis transfusions given to 591 patients from a pool of up to 870 community donors over a 3-year period were analyzed (108). On average, these patients required eight donors to support them for their usual 1-month period of thrombocytopenia. It was estimated that 75% of the patients would have a 97% chance of being supported at the B2 level or better from a donor pool size of 1500. These donor pool size estimates were based on several factors: the average number of patients supported at any one time; the minimum donation interval allowed for donors; the average patient transfusion frequency; the level of donor commitment; the average number of donors contacted before a donor was scheduled; the HLA phenotypes of patients and donors; and the minimum acceptable HLA-match grade for donors. Although much larger donor pools will clearly allow better HLA matches to be obtained, there is no evidence from transfusion data to suggest that match grades better than B2 provide any better likelihood of improved platelet increments. In addition, the costs of maintaining large HLA-typed apheresis donor panels may be prohibitively expensive considering the initial costs of HLA typing and the subsequent costs of replacing the approximately 10% of donors who are lost yearly for multiple reasons. However, modest-sized donor pools have been documented to be cost effective (109).

Platelet-Specific Antigen Matching. In the experience of the author and coworkers, patients with platelet-specific alloantibodies are most often found among patients who are highly refractory to all platelet donors, including those who are HLA well matched (17). In seven studies (110), the failure rate of HLA-A–matched platelet transfusions in clinically stable thrombocytopenic patients averaged 19%; 41 of 212 HLA-A–matched transfusions were incompatible (Table 6). Unfortunately, there are not enough platelet-specific antisera available to type community donor platelet apheresis panels for these antigens. Therefore, the best approach to finding compatible donors for patients alloimmunized to platelet-specific antigens is within their family. Using platelet-specific antigen-typed donor panels, the specificity of the alloantibody can often be identified, and then the family can by typed for the relevant antigen. If this degree of sophisticated antigen-antibody testing is not available, either platelet

Table 6 Failure Rate of HLA-A–Matched platelets

Reference	No. Refractory	No. Tested (%)
Brand et al. (8)	12/31	39
Duquesnoy et al. (102)	5/47	12
Gmur et al. (111)	1/18	6
Kickler et al. (112)	10/45	22
Lohrman et al. (113)	2/11	18
Slichter (114)	2/11	18
Tosato et al. (92)	9/49	18
Total	41/212	19

cross-match testing with available family members can be performed to select donors or, alternatively, family members can be transfused to determine compatibility. However, such patients are likely to have formed HLA antibodies as well as platelet-specific alloantibodies, and so family members may also have to be HLA compatible to obtain a good platelet increment.

Of significant interest, a recent publication suggests that it may now be possible to type for platelet-specific antigens using allele-specific oligonucleotide probes (115). Availability of this new technology may permit an alternate method of typing both patients and potential donors for platelet-specific antigens without the requirement for platelet-typing sera.

2. Cross-Match Testing

Because of the not infrequent occurrence of poor responses to HLA-selected donor transfusions and the costs to both the patient and donor of an unsuccessful transfusion, there has been a great deal of interest in determining whether platelet cross-match tests can improve the donor selection process. One of the first questions regarding platelet cross-match testing is the source of donor platelets to be used. Although platelets can be obtained from family members for cross matching, this discussion will focus on using cross-match tests to select compatible unrelated donors. There are three possible unrelated donor sources: (1) HLA-typed community donors, (2) random-donor apheresis platelets, and (3) random-donor platelet concentrates. Each of these approaches has both potential benefits and problems associated with its use. For example, selecting potential donors first on the basis of their HLA matching with the patient represents an attractive approach. However, this requires maintaining stored platelet samples on the HLA-typed donors to be used for cross-matching. There are a variety of techniques available to store platelets, but antigen reactivity is lost over time with many (116–124). In addition, to prepare and store platelet samples on a large number of donors is a time-consuming and costly endeavor. Many blood centers are now collecting single random-donor apheresis platelets to supplement platelet inventory needs that are usually met by pooling platelet concentrates harvested from routinely donated units of blood. Such random-donor apheresis units are potentially available for platelet cross-match testing. In addition, it is possible to cross match routinely prepared random-donor platelet concentrates and pool a sufficient number of compatible concentrates to constitute a transfusion dose.

Indeed, all of these potential donor sources have been tested using a variety of platelet and lymphocytotoxic antibody assays to predict compatibility, and these assays have been correlated either retrospectively or prospectively with transfusion outcome (6,8,9,89,111,112, 114,116–119,125–146). In the majority of these studies, the donors were selected based on HLA typing, and the platelet cross-match testing was done retrospectively to correlate the results of antibody testing with transfusion results. However, some recent studies have performed prospective cross-match testing with both HLA-selected apheresis donor platelets (136), random single-donor apheresis platelets (137,138), and random-donor platelet concentrates (132, 139,146). Most of these studies excluded thrombocytopenic patients who were known to have any adverse clinical factors that might affect their transfusion response. This approach obviously provides the best information on the reliability of the cross-match test to predict transfusion outcome. However, it does not deal with the practical realities of trying to determine the efficacy of these cross-match tests to predict transfusion outcome in the variety of clinically ill as well as stable thrombocytopenic patients who require platelet support. Fortunately, this problem has recently been addressed by several investigators (6,9,89,117,135). Although the predictability of the assays is clearly less when all thrombocytopenic patients are included, even in unscreened patients, transfusion responses can be predicted 60–85% of the time versus 80–100% of the time in patients selected as clinically stable. The predictability of the cross-match tests not only depends on the condition of the patient at the time of the transfusion but also on the cross-match assay used. The major use of the cross-match test is to prevent the transfusion of cross-match–incompatible donors from whom the recipient rarely receives an increment; i.e., there are very few false-positive cross-match test results. In contrast, when all thrombocytopenic transfused patients are analyzed, the incidence of false-negative cross-match test results is quite high. This suggests that a negative cross-match test does not preclude a poor transfusion response mainly because many of these patients will have clinical factors that will compromise their response to any platelet transfusion.

From a cost-effectiveness standpoint, it has been suggested that cross-matching random-donor platelet concentrates and pooling compatible units to constitute a transfusion dose can easily be justified (147). Except for very highly alloimmunized patients with antibodies to almost all members of a screening panel, a pool of compatible donors can usually be found in a random population. However, for highly immunized patients, only 4–5% of the donors may be compatible (132,139,146). Therefore, screening the large number of donors required to find compatibility for these types of patients may not be cost effective.

One of the biggest problems with platelet cross-match testing is the lack of a uniform test procedure. There are almost as many platelet antibody assays used as there are investigators working on the problem of platelet-compatibility testing. Until some standardization is developed in the field, it will remain difficult to interpret results achieved in different laboratories. However, there is increasing evidence that these assays can predict platelet compatibility, and their biggest use may well be to select compatible donors from among non–HLA-typed donors—either random apheresis donors or random platelet concentrates. Either of these strategies will avoid the necessity of maintaining costly HLA-typed apheresis panels and calling in specially selected donors. However, these cross-match selection techniques require additional validation in larger platelet transfusion trials.

B. Reversal of Platelet Alloimmunization

Even using the best available methods of preventing platelet alloimmunization, some patients will still become immunized. In addition, those individuals with prior antigenic exposures through pregnancy or because of earlier transfusions that were not modified to reduce their immunogenicity will likely become alloimmunized in spite of any preventative measures. For some of these alloimmunized patients, compatible platelet donors will not be identified using either antigen-matched donors or by using platelet cross-match testing. For these patients, it is important to determine whether there are techniques available to temporarily or permanently reverse an already-established immune response.

1. Spontaneous Antibody Loss

It has been well-documented that many patients will lose their antibodies over time often in spite of continued platelet and RBC transfusions, and thus active approaches to alloimmune reversal will not be required for these individuals. Overall, in six studies, antibody loss was documented in 144 of 340 patients (42%) (Table 7) (24,25,27,28,30,31). In one study, none of seven aplastic patients versus 10 of 20 (50%) leukemic patients lost their antibodies, suggesting there may be an influence of chemotherapy on antibody loss (24). However, the same phenomenon of antibody loss has been observed in patients on renal dialysis receiving repeated transfusions of whole blood or packed cells (148), in patients in complete remission from acute leukemia who are receiving immunotherapy with allogeneic myeloblasts and BCG (bacille Calmette-Guérin [vaccine]) (149), and in volunteers taking part in a planned immunization program involving weekly transfusions of whole blood (150). In addition, although there

Table 7   Antibody Loss

Reference	No. lost/No. tested	(%)
Leukemia		
Tejada et al. (28)	7/7	100
Holohan et al. (24)	10/20	50
Lee et al. (25)	80/234	34
Murphy et al. (30)	30/37	81
McGrath et al. (31)	10/15	67
Pamphilon et al. (27)	7/20	35
Total	144/333	43
Aplasia		
Holohan et al. (24)	0/7	0

is some variability in the data, approximately equal numbers of patients lose antibodies over time whether they are continuing to receive transfusions or not. There is also some evidence that individuals who have not been previously exposed to incompatible antigens by prior pregnancies or transfusions tend to lose their current transfusion-induced antibodies more frequently. Five of 10 patients (50%) with prior antigen exposure lost their antibodies compared with 25 of 27 (93%) with no prior antigenic exposure (30). In another study, the type of prior antigen exposure also affected antibody loss (31). If the patient had a history of both prior pregnancies and transfusions, only one of five (20%) lost their antibodies, whereas antibodies resolved in all nine (100%) with a history of only one type of exposure; i.e., either prior transfusions or pregnancies.

Of great practical importance, once antibodies disappear, patients may regain their responsiveness to random-donor platelet transfusions. For example, of 34 patients who lost their antibodies, all had good initial responses to reinstitution of random-donor platelet transfusions, and 21 of 34 (62%) never again became platelet refractory even with multiple additional transfusions (25). These data clearly suggest that a prudent strategy is to serially measure antibodies over time in platelet-refractory patients, with the goal of returning those patients who lose their antibodies to random-donor platelet therapy.

2. Intravenous IgG

There are numerous studies indicating the efficacy of treating autoimmune thrombocytopenic purpura with IV IgG (151–153). However, the effectiveness of this therapy in treating patients with alloimmune platelet destruction has yielded conflicting data. Some studies have shown an improved response to previously incompatible donor platelets in at least some treated patients (154–160), whereas other patients have shown no response (161–163). In 17 patients documented to be platelet alloimmunized both by antibody measurements and by transfusion responses, there was no improvement in posttransfusion platelet increments to pooled random-donor platelets—regardless of whether they received IV IgG prepared by Sandoz or Cutter (162,163). The test platelets were not given until after the course of IV IgG therapy (0.4–0.6 mg/kg for 5 days) had been completed to prevent platelet antibody adsorption by the transfused platelets. Similar doses of IV IgG were also given in a randomized placebo-controlled trial in which platelets from the same random apheresis platelet donor were given pre- and posttreatment. A significant increase in platelet counts was found in the seven treated patients compared with the five control patients at 1 hr posttransfusion (CCIs of 8413 versus 1050×10^9/L, respectively; $p < 0.007$) (157). Although platelet increments were improved, platelet survival was increased in only one of the treated patients. These study patients were carefully selected to have no adverse clinical factors that might influence their transfusion response, and they had documented responses to HLA-matched platelets but not to random-donor platelets, confirming the alloimmune nature of their platelet destruction.

In two other studies (158,161) patients were not selected to exclude clinical factors that might effect transfusion responses. In both of these studies, patients were refractory to pooled random-donor platelets and remained so after therapy. In one of these studies, responses were also not improved with HLA-selected donor transfusions (161), but they were improved in the other study, and these responses were maintained for weeks to months after therapy was stopped (158). In the latter study, both the recovery and survival of the HLA-selected donors' platelets were increased in 6 of 10 patients (158). Unfortunately, the very high cost of this therapy makes it imperative that methods be developed to preselect those patients who may benefit, at least transiently, from this treatment.

There are several postulated mechanisms of action of IV IgG. Improvements in platelet transfusion responses may be related to therapy-induced decreases in platelet antibody production (164), or the IV IgG may have been given fortuitously at the time when some patients were already spontaneously losing their antibodies. Alternatively, it is possible that the antibody was adsorbed by the patient's concurrent platelet transfusions (165). However, the rapid response to IV IgG observed in successfully treated patients suggests that suppression of alloantibody production is an unlikely mechanism. IV IgG may also induce a transient blockade of mononuclear phagocytic Fc receptors, and, consequently, the lifespan of transfused platelets may be prolonged. Last, the high amounts of serum IgG could induce a nonspecific protective platelet coating and/or a splitting of previously bound alloantibodies from the platelet surface and, thereby, protect the platelets from immune damage. Replacement of platelet-bound alloantibodies following incubation with IgG in vitro has been demonstrated (166).

In summary, the accumulated data indicate that there will be little or no improvement to random-donor platelet transfusions after IV IgG therapy, whereas there may be an improvement in both recovery and survival of HLA-selected donor platelet transfusions. However, improved platelet survivals may only occur after higher than usual doses of IV IgG therapy are given over an extended time. At present, IV IgG infusions should be given only to patients who are refractory to all forms of platelet therapy and who have such severe bleeding manifestations that an expensive therapeutic trial is warranted to prevent significant hemorrhage-related morbidity and mortality.

3. Plasma Exchange

In theory, it is possible to remove alloantibodies by a plasma-exchange procedure. However, as most alloantibodies are IgG and these antibodies are distributed within both the intra- and extravascular spaces, complete removal will be extremely difficult. In addition, unless concurrent immunosuppressive therapy is used to at least impair, if not prevent, additional antibody formation, the therapy will at best be only transiently successful.

Eighteen patients with aplastic anemia or acute leukemia who were refractory to pooled random-donor platelets underwent a plasma-exchange procedure either before or after bone marrow transplantation (167). Patients with aplastic anemia received both cyclosporine and cytoxan as pretransplant conditioning therapy to permit allogeneic marrow engraftment, whereas those with acute leukemia received both cycloplasphamide as well as total body irradiation. In these patients, improved postexchange platelet responses were directly related to the volume of plasma removed. Those patients who had the best postexchange platelet responses had three daily, 10-L plasma exchanges. Of the 13 patients with documented lymphocytotoxic antibodies preexchange, 8 (62%) responded, whereas only 1 of 5 (20%) without antibodies showed any improvement. Overall, 11 of the 18 patients (61%) showed improved responses to platelets from random or related donors. Nine of 14 patients (64%) benefited from pretransplant plasma exchange, and only 1 of 4 (25%) benefited when the procedure was performed posttransplant. In general, the response to transfused platelets was better with HLA-selected community donors or family member platelet transfusions than it was with pooled random-donor platelet concentrates. As with IV IgG therapy, this approach is an expensive, time-consuming procedure and should be used only for patients who have evidence of alloantibodies, who are not otherwise supportable by platelet transfusions, and who have life-theatening bleeding problems.

4. Antibody Adsorption by Transfused Platelets

In a rabbit platelet transfusion model, donor platelets equivalent to 40–60% of the total platelet mass of the recipient rabbit were transfused (165). Following this massive platelet infusion, platelet antibody titers decreased with the subsequent survival of antibody-incompatible donor platelets. However, serial tests showed that the antibody titer began increasing again within a few hours of the infusion, suggesting the benefit would be transient. The massive platelet transfusions apparently did not produce their affect by blocking the reticuloendothelial system as infusing rabbit red cell ghosts or latex particles to produce reticuloendothelial blockade did not produce an improved response to incompatible donor platelets. The investigators used the same approach in two patients with aplastic anemia who were refractory to pooled random-donor transfusions (165). Following the administration of 20 U of pooled platelets, the next platelet infusion was associated with an improved response. Because of the expected transient and incomplete nature of the antibody removal achieved by platelet immunoadsorption, this procedure should be attempted only in critical patient situations.

5. Drugs

There is evidence that certain immunosuppressive drugs may be able to reverse platelet alloimmunization. However, as antibodies are frequently lost spontaneously in patients, attributing antibody loss to drug therapy must be done with reservation. In contrast, in the animal transfusion trials (to be discussed), spontaneous improvements in platelet responses over time have not been observed.

Cyclosporine A. In a preliminary report (168), cyclosporine A in a total dosage of 20 mg/kg/day was given to six dogs that were refractory to platelets from a single random-donor dog. In three of the six dogs, the incompatible donor dog's platelets showed significant improvements in both recovery and survival by the second to third week of treatment. In serum samples that were analyzed for cyclosporine A levels at study termination, the improved platelet increments were found only in the three dogs that achieved adequate drug levels. In the future, if drug levels are continuously monitored during drug therapy with appropriate dose adjustments to maintain levels, more responders should be seen.

In addition, there are three reported cases of patients treated with cyclosporine A who showed improved platelet responses (169–171). There is also a study in six uremic patients awaiting renal transplantation showing a substantial drop in lymphocytotoxic antibody titers (p <0.006) with a combination of cyclosporine and plasma exchange (172). However, the pattern of antibody reactivity with panel lymphocytes was unchanged.

Antithymocyte Globulin (ATG). Immunized dogs given a combination of antithymocyte serum and procarbazine showed reversal of platelet alloimmunization in two of three treated recipients (33).

Four patients with anti-HLA antibodies who were refractory to pooled random-donor platelets received ATG therapy as treatment for aplastic anemia. Three of the four patients lost their HLA antibodies and became responsive to pooled random-donor platelet transfusions. Two patients lost their antibodies within 1 month of starting therapy and the third within 3 months (173).

Vincristine/Vinblastine. There is a single case report of an infant with severe aplastic anemia who was alloimmune refractory to both random and HLA-matched platelet transfusions who showed consistently good responses to HLA-matched transfusions during viscristine therapy (174). The authors postulated that the therapy was effective owing to a selective inhibition of macrophage function following phagocytosis of platelets that had bound vincristine. This hypothesis is supported by another study in which a patient with aplastic anemia, who was alloimmune refractory to random donor platelets, was given donor platelets loaded with vinblastine. After the transfusion of the vinblastine-loaded donor platelets, unmodified random donor platelet transfusions gave excellent posttransfusion platelet increments (175).

In summary, there is preliminary evidence that some immunosuppressive drugs may improve responses to random-donor or HLA-matched platelet transfusions in alloimmunized platelet refractory recipients. Unfortunately, any improvement in platelet responses usually requires at least 2–3 weeks of drug administration, and, therefore, this approach will not be appropriate for patients who are in immediate need of effective platelet support. However, for some patients who are expected to be chronically thrombocytopenic because of a damaged marrow, trials of these immunosuppressive drugs may be indicated.

6. Modification of the Transfused Platelets

Administration of Antibody-Coated Platelets. Rats were sensitized by whole blood transfusions, and antibody was obtained from the sensitized recipients and preincubated with the donor rats' platelets prior to transfusion. Three of five control rats given no additional transfusions after whole blood-induced sensitization lost their lymphocytotoxic antibodies during a 20-week observation period, as did three of five other control rats given non–antibody-coated donor platelet transfusions (176). All seven rats given antibody-coated donor platelets lost their lymphocytotoxic antibodies, and they did so at a faster rate than the control rats ($p < 0.02$). In vitro studies have shown a profound inhibitory effect of antigen-antibody complexes on B-lymphocyte proliferation after attachment of the complexes to Fc receptors on the surface of B cells.

Acid Treatment of Donor Platelets. Treatment of random donor platelets with a solution of citric acid removes HLA antigens. Two transfusions of acid-treated platelets gave acceptable CCIs in an alloimmunized platelet-refractory patient (177). Acid-eluted platelets were compatible in a platelet cross-match test, whereas they had been incompatible when tested before elution. Autologous platelet recovery and survival measurements of acid-treated platelets in two normal volunteers gave the same recovery values as untreated platelets, whereas survivals were reduced by 16% from baseline values.

REFERENCES

1. O'Connell B, Lee EJ, Schiffer CA. The value of 10-minute post-transfusion platelet counts. Transfusion 1988; 28:66.
2. Hanson SR, Slichter SJ. Platelet kinetics in patients with bone marrow hypoplasia: Evidence for a fixed platelet requirement. Blood 1985; 66:1105.

3. Harker LA. The role of the spleen in thrombokinetics. J Lab Clin Med 1971; 77:247.
4. Yankee RA, Grumet FC, Rogentine GN. Platelet transfusion therapy. The selection of compatible donors for refractory patients by lymphocyte HLA typing. N Engl J Med 1969; 281:1208.
5. Bishop JF, McGrath K, Wolf MM, et al. Clinical factors influencing the efficacy of pooled platelet transfusions. Blood 1988; 71:383.
6. McFarland JG, Anderson AJ, Slichter SJ. Factors influencing the transfusion response to HLA-selected apheresis donor platelets in patients refractory to random platelet concentrates. Br J Haematol 1989; 73:380.
7. Hogge DE, Dutcher P, Aisner J, Schiffer CA. Lymphocytotoxic antibody is a predictor of response to random-donor platelet transfusion. Am J Hematol 1983; 14:363.
8. Brand A, van Leeuwen A, Eernisse JG, van Rood JJ. Platelet transfusion therapy. Optimal donor selection with a combination of lymphocytotoxicity and platelet fluorescence tests. Blood 1978; 51:781.
9. Kakaiya RM, Gudino MD, Miller MV, et al. Four crossmatch methods to select platelet donors. Transfusion 1984; 24:35.
10. Daly PA, Schiffer CA, Aisner J, Wiernik PH. Platelet transfusion therapy. One-hour-post-transfusion increments are valuable in predicting the need for HLA-matched preparations. JAMA 1980; 243:435.
11. Mueller-Eckhardt C, Kiefel V, Santoso S. Recent trends in platelet antigen/antibody detection. Blut 1989; 59:35.
12. Schwartz KA. Platelet antibody: Review of detection methods. Am J Hematol 1988; 29:106.
13. Liebert M, Aster RH. Expression of HLA-B12 on platelets, on lymphocytes, and in serum: A quantitative study. Tissue Antigens 1977; 9:199.
14. Schiffer CA, O'Connell B, Lee EJ. Platelet transfusion therapy for alloimmunized patients: Selective mismatching for HLA-B12, an antigen with variable expression on platelets. Blood 1989; 74:1172.
15. Aster RH, Szatkowski N, Liebert M, Duquesnoy RJ. Expression of HLA-B12, HLA-B8, Bw4, and w6 on platelets. Transplant Proc. 1977; 9:4.
16. Szatkowski NS, Aster RH. HLA antigens of platelets. IV. Influence of "private" HLA-B locus specificities on the expression of Bw4 and Bw6 on human platelets. Tissue Antigens 1980; 15:361.
17. Slichter SJ, Teramura G. Frequency of platelet-specific alloantibodies in platelet refractory thrombocytopenic patients (abstr). Blood 1988; 72(suppl 1): 286a.
18. Schiffer CA. Management of patients refractory to platelet transfusion—An evaluation of methods of donor selection. Prog Hematol 1987; 15:91.
19. Saji H, Maruya E, Fuji H, et al. New platelet antigen, Sib[a], involved in platelet transfusion refractoriness in a Japanese man. Vox Sang 1989; 56:283.
20. Iikeda H, Mitani T, Ohnuma M, et al. A new platelet-specific antigen, Nak[a], involved in the refractoriness of HLA-matched platelet transfusion. Vox Sang 1989; 57:213.
21. Langenscheidt F, Kiefel V, Santoso S, Mueller-Eckhardt C. Platelet transfusion refractoriness associated with two rare platelet-specific alloantibodies (anti-Bak[a] and anti-PL[A2]) and multiple HLA antibodies. Transfusion 1988; 28:597.
22. Kickler T, Kennedy SD, Braine HG. Alloimmunization to platelet-specific antigens on glycoproteins IIb-IIIa and IB/IX in multiply transfused thrombocytopenic patients. Transfusion 1990; 30:622.
23. Pegels JG, Bruynes ECE, Engelfriet CP, von dem Borne AEGKr. Serological studies in patients on platelet- and granulocyte-substitution therapy. Br J Haematol 1982; 52:59.
24. Holohan W, Terasaki PI, Diesseroth AB. Suppression of transfusion-related alloimmunization in intensively treated cancer patients. Blood 1981; 58:122.
25. Lee EJ, Schiffer CA. Serial measurement of lymphocytotoxic antibody and response to nonmatched platelet transfusions in alloimmunized patients. Blood 1987; 70:1727.
26. Ford JM, Brown LM, Cullen MH, et al. Combined granulocyte and platelet transfusions. Development of alloimmunization as reflected by decreasing cell recovery values. Transfusion 1982; 22:498.

27. Pamphilon DH, Farrell DH, Donaldson C, et al. Development of lymphocytotoxic and platelet reactive antibodies: A prospective study in patients with acute leukemia. Vox Sang 1989; 57:177.
28. Tejada F, Bias WB, Santos GW, Zieve PD. Immunologic response of patients with acute leukemia to platelet transfusions. Blood 1973; 42:405.
29. Howard JE, Perkins HA. The natural history of alloimmunization to platelets. Transfusion 1978; 18:496.
30. Murphy MF, Metcalfe P, Ord J, et al. Disappearance of HLA and platelet-specific antibodies in acute leukaemia patients alloimmunized by multiple transfusions. Br J Haematol 1987; 67:255.
31. McGrath K, Wolf M, Bishop J, et al. Transient platelet and HLA antibody formation in multitransfused patients with malignancy. Br J Haematol 1988; 68:345.
32. Slichter SJ, Deeg HJ, Kennedy MS. Prevention of platelet alloimmunization in dogs with systemic cyclosporine and by UV-irradiation or cyclosporine-loading of donor platelets. Blood 1987; 69:414.
33. Slichter SJ, Weiden PL, Kane PJ, Storb RF. Approaches to preventing or reversing platelet alloimmunization using animal models. Transfusion 1988; 28:103.
34. Schulman NR. Immunological considerations attending platelet transfusions. Transfusion 1966; 6:39.
35. van de Wiel TWM, van de Wiel-Dorfmeyer H, van Loghem JJ. Studies on platelet antibodies in man. Vox Sang 1961; 6:641.
36. Dutcher JP, Schiffer CA, Aisner J, Wiernik PH. Alloimmunization following platelet transfusion: The absence of a dose-response relationship. Blood 1981; 57:395.
37. Sintnicolaas K, Sizoo W, Haije WG, et al. Delayed alloimmunization by random single donor platelet transfusions. Lancet 1981; 1:750.
38. Kakaiya RM, Hezzey AJ, Bove JR, et al. Alloimmunization following apheresis platelets vs. pooled platelet concentrate transfusion—A prospective randomized study (abstr). Transfusion 1981; 21:600.
39. Gmur J, von Felten A, Osterwalder B, et al. Delayed alloimmunization using random single donor platelet transfusions: A prospective study in thrombocytopenic patients with acute leukemia. Blood 1983; 62:473.
40. Slichter SJ, O'Donnell MR, Weiden PL, et al. Canine platelet alloimmunization: The role of donor selection. Br J Haematol 1986; 63:713.
41. Slichter SJ. Prevention of platelet alloimmunization. In: Murawski, ed. Transfusion Medicine: Recent Technological Advances. New York, Alan R Liss, 1985;83.
42. Surgenor DM, Wallace EL, Hao SHS, Chapman RH. (1990). Collection and transfusion of blood in the United States, 1982–1988. N Engl J Med 1990; 322:1646.
43. Dunstan RA, Simpson MB, Rosse WF. Origin of ABH antigens on human platelets. Blood 1985; 65:615.
44. Lee EJ, Schiffer CA. ABO compatibility can influence the results of platelet transfusion. Results of a randomized trial. Transfusion 1989; 29:384.
45. Carr R, Hutton JL, Jenkins JA, Lucas GF, Amphlett NW. Transfusion of ABO-mismatched platelets leads to early platelet refractoriness. Br J Haematol 1990; 75:408.
46. Messerschmidt G, Makuch R. Appelbaum F, et al. A prospective randomized trial of HLA-matched versus mismatched single-donor platelet transfusions in cancer patients. Cancer 1988; 62:795.
47. Murphy MF, Metcalfe P, Thomas H, et al. Use of leukocyte-poor blood components and HLA-matched-platelet donors to prevent HLA alloimmunization. Br J Haematol 1986; 62:529.
48. Welsh J, Burgos H, Batchelor JR. The immune response to allogeneic rat platelets; Ag-B antigens in matrix form lacking Ia. Immunology 1977; 7:267.
49. Batchelor JR, Welsh KI, Burgos H. Transplantation antigens per se are poor immunogens within a species. Nature 1978; 273:54.
50. Claas FHJ, Smeenk RJT, Schmidt R, et al. Alloimmunization against the MHC antigens after platelet transfusions is due to contaminating leukocytes in the platelet suspension. Exp Hematol 1981; 9:84.

51. Fisher M, Chapman JR, Ting A, Morris PJ. Alloimmunization to HLA antigens following transfusion with leukocyte-poor and purified platelet suspensions. Vox Sang 1985; 49:331.

52. Petranyi GG, Padanyi A, Horuzsko A, et al. Mixed lymphocyte culture-evidence that pretransplant transfusion with platelets induces FcR and blocking antibody production similar to that induced by leukocyte transfusion. Transplantation 1988; 45:823.

53. Chambers LA, Garcia LW. White blood cell content of transfusion components. Lab Med 1991; 22:857.

54. Friedman LI, Stromberg RR. White cell counting in red cells and platelets: How few can we count? (editorial). Transfusion 1990; 30:387.

55. Schiffer CA, Dutcher JP, Aisner J, et al. A randomized trial of leukocyte-depleted platelet transfusions to modify alloimmunization in patients with leukemia. Blood 1983; 62:815.

56. Sniecinski I, O'Donnell MR, Nowicki B, Hill LR. Prevention of refractoriness and HLA-alloimmunization using filtered blood products. Blood 1988; 71:1402.

57. Andreu G, Dewailly J, Leberre C, et al. Prevention of HLA immunization with leukocyte-poor packed cells and platelet concentrates obtained by filtration. Blood 1988; 72:964.

58. Oksanen K, Kekomaki R, Ruutu T, Koskimies S, Myllyla G. Prevention of alloimmunization in patients with acute leukemia by use of white cell-reduced blood components—A randomized trial. Transfusion 1991; 31:588.

59. van Marwijk Kooy M, van Prooijen HC, Moes M, et al. Use of leukocyte-depleted platelet concentrates for the prevention of refractoriness and primary HLA alloimmunization: A prospective, randomized trial. Blood 1991; 77:201.

60. Schiffer CA. Prevention of platelet alloimmunization (editorial). Blood 1991; 77:1.

61. Snyder EL. Clinical use of white cell-poor blood components. Transfusion 1989; 29:568.

62. Brand A, Claas FHJ, Voogt PJ, et al. Alloimmunization after leukocyte-depleted multiple random donor platelet transfusions. Vox Sang 1988; 54:160.

63. Englefriet CP, van Loghem JJ. HL-A in connection with blood transfusion. Haematologia 1974; 8:267.

64. Blajchman MA. The effect of leukodepletion on allogeneic donor platelet survival and refractoriness in an animal model. Semin Hematol 1991; 28:14.

65. Tucker J, Murphy MF, Gregory W, et al. Removal of graft-versus-leukemia effect by the use of leucocyte-poor blood components in patients with acute myeloblastic leukaemia. Br J Haematol 1989; 73:572.

66. Weiden PL, Flournoy N, Thomas ED, et al. Anti-leukemic effect of graft-versus-host disease in human recipients of allogeneic marrow grafts. N Engl J Med 1979; 300:1066.

67. Rebulla P, Pappalettera M, Barbui T, Cortelezzi A, et al. Duration of first remission in leukaemic recipients of leucocyte-poor blood components. Br J Haematol 1990; 75:441.

68. Lopez J, Fernandez-Villalta MJ, Gomez-Reino F, Fernandez-Ranada JM. Absence of graft-versus-leukemia effect of standard chemotherapy in patients with acute myeloblastic leukemia. Transfusion 1990; 30:191.

69. Rebulla P, Bertolini F, Parravicini A, Sirchia G. Leukocyte-poor blood components: A purer and safer transfusion product for recipients? Transfus Med Rev 1990; 4(suppl 1):19.

70. Lindahl-Kiessling K, Safwenberg J. Inability of UV-irradiated lymphocytes to stimulate allogeneic cells in mixed lymphocyte culture. Int Arch Allergy 1971; 41:670.

71. Slichter SJ. UV irradiation: Effects on the immune system and on platelet function, viability, and alloimmunization. In: Sibinga CTS, Kater L, ed. Advances in Haemapheresis. Proceedings of the Third International Congress of the World Apheresis Association. Dordrecht, The Netherlands, Kluwer Academic, 1991:205.

72. Pamphilon DH, Potter M, Cutts M, et al. Platelet concentrates irradiated with ultraviolet light retain satisfactory in vitro storage characteristics and in vivo survival. Br J Haematol 1990; 75:240.

73. Andreu G, Boccaccio C, Lecrubier C, et al. Ultraviolet irradiation of platelet concentrates: Feasibility in transfusion practice. Transfusion 1990; 30:401.

74. Buchholz DH, Miripol J, Aster RH, et al. Ultraviolet irradiation of platelets to prevent recipient alloimmunization (abst) Transfusion 1988; 28:26S.

75. Capon SM, Sacher RA, Deeg HJ. Effective ultraviolet irradiation of platelet concentrates in teflon bags. Transfusion 1990; 30:678.
76. Nemo GJ, McCurdy PR. Prevention of platelet alloimmunization (editorial). Transfusion 1991; 31:584.
77. Oh JH, McClure HM. Lymphocytotoxic antibodies induced by fresh blood, stored blood, and platelets in Rhesus monkeys. Transplant Proc 1982; 14:410.
78. Prince HE, Arens L. Effect of storage on lymphocyte surface markers in whole blood units. Transplantation 1986; 41:235.
79. Sherman ME, Dzik WH. Stability of antigens on leukocytes in banked platelet concentrates: Decline in HLA-DR antigen expression and mixed lymphocyte culture stimulating capacity following storage. Blood 1988; 72:867.
80. Vliet WC, Dock NL, Davey FR. Factors in the liquid portion of stored blood inhibit the proliferative response in mixed lymphocyte cultures. Transfusion 1989; 29:41.
81. Susal C, Terness P, Opelz G. An experimental model for preventing alloimmunization against platelet transfusions by pretreatment with antibody-coated cells. Vox Sang 1990; 59: 209.
82. Sharpe RJ, Schweizer RT, Moore RE, et al. Evidence that cyclosporine-incubated platelets retain function and release cyclosporine. Transplantation 1985; 40:102.
83. Kelton JG, Hamid C, Aker S, Blajchman MA. The amount of blood group A substance on platelets is proportional to the amount in the plasma. Blood 1982; 59:980.
84. Lewis JH, Draude J, Kuhns WJ. Coating of "O" platelets with A and B group substances. Vox Sang 1960; 5:434.
85. Aster RH. Effect of anticoagulant and ABO incompatibility on recovery of transfused human platelets. Blood 1965; 26:732.
86. Pfisterer H, Thierfelder S, Stich W. ABO Rh blood groups and platelet transfusion. Blut 1968; 17:1.
87. Skogen B, Rossbo Hansen B, Husebekk A, et al. Minimal expression of blood group A antigen on thrombocytes from A2 individuals. Transfusion 1988; 28:456.
88. Duquesnoy RJ, Anderson AJ, Tomasulo PA, Aster RH. ABO compatibility and platelet transfusions of alloimmunized thrombocytopenic patients. Blood 1979; 54:595.
89. Heal JM, Blumberg N, Masel D. An evaluation of crossmatching, HLA, and ABO matching for platelet transfusions to refractory patients. Blood 1987; 70:23.
90. Brand A, Sintnicolaas K, Claas FHJ, Eernisse JG. ABH antibodies causing platelet transfusion refractoriness. Transfusion 1986; 26:463.
91. Freireich EJ, Kliman A, Gaydos LA, et al. Response to repeated platelet transfusion from the same donor. Ann Intern Med 1963; 59:277.
92. Tosato G, Appelbaum FR, Diesseroth AB. HLA-matched platelet transfusion therapy of severe aplastic anemia. Blood 1978; 52:846.
93. Shulman NR. Immunological considerations attending platelet transfusion. Transfusion 1966; 6:39.
94. Dunstan RA, Simpson MB, Rosse WF. Le^a blood group antigen on human platelets. Am J Clin Pathol 1985; 83:90.
95. Dunstan RA, Simpson MB, Rosse WF. Presence of I/i antigen system on human platelets. Am J Clin Pathol 1984; 82:74.
96. Dunstan RA, Simpson MB, Rosse WF. Presence of P blood group antigens on human platelets. Am J Clin Pathol 1985; 83:731.
97. Dunstan RA, Simpson MB, Rosse WF. Erythrocyte antigens on human platelets: Absence of Rhesus, Duffy, Kell, Kidd, and Lutheran antigens. Transfusion 1984; 24:243.
98. Svejgaard A, Kissmeyer-Nielsen F, Thorsby E. HL-A typing of platelets. In: Terasaki, ed. Histocompatibility Testing 1970. Copenhagen, Munksgaard, 1970:160.
99. Duquesnoy RJ, Filip DJ, Tomasulo PA, et al. Role of HLA-C matching in histocompatible platelet transfusion therapy of alloimmunized thrombocytopenic patients. Transplant Proc 1977; 9:1829.
100. van Rood JJ, van Leeuwen A, Keuning JJ, et al. The serological recognition of the human MLC determinants using a modified cytotoxicity technique. Tissue Antigens 1975; 5:73.

101. Yankee RA, Graff KS, Dowling R, et al. Selection of unrelated compatible platelet donors by lymphocyte HLA matching. N Engl J Med 1973; 288:760.

102. Duquesnoy RJ, Filip DJ, Rodey GE, et al. Successful transfusion of platelets "mismatched" for HLA antigens to alloimmunized thrombocytopenic patients. Am J Hematol 1977; 2:219.

103. Oldfather SW, Mora A, Phelan D, et al. The occurrence of crossreactive "public" antibodies in the sera of highly sensitized dialysis patients. Transplant Proc 1983; 15:1212.

104. Schwartz BD, Luehrman LK, Rodey GE. Public antigenic determinant on a family of HLA-B molecules. Basis for crossreactivity and a possible link with disease predisposition. J Clin Invest 1979; 64:938.

105. Slichter SJ. Transfusion and bone marrow transplantation. Transfus Med Rev 1988; 2:1.

106. Duquesnoy RJ, Vieira J, Aster RH. Donor availability for platelet transfusion support of alloimmunized thrombocytopenic patients. Transplant Proc 1977; 9:519.

107. Schiffer CA, Keller C, Dutcher JP, et al. Potential HLA-matched platelet donor availability for alloimmunized patients. Transfusion 1983; 23:286.

108. Bolgiano DC, Larson EB, Slichter SJ. A model to determine required pool size for HLA-typed community donor apheresis programs. Transfusion 1989; 29:306.

109. McFarland JG, Larson EB, Hillman RS, Slichter SJ. Cost-benefit analysis of a platelet-apheresis program. Transfusion 1986; 26:91.

110. Schiffer CA. Management of patients refractory to platelet transfusion—An evaluation of methods of donor selection. Prog Hematol 1987; 15:91.

111. Gmur J, von Felten A, Frick P. Platelet support in poly-sensitized patients: Role of HLA specificities and crossmatch testing for donor selection. Blood 1978; 51:903.

112. Kickler TS, Braine H, Ness PM. The predictive value of crossmatching platelet transfusions for alloimmunized patients. Transfusion 1985; 25:385.

113. Lohrmann HP, Bull MI, Decter JA, et al. Platelet transfusions from HLA compatible unrelated donors to alloimmunized patients. Ann Intern Med 1974; 80:9.

114. Slichter SJ. Selection of compatible platelet donors. In: Schiffer CA, ed. Platelet Physiology and Transfusion. Washington, DC, American Association of Blood Banks, 1978:83.

115. McFarland JG, Aster RH, Russel JB, et al. Prenatal diagnosis of neonatal alloimmune thrombo-cytopenic using allele-specific oligonucleotide probes. Blood 1991; 78:2276.

116. McFarland JG, Aster RH. Evaluation of four methods for platelet compatibility testing. Blood 1987; 69:1425.

117. Tamerius JD, Curd JG, Tani P, McMillan R. An enzyme-linked immunosorbent assay for platelet compatibility testing. Blood 1983; 62:744.

118. Kickler TS, Braine HG, Ness PM, et al. A radiolabeled antiglobulin test for crossmatching platelet transfusions. Blood 1983; 61:238.

119. Millard FE, Tani P, McMillan R. A specific assay for anti-HLA antibodies: Application to platelet donor selection. Blood 1987; 70:1495.

120. Kiss JE, Salamon DJ, Wilson J, et al. Suitability of liquid-stored donor platelets in platelet compatibility testing. Transfusion 1989; 29:405.

121. Schiffer CA, Young V. Detection of platelet antibodies using a micro-enzyme-linked immunosor-bent assay (ELISA). Blood 1983; 61:311.

122. Pollack MS, Zaroulis CG, Klainbard J, et al. Retention of HLA antigens on previously frozen human platelets. Transfusion 1980; 20:458.

123. Helmerhorst FM, ten Berge ML, van der Plas-van Dalen CM, et al. Platelet freezing for serological purposes with and without a cryopreservative. Vox Sang 1984; 46:318.

124. Lizak GE, Grumet FC (1979). Storage of reagent platelets for anti-platelet antibody testing in the ^{51}Cr platelet lysis assay. J Clin Pathol 1979; 32:191.

125. Yam P, Petz LD, Scott EP, Santos S. Platelet crossmatch tests using radiolabeled staphylococcal protein A or peroxidase anti-peroxidase in alloimmunized patients. Br J Haematol 1984; 57:337.

126. Ware R, Reisner E, Rosse W. The use of radiolabeled fluorescein-labeled antiglobulins in assays to predict platelet transfusion outcome. Blood 1984; 63:1245.

127. Wu KK, Hoak JC, Koepke JA, Thompson JS. Selection of compatible platelet donors: A prospective evaluation of three cross-matching techniques. Transfusion 1977; 17:638.

128. Herzig RH, Terasaki PI, Trapani RJ, et al. The relationship between donor-recipient lymphocytotoxicity and the transfusion response using HLA-matched platelet concentrates. Transfusion 1977; 17:657.

129. Cook LO, Miller WV. In vitro tests for platelet compatibility. Vox Sang 1981; 40:247.

130. Waters AH, Minchinton RM, Bell R, et al. A cross-matching procedure for the selection of platelet donors for alloimmunized patients. Br J Haematol 1981; 48:59.

131. Myers TJ, Kim BK, Steiner M, Baldini MG. Selection of donor platelets for alloimmunized patients using a platelet-associated IgG assay. Blood 1981; 58:444.

132. Freedman J, Hooi C, Garvey MB. Prospective platelet crossmatching for selection of compatible random donors. Br J Haematol 1984; 56:9.

133. van der Velden KJ, Sintnicolaas K, Lowenberg B. The value of a ^{51}Cr platelet lysis assay as a crossmatch test in patients with leukaemia on platelet transfusion therapy. Br J Haematol 1986; 62:635.

134. Brubaker DB, Duke JC, Romine M. Predictive value of enzyme-linked immunoassay platelet crossmatching for transfusion of platelet concentrates to alloimmunized recipients. Am J Hematol 1987; 24:375.

135. Kieckbusch ME, Moore SB, Koenig VA, DeGoey SR. Platelet crossmatch evaluation in refractory hematologic patients. Mayo Clin Proc 1987; 62:595.

136. McGrath K, Holdsworth R, Veale M, et al. Detection of HLA antibodies by platelet cross-matching techniques. Transfusion 1988; 23:214.

137. Kickler TS, Ness PM, Braine HG. Platelet crossmatching. A direct approach to the selection of platelet transfusions for the alloimmunized thrombocytopenic patient. Am J Clin Pathol 1988; 90:69.

138. Rachel JM, Summers TC, Sinor LT, Plapp FV. Use of a solid phase red blood cell adherence method for pre-transfusion platelet compatibility testing. Am J Clin Pathol 1988; 90:63.

139. Freedman J, Garvey MB, Salomon de Friedberg Z, et al. Random donor platelet cross-matching: Comparison of four platelet antibody detection methods. Am J Hematol 1988; 28:1.

140. Filip DJ, Duquesnoy RJ, Aster RH. Predictive value of crossmatching for transfusion of platelet concentrates to alloimmunized recipients. Am J Hematol 1976; 1:471.

141. Tosato G, Appelbaum FR, Trapani RJ, et al. Use of in vitro assays in selection of compatible platelet donors. Transfusion 1980; 20:47.

142. Radvany R, Green D, Rossi EC, et al. Efficacy of matched platelet transfusions from unrelated donors. Transplant Proc 1977; 9:513.

143. Hecht T, Wolf JL, Mraz L, et al. Platelet transfusion therapy in an alloimmunized patient. The value of crossmatch procedures for donor selection. JAMA 1982; 248:2301.

144. Rachel JM, Sinor LT, Tawfik OW, et al. A solid-phase red cell adherence test for platelet crossmatching. Med Lab Sci 1985; 42:194.

145. Shibata Y, Juji T, Nishizawa Y, et al. Detection of platelet antibodies by a newly developed mixed agglutination with platelets. Vox Sang 1981; 41:25.

146. O'Connell BA, Schiffer CA. Donor selection for alloimmunized patients by platelet cross-matching of random-donor platelet concentrates. Transfusion 1990; 30:314.

147. Freedman J, Gafni A, Garvey MB, Blanchette V. A cost-effectiveness evaluation of platelet crossmatching and HLA matching in the management of alloimmunized thrombocytopenic patients. Transfusion 1989; 29:201.

148. Opelz G, Mickey MR, Terasaki PI. Blood transfusions and unresponsiveness to HLA. Transplantation 1973; 16:649.

149. Klouda PT, Lawler SD, Powles RL, et al. HLA antibody response in patients with acute myelogenous leukaemia by immunotherapy. Transplantation 1975; 19:245.

150. Ferrara GB, Tosi RM, Azzolina G, et al. HLA responsiveness induced by weekly transfusions of small aliquots of whole blood. Transplantation 1974; 17:194.

151. Schmidt RE, Budde U, Broschen-Zywietz C, et al. High dose gammaglobulin therapy in adults with idiopathic thrombocytopenic purpura (ITP) clinical effects. Blut 1984; 48:19.

152. Imbach P, Barandun S, d'Apuzzo V, et al. High-dose intravenous gammaglobulin for idiopathic thrombocytopenic purpura in childhood. Lancet 1981; 1:1228.

153. Fehr J, Hofman V, Kappeler U. Transient reversal of thrombocytopenia in idiopathic thrombocytopenic purpura by high-dose intravenous gammaglobulin. N Engl J Med 1982; 306: 1254.

154. Kekomaki R, Elfenbein G, Gardner R, et al. Improved response of patients refractory to random-donor platelet transfusions by intravenous gamma globulin. Am J Med 1984; 76:199.

155. Bierling P, Cordonnier C, Rodet M, et al. High dose intravenous gammaglobulin and platelet transfusions in leukaemic HLA-immunized patients. Scand J Haematol 1984; 33:215.

156. Junghans RP, Ahn YS. High-dose intravenous gamma globulin to suppress alloimmune destruction of donor platelets. Am J Med 1984; 76:204.

157. Kickler T, Braine HG, Piantadosi S, et al. A randomized, placebo-controlled trial of intravenous gammaglobulin in alloimmunized thrombocytopenic patients. Blood 1990; 75:313.

158. Ziegler ZR, Shadduck RK, Rosenfeld CS, et al. High-dose intravenous gamma globulin improves responses to single-donor platelets in patients refractory to platelet transfusion. Blood 1987; 70:1433.

159. Atrah HI, Sheehan T, Gribben J, et al. Improvement of post platelet transfusion increments following intravenous imunoglobulin therapy for leukaemic HLA-immunized patients. Scand J Haematol 1986; 36:160.

160. Becton DL, Kinney TR, Schaffee S, et al. High-dose intravenous immunoglobulin for severe platelet alloimmunization. Pediatrics 1984; 74:1120.

161. Knupp C, Chamberlain JK, Raab SO. High-dose intravenous gamma globulin in alloimmunized platelet transfusion recipients. Blood 1985; 65:776.

162. Lee EJ, Norris D, Schiffer CA. Intravenous immune globulin for patients alloimmunized to random donor platelet transfusion. Transfusion 1987; 27:245.

163. Schiffer CA, Hogge DE, Aisner J, et al. High-dose intravenous gammaglobulin in alloimmunized platelet transfusion recipients. Blood 1984; 64:937.

164. Nilsson IM, Sundqvist SB, Ljung R, et al. Suppression of secondary antibody response by intravenous immunoglobulin in a patient with a haemophilia B and antibodies. Scand J Haematol 1983; 30:458.

165. Nagasawa T, Kim BK Baldini MG. Temporary suppression of circulating antiplatelet alloantibodies by the massive infusion of fresh, stored, or lyophilized platelets. Trans- fusion 1978; 18:429.

166. Kekomaki R, Myllyla G. Effect of normal serum on the binding of specific antibodies and platelet-unrelated immune complexes to human platelets. Scand J Immunol 1979; 9:527.

167. Bensinger WI, Buckner CD, Clift RA, et al. Plasma exchange for platelet alloimmunization. Transplantation 1986; 41:602.

168. Slichter SJ, Deeg HJ, Storb R. Prevention and reversal of platelet alloimmunization with cyclosporine A (abstr) Blood 1981; 51(suppl 1):186a.

169. Yamamoto M, Ideguchi H, Nichimura, J et al. Treatment of platelet-alloimmunization with cyclosporin A in a patient with aplastic anemia. Am J Hematol 1990; 33:220.

170. Tilly H, Azagury M, Bastit D, et al. Cyclosporin for treatment of life-threatening alloimmunization. Am J Hematol 1990; 34:75.

171. Beris P, Dornier C. Prevention and circumvention of refractoriness to platelet transfusions: Interface between preparative and therapeutic apheresis. In: Nydegger, ed. Therapeutic Hemapheresis In The 1990s: Current Studies In Hematology and Blood Transfusion. Basel, Karger, 1990:267.

172. Swanepoel CR, Cassidy MJD, May M, et al. Reactivity of pretransplant cytotoxic antibodies to a selected HLA panel is not influenced by cyclosporin A, with or without plasma exchange. J Clin Apheresis 1991; 6:28.

173. Sabbe LJM, Claas FHJ, Haak HL, et al. Anti-thymocyte globulin (ATG) can eliminate platelet refractoriness. Blut 1981; 42:331.

174. Bruggers CS, Kurtzberg J, Friedman HS. Vincristine therapy for severe platelet alloimmunization. Am J Pediatr Hematol/Oncol 1991; 13:300.

175. Wong P, Hiruma K, Endoh N, et al. Vinblastine-loaded platelet transfusion in an alloimmunized patient. Br J Haematol 1987; 65:380.

176. Oh JH, Whelchel JD. Reversal of blood-induced sensitization by antibody-coated platelets. Transplant Proc 1991; 23:316.

177. Shanwell A, Sallander S, Olsson I. et al. An alloimmunized, thrombocytopenic patient successfully transfused with acid-treated, random-donor platelets. Br J Haematol 1991; 79:462.

V

The Effect of Transfusion on the Immune Response

22

Transfusion-Induced Graft-versus-Host Disease

KATHLEEN SAZAMA
University of California, Davis
Sacramento, California

PAUL V. HOLLAND
Sacramento Medical Foundation
Sacramento, California

I. INTRODUCTION

Transfusion-induced graft-versus-host disease (TI-GVHD) is a potential complication of any blood transfusion when a component containing viable immunocompetent lymphocytes is transfused into a recipient who is incapable of effectively resisting engraftment. Implicated components include whole blood and packed red blood cells (RBCs) (1–8), platelet concentrates (9,10), granulocytes from normal donors (9,11–17), granulocytes from chronic myelogenous leukemia (CML) donors (18–19), fresh plasma (1,20–24), and even previously frozen, deglycerolized RBCs (25,26) alone or in combinations (9,19,27–29). Reviewers of TI-GVHD prior to 1990 (30–40) suggested that immunosuppression or immune incompetency of the recipient was a necessary antecedent for TI-GVHD. However, recent reports of TI-GVHD in persons with no apparent immune incompetency (17,41–78) raise suspicion about the absolute requirement for recipient immunocompromise (79–82). The reports of GVHD after syngeneic and autologous bone marrow transplantation (83) are probably different from TI-GVHD because of functional immunosuppression due to chemotherapy with or without irradiation. There have been at least 65 recent reports (not including abstracts) published in English of recipients who have developed TI-GVHD (Table 1).

Transfusion-induced-GVHD continues to be reported in instances where altered immunity probably is a primary factor: 5 cases in premature and full-term neonates (74–78); 3 cases of severe combined immunodeficiency (SCID) (71–73); 5 cases of Hodgkin's disease (64–66); 4 cases of lymphoma and leukemia (67–69); 2 cases due to other immunological causes (52,70); and 16 cases of various malignancies (17,42,48,53–59). Additionally, there are reports of TI-GVHD in situations in which immunosuppression may be present (1 case at delivery) (70) and where it is not considered to be a major factor: 25 cases after cardiovascular surgery (41–50), 2 cases after elective cholecystectomy (49,51), and 1 case after amputation for diabetic gangrene (42). Efforts to explain these new reports focus on both transfusion-induced and transplantation-related GVHD and the histocompatibility between donor and recipient.

The first recognition of GVHD as a complication (frequently fatal) of blood transfusion occurred relatively recently. Although experimental GVHD was well known by the mid-1960s, especially followed transplantation of various tissues and organs (84), human TI-GVHD was

Table 1 Clinical Features of TI-GVHD Cases Reported Since 1988

Age	Sex	Diagnosis	Component(s) Received	Date of Symptom Onset	Signs Symptoms	Daignosis Procedures(s)	Outcome	Ref. No.
1. Lymphomas and leukemias								
Child	NS	Hodgkin's disease IA, CR	NS	8 d	R/D, ↑LFTs	Autopsy	Fatal	64
Child	NS	Hodgkin's disease IA, CR	NS	8 d	R/D, ↑LFTs	Autopsy	Fatal	64
20 yr	F	Hodgkin's disease NS IIA	2U PRBC + multiple platelets	9 d	F/R/D, ↑LFTs	Skin Bx BM Bx	Fatal 29 d	65
31 yr	F	Hodgkin's disease NS IIIB	14 U platelets + 3 U PRBC	7 d	R/D, ↑LFTs, ↓cells	Skin Bx BM Bx HLA typing	Fatal 48 d	66
14 yr	M	Hodgkin's disease IVB	1 U PRBC (mother) + 11 U platelets	4 d	F/R/D, ↑LFTs	Skin Bx BM Bx HLA typing	Fatal 22 d	65
67 yr	F[a]	Diffuse mixed lymphoma, IIIA	Leukocyte filtered blood (many)	?	?	?	Fatal	67
?	?	Lymphoma	Platelets (father)	?	?	?	?	68
?	?	Lymphoma	Platelets (father)	?	?	?	?	68
7 yr	F	Acute stem cell leukemia	2 U PRBC + WBC	2 wk	F/R/D, ↑LFTs, seizures	BM Bx	Fatal 6 wk	69
2. Immune deficiency								
55 yr	M	T-cell chronic lymphocytosis	4 U PRBC	2 wk	R/D, dyspnea, vomiting	Skin Bx	Fatal 54 d	70
4.5 yr	M	Purine nucleotide phosphorylase deficiency, ?SCID	5 U platelets	4 d	R/D, DIC	Skin Bx	Fatal 17 d	71
6 mo	M	SCID	?	2 d	R, ↑LFTs	Skin Bx HLA typing BM Bx	Fatal 15 d	72
2 mo	M	SCID	?	2 mo	R, ↑liver and ↑LN	Novel "T" cells	Surviving	73

3. Prematurity/neonates

Patient	Sex	Condition	Transfusion	Onset	Clinical	Diagnosis	Outcome	Ref
NB	F	Prematurity	WBC from father	30 d	R/D, ↓ PMNs, ↑ LFTs	Skin Bx, BM Bx	Fatal 46 d	74
Premie 855 g	F	Prematurity	114 ml PRBC	47 d	R/↑ liver, ↑ LFTs, ↓ cells	Skin Bx	Fatal 83 d	75
FT	M	ECMO for meconium asp	19 components	17 d	F/R/D, ↑ liver, ↑ LFTs	Skin Bx	Fatal 19 d	76
Premie 770 g	M	Prematurity 26 wk	ExTx—400 ml PRBC, platelets, plasma	20 d	F/R, ↑ liver	Skin Bx	Fatal 37 d	77
Premie 1220 g	M	Prematurity 28 wk	Numerous Tx: WB, PRBC, platelets, WBC	5 mo	↓ cells, ↑ LFTs	Autopsy	Fatal 5 mo	78

4. Operative conditions—vascular

Patient	Sex	Condition	Transfusion	Onset	Clinical	Diagnosis	Outcome	Ref
62 yr	M[a]	AA	?	?	F/D, ↑ LFTs, ↓ cells	Skin Bx	Fatal 19 d	49
63 yr	M[a]	AAA postop	2200 ml "fresh blood" + 30 U FFP	13 d	F/R, ↑ LFTs, ↑ liver	HLA typing, Skin Bx	Fatal 24 d	41

5. Operative conditions—coronary and cardiac

Patient	Sex	Condition	Transfusion	Onset	Clinical	Diagnosis	Outcome	Ref
59 yr	M[a]	CABG	4200 ml "fresh blood," 700 ml FFP, 20 U platelets	6 d	F/R, ↓ cells	Clinical Dx	Fatal 19 d	41
60 yr	M	AC bypass	2600 blood + 400 FFP	10 d	F/R	Clinical Dx	Fatal 23 d	42
76 yr	M	AC bypass	600 ml "fresh" + 800 ml "stored" blood	16 d	F/R	Clinical Dx	Fatal 23 d	42
67 yr	M[a]	CABG	Liberal use of "fresh" blood	10 d	F/R, ↑ LFTs, ↓ cells	Skin Bx	Fatal 17 d	43
67 yr	F[a]	CABG	"	13 d	"	(HLA typing) (BM Bx)	Fatal 22 d	43
61 yr	M[a]	CABG	"	10 d	"	"	Fatal 17 d	43
70 yr	M[a]	CABG	"	14 d	"	"	Fatal 34 d	43
68 yr	M[a]	CABG	"	12 d	"	"	Fatal 25 d	44
44 yr	M[a]	DVR	"	11 d	"	"	Fatal 28 d	44
63 yr	M	CABG	6 U PRBC (11 d old)	14 d	F/R/D, ARDS, ↑ LFTs	Skin Bx, BM Bx, Autopsy and HLA typing	Fatal 14 d	45
69 yr	M[b]	CABG (emergency)	2 U "fresh" WB from sons	18 d	F/R/D, tachypnea, icterus	HLA typing = 1 son was HLA homozygous	Fatal 22 d	46

(continued)

Table 1 Continued

Age	Sex	Diagnosis	Component(s) Received	Date of Symptom Onset	Signs Symptoms	Diagnosis Procedures(s)	Outcome	Ref. No.
51 yr	M[b]	CABG (elective)	2 U "fresh" WB from daughters	12 d	F/R/chills, icterus, ↓ cells	BM Bx Skin Bx Autopsy/HLA typing	Fatal 34 d	46
63 yr	M	CABG	2 U "fresh" PRBC	12 d	R/F/D/N/V	BM Bx Skin Bx	Fatal 26 d	47
66 yr	F[a]	A/C bypass +	2440 "fresh blood" (male donors)	8 d	F/R, ↑ LFTs, ↓ cells	Autopsy Skin Bx	Fatal 16 d	48
52 yr	M[a]	CABG	3600 ml "fresh blood"	?	F/D, ↑ LFTs, ↓ cells	Skin Bx	Fatal 14 d	49
68 yr	M[a]	CABG	3400 ml "fresh blood"	?	F/D, ↑ LFTs, ↓ cells	Skin Bx	Fatal 23 d	49
48 yr	M[a]	OHS	3400 mL "fresh blood"	?	F/R, ↑ LFTs, ↓ cells	Skin Bx	Fatal 25 d	49
48 yr	M[a]	CABG	400 ml "fresh" blood	?	F/R, ↑ LFTs, ↓ cells	Skin Bx	Fatal 29 d	49
77 yr	M[a]	CABG	?	?	F, ↓ cells	Skin Bx	Fatal 14 d	49
70 yr	F[a]	CABG	11200 ml "fresh" blood	?	F, ↓ cells, ? ↑ LFT	Skin Bx	Fatal 28 d	49
38 yr	M[a]	CABG	3500 ml "fresh" blood	?	F, ↓ cells, ? ↑ LFT	Skin Bx	Fatal 18 d	49
58 yr	M	Mitral commissurotomy	2 U (400 ml each)—1 U from son	10 d	F/R, ↑ LFTs	Skin Bx BM Bx HLA typing of son	Fatal 18 d	50
52 yr	M	MI →Bypass	2600 ml + 2400 ml WB	7 d	F/R	Clinical Dx	Fatal 19 d	42
56 yr	M	Amputation for diabetic gangrene	400 ml "fresh" blood	11 d	F/R	?	Fatal 24 d	42
72 yr	M[a]	Elective cholecystectomy	600 ml "fresh blood"	?	F/D, ↑ LFTs, ↓ cells	Skin Bx	Fatal 35 d	49

6. Operative conditions—other

52 yr, F[a]	Elective cholecystectomy	3 U PRBC	10 d	F/R/D, ↑LFTs, pulm. infil.	HLA typing of family	Fatal 28 d	51
7. Inflammatory states							
49 yr, F	Inflammatory bowel disease	2 U PRBC	?	D	Skin Bx	Survived	52
8. Malignancies							
53 yr, M	Lung CA	11U LR-PRBC + 4U SD Plts	1 d	F/R/D	Autopsy	Fatal 10 d	53
55 yr, M	Lung CA	6U LR-PRBC + 4U SD plts	1 d	F/R	Autopsy	Fatal 13 d	53
53 yr, M	Lung CA	6U plts	11 d	F/R	Skin Bx	Fatal 26 d	53
30 yr, F	Immunoblastic sarcoma	5U WBC from mother, maternal aunt, HLA-identical sibling (kidney donor)	14 d	N/V/D/F/R	Skin Bx	Fatal 7 wk	17
73 yr, M[a]	Squamous cell CA, neck	5400 ml blood (2000 "fresh" blood)	10 d	F/R, ↑LFTs, ↓cells	Skin Bx, liver (autopsy)	Fatal 20 d	54
53 yr, M[a]	Resection of esophageal CA	1200 ml "fresh" blood	10 d	R/F/D, ↑LFTs, ↓cells	HLA typing	Fatal 19 d	55
58 yr, M[a]	Resection of esophageal CA	2000 ml "fresh" blood + 200 ml "stored" blood	12 d	F/R	Clinical Dx	Fatal 23 d	42
74 yr, M	Gastric CA	600 ml "fresh" blood	8 d	F/R	Clinical Dx	Fatal 21 d	42
55 yr, F	Biliary CA	2400 ml PRBC ("fresh") + 2000 FFP	8 d	F/R	Clinical Dx	Fatal 18 d	42
55 yr, M[a]	Cholangio CA	1590 ml PRBC ("fresh")	13 d	F, ↑LFTs	HLA typing BM Bx	Fatal 24 d	56
63 yr, M[a]	Colon CA	3940 ml fresh blood	7 d	F/R, ↑LFTs	HLA typing	Fatal 25 d	56
69 yr, F[a]	Colon CA—colectomy	4 U PRBC from family (daughter is haplotype homozygous)	9 d	F/R/D, ↑LFTs, ↓cells	Skin Bx, autopsy, HLA typing	Fatal 15 d	57
72 yr, F[c]	Renal cell CA (postop)	7 U PRBC (2 from daughters)	12 d	F/R, vomiting, ↓cells	HLA typing Skin Bx Autopsy	Fatal 20 d	58

(continued)

Table 1 Continued

Age	Sex	Diagnosis	Component(s) Received	Date of Symptom Onset	Signs Symptoms	Daignosis Procedures(s)	Outcome	Ref. No.
73 yr	M	Prostate CA	4 U autologous + 1 U from grandson	12 d	R, ↓ cells, mental changes	Skin Bx BM Bx HLA typing Autopsy	Fatal 32 d	59
56 yr	F[a]	Cervical CA	7U PRBC (3 female, 4 male) stored 3 d	6 d	R/F, ↑LFT, ↓ cells	Autopsy	Fatal 17 d	48
25 yr	F	Ovarian CA	9U LR-PRBC, 4U WBC, 2U SD platelets	?	?	Autopsy	Fatal ?	53
9. Other								
22 yr	F[a]	Pregnancy	2 U PRBC	15 d	R/F, ↓ cells	BM Bx	Fatal 28 d	70
54 yr	F[a]	Upper GI bleed	8 U PRBC (2 d old)	10 d	F/R, N/V/D, seizures	BM Bx HLA typing	Fatal 16 d	63

Abbreviations:AAA, abdominal aortic aneurysm resection; AC, aortocoronary bypass; ARDS, adult respiratory distress syndrome; Asp, aspiration; BM, bone marrow; Bx, biopsy; CA, carcinoma; CABG, coronary artery bypass graft; CR, complete remission; D, diarrhea; DIC, disseminated intravascular coagulation; DVR, dilated ventricular resection; DX, diagnosis; ECMO, extracorporeal membrane oxygenation; ExTx, exchange transfusion; F, fever; FFP, fresh frozen plasma; FT, full term; GI, gastrointestinal; HLA, human leukocyte antigen; LFTs, liver function tests; LN, lymph nodes; LR, leuko-reduced; MI, myocardial infarction; N, nausea; NB, newborn; NS, nodular sclerosing; OHS, open-heart surgery; PMN's, polymorphonuclear leukocytes; PRBC, packed red blood cells; R, rash; SCID, severe combined immunodeficiency; SD, single donor; Tx, transfusions; U, unit; V, vomiting; WB, whole blood; WBC, white blood cell.

[a]Japanese.
[b]Jewish.
[c]Married to first cousin.

not. The first such report in the English-language literature occurred in 1965 (1), which described two infants, 8 and 3.5 months of age, whose treatment for severe progressive vaccinia necrosum consisted in part of transfusion of leukocyte-rich plasma in one case and exchange transfusion with fresh whole blood in the other. Both infants developed "erythrodermia," hepatomegaly, and fatal aplastic anemia. Further evaluation disclosed that one infant probably was immunodeficient with Swiss-type agammaglobulinemia with alymphocytosis. However, the older infant had no evidence of immunosuppression. Subsequently, more than 115 cases of TI-GVHD have been published in English (Tables 1 and 2) (1,3,5–7,9–13,15–17,19–23,27–29,64,85–101).

II. PATHOGENESIS OF GVHD

Although the mechanism of human TI-GVHD has not been fully elucidated, numerous investigations focusing on both defects or alterations in the host and characteristics of the graft are beginning to provide some insight (102,103). The three prerequisites for the development of GVHD have classically been stated as: differences in tissue histocompatibility, chiefly in the major histocompatibility complex (MHC), between the donor and the recipient; the presence of immunocompetent cells in the graft; and an inability of the host to reject the graft (104). Thus, classic immunology would require, for successful engraftment, that the immunologically and mitotically competent mature T lymphocytes from the donated blood component encounter an absent or attenuated immune response (or immunological tolerance) by the recipient's immune system (105–107). Reports of GVHD following autologous bone marrow transplantation (83) challenge the classic theory, however. Although subsequent investigators have attributed these unusual cases to an autoreactive T cell controlled by an autoregulatory T cell

Table 2 Clinical Features of Patients with Posttransfusion GVHD (up to 1988)*

Diagnosis	Age	Product transfused[a]	Outcome[b]	Ref. No.
Neonates				
1. Prematurity	28-wk gestation	600 ml WB ExTx[d]	Death, 120	85
2. Prematurity	33-wk gestation	ExTx (×2)	Death, 36	28
3. HDN[3]	32-wk gestation	IU Tx (600 ml PRBC), ExTx (1000 ml WB)	Death, 21	86
4. HDN	33-wk gestation	IU Tx (×3), ExTx (×6)	Death, 91	87
5. HDN	36-wk gestation	IU Tx (230 ml PRBC), ExTx (×5)	Death, 12	27
6. HDN	36-wk gestation	IU Tx (220 ml PRBC), ExTx (×2)	Death, 19	27
7. HDN	Term	ExTx (1500 ml WB)	Death, 20	86
8. HDN	Term	ExTx (×1)	Death, 80	88
Congenital immunodeficiency syndromes				
9. SCID[e]	1 mo	105 ml PRBC	Death, 30	89
10. SCID	3 mo	50 ml WB	Death, 17	22
11. SCID	3 mo	WB, 2U	Death, 20	90
12. SCID	3.5 mo	5000 ml WB (ExTx)	Death, 17	1
13. SCID	4 mo	WB, 1 U; PRBC, 2 U	Death, 16	5
14. SCID	5 mo	WB, 1 U	Death, 12	91
15. SCID	8 mo	750 ml BC.	Death, 14	1
16. SCID	11 mo	125 ml WB	Death, 28	92

(continued)

Table 2 Continued

Diagnosis	Age	Product transfused[a]	Outcome[b]	Ref. No.
17. SCID	18 mo	200 ml PRBC	Death, 15	3
18. SCID	5 mo	Fresh plasma	Death, 14	22
19. SCID	11 yr	Fresh plasma	Chronic GVHD	21
20. Wiskott-Aldrich syndrome	32 mo	Fresh plasma	Death, 30	20
21. Nezeloff-s syndrome	3.5 mo	Fresh plasma, 4 U	Death, 27	23
Lymphoma				
22. HD, III$_A$[e]	6 yr	WBC, 3 U	Death, 29	16
23. HD, III$_A$	18 yr	PRBC, 2 U	Death, 25	6
24. HD, II$_A$	21 yr	PLT, 6 U	Death, 27	93
25. HD, III$_A$	30 yr	PLT, 4 U	Death, 27	10
26. HD, IV$_B$	37 yr	PRBC, 2 U; PLT, 8 U	Death, 33	93
27. HD, III$_A$	58 yr	PRBC, 2 U	Death, 47	94
28. HD, I$_A$	12 yr	PRBC, 2 U	Death, 21	64
29. HD, I$_A$	10 yr	PRBC, 2 U; PLT, 4 U	Death, 30	64
30. NHL[e]	6 yr	150 ml BC	Death, 13	12
31. NHL	30 yr	WBC, 5 U	Death, 27	15
32. NHL	30 yr	WBC, 5 U	Death, 63	17
33. NHL	34 yr	WBC	Death, 14	95
Acute leukemia				
34. ANLL[e]	6 yr	PRBC, 2 U; WBC, 2 U; PLT, 4 U	Alive, chronic GVHD	9
35. ANLL	15 yr	WB, 4 U; PLT, 3 U	Death, NS	96
36. ANLL	19 yr	Washed RBC, 4 U; PLT, 1 pack	Death, 25	29
37. ANLL	38 yr	Washed RBC, 12 U; PLT 14 U, WBC, 12 U	Alive	29
38. ANLL	45 yr	PRBC, 2 U; WBC, 3 U	Death, 25	19
39. ANLL	49 yr	WB, 4 U; BC, 40 U	Death, 19	96
40. ANLL	49 yr	BC, 40 U	Death, NS	96
41. ANLL	50 yr	WBC, 10 U; PLT, 2 packs	Death, 19	11
42. ANLL	60 yr	PRBC, 4 U; WBC, 2 U; PLT, 5 packs	Death, 18	19
43. ALL[e]	5 yr	Whole Blood, 5 U	Alive, chronic GVHD	97
44. ALL	5 yr	WBC, 2 U	Alive	98
45. ALL	7.5 yr	WBC, 2 U	Death, 19	13
46. ALL	10 yr	WBC	Alive, chronic GVHD	97
47. ALL	20 yr	WB, 2 U; PRBC, 2 U; PLT, 2 U	Death, 21	99
Solid tumors				
48. Neuroblastoma	2 yr	PRBC, 1 U	Death, 21	7
49. Neuroblastoma	2 yr	PRBC, 1 U	Death, 15	100
50. Rhabdomyosarcoma	9 yr	PRBC, 2 U; PLT, 5 U	Death, 32	101
51. Glioblastoma	59 yr	BC, 8 U	Death, 12	16

[a]Includes only blood products derived from normal donors.
[b]Refers to interval from first transfusion to death, in days.
[c]PRBC, packed red cells; WB, whole blood; WBC, white blood cells; BC, buffy coat cells; PLT, platelet concentrates.
[d]ExTx, exchange transfusion; IU Tx, intrauterine transfusion.
[e]HDN, hemolytic disease of the newborn; NAIT, neonatal alloimmune thrombocytopenia; SCID, severe combined immunodeficiency disease; HD, Hodgkins' disease; NHL, non-Hodgkin's lymphoma; ALL, acute lymphocytic leukemia; ANLL, acute nonlymphocytic leukemia.
Source: Based on data from Ref. 34, Table 1.

(80) or to possible receipt of nonirradiated blood cells during bone marrow harvesting (108), experimental data provide fascinating new information regarding this process.

A. Acute GVHD

Two types of acute GVHD have been defined by investigational studies. One model involves the action of irradiation and cyclosporine A during experimental bone marrow transplantation and the other is the transfusional model that is experimentally best represented by the parent to first-generation offspring (P to F_1) transfusion situation in which HLA homozygosity is the major determinant (46) (Fig. 1). In both models, a two-phase event is postulated to result in the clinical picture of acute GVHD, but only the TI-GVHD model will be discussed further.

TI-GVHD Model

The classic experimental model of HLA-homozygous TI-GVHD is seen in murine transfusions from parents into F_1 hybrid offspring. The F_1 hybrid offspring (ab) of the mating of two different strains (aa × bb) of congenic mice (mice that are all genetically identical) will fail to reject transfused or transplanted cells from either parent with whom it shares a haplotype. However, lymphocytes from either parent can reject the F_1 hybrid recipient because they recognize as foreign the HLA haplotype donated by the other parent (aa→ab or bb→ab). This reaction is dependent on activation of donor CD4+ and CD8+ T cells that in turn cause profound immune suppression of the host's immune system and extensive donor lymphoid repopulation of the host (109,110). This effect can be enhanced experimentally by pretreatment of the donor with pertussis vaccine (111).

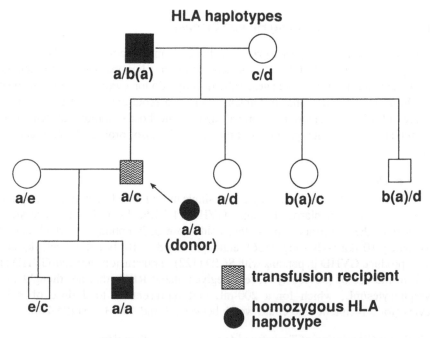

Figure 1 Prototypic family pedigree of recipient with TI-GVHD caused by HLA-homozygous blood. Note: Close family members are more likely to be HLA homozygous than the general population (except when specially HLA selected).

Primary event. The primary event in the TI-GVHD model appears to be the activation of effector mechanism(s) that cause acute GVHD tissue destruction. T cells from the transfusion graft may react with either class I (33) or class II (109) alloantigens in the recipient. Class II antigens are present on antigen-presenting cells (APCs) (macrophages, monocytes, epidermal Langerhans' cells, vascular endothelial cells, and dendritic cells in lymphoid organs), on B lymphocytes, on thymic epithelial cells, and on activated T lymphocytes (112). It is the CD4+ T lymphocyte that recognizes class II HLA differences, whereas CD8+ T lymphocytes apparently are responsible for GVHD when HLA class I alloantigens stimulate the reaction (113–115). When complete MHC differences exist (both class I and class II foreignness), either CD4+ or CD8+ cells can apparently initiate GVHD (116).

Murine Data. In mice, activated donor T cells stimulate both splenic macrophages and natural killer (NK)–like cells. The activated splenic macrophages produce prostaglandin E_2, which suppresses CD4+ T lymphocytes (117,118). The other crucial cell during this early phase in experimental studies is a specifically induced cell of donor origin that exhibits NK cell activity (103). The origin of this inducible NK cell is not completely defined but may arise from a class of newly described T cells bearing the gamma/delta T-cell receptor (119). The main function of cells with the gamma/delta receptor is thought to be surveillance of epithelial cells and all rapidly proliferating cells, such as stem cells, which are usually the target of GVHD.

Target organs in which destructive changes are seen during TI-GVHD include skin, thymus, gastrointestinal tract, liver, spleen, and bone marrow. The gamma/delta receptor–bearing (NK) T cell differs from T cells bearing the alpha/beta receptor that participate in the activation phase. The peak of these NK cells coincides with maximum tissue damage, particularly thymic and bone marrow stroma injury (120). Soon after NK injury begins, there is a profound decrease in T cells, particularly T-helper cells, and of B cells owing to the thymic and bone marrow damage of TI-GVHD.

B. Requirements for Producing Human Disease

Transfusion of donor lymphocytes capable of dividing and responding to the recipient of a cellular component initiates TI-GVHD. The activated donor lymphocytes proliferate as clones and, in turn, activate host macrophages; subsequently, donor cytotoxic cells are distributed to all cells bearing MHC antigens. In humans, there is a requirement that the donor lymphocytes (1) are sufficiently numerous to prevail against the host's immune system, (2) persist in host circulation for some period of time, and (3) also proliferate and activate host macrophages.

1. Number of Donor Lymphocytes

There are sufficient numbers of lymphocytes in a single unit of blood, in platelets, in granulocyte concentrates, and in fresh plasma to cause GVHD (4,34,66,121). For a successful human TI-GVH reaction, there appears to be a "threshold" dose of lymphocytes, which is thought to be approximately 10^7/kg body weight (36), although only 8×10^5 lymphoid cells/kg have been sufficient to produce GVHD in persons with SCID (122). Transfusion-induced-GVHD has been reported from the use of previously frozen, deglycerolized RBCs that are thought to contain $<10^7$ lymphocytes/mL, which for a 200-mL unit represents a total dose of $<2 \times 10^9$ lymphocytes (for a recipient who could weigh between 2 and 100 + kg) (25,26).

2. Survival and Circulation of Transfused Lymphocytes in Recipient

An additional requirement for initiating TI-GVHD is that lymphocytes from the transfused component must remain in the host's circulation sufficiently long to recognize the "foreign"

HLA class I and/or II antigens of the host and undergo mitosis. Lymphocytes stored up to 3 weeks in acid citrate dextrose (ACD)) are capable of mitosis in vitro (123). Recipients of numerous transfusions have been shown to experience a rise in the number of circulating atypical lymphocytes, most of which demonstrate the recipient karyotype but some of which are of donor origin (124). Lymphocytes in stored blood reportedly may circulate for at least 7 days after transfusion of whole blood into adult immunocompetent recipients (4) and for up to 6–8 weeks after neonatal exchange transfusion from unrelated donors but for more than 2 years after maternal-derived intrauterine transfusion (2). The difference between adults and neonates may reflect lack of recognition by donor lymphocytes in the neonates, possibly due to HLA similarities (125) and/or insufficient numbers of lymphocytes in washed blood components to be measured (126).

3. Proliferation of Donor Lymphocytes

Lymphocytes retain their mitotic capability for 17–22 days at 4°C (127,128). However, lymphocytes stored for more than 10 days reportedly lose their immunocompetence (129). Many reports of TI-GVHD involve transfusion of blood components that are less than 2 days old (see Table 1).

III. TRANSFUSION SETTINGS

Data from various transfusion settings have provided some bases for further defining the conditions under which TI-GVHD may occur. Several suggested mechanisms of action have been postulated for TI-GVHD related to other effects of transfusions.

A. Donor-Specific Tolerance in Renal Allografts

That blood transfusions induce immunosuppression was first observed over 25 years ago when prolonged kidney graft survival was seen in transplant recipients who had received blood transfusions prior to transplant (130–132) and reduced survival was found when either no or only a few transfusions were given or only frozen blood was used (133). This phenomenon has been attributed to both B- and T-lymphocyte effects, including specific immunological changes such as the appearance of blocking and anti-idiotypic (134,135) antibodies; to T-cell effects such as clonal deletion (136,137) or clonal anergy (138) and stimulation of suppressor cells (134,139,140); to nonspecifc and specific, i.e., CD4+–mediated, and mononuclear phagocytic cell synthesis of prostaglandin E_2 (141,142); immunological downregulation by changes in the cascade of cytokine secretion (143); and to combined effects (144). Prostaglandins of the E series (PGE) participate in immune response regulation in a dose-dependent fashion. High levels of PGE_2 suppress the cell-mediated response in vivo, whereas low levels enhance it. The experimental observation that allogeneic RBCs are themselves immunosuppressive appears to be the result of downregulation of splenic suppressor cells responsible for GVHD via a prostaglandin-dependent pathway (141,145,146).

1. Role of HLA

Sharing all or part of the MHC or of minor alloantigens is sufficient to prolong allograft survival (147). When a living related donor is a full (6/6) HLA match, there is probably no need to provide donor-specific pretransplantation transfusions. Sharing one DR antigen while being mismatched for the other provides a good immunosuppressive effect with minimal risk of sensitization (148,149). More recently, induction of specific transplantation tolerance measured by reduction in frequency of cytotoxic T-lymphocyte precursors was seen in recipients of blood transfusions and subsequent renal allografts from donors with whom they shared common HLA haplotypes or at least one HLA-B and one HLA-DR antigen (137).

2. Timing of Transfusion Immunosuppressive Effect

Of particular interest is the finding that, although the specific reduction in cytotoxic T lymphocytes does not begin until 1 week posttransfusion, there is a sharp decrease in precursors to virtually undetectable levels as early as 4 weeks. Because the time of onset of TI-GVHD is frequently more than 7 days posttransfusion (see Table 1), the onset of transfusion-induced immune tolerance appears to be consistent with the reported timing of symptomatology of acute TI-GVHD. Transfusion of "fresh" or stored whole blood or RBCs was reported in 1972 to increase numbers of lymphocytes "activated" to HLA antigens 1 week after transfusion (124). This 7-day interval also coincides with a detectable increase in PGE_2 production that is thought to mediate immunosuppression after transfusion of blood (141).

Blood transfusions reportedly also prime the cytotoxic T-lymphoctye precursor (150) as well as the T-helper precursor compartment (151). However, Sachs (152) suggests that available data cannot discriminate between three mechanisms of possible specific transplantation tolerance: clonal deletion, clonal anergy, or active immunologic suppression.

B. Congenital Immunodeficiency or Immunocompromised Conditions in Patients

An immunological "welcome" to donor lymphocytes can occur whenever a host's (recipient's) own immune system is incapable of satisfactorily resisting the foreign graft, such as during chemotherapy, from underlying disease or other immunosuppression (153). Indeed, TI-GVHD was first reported in an infant with profound congenital immunodeficiency (1) (see Table 2) (3,5,20–23,89–92) and similar reports continue even today (see Table 1) (71–73).

Neonates receiving intrauterine or exchange transfusions are other examples of situations in which TI-GVHD can occasionally be seen with a congenital immunocompromised state (27,28,85–88,154). Maternal transfer of lymphocytes may (155) but usually does not result in GVHD (156) even though maternal lymphocytes can be detected up to 2 years after birth (2).

C. Acquired Conditions of Immunoinsufficiency

1. Hodgkin's Disease

Hodgkin's disease, resulting from derangement in T-cell activity, provides a particularly vulnerable condition for TI-GVHD if unirradiated blood components are used. Reports continue to appear even after recommendations to irradiate cellular blood components for these patients (6,10,16,64–66,89,90).

2. Leukemia and Lymphoma

Severe sustained leukopenia occurring during leukemia or lymphoma chemotherapy and/or radiotherapy renders these patients vulnerable to TI-GVHD. Treatment suppresses not only the marrow but the immune system as well (9,11–15,18,19,29). These patients continue to develop and frequently die from TI-GVHD when unirradiated blood components are used for treatment (6,9,10–13,15–17,64,93–99,157).

3. Other Types of Malignancy

Malignancy may arise as a result of an immune defect, but intensive chemotherapy and/or radiotherapy is more likely the reason for TI-GVHD in the relatively few patients with nonhematological malignancy with this syndrome. Transfusion-induced-GVHD has been reported in persons with neuroblastoma (7,100) and glioblastoma (16), "malignancy" (65), rhabdomyosarcoma (101), and cancers of colonic (56,57), esophageal (42,55), gastric (42), pulmonary (17,53), cervical (48), biliary tree (42,55), epidermal (54), ovarian (53), prostatic (59), and renal (58) origin. Many persons with these malignancies underwent surgery for diagnosis or treatment, so other reasons for immunosuppression may be additive. For example, a homozygous HLA haplotype in a donor that is shared by a heterozygous recipient may be the major determinant in those without chemo- or radiotherapy as the major cause of immunosuppression (Fig. 1) (also see subsequent section regarding immunosuppression during surgery).

4. HIV Infection

No cases of TI-GVHD have been reported in persons with acquired immune deficiency syndrome (AIDS). To prevent TI-GVHD, blood components transfused to patients with AIDS often may be irradiated to prevent its occurrence (158), but it is not clear why these patients do not appear to be susceptible to TI-GVHD. The requirement for host helper T lymphocytes (CD4+) to initiate or complete events necessary for TI-GVHD to occur may be unfulfilled owing to the human immunodeficiency virus (HIV) infection that markedly depletes these cells.

D. Conditions in Which Immunoinsufficiency May Occur

1. Pregnancy

There is conflicting evidence of reduced immune responsiveness during pregnancy (159) to antigens of paternal origin inherited by the fetus. However, at least one case of fatal TI-GVHD has been reported in a pregnant woman thought to have been immunocompetent prior to pregnancy (70). In such instances, the rare chance of HLA haplotype homozygosity contributing to this occurrence can be increased with the use of donors with close blood relationships or in certain ethnic groups.

2. Postoperative States

During major surgery, nonspecific immune suppression may occur, although controversy exists in the literature (44,62,160,161). Surgical stress and induction of anesthesia result in increased endogenous glucocorticoid secretion and subsequent peripheral lymphocyte depletion. Blood loss and blood transfusion depress the immune system during surgery (162), particularly shown by impaired lymphocyte function after open heart surgery (163) and increased susceptibility to infections (164,165). Because of the altered ability of the host's T lymphocytes to resist donor T-cell proliferation, one of the conditions for acute TI-GVHD exists; namely, compromise of the host's immune system (102).

It has been speculated that use of considerable quantities of fresh blood and/or racial homogeneity may be other factors (besides surgical stress and genetic mismatch at HLA) to explain the cases of "postoperative erythrodermia" (POED) in Japan that probably represents TI-GVHD (41). In fact, among Japanese surgery patients, particularly for operations involving cardiopulmonary bypass, the incidence of TI-GVHD is thought to be 1 in 300–400 (44) to 1 in 650 (166), with a mortality of 90%.

Transfusion-induced-GVHD has also been reported in patients of Jewish ancestry transfused during surgery (46,53,54,58,62). Two theories have been proposed to explain these observations: First, immunosuppression occurs as a consequence of surgery (167), and second, HLA homozygosity of the donated lymphocytes may provide a simpler means to initiate GVHD (58,79). There are numerous reports of TI-GVHD when cells for HLA-haplotype homozygotes have been transfused into recipients with shared HLA haplotype but who are heterozygous

(55,56,58,97,168,169). In most cases, the donor is a first-degree family member whose immunocompetent lymphocytes, which are fully accepted by the recipient, mount an immunological attack on the heterozygous HLA haplotype–carrying cells of the recipient (57,61,62,170) (see Fig. 1). A recent report has implicated a second-degree relative (grandchild) (59).

3. Malignancy and Other

Besides the beneficial effect of transfusion on survival of organ grafts (171,172), there is a considerable literature on the possible deleterious effect that "tolerization" by blood transfusion can have on neoplasms. Increasing risk of recurrence of neoplasm (24) and of postoperative infections in patients receiving blood transfusions, reportedly differing for homologous versus autologous transfusion, has been attributed to immunological modulation (163,164,173,174). However, this effect was not verified in persons with cervical cancer who were transfused to >12 g/dl prior to irradiation therapy (175) nor in one patient with recurrent Crohn's disease (176). Homologous plasma has recently been suggested as responsible for the immunological transfusion effect (177); e.g., RBCs resuspended in the additive solution SAG-M do not cause immunosuppression (8).

IV. CLINICAL FEATURES

Transfusion-induced-GVHD probably continues to be underdiagnosed, although exact data are not available. The reasons for underdiagnosis include lack of recognition of the clinical features of this disease, cases where all features are not present or are subclinical in presentation, and the complexity of the clinical conditions for which many patients are transfused. Where TI-GVHD is recognized, the clinical features are reasonably typical.

A. Organs Affected and Onset

The effects of transfusion-induced donor T-lymphocyte engraftment are observed in the skin, gastrointestinal tract (including the liver), thymus, lymph nodes, and bone marrow. The onset of symptoms in a patient with TI-GVHD occurs within 1–2 weeks following transfusion. The initial finding often is a fever, followed or acccompanied by an erythematous skin rash, hepatitis, diarrhea, and pancytopenia. This "syndrome" is frequently attributed clinically to drug sensitivity or to other disease conditions. The features of GVHD are seen as early as 1–3 days after birth in infants whose disease occurs as a result of intrauterine maternal lymphocyte transfer (155).

B. Course and Clinical Staging

The course of disease is almost always inexorable deterioration with marrow aplasia and predictable consequent effects. The likelihood of fatality in TI-GVHD exceeds that following bone marrow transplantation GVHD, probably because of the profound marrow effect in TI-GVHD that is not part of transplantation GVHD. Key differences in the clinical course of TI-GVHD compared with post–bone marrow transplantation GVHD are seen in Table 3. Clinical staging (+ to + + + +) of acute GVHD consists of increasing degrees of severity of involvement of skin, liver (measured by increasing levels of bilirubin), and intestinal tract (volume of diarrhea per day) (Table 4) (112).

Table 3 Key Distinguishing Features of Acute
GVHD After Transfusion (TI) and After Bone
Marrow Transplantation (BMT)

	TI	BMT
Incidence	0.1–1.0%	30–70%
Onset	2–47 days	35–70 days
Pancytopenia	Frequent	Rare
Bone marrow	Hypocellular	Not affected
Duration of illness	<54 days	Months
Mortality	87–100%	5–10%

Table 4 Clinical Staging of Acute GVHD

Stage	Skin	Liver*	Intestinal Tract
+	Maculopapular rash, 25% of body surface	Bilirubin, 34.2–51.3 μmol/L (2.0–3.0 mg/dL)	>0.5 L diarrhea per day
++	Maculopapular rash, 25%–50% of body surface	Bilirubin, 51.3–102.5 μmol/L (3.0–6.0 mg/dL)	>1.0 L diarrhea per day
+++	Generalized erythroderma	Bilirubin, 102.6–256.5 μmol/L (6.0–15.0 mg/dL)	>1.5 L diarrhea per day
++++	Generalized erythroderma with bulla formation and desquamation	Bilirubin, >256.5 μmol/L (>15.0 mg/dL)	Severe abdominal pain, with or without ileus

*Normal range, 2–18 μmol/L (0.1–1.0 mg/dl).
Source: From Ref. 112.

C. Diagnosis

1. Skin Biopsy

The pathological features seen in skin biopsies of patients with TI-GVHD include individual eosinophilic necrosis and dyskeratosis of epidermal cells, satellite cell necrosis, basal lique-faction degeneration, and scanty mononuclear cell infiltration into the dermis (178,179). Suppressor/cytotoxic T lymphocytes have been found to predominate in the epidermis with loss of Langerhans' cells (42). This histopathological picture of TI-GVHD is similar to that seen in toxic epidermal necrolysis (TEN) except that in TEN the majority of infiltrating cells are helper/inducer cells (CD4+) (180) or macrophages (181). Also, in a newborn with congenital anomalies who was HLA-identical to his mother, the skin biopsy showed similar features to GVHD but included a novel T-lymphocyte cell line lacking both CD4 and CD8 (73). A similar reaction is seen in POED (182). Thus, in the proper clinical setting, the pathological changes described support, but are not pathognomic for, the diagnosis of TI-GVHD (93,178,183,184).

2. Cytogenetics and HLA Typing

Diagnosis of TI-GVHD can be demonstrated by cytogenetic or serological studies in the patient. Cytogenetic determination of change in karyotype (XX to XY or vice versa) has been reported (48). Also, HLA typing that documents a change in the phenotype of circulating peripheral lymphocytes, with inconsistencies in the typing with skin fibroblasts or the appearance of chimerism (6,43,46,55,56,61), is currently recommended to establish the diagnosis of TI-GVHD.

3. Thymus

The changes seen in the thymus include an effacement of the medulla, lymphocyte incursion into the medulla, medullary epithelial injury, and an ingress of macrophages laden with nuclear and cellular debris (185). There is increasing experimental evidence that immunodeficiency accompanying GVHD may be the result of injury to thymic epithelium, similar to that seen in the thymic dysplasia of severe combined immunodeficiency. The loss of the maturational microenvironment of the thymus may result in profound and permanent loss of T-cell function (69).

4. Gut

Experimental studies in mice show three alterations: (1) donor T-cell infiltration, both Lyt2+ and L3T4+, predominating in the crypt region; (2) acceleration of the epithelium renewal; and (3) increased epithelial Ia expression (186). Similar histopathological changes have been reported in a person with variable immunodeficiency (52).

V. TREATMENT AND PREVENTION

A. Treatment

Therapeutic interventions for GVHD following transfusion are evolving, benefiting from the more intensive studies relating to GVHD following allogeneic bone marrow transplantation. Recently, thalidomide was granted orphan drug status by the U.S. Food and Drug Administration (FDA) for use in GVHD following allogeneic bone marrow transplantation (187). However, because thalidomide appears to be useful only for *chronic* GVHD, its application in TI-GVHD is unlikely (188). A novel therapy formed by conjugating ricin A with specific monoclonal antibodies looks promising as an anti–T-cell immunotoxin (189).

B. Prevention

For TI-GVHD, although there are some promising new experimental treatments, including use of antithymocyte globulin (45,190), prevention is far more important (191–193). Prevention requires inactivation or removal of immunocompetent lymphocytes from the transfusion component. With irradiation, lymphocytes can be prevented from undergoing mitosis, without which TI-GVHD cannot occur. This destruction of mitotic capability remains the mainstay of most preventive regimens, although controversy about use of irradiation and possible long-term mutagenicity or carcinogenicity of irradiated components remains (194,195). The special needs for transfusion of infants and neonates also require additional data (196–199). A recent report of TI-GVHD following transfusion of blood components irradiated at 2000 rad (20 Gy) is unsettling (200), raising questions about whether 2000 rad is an effective dose or whether irradiation actually occurred and, if so, whether it had been properly delivered.

1. Irradiation

γIrradiation.   Most institutions that irradiate blood components use γ irradiation from specially designed cesium-containing sources or by exposure to cobalt-containing radiation therapy instruments. However, the dose of γ irradiation remains debatable. Reports of successful inhibition of lymphocyte mitosis with doses of 1500–5000 rad (15–50 Gy) can be found. (In a recent survey of blood centers and transfusion services irradiating cellular blood components,

42.3% used 15 Gy, 31.8% used 15.01–25.0 Gy, 22.8% used 25.01–35.0 Gy, and 3.1% used >35.01 Gy) (201).

The adverse effect of the irradiation on other cellular constituents is the subject of ongoing research, for both dose and postirradiation storage stability (62,202–210). Postirradiation RBC damage, evidenced by leakage of intracellular potassium, continue to raise concerns (207).

Despite the publication of standard guidelines for current practice nearly 6 years ago (36,204), at least 31% of institutions responding to a recent survey do not provide irradiated components for recipients with congenital immunodeficiency syndromes, 49% do not irradiate components transfused to persons with leukemia and an astounding 66% do not irradiate blood components transfused to persons with Hodgkin's disease (201). Although the risk may be small (0.5–1.0%) in these clinical conditions, the devastating consequences of TI-GVHD would seem to merit more widespread prevention measures.

Ultraviolet (UV) Irradiation. In murine models, Poljak and Hadzija (211) demonstrated that infusion of mice with UV-irradiated RBCs containing disparate HLA class I antigens resulted in subsequent tolerance of transfused cells, whereas the use of UV-irradiated spleen cells containing different HLA class II antigens elicited not tolerance but rather sensitization. Similar results have been reported in a canine model (212). Platelets UV-irradiated at a dose of 1782 J/m^2 show no loss of activity in vitro (213). How useful UV irradiation will be for routine component preparation to avoid TI-GVHD remains to be seen.

2. Filtration

The alternative to irradiation of blood components is to remove the lymphocytes by physical means; e.g., filtration. Newer methods can achieve a significant (2–3 log) reduction in the lymphocyte count, but this measure has apparently not prevented at least one case of TI-GVHD (67).

Investigators will continue to provide further definition of the intriguing immunological events surrounding TI-GVHD, perhaps even renaming it (214). With better understanding, newer treatments and continued identification of situations that place recipients at risk for this nearly universally fatal disease will evolve (215–217). In the interim, recognition of patients at risk and those situations where donors are more likely to share their HLA homozygous haplotype with a recipient (family donors or persons deliberately selected for provision of HLA-matched apheresis components) should prompt irradiation of cellular blood components to reduce, if not eliminate, the risk of TI-GVHD.

REFERENCES

1. Hathaway WE, Githens JH, Blackburn WR, et al. Aplastic anemia, histiocytosis and erythrodermia in immunologically deficient children. N Engl J Med 1965; 273:953–958.
2. Hutchinson DL, Turner JH, Schlesinger ER. Persistence of donor cells in neonates after fetal and exchange transfusion. Am J Obstet Gynecol 1971; 109:281–284.
3. Roberton NRC, Berry CL, Macaulay JC, Soothill JC. Partial immunodeficiency and graft-versus-host disease. Arch Dis Child 1971; 46:571–574.
4. Schechter GP, Whang-Peng J, McFarland W. Circulation of donor lymphocytes after blood transfusion in man. Blood 1977; 49:651–656.
5. Niethammer D, Goldmann SF, Flad HD, et al. Graft-versus-host reaction after blood transfusions in a patient with cellular immunodeficiency: The role of histocompatibility testing. Eur J Pediatr 1979; 132:43–48.

6. Dinsmore RE, Straus DJ, Pollack MS, et al. Fatal graft-versus-host disease following blood transfusion in Hodgkin's disease documented by HLA typing. Blood 1980; 55:831–834.

7. Woods WG, Lubin BH. Fatal graft versus host disease following a blood transfusion in a child with neuroblastoma. Pediatr 1981; 67:217–221.

8. Nielsen HJ, Hammer JH, Moesgaard F, Kehlet H. Comparison of the effects of SAG-M and whole-blood transfusions on postoperative suppression of delayed hypersensitivity. CJS 1991; 34:146–150.

9. Cohen D, Weinstein H, Mihm M, Yankee R. Nonfatal graft-versus-host disease occurring after transfusion with leukocytes and platelets obtained from normal donors. Blood 1979; 53:1053–1057.

10. von Fliedner V, Higby DJ, Kim U. Graft-versus-host reaction following blood product transfusion. Am J Med 1982; 72:951–961.

11. Ford JM, Lucey JJ, Cullen MH, et al. Fatal graft-versus-host disease following transfusion of granulocytes from normal donors. Lancet 1976; 2:1167–1169.

12. Betzhold J, Hong R. Fatal graft-versus-host disease after a small leukocyte transfusion in a patient with lymphoma and varicella. Pediatrics 1978; 62:63–66.

13. Rosen RC, Huestis DW, Corrigan JJ. Acute leukemia and granulocyte transfusion: Fatal graft-versus-host reaction following transfusion of cells obtained from normal donors. J Pediatr 1978; 93:268–270.

14. Ford JM, Cullen MH, Oliver RTD, Lister TA. Possible prolongation of remission in acute myeloid leukemia by granulocyte transfusions. N Engl J Med 1980; 302: 583–584.

15. Weiden PL, Zuckerman N, Hansen JA, et al. Fatal graft-versus-host disease in a patient with lymphoblastic leukemia following normal granulocyte transfusion. Blood 1981; 57:328–332.

16. Schmidmeier W, Feil W, Gebhart W, et al. Fatal graft-versus-host reaction following granulocyte transfusion. Blut 1982; 45:115–119.

17. Tolbert B, Kaufman CE, Burgdorf WHC, Brubaker D. Graft-versus-host disease from leukocyte transfusions. J Am Acad Dermatol 1983; 9:416–419.

18. Burgess MA, Garson OM. Homologous leukocyte transfusion in acute leukaemia with cytogenetic evidence of a myeloid graft. Med J Aust 1969; 3:1243–1246.

19. Lowenthal RM, Menon C, Challis DR. Graft-versus-host disease in consecutive patients with acute myeloid leukemia treated with blood cells from normal donors. Aust NZ J Med 1981; 11:179–183.

20. Douglas SD, Fudenberg HH. Graft versus host reaction in Wiskott-Aldrich syndrome: Antemortem diagnosis of human GvH in an immunologic deficiency disease. Vox Sang 1969; 16:172–178.

21. Rubinstein A, Radl J, Cottier H, et al. Unusual combined immunodeficiency syndrome exhibiting kappa-IgD paraproteinemia, residual gut-immunity and graft-versus-host reaction after plasma infusion. Acta Paediatr Scand 1973; 62:365–372.

22. Park BH, Good RA, Gate J, Burke B. Fatal graft-vs-host reaction following transfusion of allogeneic blood and plasma in infants with combined immunodeficiency disease. Transplant Proc 1974; 6:385–388.

23. McCarty JR, Raimer SS, Jarratt M. Toxic epidermal necrolysis from graft-vs-host disease: Occurrence in a patient with thymic hypoplasia. Am J Dis Child 1978; 132:282–284.

24. Marsh J, Donnan PT, Hamer-Hodges DW. Association between transfusion with plasma and the recurrence of colorectal carcinoma. Br J Surg 1990; 77:623–626.

25. Crowley JP, Skrabut EM, Valeri DM. Immunocompetent lymphocytes in previously frozen washed red cells. Vox Sang 1974; 26:513–516.

26. Crowley JP, Wade PH, Wish C, Valeri CR. The purification of red cells for transfusion by freeze-preservation and washing. V. Red cell recovery and residual leukocytes after freeze-preservation with high concentrations of glycerol and washing in various systems. Transfusion 1977; 17:1–7.

27. Parkman R, Mosier D, Umansky I, et al. Graft-versus-host disease after intrauterine and exchange transfusions for hemolytic disease of the newborn. N Engl J Med 1974; 290:359–363.

28. Seemayer TA, Bolande RP. Thymic involution mimicking thymic dysplasia. Arch Pathol Lab Med 1980; 104:141–144.

29. Schmitz N, Kayser W, Gassmann W et al. Two cases of graft-versus-host disease following transfusion of nonirradiated blood products. Blut 1982; 44:83–88.
30. Gatti RA, Kersey JH, Yunis EJ, Good RA. Graft-versus-host disease. Prog Clin Pathol 1973; 5:1–18.
31. Brubaker DB. Human post-transfusion graft-versus-host disease. Vox Sang 1983; 45:401–420.
32. Pflieger H. Graft-versus-host disease following blood transfusions. Blut 1983; 46:61–66.
33. Wick MR, Moore SB, Gastineau DA, Hoagland HC. Immunologic, clinical and pathologic aspects of human graft-versus-host disease. Mayo Clin Proc 1983; 58:603–612.
34. Leitman SF, Holland PV. Irradiation of blood products: indications and guidelines. Transfusion 1985; 25:293–300.
35. Brubaker DB. Transfusion-associated graft-versus-host disease. Hum Pathol 1986; 17:1085–1088.
36. Leitman SF. Use of blood cell irradiation in the prevention of posttransfusion graft-vs-host disease. Transfus Sci 1989; 10:219–232.
37. Weiden P. Graft-v-host disease following blood transfusions. Arch Intern Med 1984; 144:1557–1558.
38. Farmer ER, Hood AF. Graft-versus-host disease. In: Fitzpatrick T, Eisen AZ, Wolff K, et al., eds. Dermatology in General Medicine. 3rd ed. New York, McGraw-Hill International, 1986:1344–1352.
39. Gale RP. Graft-versus-host disease. Immunol Rev 1985; 88:193–214.
40. Sullivan KM, Parkman R. The pathophysiology and treatment of graft-versus-host disease. Clin Haematol 1983; 12:775–789.
41. Haga Y, Soma Y, Kawada K, et al. Two cases of postoperative erythroderma. Keio J Med 1989; 38:177–183.
42. Hidano A, Yamashita N, Mizuguchi M, Toyoda H. Clinical, histological, and immunological studies of post-operative erythroderma. J Dermatol 1989; 16:20–30.
43. Sakakibara T, Ida T, Mannouji E, et al. Post-transfusion graft-versus-host disease following open heart surgery. J Cardiovasc Surg 1989; 30:687–691.
44. Sakakibara T, Juji T. Post-transfusion graft-versus-host disease after open heart surgery. Lancet 1986; 2:1099.
45. Prince M, Pedersen JS, Szer J, et al. Transfusion associated graft-versus-host disease after cardiac surgery: Response to antithymocyte-globulin and corticosteroid therapy. Aust NZ J Med 1991; 21:43–46.
46. Thaler M, Shamiss A, Orgad S, et al. The role of blood from HLA-homozygous donors in fatal transfusion-associated graft-versus-host disease after open-heart surgery. N Engl J Med 1989; 321:25–28
47. Arsura EL, Bertelle A, Minkowitz S, et al. Transfusion-associated graft-versus-host disease in a presumed immunocompetent patient. Arch Intern Med 1988; 148:1941–1948.
48. Matsushita H, Shibata Y, Fuse K, et al. Sex chromatin analysis of lymphocytes invading host organs in transfusion-associated graft-versus-host disease. Virchows Archiv B Cell Pathol 1988; 55:237–239.
49. Mori S, Kodo H, Ino T, et al. Postoperative erythrodermia (POED), a type of graft-versus-host reaction (GVHR)? Pathol Res Pract 1989; 184:53–59.
50. Aso T, Asano Y, Harada M, et al. Fatal graft-versus-host disease following transfusion during open heart surgery. Acta Haematol Jpn 1989; 52:1064–1071.
51. Otsuka S, Kunieda K, Hirose M, et al. Fatal erythroderma (suspected graft-versus-host disease) after cholecystectomy. Transfusion 1989; 29:544–548.
52. Lee EY, Clouse RE, Aliperti G, et al. Small intestinal lesion resembling graft-vs-host disease. Arch Pathol Lab Med 1991; 115:529–532.
53. Postmus PE, Mulder NH, Elema JD. Graft versus host disease after transfusions of non-irradiated blood cells in patients having received autologous bone marrow. Eur J Cancer Clin Oncol 1988; 24:889–894.
54. Sakai H, Miyakawa H, Daiguji Y, et al. Hepatic involvement in graft-versus-host disease associated with blood transfusion. Jpn J Med 1990; 29:633–636.
55. Ito K, Yoshida H, Yanagibashi K, et al. Change of HLA phenotype in postoperative erythroderma. Lancet 1988; 1:413–414.

56. Ito K, Fujita M, Morioka M, et al. Postoperative erythroderma with change of HLA phenotypes from heterozygotes to homozygotes: A report of two cases. Eur J Haematol 1991; 46:217–222.

57. Otsuka S, Kunieda K, Kitamura F, et al. The critical role of blood from HLA-homozygous donors in fatal transfusion-associated graft-versus-host disease in immunocompetent patients. Transfusion 1991; 31:260–264.

58. Capon SM, DePond WD, Tyan DB, et al. Transfusion-associated graft-versus-host disease in an immunocompetent patient. Ann Intern Med 1991; 114:1025–1026.

59. Petz LD, Calhoun L, Beedegrun A, et al. Fatal graft-host-versus disease caused by blood transfusion from a second-degree relative; a survey of predisposing factors. JAMA 1992 (submitted).

60. Takahashi K, Juji T, Miyazaki H. Post-transfusion graft-versus-host disease occurring in non-immunosuppressed patients in Japan. Transfus Sci 1991; 12:281–289.

61. Marcus JN. HLA-homozygous donors and transfusion-associated graft-versus-host disease. N Engl J Med 1990; 322:1004–1005.

62. Thaler M, Shamiss A, Orgad S, et al. HLA-homozygous donors and transfusion-associated graft-versus-host disease. N Engl J Med 1990; 322:1006–1007.

63. Suzuki K, Akiyama H, Takamoto S, et al. Transfusion-associated graft-versus-host disease in a presumably immunocompetent patient after transfusion of stored packed red cells. Transfusion 1992; 32:358–360.

64. Ekert H, Waters KD, Smith PJ, et al. Treatment with MOPP or CH1VPP chemotherapy only for all stages of childhood Hodgkin's disease. J Clin Oncol 1988; 6:1845–1850.

65. Decoste SD, Boudreaux C, Dover JS. Transfusion-associated graft-vs-host disease in patients with malignancies. Arch Dermatol 1990; 126:1324–1329.

66. Spitzer TR. Transfusion-induced graft-vs.-host disease. In: Burakoff SJ, Deeg HJ, Ferrara J, Atkinson K, eds. Graft-vs.-Host Disease. New York, Marcel Dekker, 1990:539–555.

67. Akahoshi M, Takanashi M, Masuda M, et al. A case of transfusion-associated graft-versus-host disease not prevented by leukocyte-depletion filters. Transfusion 1992; 32:169–172.

68. Charpentier F, Bracq C, Bonin P, et al. HLA-matched blood products and posttransfusion graft-versus-host disease. Transfusion 1990; 30:850.

69. Gartner JG. Thymic involution with loss of Hassall's corpuscles mimicking thymic dysplasia in a child with transfusion-associated graft-versus-host disease. Pediatr Pathol 1991; 11:449–456.

70. Sheehan T, McLaren KM, Brettle R, Parker AC. Transfusion-induced graft versus host disease in pregnancy. Clin Lab Haematol 1987; 9:205–207.

71. Strobel S, Morgan G, Simmonds AH, Levinsky RJ. Fatal graft versus host disease after platelet transfusions in a child with purine nucleoside phosphorylase deficiency. Eur J Pediatr 1989; 148:312–314.

72. Blomquist MD, Boggards M, Guerra Hanson IC, et al. Monoclonal anti-T cell (T12) antibody treatment of graft-versus-host disease in severe combined immunodeficiency: Targeting of antibody and activation of complement on CD8+ cytotoxic T cell surfaces. J Allergy Clin Immunol 1991; 87:1029–1033.

73. Wirt DP, Brooks EG, Vaidya S, et al. Novel T-lymphocyte population in combined immunodeficiency with features of graft-vs-host disease. N Engl J Med 1989; 321:370–374.

74. Berger RS, Dixon SL. Fulminant transfusion-associated graft-versus-host disease in a premature infant. J Am Acad Dermatol 1989; 20:945–950.

75. Funkhouser AW, Vogelsang G, Zehnbauer B, et al. Graft versus host disease after blood transfusions in a premature infant. Pediatrics 1991; 87:247–249.

76. Hatley RM, Reynolds M, Paller AS, Chou P. Graft-versus-host disease following ECMO. J Pediatr Surg 1991; 26:317–319.

77. Flidel O, Barak Y, Lipschitz-Mercer B, et al. Graft host versus disease in extremely low birth weight neonate. Pediatrics 1992; 80:689–690.

78. Jequier S, Azouz EM. Cholecystitis in an infant with aplastic anemia and graft-versus host reaction. J Clin Ultrasound 1985; 13:424–426.

79. Ray TL. Blood transfusion and graft-vs-host disease. Arch Dermatol 1990; 126:1347–1350.

80. Vogelsang GB. Transfusion-associated graft-versus-host disease in nonimmunocompromised hosts. Transfusion 1990; 30:101–103.

81. Anderson KC, Weinstein HJ. Transfusion-associated graft-versus-host disease. N Engl J Med 1990; 323:315–321.

82. Rappeport JM. Transfusion-associated graft-versus-host disease. Yale J Biol Med 1990; 63:445–454.

83. Hood AF, Vogelsang GB, Black LP, et al. Acute graft-versus-host disease. Arch Dermatol 1987; 123:745–750.

84. Thomas ED, Storb R, Clift RA, et al. Bone-marrow transplantation. N Engl J Med 1975; 292:832–843.

85. Hathaway WE, Brangle RW, Nelson TL, Roeckel IE. Aplastic anemia and alymphocytosis in an infant with hypogammaglobulinemia: Graft-versus-host reaction? J Pediatr 1966; 68:713–722.

86. Bohm N, Klein W, Enzel U. Graft-versus-host in two newborns after repeated blood transfusions because of rhesus incompatibility. Beitr Pathol 1977; 160:381–400.

87. Naiman JL, Punnett HH, Lischner HW, et al. Possible graft-versus-host reaction after intrauterine transfusion for RH erythroblastosis fetalis. N Engl J Med 1969; 281:697–701.

88. Lauer BA, Githens JH, Hayward AR, et al. Probable graft-vs-graft reaction in an infant after exchange transfusion and marrow transplantation. Pediatrics 1982; 70:43–47.

89. Brubaker DB. Fatal graft-vs-host disease occurring after transfusion with unirradiated normal donor red cells in an immunodeficient neonate. Plasma Ther Transfus Technol 1984; 5:117–125.

90. Jacobs JC, Blanc WA, de Capoa A, et al. Complement deficiency and chromosomal breaks in a case of Swiss-type agammaglobulinemia. Lancet 1968; 1:499–503.

91. Gatti RA, Platt N, Pomerance HH, et al. Hereditary lymphopenic agammaglobulinemia associated with a distinctive form of short-limbed dwarfism and ectodermal dysplasia. J Pediatr 1969; 75:675–684.

92. Hathaway WE, Fulginiti VA, Pierce CW, et al. Graft-vs-host reaction following single blood transfusion. JAMA 1967; 201:139–144.

93. Burns LJ, Westberg MW, Burns CP, et al. Acute graft-versus-host disease resulting from normal donor blood transfusions. Acta Haematol 1984; 71:270–276.

94. Kessenger A, Armitage JO, Klassen LW, et al. Graft versus host disease following transfusion of normal blood products to patients with malignancies. J Surg Oncol 1987; 36:206–209.

95. De Dobbeleer GD, Ledouz-Corbusier MH, Achten GA. Graft-versus-host reaction. An ultrastructural study. Arch Dermatol 1975; 111:1597–1602.

96. Nikoskelainen J, Soederstrom K-O, Rajamaki A, et al. Graft-versus-host reaction in 3 adult leukemia patients after transfusion of blood cell products. Scand J Haematol 1983; 31:403–409.

97. Siimes MA, Koskimies S. Chronic graft-versus-host disease after blood transfusions confirmed by incompatible HLA antigens in bone marrow. Lancet 1982; 1:42–43.

98. Salfner B, Borberg H, Kruger G, et al. Graft-versus-host reaction following granulocyte transfusion from a normal donor. Blut 1978; 36:27–34.

99. Mutasim DF, Badr K, Saab G, Kurban AK. Graft-versus-host disease in a patient with acute lymphoblastic lymphoma. Cutis 1984; 33:206–210.

100. Kennedy JS, Ricketts RR. Fatal graft v host disease in a child with neuroblastoma following a blood transfusion. J Pediatr Surg 1986; 21:1108–1109.

101. Labotka RJ, Radvany R. Graft-versus-host disease in rhabdomyosarcoma following transfusion with nonirradiated blood products. Med Pediatr Oncol 1985; 13:101–104.

102. Arcura E, Bertelle A. Pathogenesis of acute graft-versus-host disease after open heart surgery. Med. Hypoth 1990; 31:39–42.

103. Ghayur T, Seemayer TA, Kongshavn PA, et al. Graft-versus-host reactions in the beige mouse: An investigation of the role of host and donor natural killer cells in the pathogenesis of graft-versus-host disease. Transplantation 1987; 44:261–267.

104. Billingham RE. The biology of graft-versus-host reactions. Harvey Lect 1968; 62:21–78.

105. Barnes DW, Loutit JF. Spleen protection: the cellular hypothesis. In: Bacq ZM, Alexander P, eds.

Proceedings of the Symposium held at Lidege. August–September 1954. New York, Academic Press, 1955; 134–135.

106. Fowler R, Schubert WK, West CD. Acquired partial tolerance to homologous skin grafts in the human infant at birth. Ann NY Acad Sci 1960; 87:403–428.

107. van Bekkum DW. Transfusion or transplantation? Isra J Med Sci 1965; 5:879–882.

108. Mulder NH, Elema JD, Postmus PE. Transfusion associated graft-versus-host disease in authologous bone marrow transplantation. Lancet 1989; 1:735–736.

109. Gleichmann E, Pals ST, Rolink AG, et al., Graft-versus-host reactions: Clues to the etiopathology of a spectrum of immunological diseases. Immunol Today 1984; 5:324–332.

110. Lapp WS, Ghayur T, Mendes M, et al. Functional and histological basis for graft-versus-host induced immunosuppression. Immunol Rev 1985; 88:107–133.

111. Levine S, Iwahara M. Graft-versus-host disease produced with whole blood: Enhancement by pertussis vaccination of donors. Transplantation 1969; 8:462–465.

112. Kirkpatrick CH. Transplantation immunology. JAMA 1987; 258:2993–3000.

113. Korngold R, Sprent J. Surface markers of T cells causing lethal graft-vs-host disease to Class I vs Class II H-2 differences. J Immunol 1985; 135:3004–3010.

114. Korngold R, Sprent J. T cell subsets and graft-versus-host disease. Transplantation 1987; 44:335–339.

115. Rolink AG, Gleichmann E. Allosuppressor-and allohelper-T cells in acute and chronic graft-vs-host (GVH) disease. III. Different Lyt subsets of donor T cells induced different pathological syndromes. J Exp Med 1983; 158:546–558.

116. Ferrara JLM, Burakoff HJ. Introduction. In: Burakoff SJ, Deeg HJ, Ferrara J, Atkinson K, eds. Graft-vs.-Host Disease. New York, Marcel Dekker, 1990:3–8.

117. Beavis MJ, Ross WB, Williams JD, Salaman JR. Blood transfusion and prostaglandin production by rat peritoneal macrophages. Surg Res Commun 1989; 6:223–229.

118. Elie R, Lapp WS. Graft versus host-induced immunosuppression: Mechanism of depressed T-cell helper function in vitro. Cell Immunol 1977; 34:38–48.

119. Ghayur T, Seemayer TA, Lapp WS. Histologic correlates of immune functional deficits in graft-vs.-host disease. In: Burakoff SJ, Deeg HJ, Ferrara J, Atkinson K, eds. Graft-vs.-Host Disease. New York, Marcel Dekker, 1990:109–132.

120. Stutman O, Yunis EJ, Teague PO, Good RA. Graft-versus-host reactions induced by transplantation of parental strain thymus in neonatally thymectomized F_1 hybrid mice. Transplantation 1968; 6:514–523.

121. Chambers LA, Garcia LW. White blood cell content of transfusion components. Lab Med 1991; 22:857–860.

122. Huang SW, Ammann AJ, Levy RL, et al. Treatment of severe combined immunodeficiency by a small number of pretreated nonmatched marrow cells. Transplantation 1973; 15:174–176.

123. McCullough J, Yunis EJ, Benson SJ, Quie PG. Effect of blood bank storage on leukocyte function. Lancet 1969; 2:1333–1335.

124. Schechter GP, Soehnlen F, McFarland W. Lymphocyte response to blood transfusion in man. N Engl J Med 1972; 287:1169–1173.

125. Hansen JA, Good RA, Dupont B. HLA-D compatibility between parent and child. Transplantation 1977; 23:366–374.

126. DePalma L, Duncan B, Chan MM, Luban NLC. The neonatal immune response to washed and irradiated cells: Lack of evidence of lymphocyte activation. Transfusion 1991; 31:737–742.

127. Petrakis NL, Politis G. Prolonged survival of viable, mitotically competent mononuclear leukocytes in stored whole blood. N Engl J Med 1962; 267:286–289.

128. Polesky HF, Helgeson M. Viability of lymphocytes in stored blood: Response to phytohemagglutinin and to allogeneic leukocytes. J Lab Clin Med 1970; 76:134– 140.

129. Harada M, Matsue K, Mori T, et al. Viability of lymphocytes in stored blood: their surface markers, mitogenic responses and MLC reactivity. Acta Haematol Jpn 1979; 42:30–34.

130. Dossetor JP, MacKinnon KJ, Gault MH, MacLean LD. Cadaver kidney transplants. Transplantation 1957; 5:844–853.

131. Morris PJ, Ting A, Stocker J. Leukocyte antigens in renal transplantation. 1. The paradox of blood transfusions in renal transplantation. Med J Aust 1968; 2:1088–1090.

132. Opelz G, Sengar DPS, Mickey MR, et al. Effect of blood transfusions on subsequent kidney transplants. Transplant Proc 1973; 5:253–259.
133. Opelz G, Terasaki PI. Improvement of kidney-graft survival with increased numbers of blood transfusions. N Engl J Med 1978; 299:799–803.
134. Ratner LE, Hadley GA, Hanto DW, Mohanakumar T. Immunology of renal allograft rejection. Arch Pathol Lab Med 1991; 115:283–287.
135. Singal DP, Fagnilli L, Joseph S. Blood transfusions induce antiidiotypic antibodies in renal transplant patients. Transplant Proc 1983; 15:1005–1008.
136. Terasaki P. The beneficial transfusion effect on kidney graft survival attributed to clonal deletion. Transplantation 1984; 37:119–125.
137. van Twuyver E, Mooijaart RJD, ten Berge IJM, et al. Pretransplantation blood transfusion revisited. N Engl J Med 1991; 325:1210–1213.
138. Qin S, Cobbold S, Benjamin R, Waldmann H. Induction of classical transplantation tolerance in the adult. J Exp Med 1989; 169:779–794.
139. Knulst AC, Bril-Bazuin C, Ruizeveld de Winter JA, Benner R. Suppression of graft versus host reactivity by a single host-specific blood transfusion to prospective donors of hemopoietic cells. Transplant Proc 1990; 22:1975–1976.
140. Knulst AC, Bril-Bazuin C, Savelkoul HFJ, Benner R. Suppression of graft-versus-host reactivity by a single host-specific blood transfusion to prospective donors of hemopoietic cells. Transplantation 1991; 52:534–539.
141. Shelby J, Maruschack MN, Nelson EW. Prostaglandin production and suppressor cell induction in transfusion-induced immune suppression. Transplantation 1987; 43:113–116.
142. Ross WB, Leaver HA, Yap PL, et al. Prostaglandin E_2 production by rat peritoneal macrophages: Role of cellular and humoral factors in vivo in transfusion-associated immunosuppression. FEMS Microb Immunol 1990; 64:321–326.
143. Kalechman Y, Gafter U, Sobelman D, Sredni B. The effect of a single whole-blood transfusion on cytokine secretion. J Clin Immunol 1990; 10:99–105.
144. Terness P, Kisiel U, Suesal C, Opelz G. Prevention of sensitization by transfusion with antibody-coated blood cells: specificity of suppression and transfer with serum or spleen cells. Transplant Proc 1987; 19:1414–1419.
145. Shelby J. Transfusion-induced immunosuppression. J Burn Care Rehab 1987; 8:546–548.
146. Shelby J, Marushack MM, Nelson EW. Effect of prostaglandin inhibitors on transfusion-induced immune suppression. Transplant Proc 1987; 19:1435–1436.
147. Hutchinson IV, Morris PJ. The role of major and minor histocompatibility antigens in active enhancement of rat kidney allograft survival by blood transfusion. Transplantation 1986; 41:166–170.
148. Lagaija EL, Hennemann PH, Ruigrok M, et al. Effect of one-HLA-DR-antigen-matched and completely HLA-DR–mismatched blood transfusions on survival of heart and kidney allografts. N Engl J Med 1989; 321:701–705.
149. van Rood JJ, Claas FHJ. The influence of allogeneic cells on the human T and B cell repertoire. Science 1990; 248:1388–1393.
150. Vandekerckhove BAE, van Bree S, Zhang L, et al. Increase of donor-specific cytotoxic T lymphocyte precursors after transfusion. Transplantation 1990; 48:672–675.
151. Vandekerckhove BAE, Datema G, Zantvoort F, Claas FHJ. An increase of donor-specific T helper precursors resulting from blood transfusions. Transplantation 1990; 48:987–991.
152. Sachs DH. Specific transplantation tolerance. N Engl J Med 1991; 325:1240–1241.
153. Hong R, Gatti RA, Good RA. Hazards and potential benefits of blood transfusion in immunological deficiency. Lancet 1968; 1:388–389.
154. Editorial. Lymphocyte hazards to the fetus. Lancet 1974; 1:718.
155. Grogan TM, Odom RB, Burgess JH. Graft-vs-host reaction. Arch Dermatol 1977; 113:806–812.
156. Githens JH, Muschenheim F, Fulginiti VA, et al. Thymic alymphoplasia with XX/XY lymphoid chimerism secondary to probable maternal-fetal transfusion. Pediatrics 1969; 75:87–94.
157. Berkel AI, Tinaztepe K. Graft-versus-host reaction manifested as toxic epidermal necrolysis in a patient with acute leukemia. Turk J Pediatr 1981; 23:37–41.

158. Mayer K. Transfusion of the patient with acquired immunodeficiency syndrome. Arch Pathol Lab Med 1990; 114:295–297.

159. Alanen A, Lassila O. Cell-mediated immunity in normal pregnancy and pre-eclampsia. J Reprod Immunol 1982; 4:349–354.

160. McLoughlin GA, Wu AV, Saporoschetz I, et al. Correlation between anergy and a circulating immunosuppressive factor following major surgical trauma. Ann Surg 1979; 190:297–303.

161. Quintiliani L, Buzzonetti A, DiGirolamo M, et al. Effects of blood transfusion on the immune responsiveness and survival of cancer patients: A prospective study. Transfusion 1991; 31:713–718.

162. Pollock R, Ames F, Rubio P, et al. Protracted severe immune dysregulation induced by cardiopulmonary bypass: a predisposing etiologic factor in blood transfusion-related AIDS. J Clin Lab Immunol 1987; 22:1–5.

163. van Velzen-Blad H, Dijkstra YJ, Heijnen CJ, et al. Cardiopulmonary bypass and host defense functions in human beings: II. Lymphocyte function. Ann Thorac Surg 1985; 39:212–217.

164. Tartter PI. Blood transfusion and infectious complications following colorectal cancer surgery. Br J Surg 1988; 75:789–792.

165. Murphy P, Heal JM, Blumberg N. Infection or suspected infection after hip replacement surgery with autologous or homologous blood transfusions. Transfusion 1991; 31:212–217.

166. Juji T, Takahashi K, Shibata Y, et al. Post-transfusion graft-versus-host disease in immuno-competent patients after cardiac surgery in Japan. N Engl J Med 1989; 321:56.

167. Slade MS, Simmons RL, Yunis E, Greenberg LJ. Immunodepression after major surgery in normal patients. Surgery 1975; 78:363–372.

168. Fagiolo E, D'Addosio AM. Post transfusion graft-versus-host disease (GVHD): Immunopathology and prevention. Haematology 1985; 70:62–74.

169. Kruskall MS, Alper CA, Awdeh Z, Yunis EJ. HLA-homozygous donors and transfusion-associated graft-versus-host disease. N Engl J Med 1990; 322:1005–1006.

170. Vogelsang GB. Graft-versus-host disease. Curr Opin Oncol 1990; 2:285–288.

171. Knulst AC, Bazuin C, Benner R. Transfusion-induced suppression of delayed-type hypersensitivity to allogeneic histocompatibility antigens. Transplantation 1989; 48:829–833.

172. Brunson ME, Alexander JW. Mechanisms of transfusion-induced immunosuppression. Transfusion 1990; 30:651–658.

173. Blumberg N, Heal JM. Transfusion and recipient immune function. Arch Pathol Lab Med 1989; 113:246–253.

174. Donnelly PK, Proud G, Shenton BK, Taylor RMR. Transfusion-induced immunosuppression and red cell clearance. Transfus Med 1991; 1:217–221.

175. Busch RS, Jenkin RD, Allt WE, Beale FA. Definitive evidence for hypoxic cells influencing cure in cancer therapy. Br J Cancer 37(suppl):302–306.

176. Scott ADN, Ritchie JK, Phillips RKS. Blood transfusion and recurrent Crohn's disease. Br J Surg 1991; 78:455–458.

177. Blumberg N, Heal JM. Perioperative blood transfusion and solid tumor recurrence—A review. Cancer Invest 1987; 5:615–625.

178. Sale GE, Lerner KG, Barker EA, et al. The skin biopsy in the diagnosis of acute graft-versus-host disease in man. Am J Pathol 1977; 89:621–633.

179. Spielvogel RL, Ullman S, Goltz RW. Skin changes in graft-vs-host disease. South Med J 1976; 69:1277–1281.

180. Merot Y, Gravallese E, Guillen FJ, Murphy GF. Lymphocyte subsets and Langerhans' cells in toxic epidermal necrolysis. Arch Dermatol 1986; 122:455–458.

181. Roujeau JC, Dubertret L, Moritz S, et al. Involvement of macrophages in the pathology of toxic epidermal necrolysis. Br J Dermatol 1985; 113:425–430.

182. Mori S, Kodo H, Ino T, et al. Postoperative erythrodermia (POED), a type of graft-versus-host reaction (GVHR). Pathol Res Pract 1989; 184:53–59.

183. Elliott CJ, Sloane JP, Sanderson KV, et al. The histological diagnosis of cutaneous graft versus host disease: Relationship of skin changes to marrow purging and other clinical variables. Histopathology 1987; 11:145–155.

184. LeBoit PE. Transfusion-associated graft-versus-host disease. Hum Pathol 1987; 18:414–415.
185. Seemayer TA, Lapp WS, Bolande RP. Thymic epithelial injury in graft-versus-host reactions following adrenalectomy. Am J Pathol 1978; 93:325–338.
186. Guy-Grand D, Vasalli P. Gut injury in mouse graft-versus-host reaction: Study of its occurrence and mechanisms. J Clin Invest 1986; 77:1584–1595.
187. Kaitlin KI. Graft-versus-host disease [letter]. N Engl J Med 1991; 325:357–358.
188. Ferrara JLM, Deeg HJ. Graft-versus-host disease. N Engl J Med 1991; 324:667–674.
189. Medical News and Perspectives. Application considered for immunotoxin in treatment of graft-vs.-host disease. JAMA 1991; 265:2041.
190. Wood PMD, Proctor SJ. The potential use of thalidomide in the therapy of graft-versus-host disease—A review of clinical and laboratory information. Leuk Res 1990; 14:395–399.
191. Holland PV. Transfusion-associated graft-versus-host disease: Prevention using irradiated blood products. In: Garraty G, ed. Current Concepts in Transfusion Therapy. Arlington, VA, American Association of Blood Banks, 1985:295–315.
192. Holland PV. Prevention of transfusion-associated graft-vs-host disease. Arch Pathol Lab Med 1989; 113:285–291.
193. Moroff G, Luban NLC. Prevention of transfusion-associated graft-versus-host disease. Transfusion 1992; 32:102–103.
194. Avoy DR. Transfusion-associated graft-versus-host disease in nonimmunocompromised hosts. Transfusion 1990; 30:849.
195. Lind SE. Has the case for irradiating blood products been made? Am J Med 1985; 78:543–544.
196. LeBlanc MH. Transfusion-associated graft-versus-host disease. J Am Acad Dermatol 1990; 6:1121–1122.
197. Luban NLC, Ness PM. Comment. Transfusion 1985; 25:301–303.
198. Sanders MR, Graeber JE. Posttransfusion graft-versus-host disease in infancy. J Pediatr 1990; 117:159–163.
199. Strauss RG, Barnes A, Blanchette VS, et al. Directed and limited-exposure blood donations for infants and children. Transfusion 1990; 30:68–72.
200. Drobyski W, Thibodeau S, Truitt RL, Baxter-Lowe LA. Third-party–mediated graft rejection and graft-versus-host disease after T-cell depleted bone marrow transplantation, as demonstrated by hypervariable DNA probes and HLA-DR polymorphism. Blood 1989; 74:2285–2294.
201. Anderson KC, Goodnough LT, Sayers M, et al. Variation in blood component irradiation practice: Implications for prevention of transfusion-associated graft-versus-host disease. Blood 1991; 77:2096–2102.
202. Linden JV, Pisciotto PT. Transfusion-associated graft-versus-host disease and blood irradiation. Transfus Med Rev 1992; 6:116–123.
203. Valerius NH, Johansen KS, Nielsen OS, et al. Effect of in vitro x-irradiation on lymphocyte and granulocyte function. Scand J Haematol 1981; 27:9–18.
204. Pritchard SL, Rogers PCJ. Rationale and recommendations for the irradiation of blood products. CRC Crit Rev Oncol Hematol 1987; 7:115–124.
205. Read EJ, Kodis C, Carter CS, Leitman SF. Viability of platelets following storage in the irradiated state. A pair-controlled study. Transfusion 1988; 28:446–450.
206. Moroff G, George VM, Siegl AM, Luban NL. The influence of irradiation on stored platelets. Transfusion 1986; 26:453–456.
207. Ramirez AM, Woodfield DG, Scott R, McLachlan J. High potassium levels in stored irradiated blood. Transfusion 1987; 27:444–445.
208. Button LN, DeWolf WC, Newburger PE, et al. The effects of irradiation on blood components. Transfusion 1981; 21:419–426.
209. Sazama K. The unfolding saga of blood irradiation. J Lab Clin Med 1990; 116:757–758.
210. Prodouz KN, Habraken JW, Moroff G. Resistance of platelet proteins to effects of ionizing radiation. J Lab Clin Med 1990; 116:766–770.
211. Poljak-Blazi M, Hadzija M. Role of class I and class II antigens in specific immunosuppression after transfusion of UV-radiated blood. Transplant Proc 1987; 19:4279–4280.

212. Deeg JH. Ultraviolet irradiation in transplantation biology. Manipulation of immunity and immunogenicity. Transplantation 1988; 45:845–851.

213. Kahn RA, Duffy BF, Rodey GG. Ultraviolet irradiation of platelet concentrate abrogates lymphocyte activation without affecting platelet function in vitro. Transfusion 1985; 25:547–550.

214. Bos GMJ, Majoor GD, van Breda Vriesman PJC. Graft-versus-host disease: the need for a new terminology. Immunol Today 1990; 11:433–435.

215. Anderson KC. Current Trends: evolving concepts in transfusion medicine. Transfusion-associated graft-versus-host disease: who is at risk? Transfus Sci 1991; 12:277–279.

216. Editorial. Transfusions and graft-versus-host disease. Lancet 1989; 1:529–530.

217. Meryman HT. Transfusion-induced alloimmunization and immunosuppression and the effects of leukocyte depletion. Transfus Med Rev 1989; 3:180–193.

23

Retroviral Infections and the Immune Response

HARRY E. PRINCE
American Red Cross Blood and Tissue Services
Los Angeles, California

I INTRODUCTION

Few infectious agents have had as profound an impact on the practice of transfusion medicine as human retroviruses. When it was realized in the early 1980s that human immunodeficiency virus-1 (HIV), the causative agent for acquired immune deficiency syndrome (AIDS), could be transmitted by transfusion of both cells and plasma products, transfusion scientists were forced to rethink many issues. These issues included questioning donors about lifestyle and sexual practices, implementation of new testing procedures, legal liabilities, and ethical responsibilities. A few years later, it was found that human T lymphotropic virus (HTLV), a retrovirus associated with malignancy and a neurological disorder, could also be transmitted by tranfusion. Although lessons learned from HIV were applied to HTLV in relation to transfusion medicine, this discovery nevertheless added to the complexities of supplying quality transfusion products.

Thanks in part to studies conducted by transfusion scientists in an effort to understand and eliminate transmission of these newly described infectious agents, there has been an explosion of information on the epidemiology, molecular biology, and immunology of human retroviruses. The focus of this chapter is the immune response in relation to HIV and HTLV infections. Three major issues are covered: the immune response induced by infection with HIV and HTLV, the detrimental effects of these viruses on immune system cells and their function, and the unique ability of the viruses to utilize components of a normal immune response to promote their own replication.

II. HIV INFECTION AND THE IMMUNE RESPONSE

A. Background

Infection with HIV eventually leads to destruction of the immune system, which allows the development of opportunistic infections and malignancies that are responsible for the mortality of infected individuals. The cellular reservoir for HIV is CD4-bearing cells, which include CD4 (helper/inducer) T lymphocytes and monocytes/macrophages. Virus-related destruction of CD4

T cells is the hallmark immunological change in HIV infection. Loss of CD4 cells is primarily responsible for the reduction of immune system recognition of and reactivity to other infectious agents that characterizes HIV infection (1).

AIDS was first identified in homosexually active men, and was then quickly recognized in transfusion and plasma product recipients. Transfusion of cell-associated HIV appears to be the major mode of transfusion-associated transmission. However, free virus is also infectious, and appears to be the mode of transmission reponsible for infection in recipients of plasma products (2). HIV-infected individuals almost always develop antibodies against viral proteins soon after infection. Blood centers thus routinely screen donated products for the presence of HIV antibodies, and any reactive products are destroyed.

B. Antibody Response to HIV

Individuals infected with HIV generally produce antibodies reactive with all of the HIV gene products identified. These include envelope proteins (gp41, gp120, gp160), core proteins (p15, p18, p24, p55), reverse transcriptase (*pol* gene product, generally referred to as p66/51), and regulatory gene products (3' orf, sor, tat-III) (3,4). Not surprisingly, envelope proteins are the antigens most consistently recognized by antibodies found in infected individuals (5,6).

Antibodies recognizing HIV are almost always detectable within 2 months of infection (3). Early studies following antibody responses in individuals with symptoms of primary HIV infection showed that antibodies recognizing both envelope and core proteins appear at about the same time; however, antibody-detection methods differ with regard to the antigens recognized in the first few weeks following primary infection. Generally, antibodies against envelope proteins are first detectable by radioimmunoprecipitation assays (RIPAs), whereas those against core proteins are first detectable by Western blot analysis (3). By 3 months after infection, however, antibodies recognizing both envelope and core proteins are usually detectable by Western blot analysis. The failure to detect antienvelope responses by Western blot in early infection appears to represent a technical problem in preparing blots from viral lysates; Burke et al. (7) have shown that serum samples collected early in infection that were RIPA-positive but Western blot negative for antibodies to envelope proteins were reactive in a Western blot utilizing a cloned envelope protein.

Although a robust antibody response to HIV proteins occurs following infection, the infection persists, thus indicating that the antibodies produced are, in the long-run, unprotective. However, several groups of investigators have identified low levels of antibodies that neutralize HIV infectivity in vitro (8–10). The vast majority of neutralizing antibodies are directed against the outer envelope protein (gp120) (8–10). Whether or not HIV-neutralizing antibodies play any role in retarding disease progression remains unclear; there appears to be a weak trend toward decreasing levels of neutralizing antibodies and advancing disease, but there are many exceptions (11). Characterization of neutralizing antibody responses appears to be of greater importance from the standpoint of development of a vaccine against HIV. Identification of the gp120 epitopes most important for inducing neutralizing antibodies is a major focus for researchers constructing HIV vaccines (12).

An aspect of the antibody response to HIV that may prove important in treatment and the development of a vaccine is the disappearance of certain antibody specificities with disease progression. For example, the prevalence of antibodies recognizing p24, the major core protein, decreases with disease progression (13–15). This decrease occurs concomitantly with an increase in the level of p24 antigen detectable in the circulation. The relationship between these changes remains unclear; the p24 antigenemia may interfere with the detection of p24 antibody, or the appearance of antigen may reflect decreased or discontinued production of anti-p24 with disease progression. If the latter explanation holds true, then maintenance of antibodies to p24 in infected individuals may be a goal of treatment therapies.

Similarly, antibodies that inhibit the activity of the HIV reverse transcriptase (RT) are found in essentially all asymptomatic HIV-infected individuals, but few patients with AIDS (15–17). In a 3-year longitudinal study of asymptomatic HIV-infected individuals with antibodies inhibiting RT activity, the development of AIDS was preceded by the loss of anti-RT activity (16). This decline in anti-RT activity did not reflect a general decline in antibodies recognizing the RT molecule; RT–immunoglobulin G (IgG) binding, as measured by RIPAs, did not correlate with IgG inhibition of RT activity. Likewise, there was no correlation between titers of antibodies recognizing virion structural proteins and antibodies inhibiting RT activity (15,17). Thus, it appears that reduced anti-RT activity does not merely reflect a general loss of antibody production capacity. As with p24, maintainance of anti-RT activity may prove important in arresting HIV disease progression.

Warren et al. (18), utilizing synthetic peptides to measure antibodies reactive with specific epitopes of the envelope protein (gp160), have found that the percentage of sera reactive with weakly immunogenic gp160 epitopes decreased with disease progression. In contrast, the percentage of sera reactive with immunodominant (strongly immunogenic) gp160 epitopes was unchanged. Thus, a "narrowing" of the humoral immune response to envelope protein epitopes occurs with progression of disease. This general phenomenon may also explain partially the similar findings for p24 and RT activity noted previously. As Warren et al. speculate (18), these changes may reflect decreased T-cell help for antibody production by B cells, caused in turn by impairments in T-helper (CD4) cell function (see Sect. II.F).

An aspect of the antibody response to HIV that is particularly pertinent to transfusion scientists is false-positive tests for antibodies recognizing HIV proteins. Thus, sera from some individuals are repeatedly reactive by enzyme immunoassays for antibodies recognizing HIV, but Western blot analysis reveals an indeterminate pattern. In most cases, this indeterminant pattern reflects reactivity with HIV core proteins only (19–21). Extensive studies (21,22) indicate the absence of true HIV infection in these individuals. The antibodies detected are apparently cross-reactive, but the antigens responsible for their induction remain undefined.

C. B-Cell Alterations

Although B lymphocytes are apparently not directly infected by HIV, a convincing body of work indicates that B cells are altered in association with HIV infection. A summary of the indicators of B-cell changes in HIV infection are listed in Table 1. Hypergammaglobulinemia was recognized early in the AIDS epidemic and, in general, reflects polyclonal increases in the levels of IgG and IgA (23,24). Hypergammaglobulinemia apparently reflects polyclonal activation of B cells; in support of this hypothesis, the level of B cells spontaneously secreting

Table 1 B-Cell Alterations in HIV Infection

Hypergammaglobulinemia (IgG, IgA)
Increased levels of B cells spontaneously secreting immunoglobulin
Increased levels of circulating immune complexes
Follicular hyperplasia characteristic of lymphadenopathy
Increased B-cell size
Increased percentage of activated B cells (CD71+)
Decreased percentage of resting B cells (LECAM-1+)
Increased percentage of immature B cells (CD10+)
Increased levels of autoantibodies
Decreased B-cell proliferative response to mitogens

immunoglobulin in vitro is elevated in association with HIV infection (23–25). Hypersecretion of immunoglobulin by B cells is in turn associated with increased levels of circulating immune complexes in HIV infection (26). Some of these complexes contain IgG, some contain IgA, and some contain both IgG and IgA. There also is evidence that the follicular hyperplasia characteristic of HIV-related lymphadenopathy syndrome is associated with hypersecretion of immunoglobulin by lymph node B cells (26).

Several other changes are also consistent with polyclonal B cell activation in HIV infection. Martinez-Maza et al. (25) found that there was an increase in B-cell size; further, the percentage of B cells expressing transferrin receptor (CD71, a marker of activated B cells) was increased, whereas the percentage of B cells expressing Leu-8 (LECAM-1, characteristic of resting, unactivated, B cells) was decreased. Autoantibodies such as rheumatoid factor and antinuclear antibodies are present in about 30% of sera from patients with AIDS (23); the production of such antibodies is usually indicative of polyclonal B-cell activation. In addition, autoantibodies recognizing both B and T lymphocytes are present in some HIV-infected persons (27). B cells from HIV-infected individuals generally exhibit decreased proliferative responses to B-cell mitogens like pokeweed mitogen and *Staphylococcus aureus* Cowan strain A (23). It is believed that this defect represents the inability to further stimulate B cells already stimulated in vivo.

The compelling data demonstrating polyclonal B cell activation in HIV infection in the absence of direct infection of B cells by the virus suggested that some component of the virus was able to interact with B cells without infecting them. A series of elegant studies by Fauci's group (28) confirmed this hypothesis. These investigators showed that B cells were directly activated by HIV proteins. Activation was apparent in assays measuring B-cell proliferation, as well as in assays measuring immunoglobulin production. Direct activation of B cells by viral proteins thus appears to account for most of the B-cell changes in HIV infection.

A somewhat surprising finding by Martinez-Maza et al. (25) was increased levels of B cells expressing CD10, a marker of immature B cells, in HIV infection. These investigators speculate that depletion of the pool of resting B cells by polyclonal activation induces a compensatory homeostatic release of immature B cells into the circulation. Although direct experimental evidence is lacking, it is conceivable that polyclonal activation of these immature B cells may be related to the increased frequency of B-cell lymphomas observed in patients with AIDS (25).

D. Non–MHC-Restricted Cytotoxicity

Another population of lymphocytes that exhibits alterations in HIV infection, even though they are not apparently infected by the virus, is the CD16+CD3– population, generally referred to as the natural killer (NK) cell subset. This subset can mediate two forms of cytolytic activity, neither of which involves sharing of major histocompatibility complex (MHC) antigens on effector and target cells. One form of activity is classic NK activity, which is represented by spontaneous lysis of a variety of malignant and virus-infected targets; this activity appears to be an important arm of the immune surveillance system against spontaneously arising tumors (29). Natural killer cells also mediate a second form of cytolytic activity, called antibody-dependent cellular cytotoxicity (ADCC), which requires an antibody bridge between the target cell and the NK cell. The Fab regions of the antibody recognizes antigens on the target cell, whereas the Fc region of the antibody interacts with a low-affinity Fc receptor (CD16) on the NK cell (29,30).

Because viral infections are prevalent in advancing HIV disease, several groups of investigators have characterized NK cell cytotoxicity in HIV infection. Plaeger-Marshall et al. (31) found that NK activity was intact in asymptomatic HIV-infected persons but decreased in patients with AIDS and AIDS-related complex (ARC). This defect appeared to be qualitative in nature because the levels of circulating CD16+ lymphocytes were normal in AIDS and ARC patients. These findings have been corroborated in several other studies (32–35).

The mechanism responsible for defective NK activity in HIV infection does not appear to reflect defective target cell recognition. Bonavida's group (35) at the University of California at Los Angeles have shown that the target cell–binding capacity of NK cells is intact in HIV infection. Low NK activity was rather due to defective triggering of NK cells to release their soluble cytolytic component, NK cytotoxic factor. As will be discussed below, ADCC activity of these cells was normal, indicating that their lytic mechanism was intact but not triggered by NK targets. Sirianni et al. (36) further suggest that the NK cytotoxic defect is due to an HIV-induced defect in mobilization of membrane cytoskeleton components in NK cells. They found that, under normal circumstances, polarization of tubulin occurs in both NK cells and target cells at the site of effector-target interaction. In contrast, when NK cells from HIV-infected individuals were used, no polarization of tubulin was observed in either the effector or target cell populations. The mechanism by which tubulin rearrangement defects are related to HIV infection remains unclear.

Antibody-dependent cellular cytotoxicity is apparently more pertinent than NK activity to the control of HIV infection because the target cells for these assays are either HIV-infected cells expressing HIV antigens or normal cells (usually CD4 cells) coated with HIV envelope proteins (37,38). Two parameters can influence ADCC—the presence of HIV-specific antibodies mediating ADCC activity and the presence of competent effector cells.

Assays for antibodies directing ADCC generally employ lymphocytes from uninfected donors as effector cells and patients' sera as the source of antibodies. Using these assays, antibodies mediating ADCC are detected in the early phases of HIV infection (39). There is some controversy, however, about the maintainance of these antibodies with disease progression. Some investigators found relatively constant levels of antibodies mediating HIV-specific ADCC at all stages of infection (34,40,41), whereas others found lower titers of antibodies with ADCC activity in patients with AIDS than in asymptomatic HIV-infected individuals (42,43). The source of this controversy remains unclear.

Assays for competent ADCC effector cells in HIV infection differ from the assays just described in that lymphocytes from HIV-infected persons are used as effector cells in the presence of a preparation of pooled sera containing high titers of antibodies mediating ADCC. Using these assays, one group of investigators found that ADCC effector function was comparable in patients with AIDS and controls (34,38); in contrast, another group found significant reductions in ADCC effector function in infected individuals compared to controls (32), and further found that the magnitude and frequency of dysfunction was greater among patients with AIDS than among asymptomatic persons. As above, the source of this discrepancy is unclear.

A third aspect of ADCC that appears important in relation to HIV infection is the measurement of ADCC effector cells armed with anti-HIV antibodies in vivo. These cells thus represent NK cells with anti-HIV attached to the Fc receptor, CD16. The assay for these cells armed in vivo consists of direct incubation of patient lymphocytes with HIV antigen–coated targets, without the inclusion of patient sera as a source of antibodies. Tyler et al. (32) have termed this activity cell-mediated cytotoxicity (CMC) to distinguish it from the classic ADCC activity. These investigators found that CMC declined markedly with HIV disease progression. The nature of the CMC defect, however, appeared to be cellular in some individuals and humoral in others. As evidence for a cellular defect, sera from some patients with essentially no CMC had high titers of antibodies that directed ADCC of normal lymphocytes; further, the patients' lymphocytes continued to show low ADCC in the presence of high-titer ADCC serum. Additional evidence of a cellular defect was the finding that the loss of CMC correlated with decreased

NK activity. In contrast, other patients with low CMC had competent ADCC effectors when tested with high-titer ADCC serum, but their serum contained no ADCC-directing antibodies, indicative of a humoral defect. One patient appeared to possess both cellular and humoral defects in ADCC.

Although these data taken together indicate that HIV-directed ADCC activity is present in HIV-infected individuals early in infection, whether this activity is beneficial or harmful remains to be elucidated. The ADCC-mediated destruction of infected cells expressing HIV antigens would be an obvious benefit, and therapeutic mechanisms to expand or reconsitute this activity may prove efficacious. Similarly, the finding that antibodies mediating ADCC are broadly reactive and lyse cells expressing gp120 from widely divergent HIV isolates (37) suggests that passive administration of high-titer ADCC antibodies to patients with low activity may control disease progression. However, antibody-directed ADCC may prove to be harmful if this activity destroys uninfected CD4 cells with adsorbed HIV antigens on their surface. Such a mechanism may account for the overwhelming loss of CD4 cells compared with the number actually infected in HIV disease (37). Although no data as yet have demonstrated gp120-coated but uninfected CD4 cells in HIV-infected individuals, a thorough search for such cells is mandated before therapeutic manipulation of ADCC is attempted.

E. Changes in CD4 and CD8 Lymphocyte Number and Subsets

As mentioned in the introduction, the hallmark laboratory change associated with HIV infection is decreased levels of circulating CD4 lymphocytes. This change appears both as a decreased percentage of CD4 cells within the lymphocyte population and as a decrease in the number of CD4 lymphocytes per microliter of whole blood (i.e., the absolute CD4 lymphocyte number) (44,45). It is now well-established that CD4 lymphocyte levels decrease with length of time since infection and disease progression. Representative cross-sectional data (46), shown in Table 2, demonstrated decreasing CD4 cell levels with length of time since seroconversion and a further decrease in CD4 cell levels with the development of AIDS. Similar changes have been documented in many studies (47–54).

In addition to decreased numbers of CD4 lymphocytes, most studies find increased levels of CD8 (suppressor/cytotoxic) lymphocytes in association with HIV infection (44–46,50, 52,54,55). In contrast to the characteristic changes in CD4 cell levels, the elevation in CD8 cell levels occurs early in infection and remains fairly constant throughout the course of HIV disease. Only in the late stages, usually in association with the development of AIDS, does the CD8 cell level begin to fall; most often, this CD8 cell decrease merely reflects the severe lymphopenia associated with AIDS (46).

Most of the initial studies of CD4 and CD8 cell levels were carried out in study groups stratified by severity of clinical complications, and thus reflected cases infected with the virus for several months to years. With the discovery of HIV as the cause of AIDS, the development of tests to detect antibodies to HIV, and a better understanding of the epidemiology of HIV transmission, investigators were able to document and describe a "flulike" illness occurring

Table 2 CD4 Cell Levels at Different Stages of HIV Infection

Study Group	CD4 Cell No./μl Whole Blood
Seronegative heterosexual men	909
Seronegative homosexual men	875
Short-term seropositive men	653
Long-term seropositive men	551
Persons with AIDS	190

within 1 or 2 months of exposure to HIV. This condition, termed primary HIV infection, was associated with seroconversion and unique changes in CD4 and CD8 cell levels not observed in later stages of the disease (56).

Figure 1 is a composite representation of typical changes in CD4 and CD8 cell levels, including those in the primary infection stage, for an individual who developed AIDS 4.5 years after HIV infection (56,57). Immediately after infection but prior to the development of primary symptoms and antibodies to HIV, CD4 and CD8 levels are normal. Soon after the seroconversion illness begins (usually around day 9), there is a drastic drop in the total lymphocyte count resulting in dramatic decreases in the absolute numbers of CD4 and CD8 cells; the relative percentages of CD4 and CD8 cells do not decrease during this phage, however. Around day 16 of illness, the total lymphocyte count rebounds; by this point, however, the CD8 cell number is slightly greater than the CD4 cell number, and it is significantly elevated compared with preillness values. During the next phase of illness, the CD4 cell number increases slightly, whereas the CD8 cell number skyrockets; the CD8 cell number usually peaks around 1 month after the beginning of seroconversion illness. The last phase of the primary illness is characterized by gradual stabilization of CD4 and CD8 cell numbers over the next 2–3 months; by this time, the CD8 cell count has typically stabilized at about 1000 cells/μl, and the CD4 count has stabilized at about 600 cells/μl. Over the next 2–3 years, CD4 cell levels slowly decrease and CD8 cell levels increase somewhat. Approximately 18 months before the development of AIDS, the CD4 cell count begins a percipitous decrease, falling at a much

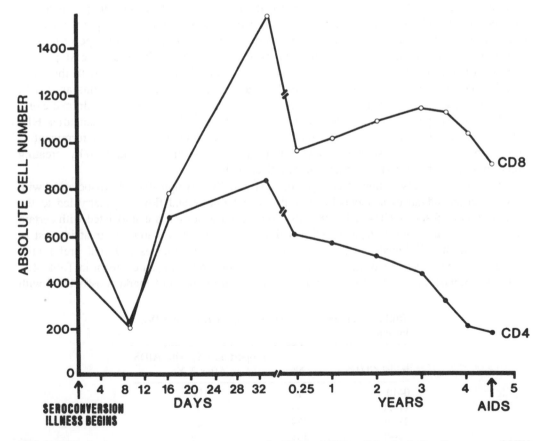

Figure 1 Composite representation of changes in CD4 and CD8 cell levels during the course of HIV disease. (Data from Refs. 56 and 57.)

faster rate than before. At about this same time, the CD8 cell increase is halted and begins to fall 6–12 months prior to the development of AIDS.

Because decreasing CD4 cell number appears to be closely associated with the development of AIDS, several different groups of investigators have explored the prognostic value of CD4 cell levels for predicting the development of AIDS. Most (58–61), but not all (62), researchers found that CD4 cell number at initial presentation was a very good predictor of survival in HIV-infected individuals. In a study of a large number of subjects, Taylor et al. (63) further found that the initial CD4 cell percentage was slightly better than CD4 cell number as a predictor of progression. As shown in Table 3, 100% of persons with initial values under 10% CD4 cells developed AIDS within 3 years compared with only 3% of persons with CD4 values greater than 40%.

Other studies have focused on the value of assessing the rates of change in CD4 cell levels over time as an indicator of HIV disease progression. Spira et al. (61) followed CD4 cell levels over a 3-year period in progressors and nonprogressors, and they found that both groups gradually lost CD4 cells; however, progressors lost, on average, 276 CD4 cells/μl over the 3-year period, whereas nonprogressors lost only 103 CD4 cells/μl. Thus, it appeared that CD4 cells were lost at a faster rate in progressors than in nonprogressors. Similar findings were obtained by Phillips et al. (64), who calculated slopes from successive CD4 cell counts for a given individual. These investigators found a unimodal distribution of negative slopes, and they suggested that AIDS developed more quickly in patients with steeper slopes.

Once the association between CD4 cell decline and the development of AIDS was established, investigators sought to determine if the pattern of CD4 cell decline provided any evidence of a codeterminant for progression to AIDS. Detels et al. (65) approached this question by carrying the slope concept a step further, calculating a series of 3-point interval slopes based on several consecutive clinic visits at 6-month intervals. Thus, the slope of a line constructed using CD4 cells levels on visits 1, 2, and 3 was compared with the slope of a line constructed using data from visits 2, 3, and 4, and so forth. Using this approach, these investigators found that slopes were level for a while but then decreased dramatically. Detels et al. suggested that this downward shift is triggered by a second event after HIV infection, thus constituting a codeterminant. The prime candidate for a codeterminant is activation of infected CD4 cells, which causes them to proliferate and thereby creating conditions favorable for HIV replication (see Sect. II.H).

After the initial description of changes in CD4 and CD8 lymphocytes in association with HIV infection, advances in monoclonal antibody technology and flow cytometry led to the description of subsets of CD4 and CD8 cells. Some of these subsets are associated with certain functional or maturational stages of CD4 and/or CD8 cells. It was thus of great interest to determine if the HIV-related changes in CD4 and CD8 lymphocytes reflected preferential changes in specific subsets of these cells. A summary of the findings are shown in Table 4.

CD4 lymphocytes can be divided into two subsets on the basis of markers associated with

Table 3 Prognostic Value of Initial CD4% in HIV Infection

Initial CD4%	N	Proportion (%) with AIDS After 3 Yr
0–10	16	100
11–20	89	40
21–30	279	20
31–40	301	9
>40	128	3

Table 4 CD4 and CD8 Subset Alterations in HIV Infection

Subset	Function/Maturational Stage	Proportional Change
CD45RA+CD4+	Naive	None
CD45RO+CD4+	Memory	None
CD25+CD4+	Memory	None
LECAM–1+CD4+	Lymph node adhesion	None
CD45RA+CD8+	Naive	Decreased
CD45RO+CD8+	Memory	Increased
LECAM–1+CD8+	Lymph node adhesion	Decreased
DR+CD8+	Immature/activated	Increased
CD38+CD8+	Immature/activated	Increased
LFA–1+CD8+	Memory	Increased density
CD11b–CD8+	Cytotoxicity	Increased
CD57+CD8+	Unknown	Increased

prior exposure to antigen. Thus, CD4 cells that have not yet interacted with the antigen they are programmed to recognize (i.e., naive CD4 cells) express CD45RA. Following interaction with antigen, CD4 cells gradually cease to express CD45RA and begin expressing CD45RO; CD45RO+CD4 cells are thus referred to as primed, or memory, cells, because they have undergone cell division as a result of interaction with antigen (66). Since memory CD4 cells show profound proliferative responses when reexposed to antigen, scientists hypothesized that the loss of antigen-specific T-cell proliferative responses in HIV infection (see next section) may reflect a specific loss of memory CD4 cells. Most investigators, however, failed to confirm this hypothesis; studies conducted by Giorgi's group (54,67), Gupta (68), and my laboratory (69) indicate that the proportion of CD4 cells expressing CD45RA (or CD45RO) is about the same in HIV-infected persons and controls; further, CD45RA+CD4 cells and CD45RO+CD4 cells are lost at similar rates with HIV disease progression. One group published conflicting data showing a selective loss of CD45RA+CD4 cells (70); however, their studies employed single-color fluorescence and an "obligate overlap" calculation method rather than dual-color cytofluorometry, as was employed in the above studies.

In light of these findings, it was somewhat surprising to find that HIV infection is preferentially associated with memory (CD45RO+) CD4 cells (71,72). Purified CD45RA+ and CD45RO+ CD4 cell subsets from uninfected persons were infected with HIV in vitro and then assayed for HIV DNA by polymerase chain reaction; memory cells contained 4 to 10 times more viral DNA than naive cells. In additional studies, higher levels of viral DNA were found in purified memory versus naive CD4 cells from HIV-infected individuals. These findings suggest that the memory CD4 cell subset should be selectively depleted in HIV infection, but this is clearly not the case. A hypothesis put forth to reconcile these discordant observations is that maintainance of a normal balance of naive and memory CD4 cells in HIV infection reflects activation-associated conversion of naive cells to memory cells during the infection process, followed by a homeostatic replacement of naive CD4 cells (71). Further work is needed to test this hypothesis.

Another marker of memory CD4 cells is CD25, the α-chain of the high-affinity interleukin-2 receptor (73). In support of the findings cited above showing a normal balance of naive and memory CD4 cells in HIV infection, the proportion of CD4 cells expressing CD25 is unchanged in HIV infection; the actual percentage of CD25+CD4 cells is decreased, however, which reflects CD4 cell depletion (74).

A third cell surface marker that can be used to determine CD4 subsets is leukocyte endothelial cell adhesion molecule 1 (LECAM-1), recognized by the monoclonal antibodies Leu-8 and TQ1. Early reports (75) suggested that LECAM-1, like CD45RA, was a marker of naive cells because it was lost following in vitro activation. More recent work has shown that LECAM-1 is an adhesion molecule that mediates lymphocyte attachment to lymph node endothelial cells (76). Because of its downregulation following cell activation, LECAM-1 expression by CD4 cells was assessed in HIV infection. The findings show that, like CD45RA, the proportion of CD4 cells expressing LECAM-1 is similar in HIV-infected persons and uninfected controls; further, both CD4 subsets defined by LECAM-1 expression were lost at similar rates in HIV disease (69,77). Thus, no subset of CD4 cells has been identified that is selectively depleted in HIV infection.

In contrast to the findings for CD4 subsets, several CD8 cell subsets, defined by expression (or lack of expression) of a second marker, are selectively altered in HIV infection. CD45RA/CD45RO expression by CD8 cells, like CD4 cells, appears to distinguish CD8 cells that have been activated previously (CD45RO+) from those that have not yet been activated (CD45RA+) (66). My laboratory has shown that the proportion of CD8 cells expressing CD45RA is decreased in HIV infection, and that this change reflected a specific increase in the absolute number of CD45RA-CD8 cells (69). Later studies confirmed that this CD45RA-CD8 subset expressed CD45RO (78). This observation suggests that the HIV-related increase in CD8 cells reflects a rise in the number of previously activated CD8 cells, perhaps generated as part of the immune response to HIV. This concept is supported by changes in CD8 subsets defined by LECAM-1 expression. LECAM-1 on CD8 cells, like CD4 cells, is lost from the cell surface following activation. Several groups have documented that the proportion of CD8 cells expressing LECAM-1 is decreased in HIV infection, reflecting a specific increase in the absolute number of LECAM-1-CD8 cells (69,70,77,79).

Other subsets of CD8 cells defined by markers associated with cell activation are altered in HIV infection; however, these secondary markers are characterized by a discontinuous bimodal expression pattern, which complicates interpretation of the cell's activation status. One such marker is HLA-DR (hereafter referred to as DR), which is found on both immature T cells (80) and activated T cells (81). Increased DR expression by T cells in association with HIV infection was reported by Prince et al. (82); Stites et al. (50) further showed that this increased DR expression was associated with CD8 cells and not CD4 cells. Several studies subsequently confirmed (67,69,79) that the absolute number of both DR-CD8 cells and DR+CD8 cells are increased in HIV infection; however, the increase in DR+CD8 cells is more marked and results in an increase in the proportion of CD8 cells expressing DR. It is unclear if these DR+CD8 cells represent immature or activated CD8 cells.

CD38 is another marker with a distribution pattern similar to that of DR; it appears on T cells in association with immaturity as well as activation (80,81). HIV-related changes in CD8 cell subsets defined by CD38 expression are similar to those characterizing subsets defined by DR expression; absolute numbers of both CD38–CD8 and CD38+CD8 cells are increased in HIV infection, with a significant increased proportion of CD8 cells expressing CD38 (46,67,69).

Whether DR+CD8 and CD38+CD8 cells in HIV infection reflect immature or activated cells is not entirely clear. Salazar-Gonzalez et al. (83) found decreased expression of ecto-5'-nucleotidase, an indicator of immaturity, in association with increased DR and CD38 expression by CD8 cells. Alternatively, Prince et al. (84) found that serum levels of soluble activation markers, including soluble CD25 and soluble CD8, were strongly correlated with DR and CD38 expression by CD8 cells in HIV infection; this finding thus suggested that DR+CD8 and CD38+CD8 cells are activated cells. Further support for this concept was presented by Desroches and Rigal (85), who found that the density of leukocyte function–associated antigen-1 (LFA-1) on CD8 cells was increased in HIV infection. Increased density of LFA-1 is associated with activation and expression of memory cell markers (86).

In order to further investigate the relationship of CD38 and DR expression by CD8 cells in HIV infection to maturational status, three-color cytofluorometric studies were recently conducted in my laboratory (78). The findings showed that (1) the HIV-related increase in CD38+CD8 and DR+CD8 cells reflects an increase in CD38+DR+CD8 cells, and (2) both naive and memory subsets of CD38+CD8 cells and DR+CD8 cells are increased in HIV infection, but the memory subset increases are more dramatic. Thus, it appears that some CD38+DR+CD8 cells represent immature CD8 cells, whereas others represent activated CD8 cells. The mechanism responsible for such a bimodal increase in CD8 cells remains unclear.

CD8 cell subsets defined by markers with no clear association with activation are also altered in HIV infection. Stites et al. (50) found that the CD11b–CD8 cell subset was selectively increased in HIV infection; Nicholson et al. (87) confirmed this. There is evidence to suggest that CD11b–CD8 cells represent cytotoxic T cells (88) rather than suppressor T cells. This suggests that the HIV-related alterations in CD8 cell subsets may reflect an adaptive response to viral challenge. The role of cytotoxic T cells in the immune response to HIV is discussed in more detail in the next section.

A final CD8 cell subset altered in HIV infection is the CD57+CD8 subset. As with some other subsets, absolute numbers of both the CD57+CD8 and CD57–CD8 subsets are increased in HIV infection (50,69,82,87,89,90). Proportional changes are less clear, however, and reflect differences in the control group used for comparison. Although the proportion of CD8 cells expressing CD57 is increased in HIV infection when compared with heterosexual controls, no significant increase is observed when compared with seronegative homosexually active men (67,69). This difference reflects a specific increase in the absolute number of CD57+CD8 cells, but not CD57–CD8 cells, in seronegative gay men (67,87). As suggested by Giorgi (67), elevation of the CD57+CD8 subset may be due to some immunostimulant common to both HIV-seropositive and HIV-seronegative gay men. Further support for this immunostimulation hypothesis comes from data (91) showing that CD57+CD8 cell levels are increased in hemophiliacs treated with clotting factor concentrate regardless of HIV antibody status.

In our three-color study of CD8 subsets in HIV infection (78), we found an increase in the percentage of CD57+CD8 cells, as expected. This increase occurred selectively in CD57+CD8 cells coexpressing DR, CD38, and CD45RO. Such a cell would thus represent an activated CD8 cell.

Although the CD8 cell subset changes described are readily identified, there appears to be little relevance of these subset alterations as predictors of HIV-related disease progression. Only CD38+CD8 subset changes appear to be related to disease severity (67,78). It will be important, however, to determine if the increase in absolute numbers of CD8 cell subsets plays any role in retarding virus replication, thus prolonging the period of latency.

F. Changes in CD4 and CD8 Lymphocyte Functions

Once scientists recognized that HIV infection was associated with opportunistic infections and CD4 cell depletion, major emphasis was placed on assessment of the immunocompetence of T lymphocytes in HIV-infected persons. The most common method for assessing immunocompetence is measurement of DNA synthesis by T cells activated with soluble antigen or nonspecific stimulators of mitosis, collectively called mitogens. Common mitogens are the plant-derived lectins phytohemagglutinin (PHA) and pokeweed mitogen (PWM), as well as monoclonal antibodies recognizing the CD3/T-cell receptor (TCR) complex. Anti-CD3 antibodies recognize the same cell surface structural complex that binds antigen, and thus in many ways represents the mitogen system most pertinent to activation events initiated by antigen.

Early studies showed that antigen- and mitogen-induced DNA synthesis by T lymphocytes was severely decreased in patients with ARC or AIDS (44,92,93). These results suggested that T cells in HIV-infected people were defective in responding to antigenic stimulation, leading to impaired clearance of organisms causing opportunistic infections.

Once decreased proliferative responses were documented in HIV infection, two major questions arose regarding this defect: (1) Did the defect reflect an abnormality of CD4 cells only or were other T cells (i.e., CD8 cells) defective as well? (2) Was the defect merely a reflection of the quantitative decrease in the percentage of lymphocytes that were CD4 cells? To answer these questions, investigators purified CD4 and CD8 lymphocyte subsets from HIV-infected persons and healthy controls and monitored antigenic/mitogenic responses in these populations. Not surprisingly, conflicting data were generated. Lane et al. (94) found that both CD4 and CD8 cells from patients with AIDS responded normally to the mitogens PHA and PWM; in contrast, purified CD4 cells from patients with AIDS did not respond to the antigen used, tetanus toxoid. (Purified CD8 cells do not exhibit antigen-specific activation either in controls or HIV-infected persons.) These results indicated a qualitative defect in CD4 cells for antigen recognition, thus suggesting that decreased antigen-induced responses of unfractionated lymphocytes did not merely reflect a quantitative reduction in CD4 cell percentage.

In contrast, similar studies by Hofmann et al. (95), detected reduced responses of purified CD4 cells and purified CD8 cells to mitogenic stimulation in HIV infection. Other studies (96,97) confirmed and extended these findings and showed that the mixed lymphocyte response (MLR) and anti-CD3 responses were decreased in purified CD4 and CD8 subsets from HIV-infected patients. Further evidence supporting a qualitative activation defect in both CD4 and CD8 populations in HIV infection came from studies of clonal expansion; Margolick et al. (98) found that both CD4 and CD8 cells from patients with AIDS had reduced proportions of clonable cells compared with health donors. Thus, most studies indicate that CD4 and CD8 cell responses to mitogen/antigen are decreased in the late stages of HIV infection.

What is the relationship of T-cell activation defects to HIV-related disease progression? Giogi et al. (54) approached this question by measuring antigen-induced proliferation of CD4 cell-enriched populations adjusted to a standard number of CD4 cells per culture well. They found that cells from almost all patients with AIDS failed to respond, whereas cells from most asymptomatic seropositive gay men tested gave normal responses. Those seropositive men whose cells were nonresponsive had a lower number of circulating CD4 cells, a longer duration of infection, and a higher likelihood of developing AIDS. Thus, development of the qualitative defect in CD4 cell activation by antigen was related to progression of HIV disease.

Clerici and Shearer (99), utilizing a different approach, measured (IL-2) production by peripheral blood mononuclear cells (PBMCs) from asymptomatic seropositive persons and activated by a variety of stimuli. Their results, summarized in Table 4, showed four distinctive patterns of responses, with a time-dependent progression from pattern 1 to pattern 4. Responsiveness to soluble antigen was lost first, indicating a loss of CD4 cell function. Loss of response to alloantigen (MLR) occurred next, indicating dysfunction of both CD4 and CD8 lymphocytes. The PHA responsiveness disappeared last, indicating severe immune dysfunction. Progression from pattern 1 to pattern 4 was predictive of a reduction in the number of circulating CD4 cells and the development of AIDS (100).

Pattern 2 of these progressive functional changes indicates selective loss of responses to recall antigens. This response requires antigen presentation by antigen-presenting cells (APCs) expressing autologous (self) HLA determinants (i.e., a self-restricted response). It is thus possible that defective responses to antigen reflect a defect in APC rather than CD4 cells. To explore this possibility, Clerici et al. (101) capitalized on the availability of a set of monozygotic twins, one HIV negative with a normal antigen response and one HIV positive with a decreased antigen response. When lymphocytes from the HIV-negative twin were mixed with APCs from

Table 5 Progressive Patterns of Lymphocyte Proliferative Dysfunction in HIV Infection

Pattern	Interleukin-2 Production in Response to		
	Soluble Antigen[a]	Alloantigen	PHA
1	+	+	+
2	–	+	+
3	–	–	+
4	–	–	–

[a]Tetanus toxoid or influenza.

the HIV-positive twin, the CD4 lymphocyte response to antigen was completely normal, indicating that the HIV-positive twin's APCs were fully functional. Thus, pattern 2 apparently reflects a defect in self-restricted antigen recognition by CD4 cells.

Soon after the description of the four patterns of responses shown in Table 5, Clerici et al. (100) found that CD4 cell activation by alloantigen is mediated by two distinct pathways. The first pathway is the strongest and constitutes what is normally considered the mechanism for MLR; CD4 cells directly recognize alloantigenic molecules on the surface of allogeneic APCs (an allorestricted MLR). The second pathway is much weaker and apparently mimics the antigenic response; alloantigen is processed and presented to CD4 cells by autologous APCs (a self-restricted MLR). Clerici et al. hypothesized that the self-restricted MLR, like the response to soluble antigen, is dysfunctional in asymptomatic seropositive individuals exhibiting pattern 2. Cell depletion experiments confirmed their hypothesis—seropositive persons with reduced antigen responses also showed reduced responses when their CD4 cells and APCs were incubated with allogeneic lymphocytes depleted of APCs (i.e., a self-restricted MLR); their allorestricted MLR was normal, however, as shown by normal responses of seropositive CD4 cells when incubated with allogeneic mononuclear cells (containing allogeneic APCs). Clerici et al. (100) suggested that differences in the density of alloantigenic epitopes on self-APCs versus allo-APCs may explain the differing results observed for the two MLR pathways. Self-APCs express processed alloantigen at a much lower density than is found on allo-APCs. The higher density may overcome the HIV-associated defect in CD4 cell recognition of alloantigen presented at low density. In support of this hypothesis, others (53) have shown that lymphocytes from asymptomatic seropositive persons do not respond to a suboptimal concentration of anti-CD3 monoclonal antibody but do respond to higher concentrations of anti-CD3. Whatever the mechanism responsible, these findings provide important additional information supporting the theory that the self-restricted CD4 cell response is the first functional defect to appear in HIV infection.

One of the mechanisms responsible for decreased T-cell activation in association with HIV infection appears related to defective transduction of activation signals from the cell surface to the cell nucleus. As just described, studies of Shearer and Clerici showed that IL-2 production in response to activating stimuli may be decreased, and that the decrease correlates with decreased DNA synthesis (101). Interleukin-2–mediated activation signals require the presence of the IL-2 receptor, which, like IL-2, is dramatically upregulated following T-cell stimulation. Several studies performed relatively early in the HIV epidemic demonstrated that the mean level of lymphocytes expressing CD25, the α-chain of the IL-2 receptor (102), was reduced in mitogen-activated cultures, and this reduced mean was associated with reduced mean levels of DNA synthesis (103–106). Additional studies conducted in my laboratory showed that (1) decreased mitogen-induced CD25 expression in HIV infection was highly correlated with decreased DNA synthesis results (107); (2) decreased CD25 expression by mitogen-activated lymphocytes reflected decreased CD25 expression by both CD4 and CD8 subsets (108); and (3) a decreased proliferative response to soluble antigen was detected by monitoring the number of CD25+ lymphocytes generated per culture (109). Other investigators found that decreased CD25 expression in association with HIV infection was significantly correlated with decreased T-cell colony growth (106,110).

Interleukin-2 production and CD25 expression are relatively late events in the activation process, occurring optimally several hours to days after activation (111). Accordingly, Hofmann et al. (112) measured a very early event in the activation process; namely, calcium influx into the cell. They found that this event was normal in cultures of cells from HIV-infected persons even though IL-2 production and CD25 expression was decreased. The step in lymphocyte activation that is defective in HIV infection is thus some point following calcium mobilization but preceding IL-2 production and CD25 expression.

Another mechanism that may be involved in defective lymphocyte activation in HIV infection is refractoriness due to prior activation. This explanation appears expecially pertinent to decreased CD8 cell activation. Pantaleo et al. (113) have shown that the DR+CD8 cell subset does not respond to anti-CD3 monoclonal antibody or PHA even in the presence of exogenous IL-2; these cells also expressed very late activation antigen-2 (VLA-2), a marker of chronic T-cell activation. Some of the CD8 cell subsets increased in HIV infection thus appear to represent CD8 cells that have been activated in vivo and are incapable of being activated further in vitro.

Recent findings from my laboratory are consistent with the hypothesis that CD8 cell subsets increased in HIV infection represent in vivo activated, terminally differentiated CD8 lymphocytes. We showed that roughly 50% of CD8 cells from HIV-infected former blood donors do not survive during a 3-day in vitro culture in the absence of any stimulant (114). Dual-color cytofluorometric analysis and subtractive calculations showed that the nonsurviving cells were preferentially found in CD8 subsets bearing phenotypes indicative of prior activation, such as DR+CD8, CD45RA-CD8, and CD38+CD8 subsets (114,115). Exogenous IL-2 did not enhance the in vitro survival of these CD8 cell subsets (115). These findings suggest that CD8 cells activated in vivo, probably in an attempt to control HIV infection, are terminally differentiated cells that do not survive during in vitro culture. These observations are of great practical importance, indicating that some of the reported defects of in vitro CD8 cell function in association with HIV infection may have simply reflected this lack of CD8 cell survival. Experimental protocols should thus include measurements of CD8 cell survival.

An unexplained paradox of decreased lymphocyte function in HIV infection is the profound immune dysfunction in light of the low number of CD4 cells actually infected by the virus (usually less than 1 in 10,000) (116). A possible explanation that has been explored by many investigators is viral protein interaction with CD4 cells in the absence of actual infection. Mann et al. (117) showed that the HIV envelope protein gp120, which contains the CD4-recognition site of the virus, inhibited PHA-induced proliferation of uninfected lymphocytes. Several subsequent studies showed that gp120 also inhibited antigen-induced proliferation of CD4 cells (118–121). Further, a recent study by Hofmann et al. (122) showed that inactivated HIV inhibited CD8 cell activation as well as CD4 cell activation by PHA; both subsets, in purified form, exhibited decreased CD25 expression and DNA synthesis in the presence of inactivated HIV.

Mechanistic studies of HIV inhibition of uninfected lymphocyte responses indicate many similarities to mechanisms involved in reduced responsiveness of lymphocytes from infected individuals. Hofmann et al. (122) found that calcium fluxes were not affected by HIV but CD25 expression was reduced. They further showed that inositol phospholipid turnover, an activation step between calcium mobilization and IL-2 production, was inhibited in uninfected lymphocytes stimulated by PHA in the presence of inactivated HIV.

One hypothesis for explaining HIV-mediated inhibition of CD4 lymphocyte activation is that the HIV envelope protein gp120 binds to CD4 molecules on uninfected CD4 cells, interfering with the interaction between CD4 and its ligand, the MHC class II molecule on APCs (123) (Fig. 2). Under normal circumstances (Fig. 2, left), the class II molecule contains the antigenic peptide to be presented to the TCR complex on CD4 cells; interaction of CD4 with a conserved site on the class II molecule stabilizes the antigen-TCR interaction needed for activation. According to the hypothesis, gp120 attachment to the CD4 molecule inhibits the CD4-class II interaction, thus preventing efficient interaction between antigen and the TCR complex (Fig. 2, right). In support of this hypothesis, gp120 blocked conjugate formation between CD4 cells and lipid vesicles bearing MHC class II (124). This mechanism does not, however, explain how HIV proteins inhibit CD8 cell activation.

In addition to inhibiting activation, HIV protein attachment to uninfected CD4 cells may also render the cells targets for immune attack. Weinhold et al. (121) have shown that activated uninfected CD4 cells incubated with gp120 serve as targets for ADCC. The concentration of gp120 needed was well below that needed to saturate all the CD4 sites. As will be discussed later, such gp120-bearing CD4 cells may also serve as targets for HIV-specific cytotoxic T lymphocytes (CTLs). It should be remembered, however, that there is as yet no evidence (125) that uninfected CD4 cells in vivo have gp120 or peptides derived from gp120 bound to them. Thus, these proposed mechanisms for decreased CD4 cell number and function caused by HIV proteins in the absence of direct infection remain speculative.

It now seems clear that at least some of the CD8 cell subsets increased in HIV infection represent HIV-specific CTLs (126). The study of CTLs is complicated by the requirements that the CTL and target cell share MHC class I antigens. To overcome this problem, investigators have developed a system whereby B-cell lines for a given individual are generated by Epstein-Barr virus (EBV) transformation of B cells. These lines are then either pulsed with synthetic peptides corresponding to HIV proteins (127) or infected with recombinant vaccinia viruses containing HIV genes. These cells are then used as targets in a chromium-release assay for measuring CTL activity in that individual. Using this approach, several groups have identified HIV-specific CTLs in fresh peripheral blood from HIV-infected individuals (127–

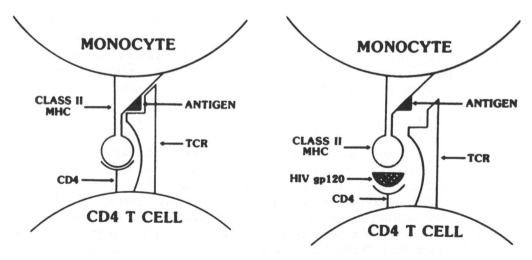

Figure 2 Possible mechanism for HIV gp120 glycoprotein inhibition of antigen-induced activation of CD4 lymphocytes. Left: Under normal circumstances, the CD4–MHC class II interaction stabilizes the interaction of the antigen-MHC class II complex with the T-cell receptor (TCR). Right: HIV gp120 interferes with the CD4–MHC class II interaction, thus inhibiting the interaction of antigen with TCR. (Derived from Ref. 123, Fig. 1.)

130). Limiting dilution analysis has shown that HIV-specific CTLs are present at high levels in HIV-infected individuals; between 0.5 and 10 HIV-specific CTLs are found per 10,000 peripheral blood lymphocytes (131). Essentially all seropositive people have CTLs specific for envelope proteins (gp120, gp160) and reverse transcriptase; only a few individuals, however, have CTLs specific for core proteins (127,129,132,133).

Longitudinal studies have shown that HIV-specific CTL activity decreases in advanced stages of HIV infection (126,130). The mechanism responsible for this decline remains unclear. Pantaleo (126) et al. have shown that the cytolytic machinery of CTLs is still intact in patients with AIDS even though HIV-specific CTL activity has been lost. This was shown using a redirected killing assay, in which murine target cells bearing Fc receptors were incubated with CTLs in the presence of anti-CD3 monoclonal antibody; the antibody formed a bridge between the CD3+ CTLs and the target cell, leading to activation of the cytolytic machinery of the CTLs.

Recent studies by French investigators (134) suggest that reduction of CTL activity with disease progression may reflect the production of an inhibitory factor by CD57+CD8 cells, which increase in parallel with reductions in CTL activity. These investigators found that supernatants from CD57+CD8 cells, but not CD57-CD8 cells, from patients with AIDS contained a potent inhibitor of CTL activity. It is unclear, however, if production of this inhibitor is related to HIV infection; studies were not conducted with CD57+CD8 cells from HIV-seronegative persons.

Another possible explanation for decreased HIV-specific CTLs in advanced HIV disease relates to the need for cytokines for efficient development of antigen-specific CTLs (135). Since CD4 cells serve as the source of these cytokines, HIV-associated CD4 cell dysfunction may explain inefficient maturation of CTLs. Evidence supporting this hypothesis was recently presented by Clerici et al. (136). They noted that lymphocytes from HIV-infected persons that did not show a CD4-proliferative response to influenza (FLU) also did not develop FLU-specific CTLs. However, if they incubated these lymphocytes with FLU in the presence of allogeneic lymphocytes, FLU-specific CTLs were generated. This finding suggested that, in the absence of allogeneic cells, FLU-specific CTL precursors were present but could not develop because the cytokines needed were absent owing to lack of CD4 cell responsiveness to FLU. However, when allogeneic cells were used to activate the CD4 cells, overriding the FLU-specific CD4 cell defect, the cytokines needed for FLU-specific CTL development were made available. These results have profound implications, suggesting that coimmunization with alloantigen may enhance antigen-specific responses in HIV-infected persons. Before implementation of such a plan, however, more work is needed to dissect the mechanisms involved and the potential drawbacks.

In addition to functioning as CTLs, CD8 cells appear to play another important role in controlling HIV infection. Walker et al. (137) showed that CD8 cells from HIV-infected individuals can inhibit HIV replication in autologous HIV-infected CD4 cells. This study came about from investigations of why virus could not be detected in cultures of cells from some individuals who were clearly infected with HIV. These investigators found that removal of CD8 cells prior to culture resulted in high levels of virus replication; readdition of CD8 cells led to a dose-dependent reduction in virus replication. The effectiveness of CD8 cell suppression of HIV replication showed great variation among individuals (138); for some people, a CD8:CD4 cell ratio as low as 0.25:1.0 effectively inhibited HIV replication, whereas for others, a 4:1 ratio was required. The mechanism responsible for this variation has not been defined.

Studies of the mechanism of CD8 cell suppression of HIV replication show that killing of infected CD4 cells is not involved. When "suppressed" CD4 cells were isolated by panning and recultured in the absence of CD8 cells, robust HIV replication occurred (139). The mechanism of suppression is thus distinct from CTL activity.

Binchmann et al. (140,141) have provided evidence that CD8 cells produce a soluble factor that is responsible for inhibition of HIV replication in infected CD4 cells. CD8 cells separated from infected CD4 cells by a semipermeable membrane were still able to inhibit HIV replication in the CD4 cells. Further studies using neutralizing antibodies showed that the inhibitory factor was distinct from interferon (INF) alpha-2, a cytokine shown previously to inhibit HIV replication. Walker et al. (142) have also detected a soluble inhibitory factor from CD8 cells. In their hands, however, CD8 cells were still much more effective than the soluble factor, leading them to suggest that two mechanisms, one involving a soluble factor and one involving cell:cell contact, may be involved in CD8 cell-mediated inhibition of HIV replication. Whatever the mechanism, it appears that the inhibitory activity is lost late in disease, allowing increased HIV replication (140,141).

G. Monocyte Alterations

During the same time period that a concerted effort was being made to define the mechanisms of CD4-gp120 interactions, it was discovered that circulating monocytes express low levels of CD4 (143). It was thus of great interest to determine if monocytes could be infected by HIV via interaction with the CD4 molecule. Several studies subsequently demonstrated that monocytes could be infected by HIV in vitro (144–146). Ho et al. (147) further showed that monocytes served as targets for HIV infection in vivo; they successfully recovered virus from cultures of monocyte-enriched cells from HIV-seropositive persons.

In contrast to CD4 lymphocytes, monocytes show a high level of resistance to the cytopathic effect of HIV (145). This difference apparently reflects restricted viral replication in HIV-infected monocytes. As a result, the infection appears to be persistent in monocytes. A logical hypothesis arising from these observations was that infected monocytes may serve as a reservoir for HIV, infecting CD4 T cells during the process of antigen presentation. Elegant studies by Mann et al. (148) confirmed this hypothesis, showing that HIV-infected monocytes could transmit the virus to T cells during the process of presenting tetanus toxoid antigen. Infectivity was inhibited by anti-CD4, anti–HLA-DR, and soluble gp120, indicating that the CD4-DR interaction critical to antigen presentation was also required for HIV transmission. These findings further pointed out that the T cells involved most actively in immune responses also are at greatest risk for infection from HIV-infected APCs.

Several studies have sought to determine if HIV-infected monocytes exhibit phenotypic and functional alterations that may explain some of the immunopathology of HIV infection. One of the most controversial issues is DR expression; some investigators have found that the percentage of monocytes expressing DR is increased in HIV infection (149), whereas others find decreased DR expression (150–152). There is general agreement, however, that those monocytes that do express DR do so at a higher cell surface density. It is also the general concensus that monocytes from HIV-infected persons are activated; an increased percentage of monocytes from persons with AIDS express CD25 (IL-2 receptor α-chain) (153), monocytes from HIV-infected persons exhibit decreased chemotaxis owing to modulation of chemotactic ligand receptors (154), monocytes from patients with AIDS spontaneously release high levels of tumor necrosis factor (TNF) (155) and IL-1 (151), and monocytes from patients with AIDS show increased cytotoxic activity against tumor cell targets (155). Further studies showed that most of these HIV-associated alterations indicative of monocyte activation could be induced by treating normal monocytes with soluble gp120 (153,154). Thus, in a manner analogous to the effects of soluble viral proteins on CD4 lymphocyte function, interaction of gp120 with CD4+ monocytes also appears to alter monocyte function.

As was discussed earlier, monocyte accessory cell function for T-cell–proliferative responses to soluble antigens appears to be intact in asymptomatic HIV-seropositive persons. Another recent study supports this hypothesis, showing that monocytes from HIV-infected individuals were able to process and present mumps antigen to mumps-specific T-cell lines (156). With disease progression and the development of AIDS, however, this monocyte activity also appears to become defective (157). Similarly, monocyte accessory cell function for some mitogenic responses, notably PWM and anti-CD3 monoclonal antibody, is also defective in the late stages of HIV disease (158,159).

As emphasized in an excellent review by Pauza (160), harboring of HIV in monocytes via persistent noncytolytic infection may explain the eventual inability of the immune response to control HIV infection. Because viral replication is restricted in infected monocytes, they probably do not display significant levels of HIV antigens on their surface. These cells are thus refractory to the HIV-specific cytolytic activities of cytotoxic T cells and cells mediating ADCC. Infected monocytes thus, in all likelihood, serve as a major reservoir of HIV, leading to persistent, ongoing infection even in the presence of a robust HIV-specific immune response.

H. Immune System Activation and HIV Infection

A truly amazing feature of HIV is its ability to take advantage of components of the normal immune response to advance its life cycle. It is now clear that CD4 T lymphocytes that have been activated by either mitogen (161,162) or antigen (163) are 10 to 100 times more susceptible to HIV infection than are resting CD4 T cells. Thus, under circumstances where antigen-specific CD4 T cells are presented antigen by HIV-infected monocytes/macrophages, the cascade of events associated with the activation of the T cell also provides for more efficient infection of the T cell by HIV.

Additional studies have demonstrated that activation also enhances viral replication in CD4 T cells already infected by HIV (164). This mechanism apparently reflects the ability of HIV to utilize factors produced by activated T cells to promote transcription of growth factors needed for the activation cascade to proceed. Activated T cells produce a protein called NF-kB, which binds to the kB elements of the IL-2 and CD25 genes, inducing transcription of these genes. The HIV genome also contains kB elements; thus binding of activation-induced NF-kB to HIV kB elements promotes transcription of HIV genes (123,165,166).

An understanding of the dual role of T-cell activation in efficiency of HIV infection and promotion of viral replication has provided insight into the mechanisms operating in two of the most common means of transmitting HIV; namely, sexual contact and transfusion. When HIV-infected seminal lymphocytes are introduced into the sexual partner, or when HIV-infected lymphocytes of donor origin are transferred to the recipient, the resulting reciprocal allogeneic stimulation activates both the infected CD4 T cells and the CD4 T cells targeted for infection. These conditions thus favor optimal HIV transmission (167).

Once the role of activation-induced transcriptional promoters in upregulating HIV gene transcription was established, it was of interest to determine if cytokines, known to enhance T-cell activation by affecting RNA transcription (123), played a role in inducing HIV expression. Fauci's group (123,168,169) approached this question by testing the ability of a variety of recombinant cytokines to induce HIV expression in chronically infected promonocyte (U1) or T-cell (ACH-2) lines (constitutive virus expression is low to undetectable in these lines). Neither IL-1, IL-2, IL-3, IL-4, platelet-derived growth factor, nor IFN-γ induced virus expression in either line. Hover, TNF-α, produced by activated monocytes/macrophages (169), induced HIV expression in both lines; additionally, IL-6 and granulocyte-macrophage colony-stimulating factor (GM-CSF) induced HIV expression in U1 cells. Enhancement of HIV expression by TNF-α apparently reflected TNF-mediated induction of a factor similar, if not identical, to NF-kB (170). This same group of investigators (171) also showed that cytomegalovirus and EBV, viruses often implicated as cofactors in triggering rapid progression of HIV disease, could induce healthy uninfected monocytes to release a factor (presumably TNF-α) upregulating HIV expression in U1 and ACH-2 cells. Interestingly, other viruses, such as herpes simplex viruses 1 and 2, hepatitis B virus, and herpes zoster virus, failed to trigger the production of this factor by monocytes. These studies provided additional evidence that events associated with immune system activation are utilized by HIV to further its replication.

As the importance of immune activation in HIV infectivity and replication become clear, investigators began to ask if the levels of soluble markers of immune activation detectable in serum were elevated in association with HIV infection. The most extensively studied serological activation markers and their cellular sources are listed in Table 6. Elevated serum levels of β_2-microglobulin (β_2M), the protein found on most nucleated cells as the constant subunit of HLA-A, HLA-B, HLA-C, were noted by Zolla-Pazner et al. (172) early in the AIDS epidemic. They further found that β_2M levels can be used as a predictor for the development of AIDS in asymptomatic seropositive individuals (172), a finding subsequently confirmed in other studies (173,174). Indeed, in one study (173), β_2M levels were a better predictor of AIDS than were CD4 T-cell levels. As suggested by the authors, β_2M may be a better predictor of progression because it reflects target cell activation in all tissues, whereas CD4 T cell levels reflect changes in only the peripheral circulation. β_2-Macroglobulin measurement also appears useful as a surrogate endpoint in therapeutic trials; HIV-infected individuals treated with azidothymidine (AZT) showed a dramatic decrease in serum β_2M levels, whereas the improvement in CD4 T-cell counts was minimal (175).

The neopterin (NEOP) level in serum is a reflection of T-cell–monocyte–macrophage interplay, being produced by macrophages activated by T-cell–derived IFN-γ (176). Like β_2M, NEOP is usually elevated at all stages of HIV infection, and there is a significant inverse correlation with CD4 cell levels (176,177). The serum NEOP level is also a powerful predictor for the development of AIDS; in most studies, CD4 T-cell levels combined with NEOP and/or β_2M levels is a better predictor than CD4 T-cell levels alone (174,176–178). A recent report from the San Francisco area showed that serum NEOP levels coupled with antibody titers to HIV p24 core protein serve as a powerful predictor of HIV disease progression (179). A high anti-p24 titer and low (i.e., normal) NEOP level at study entry had the best prognosis, with only 7% of persons developing AIDS within 54 months; in contrast, a low anti-p24 titer and elevated NEOP carried a poor prognosis, with 60% developing AIDS. As suggested by the authors, the initial immune response to virus (reflected as anti-p24 production) and virus-associated immune activation (reflected by NEOP levels) apparently represent independent components of the host response to HIV that interact to determine the clinical outcome of infection.

Serum IL-2 receptor represents soluble CD25 (sCD25) cleaved from the surface of activated lymphocytes (180). Although several studies have documented increased serum levels of sCD25 in HIV infection (181–187), the relationship of elevated sCD25 levels to CD4 T-cell levels is controversial. Some investigators, including my group, found a significant inverse correlation between sCD25 levels and CD4 T-cell levels in HIV-infected persons (184,185, 187,188), whereas others found no significant correlation (182,186). In our study (184), we

Table 6 Serologic Markers of Immune Activation Often Elevated in HIV-Infected Individuals

Marker	Cellular Source (Ref.)
β_2-Microglobulin	Activated lymphocytes (172)
Neopterin	Macrophages stimulated by IFN-gamma from activated T cells (176)
Soluble CD25	Activated lymphocytes (180)
Soluble CD8	Activated CD8+ lymphocytes (190)

found that AZT treatment profoundly reduced sCD25 levels, as was previously reported for β_2M (175); thus, we did not include AZT-treated individuals in our analysis. It is unclear if investigators finding no significant correlation also excluded such data from their analyses. Unlike β_2M and NEOP, sCD25 levels appear of limited value for predicting the development of AIDS (174,189).

The most recently described serological activation marker is soluble CD8 (sCD8), which is released from the surface of activated CD8 cells (190). Serum levels of sCD8 are elevated at all stages of HIV infection (191). Nishanian et al. (192) showed that sCD8 levels were predictive of HIV disease progression; particularly early in infection, the CD4 cell level combined with the sCD8 level was a better predictor of AIDS than the CD4 level alone. Recent studies by Osmand et al. (189) confirm these findings. Although sCD8 levels are not significantly correlated with circulating CD8 cell levels (188,191–193), they do show a significant inverse correlation with CD4 T-cell levels (188,189). Thus, CD8 cell activation and CD4 T-cell destruction in HIV infection appear related, but the nature of the relationship remains unclear. Because optimal CD8 cell activation requires cytokines from activated CD4 T cells (194), activation events leading to cytokine production by CD4 cells and activation of CD8 cells would be expected to be cytotoxic for the activated HIV-infected CD4 T cell; the net result would thus be activated CD8 cells (and sCD8 production) in light of CD4 T-cell destruction. Alternatively, the relationship may be more direct, perhaps reflecting CD4 cell destruction by activated cytotoxic CD8 cells.

In a recent study conducted in my laboratory, we sought to determine the relationships among these four serological activation markers in HIV infection. In other words, are the individuals showing increased β_2M levels the same individuals showing increased sCD8 levels, and so forth? In pairwise comparisons, each of the four serological markers showed significant correlation with the other three markers, indicating that production of all four markers is probably interrelated (188). Two recently published studies confirm these findings (189,192). Since cell-associated activation markers in HIV infection appear restricted to the CD8 lymphocyte subset (see Sect. II.E), we further asked if increased levels of the soluble activation markers were related to increased levels of activated CD8 cells in HIV infection. Our findings showed that all four serologic markers were significantly correlated with the proportion of CD8 cells expressing the activation marker CD38; further, levels of β_2M and sCD25 (but not NEOP and sCD8) were significantly correlated with the proportion of CD8 cells expressing DR (188). Thus, it appears that activated CD8 cells are responsible, at least in part, for the elevated levels of serological activation makrers that characterize HIV infection.

III. HTLV INFECTION AND THE IMMUNE RESPONSE

A. Background

Another group of retroviruses that has had a major impact on transfusion medicine is the human T lymphotropic virus (HTLV) group. Two types of HTLV, HTLV-I and HTLV-II, have been identified; these two types are quite similar, exhibiting 65% DNA sequence homology when analyzing provirus (195). HTLV-I is endemic to southwestern Japan, the Caribbean basin, the Southeastern United States, and sub-Saharan Africa (196). This virus has been linked to adult T-cell leukemia (ATL) and a neurological disorder referred to as HTLV-associated myelopathy/tropical spastic paraparesis (HAM/TSP) (197,198). However, the factors regulating the development of disease in HTLV-I–infected individuals are unclear. Estimates of the proportion of infected persons that will develop disease range from 2–5% for ATL (199–201) and 0.25–1.0% for HAM/TSP (198,202). Thus, greater than 90% of individuals with HTLV-I infection remain asymtpomatic throughout their lifetime.

HTLV-II is endemic among intravenous drug users in the United States (203,204), apparently owing to needle sharing. Recent findings also indicate that HTLV-II is endemic among Native American populations of the southwestern United States (205); these individuals, however, apparently acquired the infection via vertical or sexual transmission rather than through intravenous drug use. HTLV-II has not been clearly linked to any disease. A few cases of atypical hairy cell leukemia have been associated with HTLV-II infection (206,207); however, there is no evidence of increased risk of hairy cell leukemia or related malignancies in a geographical area where HTLV-II is endemic among Native Americans (205).

Abundant evidence indicates that both HTLV-I and HTLV-II can be transmitted by transfusion (208–210). Unlike HIV, however, HTLV transmission requires transfer of cellular blood products; plasma products do not transmit HTLV (211–213). Studies from Japan indicate that HTLV-I is transmitted at 63% efficiency (214); data for transmission efficiency of HTLV-II are not available, but the assumption is a rate similar to that of HTLV-I. Transmission of HTLV requires relatively fresh blood products. Donegan et al. (215) found that HTLV transmission was almost always limited to recipients receiving platelets or packed RBCs stored less than 8 days. Apparently, the HTLV-infected lymphocytes do not survive in RBCs stored for longer time periods (211).

Blood banks and transfusion centers now routinely test donor sera for HTLV antibodies as evidence of infection. The enzyme immunoassay utilized does not distinguish between HTLV-I and HTLV-II. In Los Angeles and other large US metropolitan areas, the most prevalent risk factor of seropositive donors is intravenous drug use or sexual contact with a drug user (216), suggesting a predominance of HTLV-II infection. Typing studies utilizing the polymerase chain reaction and/or synthetic peptide reactivity have confirmed this hypothesis (204,217).

B. Immune Response to HTLV

HTLV-infected individuals generally develop antibodies against envelope (gp61/68, gp71), core (p19, p24), and regulatory (Tax) proteins (218). The gp61/68 protein represents the major uncleaved envelope protein, and consists of a gp46 exterior component and a gp21 transmembrane component. A study of reactivity of sera from recent seroconverters with recombinant evelope peptides has shown that the C terminal region of gp46 represents a major immunogenic domain; whereas none of eight sera reacted with the N terminal half of gp46, seven of eight reacted with the middle region of gp46, and all eight reacted with the C terminal region. Accordingly, a recombinant protein consisting of this C terminal region coupled to gp21 (referred to as p21e) is now used in confirmatory tests for HTLV infection (218).

As mentioned earlier, type-specific peptides have been defined which allow HTLV-I infection to be distinguished from HTLV-II infection (219,220). These peptides represent epitopes that reside mainly in a 69–amino acid sequence bounded by two cysteine residues in the middle of the exterior envelope proteins of HTLV-I and HTLV-II (221).

Reactivity in the enzyme immunoassay used for screening occasionally gives an indeterminate result in confirmatory tests. At least some of this indeterminate reactivity can be caused by antibodies to *Plasmodium falciparum*, an etiological agent for malaria (222). Blocking studies showed that malarial antibodies cross-react with the HTLV-I p19 protein. HTLV-I seroprevalence studies in geographical areas where malaria is endemic must therefore include careful confirmatory studies to avoid an overestimation of prevalence.

The cellular immune response to HTLV is just beginning to be defined. CD8+ cytotoxic T cells are found in fresh PBMCs from patients with HAM/TSP but not from asymptomatic carriers (223). These cells predominantly recognize the Tax protein, but some envelope reactivity was also noted. These investigators also found evidence of CD4+ cytotoxic cells directed against the gp46 envelope protein in patients with HAM/TSP (224). However,

generation of these cells required repeated stimulation of HAM/TSP PBMCs with autologous T-cell lines expressing HTLV.

C. Characteristics of Infected Lymphocytes

Clues to the type of lymphocytes subject to HTLV infection came from studies of the malignant cell in ATL associated with HTLV-I infection. The ATL cell is a CD4+ T cell with a memory (CD29+CD45RA–) phenotype (225); this cell also constitutively expresses CD25, the low-affinity chain of the IL-2 receptor (226). Dysregulation of CD25 expression appears to be a direct result of HTLV-I infection; the HTLV-I Tax protein induces kB-specific proteins that bind to kB enhancer elements of both the CD25 and IL-2 genes, upregulating their transcription (227). Thus, the immortalized state of the ATL cell probably reflects an autocrine growth system involving IL-2 and its receptor.

Polymerase chain reaction studies have shown that HTLV-I infection in patients with HAM/TSP and asymptomatic carriers is also confined to memory CD4 T cells (CD4+ CD45RO+) (228). Provirus was not detected in B cells, NK cells, CD8 cells, or monocytes. It is estimated that as many as 15% of mononuclear cells from patients with HAM/TSP and 2% of mononuclear cells from asymptomatic carriers carry provirus (228,229). The restriction of provirus to memory CD4 cells suggests that CD4 cell activation may play an important role in HTLV-I infection, similar to the situation for HIV (see Sect. II.H).

The cellular reservoir for HTLV-II has not been delineated. Since both CD4+ and CD8+ lines expressing HTLV-II were derived from the rare HTLV-II–seropositive patients with hairy cell leukemia, both cell types may be infected (207).

Because CD25 expression is central to HTLV-I–associated ATL, several groups have measured soluble CD25 (sCD25) in HTLV-I infection. All studies have documented increased serum levels of sCD25 in patients with ATL and patients with HAM/TSP (230–233). Data for sCD25 levels in asymptomatic carriers are conflicting, however. Two studies, including one from Japan where carriers are essentially all seropositive for HTLV-I (231,233), found an increased mean level of sCD25; in contrast, another study from Japan found normal sCD25 levels in asymptomatic carriers (230). Prince et al. (217) found normal sCD25 levels in asymptomatic HTLV-seropositive blood donors from Los Angeles, a group consisting mostly of HTLV-II–infected persons. It thus remains unclear if increased sCD25 production characterizes asymptomatic HTLV infection.

D. Lymphocyte Subset Changes

Studies of lymphocyte subsets in HTLV-infected groups have been limited to patients with HAM/TSP and asymptomatic carriers because dramatic expansion of the malignant cell in ATL confounds measurement of other cells. Itoyama et al. (234) found that the overall percentages of CD4 and CD8 cells were normal in patients with HAM/TSP; however, the percentages of CD29+CD4, DR+CD4, and DR+CD8 cells were increased. Further, the percentage of CD25+ cells was significantly increased. These changes suggest increased levels of activated CD4 and CD8 T cells in association with HAM/TSP.

Data for lymphocyte subsets in asymptomatic carriers are conflicting and complicated (Table 7). A study from Japan, representing HTLV-I carriers, found no changes in the percentage of CD4 or CD8 cells, but identified a subtle yet significant increase in CD25+ cells (235). deShazo et al. (236), studying intravenous drug users (presumably infected with HTLV-II), found normal levels of CD4 cells, CD8 cells, and B cells; however, the percentage of CD29+CD4 cells was increased. Fletcher et al. (237) also found increased levels of CD29+CD4 cells in seropositive blood donors (presumably HTLV-II infection) from Miami, Florida, and further noted increased absolute levels of T cells, NK cells, CD45RA+CD4 cells, and DR+CD8 cells. Rosenblatt et al. (238) studied HTLV-II–infected intravenous drug users and found normal levels of T cells, CD4 cells, CD8 cells, B cells, NK cells, CD25+ cells, and DR+CD8 cells. Prince et al. studied HTLV-seropositive donors from Los Angeles (mostly HTLV-II) and also found normal levels of T, CD4, CD8, B, CD45RA+CD4, DR+CD4, and DR+CD8 cells (239) but a decreased percentage of NK cells (240). Thus, most investigators agree that the percentages of T, CD4, CD8, B, NK, and CD25+ cells are normal, and that CD29+CD4 cells are increased in association with asymptomatic HTLV infection. Conflicts arise, however, when examining CD45RA+CD4 and DR+CD8 cells.

In an effort to clarify these conflicts, my laboratory has reassessed lymphocyte subsets in asymptomatic seropositive blood donors (mostly HTLV-II). In contrast to our earlier study that utilized a Spectrum III flow cytometer (Ortho Diagnostics, Westwood, MA) (239), this study utilized a FACScan flow cytometer (Becton Dickinson Immunocytometry Systems, San Jose, CA) , which offers superior sensitivity for detecting dim fluorescence (240). We also employed a newly available monoclonal antibody defining memory T cells, CD45RO (66). This marker defines a population similar, but not identical, to the population defined by CD29 expression. The results are summarized in Table 8. In support of our previous findings, the percentages of T, CD4, CD8, and B cells were normal in the HTLV group; likewise, the CD45RA+CD4

Table 7 Lymphocyte Subsets in Asymptomatic HTLV Carriers

	References				
Parameter	235	236	237	238	239,240
Predominant HTLV type studied	I	II	II	II	II
T cells	ND[a]	Normal	Normal	Normal	Normal
CD4 cells	Normal	Normal	Normal	Normal	Normal
CD8 cells	Normal	Normal	Normal	Normal	Normal
B cells	ND	Normal	ND	Normal	Normal
NK cells	ND	Normal	High	Normal	Low
CD29+CD4+ cells	ND	High	High	ND	ND
CD45RA+CD4+ cells	ND	Normal	High	ND	Normal
DR+CD8+ cells	ND	ND	High	Normal	Normal[b]
CD25+ cells	High	ND	ND	Normal	Normal

[a]ND, not done.
[b]Increased in a later study, see Table 8.

Table 8 Selected Lymphocyte Subset Values Determined Using a FACScan Flow Cytometer

Cell Subset	Control (N = 20)	HTLV (N = 20)
T	72 ± 7	75 ± 7
CD4	48 ± 9	49 ± 8
CD8	26 ± 5	28 ± 9
B	13 ± 7	12 ± 4
CD45RA+CD4+	24 ± 8	24 ± 8
CD45RO+CD4+	34 ± 8	35 ± 8
DR+CD4+	3.6 ± 1.4	4.8 ± 1.5[a]
DR+CD8+	3.8 ± 2.5	8.0 ± 5.4[a]

[a]Significantly different from control value (P < 0.05, Mann-Whitney U test).

population was unchanged. We also found that the percentage of CD45RO+CD4 cells was unchanged in the HTLV group. In contrast to our previous findings, however, the percentage of DR+CD8 cells was significantly increased in the HTLV group; further, the percentage of DR+CD4 cells was subtly but significantly increased. The identification of an increased percentage of DR+CD8 cells was directly attributable to improved fluorescence detection by the FACScan; the specimens with increased DR+CD8 values on the FACScan gave normal values when analyzed on the Spectrum III (e.g., a sample with 11% DR+CD8 cells using the FACScan gave only 4% DR+CD8 cells using the Spectrum III). Thus, differences in instrumentation may partially explain the conflicting data in the literature for certain subset changes in HTLV infection.

E. Spontaneous Lymphocyte Proliferation

An intriguing in vitro immunological phenomenon associated with HTLV infection is spontaneous lymphocyte proliferation (SLP). As first described by Yasuda et al. (235), PBMCs from asymptomatic HTLV-I carriers cultured in vitro in the absence of exogenous stimuli spontaneously proliferated and produced CD25+ blastoid cells. Several subsequent studies confirmed this finding (241), and further revealed that PBMCs from essentially all patients with HAM/TSP also exhibit SLP (234,242–244); however, this phenomenon is not observed in ATL. Several recent studies, including those from my laboratory, have demonstrated that SLP also characterizes asymptomatic HTLV-II infection (245–247). It appears, however, that PBMCs from only about 50% of asymptomatic HTLV-I or HTLV-II carriers exhibit SLP (217). In a search for immunological correlates with SLP, the only significant difference we could identify related to circulating levels of HTLV antibodies; asymptomatic carriers exhibiting SLP had, on average, much higher levels of anti-HTLV in their serum when compared with carriers not exhibiting SLP (217). Since studies in patients with HAM/TSP show that high anti-HTLV titers are related to viral load, and all patients with HAM/TSP patients exhibit SLP, it is possible that SLP is thus related to viral load (217,229).

What cells are activated during SLP? In my laboratory, we approached this question by assessing lymphocyte markers on activated (CD25+) cells from 7-day cultures using two-color flow cytometry. Our findings (248) showed that CD8 cells and NK cells (CD16/56+) were preferentially activated during SLP. CD4 cells also showed evidence of activation but not to the same extent as CD8 and NK cells; there was no evidence of B-cell activation. These findings are consistent with those of Yasuda et al. (235), who found that the blastoid cell population in cultures showing SLP was enriched for CD8 cells.

We have recently begun studies to determine if CD4 cells are required for CD8 and NK cell activation during SLP. Our preliminary results (Table 9) indicate that highly purified CD8 cells and NK cells (containing some dimly positive CD8 cells) show SLP in the absence of CD4

Table 9 Spontaneous Lymphocyte Proliferation by Purified Lymphocyte Subsets[a]

Donor	PBMC	CD4	CD8	NK
Control	688	355	56	53
Control	823	119	81	107
HTLV+	18512	312	8425	943
HTLV+	3783	536	13941	5330

[a]Cultures of purified subsets were supplemented with 20% autologous monocytes. Data represent counts per minute in cultures pulsed with [3H]thymidine for 4 h on day 7 of culture.

cells. In contrast, highly purified CD4 cells show little, if any, proliferation. CD4 cell activation as part of SLP in PBMCs may thus reflect a bystander response to cytokines released by proliferating CD8 and/or NK cells.

The mechanisms for inducing and regulating SLP remain poorly defined. One possible mechanism is mitogenic activation of lymphocytes by HTLV proteins. Gazzalo and Duc Dono (249,250) have shown that inactivated HTLV-I particles stimulate proliferation of normal T cells. Both CD4 and CD8 T cells were activated, and the response was independent of accessory cells (i.e., monocytes). Serum from a healthy HTLV-I carrier, as well as a monoclonal antibody against the envelope gp46 molecule, inhibited activation. Further, monoclonal antibodies against the T-cell surface marker CD2, but not CD3, inhibited activation. These findings suggest the hypothesis that HTLV envelope protein, released at low levels during in vitro culture of PBMCs from HTLV-infected persons, may act as a mitogen that induces lymphocyte activation.

Data from my laboratory, however, indicate that SLP differs in many aspects from the HTLV-induced mitogenic response just described, providing indirect evidence against a mitogenic effect of envelope protein in SLP. These differences are summarized in Table 10. First, unlike the mitogenic response induced by inactivated HTLV, SLP is dependent on accessory cells. For a group of six individuals showing SLP, the mean proliferative response of PBMCs was 19,779 counts per minute (cpm) ± 6889, whereas the response of monocyte-depleted cultures was 770 cpm ± 822; on readdition of monocytes, the response was restored to a mean value of 17,348 cpm ± 12,709. These findings confirm and extend those of Itoyama et al. (243). Second, as presented in Table 9, purified CD4 cells show little activation in SLP but are efficiently activated by HTLV particles. Third, sera from asymptomatic HTLV-I and HTLV-II carriers with high titers of anti-HTLV do not inhibit SLP even when present as 25% of total culture volume. Fourth, monoclonal antibodies against HTLV-I envelope and core proteins do not inhibit SLP when compared with a monoclonal antibody against HIV envelope protein. Additional evidence against a mitogenic effect being responsible for SLP was presented by Lal and Rudolph (247), who found no HTLV antigen in supernatants of cultures showing SLP. Further, we found that supernatants from monocyte-depleted cultures (thus not showing proliferation) of proliferation-positive PBMC did not stimulate proliferation of normal PBMCs, arguing against a stimulant (e.g., envelope protein) being secreted by HTLV-infected cells in culture.

An alternative explanation for SLP suggested by Tendler et al. (244) involves Tax expression by infected cells in the absence of envelope or core gene expression. These investigators found small but detectable quantities of Tax mRNA in lymphocytes from HAM/TSP patients exhibiting SLP. As mentioned previously, Tax can upregulate IL-2 and CD25 gene expression via their kB enhancer elements. In this sense, Tax resembles the Tat protein of HIV. Both Tax and Tat apparently induce TNF-α, which in turn induces CD25 gene expression via nuclear proteins reactive with the kB enhancer element. In support of this hypothesis, Lal and Rudolph (247) found elevated levels of TNF-α in supernatants of PBMCs undergoing SLP. Thus, SLP may reflect Tax-mediated dysregulation of IL-2 and CD25 expression resulting in polyclonal T-cell activation. This hypothesis fails to explain why CD8 cells are

Table 10 Differences in the Mitogenic Effect of HTLV Particles and Spontaneous Lymphocyte Proliferation (SLP)

Characteristic	HTLV Particles	SLP
Accessory cell independent	Yes	No
Activation of purified CD4 cells	Yes	No
Inhibited by sera containing HTLV antibodies	Yes	No
Inhibited by monoclonal antibodies against HTLV	Yes	No

preferentially activated in SLP, however. At least for HTLV-I infection, CD8 cells apparently do not carry viral genome, and thus should not carry the pX gene encoding for the Tax protein (228). Perhaps Tax protein produced by infected CD4 cells can be taken up by CD8 cells, where the protein then initiates the hypothesized activation cascade leading to SLP. Much more work is obviously needed to dissect the mechanisms involved in HTLV-associated SLP.

REFERENCES

1. Ho DD, Pomerantz RJ, Kaplan JC. Pathogenesis of infection with human immunodeficiency virus, N Engl J Med 1987; 317:278.
2. Gallo RC. HIV—the cause of AIDS: an overview of its biology, mechanisms of disease induction, and our attempts to control it. Acquir Immune Defic Syndr 1988; 1:521.
3. Gaines H, Sonnerborg A, Czajkowski J. et al. Antibody response in primary human immuno-deficiency virus infection. Lancet 1987; i:1249.
4. Ganchini G, Robert-Guroff M, Aldovini A, et al. Spectrum of natural antibodies against five HTLV-III antigens in infected individuals: Correlation of antibody prevalence with clinical status. Blood 1987; 69:437.
5. Allan JS, Coligan JE, Barin F, et al. Major glycoprotein antigens that induce antibodies in AIDS patients are encoded by HTLV-III. Science 1985; 228:1091.
6. Barin F, McLane MF, Allan JS, et al. Virus envelope protein of HTLV-III represents major target antigen for antibodies in AIDS patients. Science 1985; 228:1094.
7. Burke DS, Brandt BL, Redfield RR, et al. Diagnosis of human immunodeficiency virus infection by immunoassay using a molecularly cloned and expressed viral envelope polypeptide. Comparison to Western blot on 2707 consecutive serum samples. Ann Intern Med 1987; 106:671.
8. Ranki A, Weiss SH, Valle S-L, et al. Neutralizing antibodies to HIV (HTLV-III) infection: correlation with clinical outcome and antibody response against different viral proteins. Clin Exp Immunol 1987; 69:231.
9. Ho DD, Rota TR, Hirsch MS. Antibody to lymphadenopathy-associated virus in AIDS. N Engl J Med 1985; 312:649.
10. Rasheed S, Norman GL, Gill PS, et al. Virus-neutralizing activity, serologic heterogeneity, and retrovirus isolation from homosexual men in the Los Angeles area. Virology 1987; 150:1.
11. Lasky LA. Current status of the development of an AIDS vaccine. CRC Crit Rev Immunol 1989; 9:153.
12. Redfield RR, Birx DL, Ketter N, et al. A phase I evaluation of the safety and immunogenicity of vaccination with recombinant gp160 in patients with early human immunodeficiency virus infection. N Engl J Med 1991; 324:1677.
13. Cao Y, Valentine F, Hojvat S, et al. Detection of HIV antigen and specific antibodies to HIV core and envelope proteins in sera of patients with HIV infection. Blood 1987; 70:575.
14. Lange JMA, Paul DA, Huisman HG, et al. Persistent HIV antigenemia and decline of HIV core antibodies associated with transition to AIDS. Br Med J 1986; 293:1459.
15. McDougal JS, Kennedy MS, Nicholson JKA, et al. Antibody response to human immunodeficiency virus in homosexual men. Relation of antibody specificity, titer, and isotype to clinical status, severity of immunodeficiency, and disease progression. J Clin Invest 1987; 80:316.
16. Laurence J, Saunders A, Kulkosky J. Characterization and clinical association of antibody inhibitory to HIV reverse transcriptase activity. Science 1987; 235:1501.
17. Chartterjee R., Rinaldo CR, Gupta P. Immunogenicity of human immunodeficiency virus (HIV) reverse transcriptase: detection of high levels of antibodies to HIV reverse transcriptase in sera of homosexual men. J Clin Immunol 1987; 7:218.
18. Warren RQ, Wolf H, Zajac RA, et al. Patterns of antibody reactivity to selected human immunodeficiency virus type 1 (HIV-1) gp160 epitopes in infected individuals grouped according to CD4+ cell levels. J Clin Immunol 1991; 11:13.
19. Tribe DE, Reed DL, Lindell P, et al. Antibodies reactive with human immunodeficiency virus

gag-coded antigens (gag reactive only) are a major cause of enzyme-linked immunosorbent assay reactivity in a blood donor population. J Clin Microbiol 1988; 26:641.

20. Leitman SF, Klein HG, Melpolder JJ, et al. Clinical implications of positive tests for antibodies to human immunodeficiency virus type 1 in asymptomatic blood donors. N Engl J Med 1989; 321:917.

21. Dock NL, Kleinman SH, Rayfield MA, et al. Human immunodeficiency virus infection and indeterminate Western blot patterns. Prospective studies in a low prevalence population. Arch Intern Med 1991; 151:525.

22. Jackson JB, McDonald KL, Cadwell J, et al. Absence of HIV infection in blood donors with indeterminate Western blot tests for antibody to HIV-1. N Engl J Med 1990; 322:217.

23. Zolla-Pazner S. B cells in the pathogenesis of AIDS. Immunol Today 1984; 5:289.

24. Pinching, AJ. Antibody responses in HIV infection. Clin Exp Immunol 1991; 84:181.

25. Martinez-Maza O, Crabb E, Mitsuyasu RT, et al. Infection with the human immunodeficiency virus (HIV) is associated with an in vivo increase in B lymphocyte activation and immaturity. J Immunol 1987; 138:3720.

26. Jacobson DL, McCutchan JA, Spechko PL, et al. The evolution of lymphadenopathy and hypergammaglobulinemia are evidence for early and sustained polyclonal B lymphocyte activation during human immunodeficiency virus infection. J Infect Dis 1991; 163:240.

27. Ozturk GE, Kohler PF, Horsburgh CR, Kirkpatrick CH. The significance of antilymphocyte antibodies in patients with acquired immune deficiency syndrome (AIDS) and their sexual partners. Clin Immunol 1987; 7:130.

28. Schnittman SM, Lane HC, Higgins SE, et al. Direct polyclonal activation of human B lymphocytes by the acquired immune deficiency syndrome virus. Science 1986; 233: 1084.

29. Lanier LL, Phillips JH, Hackett J, et al. Natural killer cells: definition of a cell type rather than a function. J Immunol 1986; 137:2735.

30. Imir T, Saksela E, Makela O. Two forms of antibody dependent cell-mediated cytotoxicity, arming and sensitization. J Immunol 1976; 117:1938.

31. Plaeger-Marshall S, Spina CA, Giorgi JV, et al. Alterations in cytotoxic and phenotypic subsets of natural killer cells in acquired immune deficiency syndrome (AIDS). J Clin Immunol 1987; 7:16.

32. Tyler DS, Stanley SD, Nastala CA, et al. Alterations in antibody-dependent cellular cytotoxicity during the course of HIV-1 infection. Humoral and cellular defects. J Immunol 1990; 144: 3375.

33. Fontana L, Sirianni MC, DeSanctis G, et al. Deficiency of natural killer activity, but not natural killer binding, in patients with lymphadenopathy syndrome positive for antibodies to HTLV-III. Immunobiology 1986; 171:425.

34. Ojo-Amaize E, Nishanian PG, Heitjan DF, et al. Serum and effector-cell antibody-dependent cellular cytotoxicity (ADCC) activity remains high during human immunodeficiency virus (HIV) disease progression. J Clin Immunol 1989; 9:454.

35. Katz JD, Mitsuyasu R, Gottlieb MS, et al. Mechanism of defective NK cell activity in patients with acquired immunodificiency syndrome (AIDS) and AIDS-related complex. II. Normal antibody-dependent cellular cytotoxicity (ADCC) mediated by effector cells defective in natural killer (NK) cytotoxicity. J Immunol 1987; 139:55.

36. Sirianni MC, Soddus S, Malorni W, et al. Mechanism of defective natural killer cell activity in patients with AIDS is associated with defective distribution of tubulin. J Immunol 1988; 140: 2565.

37. Lyerly HK, Matthews TJ, Langlois AJ, et al. Human T-lymphotropic virus IIIB glycoprotein (gp120) bound to CD4 determinants on normal lymphocytes and expressed by infected cells serves as target for immune attack. Proc Natl Acad Sci USA 1987; 84:4601.

38. Katz JD, Nishanian P, Mitsuyasu R, Bonavida B. Antibody-dependent cellular cytotoxicity (ADCC)-mediated destruction of human immunodeficiency virus (HIV)-coated CD4+ T lymphocytes by acquired immunodeficiency syndrome (AIDS) effector cells. J Clin Immunol 1988; 8:453.

39. Tyler DS, Stanley SD, Zolla-Pazner S, et al. Identification of sites within gp41 that serve as

targets for antibody-dependent cellular cytotoxicity by using human monoclonal antibodies. J Immunol 1990; 145:3276.

40. Koup RA, Sullivan JL, Levine PH, et al. Antigenic specificity of antibody-dependent cell-mediated cytotoxicity directed against human immunodeficiency virus in antibody-positive sera. J Virol 1989; 63:584.

41. Ljunggren K, Broliden P-A., Morfeldt-Manson L., et al. IgG subclass response to HIV in relation to antibody-dependent cellular cytotoxicity at different clinical stages. Clin Exp Immunol 1988; 73:343.

42. Rook AH, Lance HC, Folks T, et al. Sera from HTLV-III/LAV antibody-positive individuals mediate antibody-dependent cellular cytotoxicity against HTLV-III/LAV infected T cells. J Immunol 1987; 138:1064.

43. Ljunggren K, Bottiger B, Biberfeld G., et al. Antibody-dependent cellular cytotoxicity-inducing antibodies against human immunodeficiency virus. Presence at different clinical stages. J Immunol 1987; 139:2263.

44. Schroff RW, Gottlieb MS, Prince HE, et al. Immunological studies of homosexual men with immunodeficiency and Kaposi's sarcoma. Clin Immunol Immunopathol 1983; 27:300.

45. Fahey JL, Prince H, Weaver M, et al. Quantitative changes in T helper or T suppressor/cytotoxic lymphocyte subsets that distinguish acquired immune deficiency syndrome from other immune subset disorders. Am J Med 1984; 76:95.

46. Landay A, Ohlsson-Wilhelm B, Giorgi JV. Application of flow cytometry to the study of HIV infection. AIDS 1990; 4:479.

47. Rogers MF, Morens DM, Stewart JA, et al. National case-control study of Kaposi's sarcoma and *Pneumocystis carinii* pneumonia in homosexual men: Part 2, laboratory results. Ann Intern Med 1983; 99:151.

48. Jason J, McDougal JS, Holman RC, et al. Human T-lymphotropic virus type III/ lymphadenopathy-associated virus antibody. Association with hemophiliacs' immune status and blood component usage. JAMA 1985; 253:3409.

49. Hersh EM, Mansell PWA, Reuben JM, et al. Immunologic characterizations of patients with acquired immune deficiency syndrome, acquired immune deficiency syndrome-related symptom complex, and a related lifestyle. Cancer Res 1984; 44:5894.

50. Stites DP, Casavant CH, McHugh TM, et al. Flow cytometric analysis of lymphocyte phenotypes in AIDS using monoclonal antibodies and simultaneous dual immunofluorescence. Clin Immunol Immunopathol 1986; 38:161.

51. Lang W, Anderson RE, Perkins H, et al. Clinical, immunologic, and serologic findings in men at risk for acquired immunodeficiency syndrome. The San Francisco Men's Health Study. JAMA 1987; 257:326.

52. Goldsmith JM, Kalish SB, Ostrow DG, et al. Antibody to human lymphotropic virus type III: immunologic status of homosexual contacts of patients with the acquired immunodefic- iency syndrome and the acquired immunodeficiency-related complex. Sex Transm Dis 1987; 14:44.

53. Van Nossel CJM, Gruters RA, Terpstra FG, et al. Functional and phenotypic evidence for a selective loss of memory T cells in asymptomatic human immunodeficiency virus-infected men. J Clin Invest 1990; 86:293.

54. Giorgi JV, Fahey JL, Smith DC, et al. Early effects of HIV on CD4 lymphocytes in vivo. J Immunol 1987; 138:3725.

55. Sullivan JL, Brewster FE, Brettler DB et al. Hemophiliac immunodeficiency: Influence of exposure to factor VIII concentrate, LAV/HTLV-III, and herpesviruses. J Pediatr 1986; 108:504.

56. Cooper DA, Tindall B, Wilson EJ, et al. Characterization of T lymphocyte responses during primary infection with human immunodeficiency virus. J Infect Dis 1988; 157: 889.

57. Lang W, Perkins H, Anderson RE, et al. Patterns of T lymphocyte changes with human immunodeficiency virus infection: From seroconversion to the development of AIDS. J Acquir Immune Def Syndr 1989; 2:63.

58. Taylor J, Afrasiabi R, Fahey JL, et al. Prognostically significant classification of immune changes in AIDS with Kaposi's sarcoma. Blood 1986; 67:666.

59. Eyster ME, Gail MH, Ballard JO, et al. Natural history of human immunodeficiency virus

infections in hemophiliacs: Effects of T-cell subsets, platelet counts, and age. Ann Intern Med 1987; 107:1.

60. Nicholson JKA, Jones BM, Echenberg DF, et al. Phenotypic distribution of T cells in patients who have subsequently developed AIDS. Clin Immunol Immunopathol 1987; 43:82

61. Spira TJ, Kaplan JE, Holman RC, et al. Deterioration in immunologic status of human immunodeficiency virus (HIV)-infected homosexual men with lymphadenopathy: Prognostic implications. J Clin Immunol 1989; 9:132.

62. Weber JN, Rogers LA, Scott K, et al. Three-year prospective study of HTLV-III/LAV infection in homosexual men. Lancet 1986; 1:1179.

63. Taylor JMG, Fahey JL, Detels R, Giorgi JV. CD4 percentage, CD4 number, and CD4:CD8 ratio in HIV infection: Which to choose and how to use. J Acquir Immune Defic Syndr 1989; 2:114.

64. Phillips AN, Lee CA, Elford J, et al. Serial CD4 lymphocyte counts and development of AIDS. Lancet 1991; 337:389.

65. Detels R, English PA, Giorgi JV, et al. Patterns of CD4+ cell changes after HIV-1 infection indicate the existence of a codeterminant of AIDS. J Acqui Immune Defic Syndr 1988; 1:390.

66. Akbar AN, Terry L, Timms A, et al. Loss of CD45R and gain of UCHL1 reactivity is a feature of primed T cells. J Immunol 1988; 140:2171

67. Giorgi JV, Detels R. T-cell subset alterations in HIV-infected homosexual men: NIAID multicenter AIDS cohort study. Clin Immunol Immunopathol 1989; 52:10.

68. Gupta S. Subpopulations of CD4+ (T4+) cells in homosexual/bisexual men with persistent generalized lymphadenopathy. Clin Exp Immunol 1987; 68:1.

69. Prince, HE, Arens L, Kleinman SH. CD4 and CD8 subsets defined by dual-color cytofluorometry which distinguish symptomatic from asymptomatic blood donors seropositive for human immunodeficiency virus. Diag Clin Immunol 1987; 5:188.

70. Nicholson JKA, McDougal JS, Spria TJ, et al. Immunoregulatory subsets of the T helper and T suppressor cell populations in homosexual men with chronic unexplained lymphadenopathy. J Clin Invest 1984; 73:191.

71. Schnittman SM, Lane HC, Greenhouse J, et al. Preferential infection of CD4+ memory T cells by human immunodeficiency virus type 1: Evidence for a role in the selective T-cell functional defects observed in infected individuals. Proc Natl Acad Sci USA 1990; 87:6058.

72. Cayota A, Vuillier F, Scott-Algara D, Dighiero G. Preferential replication of HIV-1 in memory CD4+ subpopulation. Lancet 1990; 336:941.

73. Jackson AL, Matsumoto H, Janszen M, et al. Restricted expression of p55 interleukin 2 receptor (CD25) on normal T cells. Clin Immunol Immunopathol 1990; 54:126.

74. Zola H, Koh LY, Mantzioris BX, Rhodes D. Patients with HIV infection have a reduced proportion of lymphocytes expressing the IL2 receptor p55 chain (Tac, CD25). Clin Immunol Immunopathol 1991; 59:16.

75. Kanof ME, James SP. Leu-8 antigen expression is diminished during cell activation but does not correlate with effector function of activated T lymphocytes. J Immunol 1988; 140: 3701.

76. Tedder TF, Penta AC, Levine HB, Freedman AS. Expression of the human leukocyte adhesion molecule, LAM1. Identity with the TQ1 and Leu-8 antigens. J Immunol 1990; 144:532.

77. Giorgi JV, Nishanian PG, Schmid I, et al. Selective alterations in immunoregulatory lymphocyte subsets in early HIV (human T-lymphotropic virus type III/lymphadenopathy-associated virus) infection. J Clin Immunol 1987; 7:140.

78. Prince HE, Jensen ER. Three-color cytofluorometric analysis of CD8 cell subsets in HIV-1 infection J Acquir Immun Defic Syndr 1991; 4:1227.

79. Nicholson JKA, McDougal JS, Spria TJ. Alterations of functional subsets of T helper and T suppressor cell populations in acquired immunodeficiency syndrome (AIDS) and chronic unexplained lymphadenopathy. J Clin Immunol 1985; 5:269.

80. Schroff RW, Gale RP, Fahey JL. Regeneration of T cell subpopulations after bone marrow transplantation: Cytomegalovirus infection and lymphoid subset imbalance. J Immunol 1982; 129:1926.

81. Hercend R, Ritz J, Schlossman SF, Reinherz EL. Comparative expression of T9, T10, and Ia antigens on activated human T cell subsets. Hum Immunol 1981; 3:247.

82. Prince HE, Kreiss JK, Kasper CK, et al. Distinctive lymphocyte subpopulation abnormalities in patients with congenital coagulation disorders who exhibit lymph node enlargement. Blood 1985; 66:64.

83. Salazar-Gonzalez JF, Moody DJ, Giorgi et al. Reduced ecto-5'-nucleotidase activity and enhanced OKT10 and HLA-DR expression on CD8 T (suppressor/cytotoxic) lymphocytes in the acquired immune deficiency syndrome: Evidence of CD8 cell immaturity. J Immunol 1985; 135:1778.

84. Prince HE, Kleinman S, Czaplicki C, et al. Interrelationships between serologic markers of immune activation and T lymphocyte subsets in HIV infection. J Acquir Immune Defec Syndr 3:525.

85. Desroches CV, Rigal D. Leukocyte function-associated antigen-1 expression of peripheral blood mononuclear cell subsets in HIV-1 seropositive patients. Clin Immunol Immunopathol 1990; 56:159.

86. Sanders ME, Makgoba MW, Shaw S. Human naive and memory T cells: reinterpretation of helper-inducer and suppressor-inducer subsets. Immunol Today 9:195.

87. Nicholson JKA, Echenberg DF, Jones BM, et al. T-cytotoxic/suppressor cell phenotypes in a group of asymptomatic homosexual men with and without exposure to HTLV-III/LAV. Clin Immunol Immunopathol 1986; 40:505.

88. Clement LT, Dagg MK, Landay A. Characterization of human lymphocyte subpopulations: Alloreactive cytotoxic T-lymphocyte precursor and effector cells are phenotypically distinct from Leu 2+ suppressor cells. J Clin Immunol 1984; 4:395.

89. Gupta S. Abnormality of Leu 2+7+ cells in acquired immune deficiency syndrome (AIDS), AIDS-related complex, and asymptomatic homosexuals. J Clin Immunol 1986; 6:502.

90. Lewis DE, Puck JM, Babcock GF, Rich RR. Disproportionate expansion of a minor T cell subset in patients with lymphadenopathy syndrome and acquired immunodeficiency syndrome. J Infect Dis 1985; 151:555.

91. Ziegler-Heitbrock HWL, Schramm W, Stachel D, et al. Expansion of a minor subpopulation of peripheral blood lymphocytes (T8+/Leu7+) in patients with hemophilia. Clin Exp Immunol 1985; 61:633.

92. Stahl RE, Friedman-Kien A, Dubin R, et al. Immunologic abnormalities in homosexual men. Relationship to Kaposi's sarcoma. Am J Med 1982; 73:171.

93. Ciobanu N, Welte K, Kruger G, et al. Defective T-cell response to PHA and mitogenic monoclonal antibodies in male homosexuals with acquired immunodeficiency syndrome and its in vitro correction by interleukin 2. J Clin Immunol 1983; 3:332.

94. Lane HC, Depper JM, Greene WC, et al. Qualitative analysis of immune function in patients with the acquired immunodeficiency syndrome. Evidence for a selective defect in soluble antigen recognition. N Engl J Med 1985; 313:79.

95. Hofman B, Odum N, Platz P, et al. Immunological studies in acquired immunodeficiency syndrome. Functional studies of lymphocyte subpopulations. Scand J Immunol 1985; 21:235.

96. Ebert EC, Stoll DB, Cassens BJ, et al. Diminished interleukin 2 production and receptor generation characterize the acquired immunodeficiency syndrome. Clin Immunol Immunopathol 1985; 37:283.

97. Miedema F, Petit AJC, Terpstra FG, et al. Immunological abnormalities in human immunodeficiency virus (HIV)-infected asymptomatic homosexual men. HIV affects the immune system before CD4+ T helper cell depletion occurs. J Clin Invest 1988; 82:1908.

98. Margolick JB, Volkman DJ, Lane HC, Fauci AS. Clonal analysis of T lymphocytes in the acquired immunodeficiency syndrome. Evidence for an abnormality affecting individual helper and suppressor T cells. J Clin Invest 1985; 76:709.

99. Clerici M, Stocks NI, Zajac RA, et al. Detection of three distinct patterns of T helper cell dysfunction in asymptomatic, human immunodeficiency virus-seropositive patients. Independence of CD4+ cell numbers and clinical staging. J Clin Invest 1989; 84:1892.

100. Shearer GM, Clerici M. Early T-helper cell defects in HIV infection. AIDS 5:245.

101. Clerici M, Via CS, Lucey DR, et al. Functional dichotomy of CD4+ T helper lymphocytes in asymptomatic human immunodeficiency virus infection. Eur J Immunol 1991; 21:665.
102. Teshigawara K, Wang HM, Kato K, Smith KA. Interleukin-2 high affinity receptor expression requires two distinct binding proteins. J Exp Med 1987; 165:223.
103. Prince HE, Kermani-Arab V, Fahey JL. Depressed interleukin 2 receptor expression in acquired immune deficiency and lymphadenopathy syndromes. J Immunol 1984; 133: 1313.
104. Munn CG, Reuben JM, Hersh EM, Mansell PWA, Newell GR. T cell surface antigen expression on lymphocytes of patients with AIDS during in vitro mitogen stimulation. Cancer Immunol Immunother 1984; 18:141.
105. Gupta S. Study of activated T cells in man. II. Interleukin 2 receptor and transferrin receptor expression on T cells and production of interleukin 2 in patients with acquired immune deficiency syndrome (AIDS) and AIDS-related complex. Clin Immunol Immunopathol 1986; 38:93.
106. Winkelstein A, Kingsley LA, Weaver LD, Machen LL. Defective T cell colony formation and IL-2 receptor expression in HIV-infected homosexuals: Relationship between functional abnormalities and CD4 cell numbers. J Acquir Immune Defec Syndr 1989; 2:353.
107. Prince HE, John JK. Early activation marker expression to detect impaired proliferative responses to pokeweed mitogen and tetanus toxoid: studies in patients with AIDS and related disorders. Diag Immunol 1986; 4:306.
108. Prince HE, Czaplicki CD. In vitro activation of T lymphocytes from HIV-seropositive blood donors. II. Decreased mitogen-induced expression of interleukin 2 receptor by both CD4 and CD8 cell subsets. Clin Immunol Immunopathol 1988; 48:132.
109. Prince HE, John JK. Abnormalities of interleukin 2 receptor expression associated with decreased antigen-induced lymphocyte proliferation in patients with AIDS and related disorders. Clin Exp Immunol 1987; 67:59.
110. Winkelstein A, Kingsley LA, Klein RS, et al. Defective T-cell colony formation and IL-2 receptor expression at all stages of HIV infection. Clin Exp Immunol 1988; 71:417.
111. Smith KA. Interleukin 2: Inception, impact, and implications. Science 1988; 240:1169.
112. Hofmann B, Moller J, Langhoff E, et al. Stimulation of AIDS lymphocytes with calcium ionophore (A23187) and phorbol ester (PMA): Studies of cytoplasmic free Ca^{2+}, IL-2 receptor expression, IL-2 production, and proliferation. Cell Immunol 1989; 119:14.
113. Pantaleo G, Koenig S, Baseler M, et al. Defective clonogenic potential of CD8+ T lymphocytes in patients with AIDS. Expansion in vivo of a nonclonogenic CD3+CD8+ DR+CD25– T cell population. J Immunol 1990; 144:1696.
114. Prince HE, Czaplicki CD. Preferential loss of Leu 8–, CD45R–, HLA–DR+ CD8 cell subsets during in vitro culture of mononuclear cells from human immunodeficiency virus type 1 (HIV)-seropositive former blood donors. J Clin Immunol 1989; 9:421.
115. Prince HE, Jensen ER. HIV-related alterations in CD8 cell subsets defined by in vitro survival characteristics. Cell Immunol 1991; 134:276.
116. Fauci AS. The human immunodeficiency virus: Infectivity and mechanisms of pathogenesis. Science 1988; 239:617.
117. Mann DL, Lasane F, Popovic M, et al. HTLV-III large envelope protein (gp120) suppresses PHA-induced lymphocyte blastogenesis. J Immunol 1987; 138:2640.
118. Shalaby MR, Krowka JK, Hirabayashi SE, et al. The effects of human immunodeficiency virus recombinant envelope glycoprotein on immune cell functions in vitro. Cell Immunol 1987; 110:140.
119. Gurley RJ, Ikenchi K, Byrn RA, et al. CD4+ lymphocyte function with early human immunodeficiency virus infection. Proc Natl Acad Sci USA 1989; 86:1993.
120. Manca F, Habeshaw JA, Dalgleish AG. HIV envelope glycoprotein, antigen-specific T-cell responses, and soluble CD4. Lancet 1990; 335:811.
121. Weinhold KJ, Lyerly HK, Stanley SD, et al. HIV-1 gp120-mediated immune suppression and lymphocyte destruction in the absence of viral infection. J Immunol 1989; 142:3091.
122. Hofman B, Nishanian PG, Baldwin RL, et al. HIV inhibits the early steps of lymphocyte activation, including initiation of inositol phospholipid metabolism. J Immunol 1990; 145: 3699.

123. Rosenberg ZF, Fauci AS. Immunopathogenic mechanisms of HIV infection: Cytokine induction of HIV expression. Immunol Today 1990; 11:176.

124. Rosenstein Y, Burakoff SJ, Herrmann SH. HIV-gp120 can block CD4-class II MHC-mediated adhesion. J Immunol 1990; 144:526.

125. Moore JP, Blanc DF. Immunological incompetence in AIDS. AIDS 1991; 5:455.

126. Pantaleo G, De Maris A, Koenig S, et al. CD8+ T lymphocytes of patients with AIDS maintain normal broad cytolytic function despite the loss of human immunodeficiency virus-specific cytotoxicity. Proc Natl Acad Sci USA 1990; 87:4818.

127. Clerici M, Lucey DR, Zajac RA, et al. Detection of cytotoxic T lymphocytes specific for synthetic peptides of gp160 in HIV-seropositive individuals. J Immunol 1991; 146: 2214.

128. Walker BD, Chakrabarti S, Moss B, et al. HIV-specific cytotoxic T lymphocytes in seropositive individuals. Nature 1987; 328:345.

129. Walker BD, Flexner C, Paradis TJ, et al. HIV-1 reverse transcriptase is a target for cytotoxic T lymphocytes in infected individuals. Science 1988; 240:64.

130. Hoffenbach A, Langlade-Demoyen P, Dadaglio G, et al. Unusually high frequencies of HIV-specific cytotoxic T lymphocytes in humans. J Immunol 1989; 142:452.

131. Autran B, Plata F, Debre P. MHC-restricted cytotoxicity against HIV. J Acquir Immune Defic Syndr 1991; 4:361.

132. Johnson RP, Trocha A, Yang L, et al. HIV-1 gag-specific cytotoxic T lymphocytes recognize multiple highly conserved epitopes. Fine specificity of the gag-specific response defined by using unstimulated peripheral blood mononuclear cells and cloned effector cells. J Immunol 1991; 147:1512.

133. Dadaglio G, Leroux A, Langlade-Demoyen P, et al. Epitope recognition of conserved HIV envelope sequences by human cytotoxic T lymphocytes. J Immunol 1991; 147:2302.

134. Sadat-Sowti B, Debre P, Idziorek T, et al. A lectin-binding soluble factor released by CD8+ CD57+ lymphocytes from AIDS patients inhibits T cell cytotoxicity. Eur J Immunol 1991; 21:737.

135. Walker CM. How do CD8+ T lymphocytes control HIV replication in vivo? Res Immunol 1989; 140:115.

136. Clerici M, Stocks NI, Zajac RA, et al. Circumvention of defective CD4 T helper cell function in HIV-infected individuals by stimulation with HLA alloantigens. J Immunol 1990; 144:3266.

137. Walker CM, Moody DJ, Stites DP, Levy JA. CD8+ lymphocytes can control HIV infection in vitro by suppressing virus replication. Science 1986; 234:1563.

138. Walker CM, Moody DJ, Stites DP, Levy, JA. CD8+ T lymphocyte control of HIV replication in cultured CD4+ cells varies among infected individuals. Cell Immunol 1989; 119:470.

139. Wiviott LD, Walker CM, Levy JA. CD8+ lymphocytes suppress HIV production by autologous CD4+ cells without eliminating the infected cells from culture. Cell Immunol 1990; 128:628.

140. Brinchmann JE, Gaudernack G, Vartdal F. CD8+ T cells inhibit HIV replication in naturally infected CD4+ T cells. Evidence for a soluble inhibitor. J Immunol 1990; 144:2961.

141. Brinchmann JE, Gaudernack G, Vartdal F. In vitro replication of HIV-1 in naturally infected CD4+ T cells is inhibited by rIFN-alpha2 and by a soluble factor secreted by activated CD8+ T cells, but not by rIFN-beta, rIFN-gamma, or recombinant tumor necrosis factor-alpha. J Acquir Immune Defic Syndr 1991; 4:480.

142. Walker CM, Levy JA. A diffusible lymphokine produced by CD8+ T lymphocytes suppresses HIV replication. Immunology 1989; 66:628.

143. Stewart SJ, Fujimoto J, Levy R. Human T lymphocytes and monocytes bear the same Leu-3 (T4) antigen. J Immunol 1986; 136:3773.

144. Gartner S, Markovits P, Markovitz DM, et al. The role of mononuclear phagocytes in HTLV-III/LAV infection. Science 1986; 233:215.

145. Nicholson JKA, Cross GD, Callaway CS, McDougal JS. In vitro infection of human monocytes with human T lymphotropic virus type III/lymphadenopathy-associated virus (HTLV-III/LAV). J Immunol 1986; 137:323.

146. Crowe SC, Mills J, McGrath MS, Lekas P, McManus N. Quantitative immunocytofluorographic analysis of CD4 surface antigen expression and HIV infection of human peripheral blood monocyte/macrophages. AIDS Res Hum Retroviruses 1987; 3:135.

147. Ho DD, Rota TR, Hirsch MS. Infection of monocyte/macrophages by human T lymphotropic virus type III. J Clin Invest 1986; 77:1712.
148. Mann DL, Gartner S, Le Sane F, Buchow H, Popovic M. HIV-1 transmission and function of virus-infected monocytes/macrophages. J Immunol 1990; 144:2152.
149. Mann DL, Gartner S, Le Sane F, Blattner WA, Popovic M. Cell surface antigens and function of monocytes and a monocyte-like cell line before and after infection with HIV. Clin Immunol Immunopathol 1980; 54:174.
150. Roy G, Rojo N, Leyva-Cobian F. Phenotypic changes in monocytes and alveolar macrophages in patients with acquired immunodeficiency syndrome (AIDS) and AIDS-related complex (ARC). J Clin Lab Immunol 1987; 23:135.
151. Bender BS, Davidson BL, Kline R, Brown C, Quinn TC. Role of the mononuclear phagocyte system in the immunopathogenesis of human immunodeficiency virus infection and the acquired immunodeficiency syndrome. Rev Infect Dis 1988; 10:1142.
152. Braun DP, Kessler H, Falk L, et al. Monocyte functional studies in asymptomatic, human immunodeficiency virus (HIV)-infected individuals. J Clin Immunol 1988; 8:486.
153. Allen JB, McCartney-Francis N, Smith PD, et al. Expression of interleukin 2 receptors by monocytes from patients with acquired immunodeficiency syndrome and induction of monocyte interleukin 2 receptors by human immunodeficiency virus in vitro. J Clin Invest 1990; 85:192.
154. Wahl SM, Allen JB, Gartner S, et al. HIV-1 and its envelope glycoprotein down-regulate chemotactic ligand receptors and chemotactic function of peripheral blood monocytes. J Immunol 1989; 142:3553.
155. Wright SC, Jewett A, Mitsuyasu R, Bonavida B. Spontaneous cytotoxicity and tumor necrosis factor production by peripheral blood monocytes from AIDS patients. J Immunol 1988; 141:99.
156. Twigg HL, Weissler JC, Yoffe B, Ball EJ, Lipscomb MF. Monocyte accessory cell function in patients infected with human immunodeficiency virus. Clin Immunol Immunopathol 1991; 59:436.
157. Clerici M, Stocks NI, Zajac RA, Boswell RN, Shearer GM. Accessory cell function in asymptomatic human immunodeficiency virus-infected patients. Clin Immunol Immunopathol 1990; 54:168.
158. Shannon K, Cowan MJ, Ball E, et al. Impaired mononuclear cell proliferation in patients with the acquired immune deficiency syndrome results from abnormalities of both T lymphocytes and adherent mononuclear cells. J Clin Immunol 1985; 5:239.
159. Prince HE, Moody DJ, Shubin BI, Fahey JL. Defective monocyte function in AIDS: evidence from a monocyte-dependent T cell proliferative system. J Clin Immunol 1985; 5:21.
160. Pauza CD. HIV persistence in monocytes leads to pathogenesis and AIDS. Cell Immunol 1988; 112:414.
161. Folks T, Kelly J, Benn S, et al. Susceptibility of normal human lymphocytes to infection with HTLV-III/LAV. J Immunol 1986:136:4049.
162. Gowda SD, Stein BS, Mahagheghpour N, et al. Evidence that T cell activation is required for HIV-1 entry in CD4+ lymphocytes. J Immunol 1989; 142:773.
163. Margolick JB, Volkman DJ, Folks TM, Fauci AS. Amplification of HTLV-III/LAV infection by antigen-induced activation of T cells and direct suppression by virus of lymphocyte blastogenic responses. J Immunol 1987; 138:1719.
164. McDougal JS, Mawle A, Cort SP, et al. Cellular tropism of the human retrovirus HTLV-III/LAV. I. Role of T cell activation and expression of the T4 antigen. J Immunol 1985; 135:3151.
165. Nobel G, Baltimore D. An inducible transcription factor activates expression of human immunodeficiency virus in T cells. Nature 1987; 326:711.
166. Siekevitz M, Josephs SF, Dukovich M, et al. Activation of the HIV-1 LTR by T cell mitogens and the trans-activator protein of HTLV-I. Science 1987; 238:1575.
167. Lewis DL, Yoffe B, Bosworth CG, et al. Human immunodeficiency virus-induced pathology favored by cellular transmission and activation. FASEB J 1988; 2:251.
168. Folks TM, Justement J, Kinter A, et al. Cytokine-induced expression of HIV-1 in a chronically infected promonocyte cell line. Science 1987; 238:800.
169. Clouse KA, Powell D, Washington E, et al. Monokine regulation of human immunodeficiency virus-1 expression in a chronically infected human T cell clone. J Immunol 1989; 142:431.

170. Israel N, Hazan U, Alcami J, et al. Tumor necrosis factor stimulates transcription of HIV-1 in human T lymphocytes, independently and synergistically with mitogens. J Immunol 1989; 143:3956.

171. Clouse KA, Robbins PB, Fernie B., et al. Viral antigen stimulation of the production of human monokines capable of regulating HIV1 expression. J Immunol 1989; 143:470.

172. Zolla-Pazner S, William D, El-Sadr W, et al. Quantitation of B2-microglobulin and other immune characteristics in a prospective study of men at risk for acquired immune deficiency syndrome. JAMA 1984; 251:2951.

173. Moss AR, Bacchetti P, Osmond D, et al. Seropositivity for HIV and the development of AIDS or AIDS related condition: Three year follow up of the San Francisco General Hospital Cohort. Br Med J 1988; 296:745.

174. Fahey JL, Taylor JMG, Detels R, et al. The prognostic value of cellular and serologic markers in infection with human immunodeficiency virus type 1. N Engl J Med 1990; 322:166.

175. Jacobson MA, Abrams DI, Volberding PA, et al. Serum B2-microglobulin decreases in patients with AIDS or ARC treated with azidothymidine. J Infect Dis 1989; 159: 1029.

176. Fuchs D, Hausen A, Reibnegger G, et al. Neopterin as a marker for activated cell-mediated immunity: application in HIV infection. Immunol Today 1988; 9:150.

177. Melmed RN, Taylor JMG, Detels R, et al. Serum neopterin changes in HIV-infected subjects: Indicator of significant pathology, CD4 T cell changes, and the development of AIDS. J Acquir Immune Defec Syndr 1989; 2:70.

178. Kramer A, Wiktor SZ, Fuchs D, et al. Neopterin: A predictive marker of acquired immune deficiency syndrome in human immunodeficiency virus infection. J Acquir Immune Defec Syndr 1989; 2:291.

179. Sheppard HW, Ascher MS, McRae B, et al. The initial immune response to HIV and immune system activation determine the outcome of HIV disease, J Acquir Immune Defec Syndr 1991; 4:704.

180. Nelson DL, Rubin LA, Kurman CC, et al. An analysis of the cellular requirements for the production of soluble interleukin-2 receptors in vitro. J Clin Immunol 1986; 6:114.

181. Sethi KF, Naher H. Elevated titers of cell-free interleukin-2 receptor in serum and cerebrospinal fluid specimens of patients with acquired immunodeficiency syndrome. Immunol Lett 1986; 13:179.

182. Pizzolo G, Vinante F, Sinicco A, et al. Increased levels of soluble interleukin-2 receptor in the serum of patients with human immunodeficiency virus infection. Diag Clin Immunol 1987; 5:180.

183. Kloster BE, John PA, Miller LE, et al. Soluble interleukin 2 receptors are elevated in patients with AIDS or at risk of developing AIDS. Clin Immunol Immunopathol 1987; 45:440.

184. Prince HE, Kleinman S, Williams AE. Soluble IL-2 receptor levels in serum from blood donors seropositive for HIV. J Immunol 1988; 140:1139.

185. Reddy MM, Grieco MH. Elevated soluble interleukin-2 receptor levels in serum of human immunodeficiency virus infected populations. AIDS Res Retroviruses 1988; 4:115.

186. Lang JM, Coumaros G, Levy S, et al. Elevated serum levels of soluble interleukin 2 receptors in HIV infection: Correlation studies with markers of cell activation. Immunol Lett 1988; 19:99.

187. Honda M, Kitamura K, Matsuda K, et al. Soluble IL-2 receptors in AIDS. Correlation of its serum level with the classification of HIV-induced diseases and its characterization. J Immunol 1989; 142:4248.

188. Prince HE, Kleinman S, Czaplicki C, et al. Interrelationships between serologic markers of immune activation and T lymphocyte subsets in HIV infection. J Acquir Immune Defec Syndr 1990; 3:525.

189. Osmond DH, Shiboski S, Bacchetti P, et al. Immune activation markers and AIDS prognosis. AIDS 1991; 5:505.

190. Fujimoto J, Levy S, Levy R. Spontaneous release of the Leu-2 (T8) molecule from human T cells. J Exp Med 1983; 159:752.

191. Agostini C, Semenzato G, Vinante F, et al. Increased levels of soluble CD8 molecule in the

serum of patients with acquired immunodeficiency syndrome (AIDS) and AIDS-related disorders. Clin Immunol Immunopathol 1989; 50:146.

192. Nishanian P, Hofmann B, Wang Y, et al. Serum soluble CD8 molecule is a marker of CD8 T-cell activation in HIV-1 disease. AIDS 1991; 5:805.

193. Reddy MM, Lange M, Grieco MH. Elevated soluble CD8 levels in sera of human immunodeficiency virus-infected populations. J Clin Microbiol 1989; 27:257.

194. Nossal GJV. The basic components of the immune system. N Engl J Med 1987; 316: 1320.

195. Seiki M, Hattori S, Hirayama Y, et al. Human adult T-cell leukemia virus: Complete nucleotide sequence of the provirus genome integrated in leukemia cell DNA. Proc Natl Acad Sci USA 1983; 80:3618.

196. Green WC, Leonard WJ, Depper JM, et al. The human interleukin-2 receptor: Normal and abnormal expression in T cells and in leukemias induced by the human T-lymphotropic retroviruses. Ann Intern Med 1986; 105:560.

197. Kim JH, Durack DT. Manifestations of human T-lymphotropic virus type I infection. Am J Med 1988; 84:919.

198. Rosenblatt JD, Chen ISY, Wachsman W. Infection with HTLV-I and HTLV-II: evolving concepts. Semin Hematol 1988; 25:230.

199. Dixon AC, Dixon PS, Nakamura JM. Infection with the human T-lymphotropic virus type I. A review for clinicians. West J Med 1989; 151:632.

200. Tajima K, Kuroishi T. Estimation of rate of incidence of ATL among ATLV (HTLV-I) carriers in Kyushu, Japan. Jpn J Clin Oncol 1985; 15:423.

201. Murphy EL, Hanchard B, Figueroa JP, et al. Modelling the risk of adult T-cell leukemia/lymphoma in persons infected with human T-lymphotropic virus type I. Int J Cancer 1989; 43:250.

202. Kaplan JE, Osame M, Kubota H, et al. The risk of development of HTLV-I-associated myelopathy/tropical spastic paraparesis among persons infected with HTLV-I. J Acquir Immune Defec Syndr 1990 3:1096.

203. Lee H, Swanson P, Shorty VS, et al. High rate of HTLV-II infection in seropositive IV drug abusers in New Orleans. Science 1989; 244:471.

204. Lee HH, Swanson P, Rosenblatt JD, et al. Relative prevalence and risk factors of HTLV-I and HTLV-II infection in US blood donors. Lancet 1991; 337:1435.

205. Hjelle B, Mills R, Swenson S, et al. Incidence of hairy cell leukemia, mycosis fungoides, and chronic lymphocytic leukemia in first known HTLV-II-endemic population. J Infect Dis 1991; 163:435.

206. Rosenblatt JD, Golde DW, Wachsman W, et al. A second isolate of HTLV-II associated with atypical hairy cell leukemia. N Engl J Med 1986; 315:372.

207. Rosenblatt JD, Giorgi JV, Golde DW, et al. Integrated human T-cell leukemia virus II genome in CD8+ T cells from a patient with "atypical" hariy cell leukemia: Evidence for distinct T and B cell lymphoproliferative disorders. Blood 1988; 71:363.

208. Gout O, Baulac M, Gessain A, et al. Rapid development of myelopathy after HTLV-I infection acquired by transfusion during cardiac transplantation. N Engl J Med 1990; 322:383.

209. Hjelle B, Mills R, Mertz G, Swensen S. Transmission of HTLV-II via blood transfusion. Vox Sang 1990; 59:119.

210. Fretz C, Janlmes D, Jordan G, et al. HTLV-I transmission and myelopathy induced by blood transfusion. Transfusion 1991; 31:379.

211. Larson CJ, Taswell HF. Human T-cell leukemia virus type I (HTLV-I) and blood transfusion. Mayo Clin Proc 1988; 63:869.

212. Politis C, Papaevangelou G, Sinakos Z, et al. HTLV-I infection in multitransfused patients with thalassemia. Transfusion 1989; 29:561.

213. Canavaggio M, Leckie G, Allain JP, et al. The prevalence of antibody to HTLV-I/II in United States plasma donors and in United States and French hemophiliacs. Transfusion 1990; 30:780.

214. Okochi K, Sato H, Hinuma Y. A retrospective study on transmission of adult T cell leukemia virus by blood transfusion. Seroconversion in recipients. Vox Sang 1984; 46:245.

215. Donegan E, Busch MP, Galleshaw JA, et al. Transfusion of blood components from a donor with human T-lymphotropic virus type II (HTLV-II) infection. Ann Intern Med 1990; 113:555.

216. Williams AE, Fang CT, Slamon DJ, et al. Seroprevalence and epidemiological correlates of HTLV-I infection in US blood donors. Science 1988; 240:643.
217. Prince HE, Lee H, Jensen ER, et al. Immunologic correlates of spontaneous lymphocyte proliferation in human T-lymphotropic virus infection. Blood 1991; 78:169.
218. Chen Y-MA, Gomez-Lucia E, Okayama A, et al. Antibody profile of early HTLV-I infection. Lancet 1990; 336:1214.
219. Chen Y-MA, Lee T-H, Wiktor SZ, et al. Type-specific antigens for serological discrimination of HTLV-I and HTLV-II infection. Lancet 1990; 336:1153.
220. Lipka JJ, Bui K, Reyes GR, et al. Determination of a unique and immunodominant epitope of human T-cell lymphotropic virus type I. J Infect Dis 1990; 162:353.
221. Chen Y-MA, Zhang X-Q, Dahl CE, et al. Delineation of type-specific regions of the envelope glycoproteins of human T cell leukemia viruses. J Immunol 1991; 147:2368.
222. Hayes CG, Burans JP, Oberst RB. Antibodies to human T lymphotropic virus type I in a population from the Philippines: Evidence for cross-reactivity with *Plasmodium falciparum*. J Infect Dis 1991; 163:257.
223. Jacobson S, Shida H, McFarlin DE, et al. Circulating CD8+ cytotoxic T lymphocytes specific for HTLV-I pX in patients with HTLV-I associated neurological disease. Nature 1990; 348:245.
224. Jacobson S, Reuben JS, Streilein RD, et al. Induction of CD4+ human T lymphotropic virus type-I-specific cytotoxic T lymphocytes from patients with HAM/TSP. Recognition of an immunogenic region of the gp46 envelope glycoprotein of human T lymphotropic virus type I. J Immunol 1991; 146:1155.
225. Imamura N, Inada T, Mtasiwa DM, Kuramoto A. Phenotype and function of Japanese adult T-cell leukaemia cells. Lancet 1989; 2:214.
226. Kronke M, Leonard WJ, Depper JM, Greene WC. Deregulation of interleukin-2 receptor gene expression in HTLV-I-induced adult T-cell leukemia. Science 1985; 228:1215.
227. Greene WC, Bohnlein E, Ballard DW. HIV-1, HTLV-I, and normal T cell growth: transcriptional strategies and surprises. Immunol Today 1989; 10:272.
228. Richardson JH, Edwards AJ, Cruickshank JK, et al. In vivo cellular tropism of human T-cell leukemia virus type I. J Virol 1990; 64:5682.
229. Gessain A, Saal F, Gout O, et al. High human T-cell lymphotropic virus type I proviral DNA load with polyclonal integration in peripheral blood mononuclear cells of French West Indian, Guianese, and African patients with tropical spastic paraparesis. Blood 1990; 75:428.
230. Yasuda N, Lai PK, Ip SH, et al. Soluble interleukin 2 receptors in sera of Japanese patients with adult T cell leukemia mark activity of disease. Blood 1988; 71:1021.
231. Marcon L, Rubin LA, Kurman CC, et al. Elevated serum levels of soluble Tac peptide in adult T-cell leukemia: Correlation with clinical status during chemotherapy. Ann Intern Med 1988; 109:274.
232. Marcon L, Fritz ME, Kurman CC, et al. Soluble Tac peptide is present in the urine of normal individuals and at elevated levels in patients with adult T cell leukemia (ATL). Clin Exp Immunol 1988; 73:29.
233. Yamaguchi K, Nishimura Y, Kiyokawa T, Takatsuki K. Elevated serum levels of soluble interleukin-2 receptors in HTLV-I-associated myelopathy. J Lab Clin Med 1989; 114:407.
234. Itoyama Y, Kira J, Fukii N, et al. Increases in helper inducer T cells and activated T cells in HTLV-I-associated myelopathy. Ann Neurol 1989; 26:257.
235. Yasuda K, Sei Y, Yokoyama MM, et al. Healthy HTLV-I carriers in Japan: The haematological and immunological characteristics. Br J Haematol 1986; 64:195.
236. de Shazo RD, Chadha N, Morgan JE, et al. Immunologic assessment of a cluster of asymptomatic HTLV-I–infected individuals in New Orleans. Am J Med 1989; 86:65.
237. Fletcher MA, Gjerset GF, Hassett J, et al. Lymphocyte immunophenotypes among anti–HTLV-I/II–positive blood donors and recipients. J Acquir Immune Defic Syndr 1991; 4:628.
238. Rosenblatt JD, Plaeger-Marshall S, Giorgi JV, et al. A clinical, hematologic, and immunologic analysis of 21 HTLV-II-infected intravenous drug users. Blood 1990; 76:409.
239. Prince HE. American blood donors seropositive for human T-lymphotropic virus types I/II exhibit normal lymphocyte subsets. Transfusion 1990; 30:787.
240. Prince HE, Jackson AL. Normal expression of p55 interleukin 2 receptor (CD25) by lymphocytes

from former blood donors seropositive for human T lymphotropic viruses. Clin Immunol Immunopathol 1990; 57:459.

241. Kramer A, Jacobson S, Reuben JF, et al. Spontaneous lymphocyte proliferation in symptom-free HTLV-I positive Jamaicans. Lancet 1989; 2:923.
242. Jacobson S, Zaninovic V, Mora C, et al. Immunological findings in neurological diseases associated with antibodies to HTLV-I: Activated lymphocytes in tropical spastic para- paresis. Ann Neurol 1988; 23(suppl):S196.
243. Itoyama Y, Minato S, Kira J, et al. Spontaneous proliferation of peripheral blood lymphocytes increased in patients with HTLV-I-associated myelopathy. Neurology 1988; 38: 1302.
244. Tendler CL, Greenberg SJ, Blattner WA, et al. Transactivation of interleukin 2 and its receptor induces immune activation in human T-cell lymphotropic virus type I–associated myelopathy: Pathogenic implications and a rationale for immunotherapy. Proc Natl Acad Sci USA 1990; 87:5218.
245. Prince H, Kleinman S, Doyle M, et al. Spontaneous lymphocyte proliferation in vitro characterizes both HTLV-I and HTLV-II infection. J Acquir Immune Defic Syndr 1990; 3:1199.
246. Wiktor SZ, Jacobson S, Weiss SH, et al. Spontaneous lymphocyte proliferation in HTLV-II infection. Lancet 1991; 337:327.
247. Lal RB, Rudolph DL. Constitutive production of interleukin-6 and tumor necrosis factor-alpha from spontaneously proliferating T cells in patients with human T-cell lymphotropic virus type I/II. Blood 1991; 78:571.
248. Prince HE, Weber DM, Jensen ER. Spontaneous lymphocyte proliferation in HTLV-I/II infection reflects preferential activation of CD8 and CD16/56 cell subsets. Clin Immunol Immunopathol 1991; 58:419.
249. Gazzolo L, Duc Dodon M. Direct activation of resting T lymphocytes by human T-lymphotropic virus type I. Nature 1987; 326:714.
250. Duc Dodon M, Bernard A, Gazzolo L. Peripheral T-lymphocyte activation by human T-cell leukemia virus type I interferes with the CD2 but not the CD3/TCR pathway. J Virol 1989; 63:5413.

Index

ABH blood groups:
  Bombay and Para-Bombay phenotypes, 19–20
  decreased ABH antigens, 224–226
  H and Se blood group loci, 14–17
  molecular cloning of the H blood group
    locus, 17–18
  reactivity on cells from normal organs, 198
  structure and synthesis, 1–9
ABO antibodies:
  bacterial infections, 214–216
ABO blood group system:
  A-like antigen, 203
  A_1, 9
  A_2, 9
  A^a, 202, 509
  A^b, 202
  A^c, 202
  A^d, 202
  A_g, 224
  A_m, 224
  acquired B antigen, 229
  associations with bacteria/infection, 214–219
  associations with coagulation, 211–213
  associations with malignancy, 200–207
  cis-AB phenotype, 11
  molecular cloning of the ABO locus, 11–14
  subgroups of A and B, 9–10
ABO hemolytic disease, 566
Acanthocytosis, 181
  In(Lu) gene, 258–259
  Lu(a-b-) phenotype, 258–259
  McLeod phenotype, 258

Acetaminophen, 524
Acetylcholinesterase, 97, 101
  Cartwright antigens, 103
Acid elution test, 560
Acquired antigens, 229–232
Acquired immune deficiency syndrome (AIDS),
  216, 659
Actin, 183, 498
Actinorhodine, 544
Acute leukemia, 225, 227, 228
Acute respiratory distress syndrome, 158
ADCC, 157, 453, 465, 470, 482, 483, 663
Adenocarcinoma, 202
Adenosine triphosphate, 258
Adhesion molecules, 154, 269
  association of ABH/Lewis antigens, 204–207
  biochemistry/molecular genetics, 270
  Indian blood group, 260–270
  receptors, 27, 269
Affinity of antibodies, 342, 344, 452
AIDS-216, 659
AIDS-related complex (ARC), 284, 663
Alkaline phosphatase, 97
Alkaline phosphodiesterase 1, 97
Allele loss, 301
  mechanisms of, 301
Allelic inactivation, 300
Alloimmune hemolytic anemia, 494
Alloimmune platelet refractoriness, 598
Alloimmune response, 155
Alloimmunization, 564, 565, 573, 604
  management of, 573–579

Alpha-methyldopa, 127, 533–536, 541–542
Alveolar (lung) cells, 171
Alzheimer's disease, 172
Amaranthus caudatus, 209
Amino acid sequencing, 129
Amniotic fluid, 570
Amphotericin B, 524
Ampicillin, 524
An/Wj, 498
An^a, 54
Analytical ultracentrifugation, 344
Anaphylatoxins, 409
Anek, 40
Angina pectoris, 212
Angioimmunoblastic lymphadenopathy, 510
Anion binding, 187
Anion transport protein, 8, 176, 184, 187
Anion transport site, 185
Ankyrin, 256
Anopheles gambiae, 197
Antazoline, 524
Anti-5^b, 159
Anti-A, 151, 199
Anti-B, 151, 199
Anti-c, 128
Anti-Ch^a, 411
Anti-Chido, 279, 411
Anti-D, 109, 588
   monoclonal, 588
Anti-E, 128
anti-Fab, 501
Anti-Gd, 514
Anti-Ge^2, 72
Anti-Ge^3, 72
Anti-Gov, 151
Anti-H, 8
Anti-H(i), 274
Anti-HI, 514
Anti-HPA-1a, 150, 151
Anti-i, 219, 510
Anti-IA, 274
Anti-IB, 274
Anti-I^D, 274
Anti-idiotype, 190, 191, 501
Anti-I^F, 274
Anti-iH, 274
Anti-IH, 274
Anti-ILe^{bh}, 274
Anti-In^a, 269
Anti-IP$_1$, 274
Anti-I^T, 218, 274
Anti-K, 219
Anti-Lepore-Type Hybrids, 48
Anti-Lewis, 20
Anti-LW, 109

Anti-M, 38, 72
Anti-N, 38, 72
Anti-NA1, 159
Anti-NA2, 159
Anti-NB1, 159
Anti-NB2, 159
Anti-NC1, 159
Anti-nl, 126
Anti-O(i), 274
Anti-P, 199, 514
Anti-p, 514
Anti-P$_1$, 199
Anti-pdl, 126
Anti-P^k, 199
Anti-PI^{A1}, 529
Anti-PP$_1$P^k, 207
Anti-Pr-like, 514
Anti-Pr$_1$, 74
Anti-Pr$_2$, 74, 394
Anti-Rodgers (Rg^a), 279, 411
Anti-SCA, 498
Anti-T, 55, 67, 209
Anti-Tj^a, 207
Anti-Tn, 209
Anti-Wj, 271
Anti-Yt^a, 103
Anti-Zw^a, 150
Antibodies:
   adsorption, 618
   affinity, 452–457
   class and subclass, 450–451
   hemagglutinating, 353–360
   monoclonal (RBC), 365–385
   RBC autoantibodies, 387–399
   specificity, 452–453
Antibody-dependent cellular cytotoxicity
      (ADCC) assay, 157, 453, 465, 470, 482,
      483, 663
Anticardiolipin, 498
Anticomplement antiglobulin reagents, 423
   adverse effects of anticomplement, 424–425
   anti-C3b, 426–427
   anti-C3d, 426–427
   enhanced detection of IgG antibodies, 425–426
   monoclonal, 427
   standardization, 424
Antigen matching, 610
Antigen–antibody binding forces, 328
Antigen–antibody interactions, 327–364
   hemagglutination, 351–360
   nature of binding forces, 328–339
   thermodynamics, 339–351
Antiglobulin reagents:
   anticomplement, 423–427
   monoclonal, 379–380

Antiphospholipid syndrome, 498
Antithymocyte globulin (ATG), 618
Anton/Wj, 221, 259, 271
Aplastic anemia, 224, 228
Apronal, 524, 526
Arachis hypogaea, 120, 209
Arthrobacter ureafaciens, 69
Artocarpus intergrifolia, 209
Ascaris suum, 223
Aspergillus niger, 231
Association constants, 527
Ataxia telangiectasia, 310
Au^a, 259
Auto-anti-NA1, 159
Auto-anti-ND1, 159
Auto-anti-NE1, 159
AutoAnalyzer, 495
Autoantibodies, 126, 467
  drug-induced, 533–536
  anti-idiotype, 500–501
  IgA, 504–505
  IgG sublass, 496–497
  IgM, 505–507
  in vitro production of, 390–393
  low affinity, 501–503
  monoclonal, 390–393
  RBC, 387–399, 493–521
  Rh related, 388–389
  specificity, 387–389, 497–501
  structural analyses, 387–399
  structure of, 389–390
  V region genes, 393–394
Autoimmune chronic active hepatitis, 283
Autoimmune disease, 284
Autoimmune hemolytic anemia (AIHA), 199,
    228, 387, 436, 465, 493–521
  childhood, 515
  classification, 495
  cold agglutinin syndrome, 506–511
  direct antiglobulin test, 495
  diseases commonly associated with, 494
  IgA autoantibodies, 504
  IgG subclass of autoantibodies, 496–497
  IgM autoantibodies, 505–507
  immunological characteristics of, 494–515
  negative DAT, 501–506
  paroxysmal cold hemoglobinuria, 511–515
  serological characteristics of, 494–515
  specificity of autoantibodies, 497–501
  warm AIHA, 494–506
Autoimmune neutropenia, 157
  of infancy, 158
Autoimmune thrombocytopenic purpura,
    616
Avidity, 342

Azapropazone, 534
Aztreonam, 544

B-cell clones, 510
B-cell immunoglobulin gene, 311
B lymphocytes, 391, 535, 661, 681
  EBV transformation of, 391
  EBV-transformed B-cell clones, 390
Ba, 404
Babesia rodhaini, 279
Bacteria, 214
  Anton/Wj, 271
  blood group antigens, 214, 222
  deacetylase, 229
  I, 274
  P, 272, 274
  receptors, 219, 271–275
Bacteroides fragilis, 83, 231
Bak=Lek, 148
Band 3, 171, 498
Band 6, 498
Bandeiraea simplicifolia, 231
Basophils, 409
Bauhinea purpurea, 40
Bb, 404, 408
Benzylpenicillin, 524
Benzylpenicilloyl (BPO) determinant, 524–525
Bg antigen, 229
Biclonal gammopathy, 511
Bile duct epithelia, 209
Biphasic hemolysin, 511
Blast cells, 227
Blood group antigens:
  acquired, 229–232
  association with bacterial infection, 214–223
  association with coagulation, 211–213
  association with disease, 197–251
  association with hematological conditions,
    228
  association with immunologically important
    proteins, 269–293
  association with malignancy, 199–211
  bacterial receptors, 219–222
  biological role, 197–251
  carbohydrate associated, 1–34
  decreases and increases of, 224–229
  glycophorin associated, 35–66
  membrane abnormalities, 255–268
  parasitic infections, 222–223
  phosphatidylinositol glycan-linked proteins,
    95–108
  sialic acid-dependent, 67–93
  specific RBC membrane proteins, 257
Blood microrheology, 212
Blood transfusion, 155

Bloom's syndrome, 306
Bombay phenotypes, 16, 19
Bone grafts, 121
Bone marrow transplantation, 155
Bowman's capsule, 221
Brownian motion, 348
Burkitt's lymphoma, 202
Butizide, 524
Bw5 (B5), 280
Bystander hemolysis, 422

C1 inhibitor, 408
C2, 281, 404
C2a, 404
C2b, 404
C3, 403, 404
C3 NEF, 421
C3 convertase, 406
C3 subcomponents, 310
C3a, 404
C3b, 404, 442
C3b receptor, 410
C3b/C4b receptor, 259
C3bBb, 408
C3c, 404
C3d, 404
C3dg, 404, 410
C3f, 404, 406
C4, 279, 404
    associated with various diseases,
        283
    biochemistry, 280–281
    molecular genetics, 281–282
C4-binding protein (C4bp), 100, 408
C4 deficiency, 284
C4 isotypes, 282
C4 null genes, 283
C4A, 264, 280, 282
C4a, 404
C4A*3,*2,B*QO, 281
C4A*QO, 281, 283, 284
C4B, 264, 280, 282, 411
C4b, 404, 442
C4B*QO, 282
C4b2a, 408
C4b2a3b, 406, 408
C4B3, 283
C4d, 280
C5, 404
C5 convertase, 406
C5a, 404
C5a chemotactic receptor, 410
C5b, 404
C5b-9 MAC, 406

C6, 404
C7, 404
C8, 404
C8-binding protein (C8bp), 409
C9, 404
Cad, 57
Calcium bridging, 337
Candida albicans, 216, 231
Caprylate-dependent autoagglutinins, 531
Carbenicillin, 524
Carbimazole, 524, 526, 528, 534
Carbodiimide, 74
Carbohydrate-associated blood group antigens, 1–34
Carbromal, 524, 526
Carcinoembryonic antigen (CEA), 204
Carcinoma, 200
    of the cervix, 200
    of the colon, 200, 206
    of the female genital tract, 200
    of the gastrointestinal tract, 200
    of the stomach, 200
Cardiolipin, 498
Cartwright, 103
CD4, 659, 664, 681
CD8, 664, 668, 681
CD11, 161
CD11a, 161, 162
CD11b, 161, 162, 669
CD11c, 161
CD16, 97, 160, 447, 663
CD18, 161, 409, 443
CD21, 409
CD25, 668, 679, 681
CD29, 681
CD35, 409, 410, 442
CD38, 668
CD44, 259
CD45, 388
CD45RA, 667, 681
CD45RO+, 667, 681
CD55, 97
CD57+, 669
CD59, 97
CD64, 210–271, 445
CD557, 97
cDNA, 11
Cefamandole, 524
Cefazolin, 524
Cefotaxime, 524, 534
Cefotetan, 524, 534
Cefoxitin, 524
Ceftazidime, 524, 534
Ceftriaxone, 524
Cellular immunoassays, 465
    alloantibodies in transfused patients, 483–485

[Cellular immunoassays]
  antibody-dependent cellular cytotoxicity
    assays, 470
  autoimmune hemolytic anemia, 478–480
  characteristics of, 467–470
  chemiluminescence test, 469–470
  clinical application of, 478–485
  factors affecting, 470–472
  hemolytic disease of the newborn, 480–481
  immunological basis, 472–478
  monocyte monolayer assay, 468–469
  predicting the clinical significance of anti-
    bodies, 465–491
  rosette assay, 467–468
Central nervous system, 193
Cephalexin, 524
Cephaloridine, 524
Cephalosporins, 526
Cephalosporyl group, 525
Cephalothin, 524
Chemical mutagens, 306
Chemical mutagen-induced mutants, 308
Chemiluminescence test, 465–466
Chemotherapy, 306
Chido (Ch^a), 279–280, 484
Chimera, 14
Chloramine T, 529
Chlorinated hydrocarbons, 534
Chloroquine, 149
Chlorpropamide, 524, 531
Cholecystitis, 200
Choleithiasis, 200
Cholera, 215
Choriocarcinoma, 200
Chromosome:
  1, 100, 135, 226
  4, 305, 318
  6, 308
  7, 263
  9, 226
  11, 304
  19, 17, 26
  22, 225
  loss, 301
Chronic myeloid leukemia, 225
Chronic granulomatosis disease, 258
Chronic lymphocytic leukemia, 511
Cianidanol, 524, 526, 533, 534
Cimetidine, 540
Cis-AB phenotype, 11
Cis-linked glyoxylase I locus, 308
Cisplatin, 524, 526, 544
Citric acid, 544
Classic pathway of complement activation, 405
Cloning, 11, 17, 23

Clostridium perfringens, 69, 230
Clostridium tertium, 229
Clq, 404, 448
Clr, 404
Cls, 404
CLT, 482
Coagulation:
  association of blood groups, 211–213
Cockayne's syndrome, 310
Cold agglutinin syndrome (CAS), 387, 415, 493
  biclonal gammopathy, 511
  chronic lymphocytic leukemia, 511
  immunochemistry, 509–11
  lymphoma, 511
  macroglobulinemia, 511
  serological characteristics, 506–509
  Waldenström's, 511
Cold agglutinins, 73, 451
  immunochemistry, 509–511
  specificity, 509
Collagen, 155
Collecting ducts, 221
Colloid osmotic lysis, 417
Complement fixation, 418
Complement proteins, 404
  physical and functional properties, 404
Complement system, 99, 403, 441
  activation, 405
  alternative pathway, 403–409
  anti-C3b, 426–427
  anti-C3d, 426–427
  anticomplement reagents, 423–427
  antiglobulin reagents, 423–427
  bystander hemolysis, 422–423
  C3 NEF, 421
  C3d, 406–407, 410–414
  C3d,g, 512–514
  classic pathway, 403–409
  cold AIHA, 420
  Cromer, 275–277
  decay-accelerating factor, 275–277
  direct antiglobulin test, 420
  drug-induced immune hemolysis, 420
  fixation, 418, 529
  HEMPAS, 421
  hemolytic transfusion reactions, 421
  immunohematological diseases, 419–423
  paroxysmal cold hemoglobinuria (PCH), 420
  paroxysmal nocturnal hemoglobinuria (PNH),
    421
  platelet storage lesion, 423
  proteins regulating activation, 276, 408–409
  quantitation, 412–413
  RBC destruction, 414–419
  RBC senescence, 418–419

[Complement system]
reactive hemolysis, 422–423
receptor type 1 (CR1), 264, 278, 410, 442, 475
receptor type 2 (CR2), 410–411, 475
receptor type 3 (CR3), 161, 443, 475
receptor type 4 (CR4), 161, 475
receptors, 409–411, 441, 475
relationship to blood groups, 411–412
systemic lupus erythematosus (SLE), 420
transfusion medicine, 403–404
warm AIHA, 420
Complex model, 132
Congenital dyserythropoietic anemia, 263
Congenital spherocytosis, 228
Coronary occlusion, 212
Corrected count increment, 597
Corticosteroids, 150, 455
Corynebacterium aquaticum, 231
CR1, 100, 409, 410, 442, 475
CR2, 100, 409, 410, 475
CR3, 409, 411, 442, 443, 475
CR4, 409, 411, 475
Cr^a, 152, 484
Cranberry juice, 220
Crenation, 226
Crohn's disease, 277
Cromer antigens, 99
biochemistry/molecular genetics, 275–276
Cr$_{null}$ (Inab type), 232
serology, 275
Cross-match, 614
Cross-reactive HLA antigens, 612
Cryptantigens, 229
Cs^a, 259
Cyclic AMP, 534
Cyclic adenosine monophosphate (AMP), 534
Cyclofenil, 524
Cyclophosphamide, 310
Cyclosporin, 391, 610, 618
Cytochalasin B, 181
Cytokines, 453
Cytoskeleton, 129

D streptococcus S. faecium, 219
D, 110, 260, 404, 484, 509
immunization, 587
Dacryocytes, 226
Danazol, 455
Dantu, 48
Daudi cells, 477
Decay-accelerating factor, 97, 99
biochemistry/molecular genetics, 275–276
Delayed-type skin hypersensitivity, 210
Dexchlorpheniramine maleate, 531

Dh^a, 54
Diamond-Blackfan syndrome, 231
Diclofenac, 533, 534
Dielectric constant, 337
Diethylaminoethyl (DEAE), 529
Digestive tract, 16
Diglycoaldehyde (INOX), 524, 544
Dihydrothiazine ring, 525
Dipyrone, 524
Direct antiglobulin test:
anti-idiotype, 500–501
autoimmune hemolytic anemia, 494–497
cold agglutinin syndrome, 508
drug-induced, 524
low-affinity antibodies, 502
paroxysmal cold hemoglobinuria, 512
RBC-bound IgA and IgM, 504
small amount of RBC-bound IgG, 503
Dispersion forces, 328
DNA:
analysis, 510
damage, 315, 317
methylation, 300
repair and metabolism, 306
sequence, 11
Dolichos biflorus, 9, 230
Donath Landsteiner test, 511–515
Down's syndrome, 173
DR, 668
DR1, 282
DR3, 155, 281, 284
DR4, 283
DR6, 282
Dr^a, 152
Drug adsorption mechanism, 537
Drug-dependent antibodies:
clinical characteristics, 539–540
penicillin antibodies, 539–540
serological characteristics, 532–533; 539–540
specificity, 529–532
Drug-independent antibodies (autoantibodies), 533–536, 538
clinical characteristics, 539–540
serological characteristics, 539–540
Drug-induced immune hemolytic anemia, 494, 523–551
drugs causing, 524
mechanisms, 523–538
Drug-induced immune thrombocytopenia, 523
Drugs:
combining with RBC membrane, 526
immune response, 536–538
DRw52, 155
DRw6, 155
D^u, 110

Duchenne muscular dystrophy, 258
Duclos antigen, 43
Duodenal ulcer, 200
Dupé equation, 331
Duplication mechanisms, 301
Duzo, 147, 148
D^V, 369
Dyserythropoietic anemia, 228

e, 110, 260
E, 110, 260, 484
E. coli, 272, 274
   association with P antigen, 219–220, 272–274
E-selectin, 28
E27, 162
Early abortion, 199
Echinoccus, 223, 272
Effector cells, 470, 471
ELAM, 1, 28
ELAT, 495, 503
Electron-acceptor/electron donor, 328
Electrostatic bonds, 338, 349
Electrostatic (EL) Forces, 328, 335
Electrostatic interactions, 336
Elliptocytosis, 259
  Leach phenotype, 259
En^a, 41, 67, 260, 498
  En^{a}FR, 41
  En^{a}FS, 41
  En^{a}TS, 41
Endo-β-galactosidases, 231
Endothelial cells, 155
Enzyme-linked antiglobulin test, 495, 503
Enzyme-linked immunosorbent assay (ELISA),
   149, 368
Epidermis, 2, 16
Epithelia, 16
Epstein-Barr virus, 89
Equilibrium constants, 340
Equilibrium dialysis, 343
Erythroblastosis fetalis (see also Hemolytic dis-
   ease of the newborn), 553
Erythrocyte assays for somatic mutation, 303–
   304
  glycophorin A, 305–307
  hemoglobin, 303–304
Erythrocyte urea transporter, 261
Erythroleukemia, 263
Erythromycin, 524, 526
Erythrophagocytosis, 465
Es^a, 152
Escherichia coli O$_{86}$, 209
Eschericihia freundii, 83
Evans blue, 544
Exco-β-galactosidases, 231

Extravascular hemolysis, 435–464
  factors affecting cell clearance, 449–455

Fab domains, 528, 529
  F(ab')$_2$, 529
Factor IX, 213
Factor V, 213
Factor I, 406
Factor H, 406
Factor B, 408
Factor D, 408
Factor VIII, 213
Fanconi's anemia, 231, 306
Fasciola hepatica, 272
Fc receptors, 440, 473
  classes, 445
  FcαR, 504
  FcγR1, 444, 445
  FcγRII (CD32), 444, 446
  FcγRIII, 444, 447
  FcGran1, 160
  FcR III, 98, 160
  FcRII, 160
  FcRIII cDNA, 162
  FcRIII-1, 162
  FcRIII-B, 162
Febrile transfusion reactions, 150
Femoropopliteal artherosclerosis, 212
Fenoprofen, 524
Fetal epithelia, 209
Fibrinogen, 154
Fibroblasts, 155, 171, 192
Fibronectin, 154, 155, 448
Fimbriae, 220
FI, 79, 509
Flow cytometry, 134, 255, 303, 306, 314, 503
Fluorescence, 344
  activated cell sorting, 314
  polarization, 345
  quenching, 344
Fluorouracil (5-FU), 524
Fluorsemide, 524
Fluosol, 423
Folic acid, 544
FOMA, 376
Forssman antigen, 202
Free radical-generating systems, 178
Free energies of interaction, 340
Fuc-TIII Gene, 27
Fucoganglioside, 82
Fucosyltransferases, 2, 5, 27
Fy:-5, 132
Fy5, 264
Fy^a, 132
Fy^b, 132

G6PD Deficiency, 179
G. soja, 230
Galactosyl residues, 498
Galfenine, 533, 534
Gamma radiation, 308
Gangrene, 508
Gastric ulcer, 200
Gd, 79, 509
Gel filtration, 344
Gene conversion, 301
Gene inactivation, 301
Genomic DNA, 134
Genotoxicity assays, 299
    genetic design, 299–302
Gerbich blood group system, 35
    Ge1, 52
    Ge2, 52
    Ge3, 36, 52
    Ge4, 36, 52
    Ge, 67, 484
    Ge$_{null}$ (Leach type), 232
Giardia lamblia, 223
Glafenine, 524
Glanzmann's disease, 155
Glial cells, 171
Globoside (globotetraosyl ceramide), 207, 208,
    514
Glomeruli, 221
Glucose transport protein, 8
Glutamic acid, 544
Glutaraldehyde, 544
Glutaric acid, 544
Glyceraldehyde-3-phosphate dehydrogenase
    activity, 177
Glyceryl trinitrate (nitroglycerin), 544
Glycine soja, 230
Glycolipids, 2, 78
    changes in malignancy, 205–208
Glycophorins:
    A, 38, 42
    B, 42–44
    C, 50–54, 259
    D, 52, 259
    E, 44–45
    alloantigens, 69–73
    Lepore-Type hybrids, 46–49
    nomenclature, 36–38
    O-glycans, 54–57
    Sia-I1, Sia-b1, Sia-Ib1, 79–87
    structures and antigens, 35–66
    variants, 40
Glycoproteins (on platelets):
    GPIIIa, 152, 153
    GPIIb, 153
    GPIb/IX, 530

[Glycoproteins (on platelets)]
    GPIc/IIa complex, 155
    GPIV deficiency, 152
    GP A, 37
    GP B, 37
    GP C, 52
    GP Ib, 155
    GP Ia/IIa complex, 155
    GPA assay, 308
    GPIb/IX, 530
    GPIIb/IIIa, 530
    GPIIIa, 530
    IIIa (GPIIIa), 453
    IIb/IIIa complex, 151, 154
Glycosphingolipids, 2
Glycosylphosphatidylinositol (GPI)-linked mole-
    cule, 447
Glycosyltransferases, 12
Glyoxal, 544
Glyoxylase I gene, 308
Golgi apparatus, 12, 17
Gonorrhoea, 216
Gouty arthritis, 309
Gov, 148
Graft rejection, 199
Graft-versus-host disease (transfusion-induced),
    631
    cases reported, 632–636
    clinical features, 637–638; 644–646
    immunosufficiency, 642
    pathogenesis, 637–641
    role of HLA, 641–642
    transfusion immunosuppressive effect, 642
    transfusion settings, 641–644
    treatment and prevention, 646–647
Grandmother theory, 586
Graves' disease, 283
Group A, 211
GVHD, see graft-versus-host disease
Gy^a, 484

H blood group determinants, 1–34
    H$_1$, 202
    H$_2$, 202
    H$_3$, 202
    H$_4$, 202
    loci, 14
HAM-A, 376
Hamaker coefficient, 331
Haptens, 350, 524
    hypothesis, 527
    inhibition methods, 345
HD, 67
He Antigen, 40, 44
Heat-shock protein (HSP70), 281

Helix pomatia, 54, 230, 232
Hemabsorption tests, 149
Hematopoietic cells, 299
Hemoglobin, 303
  β-globulin gene, 304
  C, 303
  cross-linking, 178
  Köln, 179
  Leiden, 304
  S, 303
  San Jose, 304
Hemolysis, 563
  extravascular, 435, 436
Hemolytic anemia, 209, 452
Hemolytic disease of the fetus/newborn, 199
Hemolytic disease of the newborn (HDN), 109,
    451, 465, 553–595
  ABO, 566–567
  alloantibodies causing, 564–567
  amniotic fluid, 570–571
  antibodies associated with treatment, 566
  IgG subclasses, 564
  intrauterine transfusions, 576–9
  management of, 573–9
  maternal antibody titers, 569
  pathogenesis, 559–564
  percutaneous umbilical blood sampling
    (PUBS), 572–573
  prediction of severity, 480–483, 568–573
  pregnancy history, 568
  severity, 565; 567–568
  ultrasonography, 571–572
Hemolytic transfusion reactions, 199, 421
Hemolytic threshold, 542
Hemolytic uremic anemia (HUS), 230
HEMPAS, 227
Heparin, 423
Hepatocarcinoma, 318
Hepatocytes, 171, 209
Hepatoma, 171, 192
Hepatosplenomegaly, 511
Hereditary elliptocytosis (HF), 256
Hereditary erythroblastic multinuclearity, 228
Hexadimethrine bromide, 503
High-titer, low-avidity (HTLA) antibodies,
  278
HIV infection:
  antibody response, 660–661
  B cell alterations, 661–662
  β_2M, 677
  CD4, 664–675
  CD8, 664–675
  CD11, 669
  CD25, 667–668
  CD38, 668

[HIV infection]
  CD45RA, 667–668
  CD45RO, 667–668
  CD57, 669
  envelope protein gp120, 672
  gp120, 672–674
  gp160, 674
  IFN-γ, 677
  IL-2, 670–672
  IL-2 receptor, 677
  immune response, 659–678
  leukocyte endothelial cell adhesion molecule
    1 (LECAM-1), 668
  monocyte alterations, 675–676
  neopterin, 677
HLA, 599, 603, 641
  1a, 155
  1b, 155
  A1, 155
  A2, 308
  A3, 308
  A allele loss, 308
  allele loss, 314
  antigens, 612
  assay, 308
  B, 307
  B8, 122, 280, 281, 284
  B12, 280
  B35, 282
  B44, 282, 283
  B60, 280
  C, 307
  class I, 147
  class II, 147
  cross-reactive, 612
  DR3, 155, 284
  DRw52a, 155
  gene, 307
  HL-A3, 120
  matched donors, 612
  matched platelets, 151
  matching, 611
  somatic mutagenesis assay, 307
Hodgkin's disease, 203
Homologous restriction factor (HRF), 409
HPRT clonogenic assay, 310
HRF20, P18, 409
Human T lymphotropic virus (HTLV):
  characteristics of infected lymphocytes, 680–
    684
  immune response, 678–684
  lymphocyte subset changes, 680–684
  spontaneous lymphocyte proliferation, 682–
    684
HTLV-II, 679

Human monocyte system HMA-1, 156
Human platelet antigen (HPA), 147
    HPA-1, 148
    HPA-2, 148
    HPA-3, 148
    HPA-4, 148
    HPA-5, 148
Human trophoblasts, 200
Humk v 325, 510
Hut, 40
Hy/Gy^a blood group antigens, 104, 484
Hybridoma technique, 390
Hydatid cyst fluid, 223
Hydatidiform mole, 200
Hydralazine, 524
Hydrochlorothiazide, 524
Hydrogen-bonding interactions, 332
Hydrophobic sites, 334
Hydrops fetalis, 554
Hydroxybenzoic acid, 531
Hyperthyroidism, 528
Hypoplastic anemia, 231
Hypoxanthine guanine phosphoribosyl trans-
    ferase (HGPRT), 309, 366
Hysteresis, 348

I antigen, 79, 80, 259, 260, 509, 510
    biochemical pathway, 273
    mycoplasma, 274–275
IA, 509
IB, 509
Iberis amara, 40
Ibuprofen, 524
iC3b, 404, 406, 442
Icterus gravis, 553
IFC, 152
IFN-γ, 677
IgA, 450
IgA nephropathy, 283
IgG subclasses, 416, 446, 449, 475–477,
    564
    IgG1, 416, 450
    IgG2, 416, 450
    IgG3, 416, 450
    IgG4, 416, 450
iH^a, 509
Ii antigenic determinants, 79
IL-2 receptor, 670, 677
Illegitimate (incompatible) antigens, 201–211
Immune adherence (C3b) receptors, 410
Immune complex theory, 528
Immune complexes, 283
Immune hemolytic anemia, 494
    classification of, 494
    drug-induced, 523–551

Immune response, 523, 536, 659
    drugs, 523–538
    HIV infection, 659–678
    retroviral infections, 659–667
    Rh, 561
Immune thrombocytopenia, 523
    drug-induced, 523
Immunoblotting, 149
Immunofluorescence, 149
Immunogenicity, 603
Immunoinsufficiency, 642
Immunoprecipitation, 149
Indian blood group (In^a, In^b), 269–271
INF-γ, 453
Infectious mononucleosis, 219
Inflammatory synovitis, 271
INOX, 544
Insecticide, 532
Insoluble antigen, 344
Insulin, 524
Insulin-dependent diabetes, 283
Integrins, 154
Intercellular distance, 355
Interfacial free energies, 345
Interfacial tensions, 331
Interferon gamma, 446, 453
Interleukin-2, 672
Interleukin-6, 453
Intravascular hemolysis, 414, 415, 435
Intravenous gamma globulin, 150, 454, 574,
    616
Iodipamide (Cholografin), 544
Ionic strength, 369
Ionizing radiation, 315
Isoniazid, 524
I^T, 509

Jk^a, 260, 484
Jk^b, 219, 484
JMH, 103, 484
Jr^a, 484
Ju antigen, 88, 509
Juvenile dermatomyositis, 283

K, 484
K13, 498
Kell antigens, 258
Kernicterus, 553
Kidney, 171, 172
Kidney urea transporter, 261
Kn^a, 259, 484
Knisocytes, 226
Knops/McCoy blood group antigens, 100, 264
    biochemistry/molecular genetics, 278–279
    CR1, 264, 278
    serology, 273–278

Ko, 258
Ko=Sib, 148
Kp^a, 264
Kp^b, 260, 484
Kupffer cells, 415, 440
Kx, 258
K$_x$^{a}, 498

L-selectin, 28
Laminin, 155
Lan, 484
Latamoxef, 524, 533, 534
Law of mass action, 346
Le^a, 20
Leach phenotype, 53, 259
  elliptocytosis, 259
Le^b, 20
Legionella pneumophilia, 279
Leishmania, 223
Lens culinaris lectin, 53
Lepore-Type Hybrids, 45
Leprosy, 216
Lesch-Nyhan syndrome, 309
Leu-8, 668
Leu-CAM, 161
Leukemia:
  association with depressed RBC antigens,
    224–226
  association with depressed WBC antigens,
    227–228
Leukocyte adhesion family of receptors,
  444
Leukocyte adhesion molecule, 154
Leukocyte common antigen, 388
Leukocyte endothelial cell adhesion molecule 1
  (LECAM-1), 668
Leukocyte function-associated antigen-1 (LFA-
  1), 154, 161, 444, 668, 669
Leukocyte-poor blood products, 607
Leukocyte reduction, 603
Leukocytes, 127
  decreased blood group antigens, 227–228
Leukopenia, 209
Levodopa, 524
Lewis Acid-Base (AB) Forces, 332
Lewis blood groups, 1–34, 509
  association with malignancy, 201–207
  Le^x, 24, 202–207
  Le^y, 202–207
  molecular cloning of Lewis blood group
    locus, 23–27
  structure and biosynthesis, 21–24
LFA-3, 101
Li antigen, 87, 509

Lifshitz-van der Waals (LW) forces, 328
Liley zone, 570
Lipid bilayer, 255
Listeria monocytogenes, 217
Liver:
  blood flow through, 438
  physiology and structure, 439–440
Low-density lipoprotein, 449
Lud antigen, 87, 509
Lumbricus terrestris, 223
Lupus anticoagulant, 498
Lutheran system, 259
  In(Lu) gene, 258
  Inab phenotype, 101
  Lu(a-b-) phenotype, 258
  Lu1, 271
  Lu^b, 484
  Lu$_{null}$(InLu type), 232
  Para-Lutheran, 271
LW, 116
LW^a, 260, 509
LW^{ab}, 484
LW bonds, 338
Lymphadenopathy, 511
Lymphocyte assays, 307
  hypoxanthine-guanine phosphoribosyltrans-
    ferase, 309–311
  major histocompatibility locus, 307–309
Lymphocytes, 171, 467, 664
  EBV transformation, 391–393
  homing receptor, 270
Lymphoid cells, 171, 192
Lymphoma, 511
Lymphoproliferative syndromes, 510
Lymphosarcoma-cell leukemia, 227

MAC-inhibitory factor (MACIF), 409
Macrophages:
  cell destruction, 435–464
  complement receptors, 441–444
  IgG Fc receptors, 444–447
MAD-2, 369
Major histocompatibility locus, 307
Major intrinsic protein (MIP), 261
Malaria:
  association with blood group antigens, 222–
    223
Maleic acid, 544
Malignant cells:
  ABH/Lewis/Ii blood group antigens, 201–
    204
  loss of ABH antigens, 201
  P and Forssman antigens, 207–208
  T and Tn antigens, 209–211
Malignant lymphoma, 224

Mart^a, 161, 162
Mast cells, 409
M^c, 40, 41
McCoy, 259, 264, 484
McLeod Phenotype, 232, 258
    acanthocytosis, 258
    chronic granulomatosis disease, 258
    Duchenne muscular dystrophy, 258
    XK gene, 258
Me, 509
Medicago disciformis, 231
Mefenamic acid, 524
Megalobastic anemia, 229
Melanesians, 218
Melibiose, 219
Melphalan, 524
Membrane attack complex (MAC), 405, 406,
    408
Membrane cofactor protein, 100
Membrane inhibitor of reactive lysis (MIRL),
    409
Membranoproliferative glomerulonephritis, 421
Menadiol sodium diphosphate (Synkayvite),
    544
Mephenytoin, 523
MER2, 259
Mesantoin, 523
Mesothelia, 209
Metabolite, 525
Methadone, 524
Methicillin, 524
Methimazole, 528
Methotrexate, 524
Methyldopa, 127, 524, 533–536, 541–542
Methysergide, 524
M^g, 40, 41
Mi.I, 40
Mi.II, 40
Mi.VII, 40
Mi.VIII, 40
Mi^a, 40
Microcalorimetry, 345
Mimicking antibody, 227
MIRL, 98
Mitotic recombination, 300, 301
Mixed agglutination, 149
M^{k}M^k, 223
MNSs system, 35, 67
    s, 43, 260
    S, 36, 43, 260
Modifier gene, 120
Moluccella laevis, 40
Monoclonal antibodies, 71, 365, 455
    ABO typing reagents, 374–375
    anti-D, 588

[Monoclonal antibodies]
    anti-D typing reagents, 376–379
    antiglobulin reagents, 379–380
    anti-Jk^a, 381
    anti-Jk^b, 381
    anti-Le^a, 380
    anti-Le^b, 380
    anti-M, 380
    characterization of, 369–370
    diagnostic reagents, 373–381
    production of, 365–369
    to red blood cell blood group antigens, 365–
    385
    Rh antibodies, 128
    therapeutic products, 381
Monoclonal antibody immobilization of neutro-
    phil antigens (MAINA), 157
Monoclonal antibody immobilization of platelet
    antigens (MAIPA), 149
Monoclonal antibody radioimmunoassay
    (MARIA), 149
Monocyte monolayer assay (MMA), 468–469,
    481, 484
Monocytes, 440–448, 467, 675
    complement receptors, 441–444
    IgG Fc receptors, 444–447
Mononuclear phagocytic system (MPS), 435–
    461
Mutation, 300
M^v, 40, 44
Mycobacterium leprae, 279
Mycoplasma pneumoniae, 82
    I, 274
Myelofibrosis, 226
Myeloid metaplasia, 226
Myelomonocytic leukemia, 226
Myeloproliferative disorders, 224, 228
Myocardial infarction, 211
Myxoviruses, 69
M^z, 48

N antigen, 43, 509
N-acetylneuraminic acid, 68
NA system antigens, 159
    NA1, 157
    NA2, 157
    null, 157
    null phenotype, 160
Nafcillin, 524
Nak^{a}antigen, 148, 152
Natural killer (NK) cells, 446
NB system antigens, 159
Neisseria gonorrhoeae, 215
Neo-antigen, 172
Neolacto Series (type 2) Chain, 78

Neolactooctasylceramide, 82
Neonatal alloimmune neutropenia, 98, 157
Neonatal alloimmune thrombocytopenia, 150
Neopterin (NEOP), 677
NeuAc, 68
NeuNAc, 36, 68
Neucleated cells, 192–193
  band 3, 192–193
Neuraminic acid, 67
Neuraminidase, 69
Neurons, 171
Neutrophil alloantigens, 156–162
  clinical importance, 157–158
  glycoprotein localization, 159–161
  Mart^a, 156
  methods to characterize, 157
  molecular nature, 162
  NA1, 156
  NA2, 156
  NB1, 156
  NB2, 156
  NC and NC antigens, 161
  NC1, 156
  ND1, 156
  NE1, 156
  9^a (HMA1), 156
  9^b (HMA2), 156
  Ond^a(E27), 156
  Ond and Mart antigens, 161
  soluble NA antigen, 161
Neutrophils:
  agglutination, 157
  alloantibodies, 157–158
  alloantigens, 156–157
  cytotoxic test (NCT), 157
  immunofluorescence test (NIFT), 157
New World monkeys, 130
Nijmegan breakage syndrome, 307
Nitrofurantoin, 531
NK cells, 447, 663, 681
Nomifensine, 524, 531, 534
Nonimmunological adsorption of protein onto
    RBCs, 542
Nucleated cells, 192
Nucleoprotein, 535

O-Glycans, 54
Ol^a antigen, 120
Old World monkeys, 130
Oligosaccharides, 2
Om, 509
Oncogenes, 316
Oncogenesis, 202
Ond^a, 161, 162
Ontogenesis, 202

Opsonic index, 467
Organ transplantation, 155
Osteoarthritis, 271
Osteoclasts, 155
Ovalocytosis, 182, 227

p phenotype, 207
P system antigens, 127, 404, 509
  biochemical pathway, 273
  E. coli, 219–220, 272–274
  P^K, 514
  PP$_1$P^K, 514
p-aminosalicylic acid, 524
p-azobenzoate, 525
P-selectin, 28
P$_1$, 259
Pamoic acid, 544
Pancytopenia, 523
Para-Bombay phenotype, 16, 18, 19
Paraben, 531
Paragloboside, 208
Parasites, 222
  Ascaris suum, 223
  blood groups antigens, 222–223
  Echinococcus, 222
  Giardia lamblia, 222
  Hydatid cyst fluid, 222
  Leishmania, 222
  Lumbricus terrestris, 222
  Plasmodium falciparum, 222–223
  Plasmodium knowlesi, 222–223
  Plasmodium vivax, 222–223
Parotid gland, 14
Paroxysmal cold hemoglobinuria (PCH), 272,
  ′ 420, 493
  biphasic hemolysin, 512–515
  Donath Landsteiner test, 511–515
  serological characteristics of, 511–515
Paroxysmal nocturnal hemoglobinuria, 98,
  262–263
Partial D, 118
Partial lipodystrophy, 421
Passenger lymphocyte syndrome, 422
Pasteurella pestis, 214
PEG, 503
Pen=Yuk, 148
Penicillins, 526
  allergy, 540
  antibodies, 539
  penicillin-G, 524
  Penicilloyl group, 525
  Penicillic acid, 544
Peptic (gastric and duodenal) ulcer, 211
Peptide antibodies, 185
Peptide mapping, 129

Percutaneous umbilical blood sampling (PUBS), 150, 572
Perfluorocarbon blood substitute, 423
Periodate, 74
Peripheral nervous system, 16
Pernicious anemia, 200
Phagocytosis, 172, 440, 465
  collagen, 448
  factors affecting cell clearance, 449–455
  fibronectin, 448
  platelet-activating factor (PAF), 448
Phenacetin, 524, 534
Philadelphia (Ph^1)-positive chromosomes, 226
Phopholipase A$_2$, 128, 129
Phosphatidylinositol glycan-linked proteins, 95
  acetylcholinesterase, 103
  blood group antigens, 98–99
  Cartwright antigens, 103
  Cromer antigens, 99–101
  decay-accelerating factor, 101–103
  hematopoietic cells, 97–98
  Hy/Gy protein, 104
  JMH protein, 103–104
  paroxysmal nocturnal hemoglobinuria, 98
  structure and synthesis, 95–97
Phosphatidylserine (PS) flippase, 133
Phospholipid, 498
Phototherapy, 575
Phthalic acid, 544
Phytohemagglutinin (PHA), 535, 669
Picric acid, 544
Pili, 220
Placental syncytiotrophoblast, 171
Plague, 214
Plasma exchange, 574, 617
Plasmapheresis, 159
Plasmodium falciparum, 222
Plasmodium knowlesi, 222, 262
Plasmodium vivax, 222, 262
Platelet antibodies:
  detection, 149
  specificity, 151
Platelet alloimmunization, 599, 610, 615
  management of, 610–619
  prevention of, 599–610
  reversal of, 615–619
Platelet antigens, 149
  clinical importance, 150
  glycoprotein localization, 151
  molecular genotyping, 153–154
  type and characterize, 149
Platelet specific antigens, 147
  alloimmune response, 155–156
  Bak, Lek, 148–149
  Bak^a=Lek^a, 148–149

[Platelet specific antigens]
  Bak^b, 148–149
  Br, Hc, Zav, 148–149
  Duzo^a, 148–149
  glycoprotein localization, 151–152
  Gov^a, 148–149
  Gov^b, 148–149
  Ko, Sib, 148–149
  matching, 613–614
  molecular nature, 152–153
  Nak^a, 148–149
  Pen, Yuk, 148–149
  Pl^{E1}, 148–149
  Pl^{E2}, 148–149
  Pl^{T1}, 148–149
  Yuk^a, 148–149
  Zw, Pl^A, 148–149
  Zw^b=Pl^{A2}, 148–149
Platelets:
  abnormal responses, 598–599
  ABO compatibility, 602–603
  activating factor (PAF), 448
  alloantibodies, 599
  alloantigens, 147
  alloimmune refractoriness, 597–627
  cross-match, 614–615
  HLA compatibility, 603
  leukocyte reduction, 603–607
  prevention of alloimmunization, 599–610
  recovery, 597
  refractoriness to transfusion, 597–627
  responses, 598
  storage lesion, 423
  surface-bound complement, 451
  surface-bound IgG, 451
  survival, 598
  Pl^E, 147, 148
  Pl^T, 148
  ultraviolet irradiation (UVR), 607–609
Pneumococcus antisera, 88
Pneumococcus type XIV, 274
  I, 274
Podophyllotoxin, 524, 533
Pokeweed mitogen (PWM), 535, 669
Polar Acid-Base (AB) Forces, 332
Polyagglutinable RBCs, 230
Polybrene, 230, 503
Polycythemia, 226
Polyethylene glycol (PEG), 503
Posttransfusion purpura, 150, 422
Pr, 54, 498, 509
  Pr$_1$, 67, 74
  Pr$_{1d}$, 75
  Pr$_{1h}$, 75
  Pr$_2$, 74, 75, 394

Pr$_3$, 74
Pr$_{3d}$, 75
Pr$_{3h}$, 75
Pr$_a$, 75
Pr^M, 71, 75
Pr^N, 71
Preleukemia, 224
Primary sensory neurons, 16
Pro-C4, 280
Probenecid, 524
Procainamide, 524, 535
Promethazine hydrochloride, 574
Protectin, 409
Protein A-sepharose beads, 528
Protein 4.1, 498
Protein 4.2, 256
Protein losing enteropathies, 232, 277
Proteus mirabilis, 219
Protozoal infections, 422
Psoriasis, 283
Pyelonephritis, 219, 220, 274
Pyramidon, 524

Quantitative hemagglutination, 343
Quinidine, 524
Quinine, 524

Raddon Lane, 40
Radioimmunoassay (RIA), 529
Radioimmunotherapy, 310
Ranitidine, 524
Raynaud's phenomenon, 508
RBC membrane abnormalities, 255, 261
  shape changes, 258
  spiculation, 359
RDE (receptor-destroying enzyme), 69
Reactive hemolysis, 422, 504
Reactive lymphocytosis, 227
Recognition molecules, 334
Reed-Stenberg (RS) cell, 203
Refractoriness to platelet transfusions, 597–
    627
  definition, 598
  management of alloimmunization, 610–615
  prevention of alloimmunization, 599–610
  reversal of alloimmunization, 615–619
Refractory anemia, 224, 228
Renal dialysis, 40
Renal transplantation, 121
Respiratory tract, 16
Reticuloendothelial system (RES), 414, 436,
    440, 449
  enhanced function, 453–454
  factors affecting cell clearance, 449–555
  impaired function, 454–455

macrophages and monocytes, 440–448
organs involved, 436–440
Retinoblastoma locus, 316
Retroviral infections:
  antibody response, 660–661
  β_2M, 677
  CD4, 664–675
  CD8, 664–675
  CD11, 669
  CD25, 667–668
  CD38, 668
  CD45RA, 667–668
  CD45RO, 667–668
  CD57, 669
  HTLV, 678–684
  HTLV-I, 678–684
  HTLV-II, 678–684
  human immunodeficiency virus-1 (HIV),
    659–678
  IFN-γ, 677
  IL-2, 670–672
  IL-2 receptor, 677
  immune response, 659–667
  leukocyte endothelial cell adhesion molecule
    1 (LECAM-1), 668
  monocyte alterations, 675–676
  neopterin, 677
Reverse transcriptase inhibitor, 544
Rg1, 280
Rg2, 280
Rh blood groups, 109–145, 555–559
  antigens and phenotypes, 109–120
  antigens of very high incidence, 113–114
  antigens of very low incidence, 114–116
  autoantibodies, 125–127
  biochemistry of the Rh proteins, 127–133
  C,c,E, and e, 110–113
  cE(Rh27), 113
  CE(Rh22), 113
  C^G, 113
  clinical relevance of Rh antibodies, 123–
    125
  cluster model, 132
  D variants, 117–119
  D^u phenotype, 117
  f(ce,Rh6), 113
  G, 113
  function of the Rh proteins, 133–134
  gene frequencies, 557
  genetics, 134
  glycoproteins, 130
  hemolytic disease, 563, 568
  immune globulin (RhIG), 120, 581
  immunogenicity of D, 120, 123
  immunogenicity of D^u, 122–123

[Rh blood groups]
  incidence of Rh genes, 112
  nonglycosylated Rh proteins, 128–129
  Rh^A, 119
  Rh^B, 119
  Rh^C, 119
  Rh^D, 119
  rhi(C3,Rh7), 113
  Rh_{mod}, 119–120, 232
  Rh_{null}, 43, 119–120, 232
  suppresors of Rh, 119–120
  terminologies and antigen frequencies, 111
  variant Rh antigens, 116
Rh immunization, 559, 561, 562, 579, 581,
    584, 588
  augmentation, 586
  clinical studies, 561–562
  dose of Rh antigen, 561–562
  during pregnancy, 562; 584–586
  frequency, 561–562
  monoclonal anti-D, 588
  pathogenesis, 559–563
  prevention, 579–588
  RhIG prevents, 581–583
  suppression of weak D immunization, 587–
    588
Rh prophylaxis, 580, 583, 585
  antenatal, 585–586
  clinical trials, 580–581
Rheumatic disease, 200
Rheumatoid arthritis, 271, 283, 454
Rifampicin, 524, 531
Risk analysis, 317
Rodgers, 279
  serology, 279–280
Rosette assay, 467–468
Rosettes, 465, 528
Rubella virus, 89
R_x, 498, 509

Sa, 75, 509
Salis, 270
Salmonella, 215
Salvia sclarea, 209, 230
Sc1, 260, 498
Sc3, 498
SCA, 498
Schiff's base, 544
Schistosoma mansonti, 277
Schistosomiasis, 523
Schlepper, 524
Sd^a, 127, 484
Secretor (Se) locus, 2, 14–17
Sedimentation velocity, 351
Sedormid, 526

Selectins, 28, 207
Senescent cell antigen, 171–196, 498
  anion and glucose transport, 180
  band 3 mutations/alterations, 179–182
  band 3 product, 175–176, 179–193
  cellular and molecular biology, 171–193;
    182–192
  chemical models, 178–179
  isolation, 174
  mechanism of removal, 172–174
  on nucleated cells, 174–175
Serratia marscescens, 231
Serum alkaline phosphatase, 213
Serum cholesterol, 211, 212
Shigella, 215
Sialic acid, 36, 67
  dependent RBC antigens, 67–93
  in glycophorin alloantigens, 69–73
  structure and nomenclature, 67–69
Sialidase, 69
Sialidase-sensitive determinants, 506
  Sia-b1, 79, 80
  Sia-bI, 80
  Sia-I1, 79, 80
  Sia-Ib1, 79
Sialoautoantigens, 73
  glycophorin, 73–79
  immunobiologic relevance, 88–89
Sialoglycolipids, 77, 78
Sialoglycoproteins, 35
Sialyl-Le^a, 26, 206
Sialyl-Le^x, 26, 206, 207
Sialyl-Tn, 55
Sialyltransferases, 71
Sickle cell anemia, 171, 228, 498
Sideroblastic anemia, 229
Sjögren's syndrome, 283, 454
Skeletal proteins, 256
  ankyrin, 256
  band 7, 256
  protein 4.1, 256
  protein 4.2, 256
  spectrin, 256
SI^a, 259, 264, 484
Smallpox, 214
Smooth muscle cells, 155
Sodium azide, 531
Sodium dodedylsulfate-polyacrylamine gel elec-
    trophoresis (SDS-PAGE), 149, 529
Sodium iodomethamate (Iodoxyl), 544
Sodium pentothal, 524
Somatic cell culture, 315
Somatic cell genetics, 315
Somatic mutation, 299, 312, 315
  detection and quantitation, 299–323

Somatic segregation, 302
Specificity, 451
Specific red cell adherence, 201
Spectrin, 183, 256, 498
Spherocytosis, 133, 256
Spleen, 436
  blood flow, 437
Spontaneous agglutination, 507
Spontaneous antibody loss, 615
Spontaneous lymphocyte proliferation, 682
Squamous epithelial, 171
SSEA-1 antigen, 24
St^a, 48, 264
Staphylococcal protein A, 423, 529
Stibophen, 523, 544
Stomatocytes, 133, 256
  Rh$_{null}$/Rh$_{mod}$, 260–261
Stored cell autoantibody, 498
Streptococcus MG, 217
Streptomycin, 524, 526, 531, 534
Subacute sclerosing panencephalitis, 283
Sublingual glands, 14
Submaxillary glands, 14
Sulphonamides, 524
Suppressor T-cell, 534
Suramin, 544
Synthetic peptides, 182, 184
Systemic sclerosis, 283
Systemic lupus erythematosus (SLE), 264,
    283–284, 420, 454
  Chido-negative, Rodgers-negative phenotype,
    264
  McCoy, Knops, SI^a, Yk^a negative, 264

T antigen, 36, 67
  acquired, 230
  association with malignancy, 209–211
  immune response, 209–211
T cells, 313, 446, 535, 681
TQ1, 668
T-cell receptor gene, 311
T-cell receptor, 313
T-cell-derived growth factors, 391
T-transformed RBCs, 231
Target cells, 471
Tat, 683
Tax, 683
Tc^a, 152, 484
Tc^b, 152
Tc^c, 152
Temperature, 350
Teniposide, 524, 533, 534
Terephthaldicarboxaldehyde, 544
Terephthalic acid, 544

Terminal pathway, 405
Tetracycline, 524
Th, 230
Thalassemia, 228
Thermodynamics, 339
Thiopental, 524, 531
Thrombocytopenia, 209, 451
Thrombosis, 211
Thymocytes, 449
Tissue cells, 127
Tj(a-), 514
Tn antigen, 36, 55, 203, 230
  association with malignancy, 209–211
  immune response, 209–210
TNF-α, 683
Tolbutamide, 524, 526
Tolmetin, 524, 529, 533, 534
Transfusion reactions, 147
Transfusion-induced acute lung injury
    (TRALI), 158
Transfusion-induced graft-versus-host disease,
    631–657
  cases reported since 1988, 632–66
  clinical features, 637; 644–646
  immunosufficiency, 642
  pathogenesis, 637
  role of HLA, 641–642
  transfusion immunosuppressive effect,
    642
  treatment and prevention, 646–647
Transient erythroblastopenia, 229
Transmembrane proteins, 256
  band 3, 256
  glycophorin C and D, 256
  Kx polypeptide, 256
  Lutheran polypeptide, 256
  Rh polypeptides, 256
Transplacental fetal hemorrhage, 583
Transplacental hemorrhage, 560
  massive, 583–584
  prevalence, 560
Triamterene, 524
Trimellitic anhydride, 524
Trypanosoma cruzi, 279
Tuberculosis, 216
Tumor antigens, 198, 201
Tumor necrosis factor (TNF), 207, 281
Tumor suppressor genes, 316
Two-color fluorescence, 305
Tx, 230, 232
Type 1 chain, 2
Type 2 chain, 2
Type 3 chain, 2
Type 4 chain, 5
Type XIV, 88

U, 43, 260
U937 cells, 467
Ultrafiltration, 343
Ultrasonography, 571
Ultraviolet irradiation, 607
UMC, 152
Urea transport, 261
  Jk(a-b-) phenotype, 261
Urinary tract, 16
U^x, 43
U^z, 43

VA, 230, 232
Valency, 339
van der Waals-London forces, 328, 535
Variable region genes, 389, 393
  V_H, 393, 510
  V_H4.21, 394, 510
  V_HI, 510
  V_HII, 510
  V_HIII, 510
  V_HVI, 510
  V_KII, 510
  V_KIII, 393
  V_L, 393
Varicella virus, 89
Vel, 484
Very late antigens, 154
Vibrio cholerae, 69, 230
Vicia cretica, 230
Vicia graminea, 40
Vicia hyranica, 231
Vincristine/vinblastine, 619
Vitamin E, 176
Vitronectin, 154
Vitronectin receptor, 155

VLA-2($\alpha_2\beta_1$), 155, 672
VLA-5 ($\alpha_5\beta_1$), 155
VLA-6 ($\alpha_6\beta_1$), 155
Vo, 79
Vo^a, 509
von Willebrand factor (vWF), 154, 213
Vw, 40

Waldenström's macroglobulinemia, 511
Warm autoimmune hemolytic anemia
    (WAIHA), 494–506
Werner's syndrome, 307
WES^a, 152
WES^b, 152
Wild-type allele, 301, 303
Wiskott-Aldrich syndrome, 394
Wound healing, 205
Wr^b, 36, 41, 264, 498

X chromosome, 119, 258
X-linked gene, 300
X-rays, 308
Xeroderma pigmentosum, 310
Xg^a, 260, 493
XK gene, 258
X^Q, 120

Yanomama indians, 218
Yaws, 216
Yk^a, 259, 264, 484
Yt^a, 484
Yus, 52, 259

Zomepirac, 524, 534
Zw, 148